D1609559

Experimentation with Human Beings

Experimentation with Human Beings

The Authority of the Investigator,
Subject, Professions, and State
in the Human Experimentation Process

Jay Katz, *Yale University*

with the assistance of
Alexander Morgan Capron
and **Eleanor Swift Glass**

RUSSELL SAGE FOUNDATION
NEW YORK

PUBLICATIONS OF RUSSELL SAGE FOUNDATION

Russell Sage Foundation was established in 1907 by Mrs. Russell Sage
for the improvement of social and living conditions in the United States.
In carrying out its purpose the Foundation conducts research
under the direction of members of the staff or in close collaboration
with other institutions, and supports programs designed to develop
and demonstrate productive working relations between
social scientists and other professional groups.
As an integral part of its operations, the Foundation from time to time
publishes books or pamphlets resulting from these activities.
Publication under the imprint of the Foundation
does not necessarily imply agreement by the Foundation, its Trustees,
or its staff with the interpretations or conclusions of the authors.

Russell Sage Foundation
230 Park Avenue, New York, N.Y. 10017

Library of Congress Catalog Card Number: 70–188394
Standard Book Number: 87154–438–5
Printed in the United States of America by Connecticut
   Printers, Inc., Hartford, Connecticut

First Printing—August 1972
Second Printing—December 1973

To My Father

Preface

Shortly after joining the Yale Law School faculty thirteen years ago, I came upon the Nuremberg proceedings against the Nazi physicians in a casebook on criminal law then being written by my colleagues Richard C. Donnelly, Joseph Goldstein, and Richard D. Schwartz.[1] The excerpts they had selected, and the voluminous trial transcripts which I read later on, recounted in sickening detail the "medical experiments" conducted in the concentration camps "with unnecessary suffering and injury and . . . very little, if any, [protection of subjects from] injury, disability, or death."[2] In reflecting on these documents I increasingly thought that the victims of those investigations deserved a thoroughgoing exploration of the entire human research process in order to impede a repetition of such atrocities. Yet had I begun to work on this book then, my preoccupation with and intense feelings about the concentration camp experiments would have dominated it and limited its value. Investigators would have felt unfairly compared to the lowest common denominator in their ranks and, even more important, students of human experimentation, reacting to the unparalleled cruelty of those studies, would have been tempted either to condemn the entire research process or to deny that the exploitation of research subjects, as revealed at Nuremberg, is an ever-relevant problem for human experimentation. Thus, as I read more about research with human beings and began to teach a seminar on the topic, I realized that if a book were to result, it should be designed to provide a climate for the scholarly analysis of the human experimentation process. Only a thoughtful and persistent educational effort, for which this volume seeks to furnish a set of materials, can bring about real change in long-standing practices and thereby give some meaning to the suffering of those who were harmed by human experimentation against their will.

As I became increasingly involved in the world of law, I learned much that was new to me from my colleagues and students about such complex issues as the right to self-

---

[1] *Criminal Law,* New York: The Free Press (1962).
[2] Judgment of Beals, Sebring and Crawford, JJ. at pp. 305–306 *infra.*

determination and privacy and the extent of the authority of governmental, professional, and other institutions to intrude into private life. Although these issues affect the interactions of physician-investigators with patient-subjects and of the professions as a whole with the research process, they had rarely been discussed in my medical education. Instead it had been all too uncritically assumed that they could be resolved by fidelity to such undefined principles as *primum non nocere* or to visionary codes of ethics.

I also came to face the same issues personally in reviewing my own research on hypnotic dreams. I had abandoned these investigations a few years before coming to the law school because of an uneasy concern, not fully conscious at the time, about their possible psychological reverberations, however helpful or harmful, in my volunteer subjects. What troubled me was not so much the nature of the project but rather that, before proceeding, I had not posed for myself many more questions about the extent of my personal and professional duty to discuss with my subjects the impact such investigations might have on them.

Thus, in reflecting about the revelations at Nuremberg, my own education and my research experience, I realized that medicine has neglected to address itself to an important educational task. My subsequent contact with professionals from other disciplines made me aware that they too have much to learn from the exploration of the questions posed by human experimentation, for that exploration would lead them to confront similar long neglected issues in their professional interactions with human beings, be they called clients or patients rather than subjects. Lawyers have a special obligation to study these problems because they may come before courts in an increasing number of cases, and their judicial resolution would benefit from prior legal scholarship. Moreover, there is a pressing need for lay readers and public officials to become aware of these issues, and the references throughout this volume to "students of human experimentation" include such readers as well as those involved in classroom study.

Because the study of human experimentation, by the very nature of its intricate and delicate subject matter, evokes strong emotions, I found it necessary, as will the reader, to remain alert to the impact of deeply held convictions and value preferences. They need not be brushed aside, but must be identified so that they can be examined and assigned their proper place in the analysis of these issues. Otherwise the questions posed will remain distorted and obscure the problems which require decision. Furthermore, the reader who immerses himself in these materials will soon learn, as I did, that there are no easy answers to the questions raised by human experimentation in which, as in all human endeavors, a variety of values, interests, and costs press for recognition. Thus, the reader will be disappointed if he expects "correct" or "ethical" solutions to leap off the pages of this volume. Yet since choices have to be made and prices have to be paid, it is at least possible to try to do so more thoughtfully and with greater conscious recognition of the values to be preferred or to be neglected. It is to these goals that this volume speaks.

In light of these personal and scholarly considerations, I began work on the book seven years ago with my colleague and friend Richard C. Donnelly. His tragically premature death, shortly after we had embarked on our initial explorations, made me proceed alone, though in recent years with the able assistance of Alex Capron and Eleanor Glass. And, from the beginning, an ever-renewing collaboration was established with my students at the Yale Law School who contributed much to the development and revision of the book's many drafts.

The book presents materials from many sources, organized around an analytical framework which is explained in the introduction to the volume. That introduction and those provided at the beginning of every Part and chapter, as well as for certain sections within chapters, are intended to raise some of the questions which students should entertain in examining the materials that follow. Beyond such aids the book is deliberately designed to permit students and teachers to come to their own conclusions about the ordering of the human experimentation process.

Though the volume is conceived along the general lines of a law school casebook, it is not intended solely, or even primarily, for students of law. It is addressed to students, both graduate and undergraduate, of many disciplines. The legal "case method" has been transplanted successfully to other settings before. The use of clinical cases to instruct medical students originated in a suggestion made at the turn of the century by Dr. Walter B. Cannon, then a student at the Harvard Medical School. Impressed by his law school roommate's enthusiasm for the case method of instruction at the Harvard Law School, Cannon urged his professors to adopt the system for medical teaching.[3] Under the leadership of Dr. Richard C. Cabot, the "Clinicopathological Conferences" became an integral part of medical education, both for Harvard students and, through their weekly publication in *The New England Journal of Medicine,* for students and practitioners around the world. If students and teachers of human experimentation outside the law find the present adaptation of the case approach a useful one, they may wish to employ it more widely in place of the didactic method, still all too prevalent within many disciplines. Even more important, I hope that this volume will stimulate the kind of interdisciplinary teaching I have found so gratifying.

The work on this book has been assisted by an appropriation from Russell Sage Foundation, and I am grateful to its president, Orville G. Brim, Jr., whose encouragement and interest went far beyond financial support. Another study undertaken pursuant to a grant from the National Center for Health Services Research and Development[4] has also contributed substantially to the analysis developed in this volume. Over the years Dean Louis H. Pollak and his successor Abraham S. Goldstein have not only provided additional funds but also the academic atmosphere in which I could feel happily at home. I have profited from the critical stimulation of friends and colleagues, most particularly Robert C. Arnstein, Alexander M. Bickel, Renée C. Fox, Joseph Goldstein, Quintin Johnstone,

---

[3] "Undoubtedly the most brilliant example thus far of the use of cases in education is seen in the study of law. The change from the textbook to the case system wrought out in the Harvard Law School has been called America's greatest contribution to educational reform. The newer method has roused an ardor and a keenness of interest among the students such as was never known before. They learn their law not by dreary grubbing at text-books or lecture notes, but by vigorously 'threshing out a case' with one another." W. B. Cannon: "The Case Method of Teaching Systematic Medicine," 142 *Boston Medical and Surgical Journal* 31, 36 (1900). *See also* W. B. Cannon: "The Case System in Medicine," *ibid.* at 563.

[4] "Social Factors Affecting the Modern Treatment of Catastrophic Diseases," Contract No. H.S.M. 110–69–213, Health Services and Mental Health Administration, Department of Health, Education and Welfare.

Joseph Katz, Arthur A. Leff, Charles E. Lindblom, Leon Lipson, Ernst Prelinger, Roy Schafer, Vaughn Stapleton, and Stanton Wheeler. I am especially indebted to Douglas Rosenthal who read the entire manuscript and made valuable suggestions which are reflected throughout the book. Among the many students who have played a special role in the preparation of this volume I thank Robert Carter, Julian Fisher, Ronnie F. Heyman, Alan Meisel, John C. Ladd and Leonard S. Spector.

I am particularly grateful to Brad Gray, Ernst Prelinger, Derek DeS. Price, and Charles L. Remington for contributing articles specifically written for this book. Though I do not acknowledge them by name, I also wish to express my thanks to the authors who gave permission to print unpublished manuscripts or to reproduce excerpts from their writings. Among the latter I am specially appreciative of those who, in the spirit of free inquiry, granted reprint permission even though they had reservations about the purpose of this volume.

I owe a great deal to the assistance of the staff of the Yale Law School library, particularly Robert E. Brooks, Arthur Charpentier, Gene Coakley, James M. Golden, Isaiah Shein, Solomon C. Smith, and Iris Wildman. They met my unending requests for books and magazines, sometimes most difficult to locate, with gracious and dedicated efforts which speeded this venture to completion.

I thank my secretary Kathy Lewis for her expert and cheerful typing of numerous drafts of the manuscript; Elizabeth Albert, Elsa Dixler, Dorothy Egan, Isabel Malone, Doris Moriarty, Walter Moriarty, and Kathy Murray for their assistance in preparing the manuscript for publication; Janet Turk for her skillful copyediting and preparation of the index; and Jean Yoder and William Bennett of Russell Sage Foundation for the thoughtful and understanding direction they gave to the production of this volume.

I have saved for the end two most important acknowledgements: First, my gratitude to my wife Esta Mae and my children Sally, Daniel, and Amy who over the years, with minimal complaints, allowed me the time to work on this book. Their feelings for me and my work made the completion of this book possible, and I am grateful for their understanding collaboration. Finally, I thank Eleanor Glass and Alex Capron who have worked closely with me over the years. Eleanor assisted me most with earlier drafts when we were still searching for materials and trying out a variety of organizing schemes. Alex, for the last year and a half, has involved himself in this book with an intensity and intellectual support which significantly affected its final shape. It was during this period of time that in daily meetings we edited and re-edited the selections, refined and substantially reworked the book's conceptual framework, and wrote the textual introductions. My debt to him is great. My appreciation to both is reflected on the title page.

J. K.

New Haven, Connecticut
January 1972

Condensed Table of Contents

Analytical Table of Contents

Introduction 1

Part One

An Introduction to the Human Experimentation Process 7

Chapter One. THE JEWISH CHRONIC DISEASE HOSPITAL CASE 9

Chapter Two.   THE WICHITA JURY RECORDING CASE   67

Chapter Six.   WHAT CONSEQUENCES TO SUBJECTS SHOULD AFFECT THE AUTHORITY OF THE INVESTIGATOR?   323

Part Three

The Authority of the Subject as Guardian of His Own Fate   521

Chapter Eight.   WHAT ARE THE FUNCTIONS OF INFORMED CONSENT?   523

Chapter Nine.   WHAT LIMITATIONS ARE INHERENT IN INFORMED CONSENT?   609

Part Four

The Authority of Professional and Public Institutions   725

Chapter Eleven. EXPERIMENTATION WITH VOLUNTEERS AND PATIENT–SUBJECTS   727

Chapter Twelve. EXPERIMENTATION WITH UNCOMPREHENDING SUBJECTS   955

Chapter Fourteen. EXPERIMENTATION WITH DYING SUBJECTS 1053

Introduction

When science takes man as its subject, tensions arise between two values basic to Western society: freedom of scientific inquiry and protection of individual inviolability. Both are facets of man's quest to order his world. Scientific research has given man some, albeit incomplete, knowledge and tools to tame his environment, while commitment to individual worth and autonomy, however wavering, has limited man's intrusions on man. Yet when human beings become the subject of experimentation, allegiance to one value invites neglect of the other. At the heart of this conflict lies an age-old question: When may a society, actively or by acquiescence, expose some of its members to harm in order to seek benefits for them, for others, or for society as a whole?

Recent experience with human experimentation in a variety of disciplines has prompted renewed concern among the professions and the public that the present regulation of the research process is unsatisfactory. Some critics call for increased governmental controls, more detailed codes of ethics, more powerful professional review committees, or more active participation of nonscientists in research decisions. Others fear that involvement of outsiders or more stringent controls will "put a ceiling price on truth" and dry up all reservoirs of creativity and scientific progress. Yet perhaps the most pervasive viewpoint is that experimentation cannot be rationally controlled. Before accepting any of these judgments it is the task of the student of human experimentation to seek answers to three questions: (1) What limits, if any, should be placed on scientific inquiry, and what implications do these limits have for

1

society's democratic and egalitarian aspirations? (2) Who should have the authority to formulate these limits? (3) By what means should they be imposed?

In searching for answers to these questions, this book examines and evaluates the authority which should be vested in each of the chief participants in the human experimentation process—the *investigator* who initiates and conducts the experiment, the human being who is its *subject*, and the *professions* and the *state* which appraise, support, or restrict research. These participants provide the book with its structural framework. Following Part One, which presents an introductory view of the problems raised by experimentation with man, the three succeeding Parts scrutinize, respectively, the roles of investigator, subject, and professional and public institutions. The participants are introduced in this sequence in order first to evaluate the problems which arise if total authority is assigned to investigators and to identify their special qualifications and values, then to examine the competence of subjects (and their parents, spouses, or guardians) to collaborate in decisionmaking, and finally to explore the capacity of the professions and the public to play a role in the experimentation process. All the participants have unique and conflicting constellations of motivations, capacities, and value preferences by which they chart their courses. Therefore, to analyze the tensions which arise between the participants over the objectives and conduct of research, one must not only identify each actor's values but also assess his capacity and willingness to act upon them.

To sharpen the analysis, the book also adopts a functional framework based on what are seen as three basic stages in the process of making decisions about human experimentation—the *formulation* of research policy, the conduct and supervision of research which comprise its *administration*, and the *review* of research and its consequences. This complementary approach is grounded in the assumption that the authority to be assigned to each participant is not identical throughout the human experimentation process. We suggest, instead, that the nature and extent of this authority ought to be shaped and defined by the different issues and particular problems which require resolution at the three stages of the process. For example, investigators have asserted that the conduct of research should be left largely to their discretion once they have fulfilled certain obligations toward their subjects. Whatever the merits of this claim, it need not suggest that they should be given similar authority over the formulation of research policy or the review of the research enterprise.

Human experimentation cannot be analyzed in isolation, however, for inherent in its dynamics are several ubiquitous forces which shape all social interaction—man's quest for knowledge and mastery, his willingness to risk human life, and his readiness to delegate authority to professionals and to rely on their judgment. These general themes are first examined in Part One, and their importance to a definition of the participants' roles continually reemerges in Parts Two and Three. In those Parts, we have employed the structural and functional frameworks to highlight a number of issues which must be scrutinized if the student is to move toward increasingly precise conclusions about the authority that should be assigned to investigators and subjects. Thus Parts Two and Three are organized around such tasks as identifying categories of harm and other significant elements in experimental interventions (*e.g.*, the investigator's attitude toward and method of selecting subjects and his ability to predict the consequences of his work), as well as examining the extent and limits of man's capacity for insightful self-determination. In Part Four the structural-functional matrix becomes the explicit frame of reference, for the student must not only evaluate the role of the professions and the state but also integrate this evaluation with his prior analysis of the role of investigators and subjects. While this framework and the issues it highlights (*e.g.,* the definition of "harm") have proved to be useful analytic tools, they are nothing more than that. None of the problems for decision can be neatly confined either to a single participant or to a single stage in the process. Problems about the role of each participant must be re-examined in light of the capacities and incapacities of the other participants to make decisions. Similarly, the student's conclusions about problems of administration will need to be rethought in light of his examinations of, and conclusions about, formulation and review mechanisms. Thus the evaluation of the authority of each decisionmaker at each point in the process ought ideally to rest on an analysis of the roles played by all decisionmakers at all points in the process. In the end, the student of human experimentation may also wish to reappraise the conceptual categories proposed in this book.

In selecting the materials for this volume we have not been constrained by a single definition of what constitutes human experimentation. Consequently, a threshold question must be posed: What is human experimentation, and for what purposes should it be defined? The ambit of experimentation is blurred on at least two borders: First, it may or may not include "poorly designed" or "fruitless" research. Second, an intent to give or receive "benefits" may or may not remove an intervention from the category of "experiment." The materials do not draw hard and fast lines between interventions for the "acquisition of knowledge" or for the "subject's benefit" so as to leave open the question whether the authority assigned to the participants, and any restrictions imposed upon them, in one setting should apply equally to the other.

This volume includes experimental studies from several disciplines—medicine, psychology, sociology, biology, and law—and materials from many sources—trial transcripts, congressional hearings, panel discussions, appellate decisions, administrative regulations, editorial comments, legislation, private agreements, scholarly publications, and newspaper stories. These have been interwoven with commentary from philosophy, political science, economics, genetics, medicine, anthropology, psychoanalysis, biology, jurisprudence, psychology, theology, and literature. Both the relevance and the reliability of these materials, as data and as evaluations, must be subjected to critical appraisal. Scrutinizing case studies about events in the past can sometimes seem petty, sterile, or disheartening. Yet any hope for a better and more thoughtful resolution of the issues in the future depends on our willingness to engage in unstinting examination of the past, as imperfectly as it may be recalled.

This book is addressed to students of human experimentation, be they actual or potential decisionmakers. Although the questions posed throughout this volume may seldom be raised explicitly in the course of experimentation, answers to them are implicit in all decisions concerning human research. Only by bringing these questions to a conscious level can the process be subjected to much needed scrutiny. To begin this task, the student of human experimentation may find it useful to consider the following questions:

1. What goals should man seek to achieve by scientific inquiries? Are these desirable in themselves or as means to desirable but more remote ends?

2. What value conflicts arise in the human experimentation process?

a. Under what circumstances should significance to science and society outweigh what rights of patients and subjects?

b. Who, under what circumstances and by what means, should have the authority to make decisions about experimentation in order to mediate these value conflicts?

c. What procedures will permit decisionmakers to examine advances in scientific knowledge and technique so as to minimize undesired results?

3. What interventions should be labeled "experimental"?

a. What consequences should follow the designation "experimental" and how do they differ from the consequences of other designations?

b. How do the consequences differ once investigations move from theory to studies on inanimate objects and then to experimentation with animals, investigators themselves, other individuals, groups, or society?

4. What constitutes a harmful intervention?

a. To what extent should the degree or type of harm to individuals or society affect the authority of decisionmakers?

b. To what extent is the harm of an intervention mitigated by what immediate or long-range, certain or uncertain, benefits, and to whom should benefits accrue?

c. To what extent is the harm of an intervention aggravated or mitigated by an explanation of the risks and benefits involved?

d. To what extent should knowledge or lack of knowledge about harm affect the authority of decisionmakers?

5. Under what circumstances and to what extent should the consent of the subject or patient affect the decision to intervene?

a. To what extent should the capacity of subjects or patients to comprehend, to communicate, or to make rational choices affect the validity of consent?

b. How and to what extent should this capacity be evaluated?

c. Under what circumstances should the balancing of risks and benefits be left to the persons affected and when, if ever, should other decisionmakers impose limits on risktaking?

6. To what extent and for what purposes should a coexisting intention to give or receive "benefits" affect the authority of decisionmakers?

a. Who, and by what standards, has the authority to decide whether an intervention is "beneficial"?

b. Should any constraints imposed on the participants in experimental settings apply equally to therapeutic ones?

7. What persons and institutions should have the authority to formulate, administer, and review the human experimentation process?

a. What qualifications should these participants possess at the various stages in this process?

b. What information should be supplied to these participants and by what procedures?

c. To what extent should the authority of what persons and institutions be modified once a subject is labeled "normal volunteer," "patient volunteer," or "patient-subject"; "competent," "uncomprehending," "captive," or "dying"?

      d. Who should determine the limits of experimentation and how adequate are the procedures for making such decisions?

      8. What procedures should be established for obtaining data and evaluating their relevance to decisions being made throughout the process?

If this book in some measure documents man's inhumanity to man, it only serves to remind us how pervasive that phenomenon is. Human experimentation has been severely criticized on this ground. Yet in raising questions about experimentation we do not intend to indict science or stifle research, for the failure to experiment is equally an experiment which may also have unsatisfactory consequences. The real need to which this volume speaks is for greater conscious awareness and relentless scholarly analysis of the conflicting purposes of human experimentation—protecting man, advancing science, and improving the well-being of society and future generations. Only if students and decisionmakers are prepared to sort out these conflicts and to acknowledge the reality of harm to individuals and society can they begin to formulate rules and procedures which will minimize harm without erecting insuperable impediments to the acquisition of knowledge. In addressing this task for human experimentation, significant contributions may also be made to decisionmaking in other areas of law, science, and politics, for the conflicts presented in this volume are inherent in all affairs conducted by and with man.

PART ONE

An Introduction to the Human Experimentation Process

This Part introduces the major issues raised by experimentation with human beings. Two cases, one from medicine and one from law–social science, present the chief participants in the human experimentation process—the investigator, the subject, the professions, and the state—and bring into view their expectations, capacities, and value preferences. These first two chapters should begin to raise questions about the rights and duties of each participant and about the rules and procedures for resolving conflicts among them.

Research conducted by professional investigators with human subjects is only one piece in the mosaic of ubiquitous experimentation in society, for both individuals and society continuously try out new ways of comprehending and improving the human condition. To understand the problems posed by the human experimentation process it is vital to appreciate the larger societal context in which the interactions between investigators and their subjects are embedded. Chapter Three therefore scrutinizes three sets of conflicting forces which influence human experimentation: man's quest for the extension of knowledge and technology versus his fear of the unknown; man's willingness to risk human life versus his urge to protect it; and man's readiness to delegate authority to experts versus his desire to govern his own fate.

Finally, we pause briefly in Chapter Four to examine a variety of decisionmaking theories which may serve as useful models for making decisions about human experimentation. These materials provide the background for analyzing the roles of the participants at various stages in the process as it unfolds in succeeding chapters.

Throughout we ask:

1. What are the criteria for designating an intervention an experiment? How do experiments differ from other interventions into the lives of human beings?

2. What value conflicts arise among the participants in the human experimentation process?

3. Who, under what circumstances and by what means, should have authority to make decisions about the formulation, administration, and review of the human experimentation process?

4. For what purposes is it useful to distinguish between the various stages of this process?

The Jewish Chronic Disease
Hospital Case

In July 1963, three doctors, with approval from the director of medicine of the Jewish Chronic Disease Hospital in Brooklyn, New York, injected "live cancer cells" subcutaneously into twenty-two chronically ill and debilitated patients. The doctors did not inform the patients that live cancer cells were being used or that the experiment was designed to measure the patients' ability to reject foreign cells—a test unrelated to their normal therapeutic program.

The cancer experiment engendered a heated controversy among the hospital's doctors and led to an investigation by the hospital's grievance committee and board of directors. William A. Hyman, a member of the board who disapproved of the experiment, took the hospital to court to force disclosure of the hospital's records, claiming that the directors' approval of the experiment had not been properly obtained. As *Hyman* v. *Jewish Chronic Disease Hospital* wound its way up from the trial court through two appellate tribunals, it became clear that the legal issue involved in the suit, whether a hospital director is entitled to look at patients' medical records, only provided the backdrop for the questions really at issue which concerned the duties and obligations that the various participants in the human experimentation process should have toward one another.

Subsequently, these issues were confronted more directly when the Board of Regents of the University of the State of New York heard charges brought by the attorney general against two of the doctors involved. The board imposed sanctions, under the authority given it by New York Education Law § 6514(2) to revoke, suspend, or annul the license of a practitioner of medicine upon determining "after due hearing . . . that a physician . . . is guilty of fraud or deceit in the practice of medicine [or] that a physician is or has been guilty of un-professional conduct."

In examining these materials, consider the following questions:

1. What values does human experimentation seek to implement, and are they in conflict with other values?

2. How do the participants weigh these conflicting values, and what weight should be given to these values?

3. What values are preserved or undermined by delegating decisionmaking power to each participant respectively?

4. Under what circumstances should the extent of actual or potential harm and benefit to subjects or society affect the authority of each participant in the human experimentation process?

A.
How and by Whom Should Research Policy Be Formulated?*

Letter from Chester M. Southam, M.D. to Emanuel Mandel, M.D.—July 5, 1963

I want to thank you for the courtesy shown to me and Dr. Levin on our recent visit and the interest that you showed in our proposed research collaboration. This letter is to record and perhaps clarify the principal points of that conversation.

The study we discussed would permit evaluation of the immunologic status of patients with chronic non-neoplastic diseases, as revealed by promptness of rejection of subcutaneous cancer cell homografts. My own interest in these studies stems from their importance to the understanding and possible treatment and diagnosis of cancer, but I am sure that you would have an equally great interest in their potential importance for the understanding of autoimmune and degenerative diseases and in the budding field of organ homotransplantation.

Clinical research on this phenomenon is quite new—my own work started only ten years ago—but is accelerating rapidly as would be expected from its importance and as attested by the recent entry of several hospitals and research

institutes into the fields of cancer, skin, and organ transplantation in man. To date the studies carried out by me, with numerous collaborators here and at the Ohio State University Medical School, have revealed that healthy persons reject the cancer cell homografts completely and promptly (in 4 to 6 weeks) as one would obviously predict, but many patients with widespread cancer have a delayed rejection (over 6 weeks and sometimes 3 months or more). In either group of recipients the usual reaction is development of a painless subcutaneous nodule up to 2 or 3 cm in diameter at the time of maximum development. The immunologic derangement responsible for the comparative slowness of rejection in patients with cancer is still unidentified, but the search is narrowing down and an impairment of cell-associated immune mechanisms now seems probable.

There is a gap in our data in that we have not yet studied this reaction in people who do not have cancer but who do have chronic and debilitating diseases of other kinds. I would expect that the homograft rejection reaction would be normal or near normal in such patients. This estimate is based on results of scattered studies of skin homografts by others and on our recent demonstration of intact macrophage mobilization (a non-specific cellular immunologic mechanism) in such patients, whereas in cancer patients macrophage mobilization is depressed and correlates with homograft rejection. But suppo-

---

* This is an actual record. Without indicating deletions we have edited the record primarily to reduce repetition. Some repetition was necessary, however, to allow each participant to present his own understanding of the events.

sitions are not knowledge and it is the need for direct evidence on this point that brought me to you.

We do not have patients with debilitating diseases other than cancer at Memorial or James Ewing hospitals, and therefore we are seeking collaboration in some hospital with a large population of such patients. The Jewish Chronic Disease Hospital was suggested to me as a hospital which had not only the patients but also an interest in medical teaching and research, as evidenced by the Isaac Albert Research Institute and by its teaching arrangements with Kings County Hospital.

The procedure, as I explained, requires simply the hypodermic injection of a suspension of tissue-cultured cells at two sites on the anterior thigh or arm and observation of the sites at about weekly intervals for six weeks or until regression is complete. These cells are of two or more cancer cell lines. These cancer cell lines were chosen because they have the necessary growth capacity to produce a measurable reaction. It is, of course, inconsequential whether these are cancer cells or not, since they are foreign to the recipient and hence are rejected. The only drawback to the use of cancer cells is the phobia and ignorance that surrounds the word *cancer*. It would be possible to study the same process by experimental skin grafts, but this is less satisfactory for quantitation, is much more difficult technically, and is unacceptably annoying to your patients. Other than the two hypodermic injections and observation of the reaction, the only other procedure would be drawing serum for study of antibody reactions to the trans-

planted cells at approximately two-week intervals during the observation period.

I have no hesitation in suggesting these studies since our experience to date includes over 300 healthy recipients and over 300 cancer patients, and for two years we have been doing the tests routinely on all postoperative patients on our gynecology service as a measure of immunologic status, with the collaboration of Dr. Alexander Brunschwig, chief of the gynecology service. You asked me if I obtained (written) permissions from our patients before doing these studies. We do not do so at Memorial or James Ewing hospital since we now regard it as a routine study, much less dramatic and hazardous than other routine procedures such as bone marrow aspiration and lumbar puncture. We do get signed permits from our volunteers at the Ohio State Penitentiary but this is because of the law-oriented personalities of these men, rather than for any medical reason.

Collaboration in this research effort would involve no expense to the Jewish Chronic Disease Hospital or its patients since these studies are supported by a grant from the United States Public Health Service and the American Cancer Society, and I would supply all cultures and equipment from my laboratory. On the other hand, the Jewish Chronic Disease Hospital and collaborators there would be appropriately acknowledged in such scientific papers and lay publications as may ensue, subject of course to your prior approval.

I hope that this opportunity for research continues to interest you and that you will find it possible to participate in this program.

B.
How and by Whom Should the Research Process Be Administered?

1.

Petition of William A. Hyman— December 12, 1963

To the Supreme Court of the State of New York, Kings County:

The petitioner, William A. Hyman, respectfully states as follows:

That the said Jewish Chronic Disease Hospital is governed by a board of directors.

That your petitioner is still a member of said board of directors and continues to act as such director.

That in the month of September, 1963, your petitioner was informed that injections of live cancer cells had been made and were being made into non-cancerous patients at the hospital without their consent, either written or oral, and without their knowledge of the nature of the injections and that these injections were not for purposes of therapy or treatment of patients at the hospital but were done for the purpose of determining whether cancer can be induced by injection of live cancer cells and that, furthermore, some certain medical employees of the hospital were undertaking these experiments in cooperation and in concert with certain parties not affiliated with the said hospital and that all of this was being done without the approval, sanction, authorization and consent of the proper authorities of the said hospital.

That on September 30, 1963, a meeting of the board of directors of the hospital was held at which time and place Solomon Siegel, executive director of the hospital, read a report which purported to show that these injections of live cancer cells into non-cancerous patients were done with the oral consent of these patients. Furthermore, at this said meeting of the board of directors on September 30, 1963, Benjamin Saltzman, chairman of the executive committee of the said hospital, orally reported on a hearing held by him and certain associates and stated that the injection of live cancer cells into non-cancerous patients were harmless "tests" although he admitted before the board of directors that the patients who received such injections were never informed that live cancer cells were being injected into them but rather they were told that these were skin tests.

That your petitioner strenuously opposed the acceptance of the written report of the said Solomon Siegel, executive director of the hospital, and the oral report of said Benjamin Saltzman as a whitewash which imposed upon the board of directors serious civil and perhaps criminal responsibility if the facts as reported to your petitioner were correctly stated and, accordingly, petitioner made a motion that the said report of the said Solomon Siegel be rejected and that an independent committee be appointed to make a further investigation into the circumstances attending the injection of live cancer cells into non-cancerous patients.

Although to the best of my recollection there was a second to this motion by one of the directors present, there resulted considerable disorderly conduct and confusion, and a superseding motion was made to accept the report of said Solomon Siegel but, however, in the midst of the discussions and arguments back and forth at said meeting Mr. Herman W. Shane, chairman of the board of directors, suddenly declared the meeting adjourned.

At this meeting of the board of directors, he called attention to certain of the Nuremberg trials in which Nazi doctors were found guilty and some hanged and some otherwise punished for using human beings for experimental purposes without their informed consent to and knowledge of the experiments being conducted

on them and that such practices could not and should not be tolerated by any organization.

Likewise, when the attention of the directors present at this meeting was called to the fact of the responsibility devolved upon the board of directors, under the circumstances, the suggestions were disregarded and even ridiculed.

The question that he raises is whether those directors who voted to adopt that whitewash report of Mr. Siegel's would permit themselves to be used for experimental purposes. Will these directors who voted for this whitewash report consent to having injections of live cancer cells made into their bodies to see if cancer can be induced in their bodies?

That petitioner, in order to protect the integrity of the hospital and to terminate any possible abuses that may have arisen and to avoid injury to any patients and possible liability therefor on the part of the hospital and of the directors, requested the secretary of the hospital to furnish petitioner, at his expense, with a copy of the minutes of the meeting of the board of directors.

That petitioner's aforesaid request was ignored.

That petitioner wishes to be fully informed of all actions taken by the board of directors of the Jewish Chronic Disease Hospital and by all committees therein relative to the investigations of the complaints made and relative to the findings upon such investigations and to be fully informed of all the facts pertaining to the injection of live cancer cells into patients at the hospital, and petitioner, who has been associated with the said hospital for many years in various capacities, believes that it is his obligation as a director of said hospital to inquire into such happenings, and to ascertain all the facts, and to take adequate steps to protect the patients of the hospital and the good name and reputation of the hospital and of the directors and of the physicians connected with the hospital, and to avoid any possible liability on the part of the hospital and of the directors as a result of any injury that may be suffered by any patient as a result of said injections.

That the Jewish Chronic Disease Hospital, through its executive director and medical director, have contended that although the patients gave no written consent to the injections they gave their oral consent; but said contention is false and entirely without any basis in fact because some of the patients were in such mental and physical condition that they could neither know and understand the nature of the injections and the danger involved, nor consent to such injections, and other patients could speak only Yiddish, whereas Dr. Custodio could not speak one word of Yiddish, and, therefore, could neither ask for nor obtain oral consents.

That your petitioner has exhausted the remedy of requesting access to and examination and copies of the minutes of the meetings of the board of directors and the reports by Mr. Siegel and Dr. Abramson and the patients' charts and records and the other papers and documents pertaining to the experimental injection of cancer cells into non-cancerous patients, and by refusing petitioner's requests therefor the board of directors of said hospital have failed, neglected and refused to perform a duty enjoined upon them.

Wherefore, your petitioner respectfully prays that pursuant to Article 78, C.P.L.R., an order be made granting the inspection of the books, records, papers and documents sought by the petitioner herein, and granting such other and further relief as to the court may seem just and proper.

2.

Affidavits for Petitioner

a.

David Leichter, M.D.*— September 12, 1963

My name is David Leichter. I am a duly licensed physician in the State of New York having received my license in 1958 in New York State.

I have been associated with the Jewish Chronic Disease Hospital since July 1, 1959, first as chief resident in medicine and since 1960 as co-ordinator of medicine and in charge of cancer therapy and research. In this capacity all projects relating to the field of cancer were within my domain.

On or about July 3, 1963, I was approached by Dr. Emanuel Mandel, who was the director of medicine and medical education of the Jewish Chronic Disease Hospital, about a project which would involve the injection of live cancer cells

---

* The affidavits of Drs. Avir Kagan and Perry M. Fersko, coordinators in the department of medicine of the Jewish Chronic Disease Hospital, are essentially similar to the above affidavit.

into non-cancer patients of our hospital. He stated that two doctors from Memorial Hospital who had done some prior experimental work in this field would supply the hospital with this cancer cell suspension and he asked me to see them and discuss taking over this project.

After this brief discussion I told Dr. Mandel that at first blush, such a project would certainly require the informed consent of the patients on whom it was to be done, and until such prior informed consent was obtained there was absolutely no reason for me to meet with these doctors from Memorial Hospital and, further, that I did not believe such consent could be obtained. By informed consent, I mean discussing the project with the patient, advising him of the dangers, if any, informing him of the agent to be used—in this case live cancer cells. It also means to me that the patient on whom the experiment is to be made must be mentally competent and aware of the full extent and dangers of such a project, and that such consent to be legal and proper would have to be obtained in writing.

On about July 31, 1963, Dr. Avir Kagan approached me and informed me that he had been requested by Dr. Mandel to conduct experiments on chronic patients of the Blumberg Building by injecting in them a suspension of live cancer cells. He told me that he had refused to become a part of this project because he could not see how the informed consent of any of these patients could be obtained once they were aware of the nature of the agent and the purpose of the project.

On or about August 15, 1963, I received a telephone call at my home from Mr. Sol Siegel, who is the executive director of our hospital and he told me that he wanted to see me at 9 o'clock the following morning on a matter of importance.

On August 16, 1963, in his office, Mr. Siegel asked me about this cancer project and what I knew of it. I told him in detail about my first encounter with Dr. Mandel and the fact that I had refused to become a party to it because I felt that it was immoral and illegal without the prior written informed consent of each and every informed patient.

I further told him that I had been informed by Dr. Samuel Rosenfeld, the co-ordinator of medicine of the Blumberg Building, that some 18 patients in his ward had received injections of this live cancer suspension, without his knowledge, without his consent and without the patients' knowledge and informed consent, and under the auspices of Dr. Mandel and Dr. Custodio to whom he had assigned the project. He asked me some questions about the legality of Dr. Mandel's project and I told him that I had attended lectures given by Bryant L. Jones of the CCNSC (Cancer Chemo-Therapy National Service Center) whereby we were informed that it was illegal to administer experimental drugs to patients without their prior informed consent and knowledge and approval.

I also told him of the danger of rumors spreading in the hospital about giving these cancer cells to patients without their consent and the tremendous damage it could do to the reputation of the hospital and its standing in society. I also reminded him of the potential malpractice suits that might result from reactions in these patients who had received these injections. He asked me if Dr. Mandel could lose his license as a result of his action and I told him that I did not know but that it was a serious matter.

I repeated many times that I was against the project; that I had nothing to do with it; that I had not condoned it and that it was done without my knowledge and consent and against my express desires.

On or about August 26, 1963 I was informed that a meeting had been scheduled for the co-ordinators of the different divisions of the hospital to discuss this matter with Dr. Mandel and Mr. Siegel in an effort to hush it up. However, this meeting was cancelled.

On August 27, 1963 Dr. Avir Kagan, co-ordinator of the department of medicine, Dr. Perry M. Fersko, also a co-ordinator in the department of medicine, and I, in reviewing the project and our individual refusal to become a part of it and the fact that the parties responsible for it appeared to be passing the buck, thought it advisable to make our positions clear by resigning together and giving our reasons for such resignation. We realized that our position was untenable despite the fact that we had never become a party to this project and that the entire matter was unethical and immoral. Further, that if we remained, our silence or continued association with the hospital might be construed as condoning the actions of Dr. Mandel and Dr. Custodio and might be tantamount to our being co-conspirators. Therefore, on August 27, the three of us composed one letter of resignation, signed by all of us, wherein we stated the following:

We the undersigned co-ordinators in the department of medicine do hereby submit our resignations as co-ordinators, effective immediately. The reasons for our decision are based upon disagreement and opposition to certain research practices in which the department of medicine has engaged.

Our position has been stated to you. Inaction on our part might be interpreted as condoning these acts which we feel, under the circumstances, would be morally wrong.

This letter was addressed to the executive director of the Jewish Chronic Disease Hospital and copies were sent to the president of the executive board, chairman of the medical board, administrator of welfare, and the chairman of the department of medicine.

On August 28, 1963, Mr. Siegel called me in his office, advised me that he had read the resignation and attempted to intimidate me by stating that I had improperly obtained the consent of the relatives of certain cancer patients in another project involving the administration of an anti-cancer drug in cancer patients, which drug was known as Thermonycin 401.

I reminded Mr. Siegel that these were cancer patients who were actually receiving anti-cancer treatment but that these patients did not know they had cancer and that under these circumstances the law permitted us to obtain the consent of the nearest relative in an effort to save the lives of these patients, and that this situation was not in any way similar to the improper project previously described.

Mr. Siegel then attempted to claim that our resignation amounted to an abandoning of the patients. Thereupon we informed Mr. Siegel that we would be at the disposal of the hospital and the patients for any necessary treatment, free of charge and whenever required.

To date we have never been asked by anybody connected with the hospital to service such patients.

On August 29, 1963 Dr. Mandel met me at the hospital and we discussed this problem at length wherein I reiterated the fact that in my opinion the entire project was unethical and immoral and against public good and violated the rights of the patients who had not been informed of the nature of the project (i.e., the inherent dangers associated with an unknown experimental agent involving live cancer cells) and who had actually not given their informed consent. Dr. Mandel then informed me that he could not get their consent because these patients were incompetent.

I have read my statement and it is true to the best of my knowledge.

b.

Samuel Rosenfeld, M.D.—
September 12, 1963

My name is Samuel Rosenfeld. I have been a duly licensed physician in the State of New York since June, 1923.

I have been associated with the Jewish Chronic Disease Hospital for the past thirty years and have been the co-ordinator of medicine of the Blumberg Pavilion since 1956 and a visiting physician since 1945.

On Thursday, August 8, 1963, at about 10:30 A.M. while making my usual rounds in the Blumberg Pavilion, accompanied by Dr. Custodio, senior resident physician, a ward patient, Mr. Celi Stephano, stopped me, complaining bitterly of pain, and told me that he was injected under the right thigh and that that area was now swollen. He said that he had not been sick at the time he received the injection and he stated further that he knew that I had not ordered anything for him.

I inquired of Dr. Custodio, a resident in my service, and he motioned me away from the patient and then told me that he was doing experimental injections on orders from Dr. Emanuel Mandel. I was unable to pursue this subject further at the time but on the following day I again inquired of Dr. Custodio what had transpired. He told me that he was injecting material which was delivered to him by the Cancer Memorial Hospital.

On Monday, August 12, 1963, I again spoke to Dr. Custodio and he confirmed the fact that the material consisted of "cancer cells" and the project was to test the immunologic response of these patients to this agent.

On Tuesday, August 13, 1963, I was accosted by Dr. Avir Kagan, the then co-ordinator of the department of medicine, and he asked me if I was aware that Dr. Mandel had injected cancer cells in patients in my care and in my pavilion. He also spoke of other matters which made him unhappy and he told me he wished to resign. He specifically stated that Dr. Mandel had requested that he, Dr. Kagan, inject these "cancer cells suspensions" but that he flatly refused to do same.

Dr. Kagan then asked that I speak to Dr. David Leichter, who is in charge of the cancer research at our hospital, which I did, and he informed me that there was no project going on under his direction but that he had been approached by Dr. Mandel to authorize the injection of live cancer cells in chronically ill patients and that he did not consider this project feasible because of the potential danger attached to it and because the prior written consent of each patient would be required.

Dr. Kagan also told me that Dr. Perry Fersko had been requested by Dr. Mandel to give these injections but that he too had refused.

With this information on hand I felt it my duty to inform the administration of my findings as all new projects involving experimental drugs or agents, prior to their being used on patients, had to be approved by the research committee. This had not been done nor had the project received the approval of Dr. David Leichter even though this was a cancer project. In addition, it was being performed on patients for whom I am responsible in the Blumberg Pavilion, which patients had not been advised of the nature of the project nor told of its potential dangers nor had they given their prior written or oral consent. There were 18 patients in my ward who received these injections and many of them were mentally incapable of giving their consent. In my opinion this project was, therefore, both illegal and immoral and it has been conducted surreptitiously without my knowledge or consent.

In view of the fact that Mr. Sol Siegel, the executive director of the hospital, was on vacation, and Mr. Isaac Albert, the president, was seriously ill at the hospital, I contacted Mrs. Minnie Tulipan, the director of welfare and gave her all the facts and together we discussed matters further with Dr. Abraham Rabiner, patriarch of our hospital and former chief of neurology.

In the afternoon of August 14, 1963, Mrs. Tulipan told me that she had phoned Mr. Sol Siegel in Florida, had given him the facts and that he was scheduled to return on August 15, 1963.

On August 15, 1963, a patient in Ward P 6, Mr. Grossman, who had received the injection of these cancer cells was visited by three doctors from Memorial Hospital. In response to my questioning, Dr. Custodio told me that these were the doctors who were investigating the effects of the cancer cell suspension injections.

Shortly thereafter Mr. Siegel came to my home office and I informed him of the entire matter. He stated he would look into it.

On August 26, 1963, Mr. Siegel told me he was scheduling a meeting for the following day and upon inquiry as to the purpose of the meeting, I learned that in substance it was a meeting of the coordinators and his intention was to suppress this information and to take no action. I told him I would not attend this meeting as in my opinion the entire experimental project was dangerous and illegal and I would not condone what amounted to a crime. I told him that this situation was explosive, that it could result in malpractice actions and in the destruction of the reputation of the hospital. I told him in my opinion it should be handled by the board of directors and responsible physicians and that the president of the medical board and other true and loyal supporters of the hospital should be consulted.

The August 27th meeting was thereafter cancelled by Mr. Siegel.

On August 28, 1963, Mr. Siegel called me at 8:00 A.M. and told me he was going to see an important lawyer on this matter. I urged him again to make every effort to inform selective members of the board of directors of the situation since Dr. Joseph Abramson, the president of the medical board of the Jewish Chronic Disease Hospital, was not in the city.

Later the same morning, I learned that Drs. Leichter, Kagan and Fersko had resigned.

I was also told by Dr. Kagan that Dr. Mandel had called him into his office, had offered him an increase in salary and some private cases. The purpose of this effort was obvious. It was Dr. Mandel's attempt to keep Dr. Kagan and the others from talking about the project.

On August 29, 1963, I had a further discussion with Mr. Siegel who requested that I talk to Dr. Abramson who had just returned from abroad.

On August 30, 1963, at about 11:00 A.M. I discussed the matter with Dr. Joseph Abramson. After getting the entire report from me, he informed me that he would take this matter up before the grievance committee of the hospital for further evaluation.

To my knowledge no corrective action has been taken by any responsible committee or individual nor have I been asked to appear before the grievance committee or the medical board or any other responsible board of inquiry.

c.
Hyman Strauss, M.D.—November 23, 1963

I am a physician and surgeon duly admitted to practice in the State of New York specializing in gynecology and I am an attending physi-

cian in gynecology in the Jewish Chronic Disease Hospital.

On October 28, 1963, I addressed a letter to the medical board of the hospital, attention of the secretary of the executive committee which was given to that board. This letter was prompted by the horrible news that had reached me to the effect that patients in our hospital where I had been an attending physician for approximately twenty-five years were now being used for experimental purposes not associated with their therapy or their ailments, and that these experiments comprised the injection of live cancer cells into these chronic invalids at the hospital who were not informed of the fact that they were being injected with live cancer cells. As I am informed and verily believe, they were told that these injections of live cancer cells were mere "skin tests."

I am informed that no action was taken on this letter of complaint of mine. Instead, a conspiracy of silence developed in which an effort to suppress the disclosure of these practices to the membership and to the proper authorities was quite apparent.

Since no report of any proper action to correct this deplorable and outrageous situation was given to me and various other members of the medical staff, and apparently no proper and thorough investigation was made of the situation to prevent this recurrence and to prevent the practice of and to prevent the commission of these acts which belong more properly in Dachau, where for similar acts there had been prosecutions against the Nazis, I sent a copy of my letter of complaint to the Division of Professional Conduct of the New York State Education Department enclosed in my letter of October 30, 1963.

NOTES

NOTE 1.
LETTER OF HYMAN STRAUSS, M.D. TO THE MEDICAL BOARD OF THE JEWISH CHRONIC DISEASE HOSPITAL—OCTOBER 28, 1963

Inasmuch as I am unable to attend meetings at the present time for reasons beyond my control, I am obliged to write this letter as an expression of my position.

While the executive director was vacationing, an abundance of rumors found their way into medical circles. My first knowledge of this affair about cancer experimentation upon patients known to be free of malignant disease, without their fully informed written consent, came from conversations at two other hospitals in this borough. I next heard from a professor at the State University of New York, and finally a top-ranking investigator from Sloan-Kettering, a man with an international reputation, discussed this with me on the phone. I have also been questioned by laymen and clergymen not connected with our hospital. The coordinators refused to talk, indicating that they had been instructed not to say a word. Obviously, they had been successfully frightened.

Upon Mr. Siegel's return, I went to his office and asked for the truth about the matter that had already been rumored around quite a bit. He refused to make any statement but asked instead that I tell him what I had heard. Since I informed him that I was willing to discuss it only following his affirmation or denial, and since he refused to make such a statement, I left his office with the feeling that nothing could be gained and that the conspiracy of silence was continuing.

An effort to obtain an explanation from Dr. Joseph Abramson was equally unsuccessful, although instead of silence, I encountered conflicting comments. Within a period of 15 minutes, I was told first, that proper consent had been obtained in advance and duly witnessed. Next, I was told that the consent had been oral and that only some of the patients understood English. Finally, I was informed that consent was not necessary, according to Mr. Harry Albert, one of the attorneys for the hospital, and that it was unlikely that Jewish patients would agree to live cancer cell injections, especially since they were free of cancer themselves.

Finally, at the last meeting, twice when Dr. Mandel endeavored to inform the committee during his report of the resignation of the coordinators and when the question of consent was raised following a report by Dr. Slepian, the chairman arbitrarily utilized the privilege of his office to defer the discussion until the end of the meeting. The unfortunate sequence, however, was that the meeting was prolonged unduly and then abruptly and, I believe, deliberately, adjourned by the chair. This technique, I understand, was used by him at another hospital whenever he wished to stifle discussion. It might be suggested that the chairman acquaint himself with the democratic foundation of parliamentary procedure which entitles him to guide but not to dictate or interfere with full and free deliberation.

For three young coordinators to have resigned must have required some soul-searching on their parts. If undue pressures had been exerted to get them to act in ways inconsistent with their consciences, their sense of medical ethics, and in violation of the law, then their resignations, under such duress, are inacceptable. Further, men of such high ethical standards as to jeopardize their security when morality is at stake should not be lost to any hospital. Since medical liability insurance does not cover experimentation, no one has the right to demand that a physician perform any act for which he has no insurance protection without providing additional insurance which will cover him in the event of suit.

The matters at issue here are of extreme importance. A full and frank and complete hearing is absolutely necessary in order that no injustice be done to anyone. Denial of the opportunity to speak is undemocratic and should not be tolerated. All persons involved in this matter are entitled to ample opportunity to state their cases.

I therefore propose that the executive committee constitute a committee of the whole to investigate all sides in this issue. A small committee may be susceptible to instruction to act as a whitewash body. Unless we condemn what is improper, we share the guilt.

This is a medical matter and must be dealt with by medical persons. It is not within the province of the lay board of any hospital to pass upon medical ethics or to dictate what is or is not ethical in medical practice.

I feel that this is a matter involving my conscience and that no other solution can be considered satisfactorily.

NOTE 2.

LETTER OF HYMAN STRAUSS, M.D. TO DIVISION OF PROFESSIONAL CONDUCT, NEW YORK STATE EDUCATION DEPARTMENT—OCTOBER 30, 1963

The original of the previous letter was personally delivered to the secretary with the request that it be read and considered at the meeting held on October 28. I have been informed that the letter was not read and that no definitive action of any type was taken with reference to the matter described.

d.

Mendel Jacobi, M.D.—
December 11, 1963

I am a physician and surgeon duly licensed to practice medicine in the State of New York and have been practicing since 1925.

I am the consultant pathologist at the Jewish Chronic Disease Hospital.

On October 4, 1963, I examined the charts of five of the 26 patients who were subjected to the injection of live cancer cells.

In this affidavit I shall not reveal the names of the patients, but shall refer to each patient by his chart number, so as not to disclose any confidential information.

Chart No. K-14397 shows that the patient was admitted on June 8, 1962 at the age of 67. The patient had been in chronic congestive heart failure for a year and a half prior to admission. One year prior to admission he had had a cerebral vascular accident with a right hemiparesis and acute myocardial infarction. A note by the social service dated in April, 1962, describes his attitude as one of isolation, perversity and negativism with resistance to all forms of treatment. His blood urea nitrogen levels had been consistently high since admission indicating a state of chronic uremia, in which cerebration is generally poor. A psychiatric note in May, 1963, indicated that he had been in a depressive state for a year. A nurse's note dated July 16, 1963, states "Cell suspension injected into right thigh by Dr. Custodio and resident." A progress note of the same day signed by Dr. Custodio reads: "Cell suspension injected left thigh."

Chart No. 2290 shows that the patient was admitted May 21, 1941, at the age of 41, so that he is now 63 years old. The patient is a postencephalitic Parkinsonian of advanced grade who on February 19, 1963, fell while in the ward and fractured his left wrist. An undated note in the record made some ten years after his admission, when he was 52 years old, describes him as showing a marked speech defect, markedly irritable personality and one who stands in a corner and cries steadily and in a shrieking manner when his requests are not instantly carried out and that persuasion or argument was of no avail "due to the patient's low mentality and lack of insight and judgment." A note by Dr. Custodio, dated July 16, 1963, reads: "Cell suspension injected right thigh." A progress note dated September 5, 1963, notes that for two or three days he has developed hematuria. After an operation of Sep-

tember 27, 1963, it was found that he had a transitional cell carcinoma of the bladder which was resected. A consent to be photographed for moving pictures had been given by him on July 31, 1957, at which time his signature was still decipherable. Consents for cystoscopy on September 5, 1963, and for the bladder operation on September 27, 1963, were also signed by him, but with a barely legible and very scrawl-like signature. All three consents were witnessed by a person designated as his sister. However, there is no indication in the chart of any consent for the injection of the cell suspension.

Chart No. 8183 shows that the patient was admitted January 2, 1958, at the age of 38 with a diagnosis of multiple sclerosis. A history showed that in 1954 and 1955 a craneotomy and Gasserian ganglion decompression was performed twice on the right side and once on the left side. In 1957 he had been a patient in the Brooklyn State Hospital with a depressive psychosis, at which time he was unaware of his surroundings and unmanageable and his condition was diagnosed as dementia præcox. The chart shows that when admitted to the Jewish Chronic Disease Hospital in 1958 he was deemed mentally unsound and in the subsequent years his neurological status had not improved. From the beginning of 1963 onward he had repeated bouts of bilateral pneumonia and these events are specifically indicated to have occurred about May 31, 1963, and again about September 17, 1963. The chart makes no mention of any cell suspension or cell injections.

Chart No. 3762 shows the patient was admitted on June 10, 1952, at the age of 44. The diagnosis was postencephalitic Parkinsons with speech so dysarthric as to be noted "hard to understand." The chart shows he had had several falls during 1961 and 1962 on which occasions he hit his head against the ground. On May 8, 1963, there is another notation of a fall from a chair and striking his forehead on the floor. A note by Dr. Rosenfeld, the attending physician in charge, dated August 13, 1963, indicated an attempted suicide and requested psychiatric consultation. There is also a nurse's note dated August 16, 1963, that he had threatened to kill himself. The patient has been on considerable sedation throughout the years. There is no mention of cell suspension injections into this patient.

Chart No. B-15918 shows that the patient was admitted May 20, 1963, at the age of 72. The diagnosis was arteriosclerotic heart disease, coronary insufficiency, emphysema, hiatus hernia and spinal compression due to osteoporosis, with X ray showing compression fractures of the 6th, 7th and 12th dorsal vertebrae. On September 24, 1963, blood tests indicated a marked anemia and the biochemical changes of malnutrition. There are no notes of any injections of cell suspension in the chart of this patient.

I was informed by Dr. Rosenfeld that another patient who had received the cell suspension injections and who had had tabes dorsalis, central nervous system syphilis and diabetes had died. I was not able to locate the chart and have not been able to determine whether an autopsy was performed on this patient.

From my examinations of the five charts above described it is clear that these patients who were subjected to cancer cell injections were in no condition, mentally and physically, to understand the nature of the injections being given to them and to consent to such experimental injections. There was, of course, no written consent—and there is no entry in the charts of any oral consent. In fact three of the five charts do not even note the injections that were made.

3.

Answer of the Jewish Chronic Disease Hospital—January 6, 1964

The Jewish Chronic Disease Hospital herein referred to as "the hospital," by its attorney, Morris Ploscowe, for its answer to the petition herein avers as follows:

Admits that the petitioner is a director of the hospital, which is a membership corporation, and that the hospital is governed by a board of directors which presently numbers sixty.

The hospital is an institution for the care and treatment of the chronically ill, without regard to race, color or creed. The Isaac Albert Research Institute is affiliated with the hospital and has done some of the outstanding research in this country in the area of chronic diseases.

Denies that petitioner was the sole attorney for the hospital and is still one of the attorneys of record. The petitioner has never been the sole attorney for the hospital, and is not now an attorney of record.

Denies the statement that patients of the hospital were injected with live cancer cells "for the purpose of determining whether cancer can be induced." This statement is unqualifiedly false. There was absolutely no danger that any patient

would contract cancer from the subcutaneous injection given to him. Nor has any patient in fact contracted cancer or in any way been harmed by the tests administered to him. The injection was not designed to induce cancer, but to test the patient's immunologic reaction to cancer cells. The said experiment was conducted in collaboration with doctors from the Sloan-Kettering Institute. It was part of a bona fide attempt to advance human knowledge in dealing with cancer and has been financed by grants from the United States Public Health Service and the American Cancer Institute.

Admits that a board of directors' meeting was held on September 30, 1963. There were more than enough directors present for a quorum for the transaction of business.

At the said meeting, the petitioner did characterize as "whitewash" the report of Solomon L. Siegel and of the grievance committee of the medical staffs of the hospital. The said report was read at the board of directors' meeting.

The petitioner, at this meeting, did make the scurrilous analogy between Nazi experimentation at places like Dachau and the work done at the Jewish Chronic Disease Hospital with the collaboration of doctors from the Sloan-Kettering Institute and financed by United States Public Health Service funds.

The petitioner, by his emotionally rhetorical questioning at this meeting, did falsely spread the notion that the purpose of the experimentation was to see whether cancer could be induced.

The 22 members of the board of directors unanimously voted to approve the report of the grievance committee of the medical staffs of the hospital, despite the scurrilous, false and emotional statements of the petitioner. Only the petitioner dissented from this vote.

There is no truth in the petitioner's allegation that no vote was taken on the medical grievance committee report.

The documents and records which the petitioner is legally entitled to see as a director of the hospital have been mailed to him. These include the minutes of meetings of the board of directors, the report of Solomon Siegel, executive director of the hospital, the report of Dr. Joseph Abramson, the affidavit of Dr. Custodio, which were requested in the notice of motion submitted by the petitioner.

The Jewish Chronic Disease Hospital cannot legally turn over charts and records of patients, since the petitioner has not obtained the consent of such patients. The turnover of such material to the petitioner without the patients' consent is prohibited by CPLR, Sec. 4504(a), and the cases decided thereunder.

There was no attempt on the part of Isaac Albert to maintain a veil of secrecy and prevent a full disclosure of the situation, as alleged in the petition.

The petitioner is fully informed concerning the experimental work done at the hospital by the report made to the board of directors' meeting, a copy of which has been sent to him.

The right to determine whether any physician in the hospital has committed an unprofessional, illegal, or immoral act is not entrusted to any single director of the hospital, but is entrusted to various committees provided by the constitution and by-laws of the hospital, as follows:

The executive committee of the board of directors, which has full power to act on any matter requiring immediate action.

The medical conference committee, consisting of physicians, members of the staff, and directors of the hospital, which makes recommendations to the executive committee concerning medical and surgical activities of the hospital.

The medical board, which enforces rules and regulations for the proper supervision and care of patients.

The grievance committee, which has the duty to investigate "all grievances arising between members of the staff as well as the actual or alleged transgression by members of the staff."

The research committee, which has the power to review all protocols of projects submitted to it by members of the staff.

The petitioner has sought unilaterally, by a process of innuendo and slander, to arrogate to himself powers which are in the scope of the aforementioned committees of the hospital. Although not a physician, the petitioner seeks to determine what is and what is not the proper practice of medicine.

There is no individual liability of directors of a hospital for medical acts done without their knowledge.

The petition herein is not brought in good faith, but is the product of a long standing feud and vendetta which the petitioner has carried on for years against the president of the hospital, Isaac Albert.

The claim is made in these paragraphs, quoting the affidavits of various doctors, that the injections were made on patients without their consent. None of the doctors quoted was present when the injections were made, and any statement made in their affidavits concerning lack of consent is pure hearsay. Moreover, the affidavits of Doctors Custodio, Mandel and Southam, attached hereto, show that each patient was asked whether he would consent to the injection which was to be made. The injections were, in fact, made with the oral consent of the patients involved. There is no requirement in the law for written consent.

It is charged in the petition that the patients were mentally incapable of giving their consent to any injections. The refutation of this allegation is found in the affidavits of Doctors Mandel, Custodio and Abramson attached hereto. Their affidavits clearly demonstrate that these patients were not mentally incompetent to give a consent to the injections. Dr. Abramson, a neurologist and psychiatrist, who examined the affidavit of Dr. Jacobi, came to the following conclusion: "In the light of the above examination, I do not believe that any conclusion can be drawn that the five patients whose charts were examined by Dr. Jacobi were mentally incompetent."

There are charges in the above paragraphs concerning a conspiracy of silence to suppress disclosures, and to suppress facts. There has never been any such conspiracy. Nor has there been any attempt to suppress facts (see affidavits of Solomon L. Siegel and Dr. Mandel attached hereto). The complaints of the doctors whose affidavits support the petition were heard in due course by the grievance committee of the medical staff, provided for by the constitution and by-laws of the hospital. The report of the latter committee was fully discussed at the September 30, 1963 board of directors' meeting, at which the petitioner was present. All the 22 directors present, with the exception of the petitioner, voted to accept the report absolving the medical staff of any blame for alleged professional misconduct.

The charge is made that three of the doctors at the hospital (Kagan, Fersko and Rosenfeld) were asked to participate in the project by Dr. Mandel, the director of medicine, and that they refused because of either ethical grounds or because proper consents could not be obtained from the patients. The affidavit attached hereto of Dr. Mandel flatly denies that any such requests were made to these doctors.

Complaint is made that the consent of Dr. Rosenfeld was not obtained to the injections made on patients (see Fersko and Rosenfeld affidavits). Dr. Mandel, as director of medicine at the hospital, was the superior of both of the aforementioned doctors. Under the constitution and by-laws of the hospital, he did not need the consent of his subordinates for a pilot study such as the one herein under consideration.

None of the affidavits of the doctors produced by the petitioner supports the charge in the petition, that the purpose of the tests conducted at the Jewish Chronic Disease Hospital was to see whether "cancer could be induced" in any of the patients. The latter notion is a figment of the petitioner's imagination. The affidavits of Doctors Mandel, Custodio, Korman and Southam, attached hereto, make it crystal clear that no harm resulted to the patients at the hospital from the injections made on them, and no harm was expected at the time the injections were made.

For a complete and affirmative defense to the petition herein, the Jewish Chronic Disease Hospital alleges:

Upon information and belief, the petitioner has made complaints similar to those contained in his petition, to the Kings County district attorney's office, which investigates and prosecutes the commission of crime in Kings County, and to the New York State Department of Education, which has the duty of investigating and prosecuting complaints concerning breaches of medical discipline and ethics by physicians. All the doctors involved in the research and experimentation complained of have been questioned by the said public agencies. These include, Dr. Chester Southam and Arthur J. Levin of the Sloan-Kettering Institute, and Dr. Emanuel E. Mandel and Dr. D. B. Custodio of the Jewish Chronic Disease Hospital. The hospital has cooperated fully with the aforementioned public agencies in making all data available to them. Upon information and belief, the petitioner's complaints are still under advisement in the said agencies.

Wherefore, the Jewish Chronic Disease Hospital prays that the petition herein be dismissed.

4.

Affidavits for Respondent

a.

Solomon L. Siegel—January 3, 1964

I am the executive director of Jewish Chronic Disease Hospital.

The petitioner states that the injections were made in the patients at the Jewish Chronic Disease Hospital for the purpose of determining whether cancer can be induced by the injection of live cancer cells. This is an outrageous falsehood. The attached affidavits of Drs. Southam, Mandel, Korman and Custodio, and medical literature throughout the world, will support the fact that cancer cannot be induced by injection of cancer cells. It is a recognized natural phenomenon that any foreign cells injected into the human body from an outside source will be rejected. Cancer cells are no exception. The purpose of the test was to determine whether the chronically ill, debilitated patients would reject the foreign cells at the same rate as cancer patients, or at the rate associated with normal humans.

Cancer cells were used in the experiment at the hospital, because unlike other foreign cells, the resultant nodule could be measured and the rejection time could thus be determined.

It is of significance, scientifically, that the patients injected rejected the cancer cells the same as normal humans, despite the fact that these were chronically ill, debilitated patients. The problem remaining now is to isolate the immunity factor which distinguishes the normal human from the cancer victim. Such isolation would provide an important clue in the conquest of the dread disease.

It should be noted that none of the doctors who submitted supporting affidavits made the claim contained in the petition that the purpose of the tests at the hospital was to determine whether cancer could be induced. As a matter of fact, Dr. Leichter, who was familiar with problems of cancer, has admitted that the injection of the cell suspensions which were used in the project constituted no possibility whatsoever of producing cancer in the patients involved.

It is not true that the injections were made without the knowledge and consent of patients. As appears from the affidavit of Dr. Custodio, who actually administered the injections, the consent of each patient was asked for orally and obtained. Neither medical ethics nor the law require that a consent to an injection be in writing. Dr. Custodio's affidavit is better testimony as to what happened than the hearsay statements of the petition and the doctors who were not present when the injections were made. Dr. Custodio was familiar with the patients. He has been a resident physician for two years. He found no difficulty in communicating with the patients in English. Dr. Arthur Levin, from Sloan-Kettering Institute, who was present when the injections were made, is familiar with the Yiddish language and was available to talk to the patients, had this been necessary. Nor is the charge true that the patients were mentally incompetent to give their consent. Dr. Jacobi's statement concerning the mental condition of five patients, contained in his affidavit, and which is based only on an examination of their charts, is refuted by the affidavit of Dr. Joseph L. Abramson, who was president of the medical staff, and who is a consultant at the hospital in neurology and psychiatry. Dr. Abramson concluded that the charges of mental incompetence with respect to the five patients whose charts were examined by Dr. Jacobi were not justified. Dr. Jacobi did not know the number of patients involved. He stated that 26 patients were injected, whereas only 22 patients were involved in the tests at the hospital.

The fact is that neither the consent of Dr. Leichter nor Dr. Rosenfeld was required for the tests. Dr. Emanuel Mandel is the director of medicine of the hospital. He is the superior of both Dr. Leichter and Dr. Rosenfeld. Dr. Leichter was not in charge of cancer research, as claimed in Dr. Kagan's affidavit. Any project to do research required the approval of Dr. Mandel. Dr. Mandel approved the study and under the constitution and by-laws of the medical staff, he had the authority to give such approval. The said constitution and by-laws permit directors of services, without prior approval, to make pilot studies. The injection of 22 patients was such a pilot study. Dr. Mandel's only obligation was to submit a protocol to the research committee of the medical staff within 60 days.

The petitioner states that it is his obligation as a director to inquire into happenings and to ascertain all the facts and to take adequate steps to protect the patients and the good name of the hospital. Mr. Hyman is so obsessed with the notion that there has been wrongdoing at the hospital that he brushes aside the unanimous opinion of the directors who disagreed with him and of the medical grievance committee which found no wrongdoing. Moreover, he overlooks the fact that those who disagree with him are just as much interested in the welfare of the patients and the welfare of the hospital as he. One begins to wonder just how much Mr. Hyman has the interests of the hospital and patients at heart.

Mr. Hyman also overlooks an important fact: There is a basic distinction between the medical affairs of the hospital and the care of patients, on the one hand, and the administrative affairs of the hospital. It is accepted procedure in hospitals for the board of directors to detail its medical responsibilities to the medical staffs of the hospital. This is the case at the Jewish Chronic Disease Hospital. The medical and dental staffs have their own constitution and by-laws. The by-laws provide for a grievance committee to handle matters of any questionable nature. A duly appointed grievance committee considered the problems raised by the tests on the 22 patients. The grievance committee report was approved by the board of directors. Mr. Hyman wishes to set himself up as a one man court of appeal from the judgment of the grievance committee and the board of directors.

There are statements in the affidavits that Doctors Kagan and Leichter had been requested by Dr. Mandel to make injections or to authorize injections and that these doctors had refused to do so. This is contrary to the information that I received from Dr. Mandel when I made an inquiry into the matter. He stated that no such requests were made. Moreover, as the superior of the doctors, he did not need their approval to make any appropriate studies or tests. Dr. Leichter has already repudiated the statement attributed to him (see affidavit of Dr. Samuel Korman attached hereto).

Dr. Rosenfeld alleges that the project was illegal and immoral and conducted surreptitiously without his knowledge and consent. The short answer is that his knowledge and consent were not required, and it is somewhat difficult to conceive that dedicated research workers of the Sloan-Kettering Institute would be engaged in illegal and immoral practices on our patients with the consent of our director of medicine. It should be noted that Dr. Rosenfeld has a personal animus against Dr. Mandel and on more than one occasion, when I discussed the problem with him, he insisted that Dr. Mandel be discharged immediately.

Petitioner as a lawyer should know that the hospital is prohibited by law from divulging the contents of patients records which are confidential, and which records he is demanding by court order.

The petitioner has embarked upon a reckless campaign to discredit the Jewish Chronic Disease Hospital unless he has his way. The court should not assist him in his campaign. May I therefore respectfully urge the court to deny the petition herein.

b.

Emanuel E. Mandel, M.D.— December 31, 1963

I am a physician duly licensed to practice medicine in the State of New York since 1939.

I am the director of the department of medicine and director of medical education at the Jewish Chronic Disease Hospital, having held these positions since November 1961. In addition, I am a clinical associate professor of medicine at the Downstate Medical Center, State University of New York. Previously, from 1957 to 1962, I was associate professor of medicine at the Chicago Medical School and associate director of medical education at Mount Sinai Hospital of Chicago, Illinois.

The petition of William A. Hyman and the affidavits annexed thereto are replete with falsehoods, distortions, and misrepresentations. I shall try to bring these to the attention of the court.

The most shocking misstatement in Mr. Hyman's papers is the allegation that the experiment and tests conducted at the hospital were "for the purpose of determining whether cancer can be induced by the injection of live cancer cells." Similarly misleading and fallacious are references in the petition to Nazi doctors, Nuremberg trials, and Dachau methods, as well as the inane argument as to whether the directors, who voted against Mr. Hyman when the matter of the tests was being considered, would "consent to having injections of live cancer cells made into their own bodies to see if cancer can be induced in their bodies."

It should be clearly understood that there was absolutely no danger arising to patients of the hospital who received hypodermic injections of suspensions of cells obtained from cultures of human cancer tissue. The purpose of the injections (which were given to 22 patients on July 16, 1963) was to determine the mechanism and rate of rejection of the injected material by the recipients. This material represented homologous transplants, i.e., tissue of one human being transplanted into another person. While other tissue, such as normal skin muscle, could be used for the same purpose, cancer cell lines were chosen because they have the necessary growth capacity to produce a measurable reaction. "It is inconsequential whether these are cancer cells or not, since they are foreign to the recipient and hence are rejected. The only drawback to the use of cancer cells is the phobia and ignorance that surrounds the word cancer (quoted from a letter written by Dr. C. M. Southam)." Indeed, the injections could not possibly and did not "induce cancer" in any of the patients. The innuendos concerning danger to patients from "injections of live cancer cells" contained in some of the physicians' affidavits attached to the petition can be

explained only by their ignorance in the subject, unless ulterior motives were at play.

The project was undertaken because of its vital importance not only to the understanding and possible treatment and diagnosis of cancer, but also to the understanding of other diseases, particularly those of autoimmune and degenerative nature, and because of its possible contribution to our knowledge in the general field of organ homotransplantation. Tests of the nature described above had been carried on for several years on patients at Memorial Hospital in New York and on healthy prisoners at the Ohio State Penitentiary. For the past 2 years, these tests have been routinely applied to all postoperative patients on the gynecology service of Memorial Hospital as a measure of their immunologic status. These studies had revealed that healthy persons rejected cancer cell homografts completely and promptly (in 4 to 6 weeks), while patients with advanced cancer usually showed a delayed rejection (6 weeks to 3 months). The typical reaction consists in a painless subcutaneous nodule (lump) which attains a maximal size of 2 to 3 cm. in diameter and disappears within the periods noted above. The project at the hospital was designed by Dr. C. M. Southam of the Sloan-Kettering Institute to determine whether the immunologic response (rate of rejection) in chronically ill and debilitated noncancer patients was similar to that of healthy persons or conformed to that of cancer patients. Results of the project conducted at the hospital by Drs. Southam and Arthur G. Levin of The Sloan-Kettering Institute and by Dr. D. B. Custodio of the hospital clearly indicated that chronically ill, debilitated non-cancer patients reacted like normal individuals in rejecting homologous tissue cells. Hence, the delayed immunologic response of cancer patients must be attributed to the disease itself (cancer), rather than to the attendant metabolic changes (weakness, debilitation). This finding furthermore suggests that the spread of cancer in the human body is associated with an impairment of the normal immunologic defense mechanisms. If this impairment could be prevented or remedied, the spread of cancer might be halted. This discovery may prove to be of great importance in the future control of cancer.

Mr. Hyman was fully aware that the above-named investigators were not trying to "induce cancer" but that they were testing the immunologic response of our patients. This information was available from Dr. Rosenfeld's affidavit attached to the petition stating that "the project was to test the immunologic response of these patients." This is a far cry from inducing cancer in the patients. Indeed, as I stated above, there was absolutely no danger of inducing cancer by these tests.

It is charged in the petition and affidavits that the patients' consent to the skin tests had not been obtained; that many of the patients were incompetent and incapable of giving a real consent; that some of the patients did not even speak English. Please note that Dr. D. B. Custodio, senior medical resident at the hospital, voluntarily, at my suggestion, undertook this research in collaboration with the two physicians from the Sloan-Kettering Institute, Dr. Chester M. Southam and Dr. Arthur G. Levin. Each of the patients was asked by Dr. Custodio for his consent to the injections, in the presence of those other 2 physicians. Dr. Custodio had known these patients for many months and was able to communicate with them in English, despite allegations in the petition to the contrary. Obviously, Dr. Custodio was in a better position to gauge the ability of patients to comprehend the requests which were being made of them than was Dr. Jacobi who drew his conclusions concerning the patients' mental status from charts. Moreover, when personally visiting on December 20, 1963, 4 of the 5 patients listed in Dr. Jacobi's affidavit, I found each to be in satisfactory condition for comprehending or giving consent to a diagnostic test or a surgical procedure. The fifth patient had died in October following a bladder operation.

The reference in the petition and affidavits to the requirement of written consent of patients for the tests is not consistent with my understanding of the law of New York. I believe that oral consent was adequate. Such consent was obtained in every instance, in accordance with the procedure which had been in vogue at Memorial Hospital for several years. There, these tests are used as routine studies and are being considered to be even less hazardous than such other routine diagnostic procedures as bone marrow aspiration and lumbar puncture.

The petition charges that the experiments on the patients were made without the "approval, sanction, authorization and consent" of the proper authorities at the hospital. This is untrue; Drs. Southam and Levin of the Sloan-Kettering Institute were initially referred to me by Mr. Sol Siegel, the executive director of the hospital, whom they had called over the telephone about this research project. As director of medicine and of medical education of the hospital, I authorized the project after I had discussed it at great length with Drs. Southam and Levin; after I had ascertained Dr. Southam's reputation in the field of cancer research and reviewed his publication on the subject; and after I had become convinced that the proposed clinical study was likely to make a significant contribution to science without exposing our patients to any risk. Under the constitution, by-laws and rules and regulations governing the medical staff of the hospital, I had the right to engage in pilot studies and was under the obligation to inform the research committee of the hospital of such pilot studies within 60 days from the time when such project was undertaken. When complaints about the project came to the attention of the grievance committee of the medical staff at its meeting on September 7, 1963, my actions were upheld and, indeed, further studies of the same type were being encouraged by the committee. This is apparent from the annexed minutes of this meeting. Furthermore, the board of directors, at its meeting of September 30, 1963, expressed its approval, with only Mr. Hyman dissenting.

It is asserted that there may be liability on the part of the directors and the hospital because of "injuries that may be received by any patient" as a result of the injections that were made. It should be noted that no injury resulted to any patient from the injections. A small nodule (lump) formed within 2 weeks after the injection and disappeared completely not later than 2 months thereafter. This was the typical reaction which was being expected. As mentioned previously, the vital part of the project was measurement of the size of the nodule and of the time of its disappearance. With respect to the statement in Dr. Rosenfeld's affidavit that one patient complained bitterly of pain in connection with such an injection. I was advised by Dr. Custodio that this was incorrect; the patient did not complain of pain but merely inquired with respect to the lump which had formed on his thigh following the injection. This lump as well as the skin reactions in all the patients who received these tests have completely disappeared.

It is claimed that I asked three physicians at the hospital, namely, Drs. Fersko, Kagan and Leichter, to "undertake a project of injecting cancer cells" and that they all turned me down. The falsehood of this claim is, in part, proven by the affidavit concerning Dr. Leichter signed by Dr. S. Korman. The only one of those three physicians ("coordinators") to whom I suggested participation in the research project was Dr. Kagan. However, several days later, I informed Dr. Kagan that Dr. Custodio had consented to such participation so that Dr. Kagan's assistance was no longer needed. I also discussed the proposed research project with each of the other two coordinators on separate occasions in order to acquaint them with it and to obtain their respective opinions about the scientific value of the project. The opinion of each of the three physicians was indeed favorable.

The charges in Dr. Rosenfeld's affidavit that the experiment was conducted "surreptitiously" and in Dr. Jacobi's affidavit that proper notations on the patients' charts were not made are totally unwarranted and without foundation. There was no reason at all for secrecy concerning a bona fide research project which was being carried out in collaboration with one of the outstanding research institutions in the country. Dr. Custodio had been instructed by me to make appropriate entries in each of the patients' charts who received the test and, as far as I know, he complied with this instruction.

The claim contained on the last page of Dr. Rosenfeld's affidavit is completely unwarranted that I attempted to keep "Dr. Kagan and the others from talking about the project" by offering him an increase in salary and some private patients. The truth is that I reassured Dr. Kagan on August 27th that the request for an increase in salary which he had made repeatedly over the preceding 4 months would be granted. I also indicated that I would turn some of my private cases over to him and to other members of the staff in order to find more time for research. This discussion took place the day after my return from a two-week vacation, at which time I was unaware of Dr. Kagan's antagonistic attitude and of his intention to resign abruptly.

A report on this study is scheduled to be presented to the sixth Biennial International Transplantation Conference at the New York Academy of Sciences in February 1964.

c.

Deogracias B. Custodio, M.D.— January 3, 1964

I am a resident physician at the Jewish Chronic Disease Hospital. I have held this position since July 1, 1961 to June 30, 1962 and from July 1, 1963 up to date.

Some time in July of 1963 I was asked by Dr. Mandel whether I would be interested in participating in a research project which would be done at Jewish Chronic Disease Hospital with doctors from Sloan-Kettering Institute. I was told that the project was financed by a grant from the U.S. Public Health Service and that the work was being carried on under the direction of Dr. Chester Southam of Sloan-Kettering Institute. The project involved injecting patients with cancer cell suspensions in order to determine what their rate of rejection of the injected material would be. I was told that similar tests had been made on cancer patients and on healthy prisoners at the Ohio State Penitentiary. The purpose of the project was to determine whether weak, debilitated, chronically sick patients would reject this material like normal individuals or whether the rate of rejection would resemble cancer patients. I knew from my medical experience and studies that there was no possibility of any patient developing cancer as a result of these injections. The material injected was a foreign body and must by the laws of biology and medicine be rejected by the human organism.

The charge in the petition that the purpose of the injections made at the Jewish Chronic Disease Hospital was to determine whether cancer could be induced by such injections just simply is not true. Cancer cannot be induced by such injections. The purpose of the test was to determine the patients' immunological reaction to the injection of cancer cells and not "to induce cancer."

On July 16, 1963, I met with Dr. Mandel, the director of medicine of the hospital, and Dr. Chester Southam and Dr. Arthur Levin of the Sloan-Kettering Institute. Dr. Southam demonstrated the techniques of injection on three patients. I injected the other 19 patients under his general supervision. The appropriate entry showing this injection was made on the chart of each patient in accordance with proper medical practice. Before any patient was injected, Dr. Mandel obtained the oral consent from the first 2 patients and I did the oral from the next 20 patients. The patient was told that an injection of a cell suspension was planned as a skin test for immunity or resistance. The patient was also told that a lump would form within a few days which would last several weeks and gradually disappear. The patient was not told that the injection would contain cancer cells. The reason for this is that we did not wish to stir up any unnecessary anxieties, disturbances or phobias in our patients. There was no need to tell the patients that the injected material contained cancer cells because it was of no consequence to the patients.

Drs. Southam and Levin were present when I asked for the oral consent of 20 patients. Dr. Mandel obtained the consent from the first 2 patients. Dr. Mandel was present when the first 2 patients were injected as well as Dr. Southam and Dr. Levin. I had no difficulty in communicating with the patients in English. The charge that some of the patients spoke only Yiddish is not correct. Dr. Levin, I am advised, speaks Yiddish, and he could have spoken to the patients in this language had it been necessary.

Nor is there any truth in the assertion made in the petition and in Dr. Jacobi's affidavit that some of the patients were mentally incompetent to give this consent. I have known some of these patients for at least 6 months and I have no difficulty in communicating with them. In my opinion, none of the patients was mentally incompetent so that they could not give their consents to the injections.

After the injections were made, I observed the patients with Dr. Southam and/or Dr. Levin twice a week during the first 3 or 4 weeks and weekly thereafter. As expected, the lump or nodule developed and disappeared within an average period from six to eight weeks. As expected, no harm or injury occurred, as a result of these injections, to any of the patients, with the exception of the transient lump mentioned.

For my services in connection with this project I was paid the sum of $100.00 out of the research funds available to the Sloan-Kettering Institute from the U.S. Public Health Service grant.

d.

Chester M. Southam, M.D.— January 5, 1964

I am a licensed physician in the State of New York. I am employed as a full-time staff member of the Sloan-Kettering Institute for Cancer Research where I am chief of the section of clinical virology of the division of clinical chemotherapy, and chief of the section of oncogenic virology of the division of virology and immunology. I am an associate attending physician of Memorial Hospital for Cancer and Allied Diseases and an associate visiting physician of the James Ewing Hospital of the City of New York, on the chemotherapy service of the department of medicine. I am an associate profes-

sor of medicine of the School of Medicine of Cornell University. I have been with these institutions for approximately 15 years engaged in the practice of clinical medicine (medical management of cancer), medical teaching, and research in various phases of clinical and laboratory oncology.

Since 1954 one of the major types of research in which I have been engaged is the study of the relationships between immunological responses and cancer. The studies in 1954 revealed for the first time evidence of a major immunological defect in patients with advanced cancer. This was evidenced by the delayed rejection of homotransplants of neoplastic tissue-cultured human cells by such patients, in contrast to the prompt rejection which would, of course, be expected to occur since these are homotransplants (that is, these cells are foreign to the individual into whom they are injected).

A major deficiency of these investigations until the present year was the lack of direct evidence that the immunological deficiency observed in cancer patients was specifically related to cancer. Recently it was possible to establish this important point by the demonstration that patients who are chronically ill and debilitated due to various diseases other than cancer have a normal or near normal capacity to reject this same type of tissue-cultured cell transplant. This work was made possible through the collaboration of Dr. Emanuel Mandel, chief of medicine of the Jewish Chronic Disease Hospital in Brooklyn, and the cooperation of patients in that hospital.

It was possible to arrange for this collaboration because my present clinical research fellow, Dr. Arthur Levin, through personal acquaintances was able to discuss this work and the need for similar studies in non-cancer patients with persons affiliated with the Jewish Chronic Disease Hospital. Through such persons we were referred to Mr. Siegel, executive director of that hospital, who referred us to Dr. Mandel, chief of medicine, to discuss the problem and the possibility of a collaborative research project. After thorough discussion of the purpose, importance, procedures, reactions, and previous scientific publications, Dr. Mandel indicated his interest in such studies and some time later arrangements for a preliminary study were made. He was, of course, aware that homologous cells (cells from a human other than the person in whom they are injected) could not long continue to persist unless immunological reactiveness was severely impaired, and that there was no possibility of inducing cancer or causing any severe reaction in his patients.

This study was initiated on July 16, 1963, at which time each of the 22 patients was given two injections under the skin of a suspension of tissue-cultured cells of human neoplastic origin. These represented three long-established cell lines known as HEp 3, HEp 2, and RP 41. The injections were made on the anterior surface of one thigh at two sites just beneath the skin. The injections were made in the first three patients by me, as a demonstration of the technique for the instruction of Dr. Mandel and the medical resident (Dr. Custodio) who had expressed an interest in assisting in this project and who did all of the injections after my demonstration. After observing the technique, Dr. Mandel left and all of the tests on the remaining patients were done by Dr. Custodio in the presence of Dr. Arthur Levin and myself. Dr. Levin and I prepared the cell suspensions in the syringes ready for the injections and recorded details of the procedure and the patient's name in our date book. Explanations to the patient, obtaining the consents, and the writing of notes in the chart, as well as the injection itself, were the activities of Dr. Custodio. To the best of my knowledge each patient on whom these tests were done was informed that it was a test that would measure his or her reactions or defense reactions and further information was given whenever the patient wished it. To the best of my knowledge each patient did indicate his consent to this test.

The test sites were checked by Dr. Custodio and Dr. Levin at intervals of not longer than four days for the next four weeks by which time almost all reaction had disappeared. They were further checked for an additional three or four weeks until no person showed any further evidence of reaction at the test site. I, too, accompanied Drs. Custodio and Levin on three of these follow-up visits (July 19th, August 13th and August 20th).

I have seen the petition herein, in which it is charged that the purpose of the tests at the Jewish Chronic Disease Hospital was to see whether "cancer could be induced" in the patients who were injected with the cell-suspension material which was used. I wish again to assert categorically that this was not the intention of the study and that it is biologically and medically impossible to induce cancer by this means. The purpose was to test the immunological re-

sistance of these patients to cancer. No patient who was injected was harmed in the slightest by the test which was made on him, except for the lump or nodule which formed at the test site, and which disappeared within four to eight weeks. During the past 10 years, as we have seen, cancer cells have been implanted in almost 600 well persons and cancer patients. They have caused no untoward effects and have not resulted in the development of any cancers in either the well persons or those already suffering from their own cancers. The technique for measuring immune reactions is now standardized and the results are predictable. All the patients in the study undertaken at the Jewish Chronic Disease Hospital rejected the transplants as promptly as did the healthy persons. Thus it has been demonstrated that cancer patients lack an immune mechanism present in other individuals, including chronically diseased patients.

Thus the research done at the Jewish Chronic Disease Hospital has enabled us to take one more step forward in the continuing battle against cancer.

e.

Joseph L. Abramson, M.D.—
January 3, 1964

I am a physician, duly licensed to practice medicine in the State of New York since 1924. I hold the rank of consultant at Jewish Chronic Disease Hospital. I am a psychiatrist and neurologist. I was president of the medical staff of Jewish Chronic Disease Hospital from January 1, 1962 to December 31, 1963. I am consulting neuro-psychiatrist at Brooklyn Jewish and Swedish hospitals; I am a Diplomate in Neurology and in Psychiatry. I am assistant clinical professor in neurology at Downstate Medical Center; and a qualified psychiatrist in the State of New York.

Dr. Mendel Jacobi has submitted an affidavit in which he comments on the charts of five patients who allegedly were injected with cancer cells. The conclusion has been drawn from his analysis that these patients were mentally incompetent and could not give a rational consent to any injections made on them. This conclusion is not justified from the data used by Dr. Jacobi. I have examined Dr. Jacobi's affidavit and wish to make the following comments on the cases examined by him:

K14397: Does not say that he did or did not have aphasia and no indication that he did not talk or fails to understand what was said to him. Even though "perverse, negative, resistant to therapy," does not indicate that he did not comprehend. No justification for statement that "a state of chronic uremia in which cerebration is generally poor" applied in this particular case.

#2990: At age 52 a note indicates that patient had "marked speech defect, marked irritable personality—who cries steadily and in a shrieking manner." The conclusion of the examiner at the time was that "this is due to the patient's low mentality, and lack of insight and judgment." There is nothing in the above statement to justify that the patient had a low mentality. Two months after the alleged injection, the patient signed consent which was acceptable to the surgeon, for an operation on the bladder. One can obviously say, that two months before, in July, he was just as well aware of his environment, and could give consent at that time.

#8183: Admitted to Jewish Chronic Disease Hospital 1958. He had been a patient at Brooklyn State Hospital in 1957 with diagnosis of "dementia praecox." There is nothing in the chart to indicate that he was incompetent, and a diagnosis of this condition, per se, does not indicate incompetence. There is a note to the effect that the "neurologic status had not improved." There is no note in the allegation as to his mental status when he was admitted.

#3762: There is absolutely nothing in the allegation to indicate that the patient was not competent mentally even though he made a suicidal attempt one month after the alleged injection.

B15918: There is absolutely nothing in the allegation of the patient's incompetency.

In the light of the above examination, I do not believe that any conclusion can be drawn that the five patients whose charts were examined by Dr. Jacobi were mentally incompetent.

f.

Samuel Korman, M.D.— December 19, 1963

I am a physician duly licensed to practice medicine in the State of New York.

I am the associate director of the Department of Medicine of the Jewish Chronic Disease Hospital and chief of the division of neoplastic diseases in that department.

On Tuesday, December 17, 1963, between 9:30 and 10:30 A.M., I was present in the office of Dr. E. E. Mandel, director of medicine of the Jewish Chronic Disease Hospital, when he talked with Dr. David Leichter who had come to see Dr. Mandel about his reappointment to the attending staff of the hospital.

In the course of this conversation, Dr. Mandel read aloud the summary of an affidavit which Dr. Leichter had signed on September 12, 1963 pertaining to a research project that had been undertaken by Dr. Mandel in collaboration with Drs. Southam and Levin of the Sloan-Kettering Institute.

Upon listening to the reading of this summary, Dr. Leichter admitted that certain statements mentioned in the summary were untrue; to wit, that he (Dr. Leichter) had never been asked by Dr. Mandel "to undertake the project of injecting live cancer cells into non-cancer patients." Dr. Leichter further stated that he had not used the expression attributed to him in the summary that ". . . efforts were made to hush-up the complaints about the project." In addition, Dr. Leichter indicated that he (and Drs. P. M. Fersko and A. Kagan) had been quite upset at the time of their abrupt resignations from their salaried positions in the hospital (about August 27, 1963), and he conceded that they may not have used their best judgment in taking that action. Dr. Leichter also informed Dr. Mandel that he and the two doctors mentioned had made their affidavits on September 12th largely because of rumors that the hospital was going to make formal charges against them for abandonment of patients. Finally, Dr. Leichter agreed with Dr. Mandel and the undersigned that injection of the cell suspensions which were used in the project constituted no hazard whatsoever to the patients involved with respect to production of cancer.

5.

Minutes of Grievance Committee of the Medical Staff, Jewish Chronic Disease Hospital—September 7, 1963

Attendance: Drs. David Kershner, Mayer E. Ross, Harry Weiner Nathan A. Lewis (D.D.S.), Joseph L. Abramson

By Invitation: Solomon L. Siegel, executive director

Benjamin Saltzman, chairman of executive committee of board of directors

Harry B. Albert, director and hospital counsel

Absent: Dr. Samuel Millman, chairman of grievance committee

Herman W. Shane, chairman of board of directors

In the absence of Dr. Millman, Dr. Abramson presided. He opened the meeting indicating that a complaint had been brought to his attention in regard to certain research activities which had been done under instructions of Dr. Mandel, director of medicine. He read a letter of resignation by three coordinators in medicine, signed jointly by Drs. Kagan, Fersko and Leichter. (A copy of the letter is made part of these minutes). He then called upon Mr. Siegel, executive director, to relate the sequence of events leading up to his meeting.

Testimony by Solomon L. Siegel, Executive Director

He arrived at Miami Beach on vacation on Wednesday, August 14, 1963. Within an hour after checking in at a hotel, he received an emotionally frantic call from Mrs. M. Tulipan urging him to return to the hospital immediately because "something terrible has happened, which cannot be discussed on the telephone." Alarmed, Mr. Siegel arranged to return by plane and called Mrs. Tulipan at her home that evening to make arrangements to be picked up at the airport. It was during this call that Mrs. Tulipan told Mr. Siegel that "some of our patients were injected with live cancer cells" and indicated that terrible consequences would result.

Mr. Siegel arrived at the hospital Thursday afternoon and immediately saw Mrs. Tulipan. She had learned through Dr. Rosenfeld that a number of patients had been injected with live cancer cells without knowledge of Dr. Rosenfeld; that Dr. Rosenfeld learned of these injections when one of the patients called him to ask why he had been given the injection; that he then investigated and traced the injections to Dr. Custodio (resident) who gave these injections for a certain Dr. Southam and another doctor, both from Memorial Hospital who are friends of Dr. Mandel.

Under obvious emotional strain, Mrs. Tulipan practically demanded that Mr. Siegel fire Dr. Mandel at once or get his resignation. She further advised Mr. Siegel that the patients were not advised on nature of or reason for injection. She wanted to know if the medical board, research committee, or executive director knew of this project. Mr. Siegel told her he had no knowledge of this project and was quite sure neither of the other bodies had prior knowledge.

Mr. Siegel visited Dr. Rosenfeld at his private office that afternoon. He related the story substantially the same as had been presented by Mrs. Tulipan; while he had no personal reason for finding fault with Dr. Mandel, he was terribly hurt because Dr. Mandel had not discussed the project with him. He kept advising Mr. Siegel that Dr. Mandel should be fired, or that he should be forced to resign and he placed great emphasis on the fact that three coordinators had been approached by Dr. Mandel to participate in this project and each had turned it down because they told him written informed consent was required. He named Drs. Kagan, Fersko and Leichter as the individuals who had refused to participate. He also named Dr. Custodio, a resident, as the physician who had done the injections. Mr. Siegel told Dr. Rosenfeld he intended interviewing all the persons named and advised him that Dr. Mandel was on vacation and he did not feel any conclusions could be drawn without discussing the problem with Dr. Mandel. Dr. Rosenfeld kept warning Mr. Siegel that "the thing would blow up," that he'd "better get good legal advice," "that this was a terrible thing that had been done," "that he'd better fire Dr. Mandel at once," etc., etc.

The following morning, Friday, August 16, 1963, Mr. Siegel interviewed Dr. Leichter, Dr. Kagan and Dr. Custodio. Dr. Fersko was on vacation and was not available.

Dr. Leichter told him that early in July, Dr. Mandel had discussed the project with him and had advised Dr. Mandel that written informed consent was required, and that Dr. Mandel never again approached him on this matter. He was very resentful of Dr. Mandel, he did not know how many patients were injected, or who the patients were. Mr. Siegel felt the resentment and bitterness directed toward Dr. Mandel were really based on the fact that he was being superseded as chief of the cancer service by a new full-time physician (Dr. Korman) who was to join the staff as associate director of medicine. Dr. Leichter placed emphasis on his distrust of Dr. Mandel and also implied that the thing would blow up.

Mr. Siegel told Dr. Leichter that the matter of injecting the patients appeared to be in the province of the grievance committee of the medical staff and that it would be given to Dr. Abramson upon his return from vacation. He requested that Dr. Leichter not be hasty in his actions.

Mr. Siegel then met with Dr. Kagan who likewise was approached by Dr. Mandel on the proposed project. Dr. Kagan stated that he had advised him that written informed consent was required and that he did not think the patients would give such consent. Dr. Mandel never again discussed the matter with him. He had heard that injections had been given but did not know how many or to which patients. He felt this was done illegally. He appeared confused as to what course to take, feeling that knowledge that an illegal act was done implicated him and that he was morally bound to make it known. Further conversation revealed that he had other complaints against Dr. Mandel as follows:

1. He had been inveigled into using other experimental drugs without getting written consent and that he was fearful of possible damaging consequences;
2. That he wanted an appointment at the State University and did not feel Dr. Mandel was really trying to get him one.
3. That he thought he was entitled to an increase in salary and did not believe Dr. Mandel was trying to get him one.

Mr. Siegel stated he had learned that Dr. Mandel had spoken and written to Dr. Eichna at the university regarding Dr. Kagan's appointment, but that the latter had hurt his own cause when he wrote directly to Dr. Eichna without Dr. Mandel's knowledge. Dr. Eichna looked unfavorably upon such behavior.

In regard to an increase, Dr. Mandel had spoken and written to Mr. Siegel, requesting an increase for Dr. Kagan and was advised this was to be referred to the finance committee. Not believing that Dr. Mandel was trying, Dr. Kagan wrote directly to Mr. Siegel without Dr. Mandel's knowledge. Mr. Siegel looked upon this procedure with disfavor and so advised Dr. Kagan.

Mr. Siegel advised Dr. Kagan that the findings in regard to the injections would be turned over to Dr. Abramson upon his return from vacation and requested that Dr. Kagan take no hasty action. Dr. Kagan was extremely bitter toward Dr. Mandel.

Mr. Siegel then interviewed Dr. Custodio, a resident in the Blumberg Building. Dr. Custodio stated that he was engaged in a project to study the immunological response of chroni-

cally ill, debilitated patients to a cell suspension of tissue cultures taken from cancer patients. He stated he was interested in research and was glad to cooperate, since this appeared to be a worthwhile study, that he was assured by Dr. Mandel (Southam and Levin of Sloan-Kettering Institute) with absolute certainty that there could be no ill effects on the patients; that written consents were not really required bceause of the negative emotional impact of reference to "cancer"; that he had advised each patient and gotten their verbal consent, witnessed by Drs. Southam and Levin, that they would be given a skin test to determine their immunological reaction to foreign injections; that small nodules would develop and would then disappear after a few weeks; that on the advice of Dr. Mandel, he wrote into each patient's chart that a "cell injection had been given in either right or left thigh." He submitted the names of the patients who had been injected.

Mr. Siegel, after these interviews, called Mr. Samuel Bisgyer, hospital attorney, informing him of this problem and to seek his advice. Mr. Bisgyer pleaded not to get him involved, since he was not well and not really well-informed on such hospital problems.

He then called Mr. Harry Albert, an attorney on the board of directors and met with him that night. Mr. Albert thought there was no great urgency and that Mr. Siegel could return to Florida.

Mr. Siegel returned to Florida, but feeling ill-at-ease, returned the following Thursday, called Dr. Abramson's office with a message for Dr. Abramson to call Mr. Siegel immediately upon his arrival.

In frequent conversations with Mrs. Tulipan and Dr. Rosenfeld, Mr. Siegel stated he was constantly being reminded that he'd better get Dr. Mandel out of the hospital. He decided to visit Mr. Benjamin Saltzman, chairman of the executive committee, who was the next ranking officer in the absence of Mr. Isaac Albert, to acquaint him with the facts.

In the interim, Dr. Mandel returned from vacation. Mr. Siegel advised him of the nature of the problem and that he was planning to present the case to the medical staff. Dr. Mandel confidently stated that he had done nothing wrong and would gladly submit to evaluation by this body.

Dr. Abramson returned from vacation and Mr. Siegel met with him on Wednesday, August 28. Dr. Abramson already had on his desk a letter of resignation signed by Drs. Kagan, Fersko and Leichter. He readily accepted the matter as one within the province of the medical staff, felt that Mr. Siegel had handled the matter properly up to this point.

Testimony by Dr. Abramson, President of the Medical Staff

Dr. Abramson stated that he personally interviewed the doctors who had resigned. In regard to their attitude that written consent was required, he tried to allay their fears, since they had not participated in this project in any way and were in no way involved. He felt that none of the men, Drs. Kagan, Fersko and Leichter, had any substantial basis for their position, and were using this incident to support other personal complaints against Dr. Mandel. Dr. Abramson felt none of their reasons justified their actions and so advised these doctors.

Mr. Saltzman suggested that the committee consider the medical and legal aspects of the complaint, rather than the extraneous attitude of the coordinators.

Testimony by Dr. Southam

At this point, Dr. Southam of the Sloan-Kettering Institute arrived and was invited for questioning. The following facts were brought out in the questioning:

1. The work has been in progress for about 10 years, and various papers on the subject have been published in medical journals.
2. Cancer cells are used rather than other tissue cells because cancer cells are reproduced easier in measurable amounts and the rejection period is measurable.
3. In normal patients, a measurable nodule develops in about two weeks and disappears in four to six weeks. In cancer patients, the nodule might not disappear for a few months since the immunological rejection is impaired.
4. Purpose of using our patients was to determine whether the delayed rejection was unique for cancer patients only, or whether a similar reaction would be present in chronically ill patients suffering from debilitating diseases.
5. All patients injected showed the normal rejection associated with healthy individuals except one patient, and this one had a prior history of rectal surgery, based on information subsequently taken from his chart.
6. Each patient was told in advance of the test and each one consented. The word "cancer" was not used because of emotional reaction to use of word in addition to the fact that the use of cancer cells was immaterial. There was absolute certainty that there would be no permanent side effects.
7. This hospital was approached because of its reputation as a progressive medical institution interested in research and teaching, coupled with the fact that we had large numbers of debilitated patients with diseases other than cancer.
8. The tests were extremely useful. Dr. Horsfall, director of Sloan-Kettering Institute, who was never overly enthused about this project, upon hearing of the test results at our hospital, called Dr. Southam to congratulate him on his successful findings.
9. Dr. Southam's concern was for scientific progress and he would be extremely pleased if the tests could continue at our hospital.

Dr. Abramson read a notorized affidavit signed by Dr. Custodio stating that each patient had given verbal consent for the injection and that the consent was witnessed by Drs. Southam and Levin. Dr. Southam indicated that he would willingly testify that he witnessed such consent.

Testimony by Dr. Abramson (continued)

Dr. Abramson learned from Mr. Siegel that a reporter from the *World-Telegram* had called for information regarding resignation of three doctors because of certain research work. Dr. Abramson stated he saw Dr. Kagan who also stated he was approached by a man from the *World-Telegram*. He swore he gave no information and referred the reporter to officials at the hospital.

Discussion

Dr. David Kershner was highly impressed by the facts as presented. He felt the reaction of the coordinators to the project was not at all their affair, since they did not participate in the project.

He felt that it is an obligation of an institution such as ours to encourage research. We have a wealth of patient material that had never been properly utilized.

While it is advisable, wherever possible, to get written consent, it is not required by law. He suggested that use of the word "cancer" should be avoided for purpose of advancing ease of doing research projects.

Dr. Kershner stated that he was fully aware, based on his readings and clinical work, that there could not possibly be any danger to the patient in the project in question. He offered a vote of thanks to Mr. Siegel for the calm and professional manner in which the problem was handled, under very trying, emotional circumstances. He suggested that Dr. Mandel explain why the project was not handled through the research committee.

Dr. Kershner recommended the prompt acceptance of the resignations of the three coordinators and continuation of the research project, and that any calls for information from any source be referred to proper channels—Mr. Siegel, Dr. Abramson and Dr. Mandel.

Further discussion revealed that under our medical staff constitution, pilot studies may be initiated by directors of services without prior review by the research committee. However, should the director desire to continue a project, he must submit a protocol to the research committee within 60 days after initiation of the pilot study.

Dr. Mandel was called in. He indicated that in addition to the fact that this was a pilot study with a very limited number of patients, he had every intention of referring a protocol to the research committee. He admitted an oversight in not advising Dr. Rosenfeld of the study, but it was the general consensus of opinion that the director of service is not really obligated to advise all his subordinates on such matters. This question could offer no basis for charges against Dr. Mandel.

Dr. Mandel stated that the coordinators were never asked to give the injections. The projects were merely discussed with them to get their opinions. Each one thought the project had merit. It was totally untrue that they advised him that written informed consent was necessary.

He stated that only Dr. Kagan was asked if he was interested in participating, but not having gotten an answer in three days, Dr. Mandel assumed that he was too busy studying for

his board examinations and didn't want to become involved.

Mr. Harry Albert indicated that Dr. Mandel's intent should be judged in association with the very reputable Memorial Hospital and with the outstanding work done by Dr. Southam who is also associate professor of medicine at Cornell Medical School. He also questioned the involvement of Mrs. Tulipan in a complicated medical matter and strongly urged that she be forbidden to be further involved in this matter.

Dr. Abramson stated that none of the coordinators interviewed could adequately explain why Mrs. Tulipan was involved in a medical matter and why they had sent a copy of the letter of resignation to her.

Dr. Harry Weiner drew the following conclusions:
1. Dr. Mandel did not violate the constitution.
2. Resignations should be accepted.
3. A special committee should seek out facts as to who was involved in disseminating misinformation.
4. Report should be presented to medical board.
5. Responsibility for report should be the executive director's and chairman of the executive committee.

Dr. Lewis felt that the coordinators deserved to be heard. However, it was stated that they resigned without notice after being advised as to proper procedure for disposing of said matter; and that they resigned without arranging for adequate coverage of patients.

Conclusions

1. Resignations by Drs. Kagan, Fersko and Leichter were irresponsible and should be accepted.
2. There were no reasonable complaints against Dr. Mandel under the medical staff constitution.
3. A report should be submitted to medical staff.
4. All public relations matters related to this incident be referred to executive director.
5. Any medical reports resulting from the tests should be referred to research committee.
6. The scientific information resulting from this study was of outstanding significance and we should lend our support in continuing this project.

6.
Reply Affidavits for Petitioner

a.

Bernard J. Pisani, M.D.—
January 17, 1964

I was admitted to the practice of medicine and surgery in the State of New York since 1933. I have been a past president of the Medical Society of the County of New York. From 1954 to date I have served as director of obstetrics and gynecology at St. Vincent's Hospital.

The question has been put to me as to the propriety of a nontherapeutic experiment consisting of injecting live cancer cells into noncancerous patients who have not been told that this injection consists of live cancer cells and who have not given their informed consent to this experiment. (By *informed* consent is meant the voluntary agreement of a patient capable of normal comprehension, *after* this patinet has been told in lay language, the nature of the experiment, its hazards, present and potential, its complications and sequelae).

In answer to this question I state unequivocally that such an experiment, without the informed consent of the patient, is improper, unethical and immoral. Under no circumstances as a physician would I participate in or condone this type of experiment on any human being. The *known hazards* of such *experiments include growth of nodules* and tumors and may result in a *metastases of cancer* if the *patient does not reject these cells.*

In my practice of medicine and surgery and under the rules and regulations of St. Vincent's Hospital the informed written consent of the patient is required for all unusual or major procedures, therapeutic and experimental.

b.
Mendel Jacobi, M.D.—January 16, 1964

I hereby reaffirm the correctness of the statements made by me in my affidavit dated December 11, 1963.

It is stated in various affidavits filed with the answer of the respondents that the injections of cancer cells into patients at the Jewish Chronic Disease Hospital were performed merely to test the patients' immunologic reaction to these cells, not in order to determine whether cancer could be produced by such injections.

It is further stated that Dr. Mandel "was, of course, aware that homologous cells (cells from a human other than the person in whom they are injected) could not long continue to persist unless immunological reactiveness was severely impaired." Finally it is indicated that previously performed experiments had demonstrated that delayed reaction of neoplastic tissue-cultured human cell homotransplants had occurred in cancer patients "due to an impaired immunological capacity" and that "At present the only method of evaluating this type of immunologic capacity is to observe the efficiency with which homotransplants are rejected."

From these statements alone it follows that the very measure of the immunologic response the experiments performed at the Jewish Chronic Disease Hospital were to test was to be the rate of rejection of the cancerous nodule expected to develop at the injection site. If the patients' immunologic responsiveness were severely impaired —and this, from the above-quoted statement, could only have been determined after such rejection of the locally produced cancer—cancer development could have occurred. Obviously, then, saying that the injections were for the purpose of testing immunological responsiveness is merely a reverse manner of saying that it was for the purpose of establishing whether a cancer would be rejected by these debilitated patients and if so, at what rate or with what degree of completeness.

As a matter of fact, if these homotransplants were to behave as had those in cancerous patients, there was the real possibility that the locally produced cancerous nodule would grow progressively and even metastasize. In a paper published in *Science,* Dr. Southam and associates described the homotransplants of cancer cells into 14 cancer-bearing patients, noted the development of a cancer nodule at the implantation site in from 5 to 10 days after the injection, and that it attained a maximum diameter of ½ to 2 centimeters, in 1 to 2 weeks, at which time the nodules were excised completely for histologic study.

It is urged in several of the affidavits that cancer was not produced by the injections and/or that no patient was harmed in the slightest.

From one with the specific experience in the cancer field such as Dr. Southam has, or even from one who has not so limited his experience but has been in practice as long as Dr. Mandel, such statements are quite surprising in view of the fact that cancer, even when completely clin-ically eradicated by adequate and even intensive treatment, is known to recur after long periods of latency free of all evidence of cancer. It is pre-cisely for this reason that, in the field of cancer, one speaks not of cure but of 5-year, 10-year, 15-year, 20-year, etc. cure, meaning only that the cancer has not reappeared during such inter-vals. In view of the recurrence of the homo-transplanted cancer in the debilitated cancerous patients, and in view of the fact that this was deemed due to debility rather than to their in-trinsic cancer per se, and that, even now after the instant experiments, the basis for injected tumor rejection remains unknown, all that is presently warranted is the statement that the homotrans-plants of July 16, 1963 have disappeared as de-termined by local inspection and/or palpation and that some 2 months after the injections (or possibly some 5 months thereafter if the patients were re-examined at or about the date of the affidavits) no cancer is apparently pres-ent, a statement by no means equivalent to the non-development of, or freedom from, cancer in the patient.

Actually the fact that one patient, clin-ically free from evidences of cancer for the many preceding years of his hospital stay, developed overt clinical cancer of the bladder some 2 months after the homotransplants is rather dis-quieting. There is animal experimental evidence to indicate that delicate tumor-host relationship balances exist and that the growth rate of im-planted tumors may upset these balances in man-ner adverse to the animal host. In the present vague state of knowledge as to the nature of these relationships one wonders whether the very development of a tumor nodule at the site of the cancer cells injected into this patient and its sub-sequent rejection by the patient—presumably this rejection involved the patient's defense mechanisms against cancer—had, in fact, ex-hausted these defenses, and had so upset the patient's tumor-host balance to the end that the bladder cancer, previously latent (i.e. kept from growth activity by the patient's body defenses) had now attained active growth capability and overt clinical activity. If this is the patient who, according to Dr. Mandel's affidavit "died in Oc-tober following a bladder operation," this se-quence of events is even more possibly signifi-cant and disturbing.

From the above facts one must conclude that the statements anent the non-development of cancer in the patients injected on July 16,

1963 or that they were harmed in no way are presently premature and unwarranted. One pa-tient in this series is certainly dead under cir-cumstances possibly indicating at least an indirect influence of the injections; as to the others, the post-injection period will have to extend for many years before such statement can become unequivocally demonstrable. Parenthetically it should be noted that, to the best of my knowl-edge, no one other than the people involved in these injection experiments at the hospital has made an independent examination of these in-jected patients with respect to the presence of cancer or of other complications possibly se-quential to the injection, and that, if the 5 charts examined by me on October 4, 1963, are indica-tive, the records in the charts of the patients in-jected are in such a state that no conclusions as to any such developments were, or will be, pos-sible.

NOTE

CHESTER M. SOUTHAM, ALICE E. MOORE, AND
CORNELIUS P. RHOADS
HOMOTRANSPLANTATION OF HUMAN CELL LINES*

The development of human neoplastic cell lines that can be grown serially in tissue cultures and in heterologous hosts has made necessary the investigation of the capacity of such cells to grow in a homologous (human) recipient. Such studies are of fundamental importance to our knowledge of tissue transplantation and host defense mechanisms. In addition, there is the possible danger of initiating neoplastic disease by accidental inoculation during laboratory inves-tigation or by injection with such cells or cell products if they should be used for production of virus vaccine. This article is a preliminary re-port of a continuing study of (i) the persistence and growth of neoplastic human cell lines after homologous transplantation and (ii) host reac-tions to such implants.

All recipients were volunteers who were aware of the general purposes of the study and the nature of the implanted materials and who were agreeable to subsequent biopsies.

*   *   *

. . . Usually a single preparation was inoc-ulated at one or two sites, but a few recipients

---
* 125 *Science* 158–160 (1957). Reprinted by permission.

received two to four cell types simultaneously, and one received a total of seven preparations on two occasions. Complete excisional biopsies were usually performed as soon as a definitely palpable nodule appeared. In some recent studies, excision was delayed to study duration of growth and the process of regression.

Initial studies were restricted to volunteer patients with advanced incurable cancer and a very short life expectancy. Many had infectious and metabolic complications and chachexia. None had received treatment with steroid hormones, ACTH, marrow-depressing agents such as nitrogen mustard, or x-rays during the three months preceding the studies, and none received any of these treatments during the course of the studies.

Slight local induration and erythema frequently followed inoculations but subsided completely by the third day. Human embryonic fibroblasts with normal cytology were inoculated in three patients. No growth was detected, but neoplastic cells inoculated simultaneously into the same patients did grow. No other normal cells were available for study. Four epithelial cell lines of normal origin were inoculated in seven patients, usually produced nodules, and one of these recurred in one patient. These cells cannot be considered normal because they had developed neoplastic characteristics during tissue culture passage, and the nodules were histologically diagnosed as cancer.

Twenty-four homologous implantations of seven cancer cell lines (originally isolated from cancer tissues) were made in 14 cancer patients between February 1954 and July 1956. All seven lines multiplied in most of the recipients, as indicated by formation of a palpable nodule at the implantation site and by the finding of healthy cancer cells with active mitoses in the biopsies. . . . Usually the nodule appeared 5 to 10 days after implantation, reached a maximum diameter of ½ to 2 cm in 1 to 2 weeks, and was then excised completely for histologic study.

If they were not immediately excised, the implants usually regressed spontaneously and completely by 4 to 6 weeks. However, in four patients there was recurrence of cancer growth after biopsy at several implant sites. Three of these recurrences were completely removed by a repeat excision on the 19th, 42nd, and 77th days, respectively. In two patients, some of the recurrent nodules grew progressively until the patients died, 42 days and 57 days after the implantations. . . . In one of these patients, the

HEp#3 metastasized to the axillary nodes. This patient's own cancer was uterine adenocarcinoma, readily distinguished from the implanted cells, and at autopsy was found to be confined to the abdomen and perineum.

Studies to determine whether these homologous cancer cells had a similar capacity for propagation in normal healthy human beings were undertaken at the Ohio State Penitentiary in collaboration with Charles Doan and Richard Brooks and with the cooperation of John Porterfield and R. W. Alvis, warden. From a large group of volunteers, 14 were chosen for the initial study. Methods were identical with the aforementioned ones, except that only tissue cultures were used, and all studies were done simultaneously in June 1956.

There were well-defined differences in the behavior of the implants as compared with those seen in cancer patients. The initial inflammatory reaction was more marked in degree and duration, usually persisting for 1 week or more. The greatest reactions were at HEp#3 implantation sites where (in two patients) sterile abscesses formed. A firm nodule appeared at each site and reached 1 to 3 cm diameter by 14 days. By this time, erythema and edema were subsiding, and one or two nodules were excised from each volunteer. The remaining implants started to regress spontaneously by 3 weeks after implantation and were nonpalpable by 4 weeks. There has been no recurrence in the subsequent 5 months. Histologic sections of all day-14 biopsies showed a marked inflammatory reaction with mononuclear cells predominating. Aggregates of cancer cells with mitotic activity were present in only four of the 15 biopsies, and from two of these the cancer cells were reisolated in tissue culture. HcLa cells and Chang's conjunctive cells were not found in these biopsies.

Although it is tempting to postulate that the observed difference in receptivity of cancer cell homografts between normal and cancer patients is related to cancer per se, there is no present evidence against the more plausible explanation that the difference is due merely to the general debility of the cancer patients. However, no consistent differences such as uremia, hematologic abnormalities, or medications can be adduced to explain the apparent weakness of defenses in the cancer patients. Neither did the cancer patients have an "immunologic paralysis" since they did produce antibodies against viruses that were inoculated at about the same time in experimental therapeutic studies. Further studies designed to detect possible differences in cellular and humoral defense mechanisms are in progress.

*   *   *

We, as well as our collaborators, wish to express our appreciation of and admiration for these volunteers, both cancer patients and normal individuals, who, without expectation or possibility of personal gain, have made these studies possible.

*   *   *

c.
David Leichter, M.D.—January 16, 1964

In reply to the false, unwarranted accusations made against me in the answering affidavits submitted by the respondent, I wish to state the following:

As to the affidavit verified by me on September 12, 1963, I reaffirm the correctness of all my statements contained therein. The respondent seeks to impeach my credibility and the correctness of my statements by alleging that I have repudiated certain statements therein contained. This is utterly false.

7.

Rebuttal Affidavits for Respondent

a.

Chester M. Southam, M.D.—
February 4, 1964

I address myself first to the question of the measure of risk of bodily harm to the patients who were the subject of the procedures in question at the Jewish Chronic Disease Hospital. At the outset I should say that in clinical procedures neither I nor any scientist or doctor can deal in absolutes. We are always limited, at least when dealing with the human body, to speaking in terms of measurable risks. Thus while no doctor or scientist can say as to any clinical procedure, even the simplest, that there is *no possibility* of untoward results, we are constantly required, both in therapeutic and in investigative procedures, to make judgments as to whether there is any unusual risk of untoward results, and if so, the degree of that risk. In terms of this standard I unhesitatingly assert that on the basis of

present biological knowledge supplemented by clinical experience to date there was no practical possibility of untoward results to the patients who received injections of homotransplants in the form of tissue-cultured cells derived from other patients. The probability of any unforeseen deleterious consquences of this test is so extremely small as to be comparable to numerous other procedures used routinely in clinical medicine for therapeutic, diagnostic, or investigative purposes, e.g., blood transfusions, intravenous pyelograms (kidney x-rays), or tuberculin tests. The fact that these cells were tissue-cultured cancer cells did not measurably increase any risk inherent in the procedure because, being foreign to the recipient (the person injected), they bring about an immunologic reaction (defense reaction, rejection reaction) that ultimately causes their destruction and elimination.

It has been known for many years that a human being will reject cells transplanted from another human being unless both are of precisely the same genetic makeup (i.e., identical twins). In fact, intensive clinical studies are now being carried on at many research centers attempting to find methods (such as treatment with certain drugs or x-ray) to overcome this rejection reaction in the hope that diseased organs, such as kidneys, might be successfully replaced. While the precise mechanisms of cell rejection are not yet known, the fact that such mechanisms exist is beyond question. The efficiency of this type of immunological reaction can be measured in terms of the time required for complete rejection of homotransplanted cells. As yet no other method of measuring this reaction has been found, and tissue-cultured cancer cells are the only kind of cells which provide sufficient reproducibility for comparison of results in different individuals at different times.

The three lines of cells derived from human cancer which were used in the studies at the Jewish Chronic Disease Hospital were derived from tumor tissues of three patients, from 4 to 12 years ago. Since that time these cells have been cultivated in sterile bottles in the laboratory in a solution of nutrients which include salts, vitamins and blood serum. This is the process called tissue culture. After such years of growth under these artificial laboratory conditions each line of cultured cells has a high degree of uniformity and, consequently, the reaction which it will produce is highly predictable. I have had an extensive experience with each of these three cell lines in homotransplantation studies in cancer patients and in healthy volunteers during the past several years.

In the early 1950's it began to appear that the defense mechanisms (i.e., the mechanism of rejection of homotransplants) of those persons who develop cancer might be in some way impaired. The most striking indication of this was the result of clinical tests on a limited number of patients with terminal cancer as reported over the signatures of myself and Drs. Rhoads and Moore in *Science*. These were all patients suffering from advanced stages of widely disseminated cancer for whom there was no known method of treatment to either inhibit their disease or prolong their lives, each of whom died as the result of his own cancer within a relatively short time. In view of the then state of knowledge the precise details of the procedure were explained and the patients freely and readily consented.

The significant result of the test was that the rate of rejection of the foreign transplants was in all cases slower than would have been expected, indicating that there was some impairment of their immunological reaction. Because these patients had far advanced cancer before the homotransplants were injected, they did not survive for long after the tests were performed. Obviously this was not the result of the test, but rather was the reason that these particular patients were selected for these earliest tests. In no case was the patient deleteriously affected by the implants. Several patients in this initial group and in subsequent groups had not rejected their transplants in the brief interval between the start of the test and their death. In fact, at autopsy a lymph node from the armpit of one of these patients contained unrejected cancer cells of the type used for the test. (These lymph nodes are in the natural route of drainage from the forearm where the test was made in this patient.)

Prior to the publication of the article in question tests were made on a number of volunteer healthy human beings in the Ohio Penitentiary. In all such cases the foreign transplants were quickly and completely rejected, as would have been expected.

After the initial tests reported in *Science,* intensive studies were undertaken, designed to increase our body of knowledge as to the immunological reaction both of normal healthy persons and those with cancer, to homotransplants of tissue-cultured lines of human cells derived from normal and tumor tissues. Between the time of the initial tests and July 16, 1963 (the date on which the injections were made in Jewish Chronic Disease Hospital) approximately 600 persons had been studied by means of the techniques employed at Jewish Chronic Disease Hospital, approximately 300 of whom were patients with cancer and 300 healthy, normal persons. In every healthy recipient of tissue-cultured cells, these foreign transplants were rejected with uniform promptness. Some patients with cancer rejected the cells less rapidly and after significantly varying intervals of time. Patients in the earlier stages of neoplastic disease showed normal or only slightly impaired rejection reaction. Patients in the terminal stages of cancer showed the greatest deficiency in these immunological defense mechanisms (as measured by the length of time to effect rejection) and in several such persons rejection had not been accomplished in the few weeks or months that elapsed between injection of the test cells and the patient's death from his own cancer. These patients died from the effects of their own cancer before the expected ultimate rejection of the implants. The studies also demonstrated a correlation between the rate of rejection of homotransplanted cancer cells and the patient's apparent ability to restrain his own disease, thus providing additional direct evidence that patients may have immunological (defense) mechanisms to restrain their own cancer. These results, of course, give hope that, through further clinical research, methods of stimulating such mechanisms to greater efficacy can be developed.

The studies of healthy, normal persons at the Ohio Penitentiary, aside from demonstrating that the normal body will reject cancer cell homotransplants with the same efficiency as other types of homotransplants, further indicated the potentially highly significant fact that the body's rate of rejection increased with successive implantations of foreign cancer cells, suggesting long-run possibilities of building up the immunological mechanisms where deficiencies now occur. At present, studies are being continued to verify these scientific observations and to investigate their possible applicability to the treatment and prevention of human cancer. Such studies of human cancer can be accomplished only through the cooperation of patients and healthy volunteers.

Until the investigation conducted at the Jewish Chronic Disease Hospital, there was no direct clinical evidence that the impairment of the immunologic responses in patients with advanced cancer (as measured by the slow rate at which they rejected homotransplants) was associated with the fact that they had cancer rather than with the fact that they were in a debilitated state. This study provided direct clinical evidence that indeed the impairment was associated with the fact of cancer rather than general debilitation. The patients at Jewish Chronic Disease Hospital reacted in essentially the same manner as normal, healthy human beings. I want to make perfectly clear that the question in this investigation was not whether the patients would reject the tissue-cultured cancer cell homotransplants. The only question was how fast would the body mobilize its resources of rejection. Three patients known to have cancer were also included in these tests. It was expected that rejection in the three cancer patients might be delayed, consistent with our previous experience in cancer patients, but that rejection would occur after the predicted delay unless these patients succumbed very rapidly to their own cancer.

I next turn to the question of procedures. In the early stages of this clinical research and, indeed, until the last few years a full explanation was given to the patient or healthy volunteer, including the fact that the techniques employed were not designed for his own therapy, the nature of the cultured cells involved, the general purposes of the test and the expected reactions. More recently, as our body of knowledge has increased and the course of reaction to the injections became predictable, we have simply explained that the procedure was a test which had nothing to do with treatment, that it involved the injection of foreign material, described the expected course of reaction, and that its purpose was to determine the rate at which the expected nodules would develop and then regress. In all instances in which the test was done the patients have readily given their consent, and the tests were not performed if such consent was not readily given. Unless the patient inquired, we refrained from describing the precise nature of the human cells (i.e., that they had originally been derived from tumors and then grown in tissue culture) for the reason that in my own professional judgment as well as that of my professional colleagues who had followed the course of these experiments, the precise nature of the foreign cells was irrelevant to the bodily reactions which could be expected to occur.

This course was followed, I submit, not out of any disregard for the rights or best interests of the patient nor of my responsibilities as a practitioner of medicine. It was a sincere professional judgment, based upon extensive scientific and clinical experience, that the procedures involved only the same low degree of risk inherent in many routine clinical test procedures, the patient in all such cases being informed only of the facts which are important from his standpoint. I submit that but for the highly emotion-charged term "cancer cells," this conclusion would be unquestioned by those in the medical profession who are fully cognizant of the present stage of knowledge with respect to immunological reactions.

Furthermore, in my own clinical judgment —based on fifteen years of clinical management of advanced cancer patients—to use the dreaded word "cancer" in connection with any clinical procedure on an ill person is potentially deleterious to that patient's well-being because it may suggest to him (rightly or wrongly) that his diagnosis is cancer or that his prognosis is poor. Some cancer patients do not know that their diagnosis is cancer, and even those who have been informed rarely discuss it and may even deny it. It is seldom possible for the physician to be full cognizant of the cancer patient's extent of knowledge of and his attitude toward his disease. The doctor's choice of words in discussions with the patient has a great influence upon the patient's mental attitude. Since the initial neoplastic source of the test material employed was not germane to the reaction being studied and not, in my opinion, a cause of increased risk to the patient, I believe that such revelation is generally contraindicated in the best consideration of the patient's welfare and therefore to withhold such emotionally disturbing but medically non-pertinent details (unless requested by the patient) is in the best tradition of responsible clinical practice.

On these questions concerning procedure, I will readily submit to the judgment of my colleagues after they are fully informed.

b.

Frank L. Horsfall, Jr., M.D.— February 4, 1964

I am now and have been since 1937 licensed to practice medicine in the State of New York. I am now and have been since April 1, 1960 president and director and chief executive officer of the Sloan-Kettering Institute for Cancer Research, New York, New York, as well as director, Sloan-Kettering Division, Graduate School of Medical Sciences, Cornell University Medical College.

I hold now and have held since April 1, 1960 the rank of professor of medicine, Cornell University Medical College.

I have read the affidavit of Chester M. Southam sworn to February 4, 1964. I have been generally familiar with the clinical tests described therein and their results to date. I am in complete accord with the professional opinions expressed by Dr. Southam in his affidavit.

c.

Henry Thomas Randall, M.D.— February 4, 1964

I am now and have been since 1941 licensed to practice medicine in the State of New York. I am vice president for medical affairs of Memorial Hospital for Cancer and Allied Diseas and medical director of this hospital; also vice-president for clinical affairs of the Sloan-Kettering Institute for Cancer Research, and professor of surgery in Cornell University Medical College.

I have read the affidavit of Chester M. Southam sworn to on February 4, 1964. I am generally familiar with the clinical tests described therein and their results to date. I am in complete accord with the professional opinions expressed by Dr. Southam in his affidavit.

d.

Emanuel E. Mandel, M.D.— February 4, 1964

The method of obtaining the consents to the Sloan-Kettering tests, outlined in the answering papers, must be evaluated in relation to the basic medical principle that the extent of information to be imparted to the patient must be left to the judgment of the responsible physician. There are many standard techniques used by physicians for the purpose of diagnosis and treatment which may result in injury, or even death, to patients. Yet, in the interest of the patient, they are not normally preceded by any thorough-going explanations, or even by any written or oral consents (e.g., penicillin injections, the obtaining of intravenous pyelograms, "BSP" tests, X-ray treatment for non-cancerous patients, the administration of radioactive substances (iodine and phosphorus), etc.).

It must be patent that the investigative team of Sloan-Kettering and JCDH acted in full compliance with conventional procedure accepted by the medical profession at large. The injections of cell suspensions in question here

were no more hazardous than any of the above named routine tests, and, indeed, far safer than most of them or perhaps all of them. In fact, consideration was being given at the outset of this study to the possibility of adopting those injections as routine tests to uncover hidden (subclinical) cancer, since it was regarded as a routine test at Memorial Hospital (see minutes of the hearing in the offices of the New York State Education Department on December 19, 1963). For even advanced (metastatic) cancer can escape the physician's attention in a patient suffering from other chronic and debilitating disease, and even advanced cancer can, at times, be treated with success. There is no basis for the argument of Dr. Strauss and other medical witnesses that the tests were "dissociated" from the "patient's ailment and condition."

NOTE

Earl Ubell
Injecting Cancer Cells—The Case for the Defense*

Would you take an injection of a million cancer cells in your arm? The thought of it will send shudders through any normal person unfamiliar with modern biology. He thinks: what if those cells took hold and grew into a full, deadly cancer?

Yet almost every cancer biologist knows that one of the hardest biological tricks to pull is to transplant a cancer from one animal to another. And nobody has ever transplanted a cancer from one human being to another.

At the same time such experiments on human beings—injecting cancer cells—have the possibility of an enormous pay-off: a vaccine against cancer or a technique for helping the body get rid of cancer.

Given this information, one wonders why cancer injection tests on patients at the Jewish Chronic Disease Hospital in Brooklyn raised such a brouhaha. It is entirely possible that the doctors involved made a tactical error in failing to describe fully to the patients or to their families every step of the experiment. But even if they omitted the deadly word: cancer, have they hurt their volunteering patients? The answer is no.

The experiments in this field began with a question: is there something wrong with the can-

_____
* New York Herald Tribune 29, col. 5 (January 26, 1964). Reprinted by permission.

cer patient's defenses against cancer? The possibility had been raised by a whole series of tests on animals.

*   *   *

Dr. Southam induced 96 healthy men incarcerated at Ohio State Penitentiary at Columbus to volunteer with the full knowledge of what he was going to slip under their skin.

Since that time more than 300 prisoners have volunteered for the tests. In not one of them did the cancer cells become a full-blown cancer. Most of the cells died within days; in some volunteers it took a couple of weeks. When the same volunteers received additional injections, their bodies killed off the cells even more quickly.

*   *   *

But what about cancer patients? At about the same time Dr. Southam secured volunteers among the dying cancer victims at Memorial Hospital which is associated with Sloan-Kettering. Most of them were not only willing, but eager to help saying: "I know it is too late for me. Maybe this will help somebody else."

The cancer cells lived longer in the cancer victims than in the healthy volunteers. In one instance, a patient with an advanced cancer of his own died of his disease six months after receiving the injection of cancer cells. The injected cells were still alive and localized.

These tests indicated that in the cancer patient the defenses were down or at least weak. Similar results followed in almost 300 cancer patients. But none of the injected cells turned into full-blown cancers on their own.

Because of the results—namely that the injected cells never took over—Dr. Southam and his associates told their volunteers less about the nature of the injections to save them any possible anguish. Each patient was told that he was volunteering for a test, not a treatment.

Still, a basic biological issue remained open. Was the weakened defense a result of cancer or did it come simply from a person's being very sick and debilitated? Wasn't it possible that if somebody suffered a severe heart attack, say, and lost 60 pounds and was very weak, that the defenses against cancer might also be low?

It was this question which Dr. Southam tried to answer with the experiments carried out by the doctors at the Jewish Chronic Disease Hospital in Brooklyn. The results are in: these patients had the same response to the cancer cells as the healthy volunteers: the cells died in a few

days to two weeks, at most. The anti-cancer defenses were strong.

Here, then, we have a wide possibility: if there is such a biological mechanism as a defense against cancer, then it may be possible to stimulate it either before cancer strikes or perhaps even later when the cancer has taken hold.

This is the question which Dr. Southam is trying to pursue. It would be a shame if a squabble over who-told-what-to-whom should destroy a thrilling lead in cancer research.

*   *   *

8.

Sur-Reply Affidavit for Petitioner

Statements by Nathan Fink—
January 25 and February 1, 1964

[i] I, Mr. Nathan Fink, aged 73, make this statement, while a patient at the Brooklyn Chronic Disease Hospital.

Sometime in July or August of 1963, while a patient at the above hospital, two doctors visited me at my bedside and told me that I was to get an injection. This was supposedly a skin test, I was informed. They did not ask my approval nor consent.

A few days later, I detected a hardening under the top layer of my skin, in the area where I had previously been injected, my right thigh. This hardening enlarged about 2½ " in length.

During the next six or seven weeks, I was visited by these two doctors, every second or third day, at which time, one would measure the area with a ruler, and the other one would make notations in a small book. I do not know the name of these two doctors but one of the doctors, the one who made the notations in the book, was a Filipino.

Within a period of seven weeks, the hardened area seemed to have subsided, and I was informed, by the two doctors that I had a good resistance, and that the skin injection, performed upon me, had been successful.

After reading the most recent newspaper articles, about the cancer injections, performed on patients at this hospital, I now have reason to believe that I was one of the patients used as a guinea pig, in conjunction with this cancer experiment.

I again state that I was never given an opportunity by the doctors at this hospital, to accept or refuse this injection, nor was I ever told what was the actual purpose of this experiment.

[ii] I recently submitted a statement regarding an injection which I was given while a patient at B.C.D. Hospital. In that statement, I advised that I believed that this injection was a cancer experiment and that I had never given any one my oral or written consent for this experiment.

I now wish to amend this statement previously submitted. About 1 month after the injection given me in July 1963, I was approached by the same 2 doctors, at which time they suggested that I sign a blank questionnaire.

I asked what this was all about and was informed that they intended to give me a new experimental pill to pep up my appetite. They further stated that my signature was necessary for them to administer this pill. Naturally I signed this questionnaire because at this time I was actually suffering from lack of appetite.

I never was given this pill after they obtained my signature, although I asked about the pill on many occasions.

Now that I realize about the unauthorized injection given me in July 1963 and the subsequent signature taken from me, I have more reason to believe I was tricked into taking a cancer experiment with subsequent authorization.

9.

Opinions of the Court

a.

Hyman v. Jewish Chronic Disease Hospital
42 Misc.2d 427, 248 N.Y.S.2d 245
(Sup.Ct. 1964)

CONE, J.

In this article 78 proceeding the petitioner, a member of the board of directors of the respondent, seeks an order directing the respondent to permit the inspection and the making of copies by the petitioner of the minutes of the board of directors and the report of its executive director made at such meeting held on September 30, 1963, the report of Dr. Abramson made by him at the medical board meeting of October 28, 1963, the affidavit of Dr. Custodio, as well as the charts and records of the patients who submitted to the subject tests. In addition, by affidavit dated February 6, 1964, the petitioner enumerates other records that he demands access to.

It appears undisputed that the respondent, as a result of this application, has furnished the petitioner with the minutes of the board of directors, the report of the executive director and the report of Dr. Abramson, as well as the affidavit of Dr. Custodio, but refuses to turn over to the petitioner the charts and records of the patients without the consent of such patients as being precluded under section 4504(a), CPLR.

The court in making its present determination, is not passing upon the merits of the alleged improper acts or upon the technical aspects of the tests given to the patients of the respondent. It is merely called upon to determine the narrow issue as to the right of a member of the board of directors to obtain an order permitting an inspection and the making of the copies requested.

It is the well-established law of this state that a director has an absolute and unqualified right to the inspection of the corporate records regardless of his motives (*Matter of Cohen* v. *Cocoline Products,* 309 N.Y. 119; 127 N.E. 2d 906).

The basis for this premise taken by our courts is aptly stated by the court in *Cohen* v. *Cocoline* (*supra*): "In order properly to perform his directing duties, a corporate director *must, of course, keep himself informed as to the policies, business and affairs of the corporation and as to the acts of its officers.* He owes a stewardship obligation to the corporation and its stockholders, *and he may be subjected to liability for improper management during his term of office.* Because of those positive duties and potential liability the courts of this state have accorded to corporate directors an absolute, unqualified right, having its roots in the common law, to inspect their corporate books." (Emphasis supplied.)

*   *   *

Accordingly, the petition is granted . . .

b.

Hyman v. Jewish Chronic Disease Hospital
21 App.Div.2d 495, 251 N.Y.S.2d 818 (1964)

PER CURIAM.

The question presented on this appeal is whether a member of the board of directors or of the board of trustees of a hospital membership corporation is entitled as a matter of right to an inspection of medical charts of patients at the hospital. Special Term held that he is so entitled. We are of the contrary opinion.

Special Term directed that the hospital also permit petitioner to inspect records of a financial and administrative nature (e.g., books of account, fiscal records, minutes of the meetings of the board of directors, of its medical boards and committees, and rules and regulations governing the handling of patients). The hospital has acceded to such direction and has allowed petitioner to inspect such records; and such records are not involved on this appeal.

The genesis of this controversy and the facts giving rise to it may be briefly stated:

As the result of approximately ten years of research, Dr. Chester M. Southam of the Sloan-Kettering Institute for Cancer Research found that cancer patients did not have as marked a defense against cancer as did non-cancer patients. It is a biological law that human beings will reject cells which are transplanted from another human being unless both persons are of precisely the same genetic constitution (e.g., identical twins). It was found that, when a healthy individual was injected with the cancer cells of another individual, the healthy person promptly rejected the transplant, whereas when a cancer patient was injected with such foreign cancer cells, rejection of the transplant was delayed. What was not known was whether the foreign cancer cells lived longer in cancer patients (as contrasted with non-cancer patients) as the result of the pre-existing cancer or as the result of the patient's general weakness and debilitation. It was this question which Dr. Southam attempted to answer by the experiments conducted at the Jewish Chronic Disease Hospital; and it is these experiments which are involved in the present appeal.

The experiments showed that the sick and debilitated non-cancer patients had the same response to foreign cancer cells as healthy volunteers, that is, there was a prompt rejection of the transplant. This in turn opened a wide possibility that, if there be such a biological mechanism as a defense against cancer, it may be possible to stimulate it either before cancer strikes or perhaps even later when the cancer has taken hold.

The project was financed by the United States Public Health Service and by the American Cancer Society. It was undertaken by Drs. Southam and Levin of the Sloan-Kettering Institute at the Jewish Chronic Disease Hospital, with the permission of Dr. Mandel, director of the department of medicine and director of medical education of the hospital.

On July 16, 1963, under the supervision of Drs. Southam and Levin, 22 patients at the hospital were injected with foreign cancer cells on the anterior surface of one thigh at two sites just beneath the skin. The patients were not told that the injection was of cancer cells because the doctors did not wish to stir up any unnecessary anxieties in the patients. The doctors felt there was no need to tell the patients that the injected material contained cancer cells because: (a) it was of no consequence to the patients; (b) the precise nature of the foreign cells was irrelevant to the bodily reactions which could be expected to occur; (c) it was not germane to the reaction being studied; and (d) it was not a cause of increased risk to the patient.

However, the patients were told that an injection of a cell suspension was planned as a skin test for immunity or response. The patients were also told that within a few days a lump would form and would last for several weeks and gradually disappear. The patients were observed for several weeks after the injection of July 16, 1963. As expected, the lump developed and disappeared within an average period of from six to eight weeks.

The hospital and the doctors in charge of the experiment claim that each patient gave his oral consent. Petitioner, however, claims that the patients were either incompetent to give their consents or that they did not understand to what it was they were being asked to consent.

On December 2, 1963 this article 78 proceeding was instituted by petitioner to obtain the hospital records which are involved in this proceeding, as well as the hospital's financial and administrative records. The application was granted at Special Term on the ground: (a) that, regardless of his motives, a director of a membership corporation, as well as a director of a business corporation, has the absolute and unqualified right to inspect corporate records; and (b) that the disclosure of the patients' medical records to a member of the hospital's board of directors is not within the doctor-patient privilege because it is a disclosure to a member of the hospital's administration—one who has a legitimate interest in the contents of the patients' records.

In our opinion, the determination of the Special Term was improper for several reasons:

(1) Although the experiments were not conducted for the purpose of diagnosis or treatment of the patients, the results of such experiments nevertheless comprised part of the medical charts of the patients and, therefore, come

within the physician-patient privilege (*Matter of New York City Council* v. *Goldwater*).* Since the patients have concededly not waived the privilege, petitioner is not entitled to an inspection of such records.

(2) It has become a well settled rule that a director of a stock corporation is entitled to an inspection of the corporate books in order to keep himself informed as to the corporation's policies, business and activities so that he may carry out his duty to direct its affairs (*Matter of Cohen* v. *Cocoline Products, Inc.*).† The rule also applies to a membership corporation (*Matter of Davids* v. *Sillcox*).‡ However, by this rule it was never intended to permit a member of the board of directors or of the board of trustees of a hospital to inspect the medical charts of hospital patients (*Munzer* v. *State*, Ct. Cl., 41 N.Y.S. 2d 98; *Munzer* v. *Blaisdell*, 49 N.Y.S.2d 915).

(3) A corporate director is also entitled to an inspection of the corporation's books because he may be subjected to liability for improper management during his term of office (*Matter of Cohen* v. *Cocoline Products, Inc.*, 127 N.E. 2d 906). However, the possibility of petitioner's liability is here non-existent. Section 46 of the Membership Corporations Law provides that, in the absence of fraud or bad faith, the directors of a membership corporation are not personally liable for its debts, obligations or liabilities. It is only when a director personally participates in a wrongful act that he is personally liable (*Hinkle Iron Co.* v. *Kohn*, 128 N.E. 113). There is no claim of bad faith or fraud or of personal participation on the petitioner's part.

(4) The petitioner does not have the right, in his capacity as trustee or director, to act for the hospital's patients. It is only the patient or his physician who can act for the patient. No proceeding by any patient to obtain the information in question has been instituted.

(5) The hospital's future policy will be in accordance with petitioner's contention that experiments such as the one here involved should be done only with the patient's written consent after the patient has been properly informed. On September 7, 1963 the hospital's grievance committee approved the experiment. On September 30, 1963 its board of directors approved its grievance committee's report. On January 27, 1964 the hospital's research committee approved

* 31 N.E.2d 31.
† 127 N.E.2d 906.
‡ 79 N.E.2d 440.

continuance of the cancer immunization studies, but only upon the written, informed consents of the patients. Therefore, no further need for the inspection exists. It should be noted that petitioner is now in possession of the facts as to the manner in which the experiment was conducted on July 22, 1963; as to what information was given to the patients; and as to what information was not given to them.

Accordingly, the order, insofar as appealed from, should be reversed on the law and the facts, with costs; and the petitioner's application should be denied insofar as petitioner seeks the disclosure of the: (a) charts and records of patients who had been subjected to the experimental injection of live cancer cells; (b) the death certificates of any such injected patients who later died; and (c) the pathological studies, slides and laboratory data relating to all of said injected patients.

The inspection under the order (insofar as the order has not been reversed) shall proceed on twenty days' written notice or on such other date as the parties may mutually fix by written stipulation.

*   *   *

c.
Hyman v. Jewish Chronic Disease Hospital 15 N.Y.2d 317, 206 N.E.2d 338 (1965)

DESMOND, CHIEF JUDGE.

Special Term was correct in its holding that petitioner, being a director of a hospital corporation, is entitled as matter of law to an inspection of the records of the hospital to investigate into the facts as to alleged illegal and improper experimentation on patients (*Matter of Cohen* v. *Cocoline Products*, 309 N.Y. 119, 127 N.E. 2nd 906; *Matter of Martin* v. *Martin Foundation, Inc.*, 32 Misc. 2d 873, 224 N.Y.S. 2d 972).

It is argued that the data as to such experiments on patients are privileged (CPLR 4504 [a]) and that the patients have not waived the privilege. Any such confidentiality could be amply protected by inserting in the court's order a direction that the names of the particular patients be kept confidential. Actually, the supposed strict secrecy does not really exist as to qualified persons since these records have been seen, read and copied by numerous staff members and employees of the hospital and of the cooperating institution.

We are told that, since this petitioner director would not be personally liable for the wrong-doing of the hospital, he does not need such an inspection. However, the possibility of liability of the corporation of which he is a director entitles him to learn the truth about the situation on which such alleged liability may be predicated. Again, it is said that a director should not be allowed to act on behalf of the patients without their authority. We do not understand the petitioner to claim any such right of representation. He is carrying out his own duties as a director—to direct the affairs of the corporation.

It is argued, again, that an inspection is unnecessary since newly enacted rules of the hospital now require that written and informed consents of the patients be obtained before experiment. This fact, however, cannot be an obstacle to this director's effort to learn the full truth as to what has been done in the past.

No one seriously questions the right and obligation of a membership corporation director to keep himself informed as to the corporation's policies and activities so that he may do his duties and carry his responsibilities. Any necessary safeguards and protections can, in the discretion

of the Special Term, be provided by its order, including appropriate arrangements for concealing the names of individual patients if that appears to be necessary or proper. The order appealed from should be reversed, without costs, and the matter remitted to Special Term for further proceedings not inconsistent with this opinion.

SCILEPPI, JUDGE (dissenting).

I would affirm especially on the unique facts of this case: (1) The State Department of Education is inquiring into the matter; (2) the Kings County district attorney has been alerted to the situation; (3) the petitioner already knows the facts underlying his contention that the injections were given without the informed consent of the subject patients; (4) the informed consent of the patients is now required; and (5) all administrative and financial records have been ordered turned over to the petitioner. Since petitioner is already in possession of the facts as to the manner in which the experiments were conducted, no further need for the inspection exists.

C.
How and by Whom Should the Consequences of Research Be Reviewed?

1.
Informing the Board of Regents Grievance Committee for Decision

a.
Louis J. Lefkowitz, Attorney General of the State of New York
Petitioner's Post-Hearing Memorandum

IN THE MATTER
of the
Application for the revocation of the authorization and license heretofore granted to EMANUEL MANDEL, M.D. and CHESTER SOUTHAM, M.D. to practice medicine in the State of New York, and for the cancellation of their registrations as such, and for such other relief as the premises warrant.

THE STATUTES

The applicable provisions of the Education Law are as follows:
Section 6514. Revocation of Certificates.

2. The license or registration of a practitioner of medicine . . . may be revoked, suspended or annulled or such practitioner reprimanded or disciplined in accordance with the provisions and procedure of this article upon decision after due hearing in any of the following cases:
2 (a) That a physician . . . is guilty of fraud or deceit in the practice of medicine. . . .
2 (g) That a physician is or has been guilty of unprofessional conduct. As implemented and defined by the Rules of the Commissioner, filed pursuant to Statute in the Office of the Secretary of State under Title 8, part 60.1, subd. (d) 7 of the Official Compilation Codes, Rules and Regulations of the State of New York, i.e. "immoral conduct of a physician in his practice as a physician."

1. A VALID AND INFORMED CONSENT WAS NOT OBTAINED SINCE THE PATIENTS WERE NOT FULLY INFORMED OF THE NATURE AND DETAILS OF THE EXPERIMENT.

At the outset, it should be firmly understood that while we are dealing with 22 patients in a hospital, what was done to them, in the experimentation involved herein, was not done in the care or treatment of whatever illnesses or infirmities they had; and the respondents so admit.

It should also be remembered that, [all patients] had a right to expect and to demand from those charged with the administration of the hospital in its care and treatment of patients, that only those procedures and administrations of drugs that were a necessary part of their care and treatment be given and administered.

. . . An analysis of the patients selected amply illustrates that a substantial number of them had not sufficient mental or physical ability to comprehend what was being told to them or what was being done to them; and those who may have had the capacity to understand were not given the full and true nature of the experiment.

As to patient #18: Leichter had testified this patient had Parkinsons; developed lung abscess; was always running and falling against wall; had difficulty in communicating; that patient did not understand what was being explained and his speech was unintelligible. Leichter had treated this patient during the years from 1959 to 1963 and stated the patient's condition worsened with respect to July 16th. He further stated as his opinion this patient was unable to understand what an experiment of the type performed would mean.

Rosenfeld testified this patient was in a vegetative state and incommunicative the last year at the hospital; and could not have given a consent.

Southam testified this patient was in complete possession of his senses to extent he nodded agreement to permit examination at site of injection; that each time Southam saw the patient he was ambulatory, had marked shuffling gait, drooled considerably; that he did not regard the patient to be in a vegetative state, but was fully capable of understanding.

This testimony of Southam's is based upon observations made *after* injections were given. An examination of the record of this patient reveals Southam saw patient first time July 19th, then August 13, August 20 and finally October 1st.

Further, what probative weight should be given to Southam's testimony—based as it is on four visits—when it is compared to that of Leichter or Rosenfeld, doctors who have been constantly in attendance at Blumberg Building for many years prior to date of injections, and

who have seen this patient countless numbers of times, examined him and treated him?

Mandel testified he *did not* see this patient before July 16th; introduced report of psychiatrist made August 16th stating "patient is difficult to understand." Mandel stated he did not consider this a psychiatric report and that the charts were very defective. Stated he saw patient on October 5th, 1964 when the patient walked slowly, needed support, drooled a lot; tried to avoid speaking; found him fully alert and aware of place, time and what was going on and answered intelligently whatever questions were asked. Mandel submitted another psychiatric report dated October 27th, 1964 which stated patient was alert, oriented, denied hallucinations, illusions. It should be recalled that on cross-examination Mandel had testified he saw this patient *prior to* July 16th, but did not recall when; that patient drooled a lot; that patient's condition was essentially unchanged for last two or three years. Mandel could not state whether patient avoided speaking when he saw him prior to July 16th. Again, it should be recalled that Mandel, on direct examination, had testified he first saw the patient around December, 1963 and then again October 5th, 1964, and a week before he was testifying on November 4th.

Custodio testified that he did not agree with Rosenfeld's testimony concerning this patient that he was in a vegetative state and incommunicable. Custodio stated he knew patient since his service in 1961; that although patient had difficulty communicating with others who did not know him, he, Custodio, never had any difficulty and that patient understood him.

Mandel's testimony relative to this patient should be completely disregarded; he has contradicted himself as to when he first saw this patient. Even assuming he had seen the patient before July 16th, he gives no valid testimony concerning the patient's condition. As to Custodio, while he testified he disagreed with Rosenfeld's testimony he was silent as to his thoughts regarding Leichter's testimony, and it must therefore be assumed he agreed with Leichter.

It is respectfully urged, with respect to this patient, that Leichter and Rosenfeld, because of their length of service in Blumberg Building, were in a much better position to see, examine and observe this patient than were Southam (who never saw the patient before July 16th), Mandel and Custodio. Mandel's testimony is contradictory as to when he first saw the patient; at one time he testified it was October 5th, 1964; at another point in his testimony he fixed the time as at December, 1963; and still another point he stated it was *before* July 16th, but could not recall when. Custodio at least agreed the patient had difficulty communicating with others who did not know him.

It is submitted that the testimony of Leichter and Rosenfeld as to this patient should be accepted by the committee; and that a finding be made declaring this patient was incapable of understanding and thus could not have given a valid consent to participate in this experiment.

While only the records and testimony pertaining to a few patients have been shown to illustrate that the believable and probative proof established the absence of ability to understand fully the scope of the experimentation and thus give valid consent, it is by no means conceded that, in those patients not shown, there was present ability to understand and give consent.

The procedures adopted by the respondents in their conduct in pursuing the same give rise to certain compelling and important questions:

Was there any attempt on the part of Mandel, the director of medicine at JCDH, to in any way help or assist Custodio in the selection of the 19 patients in the Blumberg Building? And the answer, admittedly, was NO! Surely, this was a worth-while project—Mandel had been properly enthusiastic—but only to the extent of selecting the three cancer patients and actually being present when two of them were injected by Southam, and then Mandel left! But what of the patients in the Blumberg Building—should they have been placed at the beck and call of Custodio, or, more logically, should not this selection have been made by others more qualified, such as Rosenfeld, head of the Blumberg Building or Leichter who was not only familiar with the patients but was in charge of a cancer research project sponsored by the NIH. Was Custodio fully competent to participate in this project? On his own admission, he had never participated in such an experiment, nor had he read any literature relating to it. All he knew was what Mandel had told him. And what did Mandel know of this project? Only what Southam had told him, and the gist of what Southam told Mandel is that there was no risk to the test, that it was being done regularly at Memorial and that oral consent was sufficient with no knowledge to the patient that cancer cells were to be injected!

Why wasn't a careful screening done by both Mandel and Custodio, with a careful scrutiny of the hospital records which were available to them prior to July 16th? Why wasn't, prior to July 16th, a detailed statement prepared concerning the test, detailing each and every step of the procedures, the purposes for which the test was to be given and the names of the patients to be selected to participate? And, most important of all, why wasn't each patient informed that the injectable material was cancer cells? Why all the secrecy concerning cancer cells being injected if Mandel and Southam were so sure no deleterious effect could befall the patients? Yet Mandel had the gall to state in an affidavit submitted to the Supreme Court that everything was open and above-board!

Where was consideration shown to the patients with respect to their comfort; their freedom from unnecessary molestation and their absolute right to expect only such procedures and administrations necessary to their care and treatment? How dared Mandel introduce strangers to his hospital and to his patients and to permit these strangers to go through the various wards of the hospital, in open view of other patients? Oh, yes, those strangers were dressed like doctors—they had the long white coat commonly worn by visiting doctors; this then perhaps justified the intrusion as far as Mandel was concerned!

The haphazard method of selecting patients; the almost complete disregard of their comfort; the slip-shod manner in which the entire project was conceived and conducted, is evident throughout the record.

Southam was not concerned with whether Mandel had the right to proceed with this project without sanction or authority. Nor was he concerned with what what patients were selected; whether they were informed, and whether they were capable of giving consent. Mandel was evidently flattered that his hospital had been selected; he made no independent investigation concerning Southam or the project; he took Southam's word that no risk was involved, *although this was the first time they were engaged in performing this test upon debilitated patients;* he failed or refused to select a more capable and experienced participator than Custodio; and failed to assist and supervise the selection of patients.

And the greatest sin of all was the deliberate and willful failure on the part of the respondents herein, to inform each of the 22 patients that they were going to be injected with live cancer cells.

We are dealing with a project which admittedly was in no way therapeutic. It was, rather, an experiment relating to cancer research which had as its ultimate intention the benefit of humanity. This being the fact, it was then incumbent upon the respondents to have seen to it that ALL information connected with the experiment was given, since the patients at JCDH were being asked to become volunteers.

Respondents both admit they sanctioned and counselled the withholding from each patient the fact that the cell suspension to be used was indeed "live cancer cells." Their reasoning? They state that to release this information to the patients would cause a phobia, make them frightened, cause fear and anxiety—and this they wanted to avoid!

Every human being has an inalienable right to determine what shall be done with his own body. These patients then had a right to know what was being planned—not just the bald statement that an injection was to be given, but also the contents of the syringe: and if this knowledge was to cause fear and anxiety or make them frightened, they had a right to be fearful and frightened and thus say NO to the experiment.

Petitioner's exhibit #19, an article entitled "Problems of Informed Consent May Be Unsolvable" cites that Nuremberg Code—"the voluntary consent of the human subject is absolutely essential."

Petitioner's exhibit #6 and Resp. Southam's exhibit AA are entitled "The Normal Volunteer Program of the NIH Clinical Center" and is published by the U.S. Department of Health, Education and Welfare. Under the heading "Definitions" a distinction is made between the "normal volunteer"—a person who is judged to be in excellent health, etc., and "volunteer"—one who offers himself for a service of his own free will. Concededly, the patients at JCDH would come under the second classification. "Informed Consent" is defined as follows:

A formal, explicit, free expression of willingness to serve as a subject for research after the values and effects of such participation have been explained by the investigator and are sufficiently understood for the Volunteer to make a mature judgment.

At page 3 of the exhibit, under "Informed Consent" appears the following language:

The principal investigator *personally* provides the assigned volunteer, *in lay language* and at the level of his comprehension, with information about the proposed research project. He outlines its purpose, method, demands, inconveniences and discomforts, to enable the volunteer to make a *mature judgment* as

to his willingness and ability to participate. When he is fully cognizant of all that is entailed, the volunteer gives his *signed consent* to take part in it. (Emphasis supplied.)

It should be remembered that one of the sponsors for Southam's project and experimentation was the NIH!

How then did Southam discharge his duties and obligations to the volunteers as the principal and chief investigator in this experiment? Again, do we not see the careless and absolute disregard for the rights of the patients who were chosen to participate? While it may be argued that Southam was a stranger to JCDH and its patients and therefore relied upon Mandel, it nevertheless remains the undisputed fact that the 22 patients selected were volunteers in this project, and as to them in that capacity, Southam owed them every consideration and obligation as described by the NIH (supra). His was the duty *personally* to provide the volunteer *in lay language* at the level of his comprehension with information about the proposed research project; outlining its purpose; methods; demands; inconveniences and discomforts; so as to enable the volunteer to make a mature judgment as to his willingness and ability to participate; and only when the volunteer is fully cognizant of *all that is entailed,* does he give Southam his *signed* consent. And how did Southam discharge this duty and obligation? First, he said he left it to Mandel to decide the question of "consent" and the manner by which it was to be obtained, albeit he stressed to Mandel the method of obtaining oral consents at Memorial which, in Southam's opinion, were sufficient although the recipient of the injection was not told that cancer cells were being injected. Secondly, he said he was satisfied to have Custodio as his collaborator, despite the fact that he saw Custodio for the first time on the day of the experiment and knew nothing whatever of the latter's ability, experience or knowledge in projects of this kind. This, it is strongly urged, Southam had no right to do. As a scientist engaged in research he had the duty and responsibility for ascertaining the quality of the consent, which may not be delegated to another with impunity. This was his project, and, if it was to serve any useful purpose he should have taken and assumed full and complete authority; by having carefully screened, with Mandel, the patients that were to be selected; by having, with Mandel, spoken, in advance of the injections, to each patient, explaining in lay language at the level of the patient's comprehension, the purpose, methods, demands, inconveniences and discomforts of the proposed project.

For the record is replete with contradictory statements as to the manner by which "consents" were obtained; Mandel wasn't sure whether he had obtained so-called oral consents from one or two patients; he wasn't sure of the language he used in speaking of the project. Custodio likewise is not sure of just what words were used when speaking to the patients stating that interchangeably he used words as "immunity," "resistance" or "immunological response."

But the salient factor remains that at *no time* and to *no volunteer patient* was information given that, in truth and in fact, the cell suspension mentioned contained *live cancer cells*.

This then is the nub of the entire case. These volunteers, the 22 debilitated patients at JCDH, were not each made *"fully cognizant of ALL that is entailed"* in the proposed project. There was *missing,* deliberately and wilfully so, any statement to the effect that the injectable material contained live cancer cells. As was stated in SCIENCE, petitioner's exhibit 9, in the article entitled "Medical Ethics" and that portion under the chapter heading "Procedures not of direct benefit to the individual" found on page 1025 of the exhibit:

The common feature of this type of investigation is that it is of no direct benefit to the particular individual and that, in consequence, if he is to submit to it he must volunteer in the full sense of the word.
It should be clearly understood that the possibility or probability that a particular investigation will be of benefit to humanity or to posterity would afford no defense in the event of legal proceedings. The individual has rights that the law protects and nobody can infringe those rights for the public good. In investigations of this type it is, therefore, always necessary to ensure that the true consent of the subject is explicitly obtained.

It is therefore respectfully submitted that the respondents herein failed to secure a valid and informed consent from each of the 22 patient-volunteers to participate in the experimentation conducted at JCDH.

2. THE RESPONDENTS ARE EACH GUILTY OF EACH SPECIFICATION OF THE CHARGES.

The failure of each respondent to reveal ALL that was entailed in the experimentation to each of the volunteer debilitated patients that were selected to participate was fraudulent and deceitful. As illustrated supra, the licensees herein had no right, moral or legal, to with-

hold any information relating to the experimentation. By so doing they violated the absolute right of each patient to determine what shall be done with his own body. By withholding the fact that live cancer cells were to be injected in this experiment, they deprived each patient of their inalienable right to refuse such an injection. *No choice* was given to these volunteers.

The conduct of each respondent was unprofessional, immoral and shocking to one's sense of fairness. Mandel has testified that patients do not question procedures that are done to them in a hospital because they have confidence in the doctors and that patients tend to accept what doctors say to them. It is submitted this confidence was misplaced; that all of these patient-volunteers were duped and misled by Southam and Mandel. Surely, the image of the medical profession must be sullied in the eyes of the public, if the conduct of the respondents herein was to be sanctioned and blessed with innocence.

Again and again it must be repeated and emphasized that a human being has rights and privileges that may not be trespassed upon to any degree. How shocking indeed it would be if a person were to realize that he had no rights or privileges as to what should be done to his body, and that he was a mere "guinea pig" in the eyes of any doctor, whether scientist or researcher, who desired to perform some experimentation on him!

Such a fantastic and gruesome thought could never withstand the indignation and denial of the public.

Upon the entire case therefore it is respectfully submitted each licensee is guilty of each specification contained in the charges.

b.

Morris Ploscowe, Esq.
Brief on Behalf of Dr. Emanuel E. Mandel

THE CHARGE THAT DR. MANDEL IS GUILTY OF FRAUD AND DECEIT BECAUSE THE PATIENTS WERE NOT ADVISED "THAT LIVE CANCER CELLS WERE TO BE INJECTED IN THEIR BODIES" CANNOT BE SUSTAINED.

The reasons why the patients were not told that the injections contained tissue cultured cancer cells are not found in fraud or deceit. This is apparent from the following:

Dr. Southam was asked why he deliberately refrained from describing (the injected cells) as "cancer cells." He testified as follows:

For two reasons really. First, I saw no reason why we

should use such a word because it is not pertinent to the phenomenon which is going to follow. We are not doing something which is going to induce cancer. We are not going to do something which is going to cause them any harm; it is not going to produce a transplanted cancer. We are going to observe the growth and rejection of these transplanted cancer cells.

The fact then that they are cancer cells does not mean that there is any risk of cancer to this patient.

Now, the second point is simply that the word, "cancer," has a tremendous emotive value, disvalue, to everybody, not only to the cancer patients but to you and me. What the ordinary patient, what the non-medical person, and even many doctors whose competence in clinical medicine is great but whose knowledge of the basic science behind transplantation is not great—to them the use of a cancer cell might imply a risk that it will grow and produce cancer, and the fear that this word strikes in people is great, and I don't think I have to argue the point to make the point. I think we all recognize it. If we use words like neoplastic; if we use words like tumor, we have no problem.

. . . Many of these patients undoubtedly know deep down that they have cancer, but the great majority of them have either suppressed this knowledge from the surface or at least they are not talking about it

---

[*] CROSS-EXAMINATION OF DR. CHESTER M. SOUTHAM BY MR. CALANESE.

Q: Doctor, in Vol. 143 of *Science* which is issued February 1964 at page 551 you wrote that there was no theoretical likelihood that the injections would produce cancer. Yet, in the same article, Doctor, you stated that you were unwilling to inject yourself or your colleagues, and you stated, and I quote, "But, let's face it, there are relatively few skilled cancer researchers, and it seemed stupid to take even the little risk."

A: I deny the quote. I am sure I didn't say, "let's face it."

Q: Did you make any statement similar to that?

A: I think the philosophy is an accurate statement.

Q: What was your statement, do you recall?

A: What I am objecting to is the phrase, "let's face it." The statement that I see no reason why a doctor should necessarily serve as a recipient, this is valid, that is, this statement may validly be attributed to me.

Q: The statement, Doctor, was published by Elinor Langer in *Science* of February 7, 1964, Vol. 143, and I quote from her statement that I want to find out from you whether or not what she is quoting as coming from you is correct or not. "Southam, however, who ought to know, said in an interview with *Science* that, although there was no theoretical likelihood that the injections would produce cancer, he had nonetheless been unwilling to inject himself or

and they don't welcome conversation that brings it up. So, it is our firmly established and I feel very sound policy *not to use the word "cancer"* with the cancer patients. . . .

The position taken by Dr. Mandel and Dr. Southam in not mentioning the fact that the injections contained cancer cells is justified by medical ethics and current medical practice. Medical ethics do not require the full disclosure to a patient of all conceivable risks and all relevant information as a basis for obtaining patients' consent to a medical procedure. The amount of information imparted to a patient must bear some relation to the risk of a particular procedure. Where there is no substantial risk of harm to a patient, the information imparted to him may be kept at a minimum. We submit that in the instant case it was not necessary to tell the patient that the injections involved tissue cultured cancer cells since there was no possibility that harm could come to the patients from the said cells.[*]

It should also be noted that the amount of information which should be imparted to a patient as a prerequisite for consent to a medical

---

his colleagues, when there was a group of normal volunteers at the Ohio Penitentiary fully informed about the experiment and its possible risks and nonetheless eager to take part in it. 'I would not have hesitated' Southam said, 'if it would have served a useful purpose. But,' he continued, 'to me it seemed like false heroism, like the old question whether the General should march behind or in front of his troops. I do not regard myself as indispensable—if I were not doing this work someone else would be—and I did not regard the experiments as dangerous. But, let's face it, there are relatively few skilled cancer researchers, and it seemed stupid to take even the little risk.' "

Did you make that statement?

A: As I said before, the philosophy is correct. I do not know if I made that statement. This is reported—I remember the interview very well. I am still saying that the quotes are not necessarily correct; the philosophy is correct.

Q: That part of the quoting concerning the, "stupid to take even the little risk," do you recall that?

A: No, I don't, and this is one of the reasons that I question whether it is a true quote.

Q: Do you recall the statement that you made that there was no theoretical likelihood that injections would produce cancer?

A: This is, in other words, exactly what I have said earlier this afternoon. [From transcript of proceedings before a Subcommittee of the Committee on Grievances, Department of Education of the State of New York, September, 1964, pp. 636–638.]

or surgical procedure may be left to the sound discretion of a conscientious physician.[*] This is the import of the rules concerning the testing of drugs which is in evidence as respondent's Exhibit B, and which state that while consent should be obtained for testing of investigational drugs, the laws and the regulations make it clear

[*] EXAMINATION OF DR. EMANUEL E. MANDEL BY MR. RASHKIS, INVESTIGATOR, NEW YORK STATE DEPARTMENT OF EDUCATION.

Q: Each patient was told that an experiment to determine his immunity was to be conducted. Was each patient told that cell tissue was to be injected?
A: Yes, cell suspension was to be injected.
Q: Each patient was told this?
A: Yes, each patient was told.
Q: Did any patient ask you what a cell suspension is?
MR. PLOSCOWE: If you can recall.
A: I can't.
Q: No one asked you?
A: (No response.)
Q: Did you actually have a conversation with the patients that you spoke to them and they answered you?
A: Yes.
Q: Every patient?
A: Every patient. I asked them if they have— each and every one of them has any objection to us doing the test and they said no.
Q: Did any patient answer anything other than yes or no; that he would agree—
A: No.
Q: No patient questioned any of the terms that you used?
A: I don't remember. I don't think anyone asked.
DR. MANDEL: May I add to that?
MR. RASHKIS: Yes.
DR. MANDEL: I will say almost every day doctors come into situations where they have to ask a patient for permission to do a certain procedure, say a bone-marrow aspiration, a spinal tap, what not.
Most patients don't question these procedures; the patients have confidence in the doctors.
MR. RASHKIS: What is the purpose for the tests?
DR. MANDEL: Diagnostic nature.
MR. RASHKIS: For that particular patient?
DR. MANDEL: For that particular patient.
MR. RASHKIS: Would these patients have understood these tests were to be diagnostic in nature?
DR. MANDEL: No.
MR. RASHKIS: Is there any relevancy in the statement you made about the bone-marrow test?
DR. MANDEL: Only in terms of conversation with patients. Ordinarily they listen and tend to accept what the doctor says to them. [From transcript of proceedings before a Subcommittee of the Committee on Grievances, Department of Education of the State of New York, September, 1964, pp. 96–100.]

that if in the professional judgment of the investigator "it is not feasible or in the best interests of the subject to obtain permission, *the investigational nature of the drug need not be disclosed*." This concept of patient consent is not new, but has been part of the Code of Ethics of the American Medical Association for many years.

If, in the judgment of a conscientious physician, the investigational nature of a drug need not be disclosed, when it is tested, then there appears to be no reason why the nature of the injected material should have been disclosed to the patients at JCDH, since there was no hazard to the patients from the injections.

The following statements made by distinguished physicians in affidavits submitted on behalf of Dr. Southam, support our contention that a proper consent was obtained from the patients at JCDH in the tests conducted at JCDH and that it was not fraud or deceit not to tell the patients that the injected material contained cancer cells:

Dr. Michael J. Brennan, physician in charge of the division of oncology, Henry Ford Hospital, Detroit, Michigan, stated as follows:

. . . The need to enter into detailed description of the source and nature of a test material cannot be shown to be a part of our moral and legal duty unless it would be objectively helpful to the patient in coming to a rational and knowledgeable conclusion about the real risks of the procedure to his health.

. . . He [Southam] did not speak to these patients of giving them a treatment. He asked permission to do a test of considerable scientific import. He then faithfully explained to them the sequence of reactions which they could expect and rightly and correctly assured them of their innocuous character. He hid nothing from the patients which would have been useful to them in making a rational decision regarding the real risks of the test.

He did not mention that the test solutions were made from tissue cultures of cancer cells. This now proves to have been imprudent because of the emotional character of the response which followed revelation of that fact and the opening it gave for accusations of dishonesty and duplicity on his part. There is a difference between withholding information and giving false information but it is often overlooked. However, *the information he withheld was not needed by the patients for judging rightly that his test was safe.*

The real test of the adequacy of his description to the patients of what would happen is whether it corresponded with what did in fact happen.

It was the compassion of the good physician, not the deceit of the charlatan or the calculation of the cold experimentalist, which has laid him open to his present troubles. . . .

Dr. George E. Moore, director and chief of surgery of Roswell Park Memorial Institute of Buffalo, New York, stated as follows:

. . . For the past 4 years, I have been engaged in a similar type of project at Roswell Park Memorial Institute. My research involves the homotransplantation to patients with cancer of tissue-cultured cells derived from human cancer tissue. In my view these tests are of vital importance in the field of cancer research and it is my hope that, through the resulting increased knowledge of immunological factors relating to cancer, important strides may be made leading to possible immunization against, or treatments of, cancer. To the best of my knowledge, *there has been no practical risk of any deleterious effects upon any of the patients who served as subjects in the tests performed by me.*

The question of the type of information to be furnished a patient incident to obtaining his consent to participation in these tests was carefully explored by me in conjunction with other officials of my hospital. It was our decision that the patients would be told that their consent was sought to participation in an investigation involving the injection of live cells derived from a tumor. The word "cancer" was not ordinarily employed. In some instances the phrase "cultured cells from human tumors" was used.

While our procedures thus differ from those employed by Dr. Southam, I believe that Dr. Southam was motivated solely by his concern for the welfare of his patients; *it is clear that this is an area in which fully informed doctors acting solely for the benefit of their patients may arrive at different conclusions as to the best approach to take.* I am aware of the potentially traumatic effects which the use of the word "cancer" may produce, and for the most part, I share Dr. Southam's view that the word should be avoided in such studies since, from a scientific standpoint the general term "cancer" does not accurately reflect the nature of the biologic materials being used.

I do not believe that the differences in the procedures employed by Dr. Southam and by me cast any reflection upon the professional integrity or judgment of Dr. Southam. I believe that the factors which I know were weighed by Dr. Southam prior to making his decision make it preposterous to assert that there was any modicum of "fraud," "deceit" or "immorality" involved in his actions. . . .

Dr. Alvin L. Watne, associate professor of surgery and cancer coordinator at West Virginia Medical Center, stated as follows:

. . . In his affidavit, Dr. Southam describes the procedures which he has employed in his project relating to the study of the relationship between immunological research and cancer. I am engaged in a comparable research project. The information that we present to the patient is that this is a research project that we are conducting here in the department and that their participation is entirely voluntary. If there is any reluctance on their part, we do not press the issue. We do not use the words "cancer" or "tumor" in describing the possible transplantation. We do say that we will test the patient's ability to respond to the stimulation and that we are interested in knowing more about their particular tumor problem and that this will give us some information along that line.
. . . *I believe that the procedures described by Dr. Southam in connection with the obtaining of consents are in accord with the highest standards of the medical profession* and I subscribe to the reasons given by him for the adoption of such procedures.

Dr. I. S. Ravdin, professor of surgery and vice-president of medical affairs at the University of Pennsylvania, stated as follows:

. . . It is the considered opinion of many investigators that research in the field of host response and immune reactions is likely to provide the first important breakthrough in the treatment of malignant diseases. It is men like Dr. Southam who are best prepared to accomplish this highly desirable breakthrough.

Physicians are constantly concerned as to whether they should tell a patient that he is suffering from a malignant disease. Dr. William T. Fitts, Jr., and I studied this matter some years ago. We sent a questionnaire to members of the Philadelphia County Medical Society in order to ascertain what they did under these circumstances. *Only the dermatologists did this with any frequency.*

The question of whether a proper consent was obtained from the patients in the Southam research at JCDH was also presented to three distinguished physicians who appeared as witnesses on behalf of Dr. Mandel. Each of these physicians was asked a hypothetical question based on the facts brought out at the hearing herein which include the assumption that the patients were not told that the injections contained live cancer cells. Each of these physicians was asked the basic question, "In your opinion as an experienced and conscientious physician, do you believe that a proper consent was obtained to the aforementioned (tissue cultured cancer cells) injections?" Each of the physicians testified affirmatively that a proper consent was obtained to the injections herein.

Dr. David Kershner testified as follows:

Well, in my experience in handling surgery cases for about 40 years and the problems which we have to decide on the Malpractice and Defense Board of the State Society as well as the equal level of the county society, we talk in terms of informed consent and what is informed consent and much is made of it. I don't think any law can be laid down. I don't think we can strictly say this is informed consent and this is not informed consent and this is what you must not tell the patient. I think it has to be individualized. Patients are not all the same; they don't react the same way. But by and large, I think we can safely say that if a patient is going to be operated upon or any work is going to be done involving malignancy, and we use the word "cancer," it throws a horrible fear into the patient. . . .

Dr. Charles E. Rogers testified as follows:

The reason I say that I believe informed consent was obtained was because I don't think there was any risk involved here. It is well known that we have been trying hard to transplant tissues for a number of years and we have been failing miserably. As far as I can see, what occurred here is they wanted to find out whether there was immune response or to what degree the immune response was engendered in patients who had debilitating diseases, and since we know that we can't transplant these tissues unless we have identical twins or unless we pretreat the patient with radiation or other toxic substances, I would feel that informed consent was obtained. There wasn't a risk involved.

I base that on literature and my knowledge of the immunology such as it may be and the general knowledge I have. I just don't think there is any doubt in my mind these tissues could have possibly survived in these patients. Obviously, they didn't.

On cross-examination, Dr. Rogers was asked the following questions and gave the following answers:

MR. CALANESE: All those volunteers at Jewish Chronic Disease Hospital were not told that cancer cells were being injected.

DR. ROGERS: That isn't germane to the problem, Sir.

MR. CALANESE: As far as you're concerned?

DR. ROGERS: Yes, Sir. That is my opinion.

MR. CALANESE: Further they were told there would be no risk involved with the test they were going to be subjected to at that time.

DR. ROGERS: I think that is true in my opinion.

MR. CALANESE: That is not important as far as the patient or the volunteer is concerned?

DR. ROGERS: No, Sir. I think that you would be causing the patient undue anxiety and undue concern over a procedure that doesn't have a risk.

*　　*　　*

MR. CALANESE: It has been established here, Doctor, by the testimony so far, that all that was told to these patients is that an injection was going to be given to determine their resistance to disease and that a lump would form within a few days which would disappear within 2 or 3 weeks; that is all that was told. In your opinion, is that sufficient?

DR. ROGERS: Yes, sir, in this particular case. But, I wish to emphasize every case must be decided on its own merits. In this particular case, there was no risk and there was no need to advise the patients unnecessarily and alarm them and say these are cancer cells, you could get cancer, because the volunteer in a situation like that would be worried.

Dr. Irving Hirshleifer testified as follows:

MR. PLOSCOWE: . . . Was a proper consent obtained from the patients to the cancer injections involved in the instant proceeding?

DR. HIRSHLEIFER: Yes, sir.

MR. PLOSCOWE: Would you tell the panel the reason why you came to that opinion.

DR. HIRSHLEIFER: Well, having been in clinical investigation for many years and also having served in a teaching and training capacity and a medical school affiliated institution for many years, and having helped train many interns and residents since 1946, these were the practices which were performed in no other manner in all my experience.

MR. PLOSCOWE: When you state these were the practices, Doctor, would you be more specific, the technique of obtaining consent. That's right.

DR. HIRSHLEIFER: Yes.

MR. PLOSCOWE: Well, does it make any difference that in this particular proceeding what was done here was for the purpose of experimentation, the making of a test rather than for the therapeutic benefit of the patient?

DR. HIRSHLEIFER: These are the usual practices in hospitals where interns and residents are trained.

MR. PLOSCOWE: Can you tell me, for example, in the hospitals with which you have been associated, . . . universities and teaching institutions, are frequent tests performed on patients which have nothing to do with the therapy or treatment of the patient?

DR. HIRSHLEIFER: Yes, sir.

MR. PLOSCOWE: And is the method of consent obtained in that framework any different from the method of consent obtained here?

DR. HIRSHLEIFER: Sometimes, not to the degree that was obtained here.

MR. PLOSCOWE: Does that mean that we were more formal here?

DR. HIRSHLEIFER: Yes.

*　　*　　*

MR. PLOSCOWE: With respect to the specific project, there has been criticism of the fact that the word "cancer" was not used prior to the injection of these patients. Do you find that this is a proper subject of criticism in this particular framework?

DR. HIRSHLEIFER: No, I don't. I attempt never to use that term when conversing with a patient.

_____

[*] CROSS-EXAMINATION OF DR. EMANUEL E. MANDEL BY MR. CALANESE.

Q: Now, before the injections were made by Dr. Southam, did you personally secure the consent of any of these three patients?

A: I believe I spoke to at least one of them and this is something I cannot remember and haven't been able to remember, whether it was I or Dr. Custodio who spoke to these patients explaining what the objective was, what we were planning to do. Dr. Custodio thought it was I. It may well be.

Q: Let's take your statement that you may have spoken to at least one. Can you tell this committee exactly, to the best of your recollection today, what you told that particular patient . . . concerning this experiment?

A: I remember talking to the one that had the leukemia. I think I mentioned that earlier today, and I mentioned this morning that the patient indicated some resentment over being stuck with needles over a period of his hospitalization without evidence he was really getting better.

Q: That is what I was trying to bring out, Dr. Mandel; . . . I want you to tell this committee and this record what was said by you to this patient and what if anything was said by the patient to you.

A: It is impossible for me to do that. I can't remember it.

Q: To the best of your recollection.

A: Well, I only know I spoke to him and I recall vaguely he indicated his—the fact he was unhappy over having so many forms of treatment and diagnostic procedures and didn't think he was getting better. He showed me how he had lost weight. He showed me he had an enlarged abdomen. He had what is called ascites, free fluid in the abdomen, and I recall that I tried to reassure him.

Q: As to what?

A: As to eventual improvement, that he was going—getting better; that various procedures that have been planned for him and that have been carried out will eventually bring about his ultimate recovery.

Q: Had he told you in any manner, shape or form as to the numbers of time that tests had been made on him over a short period of time before July 16th?

A: I don't—

Q: A number of tests had been made, he was sick and tired of it, he said?

It is apparent from the aforementioned discussion that the respondents, Dr. Mandel and Dr. Southam, by failing to disclose to the patients that the cell suspension injections were cancer cells, were not guilty of fraud or deceit, but were acting in the best interests of the patients and according to accepted standards in the field of medicine.[*]

_____

A: I am sure he didn't use that expression. He was very well mannered and quite a quiet sort of fellow.

*   *   *

Q: When you spoke to him concerning this test, just exactly what did you tell him this test was and what it comprised, what the expectations were?

A: I cannot tell you exactly. I can only tell you what I told him, what has been stated a number of times; that the test was planned for the determination of his immune response or his resistance and that it would result in a lump which would disappear after a period of time, after some weeks.

*   *   *

Q: Did he ask you for any further particulars concerning the test?

A: I don't believe so.

Q: Despite the fact he made a complaint to you about too many tests having been made upon him before, you say he made no further complaint or asked you no information concerning this test?

A: He did this more in a way of general complaint and his complaint was directed primarily towards not getting better. In other words, he compared his lack of improvement with the number of procedures being applied.

Q: Was any statement made to him, Doctor, by you that this test might be of benefit to him?

A: Did I indicate that to him?

Q: Yes.

A: I am certain I didn't.

Q: Did you say anything to him, Doctor, that as part of this test, in addition to the injection and the lump that would form, that would disappear within a short period of time, that blood tests would also be taken and made?

A: I would think that I did.

Q: Don't you know?

A: I don't remember. I am quite certain this was done in every instance.

Q: You are quite sure.

A: Yes.

Q: We are speaking with respect to this specific instance, this leukemia patient. Did you tell him there would be blood tests taken?

A: I don't recall. [From transcript of proceedings before a Subcommittee of the Committee on Grievances, Department of Education of the State of New York, September, 1964, pp. 960–965.]

Even if it should be maintained that Dr. Mandel and Dr. Custodio should have told the patients that "live cancer cells" were being used in the injections despite their fear of instilling cancer phobias in the patients, there can be very little doubt that their failure to do so was an honest medical error. An honest medical error cannot be deemed fraud or deceit or "immoral conduct" of a physician.

2.

The Board of Regents Grievance Committee Makes Its Recommendations

a.

Report of the Subcommittee of the Committee on Grievances

To the Committee on Grievances:

The undersigned, subcommittee of the COMMITTEE ON GRIEVANCES duly designated to hear the charges against DR. CHESTER M. SOUTHAM and DR. EMANUEL E. MANDEL hereinafter referred to as respondents, pursuant to Section 6515 of the Education Law of the State of New York, and to report its findings and recommendation in respect to the said charges, do hereby, after due deliberation, unanimously report its findings and recommendations as provided by law as follows:

*   *   *

The findings and recommendation of Dr. Lawrence Ames, chairman of the subcommittee is as follows:

The above two physicians are charged with fraud or deceit, as well as unprofessional conduct, in the practice of medicine within the purview and meaning of the Education Law and as implemented and defined by the Rules of the Commissioner. . . .

*   *   *

Sitting as chairman of the subcommittee of the medical grievance committee hearing this case, I had full opportunity to hear all the testimony and evidence introduced by the attorneys for the respondents and by the attorney general for the petitioner.

Every opportunity was afforded both respondents and the petitioner to present their cases completely and thoroughly and there was no attempt on the part of the committee to impede or curtail the introduction of any evidence or testimony pertinent to the case. I have re-

viewed all the testimony and evidence and after a great deal of study I have come to the following conclusions:

This experiment or research project was not done for the care or treatment of any of these individuals, but rather as a non-therapeutic clinical research project.

All the patients chosen were in a very debilitated condition for that was a necessary prerequisite for this experiment.

Dr. Southam, the chief investigator, was working partly under a grant from the United States Department of Health, Education and Welfare of the Public Health Service and was governed by their rules and regulations regarding experimentation and research.

Dr. Southam was aware of the rules and regulations as set down by the Public Health Service for research and experimentation under these grants. It specifically states, "The principal investigator personally provides the assigned volunteer in lay language and at the level of his comprehension, with information about the proposed research project. He outlines its purposes, methods, demands, inconveniences and discomforts, to enable the volunteer to make a mature judgment as to his willingness and ability to participate. When he is fully cognizant of all that is entailed, the volunteer gives his signed consent to take part in it."

Dr. Southam as chief investigator and Dr. Mandel as chief of medicine of the Jewish Chronic Disease Hospital are both equally responsible for whatever took place and share equal responsibility for these acts.

The 19 patients who were chosen by Dr. Custodio were not given sufficient facts on which to base their judgment of whether or not to give consent. It is admitted that at no time were the words "cancer cell injection" ever used. Many of these 19 patients, in my opinion based on the evidence introduced, were not physically or mentally capable of understanding what was involved and therefore incapable of giving informed consent, even if such information were given to them by Dr. Custodio. The manner in which Dr. Custodio elected to choose the cases for the experiment, the very morning of the injections, and the total time consumed in giving all these injections, convinces me beyond reasonable doubt that proper informed consent could not have been obtained. It is my considered opinion that he was more interested in getting his name on a research project, than in protecting the interests of these debilitated people placed in his care and trust as senior resident at the Jewish Chronic Disease Hospital.

I find that Dr. Southam, as chief investigator, and Dr. Mandel, as chief of medicine at the Jewish Chronic Disease Hospital, did not fulfill their obligations to the people involved in this investigation, in that they did not obtain or see that the proper informed consent was obtained from these patients or those qualified to give the proper consent for them.[*]

Every human being has an inalienable right

---

[*] CROSS-EXAMINATION OF DR. CHESTER M. SOUTHAM BY MEMBERS OF THE COMMITTEE ON GRIEVANCES.

DR. HELLER: . . . the question in our minds, I believe, the committee's mind, is whether or not patients, whether they are terminal patients, patients who are socially adjusted and could be right here in a social gathering, would know the difference between a test or a treatment and whether or not they could construe, in a setting such as we have described, a test as a routine procedure within a hospital revolving about themselves and their betterment, their welfare, care and treatment?

In other words, the patients, as we have it, were not asked, "Do you know what research is? Do you know what an experiment consists of?" and we don't know what they might have answered to the question "Do you know what research is? Do you want to become a research subject?" These are the points, though they are points of semantics, yet relate to understanding of the patient. It would seem to us that cooperation depends upon the recognition of a doctor, his confidence, but not upon his understanding that this was a research project. What we are concerned with is the method of obtaining the consent, primarily. That is why I raise that question, and I would like your comment on it.

A: One of your key points, I think, is whether these patients in saying, all right, I will have a test, interpreted in this sense of something out of the ordinary, not a routine matter, test that might have been done, but a research project, an experiment.

Obviously, I cannot speak for the patients, but I think there is no question but—I am speaking now over the period of time that these tests were carried on rather than at the particular moment about which I was being questioned previously—certainly when doctors come in, two doctors known not to be associated with their hospital, it certainly was clear to most of these people, I would guess, that they know that this was something out of the routine; that this was a research, and I would not doubt at all that we used such words as research and experiment. Some patients were quite able to converse. As others, as you heard, had impaired ability to converse, but certainly those who were able to talk better, I feel confident, knew that not only that this was research involved, they probably knew that we were from a cancer re-

to determine what shall be done with his body. This, without regard as to whether he be confined to a penal institution, or free, or whether he be healthy or debilitated and confined in an institution or hospital. The same rights or priv-

---

search hospital. This is obviously opinion. This is not a statement of facts.

DR. HELLER: That is the point I am making. The ability to converse is no measure of understanding whatsoever. The most conversant patients can have the least understanding or the least competency to understand that they are being used for an experiment; that they are volunteering to do so; and that this is research; and certainly in the presence of a doctor whom they are familiar with and other doctors in white coats, confidence is automatically generated. They need no other.

My question is, isn't it an assumption on your part that these patients had understanding; they can communicate even by the visual observations of a syringe, doctor's bag, injection, they—this is part of hospital procedure. So, the communication is taken for granted. My question was, didn't you have to make an assumption that these patients understood, had understanding of the request that you were making, a request of them to volunteer as subjects for an experiment?

A: Yes. I certainly agree both in this specific instance that I was making an assumption—I think that Drs. Mandel and Custodio may be able to make a better answer to this particular point, because they know the patients better. I think it is true, also, as I think you have indicated, that we assume an understanding also when we communicate with patients, that is, I don't know if I said that clearly, but in any doctor-patient relationship there is this quality that you mentioned of the patient in a setting where he recognizes that the doctor is doing things to and for him. Undoubtedly, they associate this with what is proper. He accepts, essentially, things as being proper because they are being done under this total picture of medical doctor-patient relationship. I think that all we can do in such situations is to explain that what we are doing is not for your treatment, if necessary, to say that it makes no difference whether you have such a procedure or not. This will not influence your disease, and it will not influence your proper treatment.

DR. WIENER: Was there any deviation, as far as obtaining patients' consents here, was there any deviation from the long-standing practice of obtaining consents?

A: No, sir. There was—this was the reason that I believe that Dr. Mandel accepted this method. I had assured him that this was our established method of obtaining consents at Memorial and Ewing. [From transcript of proceedings before a Subcommittee of the Committee on Grievances, Department of Education of the State of New York, September, 1964, pp. 784–789.]

ileges must be accorded him. If they be so mentally or physically affected that they be incapable of making decisions, then the nearest of kin must be afforded the right to make this decision.

I therefore find the respondents, Dr. Southam and Dr. Mandel, both guilty beyond reasonable doubt of the charges and specifications as charged.

In considering the degree of punishment, I am considering the outstanding records of both these doctors, the high esteem by which they are held by the medical profession and scientists in general throughout the world. I also take into consideration the nature of the experiment and its purposes and I therefore recommend that they both be given a censure and reprimand.

The findings and recommendation of Dr. Saul I. Heller, member of the subcommittee is as follows:

It is my finding that Chester Southam, M.D. and Emanuel Mandel, M.D. are both guilty of each specification contained in the charges.

Just because such a project is worthy, and just because terminal patients were readily available, who were deteriorating anyhow, does not, in my opinion, warrant deceiving such patients into believing that they were submitting to ordinary and customary hospital procedure, intended to aid in the diagnosis of, or the alleviation of their particular illnesses.

This project was not even experimental therapy, although there are many inferences that it might be. In experimental therapy, patients and volunteers are selected who are able to clearly comprehend beforehand the full nature and details of the experiment, which generally are outlined on a printed form on which the patient or volunteer is asked to sign his consent. A volunteer consents after he is fully informed in lay language, that is, language that he can comprehend and this usually involves considerable thought and much discussion, with dozens of questions being asked, and fully answered over a period of time.

In my contacts with various investigators, especially during the past seven years, I was impressed by the fact that the National Institute of Health always advised the investigators to follow the above procedure in experimental therapy.

The project of Dr. Southam and Dr. Mandel at Jewish Chronic Disease Hospital was experimental research on a group of human beings, who were told that an injection was being given to them to test their immunity or resistance to

disease, and that a nodule would form and disappear. However, they were not asked to become volunteers and participate in an experiment on human beings for the purpose of furthering Dr. Southam's cancer research project. These patients and their relatives had the human right to decide what should be done with their bodies, except in a dire medical emergency.

These patients were entrusted to the care of the Jewish Chronic Disease Hospital by their relatives, who visited the patients and spoke to their doctors, and even the relatives were not informed of this research project. I cannot understand why the relatives of these patients were never informed of this experiment prior to the patients' having received the experimental injections of live cancer cells. This omission can only imply deceit, especially when one considers the procedure in any hospital, as, the unrefuted testimony of Dr. Leichter that in regard to patient No. 18, he had secured written consent from the patient's family to tap the patient's chest, and further that before administering the antibiotic drug, Terramycin 401 to patient No. 18, he also secured signed consent from the family. These procedures antedated the injections of live cancer cells.

It is only reasonable to conclude, if you must secure written consent from the family and disclose the true nature of an antibiotic, to give an antibiotic, you must disclose the true nature of the cellular material injected in this experiment, both to the patient and his family, in order to obtain informed consent, as was done by a competent resident in the case of the antibiotic, Terramycin 401. I am referring to Dr. Leichter, who in 1960 had been placed in charge of a research project sponsored by the National Institute of Health, by Dr. Goldner, the director of Jewish Chronic Disease Hospital, at that time. The competent residents at Jewish Chronic Disease Hospital were deliberately by-passed by Dr. Mandel, director at this time because he knew they would only adhere to the procedure of informed written consent.

Dr. Mandel asked Dr. Custodio, a resident who had just returned after a year's absence, if he were interested in participating in a research project which had been brought to Dr. Mandel's attention by Dr. Southam a week or so earlier. When Dr. Custodio indicated that he was interested, he was told by Dr. Mandel, "if we can get oral consents we can go ahead." He directed Dr. Custodio to prepare a list of non-cancer patients. It appears that there was no specific discussion between Dr. Mandel and Dr. Custodio of any need for their terminal patients nor their families to understand that the patients were to be used as volunteers in cancer research.

Dr. Custodio testified that he chose 19 non-cancer terminal patients, in his mind, at random, the night before the experiment; and the next morning led Dr. Southam and his assistant, Dr. Levin, to the rooms of these patients.

Dr. Southam says that an explanation of some kind was made by Dr. Custodio regarding a test to study the patient's immune reactions and that a nodule would form and later disappear.

Dr. Mandel, himself, chose three cancer patients and states he was familiar with these cases. One of these cases was scheduled for elective surgery on July 18, 1963, and such elective surgery, according to Dr. Mandel, is arranged about five days in advance, and written consent was obtained for this operation. Nonetheless, this patient was used for human experimentation just two days before this scheduled operation and died on July 19, 1963, the day after the operation.

It is obvious that this patient would never have been subjected to this experiment, had any of the 4 doctors involved in the experiment known, or cared about knowing, the status of this patient.

Another of the three cases selected by Dr. Mandel was suffering from leukemia. Dr. Mandel testified that he tried to reassure this patient that he was getting better, because the patient expressed resentment in "being stuck with needles without getting better," and compared his lack of improvement unfavorably with the number of tests. Moreover, Dr. Mandel does not remember if he explained to this leukemia patient that there would be follow-up blood tests. It does seem that this leukemia patient was led to assume that his part in this procedure was therapy for his own illness, or a diagnostic aid to help him.

I thought it necessary, in forming an opinion, to review the 19 non-cancer terminal patients, who were selected at random by Dr. Custodio in his mind the night of July 15, 1963.

The mental and physical condition of the patients renders it impossible for them to give informed consent, in terms of forming a mature judgment in a matter of one to five minutes, on a complex scientific subject. Actually they were subjected to an injection by doctors in hospital attire, and were deceived into believing that this injection was of direct therapeutic benefit to them, or was essential for their treatment. This

was evidenced by Dr. Mandel's statement that patients do not question procedures which are done in a hospital, because they have confidence in the doctors, and tend to accept what they are told. In this instance, I believe their confidence was misplaced.

I would like to re-emphasize the procedure of the experiment which illustrates that informed consents could not have been obtained, because the patients nor their families were never told the truth; in that they were being asked to submit themselves as volunteers for human experiment in the field of cancer research, on a purely research basis, and not for a direct benefit of their particular illnesses. Nor were they told the true nature of the material to be injected.

Dr. Custodio greeted the patient and in the few minutes that the doctors prepared the injections, he told the patient that this was an injection to test their immune reactions and that a nodule would form in a few days and disappear in a few weeks.

During this time, Dr. Southam was sterilizing the skin of the thigh with cotton and alcohol. If the patient appeared apprehensive, Dr. Southam would verbally reassure the patient by such remarks as, "this is cotton, this is alcohol, this is novocaine, it doesn't hurt, you've had it before." Then he would proceed with the subcutaneous injections of live cancer cells. This procedure was repeated with remaining patients, selected by Dr. Custodio. Neither Dr. Southam nor Dr. Mandel knew which patients were selected. Could this be construed as informed consent?

Dr. Mandel, medical director of Jewish Chronic Disease Hospital, was not even present at the experiment of these 19 patients, which indicates that he has shunned his responsibility to the patients entrusted to his care.

In arriving at my decision in this matter, I am extremely concerned with the fact that these chronic, debilitated, sick patients were hurriedly and unexpectedly confronted with a verbal description of a technical procedure, which, even to a normal, educated, intelligent and healthy person, would have been inadequate and untruthful. This is fraud and deceit. I also believe that the omission on the hospital charts that these patients were injected with cultured live human cancer cells constitutes fraud and deceit.

I further believe that the rights of these patients and their families were violated by the respondents in this matter; who resorted to trickery, false statement, deliberate deception. The respondents by acting in such a manner as to omit and conceal the facts of this experiment involves a breach of duty, trust and confidence to these patients, their families, and their fellowman.

The findings and recommendation of Dr. Morris F. Wiener, member of the subcommittee is as follows:

The allegation that fraud and deceit had been perpetrated upon a group of patients in the Jewish Chronic Disease Hospital by the respondents is based upon: (a). Inadequate consents having been obtained for clinical investigation in not fully disclosing the cancer-origin of the material used in certain immunologic tests, and (b). The assumption that these injections were harmful and may produce cancer.

Although no fact of personal greed on the part of either respondent was revealed, nor was any appreciable injury to any of the subject-patients clearly demonstrated, the respondents failed to obtain written or meaningful consent consistent with appropriate directive governing research projects.

The problems of informed consent are considered nebulous and insoluble by a large segment of competent medical authority. The emotional reaction to the word "cancer" very often justifies its concealment. The blind patient whose sight is restored is not informed that his or her new cornea was transplanted from a cancerous eye removed from another patient. There are other instances where significant facts are concealed from patients, concealment tolerated or condoned by both medical and civil authority.

The injection of material obtained from a culture of cancer cells is not known to cause human cancer. These diseases are the result of autonomous new-growths which develop from an unrestrained proliferation of the individual's own native body cells. Total clinical experience, notably that of surgeons and pathologists who have frequent direct physical contact with cancerous tumors, further supports the principle that cancer is not a disease that is transferable from one individual to another. The universal acceptance of pooled plasma and blood-transfusions since World War II has offered a wide experience for the possible development of cancer from one person to another, and yet not one single case has ever been recorded.

In a recent case of purported transplantation of cancer to a noncancerous patient from a cancerous patient, no analogous inference can be made. This instance was published in the *Journal of the American Medical Association,* Vol. 192: 752, 1965, the article entitled "Cadaveric Renal Homotransplantation with Inadvertent Transplantation of Carcinoma."

This article refers to the recipient of a homotransplanted kidney obtained from a patient who died of cancer and which apparently was present in the grafted organ. In order to negate the usual homograft rejection and enable the grafted kidney to survive, the patient was treated with immunosuppressive drugs for 5 months from the time of operation: Azathioprine, 100 to 300 mg. doses and Prednisone, 30 to 100 mg. daily were administered, and in addition, the grafted kidney was treated with x-radiation.

A deliberate calculated effort was made by drugs and x-ray to depress the known immune response mechanism that causes the rejection reaction. The treatment was continued until two days before death. It is obvious, and not surprising, that the immune suppression resulting from the treatment to prevent the rejection of the homotransplanted kidney also prevented rejection of the occult cancer cells within the grafted kidney.

It should be noted that the cancer cells in this case were directly transmitted as a part of a vital organized active tumor tissue from the donor to the recipient. On the contrary, in the experiment at issue, the suspension of cells used had been derived from cancer tissue which had been grown in artificial culture media for a period of 5 to 12 years. Considerable experience has shown that this artificially cultured material represents a "standardized biological," and not a biologically active organized tumor with known aggressive determinants.

With regard to the one instance of axillary metastasis following an injection of suspended tissue cultured cancer cells into the arm of one of the patients, the following points may very well be considered. The finding of extrinsic cells in lymph nodes which are not cancer and do not behave as cancer is known. In the case at issue, the presence of cancer cells in the lymph nodes may actually be a result of their passive transportation from the point of innoculation to the node. This type of passive transportation is commonly found in cases of eczematoid skin conditions, tattoo and other pigmentation. In view of the comprehensive experience involving injections of tissue cultured cells, not one case is known that resulted in cancer. The known scientific principles and abundant evidence militate against such a possibility. Delayed hypersensitivity response in healthy and in sick individuals indicates that both groups of non-cancer ill patients and healthy individuals respond immunologically like healthy patients and not like patients afflicted with advanced cancer. In other words, it was reasonable to assume confidently that prompt rejection of homographs in the aged non-cancer patients could be predictive.

This meaningful term, "practice of medicine," is well proven by the test of time since it was first mentioned by Hippocrates over 2000 years ago. It is within the profound concept of this particular specific designation that medical science has evolved. Without this functioning concept scientific medical research is imperiled. The practice of medicine throughout the centuries has been, to a great extent, a matter of trial and error, and thereby inevitably connoting clinical experimentation. The doctor-patient relationship, which is the core of the practice of medicine, is not altered by hospital practice.

If an error has, in fact, been committed, it is in an area of judgmental vagueness. "The reverse of error is not truth, but error still; truth may lie in between." The public interest may be better served by constructive suggestions aimed at greater clarification of more specific guidelines in clinical research.

However, in view of the apparent current unacceptable method of pursuing the highly laudable purpose of the research program, the respondents are found guilty of the charges herein.

I dissent from the majority opinion as to the measure of discipline. The record shows that both respondents are exceptionally well-trained and highly regarded clinical investigators, and strongly endorsed by the highest local and national medical authorities.

I, therefore, recommend no further action as to discipline be taken.

b.
Recommendations of the Medical Grievance Committee—June 10, 1965

To the Board of Regents:

I, the undersigned, secretary of the MEDICAL GRIEVANCE COMMITTEE duly appointed pursuant to the Education Law of the State of New York, do hereby certify:

1. That charges, in writing, were duly pre-ferred and filed against Dr. CHESTER M. SOUTHAM and Dr. EMANUEL E. MANDEL, duly licensed physicians of the State of New York, hereinafter referred to as respondents, wherein each respondent was charged with fraud or deceit and unprofessional conduct in the practice of medicine within the purview and meaning of Section 6514, subdivisions 2(a) and 2(g) of the said Education Law; that a copy of the said charges with notice of hearing were duly served upon each respondent, and hearings duly held thereon before a subcommittee composed of Drs. Ames, (chairman) Heller and Wiener and its written report of findings and recommendations together with a transcript of the evidence were duly transmitted to me.

2. That the said report of findings and recommendations, with the transcript of evidence, wherein it was recommended that each of the respondents, CHESTER M. SOUTHAM, M.D. and EMANUEL E. MANDEL, M.D., be found guilty of each specification of the charges herein, and further, Drs. Ames and Heller recommended that each respondent shall receive a censure and reprimand, Dr. Wiener recommends that no further action be taken as to discipline, were duly submitted to the members of the committee at a regular meeting held on June 10, 1965.

3. That, after due consideration and discussion, the vote of each member of the committee present was duly recorded as follows:

RECORD OF VOTE

MEMBER	DETERMINATION	RECOMMENDATION
DR. LAWRENCE AMES	guilty—both charges	censure and reprimand
DR. SAUL I. HELLER	same	same
DR. MORRIS F. WIENER	same	no further action
DR. FRANCIS M. BENEDETTO	same	censure and reprimand
DR. PASQUALE CARONE	same	same
DR. IRVING L. ERSHLER	same	same
DR. HENRY I. FINEBERG	same	same
DR. FRANCIS O. HARBACH	same	same
DR. SYDNEY M. KANEV	same	same
DR. JAMES C. POTTER	same	no further action
DR. SAMUEL SANES	same	same
DR. ALFRED A. SCHENONE	same	censure and reprimand
DR. SOLOMON SCHUSSHEIM	same	same
DR. HERMAN B. SNOW	same	same
DR. MILTON S. WEINBERG	same	same
DR. WILLIAM L. WHEELER, JR.	same	same
DR. FREDERICK A. WURZBACH, JR.	same	same

4. That, as appears by the aforesaid tabulation of vote, the findings and recommendations

of the subcommittee as to GUILT was thereby adopted and made the findings, recommendation and determination of the committee; and it further appears by the said tabulation of vote as to the measure of discipline that the committee recommended to the Regents by a majority vote that each respondent be given a censure and reprimand on each specification of the charges.

I FURTHER CERTIFY that annexed hereto is a true copy of the record and proceedings taken herein as follows:

1. Transcript of the evidence
2. Report, findings and recommendation of the subcommittee
3. Report, findings, determination and recommendation of committee

All of which is respectfully submitted.

Henry I. Fineberg
SECRETARY

3.

The Board of Regents' Discipline Committee Reviews the Recommendations

We are of the opinion that there are certain basic ethical standards concerning consent to human experimentation which were involved in this experiment and which were violated by the respondents. When a patient engages a physician or enters a hospital he may reasonably be deemed to have consented to such treatment as his physician or the hospital staff, in the exercise of their professional judgment, deem proper. Consent to normal diagnostic tests might similarly be presumed. Even so, doctors and hospitals as a matter of routine obtain formal written consents before surgery, and in a number of other instances, and whether or not a specific consent is required for a specific act must be decided on the facts of the particular case.

No one contends that these 22 patients, by merely being in the hospital, had volunteered their bodies for any purpose other than treatment of their condition. These injections were made as a part of a cancer research project. The incidental and remote possibility, urged by Dr. Mandel, that the research might have been beneficial to a patient is clearly insufficient to bring these injections within the area of procedures for which a consent could be implied. Actual consent was required.

What form such an actual consent must take is a matter of applying common sense to the particular facts of the case. No consent is valid unless it is made by a person with legal and mental capacity to make it and is based on a disclosure of all material facts. Any fact which might influence the giving or withholding of consent is material. A patient has the right to know he is being asked to volunteer and to refuse to participate in an experiment for any reason, intelligent or otherwise, well-informed or prejudiced. A physician has no right to withhold from a prospective volunteer any fact which he knows may influence the decision. It is the volunteer's decision to make, and the physician may not take it away from him by the manner in which he asks the question or explains or fails to explain the circumstances. There is evidenced in the record in this proceeding an attitude on the part of some physicians that they can go ahead and do anything which they conclude is good for the patient, or which is of benefit experimentally or educationally and is not harmful to the patient, and that the patient's consent is an empty formality. With this we cannot agree.

In his testimony before the subcommittee, Dr. Mandel took the position that he regards these experiments as beneficial to the patients both because the experiment might result in a diagnosis of an advanced cancer which had not been discovered by the hospital, and also because the participation in the experiment would result in extra medical attention to the patients involved and possibly other patients in the hospital. The record indicated that the only additional medical care any of these patients received as a result of this experiment was that the injections were made and they were occasionally checked thereafter as to the progress of the growth and disappearance of the nodule. The inference that participation in the experiment benefited the patients because of such additional medical care is without foundation in the record. Since the purpose of the experiment was to obtain verification of Dr. Southam's hypothesis that diseased patients would reject the implant in the same manner as healthy patients and that their rejection would not be delayed as was that of patients suffering from an advanced cancer, it is somewhat inconsistent for Dr. Mandel to say before the experiment was completed that he authorized it as a diagnostic measure. In any event, it was clearly not treatment, not experimental therapy, and not a diagnostic test which would reasonably be given to these particular patients. Nevertheless, from the manner in which they were asked for their consent and from the statement made to them that this was a test to determine their immunity or resistance to disease, the patients could naturally assume that it was being given to help in the diagnosis or treatment of their condition. They were not clearly and unequivocally asked if they wanted to volunteer to participate in an extraneous research project.

There is one point which is undisputed, namely, that the patients were not told that the cells to be injected were live cancer cells. From the respondents' standpoint this was not considered to be an important fact. They regarded the experiment as medically harmless. There was not appreciable danger of any harmful effects to the patients as a result of the injection of these cancer cells. It is not uncommon for a doctor to refrain from telling his patient that he had cancer where the physician in his professional judgment concludes that such a disclosure would be harmful to the patient. The respondents testified that they felt that telling these patients that the material did consist of live cancer cells would upset them and was immaterial to their consent. They overlooked the key fact that so far as this particular experiment was concerned, there was not the usual doctor-patient relationship and, therefore, no basis for the exercise of their usual professional judgment applicable to patient care. No person can be said to have volunteered for an experiment unless he has first understood what he was volunteering for. Any matter which might influence him in giving or withholding his consent is material. Deliberate nondisclosure of the material fact is no different from deliberate misrepresentation of such a fact. The respondents maintain that they did not withhold the fact that these were cancer cells because they thought that some of the patients might have refused to consent to the injection of live cancer cells into their bodies. This was, however, a possibility and a decision that had to be made by the patients and not for them. Accordingly, the alleged oral consents that they obtained after deliberately withholding this information were not informed consents and were, for this reason, fraudulently obtained.

Although there is conflicting testimony and evidence in this point, it is our opinion that some of these patients were in such a physical and mental condition that they were incapable of understanding the nature of this experiment or of giving an informed consent thereto. We agree with the discussion of this aspect of the case in the report of findings of Dr. Heller. We note that in no case were any relatives of any of these patients told about the experiment nor were any of these patients asked if they wished to think the matter over or discuss it with their relatives. It is noteworthy that one of these same patients was operated on two days after the injections and that prior to making the operation, which was a part of the patient's treatment, the hospital obtained two separate written consents each signed by both the patient and a relative. If there was any doubt at all concerning a patient's ability to fully comprehend and consent to this experiment, it was the duty of the physicians involved to resolve that doubt before proceeding further. Even if we accept the testimony of Drs. Mandel and Custodio as to the condition of these patients, it is still clear that there was at least a doubt as to whether or not some of them fully understood what was going on and were mentally competent to consent. We do not say that it is necessary in all cases of human experimentation to obtain consents from relatives or to obtain written consents, but certainly upon the facts of this case and in view of the fact that the patients were debilitated, the performance of this experiment on the basis of alleged oral consents from those particular patients falls short of the ethical standards of the medical profession.

We now come to the question as to the ethical responsibility of Dr. Southam for the improper conduct of this experiment. In addition to his argument that the consent obtained was proper in all respects, Dr. Southam takes the position that he was not responsible for the internal practices at this hospital. He does not remember very well exactly what was said by Drs. Mandel and Custodio while they were obtaining the consents. He realized, however, that these patients were being approached for the first time. He also knew that they were all in a debilitated condition. As a physician in charge of the experiment, it was his duty to pay enough attention to what was going on to make sure that he was dealing with persons capable of being volunteers and sufficiently informed to consent to the use of their bodies for the experiment and not merely with people who were too confused or too sick or too resigned to object to the injection. He could not avoid responsibility for the procedure followed by Drs. Mandel and Custodio when he could see and hear what was going on. He accepts responsibility for the fact that the patients were not told the material to be injected consisted of live cancer cells. He clearly indicates in his testimony that in such experiments he regards it as important to make it clear to the patients that what is being done is an experiment and is not for the treatment or diagnosis of their own condition, yet he was present, this was not adequately done, and he did not complain. A physician may not shirk his ethical responsibility or violate basic human rights so easily.

As the director of medicine at the hospital Dr. Mandel is directly responsible for the determination of the procedure followed in this experiment. His commendable desire to encourage research in the hospital cannot excuse his indifference to the rights of the patients. Although Dr. Mandel denied it, three of the physicians on his staff at the time testified that before this experiment was carried out he had discussed it with each of them and they had all individually told him that in their opinion he would be unable to obtain an informed consent from the patients. Dr. Mandel subsequently designated Dr. Custodio to carry out most of the details of the experiment and did not discuss it with those three physicians or with the staff physician who was responsible for making the normal rounds in the pavilion where the 19 non-cancer patients were housed. Dr. Mandel attempted to explain away the testimony of these four physicians by stating that they were all hostile to him. With respect to one physician who had been on the staff of the hospital for over 15 years and who held a responsible position under Dr. Mandel for over two years, and who had testified that many were physically or mentally incapable of giving an informed consent, Dr. Mandel testified that he never thought much of that doctor's ability. We believe the testimony of the other four physicians and agree with the statements of Dr. Heller in his report of findings that "the competent residents at Jewish Chronic Disease Hospital were deliberately bypassed by Dr. Mandel . . . because he knew they would only adhere to the procedure of informed written consent." Furthermore, Dr. Mandel was himself present while the first three patients were questioned and injected. The record indicates that the consents obtained from those three patients were defective in all of the respects discussed above except that they were apparently competent to have given an informed consent if they had been properly apprised of all the material facts. Dr. Mandel is equally responsible for failing to give adequate instructions to Dr. Custodio or to take any measures to assure that the other 19

patients were capable of giving an informed consent and in fact gave such consent.

An opportunity to appear before this committee was accorded to the respondents on October 5, 1965. Both respondents appeared in person. Dr. Southam was also represented by Philip Scott, John R. Hupper, and Gerald Oscar, his attorneys. Dr. Mandel was presented by Morris Ploscowe and by Irving Lattimer, his attorneys. John J. Calanese, assistant attorney general, appeared for the petitioner. This committee has given careful consideration to the entire record and to the briefs submitted to it and statements made before it.

After due deliberation and for all of the reasons discussed above it is the unanimous recommendation of this committee that the Board of Regents accept the findings of the medical committee on grievances that both of the respondents are guilty of fraud or deceit in the practice of medicine and of unprofessional conduct in the practice of medicine. It is also our unanimous recommendation that the Board of Regents modify the recommendation of said committee as to the measure of discipline, and that the medical license of each respondent be suspended for a period of one year on each specification, but that the execution of such suspensions be stayed, and each respondent be placed on probation for a period of one year upon the following terms and conditions:

1. That each respondent shall conduct himself in all ways in a manner befitting his professional status and shall conform fully to the moral and professional standards of conduct imposed by law and by his profession.

2. That so long as there is no indication of any further misconduct, each respondent may continue to practice as a physician, but that the department, upon receipt of satisfactory evidence of any such further misconduct, may forthwith terminate the stay of execution and order that the stay be vacated and the medical license of the respondent or respondents involved be suspended for a period of one year from the date of said order.

3. That any such action by the department vacating the stay of the suspension as to either or both respondents shall in no way bar further disciplinary action based upon additional misconduct.

4. That each respondent shall notify the department of any change of address or employment.

5. That upon full compliance with these

conditions for a period of one year each respondent may apply to the department for discharge from probation.

We trust that this measure of discipline will serve as a stern warning that zeal for research must not be carried to the point where it violates the basic rights and immunities of a human person.

Respectfully submitted,
JOSEPH W. MCGOVERN, CHAIRMAN
JOSEPH T. KING
CARL H. PFORZHEIMER, JR.

4.

The Board of Regents Decides

Board of Regents of the University of the State of New York
Licenses Suspended, Suspensions Stayed, Respondents Placed on Probation*

Upon the report of the Regents Committee on Discipline, made in accordance with the provisions of section 211 of the Education Law, it was

Voted, That the determination of the Medical Committee on Grievances in the matter of Chester M. Southam . . . and Emanuel E. Mandel . . . be accepted, but that the recommendation of said Committee be modified and license No. 71055 and license No. 37359 respectively, issued under date of March 21, 1951, to said Dr. Southam and December 1, 1939, to said Dr. Mandel, and their registration or registrations as physicians, wherever they may appear, be suspended for a period of 1 year on each specification, said suspensions to run concurrently from the date of the service of the order effecting such suspensions, but that the execution of

such suspensions be stayed, and each respondent be placed on probation for a period of 1 year upon the following terms and conditions:

1. That each respondent shall conduct himself in all ways in a manner befitting his professional status and shall conform fully to the moral and professional standards of conduct imposed by law and by his profession;

2. That so long as there is no indication of any further misconduct, each respondent may continue to practice as a physician, but the Department, upon receipt of satisfactory evidence of any such further misconduct, may forthwith terminate the stay of execution and order that the stay be vacated and the medical license of the respondent or respondents involved be suspended for a period of 1 year from the date of said order.

3. That any such action by the Department vacating the stay of the suspension as to either or both respondents shall in no way bar further disciplinary action based upon additional misconduct;

4. That each respondent shall notify the Department of any change of address or employment;

5. That upon full compliance with these conditions for a period of 1 year each respondent may apply to the Department for discharge from probation; and

that the Commissioner of Education be empowered to execute, for and on behalf of the Board of Regents, all orders necessary to carry out the terms of this vote.

NOTES

NOTE 1.

ELINOR LANGER
HUMAN EXPERIMENTATION—NEW YORK VERDICT AFFIRMS PATIENT'S RIGHTS*

*   *   *

[The] lawyers for Mandel and Southam raised two technical points of some interest. First, they claimed that, because "no clear-cut medical or professional standards were in force or were violated" by the two physicians, the attempt to find them guilty had an ex post facto quality. They also argued that the charges did

---

* 34 *Journal of a Meeting of the Board of Regents of the University of the State of New York* 787 (1965). [The Board of Regents consists of 15 individuals elected by joint resolution of the two houses of New York's legislature for terms of 15 years. The Regents have jurisdiction over all education in the state, public and private, and over all licensed professions excluding the law. The three Regents most intimately involved in this decision were the three members of a special committee on discipline: Joseph W. McGovern, a lawyer; Joseph T. King, a lawyer; and Carl H. Pforzheimer, Jr., an investment banker. The remaining Regents, who concurred in the decision, are drawn from a variety of business and professional interests, including law, banking, education, and philanthropy.]

* 151 *Science* 663, 665–666 (1966). Reprinted by permission. Copyright 1966 by the American Association for the Advancement of Science.

not accurately fit the case. Testimony was introduced from well-known cancer and other professional researchers, including I. S. Ravdin, vice president for medical affairs of the University of Pennsylvania, and George E. Moore, director of Roswell Park Memorial Institute, to the effect that Southam's practices did not differ dramatically from those of other researchers. "If the whole profession is doing it," one of the lawyers remarked in an interview, "how can you call it 'unprofessional conduct'?" The lawyers also argued that the "fraud and deceit" charge was more appropriate to low-brow scoundrels, such as physicians who cheat on insurance, supply illegal narcotics, or practice medicine without a license, than to their respectable and well-intentioned clients.

To all arguments of humane motivations, extenuating circumstance, conflicting testimony, or legal ambiguities, the final answer of the Regents was very simple: It is no excuse. There was never any disagreement on the principle that patients should not be used in experiments unrelated to treatment unless they have given informed consent. But in the Regents' decision, two refinements of that principle are heavily stressed. The first is that it is the patient, and not the physician, who has the right to decide what factors are or are not relevant to his consent, regardless of the rationality of his assessment. "Any fact which might influence the giving or withholding of consent is material," the Regents said. . . .

The second principle stressed by the Regents is that the physician, when he is acting as experimenter, has no claim to the doctor-patient relationship that, in a therapeutic situation, would give him the generally acknowledged right to withhold information if he judged it in the best interest of the patient. In the absence of a doctor-patient relationship, the Regents said, "there is no basis for the exercise of their usual professional judgement applicable to patient care." Southam, in an interview, disagreed. "An experimental relation has some elements of a therapeutic relationship," he said last week. "The patients still think of you as a doctor, and I react to them as a doctor, and want to avoid frightening them unnecessarily." Mandel takes a similar position. In a letter to the editor of a medical affairs newspaper he stated: "In accordance with the age-old motto—primum non nocere—it would seem that consideration of the patient's well-being may, at times, supersede the requirement for disclosure of facts if such facts lack

pertinence and may cause psychologic harm." But on this point, the Regents are clear: "No person can be said to have volunteered for an experiment unless he had first understood what he was volunteering for. Any matter which might influence him in giving or witholding his consent is material. Deliberate nondisclosure of the material fact is no different from deliberate misrepresentation of such a fact."

In closing their case, and acknowledging that the penalties imposed were severe—they might have just authorized a censure and reprimand—the Regents were pointed and succinct: "We trust that this measure of discipline will serve as a stern warning that zeal for research must not be carried to the point where it violates the basic rights and immunities of a human person."

What the impact of the case will be is by no means clear. The Regents' decision outlines clear rules for a very narrow situation and attempts to set out some broad principles as well. But it is by no means binding, and it by no means covers the variety of situations with which researchers seeking to use human subjects are faced. The question is, What will cover these situations? Codes and declarations, of which there are already several, are too general to offer specific guidance. Researchers and patients alike are too vulnerable to await a slow case-by-case accretion of specific rulings. One alternative is the development within each hospital or research institution of "ethical review committees" that could define the consent-and-disclosure requirements for each proposed experiment and see that they were adhered to. In theory, this is already taking place. During the Southam-Mandel hearings, the state attempted to prove that Southam, a recipient of an NIH grant, had violated regulations of the Public Health Service. In fact, the regulations in question govern only the normal volunteer program of the NIH Clinical Center in Bethesda. The PHS response to an inquiry from New York's Attorney General made clear that the rules were not generally applicable and stated that, "in supporting extramural clinical investigations, it is the position of the Public Health Service that proper ethical and moral standards are more effectively safeguarded by the processes of review and criticism by an investigator's peers than by regulation."

That is the theory, but the trouble is it is not yet being done. And, given the tremendous growth and variety of medical research involving human beings, if it is not done by the scientific community, someone else will start to do it. The New York Regents may be only the beginning.

NOTE 2.

AMERICAN ASSOCIATION FOR CANCER RESEARCH
MINUTES OF THE 58TH ANNUAL MEETING*

The Annual Business Meeting of Members was called to order at 5:05 P.M., April 14, 1967, at the Sherman House, Chicago, Illinois by President Kaplan. . . . Dr. Kaplan said that the two candidates for Vice-President, as selected in the recent mail balloting by members of the Association, were Drs. Leon Dmochowski and Chester M. Southam; he appointed tellers and asked them to conduct the balloting for Vice-President.

*   *   *

Dr. Kaplan announced that the tellers had informed him that Dr. Chester M. Southam had

---

been selected as Vice-President of the Association for 1967–68. . . .

*   *   *

NOTE 3.

AMERICAN ASSOCIATION FOR CANCER RESEARCH
MINUTES OF THE 59TH ANNUAL MEETING†

The Annual Business Meeting of Members was called to order at 5:10 P.M., April 12, 1968, at Haddon Hall, Atlantic City, New Jersey by Vice-President Southam. . . .

*   *   *

Dr. Southam announced that the tellers had informed him that Dr. Abraham Cantarow had been selected as the Vice-President of the Association for 1968–69. The Secretary-Treasurer said that the Board recommended that Dr. Chester M. Southam be elected President for 1968–69. When no additional nominations were made from the floor, it was moved that these two officers be declared duly elected. . . .

*   *   *

CHAPTER TWO

The Wichita Jury Recording Case

In 1954 a group of law professors and social scientists, with the approval of judges of the Tenth Judicial Circuit, recorded the deliberations of juries in six civil cases in the United States district court in Wichita, Kansas. The investigators did not inform the jurors that microphones had been concealed in the jury room. The litigants were also unaware of the research project, although their attorneys had consented to the recordings.

A year later the Internal Security Subcommittee of the Senate Committee on the Judiciary held public hearings in order to assess the impact of this experiment "upon the integrity of the jury system [which is protected by] the seventh amendment of the Constitution." These hearings led to the promulgation of a law which prohibited any recording of jury deliberations.

The duties and obligations of law professors, social scientists, judges, attorneys, and legislators towards jurors, clients, science, and society are major issues raised by the Wichita Jury Recording case. In examining these materials consider the questions raised in the introduction to the Jewish Chronic Disease Hospital case. In addition, also ask:

1. What value preferences guide the actions of the participants in the two cases toward their co-participants? What assumptions do they make about the research process?

2. Do these two cases pose different issues and, if so, why?

A.
How and by Whom Should Research Policy Be Formulated?*

1.

University of Chicago Law School Application to Ford Foundation for Support of Research on Law and the Behavioral Sciences—June 1952

The subject matter of law is human behavior. The law deals with such behavior either in problem situations or where, for one reason or another, customary behavior without the added sanction of formal rules is deemed insufficient. The law builds on assumptions about human behavior. These assumptions are important in terms of the conduct to be regulated and in terms also of the effect of the regulation. Quite apart from all this, the institution of law is to be understood and evaluated in terms of the techniques and knowledge of the behavioral sciences. Moreover, the law can furnish to the behavioral sciences a coherent set of problems which can be clearly defined and which can provide the basis for interdisciplinary research. The discipline of the law, its selection of problems and its insistence upon solutions thus can be helpful to the behavioral sciences, and anthropology, social psychology, sociology, and economic theory can aid in the realistic study of the legal system.

In the work which is set forth, legal problems are to be selected as the basis for factual research which will be helpful to the development of the law and at the same time to the development of the behavioral sciences. The specific proposal is that (a) up to three studies be selected from a limited number herein set forth for the purpose of immediate study and that (b) the staff work with an advisory group to plan a more detailed set of studies which might be undertaken. The proposal is that an adequate grant be made to the University of Chicago Law School for a 2-year period to make possible the work on the 3 studies and the planning of a more detailed program.

* Except as otherwise indicated, all materials in this chapter are reprinted from *Recording of Jury Deliberations, Hearings Pursuant to S.Res. 58 before the Subcommittee to Investigate the Administration of the Internal Security Act and Other Internal Security Laws of the Senate Committee on the Judiciary,* 84th Congress, 1st Session (1955).

* * *

Although trial by jury in both criminal and civil cases is guaranteed by the Federal and most State constitutions, the jury system has long been under attack. The continuing criticism of an institution as basic as the jury underscores the desirability of studying the actual operation of the institution. The actual impact of many legal rules depends on their application by juries. The development of many procedural rules has been profoundly influenced by the existence of the jury system and by assumptions as to how juries operate. The appropriateness of both the substantive and procedural rules thus often depends on whether the assumptions made by the law concerning the jury system are warranted. Yet most of these assumptions have not been subjected to any empirical test. The justice of the legal system as a whole and justice or injustice in particular cases often depend on the successful operation of the jury system according to the assumptions made about it.

Procedures are available for the study of the jury system. Information can be obtained as to the actual operations of the system through systematic interviews with jury members after the close of a case concerning their individual and collective patterns of decision-making, the social structure of the jury and its influence on the decisions, the role of general personality and social determinants in the patterns of cognition and judgment of jury members operating as a group in the box and in the jury room. This is one way to determine what the decision-making process and its causes have been. It is possible to test actual jurors, after the actual trial (and members of a simulated jury), to discover the impressions created by particular types of evidence, comprehension of the instructions given, and the ability to recall as influenced by the length of the trial, the order of presentation, the techniques of the lawyers, etc. Such research could determine to what extent (a) the jury conceives of its function in the same way that the formal law conceives it; (b) the jury's concept of the issues deviates from the legal concepts; (c) the jury comprehends the judge's instructions; (d) the jury comprehends the evidence in the case; (e) the jury was moved by "rational" or emotional factors rooted in personality, social background, and the social situation of the courtroom, the jury box, and the jury room discussions. This is an area also where the trial and jury system can be closely simulated; that is, mock trials created with selected juries, and the behavior of such a simulated jury can be observed under controlled conditions such as Bales has been developing in his studies of small groups. It might be added in passing that realistic studies, of discussions about real issues by groups of 12 would contribute far more to our knowledge of small group behavior in dealing with important decision-making tasks than we gain from the observation at great expense of the decision-making process of groups of students coming together for no more than an hour solving chess and arithmetic problems. There is no doubt that a sufficient number of judges and lawyers would be willing to participate in such simulated trials as to make the conditions sufficiently close to reality to be useful.

The results of such a study can have far-reaching effects on the use of the jury system and the reform of the rules of evidence. Among other problems it can help clarify are these: (1) What is the effect of interrogation of jurors by the judge rather than the attorneys; (2) what is the effect of a judge's comment on the evidence; (3) what are the advantages of oral versus written instructions to jurors; (4) to what extent are detailed regulations of admissibility frustrated by inadequate regulation of the lawyer's arguments; (5) to what extent is there an identifiable group of cases for which the jury is particularly unsuitable or for which provision should be made for special juries composed of jurors with the requisite special skills or certain personality qualities.

*   *   *

2.

Bernard Meltzer
A Projected Study of the Jury as a
Working Institution*

The proposed study of the jury system, which I have been asked to describe, is one of four projects in a research program in law and

* 287 *The Annals of the American Academy of Political and Social Science* 97–100, 102 (1953). Reprinted by permission. [Professor Meltzer was then Director of the Jury Project at the University of Chicago Law School.]

the behavioral sciences to be undertaken at the University of Chicago Law School. This research, which has been made possible by a grant from the Ford Foundation, will be conducted over a 3-year period. The program "will represent a major effort to bring to bear on the problems of law the research techniques of the behavioral sciences and, at the same time, to enrich the behavioral sciences by a study of legal institutions."

Trial by jury is a many-sided and controversial institution, which is a promising subject for interdisciplinary study. The jury plays an important role in the administration of justice. It is also a powerful symbol of our democratic faith, with an important place in our political theory. Furthermore, the jury, as an ad hoc collection of amateurs who generally must act unanimously to resolve a dispute, is a distinctive group which can be of special interest to students of small group interaction.

The jury has so often been called the "palladium of our civil rights" that this phrase has found a place in our dictionaries. At the same time, there has been continuous and lively criticism of the fitness of jury trial for some types of modern litigation. As a result, there have been significant reforms, both in this country and in England, and proposals for additional reforms.

The discussion has often involved untested assumptions about the actual workings of the institution and community attitudes toward it. In addition to such matters, which can be illuminated by empirical investigation, the debate involves fundamental and pervasive issues, such as the proper role of the expert and the amateur, the proper distribution of power between the official and the citizen, and the extent to which particular values represented by basic institutions should override any operational inefficiencies which they may involve.

Such issues cut too deep into our social fabric to be resolved by even the most comprehensive study. But a study could give us a store of reliable information about the actual workings of the jury in various contexts and the rules and usages which tend to promote or frustrate the various purposes ascribed to the jury. It could, for example, shed light on the criteria which should control eligibility for and exemption from jury service; on those rules of evidence which are based on assumptions about jury behavior; on the proper application of elastic concepts, such as "reversible error," which are also based on such assumptions. A study in addition could make clearer the actual impact of particular rules of substantive law when they are to be applied in the end by a more or less random group drawn from the community.

From the many facets of the jury system which might be examined, the following have been selected for initial emphasis in the study:

1. The functions assigned and imputed to the jury.

2. The principles, if any, on which jury trial is or is not made available to litigants; the assumptions behind the decisions of litigants to elect or to waive a jury; identifiable classes of cases in which jury trial appears to involve special inconvenience.

3. The legal rules, the administrative practices, and the litigants' choices, which determine the composition of particular juries.

4. The decisional process—the determinants of the jurors' individual judgments; the nature and effect of group deliberation.

5. Workable criteria for appraising particular verdicts.

6. The rules and usages which promote, or interfere with, informed and rational jury determinations or the efficient use of jury in adjudication.

7. The significance of the jury as a form of democratic participation—community attitudes regarding the jury.

8. The social and individual costs of the jury system in various classes of litigation.

9. A re-examination of the functions of the jury in the light of data regarding its operations.

*   *   *

. . . Since the jury room is not open to direct observation and since the general verdict, which is the usual form of a jury verdict, discloses nothing more than a general conclusion, it will be necessary to attempt to reconstruct the operations of the jury indirectly.

A variety of techniques may prove useful for this purpose. First, cases will be classified according to various criteria, which cannot be spelled out here. These cases will be studied prior to trial and observed in court by a lawyer and a social psychologist. After the jury has returned its verdict, the individual jurors will, with the permission of the courts involved, be interviewed under conditions assuring anonymity and with appropriate safeguards worked out with the courts.

These interviews will be based on two types of questions: (1) a general set of questions reflecting general presuppositions about the determinants of jury behavior in particular types of cases, and (2) a set of questions prepared by the lawyer-sociologist team based on the specific events of the trial.

These interviews should reveal the response of individual jurors to the trial; their capacity to follow and organize evidence and to understand and apply the judge's instructions; the nature and effect of the group deliberations; and the determinants of, or influential factors in, particular verdicts. These interviews should also yield data regarding the general personality and skills of the individual jurors and the impact of jury service on their attitudes regarding the jury and the administration of justice.

Some of the difficulties raised by the techniques described above deserve mention. . . .

*   *   *

[I]ndividual jurors may not be wholly aware of, or may not be able to reconstruct accurately, either their personal responses or the group activity. . . .

*   *   *

The data produced by intensive case studies of jury behavior will be supplemented by data designed to disclose the differences between judge and jury determinations. To facilitate such comparison, judges presiding over jury cases will be asked to keep records of such cases; to indicate, prior to the return of the jury verdict, the verdicts they would have reached if they had absorbed the jury function; to suggest explanations of significant differences between their "as-if" and the real verdict. In order to deepen the study of particular cases, the judges' parallel verdicts will be sought in cases which will be the subject of interviews with the jurors. In some cases, the judge may, of course, wish more time for reflection than is taken in the jury room. A record of such cases and the judge's subsequent "verdict" would be instructive.

Judges on their own initiative have in the past undertaken such comparisons, and we look forward to their cooperation in this and other phases of the study. We recognize that the judge's as-if verdict may diverge from the verdict which he might have reached if he were in fact disposing of a man's liberty or property. But the fact that judges often sit without a jury reduces this difficulty. The traditions and habits which produce the real verdict will presumably not be abandoned for the simulated verdict.

* * *

It is tempting to speculate more concretely on the final form of the study and possible impact both on the administration of justice and on legal education and research. But there has already been too much prophecy in this paper. It seems more appropriate to turn to some of the difficulties presented by the study which have general implications.

Not the least of these is a more or less explicit feeling that ignorance about the jury may be bliss. This is a curious notion in a society which is based on free inquiry and yet which is relatively uninformed about the operations of its key institutions. There is a related notion, that the examination of an important legal institution is necessarily animated by hostility to the institution, which is completely inapplicable to the projected study.

Neither of these notions should or will, we believe, be accepted by the bar, the judiciary, or the other interested disciplines. Because of their common interest in a better understanding and a continual improvement of the administration of justice, we are confident of getting their indispensable cooperation.

Any description of a plan for research is more an exercise in prophecy than in reporting. Accordingly, this prospectus is presented with the caveat that it is tentative and that my colleagues have saved their rights. This prospectus also carries with it an unrestricted invitation for critical comment. Indeed, it is the hope for such comment from lawyers and nonlawyers alike which is the primary justification for this premature delivery.

3.

Letter from Paul R. Kitch, Esq.* to Professor Bernard D. Meltzer—May 1, 1953

Your statement as to the projected study of the jury as a working institution reached my desk this week and because I have always been particularly interested in the projected research in the indicated field I am taking this opportunity to make a definite suggestion.

---

* Paul R. Kitch is a graduate of the University of Chicago Law School and an attorney in Wichita, Kansas.

For a good many years I participated in a substantial number of jury cases. As is the case with the most trial lawyers I was always interested in attempting to find out the various factors which would underlie a jury's verdict.

This office for many years consistently carried on the practice of interviewing a substantial number of the jurors who sat on each case. There was always a twofold purpose to these interviews. One, of course, was in a situation of an adverse verdict to discover if there were any grounds for charging misconduct of a jury so as to obtain a new trial. The other was to ascertain the receptiveness of jurors to certain arguments and to attempt to better evaluate the effectiveness of various approaches to a jury.

There is one conclusion which I long ago arrived at and from which I have never wavered and that is that jurors as a class are seldom accurate in their recollections as to actually what transpired in a jury room and many times intentionally deceive the interviewers in an effort to be all things to all men. In several instances we have actually examined jurors on post trial motions where there has been substantial conflict in the testimony as to what did and did not happen in the jury room. These are all matters covered by reported cases. Jurors are seldom conscious of the underlying psychological factors which have motivated their decisions.

The above paragraph is preliminary to my criticism of a so-called research project which basically is dependent upon testing methods which are unscientific to say the least. I do not mean to be critical. I only want to be constructive. Your entire paper leaves me with the clear impression that all your faculty committee has outlined is a better coordinated and obviously more efficient use of the same testing techniques that have been used by the profession for generations.

Need for true research in the indicated field is so great that it seems a shame to miss the opportunity to really make a thrilling and valuable contribution to the profession when at last some funds have been provided for the endeavor.

If the university would use the first allotment of funds for the purpose of first obtaining exact information as to what goes on in a jury room and then organizing the next step of your project on the basis of interpreting such information I am sure that you would end up with something of considerably more value than what is presently indicated.

I am certain that you could get the cooperation of various courts in permitting you to install secret transcribing devices in jury rooms so that over a comparatively short period of time you could accumulate a substantial number of actual vebatim case histories. Adequate safeguards can be arranged with the courts for the protection of the identity of the individuals involved.

Once you accumulated a sufficient body of factual information the possible uses which you could make of the material would be of inestimable value to the profession and to the public. I do not think such a study has ever been made but from the standpoint of its future public interest and public contribution I am sure that its value will be many times greater than the value of the project outlined.

*   *   *

B.
How and by Whom Should the Research Process Be Administered?

1.
Letter from Paul R. Kitch, Esq. to Orie L. Phillips, Chief Judge, Circuit Court of Appeals—November 23, 1953

You will recall that while you were in Wichita I discussed with you in a preliminary way a research project for the study of the jury system, which project is being carried out by the faculty of the University of Chicago Law School under the terms of a very liberal grant from the Ford Foundation.

A general description of the project is outlined in a pamphlet by Bernard D. Meltzer, chairman of the committee supervising the project. A copy of the same is enclosed with this letter.

The committee recognized that if a significant job is to be accomplished that it will be necessary to obtain specific and concrete information as to what actually goes on in a jury room. The only means by which the committee can assimilate scientific, accurate information concerning the actual functioning of a jury is to obtain the assistance of trial courts to the extent that actual recordings are made of a substantial number of actual jury deliberations. It is the hope of the research committee that a minimum of 500 transcriptions can be assembled over the next 3-year period.

The committee would prefer to obtain these records in the various Federal courts because of their belief that a testing program in an area where juries are generally considered to be of the highest quality would more accurately reflect the true worth of the jury system than would recordings taken from some jurisdictions where the administration of the jury system has been questioned.

The committee is quite anxious to start this project in the 10th circuit because of a belief on their part that the states represented in the 10th circuit provide more of a typical cross section of community life than most of the other circuits.

As I previously informed you Judge Hill has already indicated his willingness to assist in the proposed project provided that the matter has your preliminary approval. Once a satisfactory plan is worked out we then propose to ask the assistance of other trial judges of the circuit. We are not asking any trial judge to assume such a responsibility unless he personally desires to give his aid. However, we do feel that the project is so meritorious that we will have little difficulty in gaining the assistance of the trial judge.

Naturally it is not intended any testing methods be made of jury deliberations in criminal cases nor is it intended that such transcriptions be made of any particular case without the consent of trial counsel for the respective litigants.

It is proposed that the experimental work be carried out under very definite rules designed to fully protect all jurors against any identification.

The committee has already made preliminary experiments with various types of recording equipment. In the committee's opinion the technical aspects of this problem will be easily handled.

A formal set of rules for use of the equipment will be approved by each trial judge and, if you desire, by yourself before the project is commenced in any court. In order to be specific we have prepared the following proposed rules with the expectation that there will be suggestions made for their improvement. I will state these proposed rules specifically so that you will have something concrete to consider. They are as follows:

1. A recording microphone will be placed in each jury room. The recording instrument

with a satisfactory locking device will be placed in the judge's office or at such other place as the trial judge may designate. The trial judge will be the sole custodian of the key. The operation of the instrument will be the responsibility of the court reporter or such other person as the trial judge may designate.

2. No recordings will be made in criminal cases. No recordings will be made in civil cases without the consent of counsel for each party.

3. When a recording is taken of a jury deliberation the record will be sealed and will remain in the custody of the trial judge or such other person as he may designate until final judgment has been entered and all appeals have been terminated. When this time arises the recording will be forwarded to a person to be designated by the research committee or to such person as the circuit court may prefer to designate. A single transcription of the record will then be made. Thereafter the original recording will be destroyed. Thereafter the research committee will supervise the editing of the transcript so that all personal names or geographical references and all other identifying statements will be edited in such a way as to avoid any identification of the persons or controversies involved. The edited transcript, together with the original transcript, will then be forwarded to the clerk of the circuit court of appeals or to such other person as your court may designate for review. If such officer is satisfied that the record has been appropriately edited he will then destroy the original transcript and will return to the research committee the edited transcript. If such officer feels that further editing is necessary he shall accomplish the same, destroying both the original transcription and the suggested edited transcription, and will return to the committee the transcript as edited by such officer.

4. The entire project insofar as it involves the recording of jury deliberations will receive no publicity from any source until after the project is completed.

5. In the event that services of court reporters are required by designation of trial courts or in the event that any person is appointed by the circuit court to perform any of the duties called for hereunder such persons shall be compensated from the funds made available to the research committee in such amounts and at such times as the trial court or the circuit court may fix.

I again state the above rules are only suggestive in form and it is the desire of the committee to carry out the project under any addi-

tional restraints which the trial judges or yourself may see fit to require.

I have intentionally been very brief in the presentation. I have made no effort to outline the possible advantages of this study to the legal profession and the courts at large. Certainly the study is approached with an open mind by the research committee and there is absolutely no basis for predicting any given conclusions which can be established by the study.

If there is any reluctance on your part to approve the court's participation in this program I would be very happy to arrange for the presence in Denver of those persons who will be responsible for the carrying out of the actual project at any time which you may suggest. We are all extremely enthusiastic concerning the possible contributions to be made by this proposed study and we are very hopeful of obtaining your approval.

2.

Letter from Chief Judge Orie L. Phillips to Paul R. Kitch, Esq.—November 25, 1953

* * *

I have no objection to the project being carried out in the tenth circuit, subject to the conditions and rules set forth in your letter, with one exception.

I think it should be made plain to the jurors that while a recording is to be made of their deliberations in the jury room, it will only be released in a form which is wholly impersonal and will not disclose to the public the identity of the jurors or of the trial in which the recording was made. I think a rule should be included covering the suggestion I have made.

* * *

3.

Letter from Paul R. Kitch, Esq. to Delmas C. Hill, United States District Judge, District of Kansas—January 20, 1954

You have the original of Judge Phillips' letter giving his approval to the proposal . . . to make transcriptions of jury-room deliberations under certain conditions. . . .

However, in giving his approval to the plan Judge Phillips stated that he thought in addition to the protective measures outlined in our letter that the jury should also be advised that a transcription might be made of their jury-room deliberations.

Those in charge of the research project feel that if the jury is aware that a transcription is being made that the deliberations may be affected thereby and the accuracy of any conclusions drawn from the transcriptions will be subject to serious challenge.

They are willing to take any further measures which Judge Phillips feels to be necessary to positively guarantee the protection of the identity of the jurors. If it becomes necessary to actually advise the jury of the taking of a transcription it is doubtful if the advantages of getting the information on such a basis will justify the tremendous expense involved in the undertaking. However, I do not believe that any final decision has been reached on this point pending our efforts to obtain Judge Phillips' consent to the original plan or some modification thereof.

In addition to the above point a very realistic problem is presented and that is that few lawyers would express their consent to the making of such a transcription if the jury was to know that the same was being made.

As long as the jury does not know a transcription is being made then there is no possible basis for belief that the jury's deliberations will be affected by the making of a transcription.

If the jury is advised that a transcription is to be made of its deliberations many lawyers will feel that the jurors may not carry on their deliberations in the same manner as they would in the absence of such a transcription. Consequently any lawyer who felt he had a particularly weak case would be extremely reluctant to consent to the procedure. If the jury does not know the recording is being made we do not anticipate any difficulty in obtaining the consent of counsel in each case to the making of the transcription.

If this matter can be cleared with Judge Phillips I think that Mr. Meltzer, Mr. Kurland, and Mr. Levi are ready to take immediate steps to launch the program.

4.

Letter from Victor J. Stone to Judge Delmas C. Hill—March 18, 1954

I want to thank you most sincerely for the hospitality and cooperation that you extended to us yesterday. We were, of course, gratified to learn that you are as enthusiastic about our project as we are.

We are proceeding with our plans on the following understanding. Mr. Arents will arrange with Mr. Clark, the building supervisor, to install sound equipment necessary to do the job we have in mind. If it appears advisable, we shall have someone in Wichita to attend the machine.

It is also my understanding that we can order a copy of the trial transcript if we wish. You prefer to retain the sound tape of a deliberation until you have disposed of motions and have entered final judgment in the case. Thereupon, the tapes are to be shipped to us in Chicago, where they will be transcribed. The transcriptions will then be edited to remove any possibility of identifying the particular case. Only the edited version will ever be revealed to persons outside our immediate staff, and originals will be disposed of in accordance with your directions.

*　　*　　*

5.

Letter from Judge Delmas C. Hill to Chief Judge Orie L. Phillips— August 26, 1954

Pursuant to your request for information concerning the jury project conducted in this court during the past few months by the Law School of the University of Chicago I am happy to give you the following information.

The law school provided new equipment for the project including microphones and the recording machine itself. At project expense the microphones were installed in well-concealed places in the jury room and the machine was placed in the coat closet of my private office with proper wiring connections.

A project team was sent to Wichita by the dean of the law school with Mr. Ab Mikva, an able Chicago attorney and former law clerk to Mr. Justice Minton, as the supervisor. There were two keys to the closet which was kept locked at all times during the period the project was being carried on with one key remaining in my hands and the second key being turned over to Mr. Mikva, and at no time during the recordings was anyone permitted to listen to the same —this including myself. Mr. Mikva operated the recording machine and made such mechanical adjustments or changes on the same during the recordings as was necessary to insure proper recording but did not at any time listen to the deliberations for any other purpose.

In addition the following precautions were taken:

1. The recordings were made only in civil cases and at no time was any recording made of any criminal proceeding.

2. In each case recorded, prior to the commencement of the trial, counsel on both sides were called into my chambers and were fully advised concerning the project, and the consent of all counsel in each particular case was received before the recording of the jury deliberations was made. At this same time counsel were advised that the recordings would not be heard by anyone until after all posttrial matters were disposed of by the court and that the same would not be available to anyone for purposes of appeal.

3. No publicity of any kind or character was given to the project through the medium of the newspapers.

4. No juror had knowledge that recordings of the jury deliberations were being made so that that fact could not in any way affect the jury deliberations.

Recordings were made of jury deliberations in six civil jury trials. Two of them being automobile damage suits. Two were government land condemnation suits. One a breach of promise to marry suit and one a damage suit arising from the alleged underground seepage of water from a privately owned water reservoir.

As to all of these cases the project team was instructed by the court to do nothing with any particular recording until that case was finally disposed of by the court. At present transcripts have been made in two cases, both of which have been finally disposed of. In the two condemnation cases motions for new trials were filed and no questions raised which could in any manner be affected by these recordings as they were purely legal questions passed upon by the court during the course of the trials, and the team was permitted to make transcripts of those recordings. In the fifth case notice of appeal was given and nothing was done on this case. In the sixth case a motion for new trial is still pending and likewise nothing has been done by the team with this recording.

All of the recordings were taken back to Chicago by Mr. Mikva and placed under lock in the office of Dean Levi, but after receipt of your telephone call, I requested that they return to me all of the recordings except in the two civil cases finally completed, and also all other material they had concerning any of the incomplete cases. I have also requested copies of the transcripts in the two completed cases so that I could forward the same to you for your perusal and consideration.

In connection with these cases I permitted the team to go out and personally interview the jurors, but not until such jurors had been finally discharged from jury duty and even then without the jurors learning that any recordings had been made. I am also advised that copies of these interviews will be furnished to me so that I may forward them on to you.

Undoubtedly you also want to know the reaction of the lawyers involved in these various cases to this project and I can assure you that they were all wholeheartedly in favor of it and had a feeling that a great deal could be learned from such an experiment from which improvements could be made in our jury system.

After you called me I asked Mr. Kitch to come to my office in order that I could find out exactly what had transpired in the committee room. He stated to me that his purpose in going to the meeting was to secure the cooperation of other judges so that the project could be extended and carried on in other districts. That he did not refer to any particular district in which the project had operated but did say that it was in the 10th circuit. He also asked me to tell you that he would be very glad to fly out to Denver and talk further with you about the same if you so desired. Likewise, I would be very happy to talk with you personally about it and, of course, will give you any other desired information, and when I have received the two completed transcripts and the writeups of juror interviews, I will forward the same to you.

6.

Letter from Judge Arthur F. Lederle, American Bar Association, Section of Judicial Administration, to Paul R. Kitch, Esq.—September 22, 1954

I appreciated very much the courtesy of your attendance at our council meeting. As you perhaps know, your visit stirred up some controversy, but that is one of the things that one must expect if he is to do anything out of the regular, day-to-day routine.

I hope you will continue to maintain your

enthusiasm for your project and wish that you would continue to keep in touch with Judge Holtzoff, who is chairman of the section jury committee.

7.

University of Chicago Law School Application to Ford Foundation for Extension of Grant—December 21, 1954

On August 18, 1952, the Ford Foundation granted $400,000 to the law school of the University of Chicago "to support a research program in law and the behavioral sciences for a period of 2½ years, including about one-half year for organization and recruitment." At that time the foundation stated of the research program, "We feel that it promises to be particularly significant for the development of both law and the behavioral sciences." The research program is fulfilling the hopes and expectations held for it. This is an application for an adequate grant to insure the continuation and development of the program for a 5-year period. . . .

The program of research in law and the behavioral sciences provides for three studies to be selected for immediate and intensive study. The three studies selected and now in process are the nature and operation of the jury system; . . . The program called also for the preparation, with the help of an advisory group, and with the benefit of the experience of the present program, of an additional detailed set of possible studies. The members of the advisory group are David Cavers, Harvard Law School; Abe Fortas, Esq., Arnold, Fortas & Porter; Harold Lasswell, Yale School of Law; Robert K. Merton, Columbia University; John Ritchie III, University of Wisconsin Law School; Hon. Walter Schaefer, Illinois Supreme Court; and Hans Speier, the Rand Corp. As planned, with the help of this group, an additional detailed set of possible studies is now in preparation. The present on-going research program has been presented to this advisory group.

*   *   *

. . . The jury project has wide scope. Most emphasis has been placed on (1) problems of jury selection; (2) the effect upon the juror of the manner of his reception into the trial system; (3) the impact of the trial and of the instructions of the judge upon the jurors; (4) the nature of the jury's deliberation; and (5) a comparison of jury trials with alternative adjudicative procedures. We have been interested also in analyzing jury behavior, partly in terms of types of jurors, their beliefs, origin, economic and educational status. A considerable amount of historical, legal, and comparative law material has been prepared, both as a way of framing problems and as an aid to understanding and evaluating data.

The jury project has used a variety of techniques. Among them, it has used intensive interviews with actual jurors; the experimental jury; and questionnaires. This arrangement of technique has made it possible to try out observations from actual juror interviews by way of an experimental jury and through questionnaires. We have full files on 18 cases where we have had an observer present throughout the trial followed by intensive interviews with jurors. We have used experimental juries by recording a version of a trial, playing this version or significant modifications of it to different juries drawn from regular jury pools and under the discipline of court personnel, recording these deliberations and receiving the various verdicts. By this means it is possible to obtain data on the impact in the deliberation and on the verdict of particular evidence, modes of trial, and instructions. . . . The deliberations on the same case by different juries have provided material on the variety and recurring patterns of jury discussions with respect to the ordering of evidence and issues and the considerations of factors outside the evidence of the case. We are using a questionnaire (the judge-jury questionnaire) to determine the extent to which judges agree or disagree with jury verdicts. The questionnaire is now being filled out by more than 800 Federal and State judges in connection with jury cases as they come before the judge. Questionnaires or interviews are being used to determine further relationships between juror characteristics and votes (the criminal-juror questionnaire), the attitude of jurors toward jury service, reasons for jury waiver, and the damage expectations for jury cases in different areas of the country (regional consistency of jury verdicts).

The present work on the jury project has opened up many avenues for further investigation. We wish to continue our inquiry into the meaning to jurors of particular instructions in different type situations as, for example, the impact of various instructions on the jury, where insanity is pleaded as a defense; the effect of contributory negligence instructions, or the effect of judicial admonitions to disregard improper evidence, or to consider evidence only as impeachment testimony, or to disregard the failure of the defendant to testify in his own behalf, or to consider a confession only after it has been found by the jury to be voluntary. These are areas where the jury's felt sense of justice and its evaluation of behavior may create an application of law more meaningful than formal rules. The material on jury deliberation, now being obtained through both experimental means and the interviewing of actual jurors, will help in the present analysis of the extent to which (1) issues are understood and deliberated upon; (2) data not presented in the formal trial enter into the deliberation; (3) different types of evidence are critically evaluated; (4) the indoctrination of jurors prior to or during the trial can change juror behavior. We have prepared an experimental case to help reveal the effect upon deliberation and verdict of special interrogatories and special verdicts as means of controlling the deliberation process. The analysis of the relationship between individual juror awards and the characteristics of the jurors will give more meaning to our inquiry into the methods and the effect of the methods of jury selection. We wish to develop further the comparison to bench trials and to those relevant phases of arbitration and administrative hearings, and to obtain additional material on the impact of the jury trial in creating an image of the justice of the legal system among the jurors, the litigants, and various segments of the public.

*   *   *

8.

Letter from Chief Judge Orie L. Phillips to Paul R. Kitch, Esq.—April 14, 1955

Judge Hill talked with me on the telephone day before yesterday and advised that he would have to get consent from the lawyers in the case before the recording could be made public. He thought there would be no trouble in getting that consent.

Judge Hill also said he thought it might be better to keep anonymous the court in which the recording was made. I told him I would leave that to you and him. The important thing is to make quite clear at the outset the safeguards that

are thrown around the taking and use of the recording.

9.

Excerpts from Proceedings at the Annual Conference of the Tenth Judicial Circuit held at Estes Park, Colorado—July 7, 1955*

JUDGE HILL: [L]adies and gentlemen, one of the most precious rights possessed by the people of Anglo-Saxon nations is the right to trial by jury. That right was acquired only after years of bloodshed and is considered by all of us as one of the greatest safeguards of our individual liberties. Do we lawyers and judges follow the responsibility of the administration of the jury system as it exists today? That responsibility should never be taken lightly, but we should constantly strive to better the system by improving the efficiency of its administration. We will all agree, I am sure, that the ultimate purpose of trial by jury is the ascertainment of the truth. If we fail in any particular instance to achieve that purpose, it is not the fault of the jury system, but, rather, a deficiency in its administration, and the lawyers and judges involved must take the blame.

Down through the years the jury system has been taken for granted by both lawyers and judges, and little if no effort has been made to study the system with the view of improving its efficiency. Something over a year ago a group of Kansas lawyers in preparation for a program at the 1954 Tenth Circuit Conference carried out a most worth-while project regarding the jury system within the Federal courts of this circuit. You will all recall that project. Personally, I received a great benefit from that project and as a result changed some of my own administrative practices which I am sure has to some extent been an improvement.

The approach to this problem should be in a scientific manner and not in a hit-and-miss fashion. A study should be conducted on a nationwide basis including local, State, and Federal courts and in all geographical areas. Such a study must necessarily take a considerable time, and in the interium we should withhold our opinions, criticisms, or suggestions until such time as the study is completed. It would take

* Judge Delmas C. Hill presided and approximately 100 judges and lawyers attended this conference.

the full cooperation of the bench and bar as well as laymen and organizations interested in bettering the efficiency of the system.

In this connection we must bear in mind that the sole objective of such a study would be to better the system and not to tear it down. One of the most significant jury studies being conducted is a research project under the sponsorship of a well-known American university which includes among its activities the actual recording of jury room deliberations. Naturally, such a project must be conducted with extreme caution and with consideration for the full protection of litigants and jurors. I have requested a representative of that university to furnish me with a statement concerning the safeguards used in this connection, and I am advised by him that the following constitute a list of minimum safeguards strictly adhered to:

1. The consent of the trial judge is first obtained, and the project then conducted under such restrictions and limitations as he sees fit to use.

2. The consent of the litigants through their attorneys must be obtained.

3. That the recordings be made only in civil cases.

4. That the recordings be made only under the close personal supervision of the trial judge and not to be heard or used by anyone including the judge until after the judgment in the case becomes final.

5. The recordings when finally transcribed, then edited by the project staff to remove all geographical, personal, and other identifying references, and the original recording is then destroyed.

6. That care is exercised to prevent adverse results from such investigation and premature publicity be avoided.

7. That the product of this work be used only for scientific purposes for which it was intended.

By special arrangement with the university I referred to and with the cooperation of the project staff our program this afternoon will consist of the reproduction of one of its recordings. Before playing the reproduction we will present an abbreviated resume of the case from which the recording was made so that you may have the proper background to understand the jury deliberations as you hear them. In this connection two members of the Wichita bar will assist me. Mr. Malcolm Miller will state the case for the plaintiff, and Mr. William Tinker will state the case for the defendant. After that I will read you in substance the instructions actually given in the case which were also furnished to me by the project staff.

Let me stress the fact that the only purpose of this program is to stimulate interest amongst the bench and bar of this circuit in some sort of an effort to study scientifically the workings of the jury system toward the end that some improvement in the efficiency of the jury system in this circuit may be achieved. There are many methods by which such a study could be conducted. We are only attempting to illustrate one such method and have selected that particular method believing that it might be of interest to you.

In conclusion, let me say that as of now there are no materials available to judges, lawyers, or students of the law on the process of the workings of jury deliberations. The results of all such studies should be made available to lawyers, judges, and students of the law to the end that the efficiency of the jury system may be improved and thus our entire judicial system strengthened. . . .

* * *

JUDGE HILL: Anyone else?

JUDGE PHILLIPS: Judge Hill, I would like to have a word: It happened to be revealed at a meeting of the American Bar Association that these experiments were being carried on and a very distinguished member of the Federal Judiciary was quite critical. In fact, he condemned it severely and even went so far as to intercede with the foundation that was making some grants in aid of this project and suggested that they should withdraw their grant. As a result of that event the members of this committee asked me to present my views about the desirability and the propriety of carrying on this experiment. At first blush I had some doubts. But after carefully going over the safeguards that were thrown around the experiment I reached the conclusion that it could not do any harm, that the jury involved in the case would have no intimation or even curiosity or any idea that the recording was being made of their deliberations and that no publicity would be given to it so that juries generally might get the notion that their deliberations were being recorded so they might have some inhibitions.

I had some doubts at the beginning as to what good might come out of it after realizing they reached a conclusion that it could not be harmful. I would like to say I think there are two results that are on the credit side: One is proving, I think demonstrating, that juries generally do a good job. I think it demonstrates that. As a matter of fact, sometimes, if you ascertained the reasons or the line of reasoning that a jury goes through in reaching its verdict, you wonder what in the world they were thinking about, how they got off on this tangent or that tangent. But the thing about it is that when they get through and bring in a verdict in a vast majority of cases I think the trial judge will say the jury did the right thing. . . .

* * *

The other thing is important that Judge Murrah suggested, instructing a jury. As my good friend Mr. Rooney indicated, it is a difficult problem. No matter how you couch your language it is difficult to present a charge that will be clear and plain and intelligent to the jury. If

we discover in a particular case from one of these recordings that the jury didn't understand the charge, that on a critical issue the charge was misleading, we will avoid those mistakes in the future.

* * *

MR. GARWOOD: I would like to inquire whether these experimenters are aware of the fact that eavesdropping on juries is a criminal offense.

VOICE: May I say that eavesdropping is when you seek to use information against the individual you are eavesdropping on. It is not eavesdropping when you gather general information as to general conduct without any desire to use it against the person from whom you got the information.

JUDGE HILL: Anyone else? We will stand adjourned.

* * *

C.
How and by Whom Should the Consequences of Research Be Reviewed?

1.

Informing the United States Congress for Decision

SENATOR JAMES O. EASTLAND, chairman: This hearing has been called to make a public record of the facts behind the reports respecting the recording of the deliberations of juries, allegedly in connection with a research project financed by a grant from the Ford Foundation.

The purpose of getting the facts of this matter on record is to permit assessment of the impact of this activity upon the integrity of the jury system, as a basis for decision respecting what legislation may be necessary to protect the jury system. The Congress has an obligation in this regard, for the Congress has the duty of making all laws necessary and proper for carrying into full effect the provisions of the Constitution, and the seventh amendment of the Constitution specifically requires preservation of trial by jury, which necessarily must mean the kind of trial by jury which was in force under the common law at the time that amendment was written.

The jurisdiction of the Internal Security Subcommittee in this matter arises from the fact that anything which undermines or threatens the integrity of the jury system necessarily

affects the internal security of the United States.

The Internal Security Subcommittee has been criticized in the past for giving too much attention to matters involving subversion and subversives, and critics of the committee have pointed out that the field of internal security is not limited to matters of subversives and subversion. I suppose there may be some criticism of the subcommittee in this instance for venturing into a matter which does not appear to involve subversives or subversion. Nevertheless, I am clear in my own mind that this subcommittee does have jurisdiction to go as far as we propose to go.

* * *

My views have been especially well expressed, perhaps better than I could have done it myself, by the *Washington Post* in an editorial appearing in the issue of October 7, under the head "Jury Tapping." The *Post* said:

A jury imperatively needs to carry on its deliberations in private. When it retires to consider the evidence and arguments in a case which has been argued before it, its members must be free from any outside pressure or fear of reprisal. They must be free also to discuss the case with full confidence that what they say will not go beyond the walls of the jury room. Any impairment of this privacy not only destroys the detachment with which they ought to deliberate, but effectually deprives the litigants of their right to a fair trial. Uninhibited discussion becomes very difficult if there is fear of a concealed microphone.

It is significant, I think, that Attorney General Brownell has declared that—

We in the Justice Department are unequivocally opposed to any recording or eavesdropping on the deliberations of the jury under any condition, regardless of purpose.

*   *   *

a.

Testimony of Edward H. Levi, Dean, University of Chicago Law School— October 12, 1955

MR. SOURWINE, chief counsel: Would you give the reporter your full name, Dr. Levi?

MR. LEVI: My name is Edward H. Levi. I am professor of law and dean of the law school at the University of Chicago.

Senator, I have a statement which I think might be helpful to the committee, which I would like the privilege of making.

THE CHAIRMAN: We will put it in the record. We will put it in the record at the conclusion of your testimony.

MR. LEVI: Well—

THE CHAIRMAN: Mr. Sourwine, proceed, sir.

MR. SOURWINE: How many years have you been at the University of Chicago?

MR. LEVI: I have been at the University of Chicago on the faculty since 1936.

MR. SOURWINE: And how long have you been dean of the law school?

MR. LEVI: Since 1950.

*   *   *

MR. SOURWINE: Dean Levi, do you have any connection with the Ford Foundation?

MR. LEVI: I have no connection with the Ford Foundation other than that I am administering, that is, I am conducting a research program for which they gave the funds.

MR. SOURWINE: What was that grant from the Ford Foundation?

MR. LEVI: It was a grant of $400,000 given for research in the area of law and social sciences.

*   *   *

MR. SOURWINE: What is the nature of the project or projects under that grant?

MR. LEVI: There are three projects under that grant. One relates to the jury system. . . .

*   *   *

MR. SOURWINE: Sir, what was it hoped to learn through this project with respect to juries?

MR. LEVI: It was hoped to learn how juries operate, to what extent they understand the instructions of the judges, to what extent they are able to handle difficult problems of evidence, to what extent it might be possible to speed up the jury system, so as to avoid the clogging of the courts in the urban centers and at the same time to preserve the jury system.

THE CHAIRMAN: Now, would not the proper way to handle that, Doctor, be to confer with the jury after the verdict is rendered?

MR. LEVI: We have done so.

THE CHAIRMAN: Before it had been discharged?

MR. LEVI: We have done so. One part—

THE CHAIRMAN: Answer my question.

MR. LEVI: I am sorry, sir.

THE CHAIRMAN: Is that not the proper way to handle it?

MR. LEVI: I think that is one proper way to handle it.

THE CHAIRMAN: That is the proper way to handle it; is it not?

MR. LEVI: Senator, if what you are asking me, is, is that the only proper way, I think my answer is No, not in my judgment.

THE CHAIRMAN: Now, do you not realize that to snoop on a jury, and to record what they say, does violence to every reason for which we have secret deliberations of a jury?

MR. LEVI: Senator, on that I think that reasonable men differ. I do not.

THE CHAIRMAN: You do not think so?

MR. LEVI: I do not.

THE CHAIRMAN: You do not think that a member of a jury would frankly express his opinion? Would he hesitate to frankly express his opinion if he thought there might be a microphone hidden, taking down what they said?

MR. LEVI: I think that if he were conscious of the fact that there was a microphone, while he was conscious of it, this might result in some inhibitions.

THE CHAIRMAN: Yes. But if those things secretly happen and then it is released and the records are played before people, how is he going to know whether in that particular case there is a microphone there or not?

MR. LEVI: I agree with what you are saying, Senator. In this instance—in these instances —the records are not to be played publicly. There was to be no public discussion of it.

THE CHAIRMAN: Were they?

MR. LEVI: They were played, as I understand it—I was not there—at the conference of the Tenth Judicial Circuit by the judges. Our understanding was that this was a session at which the judges were using these recordings in order to determine whether their instructions are understood by the jury. I was told that Judge Phillips wished to have these recordings released to the judges for that purpose.

THE CHAIRMAN: Well, then, they were played before groups of people, were they not?

MR. LEVI: Senator, the answer is "Yes," they were, but not by us.

THE CHAIRMAN: Well, now, what is the reason for secret deliberations of a jury?

MR. LEVI: The reason for secret deliberations of a jury is so that the jury shall not be disturbed in its discussions, so that the discussions can be orderly and that they can state their opinions. But, Senator—

THE CHAIRMAN: Now, that is it; so that they can frankly state their opinions. That is the reason, is it not?

MR. LEVI: I believe that is right, Senator. But—

THE CHAIRMAN: Certainly. Now, that is a principal reason, is it not?

MR. LEVI: It is certainly one of the major reasons.

THE CHAIRMAN: Yes. Now, you violated that, did you not?

MR. LEVI: Senator, I beg to differ. Our recording of these deliberations was under an arrangement with the consent of the trial judge and the chief judge of the circuit—

THE CHAIRMAN: Regardless, now, of who agreed to it; regardless of who agreed to it, you still violated it, did you not?

MR. LEVI: Senator, I was trying to answer that precise point.

THE CHAIRMAN: Well, I think you go off on a question of attempting to justify it by saying—

MR. LEVI: No, sir.

THE CHAIRMAN: By saying that a judge agreed to it.

MR. LEVI: No sir. I was about to—

THE CHAIRMAN: The fact is that you violated the very reason that we have secret deliberations by juries.

MR. LEVI: What I was about to say, Sena-

tor, was that this was done under an arrangement which provided that there should be no publicity; that the recording, when transcribed, should be changed so as to remove all identifying statements, and that there shall be no release—

THE CHAIRMAN: No publicity. And practically everyone in the United States who reads the newspapers knows about this.

MR. LEVI: Yes, sir. That is what happened.

SENATOR JENNER: Who had custody of the transcriptions after they were made?

MR. LEVI: The court had custody of the transcriptions, and we had custody from the court.

THE CHAIRMAN: You had custody then?

SENATOR JENNER: Who had physical possession of the transcriptions?

MR. LEVI: I answered as I did because there was a period of time when we had custody, physical custody, and a period of time when the court had physical custody.

SENATOR JENNER: But you gave up physical custody so that they could be played at a public hearing in Estes Park, Colo.; is that right?

MR. LEVI: Not quite, sir. We gave up physical custody at the request of Judge Phillips for their playing at what we understood to be a closed session of the judges of the 10th circuit.

THE CHAIRMAN: Now, describe and explain just exactly what you did to record the deliberations of the jury in Wichita?

MR. LEVI: Senator, in order to answer that question, I have to say that the arrangements for the recordings, as I have indicated before, were set up in Wichita.

THE CHAIRMAN: By whom?

MR. LEVI: By Mr. Paul Kitch, who worked, as I understand it, with Judge Hill and obtained the consent of Judge Phillips. I was not and have never been in Wichita, but I was notified that these arrangements had been made, and after I was notified that these arrangements had been made, I sent Mr. Mikva to Wichita to carry out the arrangements with the instructions that he was to work under the direction of the trial judge.

*   *   *

MR. SOURWINE: Could you state succinctly for the record, Dean, what you hope to prove by this project?

MR. LEVI: We hope to prove, and I believe we will be able to prove, that the jury is an efficient method of deciding cases, despite the clogging of the dockets, that it can be strengthened and preserved, and that the doubts that have arisen about the jury system in various parts of this country and in the world, as for example, in England, where the jury system has been much limited, are not well established.

We wish to strengthen the jury system by this project.

*   *   *

THE CHAIRMAN: Now, did you ever discuss this in any way with the representatives of the Ford Foundation?

MR. LEVI: The representatives of the Ford Foundation? Yes, I did discuss this with the representatives of the Ford Foundation after the recordings had been made.

THE CHAIRMAN: Yes, sir. You did not before?

MR. LEVI: No, sir.

*   *   *

MR. SOURWINE: Have additional funds been requested?

MR. LEVI: Additional funds have been requested and they have been obtained. The Ford Foundation, although it has not been announced, has made a grant of $1 million, made it in August, for the continuation of the general program.

MR. SOURWINE: And that was made in August of this year?

MR. LEVI: That is right, sir.

MR. SOURWINE: Did the Ford Foundation at that time have knowledge of the fact that this project included the recording of deliberations in jury rooms?

MR. LEVI: Yes, sir.

MR. SOURWINE: It is anticipated that a report will be made of this project to the Ford Foundation?

MR. LEVI: Well, we made reports to the Ford Foundation, yes, sir.

*   *   *

MR. SOURWINE: Do you contemplate that partial disclosure of the results of this study will be permitted at any time?

MR. LEVI: You mean, of the Wichita operation?

MR. SOURWINE: Yes.

MR. LEVI: That has not been decided. The arrangement was—and I hope I may be permitted to put this in, because I want to answer it explicitly—the arrangement was that the trans-

cripts were to be so changed that there would be no identifying statements, but we have not decided whether, even though that has been done— and it has been done—this material could be disclosed, that is, in its changed form. We have never made that determination.

MR. SOURWINE: Had that editing been done, either wholly or partially, prior to the time that the recordings or portions of them were played back at Estes Park, Colo.?

MR. LEVI: I believe so.

MR. SOURWINE: Who made the selection with respect to the portion or portions to be played at Estes Park?

MR. LEVI: I do not know the answer to that question.

MR. SOURWINE: You had nothing to do with that?

MR. LEVI: No, I had nothing to do with it, and the project had nothing to do with it. We were put in a position where we were told that the chief judge of the circuit wanted the recording back, and that presumably the court had jurisdiction, and we were returning the tapes for that purpose. It was not our plan.

*   *   *

MR. SOURWINE: Do you know, sir, in how many cases the proceedings of juries or the deliberations of juries have been recorded?

MR. LEVI: You mean by us?

MR. SOURWINE: By you or anybody else, if you know of any other—

MR. LEVI: I know of no recordings by anyone else, and I am told that the Wichita operation resulted in the recording of 5 or 6 cases. I would say 6 cases, although I am told that 1 of the cases had 2 parts to it, and that makes the sixth.

*   *   *

MR. SOURWINE: All right. Was there to your knowledge any agreement that the transcription or recording of the jury's deliberations would be sealed up until all time for appeal in any individual case had passed?

MR. LEVI: I think that Mr. Kitch's letter has a statement to that effect.

MR. SOURWINE: Doesn't that statement necessarily imply the belief that what was done would have constituted ground for appeal or exception, if not concealed until the time for appeal had passed?

MR. LEVI: I should not think so, but—

MR. SOURWINE: Then why was it stipulated that it would be concealed?

MR. LEVI: I do not know. That is Mr. Kitch's letter. I would say that you were raising a legal question as to whether the consent of counsel would not operate, so that no matter whether they were looked at before or not, it would make no difference. I think the point was rather a different one, namely, that the trial judge should not be in a position of having heard the deliberations at the time when he might still be passing on motions which might relate to the case. This is my understanding.

*   *   *

NOTE

STATEMENT BY EDWARD H. LEVI, DEAN OF
THE LAW SCHOOL OF THE UNIVERSITY OF
CHICAGO—OCTOBER 12, 1955

I am happy to appear before this committee to discuss some of the aspects of the jury project now being conducted by the University of Chicago Law School and in particular that segment of the project which has recorded a limited number of actual jury deliberations.

Three points should be made. The first of these is this: A number of distinguished and able leaders of the bar believe a study of the jury system can make a substantial contribution to the administration of justice, and many of these leaders believe that such a study may properly use recordings of actual jury deliberations. The second point is that the recordings of actual deliberations were carried out under safeguards to preserve the integrity of the jury system. The third point is that the jury system is a suitable and important subject for basic study, and the study as carried out should contribute to the strengthening—and not the weakening—of this important American institution.

The leaders of the American bar who have expressed their approval of the study of the jury system include leaders in the field of legal education and research, and judges and lawyers whose distinguished positions testify to their knowledge and understanding of the need for basic research in order to improve the administration of justice.

The president, the president-elect, and five of the living past presidents since 1947 of the Association of American Law Schools have authorized the issuance of a statement in which they declare that they see great possible gain to our knowledge, to our teaching of law, to our

legal system and to our machinery of justice in a study of the jury system which includes, under safeguards, the recording of actual jury deliberations. The statement is signed by Edwin D. Dickinson, of the University of Pennsylvania; Karl N. Llewellyn, of the University of Chicago; F. D. G. Ribble, dean of the University of Virginia; Robert E. Matthews, of Ohio University; Wesley N. Sturges, of Yale University; Maurice T. van Hecke, of the University of North Carolina, and Charles B. Nutting.

The statement of the president, president-elect, and former presidents of the Association of American Law Schools is as follows:

In our opinion, a much more accurate knowledge of the actual workings of our jury system has long been needed. Such knowledge ought not only to make clearer the solid values of that system but also to suggest measures for making the system work more smoothly and effectively to achieve those values. Research into the course of actual jury deliberations is key material and the most fruitful material to further these ends. Certainly if such research is done only under supervision of the court, and if it is done only by consent of counsel on both sides, and if it is done only under the seal of professional secrecy, and if, furthermore, not even excerpts are in any event to be published without the careful and tested cutting out of each name, date, locality, or other identifying mark of any sort at all, we then see, in the recording of a body of actual jury deliberations, not only no harm or danger, but on the contrary great possible gain to our knowledge, to our teaching of law, to our legal system and to our machinery of justice.

Five judges of the Illinois Appellate Court have authorized a statement expressing their confidence that the results of the jury study should contribute to the administration of justice. Judges Hugo Friend, John G. Lewe, Roger Kiley, John V. McCormick and Ulysses S. Schwartz have authorized the issuance of this statement:

We have long been aware and have in fact worked with the jury study now being conducted by the University of Chicago Law School. We believe this to be a most important study which should have the support of both the bench and bar. In our judgment, the study is being ably conducted by able people. It deals with a most important American institution and the results of the study should contribute to the administration of justice.

*   *   *

Five former presidents of the National Conference of Commissioners on Uniform State Laws and the present chairman of the executive committee have sent messages approving of the jury study and the recording under safeguards of actual jury deliberations. These are men who have had wide experience and high position in the organized bar and who know particularly well the relationship between basic research and improvements in the administrations of justice. . . .

These statements are as follows:

HOWARD L. BARKDULL: Recording of actual jury deliberations under careful supervision of court and with consent of counsel constitutes a useful research tool in improving administration of justice. Successful operation of American courts depends on effectiveness of jury system and requires constant study for means of correcting all points of weakness or abuse. Benefits of recording greatly outweigh objections.

JAMES C. DEZENDORF: If our system of government is to be maintained and preserved we must conduct research on all phases of the judicial process. Research concerning the functioning of the jury cannot be conducted intelligently unless actual jury deliberations can be studied and reviewed.

JOE C. BARRETT: Information relating to process of jury deliberations would be of great help to trial lawyers and judges in pointing up areas wherein improvements would be made in presentation of evidence and in the court's instructions on rules of law governing the case. Recordings of actual jury deliberations should play a significant part in such a study. I am impressed with this study as a means of pointing the way for substantial improvement in the administration of justice. To be of maximum value the study should have a base sufficiently broad to demonstrate whether there is any pattern of weakness that needs correction.

* * *

b.

Testimony of Harry Kalven, Jr., Professor of Law, University of Chicago— October 12, 1955

* * *

MR. SOURWINE: Do you know anything of a condition that, in the case where the juries were deliberating, that the names of the participants in those cases were not to be disclosed?

MR. KALVEN: Yes, sir; I understand that is a very important condition they have that they not be disclosed, which would be our wish not to disclose those.

MR. SOURWINE: Who did make that condition? Did you make it, or was it made by a judge?

MR. KALVEN: I have no direct information on that. I imagine that idea would occur very quickly to both sides; that that would be quite appropriate.

MR. SOURWINE: Has that condition been adhered to?

MR. KALVEN: Very strictly, sir.

* * *

MR. SOURWINE: Do you know whether the attorneys for the parties of record in these cases gave their consent to the bugging of the jury room?

MR. KALVEN: Again, sir, I am repeating somewhat second-handed knowledge, but it was my understanding in each case they did, and they gave their consent to the judge.

MR. SOURWINE: Do you know who those various attorneys were?

MR. KALVEN: I do not of my own knowledge. Again that would seem to be an item going to identifying the cases.

MR. SOURWINE: Would you think that if you gave those names you would be identifying the cases?

MR. KALVEN: I would think so, sir.

* * *

MR. SOURWINE: [C]an you tell us briefly what you sought to learn through this project?

MR. KALVEN: Well, as I say, the answer to that is along this line. As we were making a study of the jury as such, we have our lines of inquiry, including the experimental jury routine Mr. Levi mentioned this morning, including the interviewing of jurors after trial, and getting an impression of what the trial was like; what their impressions were like, and so forth. And the chief need that we felt that we had—and we think we have now—is to have some final way of corroborating the reality, both of the experimental work and completeness and reality of the interview after trial.

The point, sir, was that a limited number of real recordings kept with all proper precautions would give us in a sense a final test, as I say, of the realism of what we are doing.

MR. SOURWINE: You were actually primarily concerned with testing the realism of these moot juries that you had set up?

MR. KALVEN: I think that is the easiest way to put it.

MR. SOURWINE: Whose deliberations you had recorded?

MR. KALVEN: That is right; you can recognize that a device like this quickly meets the objection that it looks interesting, but do real juries act like that.

MR. SOURWINE: Did the moot jury cases contain the same components of the case which were actual, and which you recorded?

MR. KALVEN: To some degree; not in fact as much as I wished they had, just as a matter of method, but they contain the same kinds of problems.

MR. SOURWINE: How did you accomplish that? Were you able to select cases which did contain those problems, or did you construct your moot cases, so as to match?

MR. KALVEN: We constructed our moot cases to—the matching is not very close, sir. I would rather not come too close to the content of the actual cases, but I think you can anticipate it would not be hard to have some common issues on the civil side of jury cases.

*   *   *

MR. SOURWINE: Do you know of the recording of the deliberations of juries in any courts, except in these 5 or 6 cases in Wichita?

MR. KALVEN: No, sir; I do not.

MR. SOURWINE: Were these five recordings in the Federal court in Wichita the only recordings of jury proceedings which were planned as a part of your project?

MR. KALVEN: Yes, sir. This is the ambiguity about whether it is 5 or 6 Mr. Levi mentioned this morning.

MR. SOURWINE: You had no plan at any time to record a larger number?

MR. KALVEN: Well, there is the original correspondence, sir, from which Mr. Kitch—perhaps Mr. Kitch can talk to that point later—in which he proposed the matter to Judge Phillips; he mentioned a large number of cases, but it was a much larger number, I think, sir, than anyone on our side had committed themselves of doing; and it was at that time, with the understanding that the juries would be told about it, and Judge Phillips had no objection to that.

MR. SOURWINE: Whose side was Kitch on?

MR. KALVEN: I think on his own side, sir. He was interested in this as an independent lawyer.

MR. SOURWINE: Was he ever on the payroll of the University of Chicago?

MR. KALVEN: No, sir, not to my knowledge.

MR. SOURWINE: Ever on the payroll of this project?

MR. KALVEN: No, sir.

MR. SOURWINE: Did he receive any compensation for the work he did, so far as you know?

MR. KALVEN: Just our thanks, I think, sir.

*   *   *

THE CHAIRMAN: Mr. Kalven, do you believe in the American jury system?

MR. KALVEN: I do, very much, sir. That is the reason why I am interested in the study.

THE CHAIRMAN: Yes, sir. Do you believe that juries should deliberate in secret?

MR. KALVEN: I think on the balance, it is better, sir, if they deliberate with an assurance of privacy.

THE CHAIRMAN: Do you believe that the American jury system is one of the greatest safeguards of human liberty?

MR. KALVEN: I think I would say, "Yes, sir," to that.

*   *   *

THE CHAIRMAN: What would happen to that great safeguard if a jury's deliberations were "bugged"?

MR. KALVEN: Well sir, I think it makes a good deal of difference who does the bugging, under what circumstances. I agree that if all juries were conscious of the fact that their deliberations might be recorded, if you will permit the phrase, by anyone whomsoever and for any purpose—

THE CHAIRMAN: It would affect them?

MR. KALVEN: I think that is right. I think that is almost irrelevant.

THE CHAIRMAN: And yet you say, for a jury, if they were conscious of the fact—well, do you not know that if it is done in some cases, that every juror is going to think, well, maybe there is a microphone in this room?

MR. KALVEN: I do not think so, sir. May I make one statement?

THE CHAIRMAN: You do not?

MR. KALVEN: The statement is this—

THE CHAIRMAN: Answer my question.

MR. KALVEN: The answer is, no, sir.

THE CHAIRMAN: You do not think that?

MR. KALVEN: No, sir. May I amplify my answer?

THE CHAIRMAN: Certainly.

MR. KALVEN: I think the only two points to be made here are these: The first point, it was not contemplated it would be having the degree of publicity there presently is about this. As Mr. Levi said this morning, it was not clear what final disposition would be made of these.

THE CHAIRMAN: Do you not realize that a procedure, so at variance with the American system of government, is bound to be widely known?

MR. KALVEN: I do not think so, sir. This procedure—this was done 15 months ago—it seems to me it has been kept a pretty good secret until recently.

THE CHAIRMAN: Everybody in the country knows it now, do they not?

MR. KALVEN: Not through our efforts.

THE CHAIRMAN: Sir?

MR. KALVEN: Not through our efforts.

THE CHAIRMAN: Regardless of whose efforts, it is known, it is not?

MR. KALVEN: In any event, I would like to get to my second point, which, I think, is more relevant. What is now known is that, with the consent of the attorneys and with the consent of the judge, and for scientific purposes, a few juries may from time to time be recorded. I see no reason why that should strike any fear in the heart of any juror in America. And that seems to me, at the maximum, the threat that has been created thus far.

THE CHAIRMAN: What is the seventh amendment to the Constitution of the United States?

MR. KALVEN: It is the amendment providing for jury trial in civil cases.

THE CHAIRMAN. Certainly.

MR. KALVEN: In cases involving the Federal Government.

THE CHAIRMAN: Certainly. That means secret deliberations?

MR. KALVEN: I am not completely sure about that, sir.

THE CHAIRMAN: You are not?

MR. KALVEN: Not as a matter of technical constitutional law. As I understand it—and I do not profess to be an expert on this point—it was rather unclear at the time the Constitution was adopted just how much jury secrecy there was. And as I understand the constitutional test for the meaning of the seventh amendment, it goes back to the institution as of the time the amendment was adopted. I am not making that as a firm proposition of law, sir. It is just my impression on that point.

THE CHAIRMAN: Let me ask you this question—have you finished your answer?

MR. KALVEN: Yes, sir.

THE CHAIRMAN: Did you write a letter to President Truman, asking clemency for the atomic spies, Rosenbergs?

MR. KALVEN: I did, sir. I have the letter with me.

THE CHAIRMAN: You say you have the letter with you?

MR. KALVEN: Yes, sir.

THE CHAIRMAN: Give us a copy of the letter.

MR. KALVEN: I would be pleased to read the letter.

*   *   *

THE CHAIRMAN: Sir?

MR. KALVEN: I wrote this letter as a private citizen to the president. No copies of this letter have been given out. This copy is from my file.

THE CHAIRMAN: Do you not know that the *Daily Worker* knew about it?

MR. KALVEN: The only way I know is that Fulton Lewis, Jr., had it on his broadcast the other night. I have no idea how the *Daily Worker* knew about it.

THE CHAIRMAN: Have you read the *Daily Worker*?

MR. KALVEN: No, sir; I have never read the *Daily Worker*.

*   *   *

SENATOR JENNER: Going back to the seventh amendment to the Constitution, Mr. Kalven, you expressed an opinion, I believe, to the chairman of the committee on that a while ago.

I want to ask you: Is there any question in your mind that the right of jury trial guaranteed by the seventh amendment encompasses all of the attributes of a jury trial as it was known at the time that amendment was written?

*   *   *

MR. KALVEN: I agree with you; that is the legal test of the meaning.

SENATOR JENNER: Then that being true, did not this include the absolute freedom of deliberation of the jury?

MR. KALVEN: Well, sir, I am not an expert on the law on that, as I was suggesting before. The law, so far as I know—and I hesitate to offer a judgment on the question like this—but so far as I know until immediately prior to that date—that is, the date of the adoption of the amendment—the law had been the other way. It appears to have been changed within a few years of that time.

I would gather that, if there was a question raised seriously today, there would be a real doubt at common law, that the jury had secrecy of deliberations. I do not want to make a point of that. I think it is agreed, since the amendment was adopted, it has been the spirit and principle of the amendment that jury deliberations are basically secret, with the qualification, sir, that you know this morning that, of course, it is permissible, if not—well, let me say it is permissible and certainly customary practice almost everywhere for the lawyers and newspapers to talk to jurors after cases, in that sense to find out what happened during the deliberations, and in that sense equally to upset the jurors' serenity of mind, and so forth, in terms of disclosure of the content of the deliberations being made after the deliberation is over.

SENATOR JENNER: After the deliberations have reached the final conclusion, but you know of no case except the case that you cited out in Wichita where a jury's free deliberation has been fettered by bugging a room?

MR. KALVEN: Sir, I want to again say I think this is an important distinction, and I think it is not being fully appreciated here, that the jury's free deliberation was not being fettered in that case, because the jury did not know about it. And in future cases, the jury's free deliberation is being fettered only in the sense that the juror would be concerned because again some judge, a judge who is primarily the custodian of the jury, would decide that it would be appropriate, with the consent of counsel, and for impartial scientific purposes, to again permit a recording to be made.

SENATOR JENNER: Well, since this has been so widely publicized—

MR. KALVEN: Well, sir—

SENATOR JENNER (continuing): What effect do you think it will have on the effect of free deliberation of the jury in the future?

MR. KALVEN: I think that is relatively easy to answer.

If it was correctly publicized, I think it would have virtually no effect.

SENATOR JENNER: Go ahead.

THE CHAIRMAN: What effect would bugging 500 or 1,000 jury deliberations have?

MR. KALVEN: I think it—sir, I will agree that if again the auspices are different—if the judge does not consent—I think this is a quite

improper practice, and I should think there was no doubt about it.

THE CHAIRMAN: Whether the judge consented or not, the effect on the jury would be the same, would it not?

MR. KALVEN: I should think it would not be. The judge is, as I say—the jury is regarded as an appendage of the court. It seems to me whether or not the judge consents, makes the enormous and crucial difference here.

THE CHAIRMAN: Do you not know, whether the judge consents or not, the pressure against free deliberation would be on that juror, would it not?

*   *   *

MR. KALVEN: Sir, it depends entirely on whether the court has consented for impartial, scientific purposes, or not.

THE CHAIRMAN: Is it not true—is it not true that you have planned to bug the deliberations of juries in 500 to 1,000 cases?

MR. KALVEN: No, sir; it is clearly not. I understand—

THE CHAIRMAN: That is not true?

MR. KALVEN: That is not true, sir. Let me explain the answer. There is this proposal. Mr. Kitch can talk to this, as I say. Mr. Kitch, I think, will indicate more ambition about this in some ways than we had, but the proposal was that—stating a number as large as 500, with the condition that the jury know about it. At no time, when that condition was removed, was it ever contemplated to do more than a handful of cases.

THE CHAIRMAN: No more than a handful of cases?

MR. KALVEN: That is right, sir; and to do them for the sake of evaluating our other observation work on the jury.

THE CHAIRMAN: I am going to read to you from a speech made today in St. Paul, Minn., by the Assistant Attorney General, Warren E. Burger. I want you to state then whether his statements are true or false:

A Justice Department official charged today that the University of Chicago Law School plans to eavesdrop on 500 to a thousand juries during its research project into the American jury system. The planting of the microphone in Wichita, Kans., jury room was only the first step in a study of "very sweeping proposals."

MR. KALVEN: Sir, I would say that the statement is truly false. The Department of Justice has good reason to know what the facts are.

SENATOR JENNER: May I ask a question, Mr. Chairman?

THE CHAIRMAN: Yes, sir.

SENATOR JENNER: Why is your study only concerned with civil procedure? Are you not interested in a scientific study of criminal procedure?

MR. KALVEN: We are studying criminal cases, too.

SENATOR JENNER: Why did you only bug civil trials; why did you not bug some criminal trials?

MR. KALVEN: I will confess, sir, because of a generally recognized difference between criminal and civil cases; and because of the generally recognized importance of the jury on the criminal side we, perhaps, had some additional hesitation about that.

SENATOR JENNER: Then your scientific study would be lopsided, in any event; would it not? You would not know what a jury was thinking on a criminal trial, but you would know everything connected with the civil trial—would that not be one-sided—this is to be an objective study, was it not; you are supposed to bring in all juries, both criminal and civil.

MR. KALVEN: That is right, sir. And we had not decided definitely the question raised about whether it would be appropriate to do it in a criminal case. Personally, I would think so.

*   *   *

SENATOR JENNER: Do you plan to go on with that in criminal procedures?

MR. KALVEN: We have had no immediate plans for some time now to go ahead. We are digesting the material that we have. I would not say that we are foreclosing the possibility of doing additional work like this, if the opportunity, with the consent of the court, with appropriate safeguards, arises.

SENATOR JENNER: In other words, then, everybody is on notice in this country that, sometime in the future, a criminal jury may be bugged for the scientific study of the research fund granted to the University of Chicago; am I to understand that?

MR. KALVEN: Sir, again they are on notice that if a court deems it appropriate, and if we deem it worthwhile, from the point of view—from our research at that time, that the possibility is considered.

SENATOR JENNER: That is all I want to know. Go ahead.

MR. SOURWINE: Will you clarify your testimony of a moment ago. Did I hear you correctly? I thought I heard you state that, at no time after the condition that juries should be advised was withdrawn, was there any consideration of eavesdropping on more than a very few, a handful, of cases; is that right?

MR. KALVEN: That is my understanding, sir.

*   *   *

I am not sure that everyone on the project sees exactly as I do on this, since I am making two statements. One is that in terms of our actual plans there were no plans to do this again in the immediate future. Secondly, my own point of view about this, which I am not sure is, as I say, completely a unanimous one, is that I would be in favor of doing this in a very limited additional number of cases.

MR. SOURWINE: But you are testifying now that, after the Wichita cases, there might have been consideration to doing it in some other cases?

MR. KALVEN: That is right, sir. And that remains true today.

*   *   *

THE CHAIRMAN: That is over the next year, you say?

MR. KALVEN: No. Over the next year, sir, if our plans had gone as projected, I think it is very doubtful we would have done any more cases. There were no concrete plans for doing any.

THE CHAIRMAN: I will guarantee you that you will not do any bugging after Congress passes some legislation.

MR. KALVEN: I admit, sir, the situation has changed somewhat.

THE CHAIRMAN: I will say it has.

MR. SOURWINE: Professor Kalven, if I heard you correctly, you used the phrase, "the generally recognized importance of the jury in criminal trials"?

MR. KALVEN: That is right.

MR. SOURWINE: Would you say the importance of the jury in civil cases is not generally recognized?

MR KALVEN: No, sir. I would say that the importance of the jury in criminal cases is recognized more widely; that I really have an eye to the fact that in many areas of civil litigation, as you know, the jury is very frequently waived now by the parties. We have the phenomenon in England of having the jury almost disappear in personal-injury litigation. And as I read the literature, it seems to me that while some people have been willing to say that the jury may not be the most effective institution on the civil side, I have never seen anyone make that statement on the criminal side, because I think its role is different.

I think, in that sense, it has a more important role on the criminal side, and that is the difference I was referring to.

* * *

MR. SOURWINE: Mr. Kalven, where are the recordings that were made of the jury deliberations in Wichita; do you know?

MR. KALVEN: Not precisely, sir. To my knowledge, they are stored in two rooms in the basement of the law school. Mr. Strodtbeck is the direct custodian of this, and I think could testify more directly to that.

MR. SOURWINE: Do you know who had access to them?

MR. KALVEN: Only two people—Mr. Strodtbeck's staff—Mr. Strodtbeck himself and, of course, I would have, whenever I would want to see them. They are under lock and key, the recordings themselves. And I think Mr. Strodtbeck could describe a little more vividly, sir, than I can, the precise security measures that have always been taken with these materials.

MR. SOURWINE: Can you tell us when and where any of these recordings have been played?

MR. KALVEN: Sir, except for performances to ourselves, for our own purposes, the only occasion I know of is the Estes Park meeting of the judges of the Tenth Judicial Circuit.

MR. SOURWINE: Who do you mean, "to ourselves"?

MR. KALVEN: The immediate—not more than a group of 5 or 6 people.

MR. SOURWINE: Who are those persons?

MR. KALVEN: I think it would be fair to say anyone on the staff at this point might, if circumstances warranted, hear the materials. I do not know that they have. They have all had contact with them.

MR. SOURWINE: How many persons are on the staff at this moment?

MR. KALVEN: I think 13. I thought you might ask that.

MR. SOURWINE: You said 5 or 6 persons a moment ago. Did you mean different groups of 5 or 6 now, and 5 or 6 later?

MR. KALVEN: I mean, sir—no, sir; I mean on this count, sir, there are 10 people at the moment. The problem about counting them, sir, is

that we have a fair amount of part-time help that is at a relatively junior level, and it is a question whether you include those on the staff or not, but any of the senior members of the staff, I am sure, would have access to this material.

* * *

MR. SOURWINE: Do you know, Mr. Kalven, about an agreement that transcripts of recordings of jury's deliberations would be sealed up until all time had elapsed for appeal from the individual case?

MR. KALVEN: I know, sir; there is some provision for that. Then, I am not familiar as of my own knowledge with that. Again, I think, Mr. Strodtbeck could talk—

MR. SOURWINE: Do you see in such a provision any implication that what was done would have constituted a ground for appeal or exception if it had not been sealed until the time of appeal had passed?

MR. KALVEN: I think, as Mr. Levi said, that since the counsel had consented to the whole arrangement, anyway, it would be a peculiar ground for appeal; that the judge, perhaps—I think, this is his own idea—perhaps was a little uneasy about his having access to this material until that had happened.

MR. SOURWINE: Have you stated, sir, publicly, that the United States attorney had agreed to the jury bugging in each instance?

MR. KALVEN: I did, sir, in the one public statement we have made, make a statement saying that all the parties to the case, I mean, that counsel for all parties to the case had agreed, including the United States attorney. I believed that to be true at the time, sir. I understand, sir, that might have been a mistake. The man actually in charge of the case was an assistant United States attorney, sir.

The intention of our statement was that the lawyer handling the Government's case had consented on behalf of the government.

MR. SOURWINE: You were quoted as having said that the thing had been cleared with the United States attorney, and I am just asking you whether you had said that.

MR. KALVEN: I think my statement is unfortunately a little ambiguous on that, sir, but I think the clear intention of it was that whoever was the lawyer for the government in the csae involved had consented, and I understand that to be the fact.

MR. SOURWINE: Who was the lawyer for the government who consented?

MR. KALVEN: I am not sure I know the name, sir. I think it was Mr. Cowger.

* * *

MR. SOURWINE: The Senator mentioned a moment ago, or you mentioned, Mr. Vishinsky. Have you ever read the *Law of the Soviet State* by Andre Vishinsky?

MR. KALVEN: No; I have never. . . .

MR. SOURWINE: Do you consider it an authoritative legal work?

MR. KALVEN: Not having read it, sir, I really do not have an opinion on it.

MR. SOURWINE: Do you agree with this quotation from Vishinsky's book, page—

MR. KALVEN: I doubt it.

MR. SOURWINE: (*reading*):

The classical form of the bourgeois court is the "court with jury" (a court with participation of sworn assessors) existing in the capitalist countries that preserve the bourgeois democratic forms of state order. In such a court the jurors (ordinarily 12) decide the guilt of the accused, and on the basis of that verdict, permanent judges (appointed by state authority) apply the law, and designate the punishment.

In its modern form, such a court was created by the bourgeoisie in consequence of its victory over feudalism and was progressive as compared with bureaucratic and caste courts of the noble landowner state. While bourgeois democracy flourished, such a court undoubtedly served as a bulwark of the political freedoms proclaimed by the bourgeoisie at the time of its triumph over the power of the feudal monarchy. But jurors are now, as they were formerly, the bulwark of that order of social relationships which rests on private capitalist property. The class character of such a court is an index as well of the class direction of the justice to which the jury gives effect.

Chosen chiefly from the circles of the middle and petty bourgeoisie, and predisposed by their own social position to see the buttressing of the existing social order as their function, jurors are captivated by the views even as to concrete matters, enunciated by the press, which is in the hands of the biggest capitalists.

MR. KALVEN: What was the question, now, sir?

MR. SOURWINE: The question is whether you agree with that statement or not?

MR. KALVEN: Insofar as I understand it, I do not agree with it.

MR. SOURWINE: You do know whether the Soviet courts have a jury system?

MR. KALVEN: I know absolutely nothing about the jury system in the Soviet courts.

MR. SOURWINE: Do you believe that the American jury system is superior to the Soviet court system?

MR. KALVEN: Yes; I certainly do, sir.

MR. SOURWINE: Do you agree with Engels as quoted by Vishinsky on page 507, that—"the English court of jurors, as the most developed, is the culmination of juridical falsehood and immorality"?

MR. KALVEN: No, sir.

MR. SOURWINE: Were you, Professor Kalven, ever a member of the committee to secure justice for the Rosenbergs?

MR. KALVEN: No, sir; I was not.

MR. SOURWINE: Were you a member of the Chicago Committee to Secure Justice for the Rosenbergs?

MR. KALVEN: No, sir; I was not.

MR. SOURWINE: Did you attend a meeting of that committee in November 1952?

MR. KALVEN: I am not sure, sir, whether one of those occasions might not have been sponsored in part by that. I would not say to that, categorically, no.

* * *

MR. SOURWINE: . . . Are you familiar or have you read the case of *McDonald and United States Fidelity and Guaranty Company* v. *Pless?*

MR. KALVEN: I am familiar with the general ruling in that case, sir, although—

MR. SOURWINE: Did you know that the court said in that case:

If evidence thus secured could be thus used, the result would be to make what was intended to be a private deliberation (by the jury) the constant subject of public investigation—to the destruction of all frankness and freedom of discussion and conference (in the jury room).

For while it may often exclude the only possible evidence of misconduct, a change in the rule would open the door to the most pernicious arts and tampering with jurors. The practice would be replete with dangerous consequences. It would lead to the grossest fraud and abuse and no verdict would be safe.

MR. KALVEN: I think there are two points to make about that, sir. One is, that is not the unanimous rule in the United States on the point of whether a jury verdict may be impeached by testimony as to what went on in the deliberations.

The second point is, that it seems to be quite a different question than the one we are involved with here, because it involves the adversary use by the parties themselves of this material to harass the jurors, to prolong the litigation, et cetera.

MR. SOURWINE: I only asked if you were familiar with that as a preface to asking you whether you agree with—

MR. KALVEN: I think if the question, sir, is whether the jury deliberations should be totally open to counsel thereafter, on any grounds whatsoever, to seek to impeach the verdict, I certainly agree with it, sir. It is a question whether, for example, quotient verdicts should be impeachable by testimony that this was the way in which the verdict was arrived at in the deliberations. I am not sure that I have made up my mind on that question. As you know, there are jurisdictions in which that is the rule.

MR. SOURWINE: It was the sense of the court in this particular case, was it not, that the inviolability of the proceedings in the jury room was so important that even, for the sake of helping to do justice to the litigants, a juror should not be permitted to testify as to what took place in the jury room?

MR. KALVEN: I think, sir, that the court also had in mind the point that has no relevance to our study, and that is that they were interested to putting an end to litigation, and the peculiar way we put the jury under surveillance, if the parties themselves could interrogate them as to what went on in the deliberations, and seek to make an adversary use of it.

The general policy that is indicated by the court in that sense, I agree with.

MR. SOURWINE: Are you familiar with the case of Clark v. United States (289 U.S.)?

MR. KALVEN: I have seen references to the case, sir. I am not directly familiar with it. I know it is another case in this general area.

MR. SOURWINE: In which it was held that— freedom of debate might be stifled and independence of thought checked if jurors are made to feel that their arguments and ballots were to be freely published to the world.

MR. KALVEN: Sir, is this not the opinion of Judge Cardozo?

MR. SOURWINE: Yes.

MR. KALVEN: To pay for one quotation with another, I understand that he goes on with an example, which I admit, of a possibility of evidence being the juror was bribed. This evidence was not available. This is paying too high for a juror for serenity of mind.

MR. SOURWINE: My question was whether you agree with the passage which I read to you.

MR. KALVEN: Yes, sir; in general we have

no dispute with you, sir, as to the importance of generally keeping the deliberations of juries confidential. We do not regard what we did as violating that principle.

MR. SOURWINE: I will ask you just about one more case:

Are you familiar with the case of Remmer v. The United States in title 347, United States Reports?

MR. KALVEN: No, sir.

MR. SOURWINE: In that case it was held that—a juror must feel free to exercise his functions without the FBI or anyone else looking over his shoulder. Would you agree with that?

MR. KALVEN: Yes, sir.

* * *

c.

Testimony of Logan Green, Esq., Garden City, Kansas—October 12, 1955

* * *

MR. SOURWINE: Mr. Green, were you ever involved in a case in which you were asked to consent to the recording, unbeknownst to the jury, of deliberations in the jury room?

MR. GREEN: Yes, sir; I was.

MR. SOURWINE: How was that matter first broached to you?

MR. GREEN: Well, we were preparing to try a case in Federal court, in Wichita, and the court called us in chambers and informed us.

THE CHAIRMAN: What court was that?

MR. GREEN: That was Judge Delmas C. Hill.

MR. SOURWINE: When you say he called "us in chambers"—you mean he called you and opposing counsel about the matter, both?

MR. GREEN: He called counsel for both parties to the lawsuit; yes, and informed us that there was a team of some kind present from the University of Chicago, as I recall, who desired to place a recording machine in the jury room during their deliberations in that case, and he asked us if any of us objected to that procedure.

Do you want me to go ahead?

MR. SOURWINE: Did you both say that you did not object?

MR. GREEN: Counsel for both sides said that they had no objection.

MR. SOURWINE: Did you feel, sir, speaking just for yourself, that you could afford to object to a project which the judge told you he had already approved?

MR. GREEN: Well, frankly, I didn't give the matter too much thought right at that time. We were preparing to select a jury, and I had a lawsuit to try, and I didn't give it as much thought as I would now.

MR. SOURWINE: Have you given the matter thought since that occasion, sir?

MR. GREEN: Yes, sir; I have since the publicity has arisen.

MR. SOURWINE: If a similar proposal should be made to you now, would you consent to it?

MR. GREEN: I do not think I would.

MR. SOURWINE: Mr. Chairman, I will state that I have been in telephonic contact with a number of the attorneys who were counsel in cases of this nature in Wichita. They all tell substantially the same story. I have suggested that Mr. Green be subpenaed, and I think that we can establish from the testimony of Mr. Kitch when he comes to the stand that this was the practice uniformly followed in each of the cases.

*   *   *

d.

Testimony of Fred L. Strodtbeck, Associate Professor of Sociology, Law School, University of Chicago—October 13, 1955

MR. SOURWINE: Give your full name, your business or profession and your address.

MR. STRODTBECK: Fred L. Strodtbeck. I am now employed as an associate professor of sociology in the law school, in the department of sociology, of the University of Chicago.

MR. SOURWINE: How long have you been there employed?

MR. STRODTBECK: Since September 1953.

MR. SOURWINE: Mr. Strodtbeck, will you tell us what your connection has been with the project for investigation of the jury system which involved the recording of the deliberations of some juries in Wichita?

MR. STRODTBECK: I think I should first state that I [came] to the project with a primary responsibility for the experimental study of jury processes. Now related to the experimental study of jury processes was this corroboratory operation which involved the recording of an actual deliberation.

*   *   *

As a part of our specialty in the study of small groups, we very, very frequently record many types of conferences and deliberations. That is the objective of our work, to capture the ongoing interaction process between persons, and then study them.

In doing this we have come to learn that it is very difficult to identify individually the voices of a large number of persons when they do participate in the type of deliberation which characterizes a jury deliberation.

MR. SOURWINE: How did you solve that problem in the jury room in Wichita?

*   *   *

MR. STRODTBECK: In the operation of making the transcription we, by piecing together the information we have, by listening to the way in which they refer to one another by name, identify the seat positions, and list them by numbers 1 through 12 around the table. These numbers are then given names, which are alphabetically discriminated.

The first man's name always begins with A, the last person's name begins with the twelfth letter from A.

In all of our subsequent transcriptions, our identifications of persons are carried out by these pseudonyms, and obviously we have in our files a key which would relate the pseudonyms to the interviewed protocols, so that the full set of information may be collated in our ultimate scientific study.

MR. SOURWINE: So that you do know and would be able to tell actually who the juror was who said a certain thing?

MR. STRODTBECK: Without question.

MR. SOURWINE: Do you see anything wrong in that?

MR. STRODTBECK: No.

MR. SOURWINE: Did you ever have anything to do with securing permission for the placing of these microphones in jury rooms?

MR. STRODTBECK: I definitely did not.

*   *   *

I knew that permission had been received from Mr. Cowger. I did not know that his position was assistant in contrast to some other rank. I did know that he was a representative of the government.

MR. SOURWINE: How did you know that permission had been secured from him?

MR. STRODTBECK: I talked to him personally.

MR. SOURWINE: And what did you say to him?

MR. STRODTBECK: After the trial, we were

particularly interested to find out something of the nature of the problems confronting the government attorney, in a case of the sort that he had engaged in.

The full scientific utilization of this material required that we know something of the strategy for the various acts which are a part of the presentation of the government's case, in an action of this type. He was very helpful in discussing the difficulties of the work and the reasons for his objecting at certain times and not having objected at other times. This was all a part of our investigation.

MR. SOURWINE: Do you mean that you discussed with him the recording of the proceedings of several juries in several different cases?

MR STRODTBECK: I did not discuss with him, at any time, the recordings of any of the deliberations which we had taken. I discussed with him his tactics in the particular case which we had observed, which we subsequently recorded the deliberations of, and which we subsequently interviewed the jurors who had participated in it.

Now, concerning the number of cases, some confusion arose in his testimony, and I believe that I can understand why it was. There were 5 actions involved in the two cases which occurred simultaneously. The 2 cases, in order to simplify the task for the jury, were broken in 2 sets, such that 3 actions occurred in 1 of the cases, and 2 actions in a subsequent case.

Mr. Cowger was very helpful working with Judge Hill to incorporate an experiment of this sort into the two sets of cases.

In one instance, the instructions were sent into the deliberation room, and in the other instance they were not. And, although I have not processed the materials in my own files, I believe that, in one instance, instructions concerning the quotient verdict were given, whereas in other instances the instructions concerning the quotient verdict were not given.

And I believe that this instruction is one which may or may not be given in such cases, in the Kansas jurisdiction.

*   *   *

MR. SOURWINE: These microphones were concealed, were they not?

*   *   *

MR. STRODTBECK: I understand, in keeping with our desire simply to not identify the cases, that it is possible for us to describe that the microphones were placed on the walls and were disguised as a part of the heating apparatus in the room.

MR. SOURWINE: Where were your wires run to your recorder?

MR. STRODTBECK: The deliberation room is immediately above the judge's chamber. The wires were run through the walls into a cloak closet off of the judge's chamber.

MR. SOURWINE: While these proceedings were being recorded, was the recorder attended?

MR. STRODTBECK: No. As soon as a deliberation was begun, we had our materials arranged in such a way that the recorder would run for a long period of time. The judge would admit perhaps one of our representatives to his chambers. They would unlock the closet in which the machine was located. The machine would be started, and then the chambers would be vacated. The person would go upstairs, and the deliberation would begin.

MR. SOURWINE: Then, nobody heard these deliberations?

MR. STRODTBECK: Not at the time they were being recorded, there was no monitoring whatsoever.

*   *   *

MR. SOURWINE: . . . I want to find out if there was any general procedure for editing either the original or the duplicate.

MR. STRODTBECK: No.

MR. SOURWINE: Have all the originals been preserved intact?

MR. STRODTBECK: Yes.

MR. SOURWINE: Have all of the so-called "duplicates" been preserved intact?

MR. STRODTBECK: Oh, yes.

MR. SOURWINE: Did you in some instances make further rerecordings from the duplicates?

MR. STRODTBECK: Yes.

MR. SOURWINE: In how many instances was that done?

MR. STRODTBECK: Just one.

*   *   *

MR. SOURWINE: . . . Will you tell us what security provisions you have been applying to the recordings, the duplicate recordings, the second duplicate recordings played at Estes Park, and the transcriptions and protocols that you have told us about?

MR. STRODTBECK: Yes; I believe I can outline the system in general.

I have treated these materials which come

from our interviews and from the recordings, as if they were confidential materials. By that I mean that whenever they are withdrawn from our files, care is taken to see that the person who withdraws the materials has a limited and specific use to make. The materials which carry identification of places are always separated from those materials which have been masked for the purposes of our subsequent study.

In all instances, our materials are kept under lock, and under conditions of surveillance, which would insure that they would not circulate.

There is one exception to this, and this was a part of the presentation of the Estes Park material. In order to have as realistic as possible a background for the appreciation of the deliberation, the masked protocols of this particular case were made available to Judge Hill who, in turn, permitted them to be read by the two lawyers who made the facts statement prior to the presentation of the deliberation.

MR. SOURWINE: They were lawyers who had had nothing to do previously with the case?

MR. STRODTBECK: That is right—nothing whatsoever.

MR. SOURWINE: And were the protocols shown to them—the protocols which had been edited some?

October 25

MT. STRODTBECK: Exactly.

MR. SOURWINE: So that you could not identify the case?

MR. STRODTBECK: Exactly.

*   *   *

MR. SOURWINE: Are the recordings kept in a safe?

MR. STRODTBECK: No; they are kept in a locked file.

MR. SOURWINE: In your office?

MR. STRODTBECK: Not in my office, but in offices which are a part of my operation.

THE CHAIRMAN: Why did you use the name "Mr. X?"

MR. STRODTBECK: At the Estes Park presentation, and this question is very important, sir, we did not identify the university. We did not identify the locale in which the recordings had been made.

And, in view of the fact that I was completely unknown to members attending the judicial conference, I could appear there, could make this presentation without in any way compromising the security that we have thrown around this entire operation.

THE CHAIRMAN: Why did you use the name "Mr. X?"

MR. STRODTBECK: I did not use the name "Mr. X." Judge Hill, in introducing me, indicated that there was a representative of the project here. And he, jokingly, as an aside, said, "Perhaps we will call him Mr. X," and that name was given to me. I did not use it. . . . The importance of maintaining the security of the location of these materials is an absolute essential for their scientific use. We do not want these materials at any time to become a part of adversary differences between the participants, and the notion of maintaining this security is a part of just standard scientific caution which would be made in using materials of this sort. It would be the same if there were confidential materials from medical records, sir.

*   *   *

MR. SOURWINE: Do you know anything about any plan under consideration at any time by the University of Chicago to record 500 or any other larger number of jury deliberations?

MR. STRODTBECK: I do know this, I have at some point seen a letter—I believe you requested this letter the other day—in which, in the original negotiations between Mr. Kitch and Judge Phillips, the reference to some number of observations was made. I do know that that letter occurred probably in November of 1953.

This particular project came to my attention and began to have serious consideration by our research staff after January 1954. As soon as this more serious consideration by our research staff began, it then became apparent that unless we had an observer present to see the trial and unless we take pains to interview all 12 of the jurors, then it would not be possible to make the full scientific exploitation of the recording.

As soon as this was clear, the notion of any large number of transcriptions of actual deliberations was obviously and physically impossible. And so I am certain that at no time since my own active participation in this project has the notion been present among any of our research staff that anything more than a very limited number of recordings would be made.

You can appreciate that, given the interviews with 12 jurors, given the text of the deliberation, given a digest of the trial, you have there, by the time this is synthesized and written out, more than enough for a regular-sized volume, and it is impossible to digest and assimilate more than a very, very small number of such sets of empirical materials.

*　　*　　*

e.
Testimony of Paul Richard Kitch, Esq., Wichita, Kansas—October 13, 1955

SENATOR JENNER: Will you state for the record your full name?

MR. KITCH: My full name is Paul Richard Kitch.

SENATOR JENNER: And your business or profession?

MR. KITCH: I am a lawyer.

SENATOR JENNER: Where do you reside, sir?

MR. KITCH: I reside at Wichita, Kans.

*　　*　　*

MR. SOURWINE: Are you connected in any way with the University of Chicago?

MR. KITCH: I am not, other than that I am a graduate of the university, if that constitutes a connection, of which I am very proud.

MR. SOURWINE: Have you ever been employed by the University of Chicago?

MR. KITCH: I have never been employed by the University of Chicago except in the capacity of a waiter, if I may be frank about it.

MR. SOURWINE: Have you, sir, ever acted for the University of Chicago?

MR. KITCH: I have acted only in a way you would have to let me explain because there are factors involved in it.

In looking back over the correspondence, I understand why you talk about my being an agent for the university.

This matter originated with a bar committee. The original idea was our idea, and I happened to be interested enough, as a fellow who went to Chicago, having heard that they had funds available, to see the project.

MR. SOURWINE: What was that bar committee, Mr. Kitch?

MR. KITCH: It started off originally as a public relations committee of the Wichita Bar Association. . . .

*　　*　　*

There had appeared a series of articles in the local paper written, ghost written, at least, for several well-known trial attorneys in the country, in which the feature of these articles was the tricks which these attorneys used from time to time, as though the trial of a lawsuit before a jury were a matter of trickery, and that the litigant who eventually won the lawsuit was the man who was able to hire a lawyer that could outtrick the jury.

MR. SOURWINE: Where did you say this appeared?

MR. KITCH: This appeared in a local Wichita paper, and as to which one, it is my recollection it was the *Wichita Beacon*. That is what precipitated the meeting of the public relations committee.

*　　*　　*

[T]he upshot of this committee action was the fact that, if there could be some way to combat this kind of publicity, to tell the American public how good the jury system was, instead of how bad it was, that it would be a fine thing, and that was the origin and nucleus of this particular survey.

That led up to this proposition. Mr. Stanley first took it up with some persons on the university staff—as to who, I do not know—at least, the dean reported to me that he had taken up the idea and suggested that I come up and talk about it. And I came up, and I talked to Mr. Levi.

He was a classmate of mine. And I told Mr. Levi that here was an opportunity to do some practical research where the definite advantage that would come from it could be pinpointed, in a practical utility to the profession, instead of dealing with my old criticism of law professors of getting unreal and theoretical, that here was a chance to sink their teeth into something.

He was very reluctant. In fairness to Ed, I have to say that I sold Ed on the possibilities, and this public relations committee sold him on the possibilities.

To get out from under any commitment on it, he said, "Well, I can see that it has got merit," but he said, "How are you going to get permission to do this sort of thing?"

He passed the buck back on that. I was ready. I said, "The bar association will back me on it, and I will guarantee to you that we will find judges in Kansas who will give you this kind of consent."

The next thing I knew, one of the staff members wrote me and said that if we could get the consent, they would be interested.

Now, there were numerous negotiations.

This was not a one-letter proposition or an overnight proposition or a one-day proposition. I talked to numerous of the trial lawyers in Wichita about it. The nucleus of the bar in Wichita has been solidly behind this. There has been no secretiveness about it. It has simply been information that has been kept by the profession.

MR. SOURWINE: You mean the bar of Wichita generally was consulted about the recording of jury deliberations?

MR. KITCH: Well, that portion of the bar of Wichita that engages in trial practice to any extent at all were all consulted, with the mass effort originating there.

MR. SOURWINE: You consulted every trial lawyer in Wichita?

MR. KITCH: I would not make that broad a statement, of every trial lawyer, because I know some fellows that may think they are trial lawyers, and I may not think they were.

MR. SOURWINE: That is why I asked the question, because I think your previous statement made it pretty clear that you had consulted everyone who participated in trial work at all. That would mean all trial lawyers.

MR. KITCH: Well, in any substantial amount. Let us say that.

MR. SOURWINE: I thought that was what it was.

MR. KITCH: Yes, that is what I mean by it. Now, that is where it started.

MR. SOURWINE: Did they know how many cases had been recorded?

MR. KITCH: Well, now, you understand, none had been recorded at the time I am talking about. We were talking about getting an opportunity to get somebody to finance this project for us.

MR. SOURWINE: You said it has been common knowledge in Wichita. Do the substantial trial lawyers in Wichita all know now that it was done?

MR. KITCH: Oh, yes.

MR. SOURWINE: Did they know before it broke in the newspapers?

MR. KITCH: Yes. That is what I am telling you.

MR. SOURWINE: Did they know in how many cases it was recorded?

MR. KITCH: They would not know the exact number, and I did not, either, because once we set it up—

MR. SOURWINE: Did they know the project had been ended?

MR. KITCH: Had been ended?

MR. SOURWINE: Yes; that there would be no more recordings.

MR. KITCH: No, because we still hope there will be.

MR. SOURWINE: All right. Go ahead.

MR. KITCH: And I will make clear on that point that, for a minute, I am not receding from the desire of the bar, and I may say it is now the 10th circuit. I think I can speak for the great majority of the trial lawyers in the 10th circuit, that we want this carried on.

Now, as to any specific number, we do not profess to be experts in research, but we want it done in a sufficient number of cases that it can be said to be a fair sampling of what the jury system actually can accomplish.

MR. SOURWINE: How many cases would that take?

MR. KITCH: In my opinion, it would take a minimum of 100 cases. I do not think you can sample six jury deliberations and arrive at any final conclusion, and I do not think you do, either. I think you would criticize a study that was based on the six juries.

Now, there is one more conclusion about this agency matter that I have got to get in here, because, having taken this up, not only with Judge Phillips but with several others of the circuit judges who expressed enthusiasm, and, from your experience with the bar, you know what trouble you get into if you ever have an idea— the next thing you do is, someone else has an idea by which you work for them.

Judge Phillips came up with the idea that while we were waiting on this, instead of waiting, we had better get to work. And the next thing I knew, and before this project, the recording project got under way, I was heading up the 10th circuit committee for a study of the jury system then and there, which resulted in sending out rather extensive questionnaires to 1,400 jurors, every juror who had served in the circuit during the past year, and then putting those results together in order to report to the judicial conference.

That report was printed. But when you start pinning my expressions of opinion down to Mr. Levi or to Judge Phillips, you have got me in so many different capacities that at any given moment, very frankly, I don't know—I mean, it would be unfair to reflect my opinion at any time to those gentlemen or to put my words in their mouths if you get the point.

*   *   *

Now, yesterday, the question was asked by the Senator. He said, "Well, now, do you know of any immediate threat to the jury system?"

Naturally we do not know of any immediate threat to the jury system. But if you will study the figures, you will find that institutions do not die by some sudden attack. They die by the gradual lack of confidence, the gradual lack of appreciation, the very thing I am talking about—these newspaper articles, that there is always trickery.

They lose confidence in it, and you have to offset that. And to document that, in this very survey that I am talking about, not conducted by the law school, but conducted by our committee, the surprising thing that we find in there, and not having it with me today I do not want to quote the exact figure, but somewhere from 30 to 40 percent of those jurors who filled out that questionnaire reported that if they themselves were involved in litigation, they would prefer to have their cases tried through the judges.

Fifty years ago, if you had put that kind of questionnaire out, you gentlemen know yourselves what kind of response you would have gotten, because at that time the confidence in the jury system was more dominant, and our Constitution was aimed at the fact of preserving that right.

And here you have got a substantial number of jurors that have come in and experienced their service in the courts and they go out and they say next, "If I have litigation of my own, I prefer to have the judge try it."

So we cannot deal up high. We have got to get down to these concrete problems of the profession to make this jury trial so that it actually accomplishes for the jury system what I might say the Federal rules have accomplished for Federal procedure.

That is the best analogy that I know of.

*   *   *

[W]ith 1 or 2 exceptions, every judge that first heard it was violently opposed to it. They would say, "Why, we can't possibly do that." And with one exception, every judge that I have presented it to since, after study, changed their minds and have given tentative approval to it.

To get the background of this, I want you —I mean, you were talking about legislation about it. I would like to have you come out to the 10th circuit, and not talk just to one judge, but talk to every judge in the 10th circuit about it.

*   *   *

MR. SOURWINE: Mr. Kitch, you stated quite clearly and quite convincingly your own purpose in all this as being to defend and improve the jury system. Are you quite sure that the project as undertaken and carried out by the University of Chicago and as financed by the Ford Foundation has exactly the same purpose and not others?

MR. KITCH: I am 100 percent convinced of that, and I have seen these boys every day work on it. There is no question in the world in my mind about that.

MR. SOURWINE: You have worked with them closely on this matter all the time?

MR. KITCH: When I say I have worked with them closely, I have kept in contact, and the boys that have come down in Wichita, for instance, I have tried to make some effort to see that they were entertained and some kind of attention given to them from the graduates of the school.

*   *   *

MR. SOURWINE: Now, did you have anything to do with the preparation of any presentation made by the university or in their behalf to the Ford Foundation seeking additional funds for this project?

MR. KITCH: No, not at any time; I never had any participation in that.

MR. SOURWINE: Did you ever have any contact, directly or indirectly, with the Ford Foundation about this project?

MR. KITCH: None whatever, and I know generalities only, what I read in the paper.

MR. SOURWINE: Now, when you went out to secure permission for the project—and you did that, did you?

MR. KITCH: Yes; I did.

MR. SOURWINE: Did you do that with the understanding you were seeking this permission for the University of Chicago?

MR. KITCH: No; I didn't, I did it—the idea I was going to prove to them was it could be done.

MR. SOURWINE: Now, did you understand that if you got their permission, that they would do it?

MR. KITCH: Not with any finality.

MR. SOURWINE: Had they told you that if they got the permission they would go ahead?

MR. KITCH: No, after I got—you could check the lapse of time, there was still quite a problem, and I had had considerable trouble getting them to move. . . .

* * *

MR. SOURWINE: Have you been connected in an attorney-client relationship in a case in which the proceedings of a jury were recorded?

MR. KITCH: My firm was counsel in one of the particular cases. I didn't—the fact of the matter is, I didn't know about it at the moment, but one of the men in the office reported to me that he had been requested to give his consent and he had given it.

MR. SOURWINE: You say you didn't know at the time?

MR. KITCH: That it was going to be recorded?

MR. SOURWINE: You did not know at the time your firm was connected with that case?

MR. KITCH: Well, I didn't know what cases were going to be recorded. Once the project was set up, I stayed clear away from it.

MR. SOURWINE: Are you presently connected in an attorney-client relationship with any of the cases in which the jury deliberations were recorded?

MR. KITCH: Well, yes, we still, the case—I don't know whether it is on appeal before the circuit court or not, but I was—my firm represented the plaintiff in the case.

MR. SOURWINE: Does the question of the jury's deliberations having been recorded have any place in the appeal procedure in that case?

MR. KITCH: In the what—appeal procedure?

MR. SOURWINE: Appeal procedure, yes.

MR. KITCH: No.

MR. SOURWINE: Was that fact mentioned at all in the appeal?

MR. KITCH: None whatever.

MR. SOURWINE: It was not disclosed?

MR. KITCH: Well, now, wait a minute. What fact mentioned—that I was connected with the case?

MR. SOURWINE: No, the fact that the jury in that case had its deliberations—

MR. KITCH: No.

MR. SOURWINE: (continuing): Listened in upon?

MR. KITCH: No. The circuit court wouldn't know that.

MR. SOURWINE: Does the client of either counsel in that case, as far as you know, know that?

MR. KITCH: You had Mr. Green yesterday.

I did not ask him whether he had taken it up with his counsel or not. I talked with him briefly—

MR. SOURWINE: Were you his adversary in that case?

MR. KITCH: Yes. Of course, I, a while ago, inadvertently identified one case. I am sorry I have not hid that, but as long as—

MR. SOURWINE: Do you know if he has advised his client that was the case?

MR. KITCH: No, I don't know, but Mr. Newkirk told me he had taken it up with his clients.

MR. SOURWINE: He did take it up with his client?

MR. KITCH: Or, my client—don't get me wrong—it is the firm's clients—

MR. SOURWINE: Well, but it is your firm's client; he doesn't know about it?

M. KITCH: That is right. The point I want to make is that Don Newkirk is a member of my firm. I wasn't trying to create the impression I was in any way trying to shift it over to him.

MR. SOURWINE: Was there any understanding in connection with the permission granted for this project on the question of whether clients would be advised with respect to the recording of the jury's deliberations?

MR. KITCH: No, there was not.

MR. SOURWINE: That was left in each case to the discretion of counsel?

MR. KITCH: That is—I assume so, because I did not cover that on the proposed rule—

MR. SOURWINE: Counsel were not cautioned to keep this confidential?

MR. KITCH: Oh, yes; they were cautioned to keep this confidential.

MR. SOURWINE: Well, would keeping it confidential permit them to tell their clients?

MR. KITCH: Yes, it would. There is no such thing as matters—I mean, I have never heard of a matter between an attorney and a client that was confidential.

MR. SOURWINE: Did you hear the testimony this morning of Mr. Mikva, that in his opinion if a client did not know that counsel had agreed to the recording of the jury's deliberations, and subsequently learned it he would, nevertheless, be bound by the attorney's waiver and would not be able to secure any—

MR. KITCH: I heard that.

MR. SOURWINE: Would you agree with that?

MR. KITCH: Definitely.

MR. SOURWINE: Do you think that counsel

could foreclose the client from his rights in a case like that?

MR. KITCH: Definitely.

MR. SOURWINE: I take it you do not think that agreement in any way constitutes improper conduct by counsel.

MR. KITCH: None whatever.

MR. SOURWINE: You think that the right of the client to free and full and unfettered deliberation in the jury room is a right that counsel may waive, and he can do that without his client's consent and without his knowledge, without constituting misconduct on the part of counsel?

MR. KITCH: I do.

Of course, you have stated that in an argumentative way. Counsel can waive jury, and I can give you all kinds of cases on it, and once counsel waives the jury, he gives away a right entirely, and there is no recourse merely because he did not consult the client; the law is very clear on that. I am talking about civil cases—you understand, there is a difference between criminal and civil.

*　　*　　*

MR. SOURWINE: Is there any connection between this project for recording the deliberations of juries and any project you know of approved by the bar association, relating to it?

MR. KITCH: Yes; there is a connection.

MR. SOURWINE: What is the connection?

MR. KITCH: You have got various bar groups that want to be kept informed on the progress, as to whether you are able to do it, make advances in it—

MR. SOURWINE: You mean, there are varied bar groups that know of this project for recording proceedings of juries?

MR. KITCH: Well, I wouldn't want to go quite so strong—

MR. SOURWINE: Well, your answer, sir, was—

MR. KITCH: The judicial section of the American Bar is quite familiar—that is the one that asked to be kept advised as we went along.

Now, when you talk about a bar group, the Tenth Circuit Judicial Conference is very definitely a bar group, and they are quite interested in these results and they do know about it.

In addition to that, we have a rather semipermanent committee called the jury study committee of the tenth circuit, in which I am involved and all of those members are very interested in knowing, at the appropriate time,

whether we have made progress and what they can do to help carry it on.

*　　*　　*

MR. SOURWINE: All right, sir.

I have no further questions.

MR. KITCH: Mr. Chairman, may I make a statement to explain background on the Estes Park—I think I can do it in a limited time, I mean, that has come into this hearing—

THE CHAIRMAN: Oh, sure.

MR. KITCH: We have not covered it, and a lot of responsible names have been involved.

I would like to state briefly that the origin of the Estes Park meetings arrived by reason of the fact that under the statute the Federal judges—

THE CHAIRMAN: Now, what judges?

MR. KITCH: All right—can't I just—I think I could save time if I could, if I could get off one point and then if you direct me, I will stop and start over—I mean, if you want me to start that way, I will.

THE CHAIRMAN: Well, go ahead.

MR. KITCH: A judicial conference is required by statute once a year, at which time you meet and consider ways and means of improving the administration of justice. That is just the background of it.

Judge Phillips, knowing about this project, asked me if—last summer, the request came here ahead of the meeting—if I could not get this research group to demonstrate the recording for the meeting the following summer, to pick out one of the recordings made and show the safeguards that we used and show the method of editing and then show the results that could be obtained and then let the judges discuss the whole project, the whole recording project.

I told him that I would endeavor to do so. I took that up with Dean Levi and he objected to it on the grounds he thought it was premature, that it would interfere with the research nature of the project.

I told Judge Levi—Dean Levi—that it put me in a very bad position, that if we had the cooperation of the 10th circuit and if they wanted this program for the purpose, that he was not in any position to deny it and he finally said that what he would do would be what Judge Phillips requested, that he would release an edited recording for the program but that he would have no connection with it whatever.

I went up there—runs in my mind in May,

because the program was scheduled in June, to see definitely that the prepared recording would be suitable for playing here—I mean, to be heard, and at that time they played it for me and I heard the edited version of this tape; it had been reduced to 30 minutes.

I heard it in a small room and it sounded adequate and so we put on the program.

* *

f.

Testimony of Irving Ferman, Washington Office Director, American Civil Liberties Union—October 13, 1955

MR. SOURWINE: Your full name, sir, your business or profession, and your address, please?

MR. FERMAN: My name is Irving Ferman. I speak in behalf of the American Civil Liberties Union as its Washington, D.C., director. I am also a member of the bar of the State of Louisiana.

* * *

The union is a private organization devoted to the preservation of our personal liberty. Accordingly, we are vitally interested in the matter before this committee today.

At this point I wish to emphasize my appreciation for what the lawyers and social scientists in Chicago are trying to do in bringing greater understanding to the functioning of our legal institutions.

* * *

The right to jury trial is a right immemorial to freedom. Upon it rests much of our Anglo-American judicial traditions. This right is firmly established in our Constitution in article III and the sixth and seventh amendments to the Constitution.

A basic distinction between our free society and the totalitarian societies of communism and fascism is the independence with which our society guards its judicial system.

* * *

Justice William O. Douglas in his *Almanac of Liberty* expresses the essential character of the jury as follows:

A jury reflects the attitudes and mores of the community from which it is drawn. It lives only for the day and it does justice according to its light. The groups of 12 who are drawn to hear a case make the decision and melt away. It is not present the next day to be criticized. It is the one governmental agency that has no ambition. To preserve this kind of status for our jury system, it is essential that we keep completely private what transpires in a jury room during the deliberative stage.

The fact that no coercion of a jury took place in the instant case at hand is of no significance. The fact that consent was obtained to the jury bugging from counsel of both sides as well as the court is of no significance, and, further, the fact that the present law, in a good number of jurisdictions, does not recognize merely communication with the jury even during a deliberation as presumption of improper influencing of a jury verdict is of no significance.

The fact is that the right to jury trial must mean all that it can possibly mean. This should involve the greatest assurance that the jury's impartiality will be protected from any kind of surveillance, embarrassment, or possibility of coercion.

When consent was obtained by the judge as well as counsel, little litigious opportunity was left for objections to be properly raised. Thus out of this consensual relation, there evolved the public policy limiting the secrecy of the jury room, and thus derogating from the basic fundamental right of a jury trial.

In short, any action which tends to establish even a climate injurious to the preservation of a particular personal right guaranteed by our Constitution must be challenged. To suggest the fact that a particular individual in a given situation has not been harmed is completely irrelevant, and likewise irrelevant is the fact that possible harm from future infringements resulting from practices of this kind may be outweighed by the good that could come from such practices.

We plead today that the jury room remain tightly closed forever.

MR. SOURWINE: Mr. Ferman, is there any question in your mind but that the right of jury trial guaranteed by the seventh amendment encompasses all of the attributes of a jury trial known at the time the amendment was written?

MR. FERMAN: There is no doubt in my mind.

MR. SOURWINE: Have you made any researches to determine what the attributes of a jury trial were at that time?

MR. FERMAN: No, I have not specifically.

* * *

THE CHAIRMAN: [I]s it your judgment that the judge in this case, Judge Hill, who permitted that, did not perform his duty?

MR. FERMAN: Well, Mr. Chairman, you could appreciate my feelings as a member of the bar in criticizing a gentleman on the bench.

THE CHAIRMAN: I know how we feel about criticizing judges. But—

MR. FERMAN: I think that I could appreciate the motivation of a judge and his interest in experimentation that might lead to an improvement of the jury system, but I think, on the other hand, that the duty to have remain private jury deliberations should have prevailed.

THE CHAIRMAN: Do you not think it was his duty to prohibit the bugging of these juries?

MR. FERMAN: Yes; I do.

* * *

NOTES

NOTE 1.

STATEMENT BY CHIEF JUDGE ORIE L. PHILLIPS, JUDGE DELMAS C. HILL, AND DEAN EDWARD H. LEVI—OCTOBER 25, 1955

Because certain statements have appeared in the public press with respect to the recording of the deliberations of juries in six cases in the United States district court at Wichita, Kans., which are inaccurate and misleading, Orie L. Phillips, chief judge of the Court of Appeals for the 10th Judicial Circuit, Delmas C. Hill, judge of the United States District Court for the District of Kansas, and Edward H. Levi, dean of the University of Chicago Law School, have prepared the following statement, which statement reflects the pertinent facts:

* * *

Early in February 1954, Mr. Kitch discussed with Judge Phillips the waiver of the condition that the jury be informed. Judge Phillips stated that he still was of the opinion the jurors should be informed, but that he might not object if the experiment were restricted to a limited number of cases. Thereafter, Mr. Kitch informed Judge Hill of this conversation had with Judge Phillips. On February 12, 1954, while Judge Hill was sitting in the Colorado district, he discussed the matter with Judge Phillips. Judge Phillips reiterated that he thought the recording should not be made without the

knowledge of the jurors. Judge Hill replied that Mr. Kitch was not willing to adopt the suggestion Judge Phillips had made in his letter because he thought informing the jurors might interfere with the freedom of their deliberations. Judge Hill asked Judge Phillips if he would object if a few cases were recorded following the procedures that Mr. Kitch had set forth in the rules, but without prior communication to the jurors. Judge Phillips replied that while he still adhered to the opinion the jurors should be informed, he would not object to it being tried out on an experimental basis in a limited number of cases.

* * *

In August 1954, in a conversation with Judge Phillips, Judge Hill again affirmed what he had said in July 1954. Judge Phillips stated that if any requests were made to make further recordings in the 10th circuit, it was his intention to present such requests to the Judicial Council of the Court of Appeals of the Tenth Circuit, composed of the five circuit judges, for full and careful consideration. No further requests for permission were made and no further recordings were made.

The recording of a limited number of actual jury deliberations was undertaken as an experiment in a serious manner to further an important study of a basic legal institution with the objective of strengthening and improving the jury system, and with a purpose to observe essential safeguards to protect the jurors and litigants from injury.

* * *

NOTE 2.

LETTER FROM CHIEF JUDGE ORIE L. PHILLIPS TO SENATOR JAMES O. EASTLAND— OCTOBER 27, 1955

* * *

As chief judge of the Court of Appeals of the 10th Circuit, I have no supervisory powers over district judges or district courts, except the power to assign a district judge to sit in the court of appeals, in a district other than his own in the 10th circuit, and in statutory three-judge courts.

Such supervisory powers as exist are vested in the Judicial Council of the circuit, composed of the five circuit judges. Accordingly, I conceived that I could only express my opinion and give advice. I certainly had no power officially to authorize that a recording be made or direct that it not be made.

The reasons I took and adhered to the position that the jurors involved should be advised in advance that the recording was to be made were twofold:

1. I felt that if the recordings were made, especially on the scale originally planned but not carried out, the fact that recordings were being made would inevitably become known to the public, but that the limitations and safeguards to be observed would in all probability not be fully known or understood by the general public.

As a result, future jurors might enter the jury room to deliberate on their verdict conscious of the fact that a recording might be made of the deliberations, but without any real understanding of the limited purpose for which the recording would be used and the abridgments that would be made thereof; and that such fact might inhibit full and frank discussion in the jury room.

On the other hand, if such jurors knew that such recordings were only made when that fact was made known to the jurors in advance of the making, they would not fear that such a recording might be made of their deliberations, and they would not thus be inhibited.

2. The second reason is based on what I conceive to be fair and decent.

While a recording of the jury's deliberations in a particular case, wholly unknown to the jurors, would not affect their deliberations or their verdict in that particular case, it seems to me that when jurors enter the jury room to deliberate on their verdict, rightfully believing that their deliberations and discussions will be effectively closed to any outside ears, that it would be grossly unfair to permit a recording to be made of their deliberations, even if made for what is believed to be for a worthy and useful purpose.

*   *   *

After the experimental recordings had been completed in the Federal district court at Wichita, Judge Hill and I reached a firm understanding that no further recordings would be permitted in that court.

By that time I had reached the conclusion that if any further requests were made for permission to make recordings in the courts of the 10th circuit, I would ask that matter be sub-

mitted to the Judicial Council of the circuit, with the request that it give the matter careful consideration and take such action as it deemed appropriate. I regret that I did not follow that course in the first instance. Hindsight is better sometimes than foresight. However, no requests have been made and no further recordings have been made in the 10th circuit.

I did not suggest the program that was put on at Estes Park in July 1955. Mr. Kitch's committee had participated in the program on another phase of the jury study at the Judicial Conference of the circuit in July 1954. It was well received and highly commended. When I came to prepare the program for the 1955 Conference, I asked Mr. Kitch if he desired to have his committee participate in the program. I definitely did not have the recordings in mind. However, Mr. Kitch suggested the presentation of a portion of one of the recordings and the building of a program around it. I told him it would be all right, providing the portion of the recording produced had been cut so as to render it wholly impersonal, and if the procedures followed in the making of the recording were fully stated. Mr. Kitch prepared the program and directed its presentation.

May I add that I have a high regard for Judge Hill. I am sure that it was his desire to proceed with the experiment cautiously and not to do anything that would injure litigants, the jurors involved, or the jury system, and that he was actuated by a desire to make a worthwhile contribution to the study being carried out by the law school of the University of Chicago. Moreover, he limited the recordings in his court to six cases.

*   *   *

2.

Congress Decides

Eighty-Fourth Congress, Second Session
An Act to Further Protect and Assure the
Privacy of Grand and Petit
Juries in the Courts of the United States
While such Juries are Deliberating or Voting*

*   *   *

Whoever knowingly and willfully, by any means or device whatsoever—

* Act of August 2, 1956, Ch. 879, §1, 70 Stat. 935; see 18 U.S.C. §1508 (1964).

(a) records, or attempts to record, the proceedings of any grand or petit jury in any court of the United States while such jury is deliberating or voting; or

(b) listens to or observes, or attempts to listen to or observe, the proceedings of any grand or petit jury of which he is not a member in any court of the United States while such jury is deliberating or voting—

shall be fined not more than $1,000 or imprisoned not more than one year or both.

*　*　*

NOTES

NOTE 1.

WALDO W. BURCHARD
LAWYERS, POLITICAL SCIENTISTS, SOCIOLOGISTS—
AND CONCEALED MICROPHONES*

*　*　*

. . . The fact that the persons who made the recordings were competent social scientists pursuing a serious study of an important American institution appeared to make no difference to the critics.

The attitudes of these critics reflect a basic distrust of social science and social scientists that should be of concern to persons in the field, and particularly to sociologists, who engage more extensively in research making use of techniques of this type than most other social scientists. If social research is to continue, it must have public support, which means, in part, that it must have newspaper support. The fact that the adverse criticism of editors and commentators went almost entirely unanswered in the public press[4] probably means that social scientists have not yet found an effective way of convincing the public and perhaps more important, the moulders of popular opinion of the propriety, utility, and most of all, the sincerity of their efforts. The fact that nearly three months elapsed between the playing of the recordings and the public announcement of the event implies that those members of the legal profession who heard

the records were not overly disturbed by them. . . .

*　*　*

NOTE 2.

TED R. VAUGHAN
GOVERNMENTAL INTERVENTON IN SOCIAL
RESEARCH—POLITICAL AND ETHICAL
DIMENSIONS IN THE WICHITA JURY RECORDINGS*

*　*　*

The failure to accomplish satisfactorily the stated objectives of the Hearings seems to lie in the political and ethical orientations of the Subcommittee members themselves. A principal purpose, closely related to the failure to see the objectives and its accomplishments was the initial failure to view the issue problematically. To the Subcommittee members, unaccustomed as they were to seeing things in the relative terms of science, the case presented no problem in the sense of an issue to be resolved. The only problem was that project members had violated a set of norms, and a set assumed by the senators to be superordinate to all others. And that problem could be satisfactorily solved through chastising the errant researchers and erecting obstacles to its recurrence.

*　*　*

A second source of the Hearings' shift in purpose, closely related to the failure to see the issue as problematical, was the failure to differentiate between scientific inquiry directed toward the acquisition of knowledge and nonscientific investigation of or intervention in the jury process. Committed as the Subcommittee members were to the supremacy of one set of values and norms, they could see no need for making such a distinction. They failed to consider that science is itself a system of norms with the same claims to legitimacy as other normative systems. It is true that the norms of science are not always apparent to those engaged in scientific pursuits, much less to laymen. But to assume that scientific objectives are "naturally" subordinate to other normative systems and values is to beg the crucial question.

*　*　*

The result of this failure to discriminate

* 23 *American Sociological Review* 686, 687 (1958). Reprinted by permission.

4. Members of the research team, of course, defended their actions before the Senate subcommittee, in interviews, in speeches, and in articles. At least one popular newspaper columnist, Fred Othman, had a good word to say for the use of concealed microphones. Nonetheless, the overwhelming bulk of commentary was unfavorable.

* Gideon Sjoberg, ed.: *Ethics, Politics and Social Research.* Cambridge, Mass.: Shenkman Publishing Co. 50, 60–75 (1967). Reprinted by permission.

between scientific and nonscientific investigations of the jury system was that the scientific position did not receive a fair hearing. All the potential disadvantages and possible abuses of nonscientific intrusion on the deliberative process were assumed to hold for scientific research as well. If this position were consistently taken by political authorities, a considerable amount of current social science research would be terminated.

The third source of the Subcommittee's failure to achieve its stated objectives is a natural consequence of the preceding ones. The one possibly legitimate role representatives of the state could have in the research process would be that of mediating between conflicting systems of values and norms. Not only did the Subcommittee fail in this respect, the members did not even entertain such a role as a legitimate possibility. Although the entire Hearing operated behind the facade of concern for the privacy of jurors while deliberating a case, every indication was that this was not the major concern. The Subcommittee failed to treat the matter either as an ethical concern or as a political problem in institutional relations. Certainly, the matter was not fully anticipated in the ambiguous legal traditions the Senators apparently thought they were defending.

*   *   *

The fact that political intervention in social research is a paramount issue here should not obscure the significance of the ethical dimension of the case. In this particular case, as is true of much research, political and ethical questions are intertwined in a very complex manner. . . .

. . . We neither posit simple solutions nor attempt to establish a code of ethics for scientists. We do, however, question some of the solutions that have been utilized in similar circumstances. To posit a hierarchy of values, for example, and then operate exclusively on that basis is to be unrealistic about the issue. To argue that in the final analysis one's conscience should be his guide is hardly any better, because one's decision is inevitably based on a pre-existing value system. . . .

The arguments in defense of unrestricted freedom of scientific inquiry are fairly well known to the social scientist, if only because they receive some prominence in textbooks on methodology. . . .

The immediate issue, of course, is the freedom of the scientist to investigate on-going ac-

tivities of an operating jury without pressure, constraint, or control by nonscientific agencies. Justification of this action is usually predicated on the broader norm that there should be unrestricted freedom of scientific inquiry, a norm which, in turn, rests on the value premise that men have the inherent right to know, i.e., that knowledge is always superior to ignorance and that nothing external to the object of investigation itself should influence the acquisition of knowledge. If knowledge is a value, any other circumstance which endangers its achievement, or influences its outcome in any way, is undesirable. The scientific enterprise cannot make significant advances without maximal freedom from external control. The pernicious effects of the intrusion of the special interests of political, religious, or other groups into the research process are well documented in the literature. Scientists could and should oppose actual or potential attempts by nonscientific interests to control or influence social research.

More specifically, the conventional textbook view would have it that investigation of the actual operations of the jury system, or any other basic social institution, is justified by the value of knowledge itself. It is better to know about the workings of the jury system than not to know. The same legitimacy that attaches to knowledge in a general sense legitimates the quest for knowledge in the particular case. From this perspective, the jury system has no special claim to inviolability from scientific investigation. More pragmatically, the investigation can also be legitimated on the grounds that any decision to alter or revise an institution such as the jury system should be based on the most accurate, precise information available. Such information would be available only through direct inquiry into the mechanisms of jury operations. . . . And scientific investigation poses no real threat to the integrity of the jury system because the scientist is not concerned with the action of individual jurors, only with patterns of behavior. Data obtained are treated as classes, not as individual attributes. As a professional scientist, furthermore, the social investigator is already bound to a long-standing set of rules that proscribe the revelation of anything that might identify a person and thereby possibly embarrass, harass, or otherwise do him injury or harm.

What such textbook methodology usually ignores is that the scientific ethic (values and norms) is only one in a system of many conflicting, competing ethics making up the social fabric. It tends, instead, to assume there is a hierarchy of ethics with the scientific ethic at the pinnacle. But in actual practice, especially in field research, as the Wichita case reveals, ethical issues are much more problematic. There is no natural law to which the scientist can appeal. Like others, he bases his decisions on personal predilections and particular values. But one person's predilections—be he scientist or saint—are not perforce more natural than another's. The proclivity among scientists to minimize, if not ignore, competing social ethics, and to define science in some independent sense, is quite widespread. In short, the scientist typically subscribes to the notion that the end of knowledge justifies the scientific means.

Counterposed to the scientific ethic are the values and norms of the judicial process. Advocates of this position contend that no circumstances justify the invasion of the traditional privacy and confidence of jury deliberations, for, normatively, there should be inviolable privacy of such deliberations. . . . Anything that undermines in any way the impartial nature of the jury should not be permitted. And, the argument continues, the jurors' impartiality is influenced by the actual or possible invasion of the jury room irrespective of the purpose. Any actual or potential surveillance undermines impartiality because it raises the possibility of considerations extraneous to the merits of the case itself. Obviously, impartiality is threatened if there are attempts to influence the verdict. Even if scientific investigation is not directed toward influencing verdicts, it still threatens impartiality to the extent that it introduces any question of possible embarrassment, coercion, or other such considerations into the minds of actual jurors. A jury is impartial to the extent that nothing but the consciences of the individual jurors influence its decision. Even if anonymity is assured or the members are unaware of immediate surveillance, impartiality is threatened unless the norm of inviolable privacy prevails. In terms of this principle, the matter of safeguards in scientific research is largely irrelevant. To protect the opportunity for an impartial and just verdict, secret deliberations must be preserved regardless of the ultimate value that might result from the scientific investigation of the jury system. . . .

* * *

Our own present position is that if certain general principles are accepted, the conflict of ethics neither poses a hopeless dilemma nor re-

stricts action to the alternative responses already reviewed. These basic premises include the denial of a natural ordering of ethics and the affirmation that the merits of the individual case determine the ascendancy of particular ethics for that particular case. If the assumption is granted that science is a part of the social system, an institution with values and norms not inherently superior to others, then ethical conflicts are inevitable. And they cannot satisfactorily be ignored, avoided, or suppressed.

To re-emphasize the need for a self-conscious sense of ethical responsibility in social research, we can conclude by very briefly indicating two general procedures which should be included in decision-making by social science researchers. First, a self-conscious and serious sense of reflection is needed, including detailed awareness and consideration of the points of view of respondents or other participants. Genuine understanding of another's point of view, including the basic values upon which his argument rests, may, of course, convince one completely of the merits of one's own position. But the decision is made on the basis of comparison not abstraction. Simply to assert scientific prerogatives as abstractions is to attempt an easy solution to a difficult problem. When contradictory positions are thoroughly understood, a decision can be based on the merits of the case. Such understanding need not necessarily alter research objectives, although this may well be the case, but it may force a reconsideration of means. Such a reassessment may necessitate more creative, innovative research procedure.

* * *

NOTE 3.

REGINALD ROSE
TWELVE ANGRY MEN*

[The setting is a jury room in New York City.]

* * *

#4: I think it's customary to take a preliminary vote.

#7: Yeah, let's vote, Who knows, maybe we can all go home.

FOREMAN [*From opposite end of the table.*]: It's up to you. Just let's remember we've

* William I. Kaufman, ed.: *Great Television Plays* 183–191, 196–197, 201–202, 227–228, 232 (1969). Reprinted by permission of International Famous Agency. © 1965 by Reginald Rose.

got a first-degree murder charger here. If we vote guilty, we send the accused to the electric chair. That's mandatory.

#4: I think we all know that.

#3: Come on, let's vote.

#10: Yeah. Let's see who's where.

* * *

FOREMAN: . . . nine . . . ten . . . eleven. That's eleven for guilty. Okay. Not guilty. [#8 *slowly raises his hand.*] One. Right. Okay, eleven to one, guilty. Now we know where we are. [#8 *lowers his hand.*]

#10: Boy-oh-boy. There's always one.

[#8 *doesn't look in his direction.*]

#7: So what do we do now?

#8: Well, I guess we talk.

* * *

#10: All right, then you tell me. What are we sitting here for?

[#8 *looks at him, trying to phrase the following. They wait.*]

#8: Maybe for no reason. I don't know. Look, this boy's been kicked around all his life. You know, living in a slum, his mother dead since he was nine. He spent a year and a half in an orphanage while his father served a jail term for forgery. That's not a very good headstart. He's a wild, angry kid and that's all he's ever been. You know why he got that way? Because he was knocked on the head by somebody once a day, every day. He's had a pretty terrible nineteen years. I think maybe we owe him a few words. That's all. [*He looks around the table, #9 nods slowly.*]

#10: I don't mind telling you this, mister. We don't owe him a thing. He got a fair trial, didn't he? What d'you think that trial cost? He's lucky he got it. [*Turning to #11.*]: Know what I mean? [*Now looking across table at #'s 3, 4, 5.*] Look, we're all grown-ups in here. We heard the facts, didn't we? [*To #8.*] Now you're not going to tell us that we're supposed to believe that kid, knowing what he is. Listen, I've lived among 'em all my life. You can't believe a word they say. You know that. [*To all.*] I mean they're born liars.

* * *

#3: Okay. Now here's what I think, and I have no personal feelings about this. I'm talking about facts. Number one: let's take the old man who lived on the second floor right underneath the room where the murder took place. At ten minutes after twelve on the night of the kill-

ing he heard loud noises in the apartment upstairs. He said it sounded like a fight. Then he heard the kid shout out, "I'm gonna kill you." A second later he heard a body fall, and he ran to the door of his apartment, looked out, and saw the kid running down the stairs and out of the house. Then he called the police. They found the father with a knife in his chest. . . .

FOREMAN: And the coroner fixed the time of death at around midnight.

#3: Right. I mean there are facts for you. You can't refute facts. This boy is guilty. I'm telling you. Look, I'm as sentimental as the next guy. I know the kid is only nineteen, but he's still got to pay for what he did.

* * *

#10 [*Impatiently in #8's direction*]: Listen, what about that woman across the street? If her testimony don't prove it, nothing does.

#11: That's right. She was the one who actually saw the killing.

FOREMAN: Let's go in order here.

[#10 *rises, handkerchief in hand.*]

#10 [*Loudly.*]: Just a minute. Here's a woman . . . [*He blows his nose.*] Here's a woman who's lying in bed and can't sleep. [*He begins to walk around the table, wiping his tender nose and talking.*] She's dying with the heat. Know what I mean? Anyway, she looks out the window and right across the street she sees the kid stick the knife into his father. The time is 12:10 on the nose. Everything fits. Look, she's known the kid all his life. His window is right opposite hers, across the el tracks, and she swore she saw him do it. [#10 *is now standing behind #6 and looking across table at #8. #10 wipes his nose.*]

#8: Through the windows of a passing elevated train.

#10 [*Through the handkerchief.*]: Right. This el train had no passengers on it. It was just being moved downtown. The lights were out, remember? And they proved in court that at night you can look through the windows of an el train when the lights are out and see what's happening on the other side. They proved it!

#8: [*To #10.*]: I'd like to ask you something. You don't believe the boy. How come you believe the woman? She's one of "them" too, isn't she?

[#10 *is suddenly angry.*]

#10: You're a pretty smart fellow, aren't you?

[*He takes a step toward #8. #8 sits calmly*

there. *#10 strides toward #8. The* FOREMAN *rises in his seat. #3 and 5 jump up and move toward #10.*]

FOREMAN [*Nervously.*]: Hey, let's take it easy.

[*#3, 5, and 10 stand behind #7. #3 and 5 have reached #10, who looks angrily at #8. #3 takes #10's arm.*]

#10 [*Angrily.*]: What's he so wise about? I'm telling you . . .

#3 [*Strongly.*]: Come on. Sit down. [*He begins to lead #10 back to his seat.*] What are you letting him get you all upset for? Relax.

* * *

FOREMAN [*To #7.*]: Okay. How about you?

#7: Me? [*He pauses, looks around, shrugs, then speaks.*] I don't know, it's practically all said already. We can talk about it forever. It's the same thing. I mean this kid is five for oh. Look at his record. He was in children's court when he was ten for throwing a rock at his teacher. At fifteen he was in reform school. He stole a car. He's been arrested for mugging. He was picked up twice for knife-fighting. He's real swift with a knife, they said. This is a very fine boy.

#8: Ever since he was five years old his father beat him up regularly. He used his fists.

#7 [*Indignantly.*]: So would I! A kid like that.

[*#3 walks over from the water fountain toward #7. He stands behind #7, talks to #8.*]

#3: And how. It's the kids, the way they are nowadays. Listen, when I was his age I used to call my father "sir." That's right. Sir! You ever hear a boy call his father that anymore?

#8: Fathers don't seem to think it's important any more.

#3: No? Have you got any kids?

#8: Three.

#3: Yeah, well I've got one, a boy twenty-two years old. I'll tell you about him. When he was nine he ran away from a fight. I saw him. I was so ashamed I almost threw up. So I told him right out: "I'm gonna make a man outa you or I'm gonna bust you in half trying." Well, I made a man outa him all right. When he was sixteen we had a battle. He hit me in the face! He's big, y'know. I haven't seen him in two years. Rotten kid. You work your heart out . . . [*He stops. He has said more than he intended and more passionately than he intended it. He is embarrassed. He looks at #8, and then at all of them. Then loud.*] All right. Let's get on with it. [*He turns and walks angrily around the table to

his seat. He sits down. #4 looks at #3 and then across the table.*]

#4: I think we're missing the point here. This boy, let's say he's a product of a filthy neighborhood and a broken home. We can't help that. We're here to decide whether he's guilty or innocent, not to go into the reasons why he grew up this way. He was born in a slum. Slums are breeding grounds for criminals. I know it. So do you. [*#5 reacts to the following.*] It's no secret. Children from slum backgrounds are potential menaces to society. Now, I think . . .

#10: [*Interrupting.*]: Brother, you can say that again. The kids who crawl outa those places are real trash. I don't want any part of them, I'm telling you.

[*The face of #5 is angry. He tries to control himself. His voice shakes.*]

#5: I've lived in a slum all my life . . .

[*#10 knows he has said the wrong thing.*]

#10: Oh, now wait a second . . .

#5 [*Furious.*]: I used to play in a back yard that was filled with garbage. Maybe it still smells on me.

#10 [*Beginning to anger.*]: Now listen, sonny . . .

[FOREMAN *has risen.*]

FOREMAN [*To #5.*]: Now, let's be reasonable There's nothing personal . . .

[*#5 shoots to his feet.*]

#5 [*Loud.*]: There is something personal! [*He looks around at the others, all looking at him. Then, suddenly he has nothing to say. He sits down, fists clenched. #3 gets up and walks to him pats him on the back. #5 doesn't look up.*]

* * *

[*The door opens. The* GUARD *enters carrying a curiously designed knife with a tag hanging from it. #4 walks into the shot and takes the knife from the guard. He turns and moves back to his seat as the* GUARD *exits. He stands behind his seat holding the knife.*]

#4 [*Leaning over to #8*]: Everyone connected with the case identified this knife. Now are you trying to tell me that it really fell through a hole in the boy's pocket and that someone picked it up off the street, went to the boy's house and stabbed his father with it just to be amusing?

#8: No. I'm saying that it's possible that the boy lost the knife, and that someone else stabbed his father with a similar knife. It's possible.

[*#4 flicks open the blade of the knife and

jams it into the table. Jurors #2, 5, 10, 11, 12 get up and crowd around to get a better look at it.]

#4: Take a look at that knife. It's a very unusual knife. I've never seen one like it. Neither had the storekeeper who sold it to the boy. Aren't you trying to make us accept a pretty incredible coincidence?

#8: I'm not trying to make anyone accept it. I'm just saying that it's possible.

[*#3, standing next to #4, is suddenly infuriated at #8's calmness. He leans forward.*]

#3 [*Shouting.*]: And I'm saying it's not possible.

[*#8 stands for a moment in the silence. Then he reaches into his pocket and swiftly withdraws a knife. He holds it in front of his face, and flicks open the blade. Then he leans forward and sticks the knife into the table next to the other. The two ornately carved knives stuck into the table, side by side, are each exactly alike. There is an immediate burst of sound in the room.*] [*Simultaneous*]

#7: What is this?

#6: What is it?

#12: Where'd that come from?

#2: How d'you like that!

[*The jurors cluster around the knives. #8 is standing away from the table, watching. #3 looks up at him.*]

#3 [*Amazed.*]: What are you trying to do?

#10: [*Loud.*]: Yeah! What's going on here? Who do you think you are?

[*#6 has taken the knife out of the table and is holding it.*]

#6: Look at it! It's the same knife!

[*#8 watches them closely, a few steps back from the group. The ad lib hubbub still goes on.*]

#4: Quiet! Let's be quiet!

[*The noise begins to subside. #4 takes the knife from #5's hand and speaks to #8, who stands at left of frame.*]

#4: Where'd you get it?

#8: I was walking for a couple of hours last night, just thinking. I walked through the boy's neighborhood. The knife comes from a little pawnshop three blocks from his house. It cost two dollars.

#4: It's against the law to buy or sell switch-blade knives.

#8: That's right. I broke the law.

*　　*　　*

#3 [*Shouting.*]: . . . Now, listen to me, you people! I've seen all kinds of dishonesty in my day . . . but this little display takes the cake! [*#3 strides swiftly toward #8. He reaches him, waves his hand in #8's face.*] You come in here with your heart bleeding all over the floor about slum kids and injustice, and you make up some wild stories, and all of a sudden you start getting through to some of these old ladies in here! Well, you're not getting through to me! I've had enough! [*To all.*] What's the matter with you people? Every one of you knows this kid is guilty! He's got to burn! We're letting him slip through our fingers here!

#8: [*Calmly.*]: Slip through our fingers? Are you his executioner?

#3 [*Furious.*]: I'm one of 'em.

#8: Maybe you'd like to pull the switch.

#3 [*Shouting.*]: For this kid? You bet I'd like to pull the switch!

#8: I'm sorry for you . . .

#3: Don't start with me now!

#8: What it must feel like to want to pull the switch!

#3 [*Raging.*]: Listen, you shut up!

#8 [*Baiting him.*]: Ever since we walked into this room you've been behaving like a self-appointed public avenger!

#3 [*Loud.*]: I'm telling you now! Shut up!

#8: You want to see this boy die because you personally want it, not because of the facts.

#3 [*Roaring.*]: Shut up!

#8: You're a sadist . . .

[*The jury groups around #3 and 8.*]

#3 [*Roaring.*]: Shut up! [*And he lunges wildly at #8. #8 holds his ground as #3 is caught by many hands and held back. He strains against the hands, his face dark with rage.*] Let me go! I'll kill him! I'll kill him!

#8 [*Calmly.*]: You don't *really* mean you'll kill me, do you?

*　　*　　*

NOTE 4.

HARRY KALVEN, JR. AND HANS ZEISEL
THE AMERICAN JURY*

*　　*　　*

The jury study has had one special burden to bear along with all the customary difficulties of large-scale research. At one point one of its research approaches generated a national scandal. As one of several lines of approach, it

* Boston: Little Brown and Co., vi–vii (1966). Reprinted by permission.

was decided to obtain recordings of actual jury deliberations, partly to learn whether post-trial interviews with jurors permit reconstruction of the events of the jury room. The move was undertaken, with the consent of the trial judge and counsel, but without the knowledge of the jurors, in five civil cases in the federal district court in Wichita, Kansas. Although extensive security measures were taken to insure the integrity of the effort, when the fact became public in the summer of 1955, there followed public censure by the Attorney General of the United States, a special hearing before the Sub-Committee on Internal Security of the Senate Judiciary Committee, the enactment of statutes in some thirty-odd jurisdictions prohibiting jury-tapping, and for a brief, painful moment, widespread editorial and news coverage by the national press.

None of the Wichita data are included in this book, nor will they be included in future books. We note the episode here simply to make clear to that man who would say, "That's all very interesting, professors, but did you ever hear a real jury deliberate?" that the answer is Yes, and to point out that one of the distinctions of the jury study is that it is a research project that has a Purple Heart.

*　　　*　　　*

CHAPTER THREE

The Impact of Societal Dynamics on Human Experimentation— Extending Knowledge, Risking Life, and Relying on Professional Authority

The Jewish Chronic Disease Hospital and Wichita Jury Recording cases provoked intense, though short-lived, debates about the nature and extent of the authority of investigators to intervene in subjects' lives, to expose them to risks, and to tamper with the fabric of professional and societal institutions. In partial defense to considerable criticism, the investigators argued that the need to acquire knowledge for the benefit of individuals and society required such interventions. More specifically, the scientists believed that the injection of "cancer cells" in debilitated subjects and the recording of jury deliberations were the next logical experiments that needed to be performed and that, as the experts in these fields, they had no choice but to carry out their research despite the risks involved.

The materials in this part are designed to explore these assertions by focusing on three issues which surfaced repeatedly in the arguments about the propriety of the two experiments: (1) the need of individuals and society continually to extend the frontiers of knowledge and technology; (2) the inevitability of injury to life and limb in all human endeavors; and (3) the need and wish to rely on the expertise of professionals. As the case studies suggest, however, three opposing motivations which also have deep roots in man and society brake these forces: (1) man's fear of the unknown and his desire to perpetuate the status quo; (2) man's belief in the paramount value of every human life; and (3) man's desire to control those decisions which affect his life.

These conflicts, between man and man as well as man and society, are presented in this section in their broadest possible context. They will recur, in varying guises, throughout this volume. The tension between self-determination and delegation of authority to experts, for instance, underlies much of the analysis of the role and authority of experimental subjects presented in Part Three. The three forces are highlighted in this chapter because a better perspective on the remainder of the book can be achieved through a prior appraisal of society's overall attitudes toward the acquisition of knowledge, the balancing of risks and benefits, and the reliance on professional authority.

A.
Man's Quest for Knowledge and Mastery

The assertion has been made that two basic characteristics underlie the origin and growth of science and technology: "the need to control the workings of nature for our welfare and the simple, irreducible need to understand the world about us and ourselves."* This proposition in turn raises a fundamental philosophical question: "What must nature, including man, be like in order that science be possible at all?"†

The materials in this section suggest that science and technology have always advanced in a relentless fashion, driven by scientists' "curiosity" and "urge for discovery" and by technologists' wish to satisfy human "wants" and "needs." Moreover, the concept of progress, which has had a powerful impact on the Western world ever since the seventeenth century, has reinforced the quest for the extension of knowledge and technology which is so manifest in contemporary society. These assumptions raise questions about the rationality of attempting to impose controls on science and technology in general and on human experimentation in particular.

In studying these materials, consider the following questions:

1. What values does man seek to maximize by scientific and technological advances? Are these values in conflict with other individual and societal values?

2. Can and should science and technology be controlled?

3. What are the distinctions between science and technology, and how relevant are they to resolving the problems raised by human experimentation?

4. What consequences should follow once investigations move from theory to studies on inanimate objects and then to experimentation with animals, investigators themselves, other individuals, groups, or society at large?

---

* J. A. Mazzeo: *The Design of Life.* New York: Pantheon Books *xiii* (1967).
† T. S. Kuhn: *The Structure of Scientific Revolutions.* Chicago: The University of Chicago Press 172 (1962).

1.

Curiosity and Necessity

a.

Basic Human Characteristics?

George Sarton
*A History of Science**

When did science begin? Where did it begin? It began whenever and wherever men tried to solve the innumerable problems of life. The first solutions were mere expedients, but that must do for a beginning. Gradually the expedients would be compared, generalized, rationalized, simplified, interrelated, integrated; the texture of science would be slowly woven. The first solutions were petty and awkward but what of it? A *Sequoia gigantea* two inches high may not be very conspicuous, but it is a *Sequoia* all the same. It might be claimed that one cannot speak of science at all as long as a certain degree of abstraction has not been reached, but who will measure that degree? When the first mathematician recognized that there was something in common between three palm trees and three donkeys, how abstract was his thought? Or when primitive theologians conceived the invisible presence of a supreme being and thus seemed to reach an incredible degree of abstraction, was their idea really abstract, or was it concrete? Did they postulate God or did they see Him? Were the earliest expedients nothing but expedients or did they include reasonings, religious or artistic cravings? Were they rational or irrational? Was early science wholly practical and mercenary? Was it pure science, such as it was, or a mixture of science with art, religion, or magic?

Such queries are futile, because they lack determination and the answers cannot be verified. It is better to leave out for the nonce the consideration of science as science, and to consider only definite problems and their solutions. The problems can be imagined, because we know the needs of man; he must be able to feed himself and his family, to find a shelter against the inclemencies of the weather, the attacks of wild beast or fellow men, and so on. Our imaginations are not arbitrary, for they are guided by a large number of observed facts. To begin with,

* Cambridge: Harvard University Press 3–5, 16–17 (1952). Reprinted by permission. Copyright 1952, by the President and Fellows of Harvard College.

archaeologic investigations reveal monuments which help us to realize the kind of objects and tools that our forefathers created and even to understand their methods of using them, and to guess their intentions. The study of languages brings to light ancient words which are like fossil witnesses of early objects or early ideas....

In order to simplify our task a little, let us assume that the primitive men we are dealing with have already solved some of the most urgent problems, for otherwise their very existence would have remained precarious, not to speak of their progress, material or spiritual. Let us assume that they have discovered how to make a fire and have learned the rudiments of husbandry. They are already—that is, some of them are—learned people and technicians, and they may already be speaking of the good old days when life was more dangerous but simpler and a man did not have to remember so many things....

* * *

Let us consider rapidly the multitude of technical problems that early men had to solve if they wished to survive, and, later, to improve their condition and to lighten the burden of life. They had to invent the making of fire and experiment with it in various ways. Not only the husbandman but also the nomad needed many tools, for cutting and carving, flaying, abrading, smoothing, crushing, for the making of holes, for grasping and joining. Each tool was a separate invention, or rather the opening up of a new series of inventions, for each was susceptible of improvements which would be introduced one by one. In early times there was already room for key inventions, which might be applied to an endless group of separate problems and which ushered in unlimited possibilities. For example, there was the general problem of how to devise a handle and how to attach it firmly to a given tool. Many different solutions were found for that problem, one of the most ingenious being that of the Eskimos and Northern Indians, namely, the use of babiche (strings or thongs of rawhide) by means of which the tool and handle are bound together; as the hide dries it shrinks almost to half its length and the two objects are inseparable. A tighter fit could hardly be obtained otherwise.

The husbandman had to discover the useful plants one by one—plants to use as food, or as drugs, or for other domestic purposes— and this implied innumerable experiments. It was not enough for him to discover a plant; he had to select among infinite variations the best modalities of its use. He had to capture animals and to domesticate the very few that were domesticable, to build houses and granaries, to make receptacles of various kinds. There must have been somewhere a first potter, but the potter's art involved the conscious or unconscious coöperation of thousands of people. Heavy loads had to be lifted and transported, sometimes to great distances. How could that be done? Well, it had to be done and it was done. Ingenious people invented the lever, the simple pulley, the use of rollers, and later, much later, that of wheels. A potter of genius applied the wheel to his own art. How could a man cover his body to protect it from the cold or the rain or the burning sun? The use of hides was one solution, the use of leaves or bark another, but nothing equaled the materials obtained by the weaving of certain fibres. When this idea occurred to a great inventor, the textile industry was born. . . .

*   *   *

Some readers will object that whatever knowledge there was, was purely practical, empirical, too raw and rough to deserve the name of science. Why should we not call it science? It was a very poor science, very imperfect, yet perfectible; our science is decidedly deeper and richer, yet the same general description applies to it—it is very imperfect yet perfectible. Or one might say: There was no pure science. Why not again? How pure must science be to be called pure? If pure science is disinterested science, knowledge obtained for its own sake without thought of immediate use, surely the early astronomers were, or might be as pure as our own. It is possible that astrologic fancies had already developed, but it is equally possible that they had not, for that would have implied a degree of sophistication which those astronomers had not yet reached. Their main reason for observing the strange behavior of certain planets may have been simply curiosity.

Curiosity, one of the deepest of human traits, indeed far more ancient than mankind itself, was perhaps the mainspring of scientific knowledge in the past as it still is today. Necessity has been called the mother of invention, of technology, but curiosity was the mother of science. The motives of primitive scientists (as opposed to those of primitive technicians and shamans) were perhaps not very different from those of our contemporaries; they varied consid-

erably from man to man and time to time and then as now covered the whole gamut from complete selflessness, reckless curiosity, and spirit of adventure down to personal ambition, vainglory, covetousness.

If research had not been inspired and informed from the beginning by a certain amount of disinterestedness and adventurousness, and by what its enemies would later call indiscretion and impiety, the progress of science would have been considerably slower than it was. The amount of knowledge attained by some primitive men can be deduced from anthropologic records and also from the amount observable in the most ancient civilizations. When man appears on the scene of history, we find him already a master of many arts, expert in many crafts, as full of lore as of cunning.

Then as now the true scientist, even as the true artist, was likely to be or to seem a bit queer and secretive; it is highly probable that his more practical neighbors already made jokes about his absent-mindedness. Of course, he was not more absent-minded than they were, but their minds were focused on different interests. He was engrossed in his own reflections; his motives being less tangible, his life seemed mysterious. Sometimes he may have wished for praise and recognition, or he may already have discovered that such praise was futile and that it was better not to try for it. If he were selfish and jealous, the primitive inventor might prefer to keep his new idea—say a better hook, or a better ax, or better materials for the making of either—to himself and his family. In almost every case the scientist or the inventor tended to be reticent. The growth of science was always entangled in psychologic and social accidents.

Not only was the development of primitive invention somewhat confidential and secret, it was also of necessity antagonistic to the regular habits and traditions that it tended to subvert. Every invention, however useful it may turn out to be (and it cannot be useful before it is used), is disturbing, and the more pregnant it is, the more disturbing. There were vested interests in prehistoric times as well as now, though they could not be described in exactly the same way and were perhaps less blatant. There was, then as now, a strong inertia impeding progress, the inertia of habit and complacency, distrust and contempt of everything novel or foreign. That inertia, however, was not simply a hindrance, but a necessity, like a flywheel or a brake, to steady and warrant mankind's invasion of the unknown. Men's resistance to new tools or new-fangled ideas was useful, because novelties should be thoroughly tested before being adopted. Every accepted tool was the fruit of a very long process of trial and error, of a very long tussle between inventors, innovators, reformers at one end and conservatives at the other. The latter were far more numerous; the former were more enthusiastic and aggressive.

*   *   *

NOTES

NOTE 1.

SIGMUND FREUD
THREE ESSAYS ON THE THEORY OF
SEXUALITY (1905) *

*   *   *

At about the same time as the sexual life of children reaches its first peak, between the ages of three and five, they also begin to show signs of the activity which may be ascribed to the instinct for knowledge or research. This instinct cannot be counted among the elementary instinctual components, nor can it be classed as exclusively belonging to sexuality. Its activity corresponds on the one hand to a sublimated manner of obtaining mastery, while on the other hand it makes use of the energy of scopophilia. Its relations to sexual life, however, are of particular importance, since we have learnt from psychoanalysis that the instinct for knowledge in children is attracted unexpectedly early and intensely to sexual problems and is in fact possibly first aroused by them.

It is not by theoretical interests but by practical ones that activities of research are set going in children. The threat to the bases of a child's existence offered by the discovery or the suspicion of the arrival of a new baby and the fear that he may, as a result of it, cease to be cared for and loved, make him thoughtful and clear-sighted. And this history of the instinct's origin is in line with the fact that the first problem with which it deals is not the question of the

distinction between the sexes but the riddle of where babies come from. . . .

*   *   *

NOTE 2.

A. V. HILL
EXPERIMENTS ON FROGS AND MEN *

Man is an inveterate experimenter. Those of us who have been small boys ourselves, or indeed are still small boys, will know what joy is found in taking an old alarm clock to bits or a bicycle to pieces, in seeing how fast we can run a hundred yards, in breeding rabbits, pigeons, or canaries, in fixing wireless apparatus together, or, when we are older, in trying a new kind of oil or petrol or even a new medicine. Boys and men, however, also girls and women, are not the only experimenters, as any who have watched a kitten or a parrot will know; and experiments made by monkeys have been scientifically studied. Man, however, is the chief experimental animal, both as experimenter and as subject. Indeed, in many of man's most joyful adventures he acts in both capacities; he makes experiments upon himself, often to his own great danger or discomfort.

To run in a Marathon race or to try to swim the Channel, to see how far one can ride a bicycle in 24 hours, to climb to 20,000 feet, to set out to walk (or to fly) to the South Pole, to make a height record in an aeroplane, to dive under the sea, all these involve trials and experiments upon oneself; which is one reason why so many apparently useless feats are performed. Every new adventure on which man has embarked throughout the ages, every change in his social, economic and political condition, has meant experiments upon his bodily frame and organization, experiments sometimes successful but often followed by disaster.

In learning the use, treatment, and preservation of food he must, unwittingly often, have made millions of experiments upon himself, thousands of them extremely unpleasant, many of them fatal. Without these experiments, however, the present order of civilization, depending as it does upon a regular supply of food, would have been impossible. When he set out to journey on the sea he experimented on sea-sickness, and later on, as his journeys lengthened, on scurvy and the need of vitamins. When he deserted a natural diet and gathered together in

---

* James Strachey, ed.: 7 *The Standard Edition of the Complete Psychological Works of Sigmund Freud.* London: The Hogarth Press and the Institute of Psychoanalysis 194–195 (1953). Reprinted by permission of Sigmund Freud Copyrights Ltd., The Institute of Psychoanalysis, the Hogarth Press, Ltd. and Basic Books, Inc.

---

* 2 *The Lancet* 261 (1929). Reprinted by permission.

cities he experimented on nutrition and the physiological effects of radiation (or its absence), with rickets as a curious result. When he began to dig deep tunnels, or to work in diving bells or diving suits, he discovered that the physical solubility of gases in his blood and tissues may affect his well-being, and he invented caisson disease. When he climbed high mountains, or went up in balloons, he discovered mountain sickness, and acclimatization to it. When he took to rapid manoeuvres in aeroplanes he found out that the human factor is a limiting one, that violent acceleration—"centrifugal force"—may play havoc with his circulation and render him suddenly unconscious. Labouring in hot mines, in extremes of climate, with excess or deficiency of sunlight; living on sterilized, preserved, or purified food; breathing quartz dust or carbon monoxide; working with materials which exert a chronic irritation on the skin, or with ultra-violet light, or with X rays and radium; in all such experiments he found limitations to his independence of his external environment; he made experiments upon himself and others, experiments involving ill-health, disaster, and death to many. Even apart from disease, from the experiments which Nature wantonly insists upon making on us, we cannot avoid making experiments on ourselves if we are to do anything new; and, even if we do nothing new, we shall probably find we must make experiments still to discover how to remain as we are.

*   *   *

NOTE 3.

DEREK J. DE SOLLA PRICE
SCIENCE SINCE BABYLON*

*   *   *

[T]he motivation for research may be an intellectual itch—indeed, the purpose of education has been defined as the business of making people uncomfortable, making them itch—but a deeper and more specific urge may have made these persons into scientists. By far the most common inner reason is that as youngsters they have wanted to be a Mr. Boyle of the Law. They seek an immortal brainchild in order to perpetuate themselves. In an age of teamwork amongst scientists, of little men working on big machines, this hallowed form of eponymic immortality is becoming insecure, and the image of really great

men and their theories has become more precious. If, however, this is becoming a problem, there is surely all the more reason to examine the process that made it possible, during the Scientific Revolution, for men to fashion bricks of science inscribed with their own names and build up, faster than ever before, an imposing edifice and superstructure of theory and experiment.

*   *   *

NOTE 4.

DEREK J. DE SOLLA PRICE
THE SCIENCE OF SCIENTISTS*

*   *   *

[S]cience seems to be its own sweet beast. It has a life and an order all of its own, intransigent to human will and desire, impervious to national origins and philosophical frameworks, unresponsive to the wishes and fears of society, sensitive only in the shortest perspective to happy accidents and creative geniuses, and responsive only parochially and temporarily to most stimuli of support and lack of support. I have, you will realize, exaggerated all these things for dramatic effect, but the general line permeates all we know of the history of science and many of the working judgments of scientists are predicated along these lines.

To put it all in another way, there is only one world to explore and discover. Moving to another analogy, there is only one proper way (at any given time) to fit together the pieces of the jigsaw puzzle. And for a last piece of picturesque theorizing about the particular go of science, one has to pick the fruit of the tree of knowledge, piece by piece, in its due ripeness.

To substantiate these generalities a little, consider the peculiar supranationality of science: Budapest and Delhi must produce the same physics as Moscow and Boston and seek the same ultimate scientific Nirvana, however different their tastes in music and philosophy and their goals in politics or economics. Temporary local deviances may exist from time to time at the research front, as when newtonians and cartesians do battle, or when a school follows Lysenko, but in the end it turns out that either you do science the one right way or you cannot pursue it at all.

Consider also the strong anticonstructionist feeling one has about scientific laws: that there is only one world there. If Crick and Watson had

---

* New Haven: Yale University Press 48 (1962). Reprinted by permission.

* 1 *Medical Opinion and Review* 88, 89–90 (1966). Reprinted by permission.

not existed, the same work would have to have been done by others; if Planck had not found his constant, it would merely have borne another name. Admittedly, there are some difficult questions—if oxygen was an element that had to be discovered early in the game, is it also true that phlogiston was similarly necessary at the time?

But in the rest of the world there is none of this simplicity: if Beethoven had not been, a unique contribution would have been lost and music might have taken a quite different path, and if Cleopatra had had a long nose or the Japanese had developed an atomic bomb, the entire course of world history could have been different.

Science seems to be so strongly ordered in all its objective certainty that one has very little chance to decide what shall be done next. One cannot, of course, predict at any time, but with all the dangers of 20/20 hindsight one can see that we can affect the order of the God-given sequence of discoveries but a little and can make only local effects in deciding that the law was due to Boyle and not to Hooke or Marriotte. Such things may be very important to Messrs. Boyle and Marriotte, or to their countries, but on the whole the juggernaut of science is little swayed.

Precisely because of this heavily impersonal inevitability of the scientific machine, and not in spite of it, we historians of science have been able to say meaningful things about the behavior of individual scientists and the forces that move them. One can see that Planck has deeper problems in attaching his name to a constant than Beethoven to a symphony. If the jigsaw puzzle is not yet ready for the piece you want to fit, no amount of inducement and support will fit it.

*   *   *

b.

Can Science and Technology Be Distinguished?

[i]
Jerome B. Wiesner
Technology and Society*

*   *   *

I would like to clear up . . . the ambiguity that exists between technology and scientific research, their objectives and their methods. This confusion is by no means surprising since modern technology has become highly dependent

upon basic scientific knowledge for much of its progress. In turn, scientific research in many fields is only possible because of the elaborate and sensitive tools that technology has made possible. The vast and powerful particle accelerators, the electron microscope with which to explore the world of cells and viruses, and the electronic computer to calculate problems which only a few years ago were beyond the scope of human comprehension, are but three of a large number of scientific tools which have extended enormously our ability to measure, observe, and understand the world around us.

This close alliance between science and technology, though relatively new, is so complete that the average person, and indeed many scientists and engineers as well, fail to distinguish any difference between them.

In the beginning, technology did not depend upon science. The inventions that provided the basis for the industrial revolution—the steam engine, the loom, the lathe, and many other machines—were invented by practical men and based upon art, observation, and common sense. In the first stage of industrialization man was exercising his ingenuity in the exploitation of the things he found around him. The factory with its power machines, its use of unskilled or semi-skilled labor doing simple repetitive operations, the utilization of raw materials like iron, coal, copper, etc., improvements in transportation growing from the development of the railroad and the steamboat are all examples of this inventiveness. Most important, of course, was that with the introduction of machines he had begun a continuing process of extending human capabilities, first by augmenting muscle power through harnessing the almost limitless energy sources found in nature, later by speeding communications by electrical means, and most recently by augmenting mental activities by the introduction of computing machines to replace human effort in menial, repetitive activities and to assist in difficult or lengthy calculations.

The fact that scientific research had little or no effect on early technology does not mean that scientists did not exist or were not working. They did and were, and during the period of the industrial revolution the foundations were laid for modern physics, chemistry, and biology. However, it was not until the middle of the nineteenth century that extensive practical use was made of the accumulating scientific knowledge. Only then did men begin to exploit the available knowledge of chemistry and electricity for useful purposes.

* Harry Woolf, ed.: *Science As a Cultural Force*. Baltimore, Md.: The Johns Hopkins Press 37–40 (1964). Reprinted by permission.

Chemists learned to synthesize organic materials and set up research laboratories for obtaining the new knowledge required to meet their applied objectives. It was in the field of chemistry that research methods were first applied in a systematic manner to develop new products. The application of electricity was more haphazard in the beginning. The scientific observations of Gilbert, Henry, and Maxwell were seized upon by the inventors of the electric motor, the electric generator, the telegraph, telephone, and other devices. Not until the end of the nineteenth century were research methods applied to the exploitation of electrical phenomena, first by Thomas Edison who, in reality, was more of an inventor than a scientist, and later by many technologists in the laboratories of such industries as the General Electric Company and the predecessors of the American Telephone and Telegraph Company. Thus, it was in these fields—chemistry and electricity—that the merger of scientific inquiry and technology first occurred, that the power of the scientific methods was applied to solving useful problems, and that the great value of the thorough understanding of physical phenomena was demonstrated. In exploiting electrical phenomena technologists deal with fields and electrons and waves which can only be observed indirectly and understood through scientific research. It is not surprising, therefore, that scientifically based industry, like the electronics industry which depends very heavily upon basic research, should be the sponsor of much fundamental research.

Modern technology still requires invention. The vacuum tube, the transistor, memory devices for computers, and new materials tailored with specific properties are all inventions. But they are inventions made by men with special knowledge who have an understanding of a scientific field and who base their inventions on an intimate familiarity with that field, just as the inventor of old called upon his first hand experience of the world he could see and feel to provide the working substance of his ingenuity.

This is the nature of modern, scientifically based technology. Clearly, the first requirement is the existence of a body of scientific knowledge. To use this knowledge as the basis for an invention in the solution of a specific problem, the technologist must have good understanding of the underlying science. Also, more likely than not, as he converges on the development of a specific device, the technologist will find that he is handicapped by the fact that the scientists who first explored the field that he is exploiting left vast areas of ignorance which must be filled before his task can be completed. These can only be filled by doing further fundamental research. Because the specific knowledge required to solve a problem is its goal, such work is often called "applied" or "directed research," though it is obvious that in another context it would be regarded as fundamental or basic research.

* * *

[ii]
Norman W. Storer
The Internationality of Science and the
Nationality of Scientists*

* * *

[W]e are concerned with the fundamental nature of the "energy" that keeps science going and with the ways in which it is channeled so that scientific activity can continue. Because science is essentially an intellectual activity rather than one that depends directly upon the exploitation of physical energy, we must agree in the beginning that this energy must be motivational in character; we bring it to mind when we ask why scientists want to engage in research and the other activities associated with it. And we must agree that its structuring is determined by the special set of norms and values that distinguish science from other sectors of society.

This definition of the problem has provided the framework for much of the "basic" research on science, beginning with Robert K. Merton's pioneering essays. . . .

. . . Merton pointed out . . . that professional recognition, the celebration by colleagues of one's scientific achievements, is the single most appropriate and legitimate reward achievement in science. Through the analysis of a series of disputes over priority in scientific discovery, . . . Merton was able to demonstrate that the receipt of professional recognition, earned by being the first to discover something, is indeed of central importance to the scientist's motivation. Even if he is reluctant to admit it, the scientist yearns for indications that his work has been accepted by his colleagues as valid and significant—indications that may range all the way from being mentioned in a footnote to being awarded a Nobel Prize. This is not to say that all research is done simply in order to gain recog-

* 22 *International Social Science Journal* 80, 83–85, 89–90 (1970). Reprinted by permission of UNESCO.

nition, but that without such feedback much of the desire to engage in research would quickly dwindle.

Why the scientist should want professional recognition is a question that has not yet been fully resolved. There are two major hypotheses at present which attempt to explain this. First, there is the proposal that the scientist is trained to want recognition during his apprenticeship in science because it certifies that he has satisfied the demanding requirements of his role: he has advanced our knowledge of some aspect of reality. A complementary hypothesis contends that the desire to create, to produce "meaningful novelty," is a basic human need and that the act of creation is not complete without the receipt of competent response to it from others. The discovery of a regular relationship between physical phenomena is a type of creativity, especially since it must be described in words or mathematical equations if it is to take its place in the body of scientific knowledge, and the person responsible for it needs the affirmation of his peers that his creation is valid and meaningful. In science, a positive response to the product of one's creativity constitutes professional recognition—and even a negative response is to be preferred over no response at all. In other contexts a person may desire affirmation of the beauty or cleverness or practical utility of what he has created, but the basic need for competent response seems to be the same in all forms of creativity.

Regardless of why the scientist desires professional recognition, it is possible now to assert that the desire for it is the normatively appropriate motive of the scientist—even though specific individuals may also find a variety of other rewards for engaging in research. This central assertion is supported by indirect evidence of several types, and the primary objection to it that remains is the problem of its apparent conflict with the idea that the scientist is disinterested, altruistic, and entirely unconcerned with fame.

Again, two different but complementary explanations have been offered for scientists' reluctance to admit their interest in receiving professional recognition. (The numerous incidents of priority conflict, together with other data showing the large proportion of scientists who admit to an occasional worry about "being scooped," are sufficient to dispose of the contention that they don't really care about this.) One explanation is that there is another norm in science which calls for humility and works to make the scientist deny his interest in receiving any

sort of reward for his achievements. The other is that since professional recognition is worthless if it is not objective—it is supposed to represent Mother Nature's judgment of the validity and significance of one's discovery, not the discoverer—the scientist hesitates to admit his interest in professional recognition because this might lead to his colleagues' bestowing it as a favor to him rather than as an impersonal evaluation of his work.

*   *   *

The description of science given . . . is of course appropriate primarily to what is called basic research—the disinterested quest for new, universally valid knowledge which is sought without regard for its possible relevance to the solution of practical problems. Applied research, on the other hand, is oriented directly or indirectly to solving "real" problems. The importance of this distinction for our purposes is that the empirical problems which beset men as physical beings, in contrast to the theoretical questions which intrigue them as intellects, are usually localized in space and time. They are related to national interests rather than scientific interests.

A problem that exists in one part of the world need not exist in other parts or at other times, so that a solution to it tends to lack the universality that characterizes answers to basic scientific questions. This means that if scientists' interests were to be guided solely by practical concerns, the consensus on what constitutes important scientific questions—which provides the foundation of the international scientific community—would immediately be shattered. And since their problems would not only be peculiar to places and times but also identified by criteria which vary from one culture to the next, the scientists of a given nation would be neither interested in nor able to contribute to the work of scientists in other nations.

Further, empirical problems do not arise in logical sequence as do the theoretical questions that occupy basic scientists, so applied research has relatively little potential for building a cumulative, generalized body of knowledge. Only coincidentally would one scientist's research have meaningful implications for another's research, so the chances for obtaining competent response to one's work from others would be drastically reduced. There is thus a considerably smaller scientific audience for achievements in applied research, and greatly diminished opportunity for the applied researcher to gain the kind of immortality that can be gained through fundamental scientific discoveries.

This means that the applied researcher must look more to non-scientists for rewards than to his colleagues, and these rewards must be something other than the competent response to creativity which is the normatively appropriate reward. They are usually money and sometimes public adulation, neither of which requires that the giver really understand what the scientist has done. The applied researcher must thus violate the norm of disinterestedness at the same time that he makes it more difficult for him to participate fully in the activities of the scientific community, and he is therefore viewed by basic scientists as threatening the moral rightness and stability of their entire enterprise. For this reason there are appreciable pressures on the young scientist not to engage in applied research. The invidious distinction between basic and applied research is obvious to any advanced graduate student and he is ordinarily trained to seek the more prestigious type of work and the sort of position in which this can be carried out with maximum facility.

Yet society's interest in encouraging and supporting science must rest ultimately on the assumption that this support will be eventually repaid in the form of solutions to pressing problems. Thus, despite the fact that it is basic research which provides the context, or the specialized universe of discourse within which the applied scientist works, there are often demands that the scientist devote himself entirely to applying his skills to one or more of the problems that his society has defined as needing solution. . . .

*　　*　　*

2.

The Impact of Values

a.

Search for Truth?

Philip Handler
An Interview*

NEWS REPORT: Do you feel any constraints should be placed on fundamental research if

---

* 19 *News Report of the National Academy of Sciences* 9 (March 1969). Reprinted by permission of the National Academy of Sciences.

there is some reason to believe that the results of that research might be harmful to society?

HANDLER: No. No constraints. Let me give you a dramatic illustration. You may know of the demonstration that one can take a fertilized frog egg, discard its nucleus and insert a nucleus from a somatic cell of some other frog, and the egg develops into a frog which is an absolutely perfect twin of the donor frog—the one that provided the transplanted nucleus. Presumably, by that technique we would make an indefinite number of perfect copies of that donor frog. It's merely a matter of time before we can switch from frogs to mammals. When we have the biological technology, we should be able to make perfect copies of the best bull or greatest cow in the world, in whatever number may be desired. This could go a long way toward improving world food production. Obviously, the next step would be man, and perhaps one day we may be able to make copies of a Bunche, Rabi, or Schirra, or of an Eldridge Cleaver, or Lew Alcindor or of any other genotype identifiable in our population.

I hope that day never comes. I can't imagine any more dangerous tool in the hands of an autocratic, dictatorial, authoritarian government. It would be the most powerful mechanism ever devised—the ultimate despoliation of the human race, degradation of the worst order. We could create an ant-like society that is utterly repugnant. The idea of exploring all of the remarkable variety in the human gene pool is far more attractive. There are all kinds of people we have yet to produce. The human gene pool is colossal in its potential variety. The other idea leads to disaster.

And yet I think there is no alternative but to go down this trail and do the biological experimentation that, one day, may offer this kind of a capability. The idea that, since we can see this end possibility, we should by fiat state, "Thou shalt not in thy laboratory do any experiment which leads down that trail," is an equally repugnant thought. That kind of censorship is as repugnant as censorship of literature in other communities and is as potentially damaging. No constraints. Utilization of scientific information is a political and social decision and we have mechanisms in our society for arriving at such decisions. Let's use those. But no constraints on dissemination of facts, the ideas people are allowed to think, or the search for scientific understanding.

Historically, there isn't much we can do in

the future that can compare to the shocks of the past. Consider the Copernican revolution, which converted this earth from the center of the universe to a tiny planet around a sun that is only a little star in the cosmos. Consider the idea of evolution which traces us to nothingness, in effect, so that man's image of himself as something created in the image of his maker has been destroyed. It is hard to think of anything that we are likely to do in the future which can conceivably be as traumatic an alteration of man's view of himself, his position in the general scheme of things as what has already happened. If we can live with these concepts, we can live with almost any other kind of information. Censorship of physics from now on can never expunge understanding of how to build nuclear weapons; censorship of biology will not abolish the knowledge which is required for biological weapons. The search for truth is man's noblest pursuit. Surely man's mind can live comfortably with the knowledge and understanding so gained without damage to man. And what better basis is there for the moral imperatives which guide our society?

NOTES

NOTE 1.

KARL W. DEUTSCH
SCIENTIFIC AND HUMANISTIC KNOWLEDGE
IN THE GROWTH OF CIVILIZATION*

. . . Science itself depends for its life on the prior acceptance of certain fundamental values, such as the value of curiosity and learning, the value of truth, the value of sharing knowledge with others, the value of respect for facts, and the value of remembering the vastness of the universe in comparison with the finite knowledge of men at any particular moment. Historically, such values have been held by outstanding scientists. One thinks of P. W. Bridgman's well-known dictum that—"in the face of the fact, the scientist has a humility almost religious"; or of Newton's description of his own work as the play of a child with pebbles on the shores of the ocean of knowledge, or his reference to the sharing of knowledge with others by describing his own achievements as being due to

his having stood "on the shoulders of giants." Beyond such evidence, it could perhaps be shown that the cumulative work of science could not go on if any of the values just listed were rejected.

As science rests on certain values, so do almost all values depend on knowledge, and thus to some extent in turn on science, if they are to proceed from the realm of words to that of action. This implies a circular chain of causation or a feedback process, as do many processes of social and cultural development. To act morally is in one sense the opposite of acting blindly. It is acting in the presumed knowledge of what in fact it is that we are doing. Almost every significant action of this kind implies serious assumptions in some field of science. To love one's neighbor requires at the very least that we find out where and who our neighbor is. If we are to respond to his needs we must first ascertain what his needs are and what action in fact is likely to be helpful to him. . . .

. . . If we evaluate an action as good on the basis of our mere surmise of the good will of its doer, therefore, we may find ourselves forced to assume that such subjective good will—as in the Kantian Imperative—must include by implication also the will to gain and apply the best available knowledge of the probable consequences of the action chosen. The duty to have good intentions, in other words, is meaningless without the duty to try to know the facts and try to foresee correctly the consequences of one's deeds, and it is this latter duty which may distinguish in practice the responsible from the irresponsible statesman, or the well-intentioned doctor from the well-intentioned quack.

Attempts at hermetic separations of science from values are thus bound to fail. Science without at least some values would come to a dead stop; ethics without at least some exact and verifiable knowledge would be condemned to impotence or become an engine of destruction. Much of the anxious discussion of international politics between statesmen and atomic scientists, or between the so-called schools of "idealism" and "realism" among political writers, hinges upon the discrepancy between the strength of the moral convictions involved and the poverty of reliable knowledge of the probable consequences of the proposed courses of action.

The relationship of science to values thus implies a double question: the mutual interrelation of science and the general values of a civilization; and the relationship of a specific state of scientific knowledge to the pursuit of

---

* Harcourt Brown, ed.: *Science and the Creative Spirit*. Toronto: University of Toronto Press 18–21 (1958). Reprinted by permission of University of Toronto Press. Copyright, Canada, 1958 by University of Toronto Press.

specific purposes or policies. The first of these problems, the general relationship of science and value, and thus to some extent of truth and goodness, leads us close to the heart of every civilization within which it is examined. If conceived as mutually incompatible, science and values may frustrate or destroy each other, dragging their civilization towards stagnation or decline. As a mutually productive and creative partnership, science and values may succeed in strengthening each other's powers in a self-enhancing pattern of growth, rendering their civilization increasingly open and able to learn from the hopes and dreams of the individuals within it, as well as from the universe around it.

This general vision of a mutually beneficial partnership becomes increasingly difficult to retain, however, as we proceed from the consideration of the growth of civilization on the grand scale to the effect of the timing of particular discoveries or innovations upon specific policies at specific times and places. Would it have been better for mankind if Einstein's principle of relativity, or Chadwick's discovery of the neutron, or Hahn's work on uranium fission had all come ten years later than they did, and no atom bomb had been available to drop on Hiroshima? Perhaps the most useful consideration in the face of questions such as these might be to realize the impossibility of foreseeing the ultimate consequences of even the smallest scientific or technological advance, as well as the inexhaustibility of most or all of the great contributions. Benjamin Franklin's answer to the question "What is the use of a scientific discovery?" consisted in asking the counterquestion "What is the use of a baby?" Just as it seems impossible to foretell the eventual good a child may do, so it is impossible to foretell what evil he may do, and our whole attitude to children is in a sense based upon the bet that the good they do will far outweigh the evil. In civilized countries we have long ago abandoned the discussion which sometimes still echoes in mythology, whether a certain child should have been killed at birth in order to forestall the harm he did in adult life. Rather we have come to center our attention on providing a family and an environment for him in which love will outweigh hate, and in which his opportunity for free and friendly growth will be the best.

If there is merit in Benjamin Franklin's argument, we might similarly decide to bet on the potential goodness rather than on the potential evil of knowledge, and concentrate on providing

a human and social environment for science in which its constructive possibilities are likely to be realized. It is possible, of course, to imagine extreme situations for some times and places in which the short-term potentialities for destruction might seem so great in the case of a particular invention or discovery, and the prevailing political régime might seem so unlikely to avoid its suicidal misuse, that a policy of temporarily restricting, delaying, or withholding such knowledge might appear as the least of several likely evils for the time being. Even granting all these assumptions, however, such a policy of fear of knowledge would have to be viewed as extremely transitory and exceptional in any modern technological civilization that is to continue to advance or indeed to survive. A civilization so prone to commit suicide that it could be saved only be concealing from it the means of its own destruction would not endure for long. Rather, for the long run and for most conditions that are likely to occur, we might do better to adopt the opposite assumption: that any modern civilization that is to endure will have to learn how to live with its new knowledge of its vast means of destruction.

*   *   *

NOTE 2.

BENTLEY GLASS
THE ETHICAL BASIS OF SCIENCE*

*   *   *

[S]cience is more than the instrument of man's increasing power and progress. It is also an instrument, the finest yet developed in the evolution of any species, for the malleable adaptation of man to his environment and the adjustment of his environment to man. If the human species is to remain successful, this instrument must be used more and more to control the nature and rate of social and technological change, as well as to promote it. In this sense, at least, science is far more than a new sense organ for comprehending the real relations of natural phenomena and the regularities we call "laws of nature." It is also man's means of adjustment to nature, man's instrument for the creation of an ideal environment. Since it is preeminently an achievement of social man, its primary function

* 150 *Science* 1254, 1255, 1258, 1260–1261 (1965). Copyright 1965 by the American Association for the Advancement of Science. Reprinted by permission.

is not simply that of appeasing the individual scientist's curiosity about his environment—on the contrary it is that of adjusting man to man, and of adjusting social groups in their entirety to nature, to both the restrictions and the resources of the human environment.

* * *

Those who distrust science as a guide to conduct, whether individual or social, seem to overlook its pragmatic nature, or perhaps they scorn it for that very reason. Rightly understood, science can point out to us only probabilities of varying degrees of certainty. So, of course, do our eyes and ears, and so does our reason. What science can do for us that otherwise we may be too blind or self-willed to recognize is to help us to see that what is right enough for the individual may be wrong for him as a member of a social group, such as a family; that what is right for the family may be wrong for the nation; and that what is right for the nation may be wrong for the great brotherhood of man. Nor should one stop at that point. Man as a species is a member—only one of many members—of a terrestrial community and an even greater totality of life upon earth. Ultimately, what is right for man is what is right for the entire community of life on earth. If he wrecks that community, he destroys his own livelihood. In this sense, coexistence is not only necessary but also right, and science can reveal to us the best ways to harbor our resources and to exploit our opportunities wisely.

. . . From the foregoing description of science as itself an evolutionary product and a human organ produced by natural selection, it may already be guessed that I do not adhere to the view that either the processes or the concepts of science are strictly objective. They are as objective as man knows how to make them, that is true; but man is a creature of evolution, and science is only his way of looking at nature. As long as science is a *human* activity, carried on by individual men and by groups of men, it must at bottom remain inescapably subjective.

* * *

From the beginning the inveterate foe of scientific inquiry has been authority—the authority of tradition, of religion, or of the state—since science can accept no dogma within the sphere of its investigations. No doors must be barred to its inquiries, except by reason of its own limitations. It is the essence of the scientific mind not only

to be curious but likewise to be skeptical and critical—to maintain suspended judgment until the facts are in, to be willing always, in the light of fresh knowledge, to change one's conclusions. Not even the "laws" of science are irrevocable decrees. They are mere summaries of observed phenomena, ever subject to revision. These laws and concepts remain testable and challengeable. Science is thus wholly dependent upon freedom —freedom of inquiry and freedom of opinion.

* * *

The scientist escapes lightly—instead of ten commandments only four: to cherish complete truthfulness; to avoid self-aggrandizement at the expense of one's fellow-scientist; fearlessly to defend the freedom of scientific inquiry and opinion; and fully to communicate one's findings through primary publication, synthesis, and instruction. Out of these grow the social and ethical responsibilities of scientists that in the past 20 years have begun to loom ever larger in our ken.

These may be considered under the three heads of proclamation of benefits, warning of risks, and discussion of quandaries. . . .

* * *

The problem of the future is the ethical problem of the control of man over his own biological evolution. The powers of evolution now rest in his hands. The geneticist can define the means and prognosticate the future with some accuracy. Yet here we enter the third great arena of ethical discussion, passing beyond the benefits of science and the certain risks to the nebulous realm of quandaries. Man must choose goals, and a choice of goals involves us in weighing values—even whole systems of values. The scientist cannot make the choice of goals for his people, and neither can he measure and weigh values with accuracy and objectivity. There is nonetheless an important duty he must perform, because he and he alone may see clearly enough the nature of the alternative choices, including laissez faire, which is no less a choice than any other. It is the social duty and function of the scientist in this arena of discussion to inform and to demand of the people, and of their leaders too, a discussion and consideration of all those impending problems that grow out of scientific discovery and the amplification of human power. Science is no longer—can never be again—the ivory tower of the recluse, the refuge of the asocial man. Science has found its social basis and has eagerly grasped for social support, and it has thereby acquired social responsibilities and a realization of its own fundamental ethical principles. The scientist is a man, through his science doing good and evil to other men, and receiving from them blame and praise, recrimination and money. Science is not only to know, it is to do, and in the doing it has found its soul.

NOTE 3.

MICHAEL POLANYI
PERSONAL KNOWLEDGE*

* * *

[S]cience may be once more discredited, as it was by St. Augustine, if it cannot avoid denaturing our conception of man. The appreciation of natural science is of recent origin and its tradition is rooted in a limited area. It is a single shoot of one civilization among many others of equal antiquity and richness. The Greeks never developed a systematic natural science, nor did Byzantium or China, despite their technological achievements. . . .

* * *

Encircled today between the crude utilitarianism of the philistine and the ideological utilitarianism of the modern revolutionary movement, the love of pure science may falter and die. And if this sentiment were lost, the cultivation of science would lose the only driving force which can guide it towards the achievement of true scientific value. The opinion is widespread that the cultivation of science would always be continued for the sake of its practical advantages. It was expected, for example, that Lysenko's theories, if false, would be soon abandoned by the Soviet Government because they could produce no useful results. This expectation overlooked the fact that such questions cannot be decided in practice. Lysenko's theories are actually the theoretical conclusions which Michurin in Russia and Burbank in the U.S. derived from their substantial successes as plant-breeders. Almost every major systematic error which has deluded men for thousands of years relied on practical experience. Horoscopes, incantations, oracles, magic, witchcraft, the cures of witch doctors and of medical practitioners before the

advent of modern medicine, were all firmly established through the centuries in the eyes of the public by their supposed practical successes. The scientific method was devised precisely for the purpose of elucidating the nature of things under more carefully controlled conditions and by more rigorous criteria than are present in the situations created by practical problems. These conditions and criteria can be discovered only by taking a purely scientific interest in the matter, which again can exist only in minds educated in the appreciation of scientific value. Such sensibility cannot be switched on at will for purposes alien to its inherent passion. No important discovery can be made in science by anyone who does not believe that science is important—indeed supremely important—in itself.

* * *

b.

Faith in Progress?

[i]
John B. Bury
The Idea of Progress*

* * *

. . . We now take [the idea of progress of humanity] so much for granted, we are so conscious of constantly progressing in knowledge, arts, organising capacity, utilities of all sorts, that it is easy to look upon Progress as an aim, like liberty or a world-federation, which it only depends on our own efforts and good-will to achieve. But though all increases of power and knowledge depend on human effort, the idea of the Progress of humanity, from which all these particular progresses derive their value, raises a definite question of fact, which man's wishes or labours cannot affect any more than his wishes or labours can prolong life beyond the grave.

This idea means that civilisation has moved, is moving, and will move in a desirable direction. But in order to judge that we are moving in a desirable direction we should have to know precisely what the destination is. To the minds of most people the desirable outcome of human development would be a condition of society in which all the inhabitants of the planet

* Chicago, Ill.: The University of Chicago Press 181–183 (1958). © Copyright 1958 by Michael Polanyi. Reprinted by permission.

* New York: The Macmillan Co. 1–7, 35–36, 43–44, 334–335, 346–347, 351–352 (1932). Reprinted by permission of the Macmillan Company. Copyright 1932 by the Macmillan Company, renewed 1960 by the Macmillan Company.

would enjoy a perfectly happy existence. But it is impossible to be sure that civilisation is moving in the right direction to realise this aim. Certain features of our "progress" may be urged as presumptions in its favour, but there are always offsets, and it has always been easy to make out a case that, from the point of view of increasing happiness, the tendencies of our progressive civilisation are far from desirable. In short, it cannot be proved that the unknown destination towards which man is advancing is desirable. The movement may be Progress, or it may be in an undesirable direction and therefore not Progress. This is a question of fact, and one which is at present as insoluble as the question of personal immortality. It is a problem which bears on the mystery of life.

Moreover, even if it is admitted to be probable that the course of civilisation has so far been in a desirable direction, and such as would lead to general felicity if the direction were followed far enough, it cannot be proved that ultimate attainment depends entirely on the human will. For the advance might at some point be arrested by an insuperable wall. Take the particular case of knowledge, as to which it is generally taken for granted that the continuity of progress in the future depends altogether on the continuity of human effort (assuming that human brains do not degenerate). This assumption is based on a strictly limited experience. Science has been advancing without interruption during the last three or four hundred years; every new discovery has led to new problems and new methods of solution, and opened up new fields for exploration. Hitherto men of science have not been compelled to halt, they have always found means to advance further. But what assurance have we that they will not one day come up against impassable barriers? The experience of four hundred years, in which the surface of nature has been successfully tapped, can hardly be said to warrant conclusions as to the prospect of operations extending over four hundred or four thousand centuries. Take biology or astronomy. How can we be sure that some day progress may not come to a dead pause, not because knowledge is exhausted, but because our resources for investigation are exhausted—because, for instance, scientific instruments have reached the limit of perfection beyond which it is demonstrably impossible to improve them, or because (in the case of astronomy) we come into the presence of forces of which, unlike gravitation, we have no

terrestrial experience? It is an assumption, which cannot be verified, that we shall not soon reach a point in our knowledge of nature beyond which the human intellect is unqualified to pass.

But it is just this assumption which is the light and inspiration of man's scientific research. For if the assumption is not true, it means that he can never come within sight of the goal which is, in the case of physical science, if not a complete knowledge of the cosmos and the processes of nature, at least an immeasurably larger and deeper knowledge than we at present possess.

Thus continuous progress in man's knowledge of his environment, which is one of the chief conditions of general Progress, is a hypothesis which may or may not be true. And if it is true, there remains the further hypothesis of man's moral and social "perfectibility," which rests on much less impressive evidence. There is nothing to show that he may not reach, in his psychical and social development, a stage at which the conditions of his life will be still far from satisfactory and beyond which he will find it impossible to progress. This is a question of fact which no willing on man's part can alter. It is a question bearing on the mystery of life.

Enough has been said to show that the Progress of humanity belongs to the same order of ideas as Providence or personal immortality. It is true or it is false, and like them it cannot be proved either true or false. Belief in it is an act of faith.

*   *   *

It may surprise many to be told that the notion of Progress, which now seems so easy to apprehend, is of comparatively recent origin. It has indeed been claimed that various thinkers, both ancient (for instance, Seneca) and medieval (for instance, Friar Bacon), had long ago conceived it. But sporadic observations—such as man's gradual rise from primitive and savage conditions to a certain level of civilisation by a series of inventions, or the possibility of some future additions to his knowledge of nature—which were inevitable at a certain stage of human reflection, do not amount to an anticipation of the idea. The value of such observations was determined, and must be estimated, by the whole context of ideas in which they occurred. It is from its bearings on the future that Progress derives its value, its interest, and its power. You may conceive civilisation as having gradually advanced in the past, but you have not got the idea of Progress until you go on to conceive that it is destined to advance indefinitely in the future. . . .

* * *

In this last stage of the Renaissance, which includes the first quarter of the seventeenth century, soil was being prepared in which the idea of Progress could germinate, and our history of its origin definitely begins with the work of two men who belong to this age, Bodin, who is hardly known except to special students of political science, and Bacon, who is known to all the world. Both had a more general grasp of the significance of their own time than any of their contemporaries, and though neither of them discovered a theory of Progress, they both made contributions to thought which directly contributed to its subsequent appearance.

* * *

[Bodin's] work announces a new view of history which is optimistic regarding man's career on earth, without any reference to his destinies in a future life. And in this optimistic view there are three particular points to note, which were essential to the subsequent growth of the idea of Progress. In the first place, the decisive rejection of the theory of degeneration, which had been a perpetual obstacle to the apprehension of that idea. Secondly, the unreserved claim that his own age was fully equal, and in some respects superior, to the age of classical antiquity, in respect of science and the arts. He leaves the ancients reverently on their pedestal, but he erects another pedestal for the moderns, and it is rather higher. . . . In the third place, he had a conception of the common interest of all the peoples of the earth, a conception which corresponded to the old ecumenical idea of the Greeks and Romans, but had now a new significance through the discoveries of modern navigators. He speaks repeatedly of the world as a universal state, and suggests that the various races, by their peculiar aptitudes and qualities, contribute to the common good of the whole. This idea of the "solidarity" of peoples was to be an important element in the growth of the doctrine of Progress.

* * *

In the sixties of the nineteenth century the idea of Progress entered upon the third period of its history. During the *first* period, up to the French Revolution, it had been treated rather casually; it was taken for granted and received no searching examination either from philosophers or from historians. In the *second* period its immense significance was apprehended, and a search began for a general law which would define and establish it. The study of sociology was founded, and at the same time the impressive results of science, applied to the conveniences of life, advertised the idea. It harmonised with the notion of "development" which had become current both in natural science and in metaphysics. Socialists and other political reformers appealed to it as a gospel.

By 1850 it was a familiar idea in Europe, but was not yet universally accepted as obviously true. The notion of social Progress had been growing in the atmosphere of the notion of biological development, but this development still seemed a highly precarious speculation. The fixity of species and the creation of man, defended by powerful interests and prejudices, were attacked but were not shaken. The hypothesis of organic evolution was much in the same position as the Copernican hypothesis in the sixteenth century. Then in 1859 Darwin intervened, like Galileo. The appearance of the *Origin of Species* changed the situation by disproving definitely the dogma of fixity of species and assigning real causes for "transformism." What might be set aside before as a brilliant guess was elevated to the rank of a scientific hypothesis, and the following twenty years were enlivened by the struggle around the evolution of life, against prejudices chiefly theological, resulting in the victory of the theory.

The *Origin of Species* led to the *third* stage of the fortunes of the idea of Progress. We saw how the heliocentric astronomy, by dethroning man from his privileged position in the universe of space and throwing him back on his own efforts, had helped that idea to compete with the idea of a busy Providence. He now suffers a new degradation within the compass of his own planet. Evolution, shearing him of his glory as a rational being specially created to be the lord of the earth, traces a humble pedigree for him. And this second degradation was the decisive fact which has established the reign of the idea of Progress.

Evolution itself, it must be remembered, does not necessarily mean, applied to society, the movement of man to a desirable goal. It is a neutral, scientific conception, compatible either with optimism or with pessimism. According to different estimates it may appear to be a cruel sentence or a guarantee of steady amelioration. And it has been actually interpreted in both ways.

*   *   *

Thus in the seventies and eighties of the last century the idea of Progress was becoming a general article of faith. Some might hold it in the fatalistic form that humanity moves in a desirable direction, whatever men do or may leave undone; others might believe that the future will depend largely on our own conscious efforts, but that there is nothing in the nature of things to disappoint the prospect of steady and indefinite advance. The majority did not inquire too curiously into such points of doctrine, but received it in a vague sense as a comfortable addition to their convictions. But it became a part of the general mental outlook of educated people.

When Mr. Frederic Harrison delivered in 1889 at Manchester an eloquent discourse on the "New Era," in which the dominant note is "the faith in human progress in lieu of celestial rewards of the separate soul," his general argument could appeal to immensely wider circles than the Positivists whom he was specially addressing.

The dogma—for a dogma it remains, in spite of the confidence of Comte or of Spencer that he had made it a scientific hypothesis—has produced an important ethical principle. Consideration for posterity has throughout history operated as a motive of conduct, but feebly, occasionally, and in a very limited sense. With the doctrine of Progress it assumes, logically, a preponderating importance; for the centre of interest is transferred to the life of future generations who are to enjoy conditions of happiness denied to us, but which our labours and sufferings are to help to bring about. If the doctrine is held in an extreme fatalistic form, then our duty is to resign ourselves cheerfully to sacrifices for the sake of unknown descendants, just as ordinary altruism enjoins the cheerful acceptance of sacrifices for the sake of living fellow-creatures. Winwood Reade indicated this when he wrote, "Our own prosperity is founded on the agonies of the past. Is it therefore unjust that we also should suffer for the benefit of those who are to come?" But if it is held that each generation can by its own deliberate acts determine for good or evil the destinies of the race, then our duties towards others reach out through time as well as through space, and our contemporaries are only a negligible fraction of the "neighbours" to whom we owe obligations. The ethical end may still be formulated, with the Utilitarians, as the greatest happiness of the greatest number; only the greatest number includes, as Kidd observed, "the members of generations yet unborn or unthought of." This extension of the moral code, if it is not yet conspicuous in treatises on Ethics, has in late years been obtaining recognition in practice.

*   *   *

[I]f we accept the reasonings on which the dogma of Progress is based, must we not carry them to their full conclusion? In escaping from the illusion of finality, is it legitimate to exempt that dogma itself? Must not it, too, submit to its own negation of finality? Will not that process of change, for which Progress is the optimistic name, compel "Progress" too to fall from the commanding position in which it is now, with apparent security, enthroned? . . . A day will come, in the revolution of centuries, when a new idea will usurp its place as the directing idea of humanity. Another star, unnoticed now or invisible, will climb up the intellectual heaven, and human emotions will react to its influence, human plans respond to its guidance. It will be the criterion by which Progress and all other ideas will be judged. And it too will have its successor.

In other words, does not Progress itself suggest that its value as a doctrine is only relative, corresponding to a certain not very advanced stage of civilisation; just as Providence, in its day, was an idea of relative value, corresponding to a stage somewhat less advanced? Or will it be said that this argument is merely a disconcerting trick of dialectic played under cover of the darkness in which the issue of the future is safely hidden by Horace's prudent god?

[ii]
Thomas S. Kuhn
The Structure of Scientific Revolutions*

*   *   *

With respect to normal science, then, part of the answer to the problem of progress lies simply in the eye of the beholder. Scientific progress is not different in kind from progress in other fields, but the absence at most times of competing schools that question each other's aims and standards makes the progress of a normal-scientific community far easier to see. That, however,

---

* Chicago: The University of Chicago Press 162–172 (1964). © Copyright 1964 by the University of Chicago Press. Reprinted by permission.

is only part of the answer and by no means the most important part. We have, for example, already noted that once the reception of a common paradigm has freed the scientific community from the need constantly to re-examine its first principles, the members of that community can concentrate exclusively upon the subtlest and most esoteric of the phenomena that concern it. Inevitably, that does increase both the effectiveness and the efficiency with which the group as a whole solves new problems. Other aspects of professional life in the sciences enhance this very special efficiency still further.

Some of these are consequences of the unparalleled insulation of mature scientific communities from the demands of the laity and of everyday life. That insulation has never been complete—we are now discussing matters of degree. Nevertheless, there are no other professional communities in which individual creative work is so exclusively addressed to and evaluated by other members of the profession. The most esoteric of poets or the most abstract of theologians is far more concerned than the scientist with lay approbation of his creative work, though he may be even less concerned with approbation in general. That difference proves consequential. Just because he is working only for an audience of colleagues, an audience that shares his own values and beliefs, the scientist can take a single set of standards for granted. He need not worry about what some other group or school will think and can therefore dispose of one problem and get on to the next more quickly than those who work for a more heterodox group. Even more important, the insulation of the scientific community from society permits the individual scientist to concentrate his attention upon problems that he has good reason to believe he will be able to solve. Unlike the engineer, and many doctors, and most theologians, the scientist need not choose problems because they urgently need solution and without regard for the tools available to solve them. In this respect, also, the contrast between natural scientists and many social scientists proves instructive. The latter often tend, as the former almost never do, to defend their choice of a research problem—e.g., the effects of racial discrimination or the causes of the business cycle—chiefly in terms of the social importance of achieving a solution. Which group would one then expect to solve problems at a more rapid rate?

*   *   *

In its normal state, then, a scientific community is an immensely efficient instrument for solving the problems or puzzles that its paradigms define. Furthermore, the result of solving those problems must inevitably be progress. There is no problem here. Seeing that much, however, only highlights the second main part of the problem of progress in the sciences. Let us therefore turn to it and ask about progress through extraordinary science. Why should progress also be the apparently universal concomitant of scientific revolutions? Once again, there is much to be learned by asking what else the result of a revolution could be. Revolutions close with a total victory for one of the two opposing camps. Will that group ever say that the result of its victory has been something less than progress? That would be rather like admitting that they had been wrong and their opponents right. To them, at least, the outcome of revolution must be progress, and they are in an excellent position to make certain that future members of their community will see past history in the same way. . . .

When it repudiates a past paradigm, a scientific community simultaneously renounces, as a fit subject for professional scrutiny, most of the books and articles in which that paradigm had been embodied. Scientific education makes use of no equivalent for the art museum or the library of classics, and the result is a sometimes drastic distortion in the scientist's perception of his discipline's past. More than the practitioners of other creative fields, he comes to see it as leading in a straight line to the discipline's present vantage. In short, he comes to see it as progress. No alternative is available to him while he remains in the field.

Inevitably those remarks will suggest that the member of a mature scientific community is, like the typical character of Orwell's *1984*, the victim of a history rewritten by the powers that be. Furthermore, that suggestion is not altogether inappropriate. There are losses as well as gains in scientific revolutions, and scientists tend to be peculiarly blind to the former. On the other hand, no explanation of progress through revolutions may stop at this point. To do so would be to imply that in the sciences might makes right, a formulation which would again not be entirely wrong if it did not suppress the nature of the process and of the authority by which the choice between paradigms is made. If authority alone, and particularly if nonprofessional authority, were the arbiter of paradigm debates, the outcome of those debates might still be revolution, but it would not be *scientific* revolution. The very existence of science depends upon vesting the power to choose between paradigms in the members of a special kind of community. Just how special that community must be if science is to survive and grow may be indicated by the very tenuousness of humanity's hold on the scientific enterprise. Every civilization of which we have records, has possessed a technology, an art, a religion, a political system, laws, and so on. In many cases those facets of civilization have been as developed as our own. But only the civilizations that descend from Hellenic Greece have possessed more than the most rudimentary science. The bulk of scientific knowledge is a product of Europe in the last four centuries. No other place and time has supported the very special communities from which scientific productivity comes.

What are the essential characteristics of these communities? Obviously, they need vastly more study. In this area only the most tentative generalizations are possible. Nevertheless, a number of requisites for membership in a professional scientific group must already be strikingly clear. The scientist must, for example, be concerned to solve problems about the behavior of nature. In addition, though his concern with nature may be global in its extent, the problems on which he works must be problems of detail. More important, the solutions that satisfy him may not be merely personal but must instead be accepted as solutions by many. The group that shares them may not, however, be drawn at random from society as a whole, but is rather the well-defined community of the scientist's professional compeers. One of the strongest, if still unwritten, rules of scientific life is the prohibition of appeals to heads of state or to the populace at large in matters scientific. Recognition of the existence of a uniquely competent professional group and acceptance of its role as the exclusive arbiter of professional achievement has further implications. The group's members, as individuals and by virtue of their shared training and experience, must be seen as the sole possessors of the rules of the game or of some equivalent basis for unequivocal judgments. To doubt that they shared some such basis for evaluations would be to admit the existence of incompatible standards of scientific achievement. That admission would inevitably raise the question whether truth in the sciences can be one.

*   *   *

These last paragraphs point the directions in which I believe a more refined solution of the problem of progress in the sciences must be sought. Perhaps they indicate that scientific progress is not quite what we had taken it to be. But they simultaneously show that a sort of progress will inevitably characterize the scientific enterprise so long as such an enterprise survives. In the sciences there need not be progress of another sort. We may, to be more precise, have to relinquish the notion, explicit or implicit, that changes of paradigm carry scientists and those who learn from them closer and closer to the truth.

It is now time to notice that until the last very few pages the term 'truth' had entered this essay only in a quotation from Francis Bacon. And even in those pages it entered only as a source for the scientist's conviction that incompatible rules for doing science cannot coexist except during revolutions when the profession's main task is to eliminate all sets but one. The developmental process described in this essay has been a process of evolution *from* primitive beginnings—a process whose successive stages are characterized by an increasingly detailed and refined understanding of nature. But nothing that has been or will be said makes it a process of evolution *toward* anything. Inevitably that lacuna will have disturbed many readers. We are all deeply accustomed to seeing science as the one enterprise that draws constantly nearer to some goal set by nature in advance.

But need there be any such goal? Can we not account for both science's existence and its success in terms of evolution from the community's state of knowledge at any given time? Does it really help to imagine that there is some one full, objective, true account of nature and that the proper measure of scientific achievement is the extent to which it brings us closer to that ultimate goal? If we can learn to substitute evolution-from-what-we-do-know for evolution-toward-what-we-wish-to-know, a number of vexing problems may vanish in the process. Somewhere in this maze, for example, must lie the problem of induction.

I cannot yet specify in any detail the consequences of his alternate view of scientific advance. But it helps to recognize that the conceptual transposition here recommended is very close to one that the West undertook just a century ago. It is particularly helpful because in both cases the main obstacle to transposition is the same. When Darwin first published his theory of evolution by natural selection in 1859, what most bothered many professionals was neither the notion of species change nor the possible descent of man from apes. The evidence pointing to evolution, including the evolution of man, had been accumulating for decades, and the idea of evolution had been suggested and widely disseminated before. Though evolution, as such, did encounter resistance, particularly from some religious groups, it was by no means the greatest of the difficulties the Darwinians faced. That difficulty stemmed from an idea that was more nearly Darwin's own. All the well-known pre-Darwinian evolutionary theories—those of Lamarck, Chambers, Spencer, and the German *Naturphilosophen*—had taken evolution to be a goal-directed process. The "idea" of man and of the contemporary flora and fauna was thought to have been present from the first creation of life, perhaps in the mind of God. That idea or plan had provided the direction and the guiding force to the entire evolutionary process. Each new stage of evolutionary development was a more perfect realization of a plan that had been present from the start.

For many men the abolition of that teleological kind of evolution was the most significant and least palatable of Darwin's suggestions. The *Origin of Species* recognized no goal set either by God or nature. Instead, natural selection, operating in the given environment and with the actual organisms presently at hand, was responsible for the gradual but steady emergence of more elaborate, further articulated, and vastly more specialized organisms. Even such marvelously adapted organs as the eye and hand of man—organs whose design had previously provided powerful arguments for the existence of a supreme artificer and an advance plan—were products of a process that moved steadily *from* primitive beginnings but *toward* no goal. The belief that natural selection, resulting from mere competition between organisms for survival, could have produced man together with the higher animals and plants was the most difficult and disturbing aspect of Darwin's theory. What could 'evolution,' 'development,' and 'progress' mean in the absence of a specified goal? To many people, such terms suddenly seemed self-contradictory.

The analogy that relates the evolution of organisms to the evolution of scientific ideas can easily be pushed too far. But with respect to the issues of this closing section it is very nearly perfect. The process described . . . as the resolution of revolutions is the selection by conflict within the scientific community of the fittest way to practice future science. The net result of a sequence of such revolutionary selections, separated by periods of normal research, is the wonderfully adapted set of instruments we call modern scientific knowledge. Successive stages in that developmental process are marked by an increase in articulation and specialization. And the entire process may have occurred, as we now suppose biological evolution did, without benefit of a set goal, a permanent fixed scientific truth, of which each stage in the development of scientific knowledge is a better exemplar.

Anyone who has followed the argument this far will nevertheless feel the need to ask why the evolutionary process should work. What must nature, including man, be like in order that science be possible at all? Why should scientific communities be able to reach a firm consensus unattainable in other fields? Why should consensus endure across one paradigm change after another? And why should paradigm change invariably produce an instrument more perfect in any sense than those known before? From one point of view those questions, excepting the first, have already been answered. But from another they are as open as they were when this essay began. It is not only the scientific community that must be special. The world of which that community is a part must also possess quite special characteristics, and we are no closer than we were at the start to knowing what these must be. That problem—What must the world be like in order that man may know it?—was not, however, created by this essay. On the contrary, it is as old as science itself, and it remains unanswered. . . .

NOTE

BERTRAND RUSSELL
THE SCIENTIFIC OUTLOOK*

*   *   *

Science in the course of the few centuries of its history has undergone an internal development which appears to be not yet completed. One may sum up this development as the passage from contemplation to manipulation. The love of

* London: George Allen & Unwin Ltd. 269–273 (1931). Reprinted by permission of George Allen & Unwin Ltd. and W. W. Norton & Company, Inc. Copyright 1931 by Bertrand Russell. Copyright renewed 1959 by Bertrand Russell.

knowledge to which the growth of science is due is itself the product of a twofold impulse. We may seek knowledge of an object because we love the object or because we wish to have power over it. The former impulse leads to the kind of knowledge that is contemplative, the latter to the kind that is practical. In the development of science the power impulse has increasingly prevailed over the love impulse. The power impulse is embodied in industrialism and in governmental technique. It is embodied also in the philosophies known as pragmatism and instrumentalism. Each of these philosophies holds, broadly speaking, that our beliefs about any object are true in so far as they enable us to manipulate it with advantage to ourselves. This is what may be called a governmental view of truth. Of truth so conceived science offers us a great deal; indeed there seems no limit to its possible triumphs. To the man who wishes to change his environment science offers astonishingly powerful tools, and if knowledge consists in the power to produce intended changes, then science gives knowledge in abundance.

*   *   *

Science in its beginnings was due to men who were in love with the world. They perceived the beauty of the stars and the sea, of the winds and the mountains. Because they loved them their thoughts dwelt upon them, and they wished to understand them more intimately than a mere outward contemplation made possible. "The world," said Heraclitus, "is an ever-living fire, with measures kindling and measures going out." Heraclitus and the other Ionian philosophers, from whom came the first impulse to scientific knowledge, felt the strange beauty of the world almost like a madness in the blood. They were men of Titanic passionate intellect, and from the intensity of their intellectual passion the whole movement of the modern world has sprung. But step by step, as science has developed, the impulse of love which gave it birth has been increasingly thwarted, while the impulse of power, which was at first a mere camp-follower, has gradually usurped command in virtue of its unforeseen success. The lover of nature has been baffled, the tyrant over nature has been rewarded. . . . Thus science has more and more substituted power-knowledge for love-knowledge, and as this substitution becomes completed science tends more and more to become sadistic. The scientific society of the future as we have been imagining it is one in which the

power impulse has completely overwhelmed the impulse of love, and this is the psychological source of the cruelties which it is in danger of exhibiting.

*   *   *

c.

Survival of Individual or Species?

[i]
Marshall Walker
*The Nature of Scientific Thought**

*   *   *

[E]thical behavior for man is that pattern of individual and collective conduct which maximizes the probability of survival of man as individual and species. This definition permits an act to be classified as ethical or unethical by examining its consequences. As time goes on and consequences become clearer, the classification of a given act in the past may change. The nuclear bombing of Hiroshima, which was intended as an ethical act (to save the lives, both Japanese and American, which would be lost in a full-scale invasion), may be classified as unethical by future historians. A classification is never certain because man is not omniscient. A man must judge whether an act is ethical or unethical in advance, hence he must try to predict the consequences. He extrapolates his knowledge of the past to predict the future. This procedure is the domain of science. His classification of acts as ethical or unethical is as reliable as his scientific predictions of future events, no more and no less. Some ethical judgments will be as "certain" as, "The sun will rise tomorrow"; others will be as uncertain as, "The probability of rain tomorrow is three out of ten.

This definition of *ethical behavior* is operationally equivalent to the traditional statement that ethical behavior is conduct according to the will of God. Religious tradition has it that God created man, encouraged him to be fruitful, and forbade suicide. Thus a pattern of behavior which maximizes man's survival is at least part of the will of God as traditionally accepted. The possibility still remains that behavior to encourage survival is not all that is necessary. It is assumed here that such items as courtesy and loving kindness, which at first appear to be op-

---

* Englewood Cliffs, N.J.: Prentice-Hall, Inc. 153–156 (1963). © 1963 by Prentice-Hall, Inc. Reprinted by permission.

tional, are positive contributions to survival probability and hence are included in the definition of ethical conduct. From this point of view the behavior of such societies as Nazi Germany does not maximize their probability of survival and leads eventually to their destruction.

Mathematicians will inquire how two different quantities, probability of individual survival and probability of species survival, can be maximized simultaneously. The quantity to be maximized is the sum of the weighted probabilities. The weighting factors must be estimated from empirical observation bearing in mind that the weighting factors have changed in the past and will probably change in the future. Different species at the present time weight the factors quite differently. Among bees and ants the survival of the species seems to be heavily weighted.

Ethical predictions take a long time to test empirically, and observations must be extended over many generations. The ethical advice, "Honor thy father and thy mother," according to tradition was pronounced by Moses acting as spokesman for the God of the Hebrews. In this case the end is stated: ". . . that thy days may be long. . . ." The conditions are not stated, but we must infer a set of conditions if the statement is to be verifiable. The assumed conditions will specify the procedure necessary for verification. Let us assume that Moses was talking to the Hebrews and that he had in mind the general conditions of Hebrew life. A predictive form of the commandment is then: "I [Moses] predict that those Hebrews who honor their fathers and mothers will increase their probability of living a long time."

This prediction is clearly based on tribal experience handed down by legend. Primitive tribes had little regard for old people; when men and women became too old to look out for themselves, they were left behind to starve when the tribe migrated. The commandment is saying, "If you honor and look after your old parents, you are setting an example for your son to follow when you yourself get old." This example illustrates clearly the concern for continued survival and the fact that obedience to this law automatically brings a probability of reward.

*   *   *

The prevalence of the verbot form of models of ethical laws has produced the illusion that there is a difference between natural laws and ethical laws. The difference is commonly stated in this way: a man can disobey the ethical law, "Thou shalt not steal," by committing a theft, but a man cannot disobey Newton's second law by any action whatever. This apparent difference disappears immediately when one regards "Thou shalt not steal" as an abbreviation for "Stealing decreases the probability of survival of man as individual and species . . ."

*   *   *

An attempt might be made to base ethical classification on the maximization of probability of individual survival alone. It seems obvious that the probability of individual survival would be increased by an individual's behavior which showed concern for the survival of others of his species. This essay does not adopt that postulate because it leads to a classification contradictory to the teaching of many ethical thinkers. Consider a man who does not believe in an afterlife, but "voluntarily" becomes a martyr to aid the survival of others of his society. Ethical teachers tend to regard this act as moral even when they have little approval for the society itself. The individual survival postulate would classify this act as unethical. The empiricist respects the judgments of many ethical teachers because he considers that these judgments are insights based on observation of society. This essay considers that the postulate of maximization of probability of survival of individual and species gives greater correspondence to the consensus of ethical teachers.

On the other hand, one might attempt to base ethical classification on the maximization of probability of species survival alone. Some insect societies appear to approach this procedure. Its success is probably due to the fact that an individual insect is not very imaginative and does not worry about his own individual future. Man, however, is very imaginative and does worry about his individual future. It seems likely that an ethic which required a man to subordinate completely his own powerful drive toward personal survival to concern for species survival alone would lead to such low morale that the survival probability of the species would be decreased by such a policy. The adoption of the postulate specifying maximization of the weighted sum of the probabilities of personal and species survival permits one to adjust the weighting factors to give maximum correspondence to the observed conditions for each species.

[ii]
*United States Atomic Energy Commission
In the Matter of J. Robert Oppenheimer*

*   *   *

DR. OPPENHEIMER: One important point to make is that lack of feasibility is not the ground on which we made our recommendations [about the hydrogen bomb].

Another point I ought to make is that lack of economy, although alleged, is not the primary or only ground; the competition with fission weapons is obviously in our minds. The real reasons, the weight, behind the report is, in my opinion, a failing of the existence of these weapons would be a disadvantageous thing. It says this over and over again.

I may read, which I am sure has no security value, from the so-called minority report, Fermi and Rabi.

The fact that no limits exist to the destructiveness of this weapon makes its very existence and the knowledge of its construction a danger to humanity as a whole. It is necessarily an evil thing considered in any light. For these reasons, we believe it important for the President of the United States to tell the American public and the world that we think it is wrong on fundamental ethical principles to initiate the development of such a weapon.

In the report which got to be known as the majority report, which Conant wrote, Du-Bridge, Buckley and I signed, things are not quite so ethical and fundamental, but it says in the final paragraph: "In determining not to proceed to develop the super bomb, we see a unique opportunity of providing by example some limitations on the totality of war and thus of eliminating the fear and arousing the hope of mankind."

I think it is very clear that the objection was that we did not like the weapon, not that it couldn't be made.

Now, it is a matter of speculation whether, if we had before us at that time, if we had had the technical knowledge and inventiveness which we did have somewhat later, we would have taken a view of this kind. These are total views where you try to take into account how good the thing is, what the enemy is likely to do, what you can do with it, what the competition is, and the extent to which this is an inevitable step anyway.

* *Transcript of Hearing Before Personnel Security Board.* Washington, D.C.: United States Government Printing Office 79–80, 249–251 (1954).

My feeling about the delay in the hydrogen bomb, and I imagine you want to question me about it, is that if we had had good ideas in 1945, and had we wanted to, this object might have been in existence in 1947 or 1948, perhaps 1948. If we had had all of the good ideas in 1949, I suppose some little time might have been shaved off the development as it actually occurred. If we had not had good ideas in 1951, I do not think we would have it today. In other words, the question of delay is keyed in this case to the question of invention. . . .

The notion that the thermonuclear arms race was something that was in the interests of this country to avoid if it could was very clear to us in 1949. We may have been wrong. We thought it was something to avoid even if we could jump the gun by a couple of years, or even if we could outproduce the enemy, because we were infinitely more vulnerable and infinitely less likely to initiate the use of these weapons, and because the world in which great destruction has been done in all civilized parts of the world is a harder world for America to live with than it is for the Communists to live with. This is an idea which I believe is still right, but I think what was not clear to us then and what is clearer to me now is that it probably lay wholly beyond our power to prevent the Russians somehow from getting ahead with it. I think if we could have taken any action at that time which would have precluded their development of this weapon, it would have been a very good bet to take that, I am sure. . . .

*   *   *

MR. GRAY: [Y]ou don't intend to have this record suggest that you felt that if those who opposed the development of the hydrogen bomb prevailed that would mean that the world would not be confronted with the hydrogen bomb?

DR. OPPENHEIMER: It would not necessarily mean—we thought on the whole it would make it less likely. That the Russians would attempt and less likely that they would succeed in the undertaking.

MR. GRAY: I would like to pursue that a little bit. That is two things. One, the likelihood of their success would we all hope still be related to their own capabilities and not to information they would receive from our efforts. So what you mean to say is that since they would not attempt it they would not succeed?

DR. OPPENHEIMER: No. I believe what we then thought was that the incentive to do it would be far greater if they knew we were doing it, and we had succeeded. Let me, for instance, take a conjecture. Suppose we had not done anything about the atom during the war. I don't think you could guarantee that the Russians would never have had an atomic bomb. But I believe they would not have one as nearly as soon as they have. I think both the fact of our success, the immense amount of publicity, the prestige of the weapon, the espionage they collect, all of this made it an absolutely higher priority thing, and we thought similar circumstances might apply to the hydrogen bomb. We were always clear that there might be a Russian effort whatever we did. We always understood that if we did not do this that an attempt would be made to get the Russians sewed up so that they would not either.

* * *

MR. GRAY: I am trying to get at at what time did your strong moral convictions develop with respect to the hydrogen bomb?

DR. OPPENHEIMER: When it became clear to me that we would tend to use any weapon we had.

MR. GRAY: Then may I ask this: Do you make a sharp distinction between the development of a weapon and the commitment to use it?

DR. OPPENHEIMER: I think there is a sharp distinction but in fact we have not made it.

* * *

MR. GRAY: Your deep concern about the use of the hydrogen bomb, if it were developed, and therefore your own views at the time as to whether we should proceed in a crash program to develop it—your concern about this—became greater, did it not, as the practicabilities became more clear? Is that an unfair statement?

DR. OPPENHEIMER: I think it is the opposite of true. Let us not say about use. But my feeling about development became quite different when the practicabilities became clear. When I saw how to do it, it was clear to me that one had to at least make the thing. Then the only problem was what would one do about them when one had them. The program we had in 1949 was a tortured thing that you could well argue did not make a great deal of technical sense. It was therefore possible to argue also that you did not want it even if you could have it. The program in 1951 was technically so sweet that you could not argue about that. It was purely the military, the political and the humane

problem of what you were going to do about it once you had it.

* * *

d.

Advancement of Social and Political Goals?

*President's Task Force on Science Policy
Science and Technology—Tools for Progress**

The Task Force recommends that the President explicitly enunciate, as a national policy, the need for vigorous, high-quality science and technology, focusing on our national goals and purposes, and recognizing the cultural and inspirational values in man's scientific progress.

The Task Force also recommends that the President call for—as one national goal—continuing leadership in science and in the technology relevant to our other national goals and purposes.

* * *

Our national progress will become ever more critically dependent upon the excellence of our science and technology. A vigorous, high-quality program aimed at advancing our scientific and technological capabilities (including the social, economic, and behavioral components) is vital to all national goals and purposes. Such a program is especially vital to our national defense and security and to our international posture generally; to our ability to negotiate properly safeguarded arms limitations; to our continued economic growth and development and to our international trade balance; to the health of business, labor, and the professions; to the quality of our environment; to the personal health and welfare of all; to the scope and quality of our educational processes; and to the culture, spirit, and inspiration of our people generally. The effectiveness of essentially all our social institutions, including particularly Government itself, is deeply influenced by the quality of our science and technology.

The Nation, therefore, has a fundamental need for excellence in science and technology. Accordingly, it also needs to insure that the effectiveness of our science and technology is not downgraded or destroyed by the unthinking or the uninformed. That is not to say that the limitations of science and technology should not be recognized. We do not suggest complacent ac-

---

* Washington, D.C.: U.S. Government Printing Office 4, 8–9, 38–39 (1970).

ceptance of the unwanted side effects of narrowly motivated or incompletely understood applications of science. Nor do we suggest that technology should dictate social purpose. On the contrary, we wish to emphasize the importance of seeking to optimize utilization of science and technology in the service of social, political, and economic goals.

Anti-Science Attitudes. The rapid rise of attitudes disdainful of science and technology, and the disillusionment of many young people with science and technology is of grave concern. The sources of these attitudes include deficiencies in the application of science and technology which should in fact be criticized and should be corrected. Inanimate technology is not of itself the problem; rather the primary need is "to conceive ways to discover and repair the deficiencies in the processes and institutions by which society puts the tools of science and technology to work." (1) The sources of the shift in attitudes toward science and technology also include widespread lack of perspective and understanding of their nature and role in past and future improvement in the human condition. The public and its elected representative must have a better grasp of both the limitations and the promise of science and technology. Priority should be given to presenting this complex matter to the public in a balanced and understandable fashion. The responsibility for achieving this understanding starts with the executive and legislative branches of the Federal government and spreads to include state and local government, universities, business and professional organizations, and other private institutions in positions of leadership.

Scientific Leadership. The scientific and technological resources of this Nation are among its most powerful tools for the achievement of our social, political, and economic purposes. The management, strength, and proper allocation of these vital resources are political responsibilities of the highest significance, with not only short-term but also very long-term implications both nationally and internationally. The leadership of today must provide the legacy for tomorrow.

The Task Force believes that one of the important national goals for which this Nation should strive is leadership and excellence in science itself—as a long-range investment in achieving the Nation's other goals, as a precursor to more directly applicable and controllable technology, and as a contribution to the culture, spirit, and inspiration of our people.

*   *   *

The United States is entering an era of profound problems as we look to the seventies and beyond. This is an era of relative strategic balance with the Soviet Union, of the emergence of Communist China as a nuclear power, of increased unrest among the non-nuclear nations and increased temptation toward confrontation and escalation, of the historic possibility of achieving verified nuclear arms limitation agreements, and of unusually intense budget pressures.

These significant new factors dictate the need for special attention to the following general aspects of science policy for national security purposes:

1. *Avoidance of technological surprise.* Technology will not stand still; on the contrary, it will likely move more rapidly. The penalty for technological surprise can be enormous.

2. *Reducing lead-time for reaction to changed circumstances.* The capability to react quickly to significantly changed circumstances—changes in perception of Soviet intentions, for example—will become even more critical than it has always been.

3. *Increased emphasis on intelligence and reconnaissance information.* In a period of relative strategic balance, it will be more important than ever to have the best possible information on what is happening behind the "Iron" and "Bamboo" curtains. The margin for error will be significantly reduced, and the premium on precision will be increased. Obviously, the need for continuing verification of nuclear arms agreements further emphasizes this point.

4. *Reduction in total costs.* The increased performance requirements for military hardware, the effects of inflation, and the budget pressures all dictate renewed attention to the matter of cost reduction.

All four of these points lead to the need for increased emphasis on research and development in relation to other competing national security activities. In guarding against technological surprise, it is vital that high-risk long-range research and development programs in critical areas be sustained. The greatest single contribution to reducing lead-times for quicker reaction to changed circumstances would be a development program which emphasizes the bringing of critical high-technology sub-elements of new weapon systems to the demonstration phase on a continuing basis. The significance of research and advanced technology for the purpose of dissolving the "Iron" and "Bamboo" curtains is apparent. Finally, direct research and development projects aimed at cost reduction are indicated: for example, development of "design for low cost" techniques, inclusion of ultimate cost in original research and development specifications, competitive research and development projects where demonstration of low cost is a primary objective.

The impact of the generally rising anti-science and anti-technology attitudes discussed previously in this report could have a particularly important effect on the correct military research and development program for the Nation. The issue of national security research in our universities, for example, has become an irrational one with many students and many faculty members alike. Attacks on the military-industrial complex have, in too many cases, become narrowly self-serving and very short range in perspective. The need for better public and Congressional understanding of both the limitations (e.g., lead-times) and the nature and importance of science and technology for national security purposes is very great indeed.

*   *   *

NOTE

DEREK J. DE SOLLA PRICE
THE SCIENCE OF SCIENCE*

*   *   *

[I] approach modern science with a mixture of doubt and hope about its analysis. On the one hand, I have grave doubts about the accuracy of our knowledge of the way in which science behaves, develops, and interacts with society; even the most able practitioners of science must surely be misled by many of the myths and idols. On the other hand, I believe that one can effectively pursue hard knowledge in this area and that such knowledge might have a rather attractive and provoking universal validity.

Yet to all this I must adduce the paradox that the new knowledge about modern science seems to be growing in the midst of strong resistance from both within and without the field of the history of science. The resistance from outside is from scientists themselves and is tradi-

tional. It has always been part of the special mystique of the scientist that he and he alone can really know about science. Only an esteemed and successful creative scientist can speak for his peers, criticize the state of science, counsel governments and universities, and guide the policies of laboratories and learned societies. An outsider must be presumed ignorant, not merely of the technical facts, but also of that special knowledge of the life of science that can only be won on its battlefields. This is in spite of the fact that creative artists have their competent art critics who may never have drawn or painted, and that practicing musicians are judged by music critics who cannot play an instrument but who wield nonetheless a pen that contributes much to the progress of their creative industry. . . .

*   *   *

3.

Curiosity and Mastery—
The Ever-Widening Net

a.

Myron G. Schultz
Daniel Carrión's Experiment*

When Carrión undertook his experiment in 1885 he was 26 years old and in his sixth year of training at the Facultad de Medicina in Lima. To qualify for his medical degree he had to prepare an original thesis, and he had devoted himself with increasing vigor during the preceding three years to a study of the epidemiology and clinical manifestations of verruga peruana. This unusual disease is manifested by multiple, nodular, vascular eruptions of the skin and mucous membranes accompanied by fever and severe rheumatic pains. Verruga peruana has existed for many centuries in the steep valleys of the Peruvian cordillera; in fact, most scholars believe that the depiction of wart-like eruptions on the *huacas,* the anthropoid ceramic artifacts of the Inca dynasty, demonstrates its pre-Columbian existence.

Carrión carefully studied nine patients with verruga peruana who were hospitalized in Lima. It was a work in which he invested his emotions as well as his intellect. As a youngster, he had

———
* John R. Platt, ed.: *New Views of the Nature of Man.* Chicago: The University of Chicago Press 49–50 (1965). Reprinted by permission.

———
* 278 *New England Journal of Medicine* 1323–1325 (1968). Reprinted by permission.

made frequent trips with his uncle, Manuel Ungaro, through the Peruvian mountains, going to and from school in Lima to his home in Cerro de Pasco. He saw people with verrugas during these trips, and this sight made a deep impression on him. He later told a classmate that through his research he hoped "to make an important contribution to aching humanity." Furthermore, an element of chauvinism crept into his work. When Dr. Izquierdo, a research worker in Chile (the country that had just defeated Peru in the so-called "War of the Pacific"), made what Carrión considered to be superficial observations on verruga peruana Carrión's wounded patriotism was inflamed. He believed that verruga peruana was a Peruvian problem and should therefore be solved by a Peruvian, not by an outsider. Carrión had the noblest of intentions, but they were paving the road to disaster.

*   *   *

Gradually, Carrión came to the conclusion that the most effective way to study the incubation period and symptomatology of verruga peruana would be to perform an experimental inoculation on himself. . . .

. . . As the months went by his determination to inoculate himself became an *idée fixe*. He repeatedly spoke of his plan to his friends and professors; they repeatedly tried to dissuade him. The final impetus came when a request was received in Lima from some important European investigators for specimens of verrugas and the Academia Libre de Medicina set up a prize competition on the subject of verruga peruana. Carrión could no longer be stopped.

On the morning of August 27, 1885, he was in the Nuestra Señora de las Mercedes ward of the Dos de Mayo Hospital. In bed No. 5 was Carmen Paredes, a 14-year-old boy with a verruga on his right eyebrow. . . . Using a lancet he had brought with him, he tried to inoculate his arm with blood taken from the verruga. . . .

*   *   *

On September 17 Carrión felt a vague discomfort and pains in his left ankle. He was not bothered greatly until two days later, when fever began. This was accompanied by strong, teeth-chattering chills, abdominal cramp and pains in all the bones and joints of his body (this mode of onset is typical of Oroya fever). . . .

Carrión told his friends that they were too worried by his illness. He said, "The symptoms I feel could not be other than those of the verruga

to which the eruption period soon will follow and all will be over."

Carrión's friends thought differently. They were impressed by the rapidity with which an anemia had developed. This is not surprising, since today it is known that the hemolytic anemia of Oroya fever can be one of the most rapidly developing and severe of any of the anemias of man. . . .

Carrión was indeed failing, but he was thinking clearly enough to say to his friends:

Up to today, I thought I was only in the invasive stage of the verruga as a consequence of my inoculation, that is, in that period of anemia that precedes the eruption. But now I am deeply convinced that I am suffering from the fever that killed our friend, Orihuela. Therefore, this is the evident proof that Oroya fever and the verruga have the same origin, as Dr. Alarco once said.

This remarkable insight expressed the essence of Carrión's experiment. He had not, as is often said, set out to prove the single etiology of verruga peruana and Oroya fever. He had merely intended to study the onset of verruga peruana; yet, when a completely different disease developed, he was able, in spite of his grave state, to grasp the full meaning of his grave experiment. In addition to demonstrating the unitary etiology of verruga peruana and Oroya fever, he demonstrated the inoculability of the disease.

Up until this time in the course of his illness, Carrión was confined to his rooming house, where he was receiving the attentions of a surrogate mother and his classmates. On October 3 he was visited by a Dr. Flores. When the doctor examined Carrión's blood under the microscope he noted that the red cells showed enlarged and altered morphology. The total red-cell count was only 1,085,000; there was also a leukocytosis. Carrión was urged by Dr. Flores to enter the hospital, where he could be given a blood transfusion, but he refused until the following day. When he finally relented and was transferred to the hospital where all was in readiness for the blood transfusion, a committee of doctors decided, inexplicably, to delay it.

In the evening he was completely delirious and rambled on about the different opinions that existed on the pathology of verruga peruana. On October 5, 39 days after the inoculation, he was in coma. Most of what he uttered was incomprehensible, but his last words were heard clearly by one of his friends. He said, *"Enrique, c'est fini."*

*   *   *

NOTES

NOTE 1.

A. J. BENATT
CARDIAC CATHETERISATION*

*   *   *

When Werner Forssmann conceived the idea of introducing a catheter into the right heart, his object was to administer emergency drugs on the operating-table in the most rapid and efficient way. He opposed intracardiac injections because of the peril of cardiac tamponade, which might arise through injuring the coronary vessels with the needle, though he does not mention whether in fact he had experienced such an accident. The first experiment was on a human cadaver, and he was amazed at the ease with which the ureteric catheter could be guided up the arm vein into the right auricle. . . . He then carried out an experiment on himself. A wide-bore needle was inserted into an antecubital vein, through which a ureteric catheter of 4-Charriére thickness was introduced and passed with great ease to a length of 35 cm. At this point, however, his colleague who performed the operation flinched and the experiment was abandoned. A week later Forssman took matters literally into his own hands. He infiltrated his left antecubital fossa with a local anaesthetic and dissected the vein. Having passed a catheter into it, he placed himself behind an X-ray screen and watched in a mirror the passage of the catheter, which he himself manipulated into the right heart. The screening plant was obviously attached to the operating-theatre where he carried out the experiment: but to get radiographs taken he had to walk, with the catheter in position, to the radiological department, which was quite a distance away. Though the journey involved climbing stairs he had no discomfort, and he mentions only an occasional sensation of warmth similar to that felt when calcium is injected.

In his report, Forssmann visualised the future applications of his method both for diagnosis and therapy. The first patient to be treated by this procedure was a woman with purulent peritonitis, who received through the catheter one litre of glucose with added adrenaline and strophanthin. After improving temporarily she relapsed and eventually died with the catheter still in the right auricle. . . .

*   *   *

Forssmann presented his paper well, performed his experiments in logical sequence, carried them out with zeal and great courage, and provided radiological evidence that the tip of the catheter had reached the right auricle. Moreover, he was the first to inject a radio-opaque substance directly into the right heart; but, though producing exemplary skiagrams of dogs, he did not succeed in obtaining contrast pictures of his own heart when he injected 'Uroselectan' through the catheter. . . .

*   *   *

NOTE 2.

G. LILJESTRAND
NOBEL PRIZE PRESENTATION
SPEECH FOR PHYSIOLOGY
OR MEDICINE (1956)*

. . . The heart is the sun of the microcosm formed by the human body, as stated already by William Harvey in his monumental treatise on the circulation of the blood. Its central role in both healthy and pathologic states is well known and is illustrated, for example, by the fact that cardiovascular diseases are at present responsible for more deaths than any other group of diseases. It is for essentially new contributions in this important field that the Nobel Prize for Physiology or Medicine has been awarded this year.

Two factors are decisive for the work of the heart. One is the pressure conditions in its various chambers. The other is the quantity of blood forced by its right side through the pulmonary vessels to its left side which, in turn, transmits the blood to all the parts of the body, to be returned once more to the right atrium. Exact data regarding these two factors have long been available through animal experiments. It has been possible to measure the pressure, after introduction of catheters connected to suitable recording instruments. . . .

As far as man is concerned, these methods were for a long time only partly applicable. Thus, it was possible to record the pressure in the peripheral arteries—and this is what is usually meant when we speak of the blood pressure—as well as in the superficial veins. These values reflect to some extent the conditions in the left ventricle and the right atrium. But measurements of the right ventricular pressure, which is of

---

* 1 *Lancet* 746–747 (1949). Reprinted by permission.

* *Nobel Lectures, Physiology or Medicine 1942–1962.* Amsterdam: Elsevier Publishing Co. 501–502, 505 (1964). Reprinted by permission. © Nobel Foundation, 1957.

essential importance for the work of the right side of the heart, was impracticable. Similarly, it was possible, for determination of the oxygen content, to take samples of the arterial blood, but not of the mixed venous blood in the right side of the heart, which gives the average value for the body as a whole. It was, in fact, necessary to resort to indirect methods. These have yielded valuable results although they have somewhat undeservedly—as is often the case—been overshadowed by the subsequent conquests. . . .

As late as 1928, there were good reasons for the statement in a textbook that in man one was naturally confined to the use of the indirect methods. Consequently, it was highly surprising when, already in the following year, Werner Forssmann at the surgical clinic in Eberswalde was able to show—by making, with the intrepidity of youth, by no means harmless experiments on himself—that a narrow catheter could be advanced from a cubital vein into the right atrium itself, a distance of almost two-thirds of a metre. Obviously, this constituted a remarkable advance. It was thereby demonstrated that, on principle, the methods well known from animal experiments could also be adapted for studies in man.

This was naturally of paramount importance for a study of pathologic changes in the circulatory system, which could be reproduced with difficulty, or not at all, in animal experiments. It also opened up better opportunities for röntgenologic examination of the right side of the heart and the pulmonary vessels, after injection of contrast medium directly into these organs. For this purpose as well, Forssmann made experiments on himself. It must have required firm conviction of the value of the method to induce self-experimentation of the kind carried out by Forssmann. His later disappointment must have been all the more bitter. It is true that the method was adopted in a few places—in Prague and in Lisbon—but on the whole Forssmann was not given the necessary support; he was, on the contrary, subjected to criticism of such exaggerated severity that it robbed him of any inclination to continue. This criticism was based on an unsubstantiated belief in the danger of the intervention, thus affording proof that—even in our enlightened times—a valuable suggestion may remain unexploited on the grounds of a preconceived opinion. A contributory cause in this substance was presumably that Forssmann was working in a milieu that did not clearly grasp the great value of his idea.

* * *

Professor Forssmann. As a young doctor you have had the courage to submit yourself to heart catheterization. As a result of this, a new method was born which since that time has proved to be of very great value. It has not only opened up new roads for the study of the physiology and the pathology of the heart and lungs, it has also given the impetus for important researches on other organs. We are glad to be able to welcome you in this country where once your ancestors worked.

* * *

On behalf of the Caroline Institute I proffer you the hearty congratulations of your colleagues on your brilliant achievements.

I now have the honour of asking you to accept the Nobel Prize from the hands of His Majesty the King.

NOTE 3.

WERNER FORSSMANN
THE ROLE OF HEART CATHETERIZATION
AND ANGIOCARDIOGRAPHY IN THE
DEVELOPMENT OF MODERN MEDICINE—
NOBEL LECTURE (1956) *

* * *

[In 1929] I carried out my first experiments in angiocardiography. Here for the first time the living heart of a dog was successfully visualized radiologically with the aid of a contrast medium. Even at that time, the complete lesser circulation in the dog could be shown with the cinematographic radioscopy according to Gottheiner.

Although no results could be attempted with human beings, because no apparatus had been devised, their possibility had at least been demonstrated in principle. Only four months after this publication, Moniz, Carvalho, and Lima were able to disclose rather better results. With them began the immense quantity of writing on angiocardiography.

Further development of technique was impeded not only by the absence of technical essentials and consequent lack of knowledge. To some outsiders, ethical considerations also weighed heavily in the balance against it. And when one thinks how hard men like Cournand

* Nobel Lectures, Physiology or Medicine 1942–1962. Amsterdam: Elsevier Publishing Co. 506, 508–510 (1964). Reprinted by permission. © Nobel Foundation, 1957.

and McMichael had to fight against such people in 1941 and later, one can perhaps understand what difficulties stood in my way twelve years before.

*   *   *

. . . Cournand and McMichael, too, . . . had strong resistance to overcome, the harder to deal with because people did not hesitate to obstruct practical research work with threadbare ethical and moral objections, such as are still occasionally raised today. But these voices also must fall silent now it has been shown how responsibly this circulation research has been conducted everywhere and with what high moral earnestness it has been applied. . . .

*   *   *

Angiocardiography, in the form in which it is practised today, is of course still burdened with risks which impose limitations on its use. Its use cannot therefore be justified for examinations which are not strictly necessary, but here, too, new possibilities can be discerned.

Further development will in many cases enable us to dispense with the massive and dangerous quantities of contrast media which at the moment we still need, and to manage instead with smaller, less harmful amounts of radioactive isotopes. . . .

From all this, we can see that modern cardiology has become something much more universal than was originally supposed.

One may compare the art of healing with a work of art, which from different standpoints and under different lighting reveals ever new and surprising beauty.

*   *   *

b.

Ronald W. Clark
JBS—The Life and Work of J. B. S. Haldane*

John Burdon Sanderson Haldane was born on November 5, 1892 . . . On both sides of the family tree his ancestors were vigorous, mentally distinguished, and toughly individualist; from them he was to draw a combination of aristocratic self-assurance, intellectual integrity, and almost endearing bloody-mindedness.

*   *   *

* New York: Coward-McCann, Inc. 11, 14, 15, 19, 25–26, 60–65 (1968). Reprinted by permission of Coward-McCann, Inc. Copyright © 1968 by Ronald Clark.

His real education came from his father, to whose example in the scientific approach to facts he owed much of his success. The education began young, and at the age of three the father was taking samples of his son's blood for investigation. A year later, both traveled to London, where John Scott Haldane was testing the atmosphere on the Metropolitan Underground. . . .

*   *   *

JBS learned more than this scientific attitude from his father. John Scott Haldane was one of those very rare men who can train themselves to ignore fear. His son, describing how his father disliked experimenting on animals and "preferred to work on himself or other human beings who were sufficiently interested in the work to ignore pain or fear," explained that his father had achieved a state in which he was almost indifferent to pain. "However," he went on, "his object was not to achieve this state but to achieve knowledge which could save other men's lives. His attitude was much more like that of a good soldier who will risk his life and endure wounds in order to gain victory than that of an ascetic who deliberately undergoes pain. The soldier does not get himself wounded deliberately, and my father did not seek pain in his work, though he greeted a pain which would have made some people writhe or groan, with laughter." . . .

*   *   *

On the wall [of Cherwell, the Haldane home in Oxford] there was worked in stone the eagle crest of the Haldanes and the single-word family motto—"Suffer." As a symbol in the life of JBS this was to have the significance of *Citizen Kane's* "Rosebud." To suffer and to endure was to seem more a natural part of life to him that it did to most men. . . .

*   *   *

John Scott Haldane's main industrial work concerned conditions in mines, and to investigate and report on these he was regularly employed by both government and industry. JBS often went, too, partly as a useful experimental animal whose reactions might be interesting, partly to be taught the facts of life. . . . JBS long remembered a pit in North Staffordshire. . . ."After a while," JBS later wrote, "we got to a place where the roof was about eight feet high and a man could stand up. One of the party lifted his safety lamp. It filled with blue flame and went out with a pop. If it had been a candle this would have started an explosion, and we should probably have been killed. But of course the flame of the explosion inside the safety lamp was kept in by the wire gauze. The air near the roof was full of methane, or firedamp, which is a gas lighter than air, so the air on the floor was not dangerous.

"To demonstrate the effects of breathing firedamp, my father told me to stand up and recite Mark Antony's speech from Shakespeare's 'Julius Caesar,' beginning 'Friends, Romans, countrymen.' I soon began to pant, and somewhere about 'the noble Brutus' my legs gave way and I collapsed on to the floor, where, of course, the air was all right. In this way I learnt that firedamp is lighter than air and not dangerous to breathe."

*   *   *

At Oxford JBS . . . decided to teach physiology, a decision which would have been recklessness in a lesser man, since he had neither degree nor other qualification in the subject. In fact Haldane, Fellow of the Royal Society and the author of more than 300 scientific papers, never did take any scientific degree, thus following his father, who never took a course in engineering but became president of the Institution of Mining Engineers.

*   *   *

Haldane's interest in a unified science course reflected his own ability to take up a new subject and worry his way quickly into its essentials. . . . With physiology, to which he now devoted himself, he had the aid of environment, since he had been brought up surrounded by the rules of the discipline. . . . John Scott Haldane had discovered that it was carbon dioxide in the human bloodstream which enabled the muscles to regulate breathing under different conditions. But it was not known whether the carbon dioxide did so by making the blood more acid, as was suspected, or by some other method. Haldane therefore taught his son the technique developed by himself of gas analysis, by which very small amounts of gas can be accurately measured. Then he gave him, together with Peter Davies, a young worker in the physiological laboratory, the task of finding how carbon dioxide did this particular job. The experiments which followed enabled JBS to make a number of useful discoveries, and they encouraged him in the practice of self-experimentation for which he was to become famous.

He and his colleague argued that if acidity of the blood was the vital factor, then an increase in the amount of alkaline sodium bicarbonate in the blood would slow down breathing, since such slowing down would help to retain more carbon dioxide and thereby retain the normal balance. The first task was therefore to discover the amount of sodium bicarbonate already in a normal person's blood. This was not easy. In fact it was three months before Haldane and Davies got their different estimates to agree. . . .

Once Haldane and Davies had finished this first part of their work, they began to use themselves as guinea pigs—for one reason which Haldane was never tired of emphasizing: neither a dog nor a rabbit nor any experimental animal other than man can "tell you if he has a headache, or an upset of his sensators of smell, both of which I obtained as symptoms during these experiments."

They wanted to see if John Scott Haldane's theory about breathing was correct, but they wanted to give a quantitative answer—to be able to state, for instance, how much more one would breathe if the alkaline reserve in the blood were increased by a stated amount. And they wanted to find out if any symptoms of certain diseases could be put down to changes in the alkalinity of the blood.

The first part of the work was fairly easy. Haldane and Davies each ate about an ounce and a half of bicarbonate of soda—and each, as expected, found that his breathing was slowed and that the carbon dioxide in the blood rose to balance the bicarbonate. Here Haldane followed what was to be his universal rule. When reporting experiments on himself, he would rarely if ever note "I felt . . ." or "I began to pant. . . ." Scientific thinking was objective thinking, and the records were couched in the impersonal form of "J. H. panting . . ." or "J. H. finding difficulty in breathing." Explaining this, JBS once wrote: "In fact, I try to think of myself as I would of anyone else. This is the essence of justice."

Getting acid into the blood was more difficult than getting it out. To start with, Haldane began by drinking hydrochloric acid; if neat, this would have been fatal, so he had to dilute it—but he diluted it so much that it failed to have much effect. He then worked out a number of chemical tricks to smuggle the hydrochloric acid into his blood disguised as something else. One method was to drink a solution of ammonium chloride. At the first attempt he dissolved five grams in 100 c.c. of water—and on drinking the solution was violently sick. He then diluted it still further and tried again; this time the trick worked, although he had to drink less than the carefully calculated amount which he estimated would kill him. The ammonium chloride, absorbed from the intestine, went to the liver, where it was turned into urea, leaving the acid behind. One or two ounces of it, JBS found, was sufficient to make him very short of breath, and after some of the experiments he panted for several days.

It had seemed unlikely that any practical results would spring from this work. However, as Appleton found when radar grew from his discovery of ionized layers in the stratosphere, the "purest" experiments can produce the most utilitarian results. So it was with this work on the acidity of the blood. Soon afterward a Continental doctor discovered that one particular kind of fit, from which some babies suffered and a few died, was caused by the extreme alkalinity of the blood. The ammonium chloride treatment was successfully used by the doctor to cure the condition. . . .

Many similar experiments followed during the next few years, some in the Oxford physiological laboratory, some in John Scott Haldane's own private laboratory at Cherwell. There was a thirteen-day experiment during which JBS drank eighty-five grams of calcium chloride dissolved in water and produced "intense diarrhoea, followed by constipation due to the formation of a large hard faecal mass. There was great general discomfort, pains in the head, limbs and back, and disturbed nights." To discover the change in the pressure of carbon dioxide in the lungs after violent exercise, he ran five times up and down a thirty-foot staircase, repeated the sequence nineteen times, and had samples of his breath taken after each. In the gas chamber of the Cherwell laboratory he recorded his own and other people's reactions to various concentrations of gas. And at Cherwell also he drank quantities of hydrochloric acid, reporting afterward that walking at three miles an hour caused severe panting and that cycling was impossible. "There were occasional slight headaches. A certain exhilaration and irritability of temper were noticed at times by myself and others, but there was no mental confusion, and the experiment was not unpleasant." In the case of the more dangerous carbon monoxide, the symptoms of poisoning were, he wrote, "the same as alcoholic poisoning, except that carbon monoxide goes a bit further. One is that you cannot walk straight

or talk straight, although you feel you are perfectly all right. If you go into a mine full of this gas with a bird in a cage, the bird gets drunk first, and then comes off its perch, and you yourself will probably feel full of beans. That is the great danger, for you tumble over, get unconscious and die."

These experiments, which had to be combined with Haldane's quota of teaching, were frequently uncomfortable, frequently unpleasant, and sometimes both. . . . But a little more information had been acquired about the way the human body works, a satisfactory conclusion for a man who could say, as Haldane did, "You cannot be a good human physiologist unless you regard your own body, and that of your colleagues, with the same sort of respect with which you regard the starry sky and yet as something to be used and, if need be, used up."

However useful it was, and of that there can be no doubt, there was a trace of exhibitionism about the way he spoke of such work, a flamboyance epitomized by his comment that the only way to test a chemical's reaction was to take ten times the dose listed as fatal in the British pharmacopoeia. . . .

*   *   *

c.

B. F. Skinner
Baby in a Box*

Since the publication of this article in the Ladies Home Journal *in October, 1945, several hundred babies have been reared in what is now known as an "Air-Crib." The advantages reported here have been generously confirmed. Although cultural inertia is perhaps nowhere more powerful than in child-raising practices, and in spite of the fact that the device is not easy to build, its use has steadily spread. The advantages to the child and parent alike seem to be too great to be resisted. One early user, John M. Gray, sent a questionnaire to 73 couples who had used Air-Cribs for 130 babies. All but three described the device as "wonderful." The physical and psychological benefits reported by these users seem to warrant extensive research.*

In that brave new world which science is

* *Cumulative Record* 419–426 (Enlarged Edition, 1959). Copyright © 1959, 1961, Appleton-Century-Crofts, Inc. Reprinted by permission of Appleton-Century-Crofts, Educational Division, Meredith Corporation.

preparing for the housewife of the future, the young mother has apparently been forgotten. Almost nothing has been done to ease her lot by simplifying and improving the care of babies.

When we decided to have another child, my wife and I felt that it was time to apply a little labor-saving invention and design to the problems of the nursery. We began by going over the disheartening schedule of the young mother, step by step. We asked only one question: Is this practice important for the physical and psychological health of the baby? When it was not, we marked it for elimination. Then the "gadgeteering" began.

The result was an inexpensive apparatus in which our baby daughter has now been living for eleven months. Her remarkable good health and happiness and my wife's welcome leisure have exceeded our most optimistic predictions, and we are convinced that a new deal for both mother and baby is at hand.

We tackled first the problem of warmth. The usual solution is to wrap the baby in a half-a-dozen layers of cloth—shirt, nightdress, sheet, blankets. This is never completely successful. The baby is likely to be found steaming in its own fluids or lying cold and uncovered. Schemes to prevent uncovering may be dangerous, and in fact they have sometimes even proved fatal. Clothing and bedding also interfere with normal exercise and growth and keep the baby from taking comfortable postures or changing posture during sleep. They also encourage rashes and sores. Nothing can be said for the system on the score of convenience, because frequent changes and launderings are necessary.

Why not, we thought, dispense with clothing altogether except for the diaper, which serves another purpose—and warm the space in which the baby lives? This should be a simple technical problem in the modern home. Our solution is a closed compartment about as spacious as a standard crib. The walls are well insulated, and one side, which can be raised like a window, is a large pane of safety glass. The heating is electrical, and special precautions have been taken to insure accurate control.

After a little experimentation we found that our baby, when first home from the hospital, was completely comfortable and relaxed without benefit of clothing at about 86°F. As she grew older, it was possible to lower the temperature by easy stages. Now, at eleven months, we are operating at about 78°, with a relative humidity of 50 per cent.

Raising or lowering the temperature by more than a degree or two produces a surprising change in the baby's condition and behavior. This response is so sensitive that we wonder how a comfortable temperature is ever reached with clothing and blankets.

The discovery which pleased us most was that crying and fussing could always be stopped by slightly lowering the temperature. During the first three months, it is true, the baby would also cry when wet or hungry, but in that case she would stop when changed or fed. During the past six months she has not cried at all except for a moment or two when injured or sharply distressed—for example, when inoculated. The "lung exercise" which so often is appealed to to reassure the mother of a baby who cries a good deal takes the much pleasanter form of shouts and gurgles.

How much of this sustained cheerfulness is due to the temperature is hard to say, because the baby enjoys many other kinds of comfort. She sleeps in curious postures, not half of which would be possible under securely fastened blankets.

When awake, she exercises almost constantly and often with surprising violence. Her leg, stomach, and back muscles are especially active and have become strong and hard. It is necessary to watch this performance for only a few minutes to realize how severely restrained the average baby is, and how much energy must be diverted into the only remaining channel—crying.

A wider range and variety of behavior are also encouraged by the freedom from clothing. For example, our baby acquired an amusing, almost apelike skill in the use of her feet. We have devised a number of toys which are occasionally suspended from the ceiling of the compartment. She often plays with these with her feet alone and with her hands and feet in close co-operation.

One toy is a ring suspended from a modified music box. A note can be played by pulling the ring downwards, and a series of rapid jerks will produce Three Blind Mice. At seven months our baby would grasp the ring in her toes, stretch out her leg and play the tune with a rhythmic movement of her foot.

We are not especially interested in developing skills of this sort, but they are valuable for the baby because they arouse and hold her interest. Many babies seem to cry from sheer boredom—their behavior is restrained and they have nothing else to do. In our compartment, the waking hours are invariably active and happy ones.

Freedom from clothes and bedding is especially important for the older baby who plays and falls asleep off and on during the day. Unless the mother is constantly on the alert, it is hard to cover the baby promptly when it falls asleep and to remove and arrange sheets and blankets as soon as it is ready to play. All this is now unnecessary.

Remember that these advantages for the baby do not mean additional labor or attention on the part of the mother. On the contrary, there is an almost unbelievable saving in time and effort. For one thing, there is no bed to be made or changed. The "mattress" is a tightly stretched canvas, which is kept dry by warm air. A single bottom sheet operates like a roller towel.* It is stored on a spool outside the compartment at one end and passes into a wire hamper at the other. It is ten yards long and lasts a week. A clean section can be locked into place in a few seconds. The time which is usually spent in changing clothes is also saved. This is especially important in the early months. When we take the baby up for feeding or play, she is wrapped in a small blanket or a simple nightdress. Occasionally she is dressed up "for fun" or for her play period. But that is all. The wrapping blanket, roller sheet, and the usual diapers are the only laundry actually required.

Time and labor are also saved because the air which passes through the compartment is thoroughly filtered. The baby's eyes, ears, and nostrils remain fresh and clean. A weekly bath is enough provided the face and diaper region are frequently washed. These little attentions are easy because the compartment is at waist level.

It takes about one and one-half hours each day to feed, change, and otherwise care for the baby. This includes everything except washing diapers and preparing formula. We are not interested in reducing the time any further. As a baby grows older, it needs a certain amount of social stimulation. And after all, when unnecessary chores have been eliminated, taking care of a baby is fun.

An unforeseen dividend has been the contribution to the baby's good health. Our pediatrician readily approved the plan before the baby was born, and he has followed the results enthu-

siastically from month to month. Here are some points on the health score: When the baby was only ten days old, we could place her in the preferred face-down position without danger of smothering, and she has slept that way ever since, with the usual advantages. She has always enjoyed deep and extended sleep, and her feeding and eliminative habits have been extraordinarily regular. She has never had a stomach upset, and she has never missed a daily bowel movement.

The compartment is relatively free of spray and air-borne infection, as well as dust and allergic substances. Although there have been colds in the family, it has been easy to avoid contagion, and the baby has completely escaped. The neighborhood children troop in to see her, but they see her through glass and keep their school-age diseases to themselves. She has never had a diaper rash.

We have also enjoyed the advantages of a fixed daily routine. Child specialists are still not agreed as to whether the mother should watch the baby or the clock, but no one denies that a strict schedule saves time, for the mother can plan her day in advance and find time for relaxation or freedom for other activities. The trouble is that a routine acceptable to the baby often conflicts with the schedule of the household. Our compartment helps out here in two ways. Even in crowded living quarters it can be kept free of unwanted lights and sounds. The insulated walls muffle all ordinary noises, and a curtain can be drawn down over the window. The result is that, in the space taken by a standard crib, the baby has in effect a separate room. We are never concerned lest the doorbell, telephone, piano, or children at play wake the baby, and we can therefore let her set up any routine she likes.

But a more interesting possibility is that her routine may be changed to suit our convenience. A good example of this occurred when we dropped her schedule from four to three meals per day. The baby began to wake up in the morning about an hour before we wanted to feed her. This annoying habit, once established, may persist for months. However, by slightly raising the temperature during the night we were able to postpone her demand for breakfast. The explanation is simple. The evening meal is used by the baby mainly to keep herself warm during the night. How long it lasts will depend in part upon how fast heat is absorbed by the surrounding air.

One advantage not to be overlooked is that the soundproofing also protects the family from the baby! Our intentions in this direction were

---

* The canvas and "endless" sheet arrangement was soon replaced with a single layer of woven plastic, which could be cleaned and instantly wiped dry.

misunderstood by some of our friends. We were never put to the test, because there was no crying to contend with, but it was never our policy to use the compartment in order to let the baby "cry it out."

Every effort should be made to discover just why a baby cries. But if the condition cannot be remedied, there is no reason why the family, and perhaps the neighborhood as well, must suffer. (Such a compartment, by the way, might persuade many a landlord to drop a "no babies" rule, since other tenants can be completely protected.)

Before the baby was born, when we were still building the apparatus, some of the friends and acquaintances who had heard about what we proposed to do were rather shocked. Mechanical dish-washers, garbage disposers, air cleaners, and other laborsaving devices were all very fine, but a mechanical baby tender—that was carrying science too far! However, all the specific objections which were raised against the plan have faded away in the bright light of our results. A very brief acquaintance with the scheme in operation is enough to resolve all doubts. Some of the toughest skeptics have become our most enthusiastic supporters.

One of the commonest objections was that we were going to raise a "softie" who would be unprepared for the real world. But instead of becoming hypersensitive, our baby has acquired a surprisingly serene tolerance for annoyances. She is not bothered by the clothes she wears at playtime, she is not frightened by loud or sudden noises, she is not frustrated by toys out of reach, and she takes a lot of pommeling from her older sister like a good sport. It is possible that she will have to learn to sleep in a noisy room, but adjustments of that sort are always necessary. A tolerance for any annoyance can be built up by administering it in controlled dosages, rather than in the usual accidental way. Certainly there is no reason to annoy the child throughout the whole of its infancy, merely to prepare it for later childhood.

It is not, of course, the favorable conditions to which people object, but the fact that in our compartment they are "artificial." All of them occur naturally in one favorable environment or another, where the same objection should apply but is never raised. It is quite in the spirit of the "world of the future" to make favorable conditions available everywhere through simple mechanical means.

A few critics have objected that they would not like to live in such a compartment themselves—they feel that it would stifle them or give them claustrophobia. The baby obviously does not share in this opinion. The compartment is well ventilated and much more spacious than a Pullman berth, considering the size of the occupant. The baby cannot get out, of course, but that is true of a crib as well. There is less actual restraint in the compartment because the baby is freer to move about. The plain fact is that she is perfectly happy. She has never tried to get out nor resisted being put back in, and that seems to be the final test.

Another early objection was that the baby would be socially starved and robbed of the affection and mother love which she needs. This has simply not been true. The compartment does not ostracize the baby. The large window is no more of a social barrier than the bars of a crib. The baby follows what is going on in the room, smiles at passers-by, plays "peek-a-boo" games, and obviously delights in company. And she is handled, talked to, and played with whenever she is changed or fed, and each afternoon during a play period which is becoming longer as she grows older.

The fact is that a baby will probably get more love and affection when it is easily cared for, because the mother is not so likely to feel overworked and resentful of the demands made upon her. She will express her love in a practical way and give the baby genuinely affectionate care.

It is common practice to advise the troubled mother to be patient and tender and to enjoy her baby. And, of course, that is what any baby needs. But it is the exceptional mother who can fill this prescription upon demand, especially if there are other children in the family and she has no help. We need to go one step further and treat the mother with affection also. Simplified child care will give mother love a chance.

A similar complaint was that such an apparatus would encourage neglect. But easier care is sure to be better care. The mother will resist the temptation to put the baby back into a damp bed if she can conjure up a dry one in five seconds. She may very well spend less time with her baby, but babies do not suffer from being left alone but only from the discomforts which arise from being left alone in the ordinary crib.

How long do we intend to keep the baby in the compartment? The baby will answer that in time, but almost certainly until she is two years old, or perhaps three. After the first year, of course, she will spend a fair part of each day in a play-pen or out-of-doors. The compartment takes the place of a crib and will get about the same use. Eventually it will serve as sleeping quarters only.

We cannot, of course, guarantee that every baby raised in this way will thrive so successfully. But there is a plausible connection between health and happiness and the surroundings we have provided, and I am quite sure that our success is not an accident. The experiment should, of course, be repeated again and again with different babies and different parents. One case is enough, however, to disprove the flat assertion that it can't be done. At least we have shown that a moderate and inexpensive mechanization of baby care will yield a tremendous saving in time and trouble, without harm to the child and probably to its lasting advantage.

d.
David M. Rorvik and Landrum B. Shettles
You Can Choose Your Baby's Sex*

* * *

Interest in choosing sex remains as high among prospective parents today as it ever was, despite the almost universal unconcern of baby doctors. And failure to produce the desired sex still creates as much anguish as it did in the past —perhaps more, since we have come to expect so much from modern medical science. . . .

One doctor who does understand the anguish of such parents is Landrum B. Shettles, M.D., Ph.D., D.Sc. (He is an assistant attending obstetrician-gynecologist at Columbia-Presbyterian Medical Center and an assistant professor of clinical obstetrics and gynecology at Columbia College of Physicians and Surgeons.) Sitting in his office, he recalls . . . when he made the discovery that may help millions select the sex of their offspring.

* * *

[A]fter examining more than 500 sperm specimens, he is convinced that . . . small, round-headed sperms carry the male-producing chromosomes, and the larger, oval-shaped type carry the female-producing X chromosomes. [I]n most cases, the round sperm far outnumbered the oval-shaped sperm.

* * *

* *Look* 86–98 (April 21, 1970). Reprinted by permission.

After making his discovery, Dr. Shettles published his findings in the scientific journal *Nature* and suddenly found himself in the middle of a controversy.

Not everybody has agreed with his findings, and he does not claim scientific infallibility. But he does stand on his record, on observations he has made in the laboratory and, most important, on his results to date. Other researchers have provided some impressive corroboration of Dr. Shettles' work.

As soon as he had made his initial discovery, Dr. Shettles had only one thing in mind: to find some means of exploiting this new knowledge to help parents choose the sex of their children. Since there definitely seemed to be a difference in the overall size of the two types of sperm, he reasoned, there must be other differences as well. Perhaps one type was stronger than the other or faster—or both. Perhaps one type could survive longer in a certain environment than the other. . . .

It seemed fairly certain that the larger, female-producing sperm (now called gynosperms) must be more resistant than the other type. Why should there be nearly twice as many of the smaller, boy-producing variety (known as androsperms) in the ejaculate of the average male if not to compensate for some inferiority in coping with the environment beyond the male reproductive tract? There may be as many as 170 boys conceived for every 100 girls, and for every 100 female births, there are about 105 male births. . . .

What accounts for the greater slaughter of androsperms within the womb? To find out, Dr. Shettles began studying the environment that exists inside the vagina and uterus at about the time of conception. . . .

* * *

Acid inhibits both gynosperms and androsperms, but it harms the androsperms first and most, cutting them out of the herd and thus out of competition. The gynosperms' greater bulk seems to protect them from the acid for much longer periods than their little brothers are able to survive.

Alkaline secretions are kind to both types of sperm and generally enhance the chances for fertilization. But in the absence of hostile acids, the androsperms are able to use the *one* advantage they have over their sisters: the speed and agility that their small, compact heads and long tails give them.

*   *   *

As a result of these findings, Dr. Shettles has formulated two procedures—one to be used if a female child is desired, the other if a male is wanted. These procedures can be used in the home *without* prior semen analysis.

The procedure for female offspring

1. Intercourse should cease two or three days before ovulation. Timing is the most important factor.
2. Intercourse should be immediately *preceded,* on each occasion, by an acidic douche consisting of two tablespoons of *white* vinegar to a quart of water. The timing might be enough to ensure female offspring, but the douche makes success all the more likely, since the acid environment immobilizes the androsperms.
3. If the wife normally has orgasm, she should try to avoid it. Orgasm increases the flow of alkaline secretions, and these could neutralize or weaken the acid environment that enhances the chances of the gynosperms.
4. The face-to-face, or "missionary," position should be assumed during intercourse. Dr. Shettles believes that this makes it less likely that sperm will be deposited directly at the mouth of the cervix, where they might escape the acid environment of the vagina.
5. Shallow penetration by the male at the time of male orgasm is recommended. Again, this helps make certain that the sperm are exposed to the acid in the vagina and must swim through it to get to the cervix.
6. No abstinence from intercourse is necessary, until after the final intercourse two or three days before ovulation. A low sperm count increases the possibility of female offspring, so frequent intercourse, prior to the final try two or three days before ovulation, cannot hurt and may actually help. This may be why Dr. Shettles says that "having girls is more fun."

The procedure for male offspring

1. Intercourse should be timed as close to the moment of ovulation as possible.
2. Intercourse should be immediately preceded, on each occasion, by a baking-soda douche, consisting of two tablespoons of baking soda to a quart of water. The solution should be permitted to stand for 15 minutes before use. This allows the soda to become completely dissolved.
3. Female orgasm is not necessary but is desirable. If a woman normally has orgasm, her husband should time his to coincide with hers or let her experience orgasm first.
4. Vaginal penetration from the rear is the recommended position. This, Dr. Shettles says, helps ensure deposition of sperm at the entrance of the womb. This is desirable because the secretions within the cervix and womb will be highly alkaline, more so even than in the vagina, in spite of the alkaline douche, and an alkaline environment is most favorable to androsperms.
5. Deep penetration at the moment of male orgasm will help ensure deposition of sperm close to the cervix.
6. Prior abstinence is necessary; intercourse should be avoided completely from the beginning of the monthly cycle until the day of ovulation. This helps ensure maximum sperm count, a factor favoring androsperms.

*   *   *

Some observers believe that our new ability to choose the sex of our children will result in a bumper crop of boys, but Dr. Shettles is personally convinced that parents will not use his techniques to produce either mostly males or mostly females. "Over the years, parents have expressed only one desire," he says, "and that is to have families that are well balanced in terms of sex. Most find an equal number of boys and girls ideal."

Many couples have told Dr. Shettles they had initially planned for a family of two children, hoping for one of each. But when both offspring turned out to be of the same sex, they made a third attempt and so on. So it is not too far-fetched to envision sex-selection making a significant contribution in the effort to control the population explosion. How much better it would be to achieve the ideal family balance in two tries instead of three or four or more or never. The advantages of sex-selection are manifest: parental satisfaction, balanced families, very possibly smaller families and, *healthier* families.

Sometimes health—or lack of it—is attached to our sex chromosomes. Only males, for example, suffer from hemophilia, the grim and often fatal "bleeder's disease." Similar hereditary, sex-linked diseases include one type of muscular dystrophy and numerous enzyme-deficiency disorders that can kill, cripple and retard for life.

Though most of these diseases remain incurable, they can be prevented if carriers of sex-linked diseases could simply avoid conceiving children of the vulnerable sex.

*   *   *

. . . For the first time in all time, parents have the opportunity to make a scientific attempt at choosing the sex of their children and to make that attempt with a high expectation of success.

e.

Sir Bernard Lovell
Man Moves into the Universe*

* * *

The scientific reasons for a manned Mars expedition are, of course, immense. . . . If replicating organisms are found to exist in the atmosphere or on the surface of the planet, unqualified support would thereby be produced for the belief that widespread development of organisms has occurred elsewhere in the universe.

The immense importance of this issue demands that the world as a whole should share the responsibility for the investigation. Contamination by human species, or by earlier rockets or satellites before the manned flights, could prejudice the entire investigation. The Soviets have not, so far, expressed their agreement with the standards suggested by the National Aeronautics and Space Administration and the Committee on Space Research of the International Council of Scientific Unions. Indeed their planetary technique, as exhibited by their investigations of Venus, allows the carrier bus to plunge to destruction in the planet's atmosphere.

The urgency of renewing attempts at a clear international understanding on these investigations arises also because of the danger of contamination on Earth by returning manned planetary probes. Even though the moon is an arid body, the Apollo program involves strict quarantine arrangements for the returning astronauts. The risks of contamination are probably negligible; nevertheless NASA has quite rightly taken

every reasonable safeguard. With Mars the risk must be far greater. The only safe assumption to make is that a spacecraft returning from Mars would probably convey entirely foreign organisms to the terrestrial environment. The consequences could be disastrous to crops or animal life unless the necessary controls can be exercised. This is manifestly an international problem, and international agreement is essential on the biological investigations to be made before a manned flight is attempted, and on the quarantine and other biological safeguards to be applied to the returning spacecraft.

* * *

NOTE

HANS JONAS
PHILOSOPHICAL REFLECTIONS ON
EXPERIMENTING WITH HUMAN SUBJECTS*

* * *

[P]rogress is an optional goal, not an unconditional commitment, and . . . its tempo in particular, compulsive as it may become, has nothing sacred about it. Let us also remember that a slower progress in the conquest of disease would not threaten society, grievous as it is to those who have to deplore that their particular disease be not yet conquered, but that society would indeed be threatened by the erosion of those moral values whose loss, possibly caused by too ruthless a pursuit of scientific progress, would make its most dazzling triumphs not worth having. Let us finally remember that it cannot be the aim of progress to abolish the lot of mortality. Of some ill or other, each of us will die. Our mortal condition is upon us with its harshness but also its wisdom—because without it there would not be the eternally renewed promise of the freshness, immediacy, and eagerness of youth; nor, without it, would there be for any of us the incentive to number our days and make them count. . . .

---

* 25 *Bulletin of the Atomic Scientists* 4, 6 (1969). Copyright © 1969 by the Educational Foundation for Nuclear Science. Reprinted by permission of Science and Public Affairs, the *Bulletin of the Atomic Scientists,* and by permission of Basic Books, Inc., publishers of Eugene Rabinowitch and Richard S. Lewis, eds.: *Man on the Moon.* New York: Basic Books, Inc. (1969).

---

* 98 *Daedalus* 245 (1969). Reprinted by permission of *Daedalus,* Journal of the American Academy of Arts and Sciences, Boston, Massachusetts.

B.
Man's Willingness to Risk Human Lives

"[W]e have become accustomed to the fact that many activities are permitted, even though statistically we know they will cost lives, since it costs too much to engage in these activities more safely or to abstain from them altogether. We have grade crossings, even though we know that with grade crossings a certain number of people will be killed each year and even though grade crossings could be eliminated relatively easily. We use automobiles— knowing that they cost us fifty thousand lives each year—because to use safer, slower means of transport would be far too costly in terms of pleasure and profits foregone. Worse even than that, we use automobiles with relatively cheap (but relatively dangerous) control systems, and so on *ad infinitum*. And we do this because we deem the lives taken to be cheaper than the costs of avoiding the accidents in which they are taken."*

The materials in this section examine risktaking in the endeavors of science and technology. The debate over the introduction of safety provisions for the coal mining industry illustrates society's refusal to eliminate known, avoidable risks because the benefits to society outweigh the estimated harm. Beyond this "calculated risk," the oral contraceptive case which appears in Chapter Eleven suggests that society is also willing to take "blind" risks with only a very rough idea of the relative benefit and harm. Another case study in this section, reconstructed from the early days of interspace exploration, illustrates the problems of making decisions about risks when neither the benefits nor the harm of an endeavor are adequately known.

Over the centuries similar dilemmas have arisen in many areas of human endeavor. "As we in our day can smile condescendingly at the primitives and ancients who practiced human sacrifice for what they considered to be the general good of the tribe or nation, future generations may ask whether we could make human sacrifice more acceptable in our day by calling it 'social cost.' "† Perhaps the materials are proof of "man's inhumanity to man," or perhaps they only provide evidence of inherent limitations in man's capacity or willingness to curtail risktaking beyond a certain point.

In studying these materials, consider the following questions:

1. What risks are, and should be, acceptable to society?

2. What values do we seek to maximize by accepting or rejecting certain kinds of risks?

3. Are these values in conflict with other individual and social values?

4. Should the fact that risks pervade all human activity make risks which occur in the pursuit of science and technology more or less acceptable?

5. What part in risk-decisions should the various participants play?

6. When should the balancing of risks and benefits be left to the person affected, and when, if ever, should society impose limits on risktaking?‡

---

* Guido Calabresi: "Reflections on Medical Experimentation in Humans." 98 *Daedalus* 387 (1969).
† Edmond Cahn: "Drug Experiments and the Public Conscience." Paul Talalay, ed.: *Drugs in Our Society*. Baltimore: The Johns Hopkins Press 260–261 (1964).
‡ The mechanisms by which society may exercise collective control over risktaking are merely touched upon here and will be enlarged upon in Part Four.

1.

The Health and Safety of Coal Miners*

a.

Statement by President Harry S. Truman upon Signing an Amendment to the Federal Coal Mine Safety Act—July 16, 1952

I have today signed S. 1310, a bill relating to the prevention of major disasters in coal mines.

This measure is a significant step in the direction of preventing the appalling toll of death and injury to miners in underground mines. These totally unnecessary and preventable accidents result in grief-stricken families as well as a shocking loss and waste of skilled manpower.

Under Public Law 49, 77th Congress, the Secretary of the Interior has been authorized to inspect coal mines to the end of making them safer places in which to work. In reporting on their inspections of coal mines, the Federal coal mine inspectors have recommended measures to correct unsafe conditions and practices, but there has been no authority to enforce these recommendations. Disaster has, in many instances, followed in the wake of repeated and unheeded warnings of impending danger.

S. 1310 will, in part, correct this situation. The measure seeks to help prevent major disasters in coal mines from five causes—explosion, fire, inundation, mantrip, or manhoist accidents. Nevertheless, the legislation falls short of the recommendation I submitted to the Congress to meet the urgent problems in this field. In particular, the bill has the following deficiencies:

1. Coal mines in which less than 15 persons are regularly employed underground are exempted from compliance with any of the mine safety provisions regardless of whether a major disaster might be imminent. This exempts a large

---

* Except as otherwise noted, all materials in this section are reprinted from the *Hearings on Bills to Improve the Health and Safety Conditions of Persons Working in the Coal Mining Industry of the United States before the Subcommittee on Labor of the Senate Committee on Labor and Public Welfare,* 91st Congress, 1st Session (1969). Members of the Subcommittee were: Senators H. A. Williams, chairman; J. Randolph; C. Pell; G. Nelson; W. F. Mondale; T. F. Eagleton; A. Cranston; J. K. Javits; W. L. Prouty; W. B. Saxbe; H. Bellmon; and R. S. Schweiker.

group of mines, many of which are hazardous and need a great deal of safety improvement. Inspections of these mines will continue under the earlier statute, but compliance with recommendations of the Federal inspectors will be on a purely voluntary basis.

2. The provisions of the legislation are directed solely toward the prevention of major disasters from the five causes mentioned heretofore. Such disasters accounted for only approximately 7 percent of the coal mine fatalities during the last 20 years. The broad phase of accident prevention in general remains the responsibility of the States in which coal is mined, despite the record to date indicating either the inability or unwillingness of the States to meet this responsibility.

3. The legislation contains several exemptions to the safety provisions particularly with regard to replacement of dangerous electrical equipment and faulty ventilation systems which have been the causes of most recent major disasters. I am advised that these exemptions were provided to avoid any economic impact on the coal mining industry, but they are so worded that the unsafe conditions and practices could continue for years before the mines would be required to comply with the law.

4. The measure contains complex procedural provisions relating to inspections, appeals, and the postponing of orders which I believe will make it exceedingly difficult if not impossible for those charged with the administration of the act to carry out an effective enforcement program. I believe that it is possible to draft simpler and more effective procedural provisions which would not adversely affect the rights of any of the parties concerned with the prevention of mine injuries and deaths.

5. The measure vests the mine safety enforcement functions directly in the Director of the Bureau of Mines. This violates the principle now established for most executive departments that functions should be vested in the department head in order to provide the flexibility of organization and clear lines of authority and accountability essential for effective administration.

. . . We will do our very best to prevent mining disasters with the authority granted in this bill but the Congress eventually will have to meet its responsibility for enacting legislation which provides tools fully adequate to prevent the great loss of life and the thousands of crippling injuries due to mine accidents.

b.

Recommendations by President Lyndon B. Johnson Urging the Enactment of the Federal Coal Mine Health and Safety Act of 1968—September 11, 1968

When President Harry Truman signed the Coal Mine Safety Act sixteen years ago, he declared that, "the legislation falls far short of the recommendation I submitted to the Congress to meet the urgent problems in this field."

The record shows just how far short that measure fell. Since 1952, over 5,500 miners have been killed on the job. Another 250,000 were seriously disabled. No one knows how many thousands more have died, their lungs blackened by the ravages of coal dust disease—pneumoconiosis.

Today, despite the safety measures on the books, coal mining remains the most dangerous and hazardous occupation for the American worker. The National Safety Council reports that of the forty major industries in this country, coal mining ranks highest in frequency and severity of death and injury.

We have succeeded in preventing many of the major coal mine disasters that took dozens of lives at a time. But coal miners are still crushed by cave-ins, burned by explosions, maimed by antiquated and unsafe equipment. They still pay with their health for the right of earning a living because the air they breathe is thick with coal dust. At the very least, one out of every ten active miners—and one out of every five retired miners—suffers from a serious respiratory disease. For the tens of thousands of miners so afflicted, the shortness of breath may shorten their lives.

Consider some of the tragedies of just the past few months:

—A massive landslide at the face of a mine in West Virginia crushed three workers to death.

—A major explosion in a Kentucky mine snuffed out the lives of a nine-man crew. The cause: the dangerous practice of hauling dynamite on a drilling machine.

—Miners in West Virginia inadvertently drilled into an abandoned water-filled mine shaft, and four were drowned.

There was nothing inevitable about these disasters. They happened because our coal mine safety laws are inadequate, and because even existing laws are all too frequently ignored.

At the present time, Federal inspectors have too little jurisdiction over the working face of the mines, where nearly half of the fatal accidents occur. They cannot tell a mine owner to shore up a sagging roof in this area. They cannot require the replacement of a potentially hazardous machine. They cannot require a reduction in the level of coal dust in the air to safe limits because the laws do not even touch on the problem of health standards. They have no jurisdiction at all over the nation's 2,250 surface mines, which account for almost 40 percent of our coal production.

Our inspectors are not even backed by effective enforcement penalties where the law does apply. It is a measure of this weakness that last year more than 80 percent of the nation's nearly 6,000 underground coal mines were in violation of one or more federal safety standards.

Today, *I urge the Congress to remedy these defects. I recommend the Federal Coal Mine Health and Safety Act of 1968.*

It is time that an enlightened and progressive nation give its coal miners a new charter of health and safety as they toil for the comfort of us all.

This Act will, for the first time:

—Extend federal enforcement to the face of mine, the area where so many deaths and injuries occur, as well as correcting 18 other specific safety omissions in the present law.

—Abolish the "grandfather clause" which allows old and unsafe electrical equipment to be used.

—Give the Secretary of the Interior authority to develop and issue safety standards as the need arises.

—Provide a way to reduce the human devastation of coal dust disease by requiring the Secretary of Health, Education and Welfare to develop health criteria, and the Secretary of the Interior, following such criteria, to issue health standards and enforce them.

—Impose meaningful and effective sanctions for failure to comply with the terms of the law: criminal penalties and higher fines for willful violations, civil penalties and injunctions to deter and stop unsafe practices.

—Apply the law's reach to surface coal mines.

—Create simplified and streamlined enforcement procedures to require quick correction of hazardous conditions.

The cost of this measure will be small. Its

benefits will be large, not only in terms of the lives it can save and the injuries it can prevent, but in practical terms of dollars and cents. Last year alone, over 1.8 million man-days were lost to the nation and the mine owners as a result of job-related deaths and injuries. Many millions of dollars in workmen's compensation payments were awarded to injured and disabled miners.

*   *   *

c.
Statement of Senator Jennings Randolph, West Virginia—February 27, 1969

*   *   *

. . . I am a prime sponsor of two of the measures on coal mine health and safety before us. On January 10, 1969, I introduced the then administration's proposed Federal Coal Mine Health and Safety Act of 1969, S. 355, a bill carefully developed over months of study and effort and refined further as a consequence of the tragic November 1968, fire and explosion at Mountaineer Mine No. 9 between Farmington and Mannington, W. Va. S. 355 is combined coal mine health and safety legislation.

On January 21, 1969, I introduced, at the request of President Boyle of the United Mine Workers of America, another measure—S. 467, proposed with the title, "Coal Mine Health Act," and considerably broader in scope than the provisions of S. 355 relating to the purpose of elim-

---

* At the time I introduced the Johnson Administration bill (January 10, 1969), I said I believed coal mine safety and coal mine health should be handled separately, but I introduced the Johnson Administration measure as a single bill, with the subject matter divided into separate titles. There seemed, on January 10, to be much closer but not complete agreement on the part of producers and miners to the safety provisions of the Administration proposal than to the health (dust control) provisions. The United Mine Workers differed sharply with the Administration's proposed legislative approach to the dust control (anti-black lung) problem. That is why the UMWA proposed and why I introduced a dust control bill.

*   *   *

There are probably opponents of health provisions of these bills (on medical and/or other technical grounds) who are not against the safety provisions.

All persons will not agree with this evaluation, but it seems to me that the prime target of all this legislation is first to recodify and modernize the mine

ination of health dangers to coal miners resulting from the inhalation of coal dust.*

*   *   *

Coal miners must have the safest attainable working conditions short of the destruction of their jobs. There must be improvement of existing conditions in the interest of arresting and, hopefully, of preventing black lung and other diseases incident to coal mining. I underscore the word "preventing" if for no other reason than to emphasize that legislation relating to compensation for claims growing out of the occupation is generally a State matter, the responsibility of the legislatures of the States.

*   *   *

d.
Statement of Senator Harrison A. Williams, Jr., New Jersey—February 27, 1969

*   *   *

The beginnings of coal mining in this country go back to 1730; our Federal Bureau of Mines was established in 1910. Yet, it was not until 1941 that the first Federal coal mine safety legislation was enacted into law . . . [Senator Randolph] was one of the chief architects of that beginning accomplishment.

In 1942, the Russell Sage Foundation published a study regarding the prevention of fatal explosions in coal mines. The authors of that

---

safety laws to mitigate against or, if possible, totally obviate, the catastrophic coal mine explosions and fires which kill and seriously injure miners and cause intensive property damage. If we can do this without encumbering the objective and delaying its fulfillment with a long and tedious controversy over dust control procedures and technology, it seems to me that we should do it.

*   *   *

Of course the "safest" mine and the "healthiest" mine is the closed one—but it does not produce the coal that is so vital to much of our country's economy—and it does not provide payrolls and livelihood for miners. The search must be for feasible ways to achieve safety and improved occupational health in active mining operations where jobs are provided. To be too reckless or too little, too late in any direction in coal mine safety and coal mine health would be catastrophic. To achieve the feasible and the "proper balance" and, at the same time, the effective will not be done easily. . . . [Letter to the Editor, *St. Louis Post-Dispatch* from Senator Jennings Randolph, February 24, 1969.]

report, commenting on title I of the Federal Coal Mine Safety Act, wrote:

. . . Undoubtedly, the record of explosions in 1940 was influential, if not the determining factor in bringing about this legislation. In this there was no departure from the usual pattern; dead miners have always been the most powerful influence in securing passage of mining legislation.

I believe the foundation referred to the great difficulty in getting the Bureau of Mines established in 1910, as well as the long history of unsuccessful efforts to enact legislation before the first breakthrough by the 1941 act.

Here we are, 27 years later, and yet another mining disaster has occurred—the Mannington-Farmington, W.Va., No. 9 mine explosions, which killed 78 men in November 1968. The stark reality contained in the Russell Sage Foundation 1942 study is as true today as it was then. Our antidisaster actions are always after the fact.

In a report from the Bureau of Mines, Department of the Interior, called "Coal Mine Fatalities of 1968," there is documented a total of 309 work fatalities in 1968. By dividing 78—the number of men killed in the Mannington explosion disaster—into 309, there was the equivalent of four Mannington disasters that year.

In 1967, the Bureau reported 220 mineworker fatalities. Despite such a large number of fatalities, the report provided the reassuring statement that there were no "major disasters" in coal mines for that year. This is because the legal definition of a major disaster means that five or more men are killed simultaneously.

As far as this Senator is concerned, these hearings must take great care to look behind and deeper than the legal definition. We must come to understand the human definition of a mine disaster. My starting point is that one man killed equals one disaster. And it seems to me that is the only definition we can in good conscience offer the widows and children of the 309 mineworkers killed in 1968.

*   *   *

. . . The largest number of underground deaths in a year are caused by roof falls in the mines. The second ranking cause is gas and dust explosions; other leading causes are haulage accidents, electrical, and machinery. Deaths from these five ranking causes of fatal accidents made up 93 percent of the total deaths in underground workings in 1968.

We have recently been made aware of the seriousness and the magnitude of the miner's occupational respiratory disease, pneumoconiosis, or 'black lung," which is caused by inhalation of coal dust. Dr. William Stewart, the Surgeon General of the United States, has said that "black lung" conservatively affects more than 100,000 soft-coal workers.

This information may be news to us but it is an old story to the coalminers. According to Dr. Lorin E. Kerr, assistant to the executive medical officer, United Mine Workers of America welfare and retirement fund, what we now know as "black lung" was called "miner's con" years ago. The first medical term was "miner's asthma"; the cause of miner's spitting, coughing, and breathlessness was unknown, so doctors used the phrase "miner's asthma" to label the condition.

After years of study and research we now call it pneumoconiosis. But call it what you will—it disables and kills.

Men die from this disease, but before they die they suffer extreme pain and shortness of breath for 15 to 20 years—many continuing to go down to the mines to work with their affliction.

The mechanization of our coal mining industry has increased the miner's chances for contracting the disease. High-powered drills, mechanized loaders, electrical cables—the whole mechanized process—creates more coal dust.

The seriousness of this problem is underscored when we consider the Surgeon General's estimate that as many as 70 percent of the 144,000 coal miners in this country are suffering from "black lung." Furthermore, pneumoconiosis is not recognized as a compensable occupational disease except in the States of Pennsylvania, Virginia, and Alabama. We just heard from Senator Randolph that it appears as though this is going to be increased by West Virginia shortly.

*   *   *

. . . It is obvious that we must have legislative standards and technical methods for controlling coal dust at safe levels.

In this otherwise dark picture there is one pleasant thought: If I read correctly the coal industry's production and fiscal reports, these hearings will not be complicated by the "bankruptcy" arguments so frequently leveled at this type legislation.

The National Coal Association calls its product "The Fuel of the Future."

In a July 1968 press release, the NCA stated

that the bituminous coal industry has recovered from its recent lean years. In 1967 it produced 551 million tons of coal and prospects were bright. Major research efforts were then underway to convert coal to competitive gasoline and pipeline gas. Major oil companies, seeing their supplies dwindling, are investing heavily in coal. The release concluded: "As America's main reservoir of energy in the years ahead, coal's prospects are glittering."

*   *   *

e.

Statement of W. A. Boyle, President, United Mine Workers of America— February 27, 1969

*   *   *

The Federal Mine Safety Act that was passed in 1941 at the insistence of the senior Senator of West Virginia, and people like him, what happened? We had to take it. It was a watered-down version of what the United Mine Workers wanted. And we accepted the 1941 law because it was better than no law at all. We had no law. And that law, Mr. Chairman, if you care to review it, provides that the Federal coal mine inspectors under the direction of the Secretary of Interior . . . had no authority whatsoever under the 1941 act except to go in and find, if the coal operator would let him go in, violations of the law, and make recommendations.

And then in 1952 we came to the Congress session after session after session during the interim period, and in 1952, after the disasters occurred in the State of Illinois and elsewhere, the Congress of the United States said it was high time that we gave these Federal inspectors some authority. They vested their men with the authority in 1952 to not only make inspections and recommendations, but to close mines and withdraw men if imminent danger existed. So we had been living with those things.

Then year after year we tried to get all mines in the United States covered by some legislation. Union mines and nonunion mines. Mines that employed from one man to 15 men were excluded. We tried to get them covered. We failed, miserably failed, before the Congress of the United States to get any consideration on that until 1966, when I appeared before both Houses.

They passed legislation then that included and protected those men who worked in mines employing less than 15 men, and it has elimi-

nated and cut down the accident rate in coal mines.

Contrary to what the coal operators who opposed that legislation at that time, contrary to what they had to say, and they tried to impress upon the Congress of the United States that the mines would close down because they were in no position to operate under those restrictive laws—I am happy to relate to you that I know of no coal mines that have been closed down by the passage of that law. But to the contrary, new mines have been opened up, both large and small.

*   *   *

As I indicated earlier, we have exercised our judgment and concluded that, if both health and safety standards are included in one bill, there will be no bill. Why do I say this? Because there are opponents who are opposed to some features of the health bill, and there are opponents who are opposed to some features of the safety bill, and, if you allow your opposition to concentrate against one bill, your prospects of success are diminished, if not completely destroyed. For these reasons, we proceeded in two directions, both with the same basic motivation, to improve the health and safety of the coal miners of the United States.

*   *   *

I direct my remarks to S. 467, the health bill pending before your committee. Before I discuss the specifics of the bill, I think it advisable to provide a historical background, particularly with comments involving coal miners' chest diseases, in general. The medical profession had concluded that, in its opinion, coal dust was not harmful to the lungs. It was their view that only exposure to silica dust was damaging to the lungs. However, in recent years, medical evidence has revealed that coal dust in the lungs does cause a major disabling disease. In fact, in recent years, there has been a rapid rise in the incidence of chest disease among coal miners and, more importantly, this incidence has developed in greater percentage among men in their forties and fifties, a most unhappy situation.

In our opinion, the increasing incidence of coal miners' dust disease has developed because of the introduction of mechanical machinery in the mines. This is particularly true when one is aware of the fact that more than 50 percent of the underground coal produced in the United States is mined by continuous-mining machinery. The coal industry was one of the first basic industries in the United States to be completely mechanized.

The union did not oppose mechanization . . . . It was the consensus of those, both on management's and on labor's side, that if there were not mechanization, there would be total elimination of coal mining in America.

However, we were not fortunetellers, nor could we look through crystal balls to realize that the introduction of machinery would increase the innumerable dust diseases which now exist. Nor did our crystal ball or our fortunetellers inform us of the other problems which would come into play, particularly involving ventilation, roof control, and methane emissions. These are things which result from experience. . . .

* * *

. . . The health bill which we offered set standards of 3 milligrams of respirable dust in a cubic meter of air. Under its provisions, the Bureau of Mines would be empowered to close a mine, or a section of a mine, where the 3 milligrams standard was being exceeded. The Bureau would inspect these mines at least once each 60 days and would take samples of the atmosphere at various locations with an instrument approved by the Bureau. The coal operators would be required to continuously monitor the coal dust levels in their mines. A permanent record of such tests would be kept for the information of the Bureau inspector.

Further, and of greatest importance, the bill sponsored by the United Mine Workers of America imposes penalties for operators who exceed the dust standards, or who fail to maintain accurate records.

* * *

. . . To our delight, we have observed that the Federal mine safety law has been enforced more effectively in the past several months than ever before in this history of the act. The credit for such enforcement belongs to the Director of the Bureau of Mines, Mr. John O'Leary. It is our fervent prayer that President Nixon will continue his appointment as Director, so that his services which he has so capably demonstrated in a short time will be continued.

* * *

Let me call to the attention of this subcommittee what happened to this coal industry of recent days. You confirmed the appointment of

a director by the name of Dr. Hibbard. He served for a short period of time with an expert on safety by the name of James Westfield—the only man in my judgment in the U.S. Bureau of Mines who was qualified on these explosions and these hazards that are found in these coal mines. To lead these rescue crews into these mines it required James Westfield.

What happened? The family became disturbed in the Department of the Interior for some reason or other. Dr. Hibbard could take it no longer, Jim Westfield could take it no longer, and they both resigned. And I was knocking on the Secretary's door repeatedly, by telephone and otherwise, asking him to appoint a new director of the Bureau of Mines. And let him tell me that I wasn't knocking on his door asking him to get a head of that department because of the condition in the coal mines of this country. And what did he do? Seven months elapsed before we had a head of that department down there. Seven months went by without a head.

* * *

SENATOR PROUTY: How effective have the State mining agencies been?

MR. BOYLE: Here is a former director of a State bureau of mines. Maybe he can answer. I refer the question to him. He will tell you.

MR. EVANS: Senator, what I am going to say I don't mean to be an indictment of every state mining department in the United States, because there are some good state mining departments in the United States. But by and large they are under the complete domination of the coal industry.

SENATOR PROUTY: Thank you.

SENATOR BELLMON: Do you mean to imply that the mine operators do not want safety?

MR. EVANS: I did not say that, Senator. I haven't indicted every coal operator in the United States. There are coal operators in the United States who are vitally interested in safety. But I am afraid that there are far too many who are not interested to the extent that they should be interested. I think that many coal miners are injured and die in mine accidents and die in mine explosions through carelessness, through neglect of mine officials, through greed, through the operators paying too much attention to production and not enough to mine safety, the general welfare of the people who work for him. I don't mean that to be indictment of every coal company in this country.

* * *

f.

Statement of Senator Jennings Randolph, West Virginia—March 7, 1969

*   *   *

Occupational health in coal mining is not likely to be as readily improvable as is the safety of operations. But in this area of concern we must make an all-out effort to find ways to prevent diseases growing out of exposure to the pollution that is an inescapable part of the industry of coal mining, at least as of the present.

We can dictate standards by law, but achieving them in practice, Mr. Secretary, will not be easy. In fact, I am not sure that the difficulties of achievement of substantially better occupational health conditions in coal mines and the cost thereof will permit coal to stay competitive in some of its present markets.

I qualify that statement—I say I am not sure. This, however, is not a reason in itself for timid or time-consuming approaches to the search for effective disease-preventing practices and equipment in the business of coal mining and in the writing of laws to require their use.

But we must look at the broad picture of humanity, technological feasibility, and economics in all of these measures. Mr. Secretary, I say to you, as I have said to others on numerous occasions, the safest coal mine and the disease-free coal mine is the one that is closed. But it is not a producer for the economy or a source of payrolls to sustain miners and their families.

*   *   *

g.

Testimony of Walter J. Hickel, Secretary of the Interior—March 7, 1969

*   *   *

The President has asked that a bill be introduced in Congress, which I understand has been identified as S. 1300. This bill would help us meet the requirements not only of today, but would give us the flexibility to take advantage of the new technologies needed to solve the problems of tomorrow. The bill differs from the existing law in a number of ways.

Briefly, it would—

Apply to all underground and surface coal mines;

Require at least three times a year the inspection of every portion of every underground coal mine;

Extend the Secretary's authority over all types of accidents, not just the disaster type such as fire, explosions, floods, et cetera;

Authorize the Secretary to propose mandatory health and safety standards for all coal mines;

Provide for review of the standards by an expanded Coal Mine Health and Safety Board;

Provide civil penalties for the violation of a mandatory standard;

Require immediate evacuation of all persons in the case of an imminent danger;

Provide for the immediate withdrawal of persons, after notice, in cases of an unwarrantable failure to comply with a mandatory health or safety standard;

Provide that all withdrawal orders remain in effect until modified or terminated by the inspector; and

Expand our research activities and capabilities.

The need for this type of legislation is unmistakable. The present law is aimed exclusively at those types of accidents in which five or more persons might die as a result of fire, explosion, flood, or other such major disaster. Statistics show that, since this law was enacted, the fatality rate for major disasters has been cut by about 50 percent. However, the statistics indicate that there has been no change in the fatality or injury rates from the day-to-day type of accidents over the past 20 years.

In 1968, 221 of the 309 fatalities were recorded as being caused by accidents not covered by the provisions of existing law. The proposal that this administration is urging Congress to approve is designed to reduce all accidents that may cause injury or death in our coal mines.

If the day-to-day accidents that cause most of our coal mine injuries and deaths are to be reduced or eliminated, we need a law that gives broad enforcement powers to the inspectors and provides stronger incentives for management and labor to improve the working conditions of the mine. We must concern ourselves with the conditions that may cause an accident that injures or kills a single miner, as well as the accidents which are classified as "disastrous" because they kill five or more.

In our opinion, the single most important feature of this bill is the provision that would require the Secretary of the Interior to develop mandatory health and safety standards for all coal mines.

The precedents for such authority are many,

and I know of no instance in which the granting of it by Congress to a regulatory agency has proved anything but highly successful. In my view, the great speed with which technology advances makes it essential that in administering coal mine health and safety laws the Secretary of the Interior has a flexibility of response to rapidly changing conditions.

Many of the interim standards contained in the administration's proposal have long been recognized as needed and desirable by industry, labor, and the Department of the Interior. They have not, however, been implemented because the authority for setting standards rests with Congress and has not been delegated to the Secretary of the Interior.

It is not practicable to expect Congress to enact specific and detailed health and safety standards. The fact that Congress has changed the coal mine safety standards only three times in the last 30 years demonstrates the inadequacy of the legislative route for establishing mine health and safety standards. We must allow sufficient flexibility in the setting of standards so that new technology can be utilized for the benefit of the miners.

There is another important safety provision in the bill which we want to call to your attention. This bill, if enacted, would eliminate the "nongassy" classification for underground mines. Since the early 1920's, stricter safety precautions have been required for the so-called gassy mines. However, experience has shown on numerous occasions the so-called nongassy mines have had gas ignitions killing and injuring miners. We believe that the distinction should be eliminated.

The elimination of this classification will, however, have far-reaching economic implications. Approximately 85 percent of the Nation's underground mines are now classified "nongassy." These mines produce about 39 percent of underground production. Their reclassification would require that they obtain certain equipment and maintain it in a satisfactory manner. This will require large new investments and increased operating costs.

In addition to the safety features, S. 1300, in an effort to combat the "black lung" disease, would establish a dust standard for underground coal mines. The legislation would, within 6 months after enactment, require that each operator maintain the atmosphere in each active working place in the mine at or below 4.5 milligrams of dust per cubic meter of air.

In those individual mines where engineering technology requires more time, the Secretary could grant, under our proposal an extension—not to exceed 6 months. We want to point out three things with regard to the short-term dust standard of 4.5 milligrams per cubic meter of air:

First, we are advised by the Bureau of Mines that the state of the art of dust control technology is not sufficiently advanced to permit an immediate industrywide imposition of a 3 standard.

Second, none of the other bills pending in the Congress establish a date certain for effectuating any dust standard.

Third, known technology can now be applied so as to achieve the recommended 4.5 standard in a relatively short period of time. The subcommittee should note, based on preliminary tests in about 20 mines, that moving to a 4.5 standard will require a reduction in dust counts in approximately 50 percent of the mines in the United States.

We have also directed the Bureau of Mines to start immediately to work with industry, equipment manufacturers, and labor to accelerate and expand research for the purpose of developing new technology which would permit a standard of 3 or lower. I am sure that the industry, the equipment manufacturers, and labor will cooperate fully with the Bureau in this endeavor.

*   *   *

Let me at this point make this administration's position very clear on the subject of a single health and safety bill versus two bills—one on health and one on safety. We recommend and strongly urge one bill covering both subjects. The health and safety of the coal miner are so closely interwoven that it is inappropriate to even contemplate their consideration as separate issues.

SENATOR WILLIAMS: . . . I have one further observation. In your statement you state an objective in making the mining industry the safest, the most healthful, and the most productive in the world. I wonder if the Department has engaged in any comparative studies in terms of safety of the mining industry in our country and the coal mining industry, say, in Great Britain, Germany, Poland, and other countries that are known to be major coal producers. And, of course, when I say safety, I mean, of course, in terms of physical safety, both the structure and in the dust and health aspects.

MR. O'LEARY [Director, Bureau of Mines, accompanying Secretary Hickel]: Mr. Chairman, we are aware of the data with regard to all activity and with regard to health and safety experience in foreign mines. I think we find two things that are significant. The productivity is perhaps a third to a fourth of that of the United States on the average in Europe and Great Britain, for example.

At the same time the safety records are significantly better than those in the United States.

*   *   *

I think there are two factors there. They are not mechanized, and they do not have thereby the inherent hazards that highly mechanized, very rapidly moving mining equipment has.

SENATOR RANDOLPH: That is exactly right.

MR. O'LEARY: At the same time, I think it is also fair to say when we were at that stage in development, that is, when we were on conventional mining techniques, that our accident rates were significantly higher than the current European experience. I think it is undeniable that there has been more attention to health and to safety in Europe.

We are finding now, however, a trend which is just beginning to appear as Europe mechanizes; the safety records are beginning to deteriorate a bit and perhaps the health records as well. This is very, very preliminary.

*   *   *

h.

Statement of John Corcoran, President, Consolidation Coal Co. and Chairman of the Board of the National Coal Association— March 12, 1969

. . . When I appeared before the Secretary of the Interior's Conference on Coal Mine Safety on December 12, 1968, I stated:

There can be no question that the health and safety of employees in the coal mining industry must be given first priority. On humanitarian grounds alone this should be self-evident.

If this is not enough, enlightened self-interest will lead us to the same inescapable conclusion.

Our trained and experienced employees constitute our most valuable resource and the protection of their health and safety is an absolute prerequisite to the successful and continued operation of our business. . . . In the regulatory area, we favor and will support any meaningful and constructive changes in laws and regulations that will improve coal mine safety.

*   *   *

Perhaps, because the demands of our utility customers are greater today than ever before, we are faced, time and again, with the charge that the coal industry places production and profits ahead of safety.

Even if we are as calloused or as unconcerned about safety as this charge would imply, the plain fact is that production, profits, and safety are so closely interrelated that one is impossible without the other.

*   *   *

While the coal industry's safety record has improved in recent years, there is no question that further improvement is needed.

In 1967, the accident frequency rate—that is, accidents per million man-hours of exposure —for the entire bituminous coal industry was 41.7 as contrasted with a frequency rate of 48.6 in 1950.

For those companies represented by the Bituminous Coal Operators Association, the accident frequency rate was 31.7 in 1967.

For comparative purposes I am advised that the preliminary 1967 frequency rate figure for all manufacturing is approximately 14.0.

*   *   *

[I]n considering specific changes, we should be certain that they are meaningful and constructive and that they truly will improve safety for it is sometimes quite easy to allow the emotion of a Farmington disaster to cloud our judgment and cause us to accept proposals that might not achieve the results all of us are seeking.

It is with this thought in mind that I would like to direct my remarks to certain general principles that are common to most of the proposed legislation, although variously expressed in the different bills.

Most of the bills before this committee provide for interim safety standards, with the right in the Secretary of the Interior to promulgate additional standards and to revise them from time to time.

I believe it would be preferable that the standards set by Congress should be mandatory, not interim, standards, and that they should continue in effect until amended by the Congress. This would insure a separation of the legislative and enforcement functions and, in the area of safety regulation, I believe this separation is important.

However, if the Congress should choose to delegate its legislative functions, I would certainly question the desirability of delegating such sweeping powers to any one individual without adequate review provisions.

In some of the proposed legislation there is not even any appeal from a standard set by the Secretary, however unreasonable or unworkable it may appear to be.

It is true that a coal operator could refuse to comply with a standard set by the Secretary under this provision, thus subjecting himself to an appealable order and having the standard reviewed in such a proceeding.

But if our objective is to see that reasonable and workable standards are set, it seems highly inappropriate that a coal operator must deliberately violate the standard in order to have its reasonableness and lawfulness properly tested.

There is now in existence a Coal Mine Safety Board of Review, a group composed of knowledgeable coal mining experts, representing the public, the men working in the mines, and the operators. This Board is already performing valuable functions under the existing law.

I would strongly recommend that it be given authority to review any proposed standards set by the Secretary before they become effective. In this way the desirability for quick action can be maintained and at the same time the propriety of proposed standards could be subjected to the scrutiny of an expert tribunal.

In addition any standards, however promulgated, should be subject to judicial review in the event their propriety is questioned.

*   *   *

i.

Statement of James R. Garvey, Vice President of National Coal Association and President of Bituminous Coal Research, Inc.— March 12, 1970

*   *   *

[T]he coal industry is not opposed to dust standards for the protection of the health of coal miners; we agree they are needed. But we do believe that a constructive and planned program should be the basis for development of such standards rather than a hasty, arbitrary selection of numbers. A planned approach can lead to the development of effective dust standards needed to protect the health of miners, while at the same time enabling industry and government to cooperate in the work necessary, not only in the resolution of such standards but also in the development of methods for control and measurement of airborne dust.

On the other hand, the arbitrary selection of standards, unsupported by substantive evidence and unaccompanied by a definitive description of sampling and measurement techniques, can only lead to confusion in the attainment of the desired health objectives.

*   *   *

High concentrations of respirable dust resulting from coal mining may very well be a health hazard, as the available evidence apparently indicates. But the level, above which adverse health effects occur, has not been determined.

It is urged that a dust standard be established in accord with the latest medical or other evidence related to dust exposure and the availability of reliable instrumentation for that dust measurement. Further, it is recommended that current technology for control of the dust generation during mining and for minimizing airborne dust distribution in possibly health-hazardous concentrations to other working places in the coal mine, plus the availability of personal protective devices for prevention of inhalation of potentially hazardous concentrations by the miner, be considered. In other words, we request that any law written take into account all the factors involved in achieving the objective, namely, health protection.

*   *   *

In most health literature relating to dust and health effects, the medical term "pneumoconiosis" appears. The word is generic, meaning dust in the lungs. Medical evidence indicates that accumulation of excessive amounts of some dusts in the lungs over a period of years may result in development of a disease which is related to the type of dust inhaled.

*   *   *

Until recently, medical authorities in this country did not recognize that the inhalation of respirable coal dust could result in a pneumoconiosis disease. It was believed that those miners who did develop disease symptoms acquired them as a result of inhalation of silica particles sometimes associated with coal dust. Since, in general, the silica content of coal dust in U.S. bituminous mines is 2 percent or less, considered to be below the value for the development of silicosis, the health problem of most bituminous coal dusts was not considered significant.

However, in the late 1930's, British medical researchers noted the prevalence of pulmonary disabilities in coal miners which was not related to the silica content of coal dust. This resulted in the instigation of a comprehensive study of the subject beginning in 1953 and still continuing.

Although the U.S. Public Health Service suspected health effects from coal dust inhalation as early as 1952, it was not until a prevalence study of coal workers' pneumoconiosis in the miners of the Appalachian region, started in 1963 and completed 2½ years later, that substantive evidence of possible health effects became available. The results of that study covering 4,000 coal miners indicated that for all working miners, 9.5 percent had X-ray evidence of pneumoconiosis, of which 6.5 percent were classified as the simple variety and 3 percent the complicated variety.

* * *

Further, the evidence of coal workers' pneumoconiosis revealed by the Public Health survey related the prevalence to years of employment in the mine, but it could not be related to coal dust concentration, because data on dust were not available. In other words, we do not know what amount of coal dust exposure causes disease. We do know that if you are exposed by working a number of years in the mine, you do have an effect.

* * *

The conclusion that the transition to continuous mining machines has caused an increase in exposure to respirable dust in coal mining operations has not been substantiated by the limited data which are available and, quite the contrary, appears to be true.

In the early 1950's the continuous mining machine was introduced in coal mining, and its use has increased ever since. There are several reasons for our belief and the belief by many other experts that such machines actually reduced the respirable dust exposure.

First of all, as has already been mentioned here this morning, high-pressure water sprays are standard equipment on almost all continuous miners and are used to allay the dust as the coal is broken from the face.

In addition, with the continuous mining machine it is usually necessary to have greater quantities of air at the face than with past mining practices. This is to dilute and carry away the methane which is liberated in increasing quantities by the more rapid rate of penetration of these machines.

Increasing air flow to control methane also reduces dust concentration by carrying it away from the face and where the men are working. We certainly do not believe that return to former mine practices is justified.

A suggestion made in one of the bills before this Congress "that all coal to be mined should be first under cut, center cut, top cut or sheared" is contrary to what evidence we have on respirable dust exposure.

Gentlemen, I believe it is of interest to note that since it apparently requires, again referring back to my medical reading, 15 to 20 years for medical evidence of pneumoconiosis to appear, at least X-ray evidence, the health data obtained by the Public Health survey in 1963 probably relate to dust concentrations associated with methods of mining prior to the introduction of the continuous miner.

* * *

NOTE

BITUMINOUS COAL OPERATORS' ASSOCIATION POSITION AS TO SUFFICIENCY OF THE FEDERAL COAL MINE SAFETY ACT—JULY 31, 1967

The considered view of the coal mine industry, as represented by B.C.O.A. and confidently that of large numbers of operators not represented by B.C.O.A., is that the 1966 Federal Coal Safety Act does not materially lack sufficiency and that present considerations for further amendments should be few, if any.

This view is in no sense negative, but rather one concluded from objective analysis of the total problem and the 20 proposals made by the Bureau.

* * *

j.

Testimony of Dr. I. E. Buff, Chairman, Committee of Physicians for Miners' Health and Safety, Charleston, W.Va.— March 13, 1969

DR. BUFF: . . . Now I want the lights out, please, and I want to show you what we are talking about.

SENATOR WILLIAMS: Is this film or slides?

DR. BUFF: Slides . . . [T]his is what you see in a coal miner, black lung. It is dead, half dead. The carbon dioxide cannot come out. There it comes in eddies. You do not get a transmission of oxygen to the carbon dioxide. So what happens. You get an individual whose brain is damaged, whose lungs are damaged, whose kidneys are damaged, whose heart is damaged, whose bones are damaged.

There is not an organ in the body that is not affected by high CO_2. What it means basically is this: You are not getting the feed line, the oxygen, to the muscle, to the tissue, and the tissue works halfway.

Well, a halfway-working liver makes you look half dead. This is the reason why people with black lung look like they have got cancer.

If I had my choice of cancer of the lung or black lung I would take cancer of the lung because you live 4 or 5 years and you die.

With this you live 15 and 20 years and you choke to death as if one takes a string and ties it around your neck, day by day, tighter and tighter, begging for a little air, just a little air.

This is a disgrace; this is terrible. It should never have existed and it should be eliminated from our people in this country.

*   *   *

[The coal miner] has nowhere to go. He has no paved streets. They are made of dirt and coal dust. His hair is terrible. His water has iron and sulfates in it and acids. And the sewerage system is something of the 17th century.

You just dump it in a creek. But there is no sewage system in very many coal mining areas in this country. They throw it out of the back yard or in the creek.

They can't get life insurance of over $1,000 or $2,000. Who would want to give it to them? Because they live 10 years less than the older population. It is risky.

Then in West Virginia last year, 1 in 300 miners was killed. This is not a good risk for an insurance company. Who would give a coal miner accident insurance?

SENATOR SAXBE: You mean on the average, 1 in 300 miners was killed?

DR. BUFF: Last year. As far as accident insurance, as of January 1969, in 1 month the West Virginia State Compensation Department reported 1,140 accidents in 1 month. Multiply this by 12 and divided into 43,000 miners and you come up with a 30 percent accident rate.

What industry in this country can even touch it? Who would give him accident insurance? That means if a man works 3 years he is bound to get hurt. And the worse thing, and I think this is what has always bothered me so

much and I know it is going to bother you, the suppression of brains in the coal mining community.

The schools are bad, the teachers are the worst that you can get, and they really do not want these people to get a high school education and go to college and become doctors, lawyers, scientists, and other things—the professions.

They want to add fodder to that machine and the women are kept ignorant. The men won't stay there without women.

At West Virginia University, two professors enlisted 25 graduate students to go into Monongalia County to help with preventing dropouts.

Do you know what happened? They asked for $3,000. The service club refused to give it to them. They went to Charleston, to a very benevolent individual; he refused.

The basic reason was that this is a bad thing to start—education at this level among the coal miners' children. But they put the money out of their own pockets for transportation and I can report to you now that students at West Virginia University are doing a great job in trying to keep these children from becoming dropouts and giving them incentives to learn.

Let us talk about the economic pressure of the coal company. If the man does not behave he gets blacklisted. If blacklisted, he can't get any job in another coal company. These are not idle remarks. They are true, it happens every day.

In some coal communities they have police departments; they remind you of the Gestapo of Germany. Let us take the medical care in a coal mining community. The medical care is second or third rate.

I want to report to you that we have had 50 meetings of miners in the state of West Virginia to educate them in what dust disease was, what it does, and how it will affect them and what they should do about it.

In the first place, we have the best educated coal miners in the United States on dust disease. They really know their stuff.

In the last fight with the legislature in order to get a compensation law, and I would like to hesitate here a minute and show you what happens in Charleston [putting on white hat].

The legislators wore the white hats when they talked to the miners and they said, "We are for you."

They went into committee and [witness puts on black hat] they put the black hat on of the coal operator. That is exactly how they voted. They tore this law to pieces.

When they came out [witness puts on white hat again] they said, "I tried but I couldn't do anything."

At these 50 meetings that I have had I would shake hands with all the coal miners. Some would have one finger missing, some two fingers, some three fingers, some could not raise their arm, some limped, some, you look on their face and you see the scars of coal mining accidents.

I would say to a man, "How old are you?" He would say, "30." I would say, "You look like 50." Another one would say he is 40. He looked like 60. They actually deteriorate earlier than other people.

* * *

[G]entlemen, I am disturbed by the fact that the Federal Government gave $63 million for coal research for new markets in 1969 and not even a million dollars for coal dust control.

Why do you give so much for the production and nothing for the man? They have also an education program because the coal miners are getting disabled at a fast rate. So they go to the high schools and they enlist these students with Federal funds for training.

I asked many high schools to give the other side of the story as far as the health of the coal miner, the fact that if he does not die in an accident he may die of black lung and that he will be sick the last 10 or 15 years of his life.

But only until recently did anyone allow me to speak and that was in Wyoming County, with three high schools.

Yet the Federal Government gave $5 million for this program.

Mr. Chairman, the Department of Education of this government wrote me and said they are interested in education, they are not interested in health. The Department of Mines wrote me and said these people will be strip miners who are trained so they do not get dust disease. This is an exaggeration.

Strip miners get dust disease the same as anyone else. . . .

Now let us get to the crux of the problem, the black lung business where there is so much argument as to how many cases are there.

I know because in previous testimony there have been some who say it is a rare disease, some say it is like phlegm in the nose and you flop it out.

But you can't do that. Because once it gets in the lungs it is progressive; 1,000 autopsies were done in the Beckley hospital. Eighty-five percent showed coal dust disease. We figure that about 50 percent of the miners eventually become disabled from this disease. It is a progressive disease.

If a man leaves a mine, 10 years later it affects him. He gets short of breath, he develops the emphysema, he develops the right heart failure and out he goes.

Of course, it is easy enough to say that mining did not have anything to do with it. But it does.

Those who do not have coal dust disease do not get right side of the heart failure. What are the symptoms? What does a coal miner look like? What does he say? He says, "I am so short of breath, I can't work like I used to. When I work real hard, why, I get dizzy."

He says, "I start coughing, I am spitting up black stuff."

He uses about 30 to 40 percent of the energy of his body in breathing while in a normal person it is 10 percent. . . .

* * *

And, there, dust. You talk about dust standards. You know it makes me smile sometimes the way you talk about 3 milligrams and about 4½ milligrams. My lord, in some of those mines it is 300 milligrams. You can't see a foot ahead of you.

So, the dust on the ground these men have told me is such they have worked in 18 inches and 20 inches of dust which should have been removed because it causes explosions and it makes people sick, humans sick, not animals, but humans.

Now the most dastardly practice in this book is working "ahead of air." That means ahead of ventilation. I should say about 90 percent of the miners have done this in time.

The reason it is bad is because they have bad lungs anyhow, they can't help it, and if you cut the oxygen down from 19½ to 18 percent the man becomes unconscious. So they are hauling him out of the mines, "heart attack, heart attack," to the hospital.

He doesn't have a heart attack, he has respiratory failure. Heart attack is not compensable, respiratory failure is. You have to be a pretty strong doctor to make a diagnosis of respiratory failure if you work for a coal company. I do not think you would be around very long.

* * *

Now I think a lot has been said about masks in the prevention of dust. I saw, Mr. Chairman, a picture of you with a mask on you yesterday.

SENATOR WILLIAMS: It was upside down.

DR. BUFF: I know that. Basically, I want to tell you that mask wouldn't help you. It is a waste of time. The particles of dust that cause pneumoconiosis, the filter in that mask will not take out because if it took that particle of dust out you could not breathe. They are the same size as air particles.

*   *   *

. . . If you cut the dust out you cut the air out. That is why these fellows start working in it and they throw it off and they say, "I can't work in this thing." It suffocates you.

They are not sick in the head. They know what they are talking about.

And then there is the other problem. Most of them have lung disease. If you cut down the oxygen supply through that mask he is going to get silly, he is going to see double. So he throws it off.

*   *   *

The people in England and the people in Czechoslovakia have a good system. We say they don't produce coal in the proportion that we produce it and that is why it wouldn't work here. No one knows. No one knows.

SENATOR EAGLETON: Are there statistics available on the incidence of black lung in Wales and in Czechoslovakia?

DR. BUFF: Yes, sir, in Wales it has been reduced from 60 to 20 percent.

SENATOR EAGLETON: What about Czechoslovakia?

DR. BUFF: It is supposed to be somewhere around 25 percent now. I do not know what it was recently but it is going down. They are very strict on this dust control.

SENATOR EAGLETON: In your opinion, what are the key things they are doing that we are not doing?

DR. BUFF: They have a system where they suck the air, when they cut the coal they cut large pieces instead of small pieces.

They have like a cyclone over the machine. It sucks back the air. It goes through a wool-cotton filter and then an electrostatic precipitator and it comes out clean.

It is a little expensive but, my lord, we are talking about human lives. We are not talking about other things.

Now if the industry itself says that they cannot reduce dust, it is not economically feasible, it will put men out of work, it will put their wives and children on the want list, I give you one answer: What is the price of a husband that is killed in an accident?

What is the price of a coal miner who chokes to death the last 10 years of his life and leaves his family and his boys to support him?

Is this fair? Let us consider another thing about economic feasibility.

The Czechoslovakian Government and the British Government compete with us a little bit in coal. We want private industry to do this but if they cannot, if they say they will not, then the government of these United States will have to do it for them.

As far as West Virginia is concerned, I am worried about the fact that when a coal miner goes into the mines you know he has no toilet. He does his business on site or up the hollow.

He breathes this stuff after it dries and he gets fungus infection in his lungs from this. I asked a couple of coal operators would they put toilets in the mines, chemical toilets?

The answer I got was "Do you know I have 300 miners? They put out 2 pounds of waste a day. That would cost me 25 cents a man or $75 a day for toilets. Do you think I'm nuts?"

*   *   *

The chief of mines of Kentucky is a coal operator. The chief of mines of West Virginia used to work for Consolidation Coal. No vested interest, just a tinge.

What we need is a rigid health and safety act with 100 percent enforcement.

We need this enforced like we do with the other agencies of the government.

We do not want any hanky-panky. We do not want an inspector coming around and letting them know 3 weeks in advance they are coming.

We do not want an inspector coming around and the superintendent meets him and says, "Don't go to mine No. 1, go to No. 9. No. 9 is cleaned up. The other is filthy."

This happened to Armco. The inspector went to one and closed the mine. I think he might have regretted that because that is an awful lot of pressure on one company. They did clean it up and, thank God, they might have saved some lives.

But we feel that the coal industry—the coal owners, because I do not think we should talk about operators or producers—I think we ought to get to the gist of it, who owns this coal.

I think the Federal Government should find out who owns the coal mines. You are jumping on the wrong guy when you jump on the operator. He leases; he takes orders. He is just a boy.

The coal owner is the boss. You know as well as I do that most big corporations do not have too much respect for state law but they do respect Federal laws.

Gentlemen, one corporation tried to play a little game with the Federal Government and the officers ended up in jail. You do not play with the Federal Government.

* * *

k.
Testimony of Donald L. Rasmussen, Chief, Pulmonary Section, Appalachian Regional Hospital, Beckley, W.Va.—March 13, 1969

During the past 6 years, I have been engaged in the evaluation of pulmonary function and work capacity in coal miners from southern West Virginia, southwestern Virginia and eastern Kentucky. I have become acquainted with the lung diseases afflicting miners and have demonstrated physical impairment in many. I have also become acquainted with some of the socio-economic consequences of the lung diseases of coal miners. The latter are responsible for suffering not only of the miner but also his family.

* * *

Among the 3,000 miners evaluated in our laboratory, approximately 50 percent have been found to have significant impairment of pulmonary capacity. An additional 40 percent show varying degrees of impairment, while 10 percent show little or no abnormality. Of interest is the fact that the x-ray findings bear little relationship to functional capacity. Thus, men whose x-ray reveals only a widespread increase in linear markings may have impairment as great as one with advanced pneumoconiosis (complicated pneumoconiosis or so-called "progressive massive fibrosis"). We are aware of men in the 70 and 80 year group with advanced penumoconiosis, who are apparently as healthy as age permits.

Our observations in Beckley have been challenged by the coal corporations and are not recognized by industry-oriented physicians nor even a number of experts in various medical schools as well as within the U.S. Public Health Service. These critics base their opinions on published medical evidence, largely that from Britain. None of the criticism is based on actual test results.

Much emphasis has recently been placed on cigarette smoking and this has been labeled as the cause of disabling lung disease in coal miners. The effects of cigarette smoking are obvious in our miners and cigarette smoking can produce measurable abnormalities, even in our subjects who have no overt bronchitis. On the other hand, the effect of working at the face in mechanized operations shows a more marked effect than any other known factor, including cigarette smoking. Workers at the face in mechanized operations appear to develop pulmonary impairment on the average 5 years earlier than all other workers within the mine. This is even more startling since certain miners in other areas are also exposed to relatively high dust concentrations.

Suggestions by the coal industry that "additional research" is warranted before dust suppression is imposed should be regarded as evidence of a total lack of regard for human life and health. We are disturbed by the increasing frequency with which we encounter men less than 40 years of age who have been employed for under 20 years who are significantly impaired or exhibit clear-cut abnormalities of pulmonary function. Almost always, these men have been employed at the working face. The majority of such men have worked on or near continuous mining machines for 3 to 10 years only, having spent the earlier years operating more conventional machines. It is our opinion, that unless immediate and rigid dust control measures are instigated, we will see a shocking increase in pulmonary disability within 5 to 10 years.

Much more research is indeed necessary in order to more clearly define the dust diseases of coal workers, and to find additional methods of safeguarding the health of miners. Methods of early detection of impaired health are required to identify those men who should be moved to non-dusty areas. Uniform workman's compensation based on objective physiologic methods should be sought, and much more effort is required to provide employment for the presently affected miners who, under present practices, are doomed to an early disability and impoverishment.

* * *

l.
Testimony of Dr. Harvey A. Wells, Coordinator, Conemangh Valley Memorial Hospital, Johnstown, Pa.—March 13, 1969

* * *

My experience in West Virginia and Pennsylvania coalfields leads me to the inescapable conclusion that the main factor that has led to the deplorable conditions in and around the mines is the fact that employers are effectively immune from suit under most state compensation acts and they are not liable for even the most callous disregard for the health and safety practices.

For example, in West Virginia, the injury from death and disease caused by gross negligence of an employer cannot be compensated by a jury unless the essential elements of first-degree murder can be demonstrated.

Relatively minor additions to the proposed Federal legislation could result in major benefit in the workplace and make it much cheaper to run a safe shop than a dangerous and unhealthy one.

What I am saying, gentlemen, is that we must give these men back the right to a jury trial. This denial has led to the deplorable conditions and if we can give them the right to go to a jury in cases where there is negligence and bad health and safety practices, we will go a long way toward the elimination of these bad practices because the man who does the wrong will have to pay the bill.

This is the American way, the way it should be done. Because of the inequities in the various states' compensation acts, the employers do not have to answer for their wrongdoings.

* * *

SENATOR EAGLETON: If a 3-milligram limit were adopted and rigorously enforced, would the incidence of black lung be reduced or would the disabling effects of black lung simply be prolonged?

What I am getting at is this, would a 3-milligram limit merely prolong the work and life expectancy of the worker but sooner or later black lung will appear in many coal miners even with the 3-milligram limit for coal miners?

DR. RASMUSSEN: I do not think anyone can answer your question specifically related to a 3-milligram level, whether continued exposure at this level would be, let us say, completely well tolerated and handled by every miner in the mine for any length of time.

We do not know the answer to this question. I think that the British experience would certainly indicate that a lower dust level than we now have would result in a much lower incidence of the disease.

I suspect that were men to remain in the mines for, say, a greater length of time that some of them would again begin to show change.

I think it is a time and dose related matter.

DR. BUFF: You asked how much money was spent by Britain. In 1967, $10 million. We spent $4½ million in 5 years. Great Britain in 1 year, $10 million. A smaller country.

SENATOR WILLIAMS: Thank you, gentlemen. We have a vote. I would like to say while we have had this remarkable testimony, Apollo 9 reentered the atmosphere and is down safe.

SENATOR RANDOLPH: I want the record to show that sometimes we do better above earth and on earth than we do under the earth.

* * *

SENATOR BELLMON: . . . As I listened to . . . [your] statement, I was impressed by the fact that Utah and Oklahoma have a great deal in common in that both of us have immense reserves of coal which are not presently being mined as much as we hope they will be in the future, and the question that comes to my mind now is the one that has crossed my mind when other witnesses have appeared, and that is this: Whether or not there is danger that in drafting safety legislation we will be so restrictive that we may limit the future development of our coal reserves and cause the cost of coal mining to go up to the point where our industries and utilities will turn increasingly to petroleum and perhaps nuclear power as a sort of energy.

As a Senator from Utah, are you concerned we need to be careful we don't go too far in this field, or do you feel there is a danger here?

SENATOR MOSS: Well, of course, it is to be hoped that the mining of coal will be economic and profitable and, therefore, this resource will be used. But I don't think that we can sacrifice any safety measure for the men who must mine the coal, in order to keep the cost down.

I think even if the resource has to stand unused, that we must not bring it out of the mines by endangering their health or periling their lives, by proceeding with less than the maximum amount of safety that we can possibly devise for the mines.

I really don't worry too much. I think the use of coal is on the increase now, and I think our energy demands are going up at such an astronomical rate that surely the coal fields will be called upon to furnish a good part of that energy. As we go forward in developing coal, I want the safety factor kept paramount. I wouldn't restrain any effort in the safety field just to keep the cost down.

* * *

m.
Testimony of Dr. William H. Stewart, Surgeon General, Public Health Service— March 18, 1969

* * *

For over 30 years, the Public Health Service has undertaken cooperative studies with the Bureau of Mines on coal miners' health problems. Not until 1963, however, did the Department first receive funds for the specific support of operations in this area. Our first major project was a prevalence study of pneumoconiosis in soft coal miners in Appalachia and other coal mining areas.

This study established pneumoconiosis among soft coal workers in the United States as an occupational respiratory disease of serious and previously unrecognized magnitude. Our research showed that one in 10 men in the mines and one in five of the former miners in Appalachia showed X-ray evidence of this chronic respiratory disease. Data from postmortem examinations would indicate an even higher prevalence of this disease.

For work periods less than 15 years underground, the occurrence of pneumoconiosis among miners appeared to be spotty and showed no particular trend. For work periods greater than 15 years underground, there was a linear increase in the prevalence of the disease with years spent underground.

The major shortcoming of this study was the lack of environmental data, especially on dust concentrations, particle size and chemical composition. For information on the relationship between environmental factors and the disease, we consulted with the British National Coal Board, which provided us with technical information indicating a straight-line relationship between the amount of dust breathed and the progression of pneumoconiosis in miners.

* * *

The United States is the only major coal-producing nation in the world which does not have an official Government standard for coal mine dust. Since Great Britain began requiring dust control efforts in the coal mines—which resulted in reduced concentration levels—there has been a substantial reduction there in the prevalence of coal workers' pneumoconiosis.

Thus, the incidence of new cases in miners has decreased from 8.1 new cases per 1,000 miners in 1955 to 1.9 new cases per 1,000 miners in 1967; the age specific prevalence of simple coal miners pneumoconiosis has also decreased as has the overall prevalence (12.5 percent in 1959–62 as compared to 10.9 in 1964–67).

An official respirable dust standard for coal mines could, in our opinion, if properly enforced, make a significant reduction in new cases of pneumoconiosis and decrease the rate of progression of old cases. Last year we concluded that sufficient data were available to recommend the adoption of an interim coal dust exposure standard for miners, pending further refinement of technical knowledge. After careful analysis of the British and Pennsylvania experiences, and after consultation with many authorities, we concluded that:

An interim standard should represent no more than a reasonable degree of risk to our miners, given our present technology, and be one that would significantly reduce the rate at which new cases of pneumoconiosis would develop in the future and old cases would progress.

On the basis of those conclusions, last December, the Secretary of Health, Education, and Welfare recommended to the Department of the Interior a Federal standard which could be used to lower respirable dust levels in coal mines. This standard called for a respirable dust level not to exceed 3.0 milligrams per cubic meter as measured by the Mining Research Establishment (MRE) horizontal elutriator instrument.

We recommended this standard in the conviction that it could, if adopted and properly enforced throughout the coal mining industry, make a significant reduction in coal miners' pneumoconiosis. This standard, if adopted and enforced, would place the United States along with other major coal-producing nations which have set health standards for dust exposures in the coal mining industry.

* * *

SENATOR RANDOLPH: Dr. Stewart, we have heard conflicting testimony as to the number of cases of coal workers with pneumoconiosis—that is a word I am having trouble with this morning. How much black lung disease is prevalent in the United States?

I recall one source made an estimation of 100,000, of 135,000 workers.

Now, does the U.S. Public Health Service have reliable statistics—I shouldn't perhaps use the word reliable—but statistics that can be presented to the subcommittee?

DR. STEWART: Yes; I have used the figure 100,000 as an estimate of pneumoconiosis that was based on the prevalence rates we found in our study of both active miners and of inactive miners. I think the difficulty arises, Senator Randolph, when people try to apply that to 135,000 active miners. We included also the inactive miners in the estimate. One out of 10 active miners, one out of five inactive miners.

The difficulty we have had is in determining how many inactive miners there are. We used a figure of 400,000 inactive miners, derived from a variety of data, in making our estimate of the cases of pneumoconiosis. In addition we know from other data, for example—the known number of disabled miners in Pennsylvania and the total man-years of mining experience between 1940 and 1955, that you can come up with a figure close to 100,000 for the total of coal miners' pneumoconiosis cases.

We also know from the disability insurance statistics of the Social Security Administration that the disability among miners from respiratory diseases is much greater than the average that you would expect.

As far as what is needed for making a decision that you have a health problem, that we need to take some preventive measures, that estimate of 100,000 cases is a perfectly good statement.

*   *   *

SENATOR EAGLETON: Doctor, do I take your testimony to mean that clearly from a medical point of view, due to research that has been made available to you, part of which the Public Health Service has participated in, that 3.0 is clearly a preferable permissible level than anything higher thereto, 4.5, or anything else you might pick out of the air?

DR. STEWART: From a medical standpoint, that is correct.

SENATOR EAGLETON: So, in terms of you as a professional physician, you would recommend, would you not, 3.0 from a medical point of view, not being a construction expert or design engineer or coal mining?

DR. STEWART: Ideally, I recommend no dust. But knowing the practicalities of the situation, you can never reach that. And this is so true of many things we do. We are always measuring the benefit and risk on so many things. The determination of that level depends on the technology of mining and the determination to reach some level.

SENATOR EAGLETON: But the health of the coal miner is going to be better protected by a 3.0 level than by a 4.5 level?

DR. STEWART: This is correct.

*   *   *

n.

Statement of Representative Ken Hechler, West Virginia—March 20, 1969

*   *   *

Whenever legislation of this nature is discussed, a lot of attention is put on the economics of the industry and what it will cost the industry to clean up the mines and take strict safety precautions. The phrase "technologically feasible" is used to describe limits beyond which some people claim it is impossible to go. There is a tendency to look at this problem in terms of certain entrenched forces and practices which some people claim are immutable. Therefore, some people claim we had better not do anything unless there is full agreement throughout the industry.

I submit that we ought to start with an entirely different premise—the individual human being. We ought to find out what is necessary to protect the life, the health, and the safety of these 144,000 human beings who work in the coal mines. And *then* we ought to go ahead bodily and take the measures necessary to protect these human beings.

I believe we can not only achieve a high degree of health and safety for the individual coal miner but also keep the industry prosperous. I am encouraged in this belief by the progressive coal operators, the new breed of young and imaginative coal operators who are convinced that this approach is not only possible but essential for the survival of the industry.

Today, more than ever before, the people of this nation are concerned with their environment —how they live, the air they breathe, and the water they drink. That is why in recent weeks over 40,000 coal miners in West Virginia, against the opposition of their own union, rose up and said: "We want something done about these conditions, and the disease of black lung from which coal miners suffer." Some observers marvelled that the miners weren't satisfied just with high wages— they wanted freedom to breathe fresh air, and they were willing to give up their pay to fight for fresh air. The old rules of economics and politics are being swept away in the surging drive for a better life, for the dignity of the individual, for the quality of life which a human being lives here on earth. The coal miner has been watching the grandeurs of science and technology bring a new life to millions of Americans, and gouge out more coal per minute, while doing nothing to improve his health and safety.

In fact, science and technology has brought greater threats to the health and safety of the coal miner.

*   *   *

The main point I want to make, Mr. Chairman, is this: year after year after year, we have compromised this issue at the expense of the human beings who suffer the consequences of injury and death in the coal mines. We have allowed loopholes to be driven into the legislation which have made a mockery of effective mine safety regulations. Down through the years, we have tolerated a Bureau of Mines which has been subservient to every special interest except the man who mines the coal. The Bureau of Mines has been moribund, a colossal failure when it came to protecting the men in the mines, production-oriented, filled with dead wood, backward and bureaucratic, stifling the initiative of any imaginative official, leaderless, having the backbone of a chocolate eclair, and rarely challenged either to do its job or seek more effective tools to do a better job.

Each of us remembers what we were doing on a red-letter day. I recall talking with two or three officials on the day of the Farmington disaster. Director O'Leary was easy to reach, and he ticked off clearly and crisply what had to be done to strengthen the enforcement of existing regulations, and what needed to be done in the future. To a friend of mine, all one official could say was: "This was a great mine, it produced 9,600 tons a day." High up in the Department of the Interior, another official warned me on November 20: "Don't let an accident like this excite you. After all, nobody did this on purpose. And please, Mr. Congressman, don't indulge in any recriminations against anybody on account of this."

*   *   *

o.
Testimony of Dr. Ian Higgins, School of Public Health, University of Michigan— March 26, 1969

*   *   *

SENATOR WILLIAMS: I wonder if our feeling, that we should make mandatory an annual physical examination, fits in here at all?

DR. HIGGINS: This is more frequent than I think is necessary. In fact, in the British mines I think the general view is about once every 5 years is probably sufficient.

The development of pneumoconiosis is so slow, given reasonably safe dust levels, that annual X-rays are unnecessary and probably not worth the cost. On the other hand, I think if one is dealing with an area where the dust levels may be less certain, which may be the case in this country, then something more frequent than 5 years might be desirable and possibly 3 years would be a safer time.

*   *   *

SENATOR WILLIAMS: Is it possible, do you think, to get what I call an early warning, to catch a man in time so that he could be withdrawn from employment at the face or maybe out of the mine altogether?

DR. HIGGINS: I think there is no doubt detecting the early X-ray changes; the early warning as you call it, is sound preventive medicine and effective.

I strongly believe, however, that compulsion should not be instituted. It may be in the man's best interests to leave the mines. If he does not want to do so, he should not be compelled to do so. I think Britain is unique in Europe in that no man is made to follow any advice he is given. The only justification for suspending him is active tuberculosis which would make him a risk to his fellows. I believe that only by stressing advice and avoiding compulsion will one get full cooperation from the miners for periodic X-rays.

SENATOR WILLIAMS: He makes the judgment, but he makes it based on information.

DR. HIGGINS: He makes it on the best evidence that can be given to him.

SENATOR WILLIAMS: We are doing this all the time, those of us who smoke. We are making a judgment.

DR. HIGGINS: That is right.

*   *   *

p.
Testimony of Cloyd D. McDowell, President, Harlan County Coal Operators Association, Harlan, Ky.—March 26, 1969

*   *   *

. . . Regarding mandatory health standards for controlling dust in underground mines, we agree that some control is needed. However, there is a greater need for research and study of this problem in order to establish all the facts pertaining to it rather than setting an arbitrary limit of 4.5 milligrams of dust per cubic meter of air, which may or may not be the proper limit.

We do know that one cigarette contains over 35 milligrams of tar and nicotine which we presume would be in the form of respirable dust if it is inhaled as smoke. Are we then expected to keep mine air purer than a room in which a cigarette has been smoked? Medical witnesses have testi-fied that they are not sure that cigarette smoking is harmful to health. Others say it is and yet not a law has been passed to prevent the sale or use of cigarettes.

A lung specialist from Great Britain visited all of the United Mine Workers' hospitals in 1958 to instruct these doctors in the diagnosis of lung diseases, including pneumoconiosis. I attended the meeting held in Harlan and heard him say that breathing coal dust would not cause coal miners' pneumoconiosis unless there was another substance present.

Dr. William H. Anderson, of Louisville, was present at this meeting and since has made a de-tailed study of coal miner's pneumoconiosis. He has testified in case after case that coal dust by itself would not cause miners' pneumoconiosis.

Coal dust per se may or may not be harmful to the health of miners, but it could be other fac-tors such as the amount of sulphur in the dust, or the silica content or some other substance. We are told that anthracite coal dust is more abrasive than bituminous and it may be for this reason that a larger number of miners are affected by dust in Pennsylvania than in other states.

We believe that the dust problem should be attacked from the standpoint of preventing dust by requiring the manufacturers of mine machin-ery to build dust-suppressing attachments on all mine equipment rather than establishing a level of dust concentration. We have had a great deal of success in preventing dust by using water sprays on coal-cutting equipment. The use of dust collectors and respirators should be required where necessary and many other means can be developed through research if funds were avail-able.

We realize that safety problems multiply in geometric ratio to the amount of coal produced in a section of a mine. The faster the coal is re-moved from the face, the greater will be the amount of dust produced. Also, the amount of methane liberated will be increased proportion-ately.

*   *   *

A mine is as safe as the people that work in the mine. No law should be passed that sets a penalty for one group of people while other peo-ple are exempted from the penalty even though they may violate the law endangering themselves and others. From my own experience I can testify that over 95 percent of the safety violations are committed by workmen and not by the operator

in our mines. However, should an official or an employee knowingly violate any law that will en-danger the health and safety of the people in the mine, he should be penalized.

*   *   *

As far as we can determine, there is no basis for setting a limit of 4.5 milligrams of allowable float dust in the mine atmosphere. We are aware of the clamor of many people who have never been in a coal mine to have something done about this problem. Long before the "black lung" issue was brought up, many of our mines had installed water on their continuous miners and were using a wetting agent such as calcium chloride and others to allay dust on their haulage roads, to im-prove vision and prevent a possible dust explo-sion.

Now I would like to state here that in our areas I know of no continuous mine machine that is being operated without water.

I do not believe that coal dust is entirely re-sponsible for all the respiratory diseases that occur in coal miners. I can say from my own ex-perience that smoking cigarettes is one of the greatest contributors to lung disease. I was reared in a coal mining town. My father was a cutting machine operator in the mines from 1913 until his retirement in 1953. He lived to be 80 years of age and was never troubled with "black lung" or any respiratory illness. He never smoked a ciga-rette in his life, which may account for his good health and longevity.

*   *   *

q.

Testimony of John F. O'Leary, Director, U.S. Bureau of Mines—May 2, 1969

*   *   *

[T]he Bureau of Mines has a research budget of around $2 million a year and most of that, I am sorry to say, is spent in testing. When I made inquiries as to the exact distribution of the budget I found perhaps $300,000 a year has been spent on the entire field of health up until now. That is why before Mannington immediately upon as-suming this office I asked for an additional mil-lion dollars. About a like amount is spent on safety. Mr. Mullins pointed out that it took us some 8 years to develop the monitor, and I want to put as a corollary to that at $50,000 a year. Now I don't know that you could have done it at $100,000 a year in 4 years but I know you could have appreciably shortened that 8-year period of time if the system had been willing to put the money to it.

I think that really brings me to a kind of sad commentary on the system that develops the technology here. In fact, the coal industry does not develop its own technology, it is developed largely externally outside the coal industry.

NOTES

NOTE 1.

LETTER FROM RUSSELL E. TRAIN, UNDER-SECRETARY OF THE INTERIOR, TO SENATOR HARRISON A. WILLIAMS, JR.—MAY 16, 1969

*   *   *

Industrial health standards cannot be based upon personal health criteria alone. Consideration must also be given to engineering feasibility.

The proposed interim standard for respirable coal mine dust is a case in point. Because of technological limitations, it is infeasible to establish a standard immediately at the level indicated to be desirable from a personal health standpoint alone. New technology is needed to achieve a better standard, and the Bureau of Mines is better equipped than any other Federal agency to move the industry in the direction of greater health as well as increased safety. . . .

*   *   *

NOTE 2.

LETTER FROM RALPH NADER TO STEWART L. UDALL, SECRETARY OF THE INTERIOR—MARCH 23, 1968

. . . I am writing in the hope that you will bring your immediate, personal attention to bear upon the tragic plight of coal miners resulting from unsafe coal mine practices. The Bureau of Mines in your Department has, under the Federal Coal Mine Safety Act of 1952, the responsibility for promoting coal mine safety and informing Congress of the need for additional legislation. As the second most hazardous occupational category in terms of disabling injuries and the first in terms of pneumoconiosis, coal mining presents a challenge to the Bureau of Mines that is readily apparent, except apparently to the Bureau of Mines.

*   *   *

The fundamental explanation for the Bureau's lassitude toward the demands of mine health and safety conditions is that it is the captive of the coal mine operators which include large steel companies who own mines. The Bureau follows the undesirable practice of holding regular private meetings with the Bituminous Coal Operators' Association (BCOA) and the United Mine Workers (UMW) and accepting the recommendations which they agree upon to transmit to Congress.

The UMW leadership has shown a consistent bias in favor of the coal operators' viewpoints toward preventive safety policy which has produced an enduring indifference towards preventive safety and health measures for their own membership and especially towards coal miners that do not happen to be unionized. Alas for the brotherhood of workers! Its rhetoric aside, the UMW leadership has been persuaded by coal management into choosing the alleged health of the industry over the health of its workers. The specious choice of jobs over more safety is drummed into UMW officers by management and the choice has been to ignore needed safety improvements and especially preventive dust control. The UMW *Journal* devotes endless space to the threat of other energy sources to coal and virtually nothing to the crucial matter of coal dust hazards. The union has built hospitals to receive the human debris from the mines but very little to push for preventive dust control and needed, but neglected, safety practices whose furtherance the rank and file entrust to their leaders.

*   *   *

NOTE 3.

LETTER FROM STEWART L. UDALL TO RALPH NADER—JUNE 12, 1968

*   *   *

. . . I am frank to confirm your general conclusion: although pneumoconiosis has been recognized for many years as a serious health problem in the coal mining industry, we have moved very slowly toward corrective measures. . . .

[O]ne of the more difficult technical handicaps in coming to grips with pneumoconiosis is that of securing accurate measurement and analysis of coal mine dust. The Bureau has not been idle in tackling this fundamental issue, having devoted extensive time and effort toward the development and testing of the required instrumentation. With that work completed, it has now begun the major survey of dust float in coal mines—a prerequisite to establishing effective standards. Even before precise scientific information is available, however, it may be possible to formulate interim guidelines and to take other steps to minimize health hazards, pending more definitive standards to be prescribed and enforced.

To be equally candid about the seriousness of pneumoconiosis, it is clear that the demonstrated incidence of this insidious and irreversible malady warrants most serious concern. A statistically reliable sample survey conducted by the Public Health Service over the years 1963–64 revealed that 9.5 percent of currently employed miners and 18.6 percent of formerly employed miners had contracted the disease. The survey also indicated that its incidence increases with years of work underground. For example, of the currently employed population in the sample, 4 percent of those with 10–19 years of underground work had the disease while 8.6 percent of those with 20–29 years' exposure were afflicted. The higher percentage among the formerly employed could support an inference that exposure has led to changes in occupation, if not to disabling illness. Only a detailed case study can reveal the true facts, however, since it is also possible to surmise that improved ventilation and other preventive measures in relatively recent years may have reduced exposure in the present mine workforce.

* * *

The role of the Bureau with respect to problems of occupational health in coal mines has remained investigative and advisory under the original Title I, and in this area the Bureau has not assumed the kind of leadership it has displayed in the field of safety. This situation is in part attributable to the existence of a division of responsibility in the area. Out of a laudable desire to avoid wasteful duplication of effort, the Bureau has operated under a long-standing agreement with the Public Health Service under which the latter agency carries on the basic research relating to occupational diseases affecting the mining industry. While we have no present intention of abandoning that arrangement, it is clear from our analysis to date that more efficient coordination and cooperative mechanisms are needed.

* * *

NOTE 4.

LETTER FROM RALPH NADER TO
STEWART L. UDALL—JUNE 27, 1968

* * *

1. Medical opinion by physicians working in the coal mine health area believe that the incidence of pneumoconiosis is considerably higher than the 1963–64 figures in your letter. Their reasoning is based on the fact that the present years are beginning to reflect the toll of the mechanization which began in the Fifties and which produces more and finer coal dust. Another reason is given by Dr. Walter A. Laquer of the Beckley (W.Va.) Appalachian Regional Hospital; namely, that many cases of pneumoconiosis are not detected by x-rays.

2. Exactly what corrective measures you have in mind were not made clear. From expressions within the Department and within the Department of Health, Education and Welfare, it is all too likely that refuge will be taken in undertaking a long range study to measure more mines for dust content and testing the required instrumentation. Fortunately, from the long experience in England and West Germany, which are far ahead of the United States in coal dust control, instrumentation and standards are available for use in this country. Action can and must be taken now, even though further research and testing be fostered. Experience in the Ontario metal mines can be utilized as well. Although the fact that some other nations have put into practice a more humane health policy than that prevailing in the United States (where apparently miners' lives are still considered cheaper than coal dust control) should be a source of shame, it can also be a spur for jettisoning any further neglect here. It is deeply dismaying to recall that the 1936 Pneumoconiosis Conference in this country concluded with recommendations which were utilized by the British and in Ontario for many years but have been ignored in this country. In some states, such as West Virginia and Kentucky, public authority has been in the grip of the coal-steel barons for so long in this area that even the pitiful human debris that mark many retired coal miners receives a disgraceful pittance of workman's compensation and that only for certain, not all, worker-related diseases. West Virginia does not recognize pneumoconiosis as a compensable disease. Can there be any conceivable excuse for permitting mining conditions that lead to the deposit of human excreta randomly to further more disease or allowing misdiagnosis of miners who collapse at work to avoid responsibility for methane and other gaseous concentrations?

The division of responsibility which you note between the Bureau of Mines and the Public Health Service does not extend to a division of responsibility over control. It is a division, if any, between control *and* research. Control remains with the Bureau and there is no exculpation derivable from any relationship with the Public Health Service which has its own immobilities and indecisions. Nothing can even partially excuse the fact that the Bureau has done nothing about controlling dust in the mines, has never once closed down a mine for dust—not gas hazard-related but lung hazard-related. The Bureau does not even have a ranking of mines in terms of dust density.

3. [Y]our reference to the Department's advising the Labor Committee of both houses of Congress, neglects to mention the insupportable delays first in sending your promised recommendations to Congress by April, not yet delivered, and second, in view of the lateness of the session and early adjournment, the Department has effectively terminated any prospect of legislation this year.

4. If these hundreds of thousands of violations of the safety code in the past decade were not deterred because the code is advisory only, what has kept the Department from working openly and vigorously to have these codes enacted into law with penalties for violation? This lassitude, to use a kind word, has turned the Department's inspection process into a tragic farce. The Department has been restricting itself to imminent disaster situations and major disasters, defined as exceeding five fatalities, and overlooking the smaller hazards that can take single lives. This same attitude has permitted the continuance of a shocking gap in the 1952 law which exempted, among others, the working face of the mine which is the area of greatest accident-injury frequency.

*   *   *

5. On page 4 of your letter discussing the 1963 Task Force on Coal Mine Safety and current findings and recommendations, some clarification is needed. It is simply not accurate to imply that "elimination of the reasonable time provisions" was a reform because replacing them was the "unwarrantable" violation proviso. This places an onerous burden on mine inspectors, hampering enforcement by requiring mine inspectors to show that all violations must be unwarrantable before penalties or a notice to abate such conditions can be imposed. This means that a withdrawal and debarment order will not be issued if the repeated violation did not arise as a consequence of a lack of due diligence on the part of the operator.

6. Last year's report, noted in your letter, capitulated to the demands of the coal mining in-

terests and became explicitly inconsistent with the recommendation in the 1963 Task Force report pertaining to nonpermissible electrical equipment. The Task Force recommended their elimination within a one year period; the 1967 report suggested a five year period to terminate—4 years later. Moreover, over the strong objections of some mining inspectors, the Bureau of Mines has allowed mine owners to move this unsafe electrical equipment into entirely different mines—often many miles away and sometimes across state lines. This is an example of the Bureau of Mines' discretion and another reason why your office should exercise a thorough supervision.

r.

Letter from Walter J. Hickel, Secretary of the Interior, to Senator Ralph Yarborough, Chairman, Committee on Labor and Public Welfare—July 17, 1969

Your committee, yesterday, requested this department's comments on the provisions of the July 9, 1969, committee print of the coal mine health and safety legislation which give us concern.

*   *   *

The Dust Standard

The panel proposed in the print should be allowed to waive the dust standard on a mine-by-mine basis for six months after the effective date of the dust standard where it determines that the procurement, installation, and associated construction of equipment and facilities necessary to attain the dust standard cannot be accomplished in the first six months after enactment.

We continue to favor the provision of S. 2405 establishing no exact date for a 2.0 standard to be reached but requiring that the Secretary establish this standard as soon as possible. With the present state of technology, it is possible to predict with the research already underway that a 3.0 standard could be attainable in three years. The attainment of a 2.0 standard, however, may depend on the outcome of research that has yet to be started and the results of which are unknown and unpredictable. If the research is extremely favorable, the time required to meet the standard could be less than 6 years. If the research fails, it may require more than the 6 years provided in the print. The print itself recognizes that it may not be possible to attain a 2.0 standard within 6 years and authorizes the Secretary to establish a new schedule specifying a later time for compliance with the 2.0 standard and requiring him to notify the Congress of such new schedule. If either House does not object by resolution within 60 legislative days, the new schedule will become effective. If the Committee insists on a 6 year schedule for the 2.0 standard, this additional authority is essential in view of the present state of technology.

*   *   *

Time Period for Making Equipment Permissible

The print provides that nonpermissible electric face equipment over 25 horsepower at nongassy mines be made permissible within 16 months after enactment, with provision for the panel to issue permits of noncompliance to use such nonpermissible equipment for up to an additional 44 months, or a total of 60 months after enactment. We understand that the Committee is considering lowering this period to a total of 48 months.

At the request of your Committee, a statistical sample was taken by our field personnel on the number and condition of existing nonpermissible equipment in use and the cost of their conversion. This sampling which was conducted in a very short time and represented, for example, in the case of nongassy small mines, only 90 out of over 2,700 such mines might suggest that the conversion of all this type equipment would be possible within 3 to 4 years. We believe that the data, because they are so limited, do not justify the selection of a specific time period. In our opinion, the time period should be left open. If the panel finds that the equipment and parts are available for the conversion in a shorter period, then we are certain the panel will not grant extensions beyond that period.

Penalties

The print establishes a criminal penalty against the miner and operator for violating knowingly a health or safety standard.

In regard to the miner, there is only one standard involving smoking or carrying matches underground which places any obligation on him. In all others, the operator is solely responsible for compliance. We believe that a criminal penalty against the miner for violating the standard is not appropriate, but we would not object to a civil penalty against the miner for violating the smoking standard since this is of serious consequences to other persons underground.

In regard to the operator, we believe that the civil penalty is sufficient, particularly when we consider the difficulty in proving a criminal violation.

*   *   *

Compensation

The print provides that, in cases where a mine or portion thereof is idled, by reason of an unwarrantable failure closing order, the miners shall be fully compensated by the operator. Similarly, under Title I of the print, the miner who is moved to another portion of the mine because of developing pneumoconiosis is guaranteed his regular rate of pay. In our opinion, both of these matters should be left for negotiation between management and labor.

Miscellaneous

*   *   *

Section 301(a) provides that a minimum of 4 inspections annually must be made of the entire underground coal mine. S. 2405 established the minimum at 3 inspections annually. We fail to see any real advantage in this requirement, particularly when it is so difficult to obtain qualified inspectors. Experience shows that at many large mines an inspection of the entire mine may run as long as a month. In our opinion, more has been gained since Farmington through the increased frequency of spot inspections, which do not, usually, cover the entire mine. Spot inspections, plus civil penalties, will be our most effective tools. On the other hand, if we find that increased full scale inspections are necessary for safety purposes, the bill provides that additional inspections can be required.

*   *   *

NOTES

NOTE 1.

LETTER FROM RUSSELL E. TRAIN, UNDERSECRETARY OF THE INTERIOR, TO SENATOR RALPH YARBOROUGH—MAY 22, 1969

*   *   *

The Department, through the Bureau of Mines, has been engaged in a program of research and development in connection with this industry since 1910. Many of the health and safety innovations in this industry were developed by the Bureau, such as the introduction of the widespread use of roof bolts. Until recently our annual research and development budget for health and safety has been about $2 million annually, a good portion of which has been devoted to "testing" rather than research. In fiscal year 1970, however, we have increased this budget substantially to $3.3 million. We recognize that there is a need for more health and safety research for this industry, but we doubt that a system which taxes the production of coal and earmarks the revenues for health and safety research is the most appropriate method to supply this need.

* * *

[O]ther dangerous industries, such as the nuclear industry which is a competitor of the coal industry, are not required to pay directly for health and safety research. The proposal might tend to confine the entire research and development effort to the government. The future research and development effort should, in our opinion, not be carried out by the government alone. Industry should be encouraged to assume, on an industry-wide basis, a greater role in this area.

Further, we believe that tax on the coal industry for health and safety research and development purposes should not be imposed without thorough study of its impact on the industry and the consideration of alternative approaches. To our knowledge, this has not been done to date.

* * *

NOTE 2.

BEN A. FRANKLIN
U.S. LAGS IN EFFORT TO IMPLEMENT MINE
SAFETY LAW*

The frequently troubled coal regions are being placed in a further state of turmoil these days as a result of lagging efforts to implement a new coal mine safety law.

The law involved is the Federal Coal Mine Health and Safety Act of 1969 . . .

* * *

The law has its partisans and detractors here, and few officials claim to be objective about it. But even many of those who make that claim say it may be trying to accomplish too much reform all at once.

The wide scope of the new law is generally welcomed by government safety men. But it is causing concern and leading to forecasts of dislocations that will cause a decline in support when coal reserves are critically short. Accordingly, the Bureau of Mines expects to begin with "token enforcement."

The coal mining industry is howling, predicting crippling reductions in fuel supplies for electric utilities and trying to negotiate last-minute relief as the new law heads toward a series of effective dates beginning April 1. The coal industry says it is working in the dark, without knowing what is expected of it.

There is disarray at the Bureau of Mines, stemming in part from a frantic bureaucratic scramble to obey the timing imposed by Congress. Some provisions of the law, which industry leaders contend will "just explode normal coal production," have a very short fuse.

The worst crisis is being caused by the fact that the most costly and controversial section of the law—language establishing for the first time strict limits on the amount of lung-damaging microscopic coal dust that will be allowed in the air that the miners breathe if the operator expects to stay in production—were required by law to be translated by government health and safety experts into precise regulations for the mine owners by Feb. 28.

They were not. A complete set of proposed dust regulations was drafted nearly on time by John F. O'Leary, who was director of the Bureau of the Bureau of Mines until he was forced out by the Nixon administration reportedly at the coal industry's insistence.

But the delay in publishing the regulations since then reflects the fact that the leaders of the mining industry have been holding closed-door conferences with government officials on the O'Leary draft.

In a letter Friday to Walter J. Hickel, the Secretary of the Interior, who has jurisdiction over the Bureau of Mines, W. A. Boyle, president of the United Mine Workers said that "we assume" the delay "is a further indication of the callous disregard for the health and safety of the coal miner."

* * *

The dust regulation deadline now is three weeks past. The O'Leary regulations, which officials in the Bureau of Mines insist "have not been substantively weakened," are still not ready

* The New York Times 15, cols. 1–2 (March 23, 1970). © 1970 by The New York Times Company. Reprinted by permission.

for promulgation in the Federal Register. As a result, other deadlines are piling up.

*   *   *

NOTE 3.

COAL MINERS TELL SENATE INQUIRY SAFETY RULES ARE BEING BROKEN*

Miners told Senator Harrison A. Williams, Jr. today that safety regulations were "constantly being broken" at a gaseous United States Steel Corporation mine near this southwestern Pennsylvania town.

Mr. Williams, Democrat of New Jersey, took members of his Senate subcommittee into the coal fields to hear the complaints of dissident miners. He talked to men preparing to enter United States Steel's Cherokee shaft in nearby Bentleyville, Pa. on the morning shift. It was the miners' first full day back on the job since a three-day strike over safety issues.

"I can see already that they're not approaching what the law requires," Mr. Williams, author of the new Coal Mine Health and Safety Act, said of Federal officials.

Mickey Britvich, of Denbo, Pa., vice president of Local 1248 of the United Mine Workers union told Mr. Williams that the government had not sent any investigators to the mine to test for gaseous conditions although the law required them to inspect one every five days.

"The safety regulations are constantly being broken," Mr. Britvich said. "We have to keep pressure on them all the time."

*   *   *

NOTE 4.

BEN A. FRANKLIN
CHAIRMEN OF TWO SENATE COMMITTEES URGE A FEDERAL INQUIRY INTO FATAL COAL MINE EXPLOSION IN KENTUCKY†

Demands for investigations to fix the cause and responsibility for the eastern Kentucky coal mine explosion that killed 38 men last Wednesday began to mount here today.

The chairmen of two Senate committees strongly urged the Interior Department to convene immediately a public hearing in eastern Kentucky in which the Bureau of Mines would take the testimony of miners, their widows [sic] and Federal mine safety officials. They asked that the hearing look into the enforcement of the new Federal Coal Mine Health and Safety Act of 1969.

The request was made in a letter to Acting Secretary of the Interior Fred J. Russell from Senators Henry M. Jackson of Washington, chairman of the Committee on Interior and Insular Affairs, and Harrison A. Williams, Jr. of New Jersey, chairman of the Committee on Labor and Public Welfare. Both Senators are Democrats.

In drafting the mine safety act, their letter said, "Congress took great care to provide you with all the necessary tools to assure safe working conditions" in the mines. It said "the public has a right to know" what caused the Kentucky disaster exactly one year after passage of the law.

*   *   *

In letters to Senator Williams and Representative Perkins, Ralph Nader, the safety advocate, charged that the Kentucky disaster showed "the Administration's continued and flagrant disregard of the coal mine health and safety law." He said that a Congressional committee should determine who was responsible for the Bureau of Mines, decision not to inspect the mine on Dec. 22, deadline for abatement of a number of previously reported safety violations.

Representative Ken Hechler, Democrat of West Virginia, speaking on the House floor, said that the White House had "lobbied behind the scenes to weaken the mine safety bill" and that the President threatened to veto it last December.

"The President is in a position now to insist that the law be enforced," Mr. Hechler declared. "Let him send out the word that if he is really interested in law and order, here is a good place to start."

2.

The Health and Safety of Astronauts

Derek J. de Solla Price
The Case of the Kamikaze Astronauts*

Like the interest displayed by Sherlock Holmes in the barking of the dog during the

---

* *The New York Times* 29, col. 1 (June 27, 1970). © 1970 by The New York Times Company. Reprinted by permission.
† *The New York Times* 34, col. 1 (January 3, 1971). © 1971 by the New York Times Company. Reprinted by permission.

* Unpublished manuscript (1970). Printed by permission of the author who retains all rights.

night, we must see some significance in the Kamikaze asronauts that did *not* participate on either side of the race for the Moon. Early in the history of the Soviet-American competition following Sputnik it must have become quite clear to both sides that one could "cheat" in the race by designing a non-return soft landing on the Moon. The economy of not carrying the fuel to blast off from the lunar surface and make the return to a soft landing on the Earth is so very great that a couple of generations of rocketry, several years of work and very many billions of dollars separate the two objectives. There seems little doubt that either side could have won by mounting a mission that would have set a live man on the surface of the Moon but left him to a certain death there sooner or later after hours or days or even weeks of useful research work as oxygen and water ran out.

Let it be said immediately the life would not have been lost in any cause so trivial as a simple winning of a race between two superpowers. An early knowledge of the nature of the lunar surface might have made unnecessary much of the subsequent effort and money, and it could even have saved the lives that were lost in working towards the objective of landing men on that hostile surface with only a good chance, but still no presumed certainty of safe return. We might even have learned enough that the decision would have been to abandon the lunar target and plan more slowly for an eventual planetary exploration of Venus or Mars a decade or so later.

Let it also be said that there must have been no dearth of ready volunteers on both sides for such a certain suicide mission. Given that it was seen as part of the glorious destiny of mankind and of high national purpose, there would have been as many ready to lay down their lives without hope. Such Kamikaze suicide volunteers have always been forthcoming in wartime and insurrection, but also for geographical exploration as well as for scientific research. The very glamour of space for a generation brought up on science fiction and the knowledge that the sacrifice would be more visible and more assured of immortal fame than almost any preceding case would clearly have produced candidates galore, including several already vetoed by the space agencies of the two nations concerned and (for what it is worth) the present writer, too.

In spite of all this it is quite clear that not only was such a mission rejected, but it seems highly probable that the possibility was rejected out-of-hand and without even fleetingly serious attention by either side. After all the fuss of leaving a dog to die in orbit, any nation that left the first man on the Moon to die would have been exhibiting a gross and utter callousness in full view of the world and in such a way that the mere scientific and moral victories over space would have become a sour prize. In retrospect however, if it is true that both nations seriously overspent at this stage and risked a considerable and lasting world reaction against science and space in this process, it might have been much wiser to permit the sacrifice of a single life in a blaze of glory instead.

NOTE

AN INTERVIEW WITH RALPH E. LAPP
THE COMING TRIP AROUND THE MOON*

*   *   *

Do you think, then, that we are taking unnecessary risks in our race to the moon?

We are pushing our luck, gambling that everything will work perfectly. NASA experts will assure you that they have thought through the risks and have planned for them. Well, they didn't in Apollo-204. They maintain they have backup systems in case there are systems malfunctions. They also contend that risk evaluation can take place at critical points in Apollo's flight path. For example, the decision to accelerate from an Earth orbit to escape velocity can be made in orbit. Likewise the decision to descend into a lunar orbit can be made when all systems have been checked out just prior to injecting into that orbit.

*   *   *

If Apollo's main engine fails to fire in a lunar orbit, what happens?

Our astronauts will be stranded in orbit.

You mean they are condemned to death?

Well, they can't get out and fix the engine. They are completely dependent on that engine firing. There is no backup there.

*   *   *

* *The New Republic* 16–17 (December 14, 1968). Reprinted by permission of THE NEW REPUBLIC. © 1968, Harrison-Blaine of New Jersey, Inc.

Has NASA studied this problem of rescue?

Yes, they did several years ago. However the study showed that it would be costly to provide for a rescue capability, and it would slow down the space program. It was abandoned. . . .

So the United States has no backup capability to rescue or relieve the Apollo crew?

No. Apollo-9 won't be ready to fly until one or two months after Apollo-8. It's not slated for a lunar goal but rather to run a 10-day earth-orbital check-out of the lunar module.

We could delay the program so that Apollo-9, configured to have a relief-capability, would be on the pad ready for launch if Apollo-8 runs into trouble.

If we can relieve the crew, either through exchange or by provisions, I'm sure that NASA would undertake heroic measures to rescue the astronauts. It would be a fantastic rescue mission and might have more impact than the original flight. At the very least we ought to be prepared to attempt a rescue.

* * *

How much does an Apollo cost?

The unit cost depends on how you distribute charges for research, development, production facilities and launch complexes. NASA gives out a figure of $349 million based on a production rate of two a year. But if you take total expenditures for manned space flight and distribute them over 11 Apollos the unit cost would be about $2 billion. Somewhere between these two values is a reasonable estimate.

* * *

If the astronauts were marooned on the moon couldn't we ferry supplies to them?

NASA has not planned to do so. I would suggest it would be better to break the trail to the moon by landing supplies in advance. Then have the LEM (lunar excursion module) descend from orbit to this site. However it would change our lunar timetable; we might not be the first on the moon.

Is advance landing of supplies practical?

NASA successfully landed five Surveyor devices on the lunar surface and many television pictures were sent back to earth. Landing a cargo would be a much simpler operation. This pathfinder payload could be fitted with a radio beacon to guide in the LEM.

* * *

3.

Risking Lives—At What Cost?

a.

Guido Calabresi
The Costs of Accidents
A Legal and Economic Analysis*

* * *

Our society is not committed to preserving life at any cost. In its broadest sense, the rather unpleasant notion that we are willing to destroy lives should be obvious. Wars are fought. The University of Mississippi is integrated at the risk of losing lives. But what is more pertinent to the study of accident law, though perhaps equally obvious, is that lives are spent not only when the *quid pro quo* is some great moral principle, but also when it is a matter of convenience. Ventures are undertaken that, statistically at least, are certain to cost lives. Thus we build a tunnel under Mont Blanc because it is essential to the Common Market and cuts down the traveling time from Rome to Paris, though we know that about one man per kilometer of tunnel will die. We take planes and cars rather than safer, slower means of travel. And perhaps most telling, we use relatively safe equipment rather than the safest imaginable because—and it is not a bad reason—the safest costs too much. It should be apparent that while some of these accident-causing activities also result in diminution of accidents—the Mont Blanc tunnel may well save more lives by diminishing traffic fatalities than it took to build it—this explanation does not come close to justifying most accident-causing activities. Railroad grade crossings are used because they are cheap, not because they save more lives than they take.

Since we are not committed to preserving life at any cost, the question is the more complex one of how far we want to go to save lives and reduce accident costs. This leads us to the second myth: that economic theory can answer the question. Just as economic theory cannot decide for us whether we want to save the life of a trapped miner, so it cannot tell us how far we want to go to save lives and reduce accident costs. Economic theory can suggest one approach—the market—for making the decision. But decisions balancing lives against money or convenience cannot be purely monetary ones, so the market method is never the only one used.

* New Haven: Yale University Press 17–20, 23–31 (1970). Reprinted by permission.

The decision to build the Mont Blanc tunnel is not based solely on whether the revenue received from tolls will pay for the construction costs, including compensation of the killed and maimed. Neither is the decision to permit prostitution based solely on whether it can pay its way. Such pure free enterprise decisions have never been acceptable and have been, in fact, rejected by even the most orthodox of classical economists, who did, however, feel it necessary to explain the rejection through the use of such terms as external social costs and benefits, concepts which are not self-defining and are in fact as narrow or as broad as any society cares to make them.

The issue, whether or not expressed in terms of hidden social costs or hidden social savings theories, is how often a decision for or against an activity should be made outside the market. Such decisions operate on the one hand to create subsidies for some activities that could not survive in the marketplace, and on the other to bar some activities that could more than pay their way. The frequency with which decisions to ignore the market are made tells something about the nature of a society—welfare, laissez faire, or mixed. It is clear, however, that in virtually all societies such decisions to overrule the market are made, but are made only sometimes.

In accident law too, the decision to take lives in exchange for money or convenience is sometimes made politically or collectively without a balancing of the money value of the lives taken against the money price of the convenience, and sometimes made through the market on the basis of such a value. The reasons for choosing one way rather than the other are not entirely reasons of principle. Great moral issues lend themselves to political determination and must be decided in whatever political way a society chooses. But whether to use rotary mowers instead of reel mowers and what method to use for making steel are questions not easily answered collectively. For one thing, they occur too frequently. Every choice of product and use involves, tacitly or otherwise, a decision regarding safety and expense. The dramatic cases can be resolved politically. We ban the general sale of fireworks regardless of the ability or willingness of the manufacturer to pay for all of the injuries resulting from their use. But we cannot deal with every issue involved in every activity through the political process. In most cases, the marketplace serves as the rough testing ground. A manufacturer is usually free to employ a process that occasionally kills or maims if he is able to show that consumers want his product badly enough to enable him to compensate the injured. Economists would say that, except in some areas where collective decisions are needed, this is the best method for deciding whether the activity is worth having. But the tautologous nature of this statement makes it clear that ultimately, we collectively, and not economics, are the boss.

In other words, although the market can help us to decide how far we wish to go to avoid accidents, it cannot solve the whole problem for us. And when we overrule the market and ban an accident-causing activity that can pay its way or subsidize an activity that cannot, we are not violating absolute laws. We are making the same type of choice between accidents and accident-causing activities that the market makes, but we are choosing, for perfectly valid reasons, to make it in a different way. We are preferring a collective approach or method (e.g. because it enables consideration of nonmoney costs which the market cannot deal with, or because in the particular instance it is cheaper) to a market approach, even though the market might allow for individual differences in tastes and desires that the collective decision might tend to ignore.

*   *   *

One final . . . word of caution may be useful. When we deal with accidents we are dealing with costs, for that is what accidents involve. We are, to be sure, also dealing with emotional and moral attitudes, but we are always dealing with these in relation to costs. If we were not, we would wish to avoid accidents "at all costs." It follows that in examining any approach to accidents we must always keep in mind the cost of establishing and effectuating the approach, as well as the benefits the approach is expected to bring about. These costs and benefits, moreover, must be compared with the costs and benefits of alternative approaches. We must, in short, always ask whether the game is worth the candle, not only in terms of the cost of the candle but also in terms of other games we might be playing.

*   *   *

What, then, are the principal goals of any system of accident law? First, it must be just or fair; second, it must reduce the costs of accidents.

Justice

Justice, though often talked about, is by far the harder of the two goals to analyze. It is often said that a particular system of accident law, be it fault, social insurance, or enterprise liability, is supported by one's sense of fairness or justice. But such statements are rarely backed up by any clear definition of what such support means, let alone by any empirical research into what is considered fair.

In fact, it is doubtful that such empirical research would tell us very much anyway. As one scholar has observed, it is much easier to describe instances of *injustice* than examples of justice. We are much surer that particular processes or results are unfair than that particular arrangements are just in some positive sense. We can readily document specific injustices that occur in existing systems, such as the fault system or workmen's compensation. But the requirements of fairness that those systems may meet are difficult to define and therefore are usually stated in generalities, in hope of striking a responsive chord. This responsive chord, however, may be an inadequate guide to what our reaction would be if the system were changed. Conversely, while it is fairly easy to argue that particular untried systems will cure current injustices, it is much harder to foresee the injustices they may create.

More important, claims that particular systems are just, like those that justice is in some sense a goal concurrent with accident cost reduction, fail to ring true. They seem to suggest that a "rather unjust" system may be worthwhile because it diminishes accident costs effectively; or, conversely, that there is one system that can be termed just to the exclusion of all others, i.e. that is supported by justice in the same sense that economic efficiency may prefer one system to all others. But the words just and unjust do not sound right to me in either of the statements. They ring true in rather different contexts, as when we say that we reject a particular system or parts of it as unjust, or that a system taken as a whole does not violate our sense of justice. This suggests that justice is a totally different order of goal from accident cost reduction. Indeed, it suggests that it is not a goal but rather a constraint that can impose a veto on systems or on the use of particular devices or structures within a given system (e.g. administrative tribunals under the fault system) even though those same structures might not be unjust in another system (e.g. administrative tribunals under workmen's compensation).

All this discussion may make the concept of justice seem both negative and elusive. But it affords no excuse for ignoring justice in discussing accident law. Our reaction to accidents is not a strict dollars-and-cents one. If it were, I doubt that we would accept railroad crossing accidents because it costs too much to eliminate grade crossings and yet spend "whatever it takes" to save a known individual trapped in a coal mine. An economically optimal system of reducing accident costs—whether decisions are made collectively, through the market, or through a combination of both—might be totally or partially unacceptable because it strikes us as unfair, and no amount of discussion of the efficiency of the system would do much to save it. Justice must ultimately have its due.

But if the elusiveness of justice cannot justify ignoring the concept, it at least justifies delaying discussion of it. The fact that what is unfair is easier to define than what is fair, like the fact that what is fair in one system may be unfair in another, indicates that it would be better to examine the requirements of accident cost reduction first and then to see how various untried methods and systems suggested by that goal compare in terms of fairness with the systems we use today—how, in other words, they comply with our general sense of fairness and whether they are more or less likely to create specific instances of injustice than the current systems. Such an approach may not lead us to the fairest systems possible but it may well indicate whether change is desirable.

Reduction of Accident Costs

Apart from the requirements of justice, I take it as axiomatic that the principal function of accident law is to reduce the sum of the costs of accidents and the costs of avoiding accidents. (Such incidental benefits as providing a respectable livelihood for a large number of judges, lawyers, and insurance agents are at best beneficent side effects.) This cost, or loss, reduction goal can be divided into three subgoals.

The first is reduction of the number and severity of accidents. This "primary" reduction of accident costs can be attempted in two basic ways. We can seek to forbid specific acts or activities thought to cause accidents, or we can make activities more expensive and thereby less attractive to the extent of the accident costs they cause. These two methods of primary reduction of accident costs are not clearly separable. . . .

The second cost reduction subgoal is concerned with reducing neither the number of accidents nor their degree of severity. It concentrates instead on reducing the societal costs resulting from accidents. I shall attempt to show that the notion that one of the principal functions of accident law is the compensation of victims is really a rather misleading, though occasionally useful, way of stating this "secondary" accident cost reduction goal. The fact that I have termed this compensation notion secondary should in no way be taken as belittling its importance. There is no doubt that the way we provide for accident victims *after* the accident is crucially important and that the real societal costs of accidents can be reduced as significantly here as by taking measures to avoid accidents in the first place. This cost reduction subgoal is secondary only in the sense that it does not come into play until after earlier primary measures to reduce accident costs have failed.

*   *   *

The third subgoal of accident cost reduction is rather Pickwickian but very important nonetheless. It involves reducing the costs of administering our treatment of accidents. It may be termed "tertiary" because its aim is to reduce the costs of achieving primary and secondary cost reduction. But in a very real sense this "efficiency" goal comes first. It tells us to question constantly whether an attempt to reduce accident costs, either by reducing accidents themselves or by reducing their secondary effects, costs more than it saves. By forcing us to ask this, it serves as a kind of general balance wheel to the cost reduction goal.

*   *   *

It should be noted . . . that these subgoals are not fully consistent with each other. For instance, a perfect system of secondary cost reduction is . . . inconsistent with the goals of reducing primary accident costs. We cannot have more than a certain amount of reduction in one category without forgoing some of the reduction in the other, just as we cannot reduce all accident costs beyond a certain point without incurring costs in *achieving* the reduction that are greater than the reduction is worth. . . .

In this sense, it may seem unwise to divide accident cost reduction into three subgoals at all. It might seem better to lump all accident costs together and concentrate on finding that point at which further accident cost reduction is not worth its costs, especially since the division of accident cost reduction into subgoals is ultimately an arbitrary one. . . .

*   *   *

One could, of course, consider the goals of accident law more broadly and ask what accident law may do to cure evils in our society that are not a result of accidents. The list of possibilities would be endless, and any analysis of accident law would be virtually impossible. Nevertheless, we should be aware that accident law, like any other branch of law, can be used to accomplish an enormous variety of goals. . . .

*   *   *

NOTE

Guido Calabresi
Reflections on Medical Experimentation in Humans*

The problem of experimentation on humans necessarily looks rather different to one who has concentrated on accident law than it does to the doctor or even to the jurisprude. The torts professor sees the possibility of a choice between the life, well-being, or comfort of a given patient and the lives or well-being of unknown future patients. He is immediately struck that the issue in medical experimentation is the risking of lives to save other lives while in accident law, almost always, the issue is the taking of lives simply because saving them costs too much.

In torts law, we have become accustomed to the fact that many activities are permitted, even though *statistically* we know they will cost lives, since it costs too much to engage in these activities more safely or to abstain from them altogether. We have grade crossings, even though we know that with grade crossings a certain number of people will be killed each year and even though grade crossings could be eliminated relatively easily. We use automobiles—knowing that they cost us fifty thousand lives each year—because to use safer, slower means of transport would be far too costly in terms of pleasures and profits forgone. Worse even than that, we use automobiles with relatively cheap (but relatively dangerous) tires, airports with relatively cheap (but relatively dangerous) control systems, and so on *ad infinitum*. And we do this because we deem the lives taken to be cheaper than the costs of avoiding the accidents in which they are taken.

From the perverse standpoint of accident

* 98 *Daedalus* 387–393 (1969). Reprinted by permission of *Daedalus,* Journal of the American Academy of Arts and Sciences, Boston, Massachusetts.

law, then, the whole fury about medical experimentation would seem to be a tempest in a teapot. Surely it is more justifiable to take some lives in order to save more lives than it is to take lives simply to save money, as we do in the accident field. But this view, I fear, is far too superficial. Even in the accident field, there are many occasions when we do treat life as a pearl beyond price. When a known individual is trapped in a coal mine, we try to rescue him at enormous money cost and even at the risk of many other lives. Yet if we always gave human life the value we give to the life of the man in the coal mine, we would surely abolish grade crossings, make cars and airports much safer, and perhaps even forbid "non-essential" driving completely. What is the meaning of this apparent paradox? And what does it tell us about medical experimentation?

The first possible explanation has to do with statistics. Somehow a man is less a man to us when he is simply a number. We know the man trapped in the coal mine, just as we often know the patient subjected to experimentation. The statistical accident victim we do not know, and so we can ignore him. But that is not in itself an adequate explanation. The statistical victim is just as real as the man in the coal mine. If we want to be fully rational, we must admit to ourselves that he has as much of a family as a known victim, that he and they suffer as much when he is killed, and that only a willful ignoring of reality enables us to treat him as less real than the man trapped in the coal mine.

But perhaps this willful ignoring of statistical victims is less foolish, though no more "rational," than it might seem at first glance. We are committed to "humanism," to the dignity of the individual, and to human life. Much of the fabric of our society depends on our belief in this commitment, as do most of our traditional and "cherished" liberties. Accident law indicates that our commitment to human life is not, in fact, so great as we say it is; that our commitment to life-destroying material progress and comfort is greater. But this fact merely accentuates our need to make a bow in the direction of our commitment to the sanctity of human life (whenever we can do so at a reasonable total cost). It also accentuates our need to reject any societal decisions that too blatantly contradict this commitment. Like "free will," it may be less important that this commitment be total than that we believe it to be there.

Perhaps it is for these reasons that we save the man trapped in the coal mine. After all, the event is dramatic; the cost, though great, is unusual; and the effect in reaffirming our belief in the sanctity of human lives is enormous. The effect of such an act in maintaining the many societal values that depend on the dignity of the individual is worth the cost. Abolishing grade crossings might save more lives and at a substantially smaller cost per life saved, but the total cost to society would be far greater and the dramatic effect far less. I fear that if men got caught in coal mines with the perverse frequency with which cars run into trains at grade crossings, we would be loath to rescue them; it would, in the aggregate, cost too much. Lest this remark seem unduly cynical, we might consider our past unwillingness to keep all but a few victims of renal failure alive by use of artificial kidneys. Until now, artificial kidneys have cost too much, and people perversely have suffered kidney failure too frequently, so even though the victim was as clearly known to those who had to decide whether to save him as is the man in the mine, the answer quite frequently was no.

It should be clear that the foregoing does not mean that individual human life is not valued highly. Nor, certainly, does it suggest that we are indifferent to when and how society should choose to sacrifice lives. Quite the contrary; it indicates that there is a deep conflict between our fundamental need constantly to reaffirm our belief in the sanctity of life and our practical placing of some values (including future lives) above an individual life. That conflict suggests, at the very least, the need for a quite complex structuring to enable us *sometimes* to sacrifice lives, but hardly ever to do it blatantly and as a society, and above all to allow this sacrifice only under quite rigorous controls. (This last desire to control individual takings and yet to keep society from being the blatant taker itself reflects a conflict of desires.) I suggest that the problem with human experimentation lies in the fact that, unlike accidents, it has seemed to be quite unamenable to most of the complex "indirect" controls over takings of lives we have so far developed in our society.

In the field of accidents, much of the control over the taking of human lives is accomplished by what economists call the market. Limbs and lives are given a money value; the activities that take lives or limbs in accidents pay the victims; and people quite coldly decide whether it is cheaper to install a safety device or to pay for the accidents that occur because the safety device is missing. Despite the enormous oversimplification of the foregoing example (the effect of "fault" in determining accident payments, for instance, is ignored), it indicates how "accidents" are controlled in an indirect fashion which, nonetheless, takes into account both the values of lives taken and the cost of saving them.

The beauty of the market device is that no one seems to be making the decisions to take lives and, therefore, no blatant infringement of the commitment to human life as sacred occurs. Moreover, when society *does* enter into the accident field directly, it is usually to impose more stringent prohibitions, regulations, or safety standards than the market would bring about. We do not allow drunken driving—any more than we allow murder—even though the drunk may be perfectly willing to compensate his victim. The consequence is that collective societal action seems always to be directed toward preserving the individual life rather than taking it, and our commitment is further strengthened. (Only a few professors worry that failure to go beyond the market in areas where the individual choice to take lives is less obvious than in drunken driving or murder is also a societal decision, but one which lets lives be taken. Such ratiocinations of professors happily do not destroy the picture of a self-contained system in which almost all collective decisions are life-saving ones.)

Other elements of accident law serve to reduce still further the blatantness of the taking. In many situations, the victim can be said to have, to some extent at least, consented to the risk. Consent is often actually very dubious. Are we, in fact, free to avoid driving cars? Is a tunnel-digger free to engage in a safer occupation? And is there any consent at all when a pedestrian is run down by a car? But these questions are neither here nor there. They would be crucial were free consent the keystone of the system (as it may have to be in medical experiments). Where, however, consent serves merely to lessen further the directness of a taking that is already controlled by a seemingly impersonal system, even semi-free consent suffices to support the belief that our society prizes individual lives above all.

The same is true about the introduction of moral elements like fault into a system of accident law. The search for a faulty party on whom damages must rest can seriously undermine the market control system I have described. For this and other reasons, fault may well be on its way out. This is especially true since too many people have come to realize that frequently the search for a faulty party in an accident is either a sham or a fraud. When people still believed otherwise, however, the semblance of a search for a faulty party served, like consent, to reinforce the belief that the level of accidents was a matter of individual choice and not something society determined.

Finally, the temporal juxtaposition of decisions to avoid accidents and lives taken serves to make "accidental" takings of lives seem less blatant. At the time a decision to adopt a safety device is to be made, the cost of the device is both present and real; the accident costs to be saved may also be statistically known; but the lives themselves are in the future and seem conjectural. Once again, if the decision is made against the device, even the individual making the decision—let alone society—does not seem to be choosing "certainly" to destroy lives.

In medical experiments, much of this process seems reversed. It is the lives to be saved by the experiment that seem future and conjectural, while the life to be risked or taken is both present and real. Most of the elements of fault are absent—the victim usually is sick through no choice or fault of his own. As a result, only the possible presence of consent seems left to lessen the blatantness of the choice to risk a life. But consent can no more do the whole job here than it can in accidents. Totally free consent is simply too rare an animal. The usual semi-free consent serves in accident situations because it reinforces an adequate system of control governing more generally when lives are to be taken, but without seeming to infringe on our basic commitment to human life. Just such a system of control is needed in medical experimentation.

Perhaps, however, we have accepted the analogy between medical experiments and accidents too quickly. It may be that the taking of lives that happens in accident situations is different in substance from the taking that occurs in medical experiments, or would occur were we to let the man trapped in a coal mine die. If there is a difference that goes beyond the matter of appearances, beyond the existence in accidents of a complex self-operating system of control, then the problem of medical experiments cannot be solved simply by devising complex, indirect control mechanisms to balance society's interest in present as against future lives.

The nub of the argument is this: The notion is incorrect that we in some sense choose the number of people who will be killed in automobile accidents by choosing a market system that will determine how much safety is worth. The notion is only made plausible by a verbal trick—by using the words "we choose" to describe both the effects of the social system in which we live and which we tolerate, but which we cannot in fact be said to choose, and events as to which we can be said to exercise purposive choice. "We" do not choose automobile accidents, the argument runs, any more than "we" choose a world in which hundreds of thousands of Indians die young of disease and lack of food. We do not choose this because the alternative is never presented in a realistic enough fashion; it is never presented so that the costs of saving the Indians are clear. The costs of saving the Indians, like the costs of avoiding automobile accidents, are the costs of moving from an existing social system to a new one. As such, they are unknown and involve a substantial risk that, whatever pattern of life the new system brings, *more* lives will be taken than in the old system. How different, the argument concludes, is this passive tolerance of the world as it is from the active choice to let someone caught in a coal mine die, or from the decision to risk an individual human life in a medical experiment.

I do not believe that this argument destroys the usefulness of the analogy between medical experiments and automobile accidents. In a way, it is no more than a mixture of two quite different points. First, a choice to save a life at the price of paying readily ascertainable costs is very different from a choice to save lives when the saving would be accomplished only by a radical restructuring of society entailing unknown costs. This point is certainly true, but does not distinguish many accident situations from medical experiments. Second, there is a genuine difference between a positive choice to subject someone to a risk or to take his life and a passive acquiescence in a system that results in lives being taken when they could be saved at ascertainable costs. This second is a distinction which, I claim, has only psychological significance. Because the choice to take lives is less obvious, it is less destructive of the essential myth that human life is a pearl beyond price.

There are, to be sure, accident situations where lives could be saved only by restructuring our whole social system. Giving up the automo-

bile altogether might be an example. It is hard to know what the full costs of that decision would be, or whether in the end the change would save or cost more lives. As such, it is fair to say that we do not choose to take lives by having automobiles in the same sense as we choose to let the man in the mine die if we fail to rescue him. But there are other situations where lives can be saved without such a radical change. Abolition of grade crossings, differently made automobiles, and more safely constructed highways—all would save lives in exchange for readily determinable costs. We can (but do not) require these. We allow their establishment to be controlled by the market. What is more, we readily observe the results of market control. We then discuss in Congress whether intervention is justified, and we often decide not to intervene. In our passivity, we are choosing to let the indirect market control method make the choice between lives and costs, and no amount of talk about merely tolerating an existing social system can change that.

But this second point may be more subtle. It may center on the fact that there is no one who can clearly be identified with the "we" in the last paragraph. No one has purposefully chosen the market method of controlling accidents, and no one, in our society, has the clear responsibility for making radical changes in the method. These facts happily leave us with the feeling that no one is directly responsible for any specific life taken and that neither as individuals nor as a society do we choose against lives in order to save money. Yet it remains true that we are unlikely to want to scrap the system of control that luckily has come into being. And to say this is precisely to say that a method which gives *satisfactory* control of the choice between lives and cost is operating without anyone bearing the onus of having purposefully chosen the method, let alone the onus of seeming to destroy individual lives for the sake of money. Since no adequate control system over medical experiments has arisen by itself, we cannot avoid the onus of working purposefully toward establishing a control system. This indicates that we will not end with so psychologically satisfactory a result as we have in the field of accidents. But, if anything, this fact heightens the need for establishing a system in which the actual choice over the taking of lives is as diffuse as possible.

Thus, the question remains as to whether or not we can find a control system in the medical experiment field that affords an adequate balancing of present against future lives and is still sufficiently indirect and self-enforcing as to avoid clear and purposive choices to kill individuals for the collective good.

b.

Edmond Cahn
Drug Experiments and the Public Conscience*

*   *   *

The thalidomide tragedy of 1962 showed that it was not only the manufacturers and dispensers of drugs who needed to reassess their moral responsibilities. It also revealed a certain disease of hypocrisy affecting large portions of the American people. The hypocrisy manifests itself in two different but related syndromes, which for purposes of convenience we can call the "Pharaoh syndrome" and the "Pompey syndrome."

When ancient Pharaoh built a pyramid, it is possible that his more methodical overseers might have reported that the cost of construction had included some thousands or hundreds of thousands of human lives. Proper accounting would have computed these lives as part of the over-all expense to the Egyptian throne; someone may even have kept comparative figures of mortalities from construction job to construction job. Be that as it may, Egyptian records do not say that anyone hesitated to expend a few, a few thousand, or a few hundred thousand workers.

Nowadays many Americans are satisfied to refer to the thalidomide episode and its consequences with some mildly regretful remarks about "the social cost of progress." To some of us, such remarks do not seem quite adequate. We suspect that it requires an authentic "Pharaoh syndrome" to convert misshapen babies with flippers for arms into mere items of "social cost." We grant, of course, that there is something conveniently impersonal about the phrase "social cost."

*   *   *

The second or "Pompey syndrome" may be even more popular in this country. I have taken the name from young Sextus Pompey, who ap-

* Paul Talalay, ed.: *Drugs in Our Society*. Baltimore: The Johns Hopkins Press 255, 258–261 (1964). Reprinted by permission.

pears in Shakespeare's *Antony and Cleopatra* in an incident drawn directly from Plutarch. Pompey, whose navy has won control of the seas around Italy, comes to negotiate peace with the Roman triumvirs Mark Antony, Octavius Caesar, and Lepidus, and they meet in a roistering party on Pompey's ship. As they carouse, one of Pompey's lieutenants draws him aside and whispers that he can become lord of all the world if he will only grant the lieutenant leave to cut first the mooring cable and then the throats of the triumvirs. Pompey pauses, then replies in these words:

Ah, this thou shouldst have done,
And not have spoke on't! In me 'tis villainy;
In thee't had been good service. Thou must know
'Tis not my profit that does lead mine honour;
Mine honour, it. Repent that e'er thy tongue
Hath so betrayed thine act; being done unknown
I should have found it afterwards well done,
But must condemn it now. Desist, and drink.

Here we have the most pervasive of moral syndromes, the one most characteristic of so-called respectable men in a civilized society. To possess the end and yet not be responsible for the means, to grasp the fruit while disavowing the tree, to escape being told the cost until someone else has paid it irrevocably; this is the Pompey syndrome and the chief hypocrisy of our time. In the days of the outcry against thalidomide, how much of popular indignation might be attributed to this same syndrome; how many were furious because their own lack of scruple had been exposed! So many did not really care, did not even want to know what the new drugs might cost in terms of human injuries and fatalities. The dispensers of thalidomide had outraged the public by breaking an unwritten law—the law against interrupting the public's enjoyment of fruits with disagreeable revelations about the tree and the soil where the fruits have grown.

. . . Posterity will not fail to recognize the Pharaoh and Pompey syndromes in the behavior of our contemporary public. As we in our day can smile condescendingly at the primitives and ancients who practiced human sacrifice for what they considered to be the general good of the tribe or nation, future generations may ask how we could make human sacrifice more acceptable in our day by calling it "social cost." . . .

*   *   *

C.
Man's Readiness to Delegate Authority to Experts

Technologically advanced societies, with their complex division of labor, accord a unique position to persons whose training qualifies them to apply specialized knowledge in the resolution of individual problems. As "professionals" they are given authoritative status to define the qualifications and rules of their discipline and to work with relative autonomy, unfettered by many forms of social control. Since most experimenters are identified with one of the traditional professions, their relationship both to society and to individual subjects is colored by prevailing attitudes toward professionals in general.

Usually, the professional's services are sought by the client. Once the client has "placed himself in the expert's hands," it is generally the expert who selects the goals and means of action and who decides how his skills can best be employed to satisfy the client's needs. Such interactions are supported by an actual willingness of the patient/client to trust his expert or by an expectation that he do so. While there are acknowledged and unacknowledged constraints on the professional, many of them seem to increase, rather than to limit, his professional autonomy. For example, licensing statutes, designed to screen out incompetent practitioners, also safeguard the profession's monopolistic power.

The materials on the authority of the professionals in nonexperimental settings are of interest to us primarily for the light they shed on experimental interventions. The differences between these two settings often become blurred. This influences not only subjects, who unlike patients have usually yielded the role of initiator to the professional, but also investigators who typically conduct themselves according to standards and habits developed in clinical settings. Thus, in seeking answers to the following questions, consider whether the characteristics of investigators differ from those of other professionals so as to alter the authority which investigators should exercise:

1. What are the distinctive qualities of professional expertise?
2. In what ways do these qualities affect the authority of the expert?
3. To what extent do the values promoted by reliance on professional expertise conflict with other values in our society?
4. How and to what extent should the authority of professionals be extended or limited?
5. To what extent are either the individual's or society's interests well served by leaving the client's protection to the professional's judgment of what is in the client's "best interests"?
6. To what extent should nonprofessionals control the actions of professionals with respect to individual problems or issues of social policy?

1.

The Professional in Society—Power and Competition

a.

Howard S. Becker
The Nature of a Profession*

* * *

Professions, as commonly conceived, are occupations which possess a monopoly of some esoteric and difficult body of knowledge. Further, this knowledge is considered to be necessary for the continuing functioning of the society. What the members of the profession know and can do is tremendously important, but no one else knows or can do these things. The archetype in this respect is medicine, which is supposed to have an absolute monopoly of the knowledge necessary to heal the sick. Healing the sick and maintaining the health of the society is seen as one of the important functions which must be performed if the society is to maintain its equilibrium.

The body of knowledge over which the profession holds a monopoly consists not of technical skills and the fruits of practical experience but, rather, of abstract principles arrived at by scientific research and logical analysis. This knowledge cannot be applied routinely but must be applied wisely and judiciously to each case. This has several consequences.

In the first place, it is supposed that only the most able people will have the mental ability and the proper temperament to absorb and use such knowledge. Therefore, recruitment must be strictly controlled, to ensure that those who are not qualified do not become members of the profession. Recruitment is controlled, first, by careful weeding out of prospective candidates, and, then, by a lengthy and difficult educational process which eliminates those who were mistakenly selected. Lengthy training is considered necessary anyway, because the body of knowledge is supposed to be so complex that it cannot be acquired in any shorter time.

Secondly, it is felt that entrance into professional practice must be strictly controlled, and that this control must ultimately lie in the hands of members of the profession itself. Difficult ob-

---

* Nelson B. Henry, ed.: *The Sixty-First Yearbook of the National Society for the Study of Education.* Chicago, Ill.: The National Society for the Study of Education 27–46 (1962). Reprinted by permission.

stacles, in the form of examinations of all kinds, must be surmounted by candidates for practice, and no one must be allowed to practice who has not so demonstrated his competence. This means that the police power of the state must be utilized, through the device of licensure procedures, to control entrance into practice. But if the knowledge monopolized by the profession is so difficult to acquire, it follows that no layman can fully acquire it and, therefore, that the governmental bodies which grant licenses must be controlled by members of the profession itself. Similarly, the approval and accreditation of educational institutions and procedures must also be done by members of the profession. In short, the professional, by virtue of the esoteric character of his professional knowledge, is free of lay control.

Finally, since recruitment, training, and entrance into practice are all carefully controlled, any member of the professional group can be thought of as fully competent to supply the professional service.

Any profession which so monopolizes some socially important body of knowledge is likely to be considered potentially dangerous. It might use its monopoly to enrich itself or enlarge its power rather than in the best interests of its clients. The symbol of the profession, however, portrays a group whose members have altruistic motivations and whose professional activities are governed by a code of ethics which heavily emphasizes devotion to service and the good of the client and condemns misuse of professional skills for selfish purposes. This code of ethics, furthermore, is sternly enforced by appropriate disciplinary bodies. Professional associations have as their major purpose the enforcement of such ethical codes.

The client, therefore, is supposed to be able to count on the professional whose services he retains to have his best interests at heart. He rests comfortable in the knowledge that this is one relationship in which the rule of the market place does not apply. He need not beware but can give his full trust and confidence to the professional who is handling his problems; the service given him will be competent and unselfish. This is conceived as necessary if the professional is to perform his work successfully. If the patient cannot trust the physician completely, he will withhold facts that might be vital in successful treatment; the lawyer cannot protect his client's interests without full knowledge of his client's affairs, and this might be withheld if the client could not trust him.

If the client is to trust the professional completely he must feel that there are no other interests which will be put before his in the performance of the professional activity. Among the other interests which might intrude are the interests related to institutions within which the professional makes his career. Thus, the ideal professional is a *private* practitioner, in business for himself, so to speak. He has no ties to a superior officer or bureaucratic system of rules; he receives his income directly from fees paid by the client, not from any third party.

A final element in the symbol of the profession is not so often mentioned in the attempts to define the term. This is the image of the profession and the professional as occupying an esteemed position in the society. Members of the professions are usually thought of, as they often in fact are, as people of sizable income and high community prestige. They are considered to be entitled to an important voice in community affairs. Professional associations are thought of as important public institutions, similarly entitled to a voice in public affairs, particularly (although not exclusively) with respect to those issues which touch on their professional concerns or competence.

The above features are the essential components of the symbol "profession." To risk repetition, this symbol does not describe any actual occupation. Rather, it is a symbol that people in our society use in thinking about occupations, a standard to which they compare occupations in deciding their moral worth. It represents consensus in the society about what certain kinds of work groups *ought* to be like, though it is not an accurate picture of any reality.

What role does this symbol play in the operation of our society and in the functioning of work groups? In the first place, the symbol can be seen as containing an ideology which provides a justification and rationale for one very important aspect of the work situation of those groups possessing the title. Professionals, in contrast to members of other occupations, claim and are often accorded complete autonomy in their work. Since they are presumed to be the only judges of how good their work is, no layman or other outsider can make any judgment of what they do. If their activities are unsuccessful, only another professional can say whether this was due to incompetence or to the inevitable workings of nature or society by which even the most competent practitioner would have been stymied. This image of the professional justifies his demand for complete autonomy and his demand that the client give up is own judgment and responsibility, leaving everything in the hands of the professional.

This analysis may lead some people to conclude that I am saying that the symbol of the profession is used simply as a device by which the self-interest of the work group can be furthered. This would be incorrect. Professional autonomy may be used strictly in the interests of the client; in fact, it is likely that without some measure of autonomy the client's interests cannot be well served. If a doctor is not free to make the diagnosis he thinks correct and prescribe the course of treatment he thinks most efficacious rather than the one the patient finds most palatable, the patient's health may indeed suffer. In short, the symbol of the profession is not merely selfish propaganda; many of the propositions contained in it are in large part true. Nevertheless, we must not forget that it is a symbol, rather than an exact description of reality, and that it may be used for political purposes.

*   *   *

If deviations from the symbol of the profession were simply the result of natural human orneriness—of Original Sin, so to speak—the sociologist would indeed be nothing but a muckraker in drawing attention to them. But the fact is that deviations from the ideal are neither random nor idiosyncratic. They do not occur because a few professionals are bad men or weak men. They occur systematically and are created by the operation of social forces. In other words, they are integral parts of the social structure of occupational life and are regarded as deviations because they are considered morally unworthy. (Not all the deviations I will speak of are so heavily morally toned, although some are.) I confine myself to a consideration of medicine and law, because these occupations most closely approach the symbol. Also, medicine and law have been much studied by sociologists, so that we have some accurate descriptions with which to compare the symbol.

Medicine and law fail to match the symbol in that neither actually holds a monopoly over its esoteric knowledge or functions. Lawyers do a great many things, but hardly any of them are not done on occasion, or, often, as full-time work, by people who are not lawyers. In fact, many lawers suffer greatly because of the competition of nonlawyers in many fields of legal work. Lawyers do tax work and draw up wills;

but accountants also do tax work, and officers of banks are quite willing and able to draw up wills. The lawyer does maintain a monopoly over one area: appearing in court to defend clients; but this represents a small part of the lawyer's work. Similarly, doctors perform the function of healing the sick. But they share this function with members of many other occupations: osteopaths, chiropractors, chiropodists, faith healers, and so on. Nor is their knowledge restricted to the circle of those who are fully trained and licensed physicians, for much of it is created by and known by nonphysicians who are scientists.

The reality differs from the symbol in another respect. All members of a profession are not equally competent to supply the *core service* —"the most characteristic professional act." This is true because of the great internal differentiation and specialization which characterize present-day professions. It is not only that there is a technical division of labor among the various specialties, although this is certainly so much the case that the services provided can only be provided by a member of a particular specialty. But beyond this we find that the specialties differ so in ideology, sense of mission, work activities, and work situation that they can most profitably be thought of as distinct occupations rather than as specialized aspects of one occupation. . . .

The relations of clients and professionals, in fact, are quite different from those specified in the symbol. Ideally, the client puts his full faith and trust in the professional whose services he uses. But this is not the way clients behave. They continually make judgments about the work and capabilities of the professionals they use. Medical patients often change doctors, and they do this because they have decided for themselves, on the basis of their own knowledge and experience or, frequently, on the advice of friends, relatives, and neighbors, that another doctor will do a better job for them. Research has shown that patients distinguish between diseases which are ordinary and everyday and therefore can be treated by any doctor (so long as he is convenient and inexpensive) and those diseases which are dramatically out of the ordinary and require the services of a doctor who can convince them, in one way or another, that he is specially good. The clients of professionals, in short, characteristically reserve a right of judgment denied to them by the symbol.

Similarly, the symbol of a work group bound by a code of ethics designed to protect the client is in some ways not a realistic description. Every profession contains unethical practitioners. This would be of small importance, as I have said, if it were simply a matter of human frailty, of weak men succumbing to temptation. But it appears that this is a chronic feature of the social structure of prestigeful occupations, another aspect of their differentiation and specialization (although in this case the differentiation takes place with respect to ethicality rather than technique). Hughes points out that lawyers deal with human quarrels:

A lawyer may be asked whether he and his client come into court with clean hands; when he answers, "yes," it may mean that someone else's hands are of necessity a bit grubby. For not only are some quarrels more respectable, more clean, than others; but also some kinds of work involved in the whole system (gathering evidence, getting clients, bringing people to court, enforcing judgments, making the compromises that keep cases out of court) are more respected and removed from temptation and suspicion than others. In fact, the division of labor among lawyers is as much one of respectability (hence of self concept and role) as of specialized knowledge and skills. One might even call it a moral division of labor, if one keeps in mind that the term means not simply that some lawyers are more moral than others; but that the very demand for highly scrupulous and respectable lawyers depends in various ways upon the availability of less scrupulous people to attend to the less respectable legal problems of even the best people.*

Very little is known about the social systems in which unethical practice is embedded; this is one of the most neglected areas in the study of professions, partly because of the practical difficulties involved and partly, I fear, because to study such problems calls attention to the disparity between symbol and reality.

Finally, professional practitioners are typically not as autonomous as the symbol would have us believe. The constraints which belie the symbol have several different sources. In the traditional pattern of private practice for a fee, professionals may be constrained by the wishes of their clients. In so far as a professional depends on his reputation among laymen for his practice, there is a continuing pressure for him to give the kind of service that, in the layman's eyes, is satisfactory. Freidson has noted that the general medical practitioner, of all physicians, is most in this position and is most likely to defer to his patients' wishes with respect to methods

---

* E. C. Hughes, *Men and Their Work*. Glencoe, Ill.: The Free Press 71 (1958).

of treatment. Depending essentially on other laymen for his referrals (standing, as Freidson says, at the apex of the "lay referral structure" which also includes friends, neighbors, relatives, and the corner druggist), the general practitioner tends to be sensitive to the demands of clients for new drugs, for instance, and to avoid procedures which may seem unnecessary and unpleasant to his patients.

*   *   *

NOTES

NOTE 1.

EVERETT C. HUGHES
MEN AND THEIR WORK*

*   *   *

An occupation consists, in part, of a successful claim of some people to *licence* to carry out certain activities which others may not, and to do so in exchange for money, goods or services. Those who have such licence will, if they have any sense of self-consciousness and solidarity, also claim a *mandate* to define what is proper conduct of others toward the matters concerned with their work. The licence may be nothing more than permission to carry on certain narrowly technical activities, such as installing electrical equipment, which it is thought dangerous to allow laymen to do. It may, however, include the right to live one's life in a style somewhat different from that of most people. The mandate may go no further than successful insistence that other people stand back and give the workers a bit of elbow room while they do their work. It may, as in the case of the modern physician, include a successful claim to supervise and determine the conditions of work of many kinds of people; in this case, nurses, technicians and the many others involved in maintaining the modern medical establishment. In the extreme case it may, as in the priesthood in strongly Catholic countries, include the right to control the thoughts and beliefs of whole populations with respect to nearly all the major concerns of life.

Licence, as an attribute of an occupation, is ordinarily thought of as legal permission to carry on a kind of work. There is a great body of jurisprudence having to do with the matter of licence, both in principle and as it occurs in various occupations. I have in mind something both

---

* Glencoe, Ill.: The Free Press 78–80 (1958). Reprinted by permission of the author who retains all rights.

broader and deeper, something that is sometimes implicit and of undefined boundaries. For it is very difficult to define the boundaries of the licence to carry on a certain kind of activity. What I am talking of is a basic attribute of society. Occupations here offer us an extreme and highly lighted instance of a general aspect of all human societies. For society, by its very nature, consists of both allowing and expecting some people to do things which other people are not allowed or expected to do. All occupations —most of all those considered professions and perhaps those of the underworld—include as part of their very being a licence to deviate in some measure from common modes of behavior. Professions also, perhaps more than other kinds of occupations, claim a legal, moral and intellectual mandate. Not merely do the practitioners, by virtue of gaining admission to the charmed circle of colleagues, individually exercise the licence to do things others do not do, but collectively they presume to tell society what is good and right for the individual and for society at large in some aspect of life. Indeed, they set the very terms in which people may think about this aspect of life. The medical profession, for instance, is not content merely to define the terms of medical practice. It also tries to define for all of us the very nature of health and disease. When the presumption of a group to a broad mandate of this kind is explicitly or implicitly granted as legitimate, a profession has come into being.

The understanding of the nature and extent of both licence and mandate, of their relations to each other and of the circumstances in which they expand or contract is a crucial area of study not merely of occupations, but of society itself. In such licences and mandates we have the prime manifestation of the *moral division of labor;* that is, of the processes by which differing moral functions are distributed among the members of society, both as individuals and as kinds or categories of individuals. Moral functions differ from each other both in kind and in measure. Some people seek and get special responsibility for defining the values and for establishing and enforcing social sanctions over some aspect of life. The differentiation of moral and social functions involves both the setting of the boundaries of realms of social behavior and the allocation of responsibility and power over them. One may indeed speak of jurisdictional disputes concerning the rights and the responsibilities of various occupations and categories of people in defining and maintaining the rules of conduct concerning various aspects of personal and social life.

* * *

NOTE 2.

EVERETT C. HUGHES
PROFESSIONS*

Professions are more numerous than ever before. Professional people are a larger proportion of the labor force. The professional attitude, or mood, is likewise more widespread; professional status, more sought after. These are components of the professional trend, a phenomenon of all the highly industrial and urban societies; a trend that apparently accompanies industrialization and urbanization irrespective of political ideologies and systems. The professional trend is closely associated with the bureaucratic, although the queen of the professions, medicine, is the avowed enemy of bureaucracy, at least of bureaucracy in medicine when others than physicians have a hand in it.

A profession delivers esoteric services—advice or action or both—to individuals, organizations or government; to whole classes or groups of people or to the public at large. . . . [T]he action—it is assumed or claimed—is determined by esoteric knowledge systematically formulated and applied to problems of a client. The services include advice. The person for or upon whom the esoteric service is performed, or the one who is thought to have the right or duty to act for him, is advised that the professional's action is necessary. Indeed, the professional in some cases refuses to act unless the client—individual or corporate—agrees to follow the advice given.

The nature of the knowledge, substantive or theoretical, on which advice and action are based is not always clear; it is often a mixture of several kinds of practical and theoretical knowledge. But it is part of the professional complex, and of the professional claim, that the practice should rest upon some branch of knowledge to which the professionals are privy by virtue of long study and by initiation and apprenticeship under masters already members of the profession.

* * *

Professionals *profess*. They profess to know

_____
* 92 *Daedalus* 655–657 (1963). Reprinted by permission of *Daedalus,* Journal of the American Academy of Arts and Sciences, Boston, Massachusetts.

better than others the nature of certain matters, and to know better than their clients what ails them or their affairs. This is the essence of the professional idea and the professional claim. From it flow many consequences. The professionals claim the exclusive right to practice, as a vocation, the arts which they profess to know, and to give the kind of advice derived from their special line of knowledge. This is the basis of the license, both in the narrow sense of legal permission and in the broader sense that the public allows those in a profession a certain leeway in their practice and perhaps in their very way of living and thinking. The professional is expected to think objectively and inquiringly about matters which may be, for laymen, subject to orthodoxy and sentiment which limit intellectual exploration. . . .

Since the professional does profess, he asks that he be trusted. The client is not a true judge of the value of the service he receives; furthermore, the problems and affairs of men are such that the best of professional advice and action will not always solve them. A central feature, then, of all professions, is the motto—not used in this form, so far as I know—*credat emptor.* Thus is the professional relation distinguished from that of those markets in which the rule is *caveat emptor,* although the latter is far from a universal rule even in exchange of goods. The client is to trust the professional; he must tell him all secrets which bear upon the affairs in hand. He must trust his judgment and skill. In return, the professional asks protection from any unfortunate consequences of his professional actions; he and his fellows make it very difficult for anyone outside—even civil courts—to pass judgment upon one of their number. Only the professional can say when his colleague makes a mistake.

The mandate also flows from the claim to esoteric knowledge and high skill. Lawyers not only give advice to clients and plead their cases for them; they also develop a philosophy of law —of its nature and its functions, and of the proper way in which to administer justice. Physicians consider it their prerogative to define the nature of disease and of health, and to determine how medical services ought to be distributed and paid for. Social workers are not content to develop a technique of case work; they concern themselves with social legislation. Every profession considers itself the proper body to set the terms in which some aspect of society, life or nature is to be thought of, and to define the general lines, or even the details, of public policy concerning it. The mandate to do so is granted more fully to some professions than to others; in time of crises it may be questioned even with regard to the most respected and powerful professions.

* * *

b.

Mancur Olson
The Logic of Collective Action*

* * *

Many of those who criticize organized labor because of the coercion entailed in labor unions are themselves members of professional organizations that depend upon compulsion as much as unions do. Many organizations representing prosperous and prestigious professions like the law and medicine have also reached for the forbidden fruits of compulsory membership. There is in fact a pervasive tendency towards compulsion in professional associations generally. "The trend," writes Frances Delancey, "is toward the professional guild." This is what many other scholars have also observed. "A characteristic of the politics of the professional association," according to V. O. Key, "is their tendency to seek the reality, if not invariably the form, of a guild system." J. A. C. Grant argues that the guild "has returned. Its purposes are the same as in the Middle Ages." The guild form of organization is often adopted not only by the ancient and learned professions, but also by undertakers, barbers, "beauticians," "cosmeticians," plumbers, opticians, and other groups interested in professional status. This adoption of the guild form of organization is evidence for the by-product theory of large pressure groups, for compulsory membership has always been, Grant points out, "the first rule" of the guild system.

The self-regulating guild with compulsory membership has reached its furthest degree of development in many state bar associations. Many state legislatures have been induced to require by law that every practicing lawyer must be a member of the state bar association. These bar associations have closed shops enforced by government, and thus should be the envy of every labor union.

The modern professional associations or guilds are moreover coming to resemble "minia-

ture governments." They have "all the types of power normally exercised by government." State governments often give the professional groups authority to govern themselves (and to a degree their clients) and to discipline any members of the profession that do not maintain the "ethical" standards the profession finds it expedient or appropriate to maintain. It follows that, even when membership in these associations is not a legal requirement, the individual in professional practice knows that he has an interest in maintaining membership in good standing with the professional association.

The advantages of maintaining membership and good relationships with a professional association may be illustrated by the fact that it was not found expedient to release the name of a doctor who had written to a congressional committee to argue that "the central organization of the AMA in Chicago has no idea what the average physician wants his patients to have." Oliver Garceau, author of the classic work on the American Medical Association, has argued that the recalcitrant doctor in trouble with organized medicine may face "a genuine economic threat." When the American Medical Association blocked the Denver city council's program for Denver General Hospital in 1945, a Denver councilman, according to *Time* Magazine, was driven to exclaim: "Nobody can touch the American Medical Association. . . . Talk about the closed shop of the AFL and the CIO—they are a bunch of pikers."

The role of coercion, even in its subtler forms, in the American Medical Association is, however, probably less important as a source of membership than the noncollective benefits the organization provides its membership. According to Garceau, there is "one formal service of the society with which the doctor can scarcely dispense. Malpractice defense has become a prime requisite to private practice." One doctor who had founded a cooperative hospital, and lost his membership in his medical society, discovered that not only had he lost his chance to have other doctors testify in his behalf during malpractice suits, but that he had lost his insurance as well. The many technical publications of the American Medical Association, and the state and local medical societies, also give the doctor a considerable incentive to affiliate with organized medicine. The American Medical Association publishes not only its celebrated *Journal,* but also many other technical periodicals on various medical specialties. Since the nineteenth century

---

* Cambridge, Mass.: The Harvard University Press 137–140 (1965). Reprinted by permission.

the *Journal* alone has provided a "tangible attraction for doctors." The importance of this attraction is perhaps indicated by a survey conducted in Michigan, which showed that 89 per cent of the doctors received the *Journal of the American Medical Association,* and 70 per cent read a state society journal, but *less than 30 per cent* read any *other* type of medical literature. The *Journal* has been, moreover, the "prime money maker of the organization." Much of the organization's revenue, according to Garceau, comes from drug companies' advertisements—advertisements which Garceau believes helped companies obtain the AMA seal of approval for their products. The conventions of the American Medical Association and many of its constituent organizations also provide technical information needed by doctors, and thus give the member a "direct return in education" for the investment in dues, just as the medical journals do.

In short, by providing a helpful defense against malpractice suits, by publishing medical journals needed by its membership, and by making its conventions educational as well as political, the American Medical Association has offered its members and potential members a number of selective or noncollective benefits. It has offered its members benefits which, in contrast with the political achievements of the organization, can be withheld from nonmembers, and which accordingly provide an incentive for joining the organization.

* * *

NOTE

WILLIAM J. GOODE
THE PROTECTION OF THE INEPT*

The dissident have throughout history voiced a suspicion that the highly placed have not earned their mace, orb, and scepter. . . . Against the grandiloquent assertion of kings that they were divinely appointed, both court jesters and the masses have sometimes laughed, and asked, where were their virtue and wisdom? . . .

. . . In our less heroic epoch, we are assured that we live in an achievement-oriented society, and the norm is to place individuals in their occupations by merit. . . .

. . . However the privileged (at all levels of privilege) do try systematically to prevent the talent of the less privileged from being rec-

---

* 32 *American Sociological Review* 5–8 (1967). Reprinted by permission.

ognized or developed. And though analysts of stratification assume that social mobility is an index of open competition, ample if unsystematic evidence suggests that both the able and the inept may move into high position.

These comments . . . describe arrangements which every social system exhibits, and which cope with a universal *system problem:* How to utilize the services of the less able?

The social responses to this problem are the resultant of two sets of factors in tension: protection *of* the inept; and protection of the group *from* the inept. In almost all collectivities . . . the arrangements for protecting the less able seem to be more pervasive, common, and effective than those for protecting the group from ineptitude. . . .

* * *

Let us . . . consider briefly some of the wide array of evidence that groups do not typically expose or expel their members for lesser achievement or talent. . . .

Almost every inquiry into the productivity of workers has shown that the informal work group protects its members by setting a standard which everyone can meet, and they develop techniques for preventing a supervisor from measuring accurately the output of each man. Higher level management has for the most part evaded such scrutiny, but industrial sociologists have reported comparable behavior there, too. The protection of one another by lower-level workers might be due to less commitment; the fact that higher-level men do the same suggests the need for a more general explanation.

All professions, while claiming to be the sole competent judges of their members' skills, and the guardians of their clients' welfare, refuse to divulge information about how competent any of them are, and under most circumstances their rules assert it is unethical to criticize the work of fellow members to laymen. Wall Street law firms try to find good positions in other firms for those employees they decide are not partnership material. When a new profession is organized, grandfather clauses permit older practitioners with less training to continue in practice without being tested. When hospitals begin to demand a higher performance standard from those who enjoy staff privileges, inevitably rejecting some, both patients and physicians object. One study of a group of physicians showed that there was little relationship between an M.D.'s income and the quality of medical care he gave to his patients.

Wherever unions are strong, foremen know that promotion by merit rather than by seniority is unwise, and in any event unusual. Many corporations do not fire their managers; they find or create other posts for them. Employees are close students of promotion behavior, and are "notoriously suspicious and cynical" about management claims that promotions are through merit. Many are not convinced the best men are at the top. More generally, members of what Goffman calls "teams" (army officers, parents, policemen, managers, nurses, and so forth) protect each other from any exposure of their errors.

* * *

Few are fired for incompetence, especially if they last long enough to become members of their work group. One consequence is that, in craft or white collar jobs, higher standards are set for obtaining a job than for performance. The result is that a high level of formal education is often necessary for jobs that any average eighth-grader could learn to perform rather quickly. Once the person enters his work group, however, the social arrangements do not permit much overt discrimination between the less able and the rest. . . .

* * *

c.

Murray T. Bloom
The Trouble with Lawyers*

* * *

It started with Ford Hoffman, a Phoenix real estate broker—a nonfirebrand and nonrevolutionary. In fact Hoffman still isn't mad at lawyers. He is still a bit incredulous that his little $4,000 routine real estate deal started the great battle.

* * *

The revolution began early in July, 1952, when Hoffman as a licensed broker drew up an agreement of sale, warranty deed, quitclaim deed and bill of sale on a property. They sound awfully impressive, but in fact they are just printed forms and filling them in took Hoffman less than fifteen minutes. He made no charge for the work, but he did get a broker's commission on the sale. It didn't even occur to Hoffman that he

* New York: Simon and Schuster 110–124 (1968). Copyright © 1968, by Murray Teigh Bloom. Reprinted by permission of Simon and Schuster.

was guilty of one of the dirtiest phrases in the legal lexicon—"unauthorized practice of law." (UPL spewed out as initials at bar association meetings makes a sneering epithet.)

* * *

Among lawyers themselves there is considerable disagreement about . . . UPL committees. Former Supreme Court Justice Wiley Rutledge, a conservative, said in 1941:

I do not like what I fear is becoming the bar's trade-union approach to the problem. . . . I doubt whether . . . it is necessary or desirable for bar associations to become closed shops, not only as to the business lawyers are now performing but as to a great deal of business which has always been done by other men, although lawyers may have been doing it for a long time.

The more orthodox view was expressed in 1951 by Edwin M. Otterbourg, a New York lawyer who was one of the pillars of the UPL committee:

Actually, unauthorized practice of law is a swindle upon the public. Whenever it takes place, some person receives either incompetent or unqualified advice, or advice which cannot be honestly disinterested. . . . Reliance upon such advice may result in irreparable injury and loss. . . .

For several months I tried to find serious instances of such injury and loss suffered by the public. I couldn't. I finally stopped trying when Professor Quintin Johnstone, of the Yale University Law School, wrote in a 1967 book: "Nor are there many instances of persons being harmed from having laymen do their legal work." Further, he went on, there is a "public benefit from much of the lay competition that now exists. Lay legal services often are performed at lower cost than if the work were done by lawyers."

In fact Ford Hoffman was simply filling out forms without extra charge—which every real estate man in the state had been doing long before Arizona became a state.

It started friendly. Hoffman was told that it was going to be a test case when the State Bar of Arizona on October 30, 1953, filed its suit against him claiming that he had practiced law without a license. At the same time a similar action was brought against five title insurance companies, since they, too, often filled out these forms in cases where real estate purchasers bought title insurance.

Superior Court Judge Henry S. Stevens ruled in favor of Hoffman and the title companies. He said real estate brokers and title companies could continue to prepare certain legal documents and perform some other services incidental to their businesses without being guilty of unauthorized practice of law.

The State Bar now carried the case to the State Supreme Court, but Hoffman, who felt he had already spent too much in defending himself, dropped out of the case. On November 1, 1961, the Arizona Supreme Court unanimously overturned the lower court ruling. Neither real estate brokers nor title companies could prepare *any* of the documents, including even the simple printed preliminary purchase agreements.

The fact that the brokers didn't get paid for the work of filling out these printed forms didn't matter, said the court. That they had been doing it unhindered for many years also didn't count. But, the court admitted, "the record does not disclose any testimony regarding specific injury to the public from [these] practices."

The court was also out to close all loopholes, such as the possibility of the brokers and title companies getting legislation giving them the right to do what they had been doing all along: ". . . although the legislature may impose additional restrictions which affect the licensing of attorneys, it cannot infringe on the ultimate power of the court to determine who may practice law."

Now what had started out as "a friendly little test case" lost all cozy amicability. The Arizona Bar, which had been supported by the American Bar Association, rejoiced at a great victory. The Arizona Association of Realtors, of which Ford Hoffman was not a member, got into the battle. This was *serious*.

Why should real estate men think their very livelihood was affected by the Supreme Court ruling?

Robert E. Riggs, now a professor of political science at the University of Minnesota, but then a young lawyer in Arizona, analyzed the realtors' problem cogently:

Although loss of the right to prepare other documents might be an inconvenience to the real estate agent, the preliminary sales agreement was vital. By it the agent obtained the signatures of both parties, binding them to the sale. Sales could be lost if a prospective buyer or seller changed his mind while waiting for a lawyer to draft the sales contract. Cost was also a consideration, since the agent might have to pay the lawyer for filling the blanks on many sales agreement forms for sales that were never consummated.

Now, too, the newspapers of Arizona began to see some of the sweeping implications of the Supreme Court decision. The Tucson *Daily Citizen*, for example, saw it as

likely to hike the cost of the average real estate deal. What is more, the ruling will put more money in the pockets of the lawyers . . . the customers are now forced to retain attorneys to represent them. . . .

But for the Arizona *Daily Star* there was an even more important issue involved: The Supreme Court, in denying the Legislature the right to determine what constitutes the practice of law, had

arrogated to itself and to members of the State Bar of Arizona a legalized special privilege that is denied all other professions. . . . Thus we see the court composed of lawyers settling it in favor of lawyers. . . . It would be just as sensible and justified if the medical doctors would demand that such specialized services as blood examinations, and microbiology, be done by licensed M.D.'s. It is now done by technicians. Nurses would be denied the right to take cardiograms, and so on. . . . It is adverse to the public interest in the additional cost it imposes on the average citizen.

*   *   *

In Arizona, as in twelve other states, the people can institute a constitutional amendment. In order to place the amendment on the regular ballot, at least 15 percent of the registered voters have to sign the initiative petition. Some 60,000 signatures would be required for such an amendment to be voted on in the November, 1962, general election. And the petitions with the names would have to be filed not later than July 6. They had four months.

*   *   *

On July 6, 1962, the real estate men filed some 107,420 signatures on their petition with the Secretary of State of Arizona. This was nearly twice as much as the needed 60,000 and represented 28 percent of the electorate. It was also the largest number of signatures ever filed on an initiative measure in the state's history. The Secretary of State assigned it a number, and now the conflict was to become the Battle of Proposition 103.

That day the *Arizona News* of Phoenix declared editorially for the real estate men.

The cost of an attorney's fee has been added to the rather heavy closing costs when a home or other piece of property changes hands. . . .
The real estate men and title companies were expected to be content with this ruling—just pass it on to the customer as manufacturers do when the

cost of a product goes up with wage or other production increases.

In taking their case to the people, the realtors are warning the public that the legal fraternity is known to be eyeing other professions from which they could collect a legal fee in every individual transaction. . . .

. . . this appears to be a case in which, unless the people speak, their rights will be submerged by the selfish demands of a profession which has demonstrated throughout the contention on this issue, that it has regard for no right but its own.

Now for the first time the Arizona Bar became worried. Promises of help were sought at the American Bar Association convention in August. There the National Conference of Bar Presidents urged the ABA to lend all possible assistance to the State Bar of Arizona in its fight against the proposed amendment. In Arizona two public relations firms and an advertising agency were taken on for the campaign.

The campaign slogans emerged quickly. The realtors chose "Protect Your Pocketbook" and "Protect Your Right to Choose," and the bar's was "Save Our Constitution." . . . The realtors got an unexpected assist from a local law journal, the *Arizona Weekly Gazette,* which carries local court announcements and news of pleadings. The *Gazette* had a long news item from Salt Lake City where an unauthorized practice of law group had cited the many professions and occupations that were currently infringing on law practice. Included were architects, "who quite generally draw construction contracts and notices of completion"; banks and trust companies, "when they go too far in estate planning"; claims adjusters, when they intervene between attorney and client; CPAs, "when they give tax advice without limitation"; life insurance brokers and salesmen, "when they give estate tax and estate planning advice"; and notaries public, who "prepare legal documents"; and, of course, real estate brokers.

The news story, widely reprinted in realtor ads, surely helped convince some of these groups that the lawyers would turn on them, too, when they had finished with the realtors.

* * *

By November 2, Election Day, there was little doubt that the realtors would win. The only real question was by how much. Even the realtors were surprised by their majority; some 236,856 voters supported them, and only 64,507 were against the amendment, a majority of nearly 4 to 1.

The postmortems for the lawyers were sobering. They knew their profession had acquired a more tarnished image. In a letter to the *Journal of the American Bar Association* in May, 1963, an Oklahoma attorney spoke for many when he wrote: "In the Arizona case it was apparent that the bar was more concerned about its loss of business than it was about public welfare. . . ."

An Arizona lawyer, Robert E. Riggs, a Mormon who had practiced in his father's law office in Tempe for a year before deciding that he would be happier teaching political science, did an analysis of the battle for the *Arizona Law Review.* "But," he told me recently, at the University of Minnesota where he is teaching, "they wouldn't print it. They felt I was too hard on the lawyers, too critical of the bar." The study, which appeared in the *Southern California Law Review,* actually was quite mild in its conclusions:

This may be a time for reappraisal, as the *American Bar Association Journal* has suggested. If such it be, this essay is a plea that the reappraisal look beyond tactics and methods to the basic premises and concepts defining the role of the legal profession in society.

In looking back on the case, Dr. Riggs still feels that "the bar is very privileged and very protective of itself." He still finds it incredible that the Arizona Supreme Court had ruled as it did in outlawing the preparation of any contracts by realtors. "How can judges be impartial vis-à-vis lawyers in a matter such as this?"

* * *

In Illinois the brokers and the lawyers were embroiled in a ten-year court battle that was finally resolved in October, 1966. Here the bar won clearly: *only lawyers* could handle the completion of all real estate transactions, regardless of size. Both the buyers and sellers had to have attorneys, and the lawyers, of course, had to be paid.

For a time the Illinois brokers thought of getting a constitutional amendment along the Arizona lines, but in Illinois a two-thirds approval of each house of the legislature is required before the proposed amendment can go on the ballot. Presumably when the brokers took a head-count of the many lawyers in the legislature, they decided the idea wasn't too practical.

The Chicago *Daily News* interpreted the lawyers' victory this way on October 27, 1966:

Don't be surprised if the final cost of buying that new house you are buying is $200 more than you figured. . . . Sources within the legal profession told the *Daily News* the agreement would primarily affect the average home buyer, who previously did not hire an attorney. He could now pay as much as $325 extra on the purchase of a $30,000 home. . . .

* * *

There are about a million new homes built in the United States each year and an estimated two to two and a half million existing homes sold—or a total of about three and a half million home sales. The increase in legal fees, if the Illinois verdict spreads, could be hefty. At a modest set of legal fees totaling only $200 per house, this would come to $700,000,000 a year added to the cost of living in a house of your own.

Fortunately, several State Supreme Courts have not seen fit to go along with the zealous unauthorized practice committees. In Michigan, Missouri, Wisconsin and Minnesota, real estate brokers are still permitted to fill in forms without the help of lawyers. These states, in effect, are following the reasoning set forth by the Minnesota Supreme Court in 1940:

It is the duty of this court so to regulate the practice of law and restrain such practice by laymen in a common sense way in order to protect primarily the interest of the public and not to hamper and burden such interest with impractical technical restraints. . . .

The rare instances of defective conveyances in such transactions are insufficient to outweigh the great public inconvenience which would follow if it were necessary to call in a lawyer to draft these simple documents.

* * *

d.

In the Matter of Community Action for Legal Services, Inc.
26 App. Div.2d 354, 274 N.Y. S.2d 779
(Sup. Ct. 1966)

* * *

BREITEL, J. Three applications on behalf of proposed corporations wishing to practice law under the provisions of section 280 of the Penal Law are pending before the court. The proposed corporations would be Community Action for Legal Services, Inc., New York Legal Assistance Corporation, and Harlem Assertion of Rights, Inc. . . . The plans are to establish neighborhood law offices and provide representation for disadvantaged members of the community, disadvantaged because of poverty and just as often because of disfavored minority status. The financial support for the programs is expected to come largely, if not exclusively, from Federal

funds under the auspices and control of the Federal Office of Economic Opportunity.

Regrettably, the present applications may not be approved by the court. In rejecting them, however, the court invites the resubmission of proposals free from the infirmities in the present applications, with the suggestion that any new applications be submitted promptly, in final form, and in succinct integrated documents.

* * *

Section 280 of the Penal Law is the governing statute making it a crime for corporations to practice law. It contains, however, an exception for charitable or other corporations which have first obtained approval by the applicable Appellate Division. It is immediately evident that the allowable practice of law by corporations is highly exceptional, permissible only in carefully circumscribed conditions consonant with the policy of limiting the practice of law to licensed professionals. This is a general principle to be observed.

Basic to the principle is that the restriction of legal practice to lawyers and the maintenance of professional standards are for the benefit of the public and not for the economic preservation or professional enhancement of the Bar. The professional standards and Canons of Professional Ethics are justifiable only as protective of the public. Inherent to the legal professional system is the direct and often summary control and discipline of lawyers by the courts. . . . No similarly direct, and rarely any summary, control over laymen exists in the courts. The direct and summary control over the members of the profession by any agency, but especially by the courts, is a unique difference distinguishing the legal profession from other professions.

The most embracive of the applications is that on behalf of Community Action for Legal Services, Inc. (CALS). CALS itself would not practice law but it would finance and control subcontractors or delegate agencies which would. . . . CALS would have a board of directors of 32 members, at least 12 of whom are to be chosen from or recommended by the New York City Council Against Poverty from "nominations made by community committees in designated poverty areas in the City." It might have as many as 35 directors who shall "in the main" be lawyers. It would have power to establish "guidelines" for the operation of legal services programs, that is, neighborhood law offices, and render advice and assistance to delegate agencies. . . . CALS would have an advisory committee on legal services with 18 members (only 6 of whom will definitely be lawyers) who would be chosen by law school deans and delegate agencies not represented on the CALS board.

*   *   *

[The court's] official concern is with the feasibility of maintaining minimal standards. The interposition of supervising licensed corporations and the unlimited power of contracting out of legal services to delegate, subdelegate, and sub-subdelegate agencies is a thicket through which none could penetrate, even if the non-lawyer controls were eliminated. Hence, recognizing the novelty and difficulty of the programs contemplated and the anticipated use of laymen by the lawyers to a degree never before countenanced in the profession, the court should not licence more than one legal assistance corporation, using Federal economic antipoverty funds, in any one area, as large as a county or at least half a county. One set of neighborhood law offices operated by one entity in such an area is both enough and all that could be responsibly supervised by any one directorate and by this court insofar as gross breaches of ethics may ever become involved. The present proposals are just unworkable because of the clumsy overlapping, excessive layers of organizations, and the built-in incentives to competitive antipoverty law offices operating in the same area.

On the basis of these remarks, the pending applications are deficient. No matter how many interpositions of corporations and boards are provided, with respect to each proposed corporation the lawyer operations would be subject ultimately to lay control. This is not permissible if the public is to be protected from abuses and if this court is to carry out its responsibility to enforce minimum standards on those over whom it has direct control. Nor does the statute permit it.

In this connection the court would have no concern, as it could not, with any council or advisory group, consisting exclusively or largely of laymen, in any legal assistance corporation, reviewing and addressing itself to broad questions of policy. But the court is concerned that such a corporation be directly controlled and supervised by lawyers summarily responsible to the court for the maintenance of professional standards. . . .

. . . Recognizing the need for diverse representation and the requirements of the Federal agency for community involvement, it is suggested that those needs be met in a council or other policy group as mentioned above and not in the board of directors or managers of law offices. This should involve no serious difficulty. The management of law offices is not something in which even involved members of the community may be deemed to be competent. No one would assume that patients are competent to tell physicians how to practice their profession. On the other hand, the competence of lay members of the community to speak for themselves on broad questions of policy affecting the community cannot be gainsaid.

At this point, it may be helpful to note that those who sponsor a legal assistance corporation need not be lawyers. But once a licensed corporation is created, it could and should be cut loose from the sponsors, if they are not lawyers or cannot meet the standards required for operation of a legal assistance corporation. This separation should apply to hiring and fiscal functions, for the power to hire and that of the purse are overwhelming. . . . In making these comments the court is not officially concerned with the efficiency, economy, or esthetics of any planned program, none of which is its proper concern. Rather it is concerned with insuring that the public will receive the best available legal services in the same way as those who retain their own private lawyers, with effective recourse to the court for gross professional failure.

*   *   *

The court, in conclusion, affirms its recognition of the importance of the programs involved. It accepts, indeed is hospitable to the view, that new institutions must be fashioned to function alongside traditional legal aid societies. It believes that such a development will involve change and enlargement in traditional concepts of professional standards, ethics, and office organization. Nevertheless, it still must require that protection of the public be the paramount and final determinant of the form and content of any institutional development of these new programs over which it has responsibilities. Certainly, factional, political, and narrow group or professional interests must be either subordinated or ignored entirely in the fashioning of these new institutions, if the service of such interests would impede the protection of the public.

*   *   *

2.

The Professional in Practice—
Traditional Concepts of Power and Authority

a.

Alexander Solzhenitsyn
Cancer Ward*

First, Ludmila Afanasyevna took Kostoglotov into the treatment room. A female patient had just emerged after her session. The huge 180,000-volt X-ray tube, hanging by wires from the ceiling, had been in operation almost nonstop since 8 A.M. There was no ventilation and the air was full of that sweetish, slightly repellent X-ray warmth.

*   *   *

She was in a hurry, not only because she wanted to get out quickly, but also because the X-ray program could not be delayed even for a few minutes. She motioned Kostoglotov to lie on the hard couch under the X-ray tube and to uncover his stomach. Then she went over his skin with some sort of cool, tickly brush. She outlined something and seemed to be painting figures on it.

After this she told the nurse about the "quandrant scheme" and how she was to apply the tube to each quadrant. She then ordered the patient to turn over onto his stomach and she brushed some more lines on his back. "Come and see me after the session," she said.

*   *   *

He went to see Dontsova. She was sitting in the short-focus apparatus room. Through her square glasses, rounded at the four corners, she was examining some large X-ray films against the light. Both machines were switched off, both windows were open and there was no one else in the room.

"Sit down," said Dontsova drily.

He sat down. She went on comparing the X-rays.

Although Kostoglotov argued with her, he did it only as a defense against the excesses of medicine, as laid out in a mass of instructions. As for Ludmila Afanasyevna herself, she inspired only confidence, not just by her masculine decisiveness, by the precise orders she gave as

---

* New York: Farrar, Straus & Giroux, Inc., Bantam Books 65–80, 85–88 (1969). Reprinted by permission of Farrar, Straus & Giroux, Inc. © Alexander Solzhenitsyn, English translation © The Bodley Head, Ltd., 1968.

she watched the screen in the darkness, by her age and her indisputable dedication to work and work alone, but also, above all, by the confident way in which, right from the very first day, she had felt for the outline of his tumor and traced its circumference so precisely. The tumor itself proclaimed the accuracy of her touch, for it had felt something too. Only a patient can judge whether the doctor understands a tumor correctly with his fingers. Dontsova had felt out his tumor so well that she didn't need an X-ray photograph.

She laid aside the X-ray photographs, took off her glasses and said, "Kostoglotov, there is too big a gap in your case history. We must be absolutely certain of the nature of your primary tumor."

When Dontsova started talking like a doctor, she always spoke much more quickly. In one breath she would leap through long sentences and difficult terms. "What you tell us of your operation the year before last and the position of the present secondaries, is in agreement with our diagnosis. However, there are other possibilities which can't be excluded, and this complicates your treatment for us. You'll understand it's impossible now to take a sample of your secondary."

"Thank God! I wouldn't have let you take one."

"I still don't understand why we can't get hold of the slides with the sections of your primary. Are you absolutely sure there was a histological analysis?"

"Yes, I'm sure."

"In that case why were you not told the result?"

She rattled on in the rapid style of a busy person. Some of her words slipped by and had to be guessed at.

Kostoglotov, however, had got out of the habit of hurrying. "The result? There were such stormy goings-on where we were, Ludmila Afanasyevna, such an extraordinary situation that I give you my word of honor. . . . I'd have been ashamed to ask about a little thing like my biopsy. Heads were rolling. And I didn't even understand what a biopsy was for." Kostoglotov liked to use medical terms when he was talking to doctors.

"Of course you didn't understand. But those doctors must have understood. These things can't be played about with."

*   *   *

"[B]ut I want to know when *I* can go back [home]". . . Kostoglotov looked at her somberly.

"You will go home," Dontsova weighed her words one by one with great emphasis, "when I consider it necessary to interrupt your treatment. And then you will only go temporarily."

Kostoglotov had been waiting for this moment in the conversation. He couldn't let it go by without a fight.

"Ludmila Afanasyevna! Can't we get away from this tone of voice? You sound like a grown-up talking to a child. Why not talk as an adult to an adult? Seriously, when you were on your rounds this morning I . . ."

"Yes, on my rounds this morning"—Dontsova's big face looked quite threatening—"you made a disgraceful scene. What are you trying to do? Upset the patients? What are you putting into their heads?"

"What was I trying to do?" He spoke without heat but emphatically, as Dontsova had. He sat up, his back firm against the back of the chair. "I simply wanted to remind you of my right to dispose of my own life. A man can dispose of his own life, can't he? You agree I have that right?"

Dontsova looked down at his colorless, winding scar and was silent. Kostoglotov developed his point:

"You see, you start from a completely false position. No sooner does a patient come to you than you begin to do all his thinking for him. After that, the thinking's done by your standing orders, your five-minute conferences, your program, your plan and the honor of your medical department. And once again I become a grain of sand, just as I was in the camp. Once again nothing *depends* on me."

"The clinic obtains written consent from every patient before every operation," Dontsova reminded him.

(Why had she mentioned an operation? He'd never let himself be operated on, not for anything!)

"Thank you! Thank you for that anyway! Even though it's only for its own protection, the clinic at least does that. Unless there's an operation you simply don't ask the patient anything. And you never explain anything! But surely X-rays have some effect too?"

"Where did you get all these rumors about X-rays?" Dontsova made a guess. "Was it from Rabinovich?"

"I don't know any Rabinovich!" Kostoglotov shook his head firmly. "I'm talking about the principle of the thing."

(It was in fact from Rabinovich that he'd

heard these gloomy stories about the aftereffects of X-rays, but he'd promised not to give him away. Rabinovich was an outpatient who had already had more than two hundred sessions. He'd made very heavy weather of them and with every dozen he'd felt closer to death than recovery. Where he lived no one understood him, not a soul in his apartment or his building or his block. They were healthy people who ran about from noon till night thinking of successes or failures—things that seemed terribly important to them. Even his own family had got tired of him. It was only here, on the steps of the cancer clinic, that the patients listened to him for hours and sympathized. They understood what it means to a man when a small triangular area grows bone-hard and the irradiation scars lie thick on the skin where the X-rays have penetrated.)

Honestly, there he was talking about "the principle of the thing!" Wasn't that just what Dontsova and her assistants needed—to spend days talking to patients about the principles on which they were being treated! Where would they find the time for the treatment then?

Every now and again some stubborn, meticulous lover of knowledge, like this man or Rabinovich, would crop up out of a batch of fifty patients and run her into the ground, prizing explanations out of her about the course of his disease. When this happened, one couldn't avoid the hard task of offering the occasional explanation. And Kostoglotov's case was a special one even from the medical point of view by virtue of the extraordinary negligence with which it had been handled. Up to the time of her arrival on the scene, when he had finally been allowed out to receive treatment, it was as if there had been a malicious conspiracy to drive him to the very borderline of death. His case was a special one too because of the exceptionally rapid revival which had begun under X-ray treatment.

"Kostoglotov! Twelve sessions of X-rays have turned you from a corpse into a living human being. How dare you attack your treatment? You complain that they gave you no treatment in the camp or in exile, that they neglected you, and in the same breath you grumble because people *are* treating you and taking trouble over you. Where's the logic in that?"

"Obviously there's no logic." Kostoglotov shook his shaggy black mane. "But maybe there needn't be any, Ludmila Afanasyevna. After all, man is a complicated being, why should he be explainable by logic? Or for that matter by economics? Or physiology? Yes, I did come to you as a corpse, and I begged you take me in, and I lay on the floor by the staircase. And therefore you make the logical deduction that I came to you to be saved *at any price!* But I don't want to be saved at any price! There isn't anything in the world for which I'd agree to pay *any* price!" He began to speak more quickly. It was something he never liked doing, but Dontsova was making an attempt to interrupt and he still had a great deal more to say on the subject. "I came to you *to relieve my suffering!* I said, 'I'm in terrible pain, help me!' And you did. And now I'm not in pain. Thank you! Thank you! I'm grateful and I'm in your debt. Only now let me go. Just let me crawl away like a dog to my kennel, so I can lick my wounds and rest till I'm better."

"And when the disease catches up with you, you'll come crawling back to us?"

"Perhaps. Perhaps I'll come crawling back to you."

"And we shall have to take you?"

"Yes! And that's where I see your mercy. What are you worried about? Your recovery percentages? Your records? How you'll be able to explain letting me go after fifteen sessions when the Academy of Medical Science recommends not less than sixty?"

Never in her life had she heard such incoherent rubbish. As a matter of fact, from the records' point of view it would be to her advantage to discharge him and make a note of "Marked improvement." This would never apply after fifty sessions.

But he kept hammering away at his point.

"As far as I'm concerned, it's enough that you've driven back the tumor and stopped it. It's on the defensive. I'm on the defensive too. Fine. A soldier has a much better life in defense. And whatever happens you'll never be able to cure me completely. There's no such thing as a complete cure in cancer. All processes of nature are characterized by the law of diminishing returns, they reach a point where big efforts yield small results. In the beginning my tumor was breaking up quickly. Now it'll go slowly. So let me go with what's left of my blood."

"Where did you pick up all this information, I'd like to know?" Dontsova frowned.

"Ever since I was a child I've loved browsing through medical books."

"But what *exactly* are you afraid of in our treatment?"

"Ludmila Afanasyevna, I don't know what to be afraid of. I'm not a doctor. Perhaps you know but don't want to tell me. For example,

Vera Kornilyevna wants to put me on a course of glucose injections. . . ."

"Absolutely essential."

"But I don't want it."

"Why on earth not?"

"In the first place, it's unnatural. If I need grape sugar, give it to me through the mouth! Why this twentieth-century gimmick? Why should every medicine be given by injection? You don't see anything similar in nature or among animals, do you? In a hundred years' time they'll laugh at us and call us savages. And then, the way they give injections! One nurse gets it right first time, another punctures your . . . your ulnary flexion to bits. I just don't want it. And now I see you're getting ready to give me blood transfusions. . . ."

"You ought to be delighted! Somebody's willing to give their blood for you. That means health, life!"

"But I don't want it! They gave a Chechen here a transfusion in front of me once. Afterwards he was in convulsions on his bed for three hours. They said, 'Incomplete compatibility'! Then they gave someone else blood and missed the vein. A great lump came up on his arm. Now it's compresses and vapor baths for a whole month. I don't want it."

"But substantial X-ray treatment is impossible without transfusion!"

"Then don't give it! Why do you assume you have the right to decide for someone else? Don't you agree it's a terrifying right, one that rarely leads to good? You should be careful. No one's entitled to it, not even doctors."

"But doctors *are* entitled to that right—doctors above all," exclaimed Dontsova with deep conviction. By now she was really angry. "Without that right there'd be no such thing as medicine!"

"And look what it leads to. You're going to deliver a lecture on radiation sickness soon, aren't you?"

"How do you know that?" Ludmila Afanasyevna was quite astonished.

"Well, it wasn't very difficult. I assumed . . ."

(It was quite simple. He had seen a thick folder of typescript lying on her table. Although the title was upside down, he had managed to read it during the conversation and had understood its meaning.)

". . . Or rather I guessed. There is a new name, radiation sickness, which means there must be lectures about it. But you see, twenty years ago you irradiated some old Kostoglotov in spite of his protests that he was afraid of the treatment, and you reassured him that everything was all right, because you didn't know then that radiation sickness existed. It's the same with me today. I don't know yet what I'm supposed to be afraid of. I just want you to let me go. I want to recover under my own resources. Then maybe I'll just get better. Isn't that right?"

Doctors have one sacred principle: the patient must never be frightened, he must be encouraged. But with a patient as importunate as Kostoglotov exactly the reverse tactics were required—shock.

"Better? No, *you won't get better!* Let me assure you"—her four fingers slammed the table like a whisk swatting a fly—"that you won't. You are going—" she paused to measure the blow—"*to die!*"

She looked at him to see him flinch. But he merely fell silent.

"You'll be exactly like Azovkin—and you've seen the condition he's in. Well, you've got the same disease as him in an almost identical state of neglect. We're saving Ahmadjan because we began to give him radiotherapy immediately after his operation. But with you we've lost two years, can you imagine it? There should have been another operation straight away on the lymph node, next to the one they operated on, but they let it go, do you see, and the secondaries just flowed on! Your tumor is one of the most dangerous kinds of cancer. It is very rapid to develop and acutely malignant, which means secondaries appear very quickly too. Not long ago its mortality rate was reckoned at 95 per cent. Does that satisfy you? Look, I'll show you . . . ."

She dragged a folder out of a pile and began to rummage through it.

Kostoglotov was silent. Then he spoke up, but quietly, without any of the self-confidence he had shown a few minutes earlier.

"To be frank, I'm not much of a clinger to life. It's not only that there's none ahead of me, there's none behind me either. If I had a chance of six months of life, I'd want to live them to the full. But I can't make plans for ten or twenty years ahead. Extra treatment means extra torment. There'll be radiation sickness, vomiting . . . what's the point?"

"Ah yes, I've found it! Here are our statistics." And she turned toward him a double page taken from an exercise book. Right across the top of the sheet was written the name of his type of tumor. Then on the left-hand side was a heading, "Already dead," and on the right, "Still alive." There were three columns of names, writ-

ten in at different times, some in pencil, some in ink. On the left there were no corrections, but on the right, crossings out, crossings out, crossings out. . . . "This is what we do. When a patient's discharged, we write his name in the right-hand list and then transfer him to the left-hand one. . . . Still, there are some lucky ones who've stayed in the right-hand one. Do you see?"

She gave him another moment to look at the list and to think about it.

"You *think* you're cured." She returned to the attack with vigor. "You're as ill as you ever were. You're no different than when you were admitted. The only thing that's been made clear is that your tumor *can* be fought, that all is not lost yet. And this is the moment you choose to announce you're leaving! All right, go! Get your discharge today! I'll arrange it for you now. And then I'll put your name down on the list—'Still alive.' "

He was silent.

"Come on, make up your mind!"

"Ludmila Afanasyevna"—Kostoglotov was ready for a compromise—"Look, if what's needed is a reasonable number of sessions, say, five or ten . . ."

"Not five or ten! Either no sessions at all or else as many as are necessary! That means, from today, two sessions daily instead of one, and all the requisite treatment. And no smoking! And one more essential condition: you must accept your treatment not just with faith but with *joy!* That's the only way you'll ever recover!"

He lowered his head. Part of today's bargaining with the doctors had been in anticipation. He had been dreading that they were going to propose another operation, but they hadn't. X-ray treatment was tolerable, it wasn't too bad.

Kostoglotov had something in reserve—a secret medicine, a mandrake root from Issyk Kul. There was a motive behind his wish to go back to his place in the woodlands—he wanted to treat himself with the root. Because he had the root, he'd really only come to the cancer clinic to see what it was like.

Dr. Dontsova saw she had won the battle and could afford to be magnanimous.

"All right then, I won't give you glucose. You can have another injection instead, an intramuscular one."

Kostoglotov smiled. "I see I'm going to have to give way."

"And please, see if you can hurry up that letter from Omsk."

As he left the room it seemed to him that

he was walking between two eternities, on one side a list of the living, with its inevitable crossings out, on the other—*eternal* exile. Eternal as the stars, as the galaxies.

The strange thing is that if Kostoglotov had persevered with his questions—What sort of injection was it? What was its purpose? Was it really necessary and morally justified?—if he had forced Ludmila Afanasyevna to explain the workings and the possible consequences of the new treatment, then very possibly he would have rebelled once and for all.

But precisely at this point, having exhausted all his brilliant arguments, he had capitulated.

She had been deliberately cunning, she had mentioned the injection as something quite insignificant because she was tired of all this explaining. Also, she knew for sure that this was the moment, after the action of the X-rays in their pure state had been tested on the patient, to deal the tumor yet another crucial blow. It was a treatment highly recommended for this particular type of cancer by the most up-to-date authorities. Now that she anticipated the amazing success that attended Kostoglotov's treatment, she could not possibly weaken before his obstinacy or neglect to attack him with all the weapons she believed in. True, there were no slides available with sections of his primary, but all her intuition, her powers of observation and her memory suggested to her that the tumor was the kind she suspected—not a teratoma, but a sarcoma. . . .

It was on this very type of tumor with precisely these secondaries that Dr. Dontsova was writing her doctoral thesis.

*　　*　　*

Today, however much she bustled about the clinic, there was something gnawing at her self-confidence, and at her sense of responsibility and authority. Was it the pain she could clearly feel in her stomach? Some days she didn't feel it at all, other days it was weaker, but today it was stronger. If she wasn't an oncologist she'd have dismissed it or else had it investigated without fear. But she knew the road too well to take the first step along it: to tell her relatives, to tell her colleagues. When it came to dealing with herself she kept herself going with typical Russian temporizing: Maybe it'll go away. Maybe it's only my nerves.

But it wasn't just that, it was something else that had been gnawing at her all day, like a splinter in the hand, faintly but persistently.

Now that she was back in her own little den, sitting at her own table and reaching out for the file on "Radiation Sickness" which the observant Kostoglotov had noticed, she realized that all day she had been more than upset, really wounded by that argument with him about the right to treat.

She could still hear his words: "Twenty years ago you gave radiation treatment to some old Kostoglotov who begged you not to do it. You didn't know about radiation sickness then!"

And in fact she was due shortly to give a lecture to the society of X-ray specialists on "The Late Aftereffects of Radiotherapy." It was almost exactly what Kostoglotov had reproached her with.

It was only recently, a year or two ago, that she and other X-ray specialists here and in Moscow and in Baku had begun to observe certain cases that could not immediately be understood.

A suspicion arose. Then it became a guess. They began to write letters to each other and to speak about it, not in lectures at this stage but in the intervals between lectures. Then somebody read a paper in an American journal, and somebody else read another. The Americans had something similar brewing. The cases multiplied, more and more patients came in with complaints, until suddenly it was all given a name: "The late aftereffects of radiotherapy." The time had come to speak of them from the rostrum and to reach a decision.

The gist of it was that X-ray cures, which had been safely, successfully, even brilliantly accomplished ten or fifteen years ago through heavy doses of radiation, were now resulting in unexpected damage or mutilation of the irradiated parts.

It was not so bad, or at any rate it was justifiable, in the case of former patients who had been suffering from malignant tumors. Even today there would have been no other solution. They had saved the patient from certain death in the only way possible; they had given large doses because small doses would not help. And if the patient reappeared today with some sort of mutilation, he had to understand that this was the price he must pay for the extra years he had already lived, as well as for the years that still remained ahead of him.

But then, ten, fifteen or eighteen years ago, when the term "radiation sickness" did not exist, X-ray radiation had seemed such a straightforward, reliable and foolproof method, such a magnificent achievement of modern medical technique, that it was considered retrograde, almost a sabotage of public health, to refuse to use it and to look for other, parallel or roundabout methods. They were afraid only of acute, immediate damage to tissue and bone, but even in those days they rapidly learned to avoid that. So—they irradiated! They irradiated with wild enthusiasm! Even benign tumors. Even small children.

And now these children had grown up. Young men and young women, sometimes even married, were coming with irreversible mutilations of those parts of the body which had been so zealously irradiated.

*   *   *

But these incidents had greatly shocked Ludmila Afanasyevna. They had left her with a gnawing feeling of deep-rooted and unpardonable guilt. And it was right there that Kostoglotov had struck home today.

She crossed her arms, hugging her shoulders, and walked round the room from door to window and back again, across the free strip of floor between the two apparatuses that were now switched off.

Was it possible? Could the question arise of a doctor's *right* to treat? Once you began to think like that, to doubt every method scientifically accepted today simply because it might be discredited or abandoned in the future, then goodness knows where you'd end up. After all there were cases on record of death from aspirin. A man might take the first aspirin of his life and die of it! By that reasoning it became impossible to treat anyone. By that reasoning all the daily advantages of medicine would have to be sacrificed.

It was a universal law: everyone who *acts* breeds both good and evil. With some it's more good, with others more evil.

*   *   *

b.

Talcott Parsons
The Social System*

*   *   *

There seem to be four aspects of the institutionalized expectation system relative to the sick role. First, is the exemption from normal social role responsibilities, which of course is relative to the nature and severity of the illness. This exemption requires legitimation by and to

_____
* Glencoe, Ill.: The Free Press 436–437, 441–443, 445–453, 463–465 (1951). Copyright © 1951 by Talcott Parsons. Reprinted by permission.

the various alters involved and the physician often serves as a court of appeal as well as a direct legitimatizing agent. It is noteworthy that like all institutionalized patterns the legitimation of being sick enough to avoid obligations can not only be a right of the sick person but an obligation upon him. . . .

The second closely related aspect is the institutionalized definition that the sick person cannot be expected by "pulling himself together" to get well by an act of decision or will. In this sense also he is exempted from responsibility—he is in a condition that must "be taken care of." His "condition" must be changed, not merely his "attitude." Of course the process of recovery may be spontaneous but while the illness lasts he can't "help it." This element in the definition of the state of illness is obviously crucial as a bridge to the acceptance of "help."

The third element is the definition of the state of being ill as itself undesirable with its obligation to want to "get well." The first two elements of legitimation of the sick role thus are conditional in a highly important sense. It is a relative legitimation so long as he is in this unfortunate state which both he and alter hope he can get out of as expeditiously as possible.

Finally, the fourth closely related element is the obligation—in proportion to the severity of the condition, of course—to seek *technically competent* help, namely, in the most usual case, that of a physician and to *cooperate* with him in the process of trying to get well. It is here, of course, that the role of the sick person as patient becomes articulated with that of the physician in a complementary role structure.

*   *   *

By the same institutional definition the sick person is not, of course, competent to help himself, or what he can do is, except for trivial illness, not adequate. But in our culture there is a special definition of the kind of help he needs, namely, professional, technically competent help. The nature of this help imposes a further disability or handicap upon him. He is not only generally not in a position to do what needs to be done, but he does not "know" what needs to be done or how to do it. It is not merely that he, being bedridden, cannot go down to the drug store to get what is needed, but that he would, even if well, not be qualified to do what is needed, and to judge what needs to be done. There is, that is to say, a "communication gap."

*   *   *

This disqualification is, of course, not absolute. Laymen do know something in the field, and have some objective bases of judgment. But the evidence is overwhelming that this knowledge is highly limited and that most laymen *think* they know more, and have better bases of judgment than is actually the case. . . .

*   *   *

[T]he situation of illness very generally presents the patient and those close to him with complex problems of emotional adjustment. It is, that is to say, a situation of strain. Even if there is no question of a "psychic" factor in his condition, suffering, helplessness, disablement and the risk of death, or sometimes its certainty, constitute fundamental disturbances of the expectations by which men live. They cannot in general be emotionally "accepted" without the accompaniments of strain with which we are familiar and hence without difficult adjustments unless the patient happens to find positive satisfactions in them, in which case there is also a social problem. The significance of this emotional factor is magnified and complicated insofar as defensive and adjustive mechanisms are deeply involved in the pathological condition itself.

The range of possible complexities in this sphere is very great. The problems are, however, structured by the nature of the situation in certain relatively definite ways. Perhaps the most definite point is that for the "normal" person illness, the more so the greater its severity, constitutes a frustration of expectancies of his normal life pattern. He is cut off from his normal spheres of activity and many of his normal enjoyments. He is often humiliated by his incapacity to function normally. His social relationships are disrupted to a greater or a less degree. He may have to bear discomfort or pain which is hard to bear, and he may have to face serious alterations of his prospects for the future, in the extreme but by no means uncommon case the termination of his life.

*   *   *

. . . There are two particularly important broad consequences of the features of the situation of the sick person for the problem of the institutional structuring of medical practice. One is that the combination of helplessness, lack of technical competence, and emotional disturbance makes him a peculiarly vulnerable object for exploitation. It may be said that the exploitation of the helpless sick is "unthinkable." That happens to be a very strong sentiment in our society, but for the sociologist the existence of this sentiment or that of other mechanisms for the prevention of exploitation must not be taken for granted. There is in fact a very real problem of how, in such a situation, the very possible exploitation is at least minimized.

The other general point is the related one that the situation of the patient is such as to make a high level of rationality of judgment peculiarly difficult. He is therefore open to, and peculiarly liable to, a whole series of ir- and non-rational beliefs and practices. The world over the rational approach to health through applied science is, as we have noted, the exception rather than the rule, and in our society there is, even today, a very large volume of "superstition" and other non- or irrational beliefs and practices in the health field. This is not to say that the medical profession either has a monopoly of rational knowledge and techniques, or is free of the other type of elements, but the volume of such phenomena outside the framework of regular medical practice is a rough measure of this factor. This set of facts then makes problematical the degree to which the treatment of health problems by applied science has in fact come to be possible. It can by no means be taken for granted as the course which "reasonable men," i.e., the normal citizen of our society will "naturally" adopt.

*   *   *

The role of the physician centers on his responsibility for the welfare of the patient in the sense of facilitating his recovery from illness to the best of the physician's ability. In meeting this responsibility he is expected to acquire and use high technical competence in "medical science" and the techniques based upon it. The first question to ask about his situation, therefore, concerns the relation of these technical tools to the tasks he is called upon to perform and the responsibilities he is expected to live up to.

In a certain proportion of cases the doctor has what may be called a perfectly straightforward technological job. His knowledge and skill give him quite adequate tools for accomplishment of his ends; it is only necessary to exercise sufficient patience, and to work steadily and competently at the task. This would, it is true, leave the "penumbra" of emotional reactions of patients and their families for him to deal with, and his own emotional reactions to such things as severe suffering and imminence of death might well pose certain problems of emotional adjustment to him. But with these qualifications it would be much like any other high level technical job.

But in common with some and not other technical jobs there is in this case a shading off into cases with respect to which knowledge, skill and resources are not adequate, with hard, competent work, to solve the problem. There are two main aspects to this inadequacy. On the one hand there are cases, a good many of them, where the upshot of a competent diagnosis is to expose a condition which is known, in the given state of medical knowledge and technique, to be essentially uncontrollable. This is true both in the individual case and generally. Though there is a fundamental relationship between knowledge and control, this is a general and not a point-for-point relationship. Optimistic biases are very general and fundamental in human social orientations, perhaps particularly in our society and certainly in relation to health. It is, therefore, very common that the initial effect of a given advance in knowledge is to demonstrate the impossibility of controlling things which were thought to be readily controllable, to expose unfavorable factors in the situation which were not previously appreciated, and to show the fruitlessness of control measures in which people had previously had faith.

*   *   *

The absolute limits of the physician's control—which of course are relative to the state of medical science at the time and his own assimilation of it—are not the only source of frustration and strain. Within these limits there is a very important area of uncertainty. As in so many practical situations, some of the factors bearing on this one may be well understood, but others are not. The exact relation of the known to the unknown elements cannot be determined; the unknown may operate at any time to invalidate expectations built up on analysis of the known. Sometimes it may be known *that* certain factors operate significantly, but it is unpredictable whether, when and how they will operate in the particular case. Sometimes virtually nothing is known of these factors, only that the best laid plans mysteriously go wrong. In general the line between the spontaneous forces tending to recovery—what used to be called the *vis medicatrix naturae*—and the effects of the physician's "intervention" is impossible to draw with precision in a very large proportion of cases.

*   *   *

The primary definition of the physician's responsibility is to "do everything possible" to forward the complete, early and painless recovery of his patients. The general effect of the existence of large factors of known impossibility and of uncertainty in the situation with which he has to cope is to impose strain upon him, to make it more difficult for him to have a "purely rational" orientation to his job than if his orientation were such as to guarantee success with competent work. This is true of his own orientation without taking account of reciprocal interactions with his patients and their intimates.

But the function of "doing everything possible" is institutionalized in terms of expectations, and these expectations are most vividly and immediately embodied, besides in the physician's own attitude system, in the attitudes of precisely this group of people. But compared to most such groups their involvement is, because of the considerations analyzed above, peculiarly intensive, immediate, and likely to contain elements of emotional disturbance which are by definition, tendencies to deviant behavior. Hence the elements of strain on the physician by virtue of these impossibility and uncertainty components of his situation are particularly great. Non- and irrational mechanisms [are] prominent in the reactions of sick people to their situations, and those of their families. In spite of the discipline of his scientific training and competence, it would be strange if, in view of the situation, physicians as a group were altogether exempted from corresponding tendencies. In fact that magic frequently appears in situations of uncertainty is suggestive. [I]t is clear from the above that quite apart from the operation of so-called psychic factors in the disease process itself, the strains existing on *both* sides of a doctor-patient relationship are such that we must expect to find, not merely institutionalization of the roles, but special mechanisms of social control in operation.

Factors of impossibility, and uncertainty in situations where there is a strong emotional interest in success, are common in many other fields of applied science—the military field is an outstandingly important example. There are, however, certain other features of the situation of the physician which are not common to many other fields which share those so far discussed. The engineer, for example, deals primarily with non-human impersonal materials which do not have "emotional" reactions to what he does with them. But the physician deals with human beings, and does so in situations which often involve "intimacies," that is, in contexts which are strongly charged with emotional and expressively symbolic significance, and which are often considered peculiarly "private" to the individual himself, or to especially intimate relations with others.

* * *

Modern developments in psychology, particularly psychoanalysis, have made us aware that in addition to resistances to access to the body, and to confidential information, anyone taking a role like that of the physician toward his patients is exposed to another sort of situational adjustment problem. That is, through processes which are mostly unconscious the physician tends to acquire various types of projective significance as a person which may not be directly relevant to his specifically technical functions, though they may become of the first importance in connection with psychotherapy. The generally accepted name for this phenomenon in psychiatric circles is "transference," the attribution to the physician of significances to the patient which are not "appropriate" in the realistic situation, but which derive from the psychological needs of the patient. For understandable reasons a particularly important class of these involves the attributes of parental roles as experienced by the patient in childhood. . . .

If all these factors be taken together it becomes clear that, in ways which are not true of most other professional functions, the situation of medical practice is such as inevitably to "involve" the physician in the psychologically significant "private" affairs of his patients. Some of these may not otherwise be accessible to others in any ordinary situation, others only in the context of specifically intimate and personal relationships. What the relation of the physician's role to these other relationships is to be, is one of the principal functional problems which underlie the structuring of his professional role.

* * *

[T]he sick person is peculiarly vulnerable to exploitation and at the same time peculiarly handicapped in arriving at a rationally objective appraisal of his situation. In addition, the physician is a technically competent person whose competence and specific judgments and measures cannot be competently judged by the layman. The latter must therefore take these judgments and measures "on authority." But in this type case there is no system of coercive sanctions to back up this authority. All the physician can say to the patient who refuses to heed his advice is "well, it's your own funeral"—which it may be literally. All this of course is true of a situation which includes the potential resistances which have been discussed above.

These different factors seem to indicate that the situation is such that it would be particularly difficult to implement the pattern of the business world, where each party to the situation is expected to be oriented to the rational pursuit of his own self-interests, and where there is an approach to the idea of "caveat emptor." In a broad sense it is surely clear that society would not tolerate the privileges which have been vested in the medical profession on such terms. The protection of the patient against the exploitation of his helplessness, his technical incompetence and his irrationality thus constitutes the most obvious functional significance of the pattern. In this whole connection it is noteworthy how strongly the main reliance for control is placed on "informal" mechanisms. The law of the state includes severe penalties for "malpractice" and medical associations have relatively elaborate disciplinary procedures, but these quite definitely are not the principal mechanisms which operate to ensure the control of self-orientation tendencies. . . .

Here it may be noted that the collectivity-orientation of the physician is protected by a series of symbolically significant practices which serve to differentiate him sharply from the businessman. He cannot advertise—he can only modestly announce by his "shingle" and the use of his M.D. in telephone directories and classified sections, that he is available to provide medical service. He cannot bargain over fees with his patients—a "take it or leave it" attitude is enjoined upon him. He cannot refuse patients on the ground that they are poor "credit risks." He is given the privilege of charging according to the "sliding scale," that is, in proportion to the income of the patient or his family—a drastic difference from the usual pricing mechanism of the business world. The general picture is one of sharp segregation from the market and price practices of the business world, in ways which for the most part cut off the physician from many immediate opportunities for financial gain which are treated as legitimately open to the businessman. . . .

[T]he definition in terms of collectivity-orientation is expected to be reciprocal. The most usual formulation for this is that the patient is expected to "have confidence" in his physician and, if this confidence breaks down, to seek another physician.

This may be interpreted to mean that the relationship is expected to be one of mutual "trust," of the belief that the physician is trying his best to help the patient and that conversely the patient is "cooperating" with him to the best of his ability. It is significant for instance that this constitutes a reinforcement of one of the principal institutional features of the sick role, the expectation of a desire to get well. It makes the patient, in a special sense, responsible to his physician. But more generally, . . . collectivity-orientation is involved in all cases of institutionalized authority, that is authority is an attribute of a status in a collectivity. In a very special and informal sense the doctor-patient relationship has to be one involving an element of authority—we often speak of "doctor's orders." This authority cannot be legitimized without reciprocal collectivity-orientation in the relationship. To the doctor's obligation to use his authority "responsibly" in the interest of the patient, corresponds the patient's obligation faithfully to accept the implications of the fact that he is "Dr. X's patient" and so long as he remains in that status must "do his part" in the common enterprise. He is free, of course, to terminate the relationship at any time. But the essential point is the sharp line which tends to be drawn between being X's patient, and no longer being in that position. In the ideal type of commercial relationship one is not A's customer to the exclusion of other sources of supply for the same needs.

* * *

NOTES

NOTE 1.

RENÉE C. FOX
EXPERIMENT PERILOUS*

* * *

[P]hysicians are confronted with two basic types of uncertainty. One of these derives from limitations in the current state of medical knowledge. There are many questions to which no physician, however well trained, can yet provide answers. The second type of uncertainty results from incomplete or imperfect mastery of available knowledge. No one can have at his command all the information, lore, and skills of modern medicine.

In turn, these forms of uncertainty to which all physicians are subject are connected with another set of problems which they also inevitably face: problems of therapeutic limitation. Since the knowledge and skills of the physician are not always adequate, there are many times when his most vigorous efforts to understand illness and to rectify its consequences are of little or no avail.

What the physician *can* do to help a patient, then, is often limited. What he *ought* to do is frequently not clear. And the consequences of his clinical actions cannot always be accurately predicted. Yet, in the face of these uncertainties and limitations, the physician is expected to institute measures which will facilitate the diagnosis and treatment of the problems the patient presents.

Largely because what the physician decides to do (and not to do) on behalf of a patient is generally based on less than perfect knowledge, it has been said that "in a sense [his] every clinical act is an investigation," and that "medical experimentation on human beings, in its broadest meaning and for the good of the individual patient, takes place continually in every doctor's office."

The rapidity with which new diagnostic and therapeutic procedures and new drugs have been appearing in the last few swiftly moving decades is also responsible for the fact that the practicing physician is often cast in the role of experimenter. It is hard for the physician simply to keep abreast of these developments, and even more difficult for him to appraise them. The available reports about their benefits and dangers are tentative and far from consistent, since only gradually, and to a considerable extent on the basis of a trial-and-error empiricism, can relatively definitive judgments about a new procedure or drug be reached. Thus, although typically, the physician in practice has published literature and the informally transmitted opinions and experiences of colleagues to inform him about the properties of new technics and drugs, the degree of uncertainty about their benefits, limitations and hazards which still remain is often large enough to warrant calling "experimental" some of the clinical trials he conducts on patients. Before he carries out such trials, the practicing physician, like the research physician, has the problem of trying to determine whether the dangers of the contemplated procedure or drug are sufficiently less than the hazards of the patient's disease, and its potential benefits sufficiently greater than both, to justify asking the patient to undergo it. If they seem to be, and he therefore decides to carry out such a procedure on a patient or administer such a drug, the practicing physician, like the clinical investigator, sometimes finds himself in a situation where the measures he employed fail to benefit the patient clinically, or have negative effects on him. Thus, physicians in practice, as well as research physicians, experience some of the uncertainties, limitations, moral ambiguities, and untoward consequences connected with the application of advanced medical knowledge and techniques to the medical problems of patients.

Not only medicine, of course, but all scientific activity has social consequences, harmful as well as beneficent. However technical or abstract the experiments which biological and physical scientists conduct in their laboratories and field stations may seem, ultimately they may affect the lives of men and women in powerful ways—both for good and for evil. The "pure" scientist, however, is in several respects further removed and better insulated from the ultimate outcome of his actions than the physician is. On the whole, his attention is confined to the test tube and microscope; his research is conducted on lifeless matter or on animals; and the social implications of what he does are for the most part indirect and long-range.

The special difficulty of the physician—the problem that distinguishes him from most other scientists, be they in the fields of pure or applied science—is that the material on which he works is the disease-stricken human being. Thus, the decisions the physician makes, the procedures he carries out, the drugs he prescribes have a proximate, visible, flesh-and-blood impact on the patients under his care. To a significant extent, whether patients get better, get worse, or whether their conditions remain stubbornly fixed is contingent upon what the physician is or is not able to do for them. Because the welfare of the patient is this directly associated with his actions, the human consequences of his uncertainty, limitation, and fallibility are more apparent to the physician than to most other scientists. It is harder for him to forget or systematically ignore the fact that what he does as a scientist makes an impact on people. Furthermore, the people whom he affects are not remote, anonymous entities. They are his patients: the individuals whom he sees, to whom he talks, and on whom he

carries out various procedures, in his office, in their homes and in the hospital.

* * *

NOTE 2.

FRED DAVIS
UNCERTAINTY IN MEDICAL PROGNOSIS, CLINICAL AND FUNCTIONAL*

Medical sociology is indebted to Talcott Parsons for having called attention to the important influence of uncertainty on the relationship between doctor and patient in the treatment of illness and disease. This is described as a primary source of strain in the physician's role, not only because clinically it so often obscures and vitiates definitive diagnoses and prognoses, but also because in an optimistic and solution-demanding culture such as ours it poses serious and delicate problems in the communicating of the unknown and the problematic to the patient and his family . . . As a ready-made explanation of a disturbing element in the relationship between doctor and patient, the concept—uncertainty—stands in danger of being applied in a catch-all fashion whenever . . . communication from doctor to patient is characterized by duplicity, evasion, or other forms of strain. That other factors, having relatively little to do with uncertainty, can also systematically generate strain in the relationship may unfortunately be ignored because of the disposition to subsume phenomena under preexistent categories.

The present paper examines the scope and significance of uncertainty as evidenced in the treatment of a particular disease. Specifically, it seeks to distinguish between "real" uncertainty as a clinical and scientific phenomenon and the uses to which uncertainty—real or pretended "functional" uncertainty—lends itself in the management of patients and their families by hospital physicians and other treatment personnel. . . .

The disease in question is paralytic poliomyelitis, and the subjects are fourteen Baltimore families, in each of which a young child had contracted the disease. These were studied longitudinally over a two-year period. . . .

* * *

[O]ne must assume that the doctor's knowledge of the disease and its physical effects is

---

* 66 *American Journal of Sociology* 41–47 (1960). Reprinted by permission.

more accurate, comprehensive, and profound than that of the parents. The problem, then, could be stated: How much information was communicated to the parents? How was it communicated? And what consequences did this communication have on the parents' expectations of the child's illness and prospects for recovery? And, since in paralytic poliomyelitis (as in many other diseases and illnesses) uncertainty does affect the making of diagnoses and prognoses, an attempt was made to assess the scope, significance, and duration of uncertainty for the doctor. This then provided some basis for inferring the extent to which the parents' knowledge and expectations, or lack thereof, could also be attributed ultimately to uncertainty.

*   *   *

[T]he pathological course of paralytic poliomyelitis is such that, during the first weeks following onset, it is difficult in most cases for even the most skilled diagnostician to make anything like a definite prognosis of probable residual impairment and functional disability. . . .

During this initial period of the child's hospitalization, therefore, the physician is hardly ever able to tell the parents anything definite about the child's prospects of regaining lost muscular function. In view of the very real uncertainty, to attempt to do so would indeed be hazardous. To the parents' insistent questions, "How will he come out of it?" "Will he have to wear a brace?" "Will his walk be normal?" and so on, the invariable response of treatment personnel was that they did not know and that only time would tell. Thus during these first weeks the parents came to adopt a longer time perspective and more qualified outlook than they had to begin with.

By about the sixth week to the third month following onset of the disease, however, the orthopedist and physiotherapist are in position to make reasonably sound prognoses of the amount and type of residual handicap. This is done on the basis of periodic muscle examinations from which the amount and rate of return of affected muscular capacity is plotted. . . .

*   *   *

By this time, therefore, the element of clinical uncertainty regarding outcome, so conspicuously present when the child is first stricken, is greatly reduced for the physician, if not al-

together eliminated.[7] Was there then a commensurate gain in the parents' understanding of the child's condition after this six-week to three-month period had passed? Did they then, as did the doctors, come to view certain outcomes as highly probable and others as improbable?

[T]he answer to these questions is that, except for one case in which the muscle check pointed clearly to full recovery, the parents were neither told nor explicitly prepared by the treatment personnel to expect an outcome significantly different from that which they understandably hoped for, namely, a complete and natural recovery for the child. This does not imply that the doctors issued falsely optimistic prognoses or that, through indirection and other subtleties, they sought to encourage the parents to expect more by way of recovery than was possible. Rather, what typically transpired was that the parents were kept in the dark. The doctors' answers to their questions were couched for the most part in such hedging, evasive, or unintelligibly technical terms as to cause them, from many such contacts, to expect a more favorable recovery than could be justified by the facts then known. As one treatment-staff member put it, "We try not to tell them too much. It's better if they find out for themselves in a natural sort of way."

Indeed, it was disheartening to note how, for many of the parents, "the natural way" consisted of a painfully slow and prolonged dwindling of expectations for a complete and natural recovery. This is ironical when one considers that as early as two to three months following onset the doctors and physiotherapists were able to tell members of the research team with considerable confidence that one child would require bracing for an indefinite period; that another would never walk with a normal gait; that a third would require a bone-fusion operation before he would be able to hold himself erect;

---

[7] As in nearly all applied fields of endeavor, medicine necessarily deals in probabilities rather than absolutes. Hence some measure of uncertainty is always present, the crucial question being the matter of degree and not the mere presence. Admittedly, no hard-and-fast lines can be drawn at the point at which uncertainty acquires therapeutic significance; but, if the concept is to have any analytical value at all, it cannot be applied to all instances of illness in which it is possible to concede the existence of some degree of uncertainty, however slight. If this were done, there would not be an instance to which it did not apply.

and so on. By contrast, the parents of these children came to know these prognoses much later, if at all. And even then their understanding of them was in most instances partial and subject to considerable distortion.

But what is of special interest here is the way in which uncertainty, a *real* factor in the early diagnosis and treatment of the paralyzed child, came more and more to serve the purely managerial ends of the treatment personnel in their interaction with parents. Long after the doctor himself was no longer in doubt about the outcome, the perpetuation of uncertainty in doctor-to-family communication, although perhaps neither premeditated nor intended, can nonetheless best be understood in terms of its functions in the treatment system. These are several, and closely connected.

Foremost is the way in which the pretense of uncertainty as to outcome serves to reduce materially the expenditure of additional time, effort, and involvement which a frank and straightforward prognosis to the family might entail. The doctor implicitly recognizes that, were he to tell the family that the child would remain crippled or otherwise impaired to some significant extent, he would easily become embroiled in much more than a simple, factual medical prognosis. Presenting so unwelcome a prospect is bound to meet with a strong—and, according to many of the treatment personnel, "unmanageable"—emotional reaction from parents. . . . Moreover, to the extent to which the doctor feels some professional compunction to so inform the parents, the bustling, time-conscious work milieu of the hospital supports him in the convenient rationalization that, even were he to take the trouble, the family could not or would not understand what he had to tell them anyway. Therefore, in hedging, being evasive, equivocating, and cutting short his contact with the parents, the doctor was able to avoid "scenes" with them and having to explain to and comfort them, tasks, at least in the hospital, often viewed as onerous and time-consuming.

*   *   *

[I]t must in fairness be recognized that there is still little agreement within medical circles on what practice should be in these circumstances. (The perennial debate on whether a patient and his family should be told that he is dying of cancer, and when and how much they should be told, is an extreme though highly relevant case in point.) And perhaps the easiest

recourse of the hospital practitioner—who, organizationally, is better barricaded and further removed from the family than, for example, the neighborhood physician—is to avoid it altogether.

Clearly, then, clinical uncertainty is not responsible for all that is not communicated to the patient and his. family. Other factors, interests, and circumstances intrude in the rendering of medical prognoses, with the result that what the patient is told is uncertain and problematic may often not be so at all. And, conversely, what he is made to feel is quite certain may actually be highly uncertain. . . .

*   *   *

NOTE 3.

WISCONSIN BAR ASSOCIATION
INTERVIEWING CLIENTS*

Most lawyers spend too much time in interviewing clients. This is very wasteful and costly to the lawyer. The use of time records will tend to regulate this difficulty. Also, the use of checklists in interviews will help to prevent drawn-out conferences with clients.

The following items will prove helpful in client interviews:

1. Develop and use definite systems for keeping interview time at a minimum. For example, upon signal, the secretary can interrupt the interview with a message requiring the lawyer's attention. Mainly, however, limitation of interview time is a matter of sticking firmly to the matter at hand and not letting the interview wander to a point where the client is giving the advice and opinion rather than receiving it.

2. Be affable and polite. Clients respond to friendly treatment and a smile.

3. Get at the client's problem immediately and stick to it. Don't bother to explain the reasoning processes by which you arrive at your advice. The client expects you to be an expert. This not only prolongs the interview, but generally confuses the client. The client will feel better and more secure if told in simple straightforward language what to do and how to do it, without an explanation of *how* you reached your conclusions.

4. Do something for your client, if possible. Perhaps a quick telephone call can be made or and on-the-spot letter dictated. A lawyer is trained in these matters and can do them easily.

---

* R.M.–11 (Sept. 11, 1959). Reprinted by permission of the Wisconsin Bar Association.

Many times a lawyer can do in minutes a job which would require hours of time and effort of the client.

5. Take every opportunity to explain in simple language the functions of various courts and the basic rules of conduct and procedure in the courts. If the client understands that not all cases are matters for long, formal jury trials, he will approach the law with less fear and trembling. The client should know that most legal matters never result in trial and that most court procedures are rather informal in nature. It is natural for persons to be more at ease when dealing with matters with which they have some basic knowledge. Therefore, for the client's peace of mind, he should be made familiar with the basic workings of the court in which his matter is being handled and of his own role in the proceedings if he is required to make an appearance in court.

6. Quit when you're ahead. When you have reached the conclusion of the conference, break it off clearly. Otherwise it will drag on as new themes and situations develop. Tactfully but clearly wind up the conference and usher the client out.

c.
Raymond S. Duff and August B. Hollingshead Sickness and Society*

*   *   *

When an individual becomes a patient he is confronted with the necessity of dealing with a physician or physicians. The association brought into existence by the mutual interest of the patient and his physician in the illness—the doctor-patient relationship—is symbolized by *sponsorship*, the method through which the physician assumes responsibility and discharges obligations to care for the patient. Sponsorship is believed to have its roots in the mutual images and expectations of patients and physicians. Ideally, the doctor-patient relationship revolves around only the sick or troubled person who is a client (patient) and the professional person (physician) whom he consults. Crucial decisions regarding diagnosis and treatment of disease should not be influenced by extraneous matters. However, physicians and patients are inextricably parts of the

society to which both belong. The broader social contexts of the patient and his family, the physician and his family, the hospital, insurance companies, the institutions of government, religion, education, and so on are related in one way or another with the interactions that take place between physicians and patients. The sick person looks to the physician for advice and help. The physician, in performing his professional role, is concerned directly with the problem the patient brings to him and indirectly with his own interests: his practice, possibly learning or research, or some combination of these pursuits. To a certain extent, therefore, each partner in this relationship must look after his own interests. The patient has an illness: the physician has a career. Each partner must make tentative judgments about the other. The patient accepts the competence of the physician to diagnose and treat his problem, and the physician accepts the sponsorship of the patient.

Reciprocal expectations between patient and physician were based upon the respective images which patients and physicians had of each other. Ward patients recognized their low status and expected to be used as teaching subjects and, to some extent, as research material. The doctors reciprocated these expectations and offered little apology since these patients, though being charged for their hospital services were not being billed for their medical care.[*] The semiprivate and private patients did not expect to be used as research subjects. Furthermore, the semiprivate and private patients were fully aware that they had physician sponsors who were responsible to them for the diagnosis and treatment of, and information, about their diseases. They expected to pay their physicians directly

---

[*] Persons who were housed on the ward accommodations seldom realized initially that they had to endure the indignities of ward treatment in order to benefit from the advances of medical technology which were probably developed in the first place on some hospital ward. They resented being passed over by powerful professors in the School of Medicine who moved around them on the wards, treated them as clinical material, and "talked their Latin" as they discussed the case with the medical students and the house staff in front of the patients. These patients and their families knew that a gulf of social distance separated them from the important figures inside and outside the hospital. They did not fully understand what went on around them, but they had an awareness of their ignorance and they were humiliated at the treatment they had to endure to get medical attention [p. 119].

---

* New York: Harper & Row 124–134, 140–145 (1968). Copyright © 1968 by Raymond S. Duff and August B. Hollingshead. Reprinted by permission of Harper & Row, Publishers, Inc.

for the personal services they had received from them.

*   *   *

Committee Sponsorship

One of the resident physicians used the term "committee doctor" when describing the physician-patient relationship in the ward accommodations. This gave us our cue for the label used here. *Committee sponsorship* was found to apply to all ward patients and to no others. . . . The patient in committee sponsorship had no single continuing doctor on whom he could depend. Care of the patient was vested in the always-present and ever-changing committee whose members—doctors at the house-staff and medical-student levels—rotated within the institution during their training years and then, in most instances, left it. These physicians and students identified professionally with the School of Medicine and looked to it primarily for aid in the development of their careers. They were most impressed and influenced by teachers and researchers who necessarily had little time for patient care and whose major interest was new knowledge through research. Learning was the overriding consideration.

In the School of Medicine, diseases were the necessary "clinical material" for the teaching and research program. In a conference room in the Medical Center, used for teaching students and house officers, a sign posted above a blackboard admonishes: "Think Pathology!" The hospital was the place in which the students and house officers saw patients. The patient was the vehicle for the study of disease. To be sure, these young physicians realized that the problems of patients were great; they realized the chief task of a physician is to treat disease, but they were students who had to learn how to become physicians before they could treat people. When we asked them about the patients, they usually knew the nature of the patient's disease and something about his ongoing treatment but they knew little about the patients as human beings; thus, our questions embarrassed them. Some told us we were choosing the less ill patients who required less time to care for or that they had been assigned to the patient in question for only a few days and had had little contact with him. One intern was more precise in his views; he ended a rather nonproductive interview with this comment: "I cannot answer your questions. You're interested in patients. I'm interested in the disease in the body in the bed."

*   *   *

Mrs. O'Pell, a 56-year-old woman of Irish birth, was selected to illustrate some facets of committee sponsorship. Mrs. O'Pell had been in reasonably good health most of her life except for her nervousness and hypochondriacal tendencies. She did not trust the general practitioners, whom she saw for these complaints, to deal with her more complicated problems. For these she went to the clinic. She considered the clinic and ward accommodations as places where poor people get care. She viewed the doctors as being much above and distant from her, and she communicated poorly with them; they responded in general by ignoring her as a person.

One week prior to her admission she had some teeth extracted under general anesthesia in this hospital. The day following the procedure, she developed pains in her chest and a sore throat. She visited the Emergency Room where some X rays were taken and "pain killers" prescribed. Still feeling ill the next day, she came again to the Emergency Room and was sent to the medical clinic for further examinations. She was sent home again although the chest pain was not alleviated. She returned the following day to the medical clinic and decided to "sit them out". . . . Finally, a doctor did see her and decided to admit her to the hospital.

Up to this point, Mrs. O'Pell had been seen by two dentists, four medical students, two interns, and one assistant resident, all of whom she viewed as inexperienced students. She attributed her illness to improper anesthesia and poor dental technique of a "young student, that Puerto Rican dentist." When she was admitted to the hospital she was seen by three more members of the committee—a medical student, an intern, and an assistant resident. The medical student spent more time with her than the others so she felt that he was her physician more than anyone else. When he left for the weekend she was worried, but she assumed that he had left orders to be carried out in his absence. The student, however, spent little time with her, knew nothing about her family, and felt he did not understand her situation well. The family, while visiting and through telephone calls to the hospital, tried to get information by seeking a doctor to answer their questions. They never succeeded in finding a doctor who would listen to them.

Mrs. O'Pell realized the doctors were teaching one another and learning on her. In her opinion the pelvic examination was "quite a production." The doctors talked to one another but not to her. Three thoracenteses were done in just this way—one doctor teaching another. She said that one doctor seemed to be especially knowledgeable about "needles," while the other one seemed to know more about examining her. . . .

Shortly after her admission to the hospital, the resident in radiology concluded from his study of the X ray that the problem was pulmonary embolus. The intern reported this diagnosis to Mrs. O'Pell explaining that a clot which had probably formed in her leg had broken off and lodged in her lungs. Although she did not tell the doctors, she was extremely frightened by this diagnosis because a close friend had died suddenly and unexpectedly of this condition.

After Mrs. O'Pell was in the hospital two days, the attending physician (a faculty member in the School of Medicine), who was introduced to her as an outstanding international authority on diseases of her kind, visited her. He examined her briefly, listened to her history, and informed her that the doctors were doing the "right things" for her. He left before Mrs. O'Pell could ask him any questions. When she asked the medical students and the intern again what her diagnosis really was, they said she had an embolus and that the attending physician concurred with their diagnosis and treatment. In reality, the attending physician thought the cause of the illness was not embolus but aspiration during the dental extraction while under general anesthesia.

*   *   *

After discharge from the hospital, Mrs. O'Pell consulted a general practitioner for his interpretation of the cause of her illness. He examined her legs carefully, found no evidence of phlebitis, and said that embolization probably did not account for the illness. This was not reassuring to Mrs. O'Pell because, although she appreciated his interest in her, she discounted his competence. She then saw another physician who told her that she was very lucky that the clot had struck her lungs instead of her heart or her brain because then she would not have survived. Thinking of illness and death, Mrs. O'Pell decided to visit Ireland, the land of her birth, while she was still able to travel. . . .

From the viewpoint of the doctors, Mrs. O'Pell was a model patient, cooperative and forbearing. She made no demands and seemed to accept without any major challenge their explanation of her illness. She responded dramatically to treatment which was most gratifying to all, and finally she was discharged as "cured" from the medical clinic. The doctors felt that they had learned much while practicing splendid medicine. They knew nothing of Mrs. O'Pell's doubts and fears about her illness. Although the pulmonary disease was treated successfully regardless of its nature, the management of this patient did involve some risks of treatment (anticoagulant therapy) which she almost certainly did not require and which was costly to her and her family. The management by the physicians had the effect of increasing the severity of her hypochondriasis; she went to more doctors, incurring higher costs, and her fears were never successfully relieved.

*   *   *

We found many handicaps to a cooperative relationship between doctors and patients in the committee sponsorship. The patients viewed themselves as uneducated and incapable of understanding the explanations of the professionals; patients often referred to the doctors "talking among themselves" and using "their Latin" or "their Greek." Most patients believed the doctors withheld information from them. Several patients told us: "Doctors have their secrets." The patients were embarrassed by their ignorance and remained silent to avoid exposure. Thus, they failed to put their questions to the doctors although they asked such questions of family members, our data collectors, and sometimes the nurses if the latter would listen. (They did not often question the nurses, however, because they thought the nurses gave them little encouragement and were probably incapable of answering them.)

These patients lacked the standing to make demands upon their physicians. They expected to be cared for by interns and medical students, yet they were resentful of being "pushed around" and ignored as individuals. Some realized that inconvenience, discomfort, and at times higher costs for decisions made in the interest of teaching and research, rather than in the interest of the patient, were necessary in order for them to get the benefits of service within the ward accommodations.

*   *   *

The unsatisfactory interpersonal relationships between sick patients and student physicians in committee sponsorship had pervasive consequences. Sometimes diagnoses were less than adequate. Patients were poorly informed and often confused. Even if the treatment was successful, the patients resented the attitudes of the hospital staff: student physicians, nurses, nursing students, aides, and so on. When the treatment was not successful, as was often the case among these very sick persons, their suspicions increased sharply. Weakened and frightened, they had to accept what was offered to them; there was almost no alternative choice. Both sponsor and patient recognized the distance between them; neither was comfortable with it, but only the patient had to endure it without hope for ameliorative change.

In summary, interest in the patient as a human being, though present occasionally in exemplary ways, could not be sustained when there was so little in common between the providers and recipients of service and when the patient was in no position to pay for the physician's time and hence make demands upon him. Interest in the disease, lack of interest in the patient, and difficulty in communication characterized the ward accommodation in which the formal learning of medical students, house officers, and senior physicians took place. The impact of these influences was noted for all ward patients.

Semicommittee Sponsorship

Semicommittee sponsorship involved a private physician nominally, but a large segment of responsibility for the diagnosis and treatment of the disease, as well as communication with the patient, was assumed by house officers. The private physician admitted the patient to the hospital and may have influenced the diagnostic and treatment choices of the timing of discharge, but he was not close to the patient or his care. The patients, the house staff, and the private physicians recognized this pattern of sponsorship. Private physicians in semicommittee sponsorship were often general practitioners, very busy internists, or surgeons who spent little time with their patients. These physicians often exhibited a lesser competence in diagnosis and treatment procedures, particularly on the medical service, than others described in the casual and committed sponsorships.

*   *   *

Committed Sponsorship

Committed sponsorship involved a determined assumption of responsibility for the patient by the physician. The physician's interest in the patient extended beyond his interest in the disease. These patients were of higher social sta-

tus and some of them treated their physicians as subordinates. The physicians showed their interest and assumed responsibility accordingly. . . .

Dr. Sail, a successful practitioner of medicine, is an example of the optimal complex of medical and social relations characteristic of committed sponsorship. He developed a hernia and was admitted by a surgeon for treatment. These two physicians had dealt with each other professionally about patients of mutual interest and had met frequently on social occasions, but they were not close friends. Dr. Sail was admitted at his convenience and placed on the operating schedule so he would get fresh staff and the first choice of anesthesiologists. The surgeon saw to it that the admissions office, the floor nurses, the house staff, the operating room staff, and the anesthesiologists were informed of the admission of his special patient. Subsequent to the operation, the surgeon visited him frequently in his room, explained all treatments that were given, and supervised them diligently. Dr. Sail was given more attention than he wanted or needed by the nurses on the floor as well as by private-duty nurses caring for other patients. (These nurses either had been his patients or had cared for his patients at another time.) Mrs. Sail was kept informed of the progress of the surgery and the course of her husband's treatment. Dr. Sail's recovery was rapid and uneventful.

*   *   *

Although committed sponsorship was almost always dictated and enjoyed by the patients, it was not always an enlightened relationship which served the patients' best health interests. For example, Mrs. Leadon was an anxious, emotionally unstable individual who had sought out the services of many physicians. In the year prior to her admission she managed to persuade the physicians to do a gastrointestinal series, two breast biopsies, and several examinations. One physician who saw her reported that her cysts were benign and, although they should be checked occasionally for any suspicious changes, they should be left alone. She was dissatisfied with his evaluation and went to see a doctor who had removed a breast cancer for a friend of hers in the recent past. She cultivated the doctor and he seemed to enjoy her company. He admitted her to the hospital for still another biopsy.

In her shopping for physicians, Mrs. Leadon revealed enough about herself to indicate that she needed medical care but never enough so that the physicians became aware that her behavior was a manifestation of an emotional disturbance. She enjoyed the physicians' examinations and discussed them freely. She told us one physician was a friend who "lives near by and does not examine me internally because he knows me too well and gets embarrassed." Mrs. Leadon enjoyed being seductive with her friends and particularly with her physicians. She not only demanded examinations but further operations. In the hospital her performance was childlike, exhibitionistic, and seductive. Although she made the most of her opportunity to perform, she was frightened of the anesthesia and surgery. She felt, however, that it was a necessary price she had to pay to be relieved, even temporarily, from the continuous adversities of her troubled life at home. The physician, in admitting her to the hospital, provided removal from the troubled home atmosphere, interest as a physician and a male, and dramatic validation of the sickness as evidenced by further surgery.

The surgical resident who saw Mrs. Leadon at admission was unaware of any of this background. He casually commented that he did not think another breast biopsy was really necessary at that time. Mrs. Leadon was infuriated; she told him to leave her room and not return. Meanwhile, her surgeon, a private practitioner, came in daily, held hands with her for a few minutes, and listened to her chat. She exhibited herself in varying ways to him, which he seemed to enjoy. Near the end of the hospitalization when she discovered the breast scar was longer than she had expected and when she was feeling very depressed at having to leave the hospital to return home, her surgeon visited and discovered her weepy mood. He put his arm around her shoulder and she immediately began to smile. He said, "You're happy; you're cheerful; you're content. We should do this more often." He joked with her for a few minutes and then left. Mrs. Leadon concluded that her surgeon was "very nice."

In talking to us Mrs. Leadon described herself as being "kind of nutty" or "mental." She discussed her favorite movie actors, all of whom were paragons of masculinity, and also she described her attraction to "powerful movies like those with miracles and the fantastic." She was extremely anxious about instruction for her children in sexual matters, courtship, and so on. She indicated her pleasure with her surgeon because

she felt he had agreed to admit her for further breast biopsies at her desire. She thought this was what he meant when he said, "We should do this more often."

Mrs. Leadon's committed sponsorship was a continuing and close one, but we have to ask *to what it was committed*. The physician failed to perceive the main problem, or he chose to ignore it. He appeared to be concerned primarily with pleasing and enjoying his appealing, seductive patient and perhaps, in part, with the promotion of his practice of surgery.

Physician-patient relationships for six of the twenty-three private patients involved in committed sponsorships were similar to the interactions that prevailed between Mrs. Leadon and her physicians. The physicians were drawn into these sponsorships by powerful patients who communicated selectively and in some instances dictated diagnosis or therapy or both. Committed sponsorship, though very favorable for some patients, was not favorable for others. It may have promoted the practices of physicians and led to at least superficial satisfaction of patients but, as we have indicated in the example of Mrs. Leadon, the relationships were often less than therapeutic.

*   *   *

[C]ommitted sponsorship offered the best opportunity for the physician and patient to join in the diagnosis and treatment of health problems. Patients and physicians in general were pleased with their relationship, but in the majority of cases committed sponsorship simply made the technical aspects of patient care more tolerable, if not pleasant, for the patients and physicians, while about 25 per cent of the committed sponsorships constituted a threat to the patient. We wish to state clearly that the *physician by himself* was never found to be entirely responsible for this threat; it is equally clear at the same time that the *patient by himself* was not fully responsible. This type of sponsorship, in which the patient demanded and paid for the physician's time, was open to influences of the patient or physician, or both, which focused on the importance of pleasantry and good manners as opposed to solving the patient's problems. In only one of the 24 cases was this sponsorship an exemplary one, devoted to the task of professional management of both technical and personal aspect of patient care. The influences and fear of mental illness, plus the narrow training and correspondingly narrow framework of medical practice, may have contributed largely to these disturbing situations. Superficially, we found little to suggest that the patients or their physicians understood these dilemmas or wanted a change in their relationships. However, in the more problematic relationships, the deeper feelings of patients indicated dissatisfaction and annoyance. They knew something was not right but they kept their feelings to themselves. They did not communicate their dissatisfaction to their spouses or to their physicians.

*   *   *

d.

L. J. Henderson
Physician and Patient as a Social System*

*   *   *

. . . A patient sitting in your office, facing you, is rarely in a favorable state of mind to appreciate the precise significance of a logical statement, and it is in general not merely difficult but quite impossible for him to perceive the precise meaning of a train of thought. It is also out of the question that the physician should convey what he desires to convey to the patient, if he follows the practice of blurting out just what comes into his mind. The patient is moved by fears and by many other sentiments, and these, together with reason, are being modified by the doctor's words and phrases, by his manner and expression. This generalization appears to me to be as well founded as the generalizations of physical science.

If so far I am right, I think it is fair to set up a precept that follows from all this as a rule of conduct: The physician should see to it that the patient's sentiments do not act upon his sentiments and, above all, do not thereby modify his behavior, and he should endeavor to act upon the patient's sentiments according to a well-considered plan. . . .

However, in this case the application of science to practice is peculiarly difficult. If I am to speak about it, I must in the first place beg explicitly to disclaim any skill of my own. . . . Accordingly, what I am now to say to you is, in the main, second-hand knowledge that I have cribbed from others. It represents, so far as I can understand what I have seen and heard, the soundest judgment, based upon experience, skillful performance and clear analysis in this field. In order to be brief and clear, I shall permit myself the luxury of plain assertion.

In talking with the patient, the doctor must not only appear to be, but must be, really interested in what the patient says. He must not suggest or imply judgments of value or of morals concerning the patient's report to him or concerning the patient's behavior. (To this there is one exception: When the patient successfully presents a difficult objective report of his experiences, it is useful to praise him for doing well what it is necessary that he should do in order to help the physician to help him.) In all those matters that concern the psychological aspects of the patient's experience few questions should be asked and, above all, no leading questions. There should be no argument about the prejudices of the patient, for, at any stage, when you are endeavoring to evoke the subjective aspect of the patient's experience or to modify his sentiments, logic will not avail. In order to modify the sentiments of the patient, your logical analysis must somehow be transformed into the appropriate change of the patient's sentiments. But sentiments are resistant to change. For this reason, you must so far as possible utilize some part of the sentiments that the patient has in order to modify his subjective attitude.

When you talk with the patient, you should listen, first, for what he wants to tell, secondly, for what he does not want to tell, thirdly, for what he cannot tell. He does not want to tell things the telling of which is shameful or painful. He cannot tell you his implicit assumptions that are unknown to him, such as the assumption that all action not perfectly good is bad, such as the assumption that everything that is not perfectly successful is failure, such as the assumption that everything that is not perfectly safe is dangerous. We are all of us subject to errors of this kind, to the assumption that quantitative differences are qualitative. Perhaps the commonest false dichotomy of the hypochondriac is the last of those that I have just mentioned: the assumption that everything not perfectly safe is dangerous.

When you listen for what the patient does not want to tell and for what he cannot tell, you must take especial note of his omissions, for it is the things that he fails to say that correspond to what he does not want to say plus what he cannot say. . . .

[B]eware of your own arbitrary assumptions. Beware of the expression of your own feel-

* 212 *New England Journal of Medicine* 819, 821–823 (1935). Reprinted by permission.

ings. In general, both are likely to be harmful, or at least irrelevant, except as they are used to encourage and to cheer the patient. Beware of the expression of moral judgments. Beware of bare statements, of bare truth, or bare logic. Remember especially that the principal effect of a sentence of confinement or of death is an emotional effect, and that the patient will eagerly scrutinize and rationalize what you say, that he will carry it away with him, that he will turn your phrases over and over in his mind, seeking persistently for shades of meaning that you never thought of. Try to remember how as a very young man you have similarly scrutinized for non-existent meaning the casual phrases of those whom you have admired, or respected, or loved.

*   *   *

NOTES

NOTE 1.

ELIOT FRIEDSON
PATIENTS' VIEWS OF MEDICAL PRACTICE*

. . . In the Family Health Maintenance Demonstration many patients would not accept the services of the social worker in spite of their need and the recommendation of the physician and nurse. In the Montefiore Hospital Medical Group a sizable proportion of patients chose to avoid services to which they were entitled by contract. A lesser but nonetheless important proportion of Demonstration patients used outside services even when they were enrolled in a program with which they expressed overwhelming general satisfaction. Analysis indicated that the patient rejected professional services when they did not fit into his scheme of things—when they were isolated from the steps he goes through in seeking help, when they contradicted his own and his lay consultants' conception of illness and treatment, when they were insulated from the way by which he and his lay consultants try to establish their reliability, and when they required him to sacrifice personal convenience. The professional expects patients to accept what he recommends on his terms; patients seek services on their own terms. In that each seeks to gain his own terms, there is conflict.

How typical of the doctor-patient relationship is conflict? The profession itself contends, as Hughes observed, "that there is no conflict of

interest or perspective between professional and client—or at least . . . none between the good professional and the good client." It may be that the professionals of the Demonstration and the Medical Group are not all they should be, but they all have excellent credentials and those observed at work seemed to possess admirable skill and conscientiousness. It may also be that patients in The Bronx are unusually demanding and arrogant, but, except for one or two, those interviewed seemed to have only the best of intentions. It is quite likely that the particular situation studied stimulated more overt conflict than is present in other situations, but the nature of the conflict itself did not seem unusual.

Struggle between patient and doctor seems to have gone on throughout recorded history. Almost 2500 years ago, the Hippocratic corpus collected doctors' complaints about the nonprofessional criteria that people used to select their physicians, criticism of patients for insisting on "out of the way and doubtful remedies" or on overconventional remedies like "barley water, wine and hydromel," and for disobeying the doctor's orders.

The patients who have left us documents often treat the physician as a potential danger to which one must respond cautiously and whom one must always be ready to evade. Patients have circulated stories about the occasions on which they successfully cured themselves, or continued to live for a long time in defiance of medical prognoses. This sort of literature may be represented by the Roman "epigram about a doctor Marcus who touched a statue of Zeus, and although Zeus was made of stone he nevertheless died," and by Benvenuto Cellini's little story:

I put myself once more under doctor's orders, and attended to their directions, but grew worse. When fever fell upon me, I resolved on having recourse again to the wood: but the doctors forbade it, saying that if I took it with the fever on me, I should not have a week to live. However, I made my mind up to disobey their orders, observed the same diet as I had formerly adopted, and after drinking the decoction four days, was wholly rid of fever. . . . After fifty days my health was re-established.

Physicians have left us instructive essays on "decorum"—practical guides to the physician for managing his relations with the patient in such a way that threats to his authority are minimized. . . .

*   *   *

Struggle between physician and patient has not been restricted to times past. [C]ontempo-

---

* New York: Russell Sage Foundation 171–175, 177–178, 180–181, 183 (1961). Reprinted by permission.

rary studies . . . reveal that elsewhere, as in The Bronx, patients do not always do what physicians tell them to do. They persist in diagnosing and dosing themselves and in assigning great weight to lay advice and their own personal dispositions. It is difficult to get them to cooperate wholly with health programs that, professionals believe, are for their own good.

That the problem continues is somewhat paradoxical, for it seems unquestionable that the medical practitioner has reached an all-time peak of prestige and authority in the eyes of the public. The physician of today is an essentially new kind of professional whose scientific body of knowledge and occupational freedom are quite recent acquisitions. His knowledge is now far more precise and effective than it has ever been in the past, since for the first time it could be said that from " 'about the year 1910 or 1912 . . . [in the United States] a random patient with a random disease consulting a doctor chosen at random stood better than a 50-50 chance of benefiting from the encounter.' " The physician has obtained unrivaled power to control his own practice and the affairs that impinge upon it, and the patient now has severely limited access to drugs for self-treatment and to nonmedical practitioners for alternative treatment. But the ancient problem continues.

*   *   *

What also happens is that more of reality than proves to be appropriate tends to be subsumed under the ordinary and commonly used categories. This again seems to be in the very nature of professional practice—if *most* patients have upper-respiratory infections when they complain of sneezing, sounds in the head, a running nose and fatigue, then an upper-respiratory infection is probably involved when *one* particular person makes the complaint. It could, indeed, be an allergy or even approaching deafness, but it is not probable—that is to say, it was not commonly the case in the past. The physician cannot do otherwise than make such assumptions, but by the statistical nature of the case he cannot help being wrong sometimes.

These problems of diagnosis are not only problems for the doctor but for the patient as well. All the patient knows is what he feels and what he has heard. He feels terrible, his doctor tells him that there's nothing to worry about, and a friend tells him about someone who felt the same way and dropped dead as he was leaving the consulting-room with a clean bill of health. For the patient the problem is, When are subjective sensations so reliable that one should insist on special attention, and when can one reasonably allow them to be waved away as tangential, ordinary and unimportant; when is the doctor mistaken? The answer to these questions is never definite for any individual case, and indeed cannot be resolved decisively except by subsequent events. All of us know of events that have contradicted the judgment of the physician, and, of course, many others that have contradicted the patient.

The situation of consultation thus proves to involve ambiguities that provide grounds for doubt by the patient. Furthermore, those ambiguities are objective. Most reasonable people will agree that the doctor is sometimes wrong, whether by virtue of overlooking the signs that convert an ordinary-appearing case into a special case or by virtue of the deficiencies of the knowledge of his time. He is less often wrong now than he was a hundred years ago, but frequency is not really the question for the individual. Even if failure occurs once in ten thousand cases, the question for the patient is whether it is he who is to be that one case, a question that no one can answer in advance. If the evidence of his senses and the evidence of his knowledge and that of his intimate consultants are contradicted by the physician, the patient may understandably feel it prudent to seek another physician or to evade the prescriptions he has already obtained.

*   *   *

[T]he well-educated patient in The Bronx [fairly well versed in modern medicine, on occasion cooperates] admirably with the physician, but on occasion he is also quite active in evaluating the physician on the basis of his own knowledge and "shopping around" for diagnoses or prescriptions consonant with his knowledge. He is more confident and cooperative in routine situations, perhaps, but he is also more confident of his own ability to judge the physician and dispose himself accordingly. A less-educated patient may be far more manageable.

The dilemma in patient education is now clear. When he lacks health education the prospective patient is unlikely to seek the aid of a professional consultant, and he is unable to give the doctor a history or cooperate with the treatment. When he is well educated the prospective patient is confident of his ability to treat himself "scientifically," and when he sees a doctor he feels more confident of his own ability to judge the doctor's services.

*   *   *

. . . In The Bronx questions arose when the consultant did not act as he was expected to, when the diagnosis seemed implausible, when the prescription seemed intolerable and unnecessary, and when "cure" was slow or imperceptible. They became pressing when the problem of consultation assumed what seemed to be serious proportions. What was needed to sustain the relationship was a stronger sort of confidence than supported initial consultation.

It may be that this stronger sort of confidence is in the minds of those who make a special connection between professions and client confidence. Certainly it is true that three of the old, established professions deal with some of the most anxiety-laden topics of existence—the body, the soul, human relations, and property. Anxiety inherent in those topics, a stronger confidence is required for entrusting oneself to doctors, clergymen, and lawyers than to plumbers, piano-tuners, and fitting-room tailors. However, we have enough evidence from The Bronx study to know that in the early stages of illness there is not enough anxiety even to motivate search for professional help. One first tries tinkering with his piano himself before deciding to call in a professional tuner; one first tries tinkering with his organs himself before calling in a doctor. In the later stages of illness, when anxiety does occur, it can as well interfere with as sustain confidence. Consultants with professional standing thus *claim* confidence, but do not necessarily get it.

NOTE 2.

MEDICAL AUDIT UNIT OF THE TEAMSTER
CENTER PROGRAM
A STUDY OF THE QUALITY OF HOSPITAL CARE
SECURED BY A SAMPLE OF TEAMSTER
FAMILY MEMBERS IN NEW YORK CITY*

* * *

The present report is a study of the quality of medical care received by . . . a sample of patients who had a claim paid by Blue Cross in May 1962 to hospitals in New York City. . . .

Based upon written consents, photostatic copies of the hospital records of 78 per cent of the original sample were obtained. The records were reviewed by thirteen clinicians with recognized professional standing in their specialties.

----

* M. A. Morehead, M.D., M.P.H., Director. New York: Columbia University School of Public Health and Administrative Medicine 7–8 (1964). Reprinted by permission.

The surveyors were asked to judge on the basis of their knowledge and experience the quality of the medical care rendered. [I]n order to assess the reproducibility of evaluation results, two surveyors independently reviewed each record. . . .

. . . Sixteen per cent of the admissions were to voluntary hospitals affiliated with medical schools, 40 per cent to voluntary hospitals with programs approved by the American Medical Association for the training of interns and/or residents. Fourteen per cent were to the smaller voluntary hospitals without approved training programs, and 24 per cent were to proprietary hospitals. Six per cent of the admissions were to municipal hospitals.

Eighteen per cent of the admissions were to the ward services of voluntary or municipal hospitals where the patients were under the care of house staff. . . .

* * *

In the opinion of the reviewing surveyors, only 57 per cent of the care given in the total of all admissions reviewed represented "optimal" medical care; 43 per cent of the care was believed to have been performed in a "less than optimal" fashion when viewed in light of the standards of present day medical practice.

There was variation by specialty in the proportion of medical care considered as "optimal" —obstetrics/gynecology, 80 per cent; general surgery, 57 per cent; pediatrics, 43 per cent; and general medicine, only 31 per cent. The other specialty areas all had a higher proportion of care considered "optimal." The handling of the ophthalmology cases was particularly outstanding; the orthopedic cases were also felt to have received a very satisfactory level of medical care.

* * *

When the findings of the quality of medical care were examined in relation to the type of hospital, the qualifications of the physicians and the type of case, it was found that the highest proportion of medical care judged as "optimal" was provided by the voluntary hospitals affiliated with medical schools, regardless of the recorded qualifications of the physicians or the type of case. Eighty-six per cent of such admissions were considered to have received "optimal" medical care. The "optimal" performance ratings decreased among the different hospital classifications so that less than half (47 per cent) of the care given in the proprietary hospitals was considered "optimal."

Sixty-six per cent of the admissions under

the care of house staff were judged as having received "optimal" care. The "optimal" performance ratings decreased by the other three classifications of physicians . . .—Class I, 65 per cent; Class II, 52 per cent; Class III, 33 per cent.

The principal reason that medical care was considered "less than optimal" was the failure to adequately determine the cause of the patients' presenting symptoms so that rational, as opposed to symptomatic, therapy could be given. Preoperative management and the techniques of the surgical procedure were important reasons in the admissions where surgery was performed and for whom care was judged "less than optimal."

* * *

NOTE 3.

CHARLES S. BRANT AND BERNARD KUTNER
PHYSICIAN-PATIENT RELATIONS IN A TEACHING
HOSPITAL*

* * *

The study was limited to the surgical service. . . . For this type of patient, hospitalization is experienced as a radical disjunction from deeply ingrained habits, life patterns and expectations.

The study procedures consisted of personal interviews with fifty patients, unselected except for diagnosis, conducted both pre-operatively and post-operatively. . . . The interviews were aimed at elicitation of feelings about hospitalization, knowledge of and attitudes toward diagnosis and contemplated surgery, and understanding of the work of physicians and nurses. A large portion of the surgical residents were also interviewed for the purpose of learning their views and attitudes concerning relationships with patients and the role of the physician in the other than purely technical aspects of patient care. A sample of the graduate nurses on the surgical service were interviewed in order to gain insight into their perceptions of the psycho-social needs of patients and to obtain their observations and impressions as to how these needs are manifested by patients, and how they are managed by physicians and nurses. Finally, direct observations were made of physician-patient interaction in treatment situations at the bedside and during ward rounds.

Some principal findings of the study may be summarized as follows:

1. Despite the acknowledged desirability of

such a procedure, rarely do the house staff physician and the patient meet in a private, unhurried conference to discuss the diagnosis and the plan of therapy. Usually, the physician informs the patient at the bedside briefly and in general terms that an operation on a given organ is necessary because it is diseased or is not functioning properly. Signed consent for the procedure is then requested.

2. Patients seldom attempt to ask the house staff physicians about the impending surgery at the time they are informed of it, yet, many patients admit that questions come to mind which they want to ask. The tendency is very common for the patient to feel that he should not "bother the doctor" by asking questions. House staff physicians interpret the silence and passivity of patients as meaning that the patients have no immediate problems, and, therefore, they see no need to elicit from patients whatever questions may be troubling them.

3. Experienced graduate nurses on the surgical wards tend to agree that patients frequently feel isolated, are often in a state of anxious uncertainty about their conditions and do not understand the events occurring in the course of their hospitalization. Patients frequently put questions to nurses about diagnosis, prognosis, tests and medications which nurses feel they are not qualified to answer, or which they feel, as nurses, they are not free to answer. When they refer these questions to house staff physicians, in some instances nurses are requested to answer the patient's questions themselves; in others, the physician may indicate he will do so himself. In the latter situation, the intention is sometimes forgotten, owing to the pace and multiplicity of tasks in the house officer's total schedule of work, and his common tendency to give low priority to talking with patients.

4. The paucity and infrequency of communication from the professional personnel about their illnesses, therapy and impending events leads patients sometimes to acquire misinformation and misinterpretations by asking questions of other patients who have seemingly similar illnesses or have had apparently similar surgery.

* * *

6. Patients rarely know in advance of normal, predictable post-operative events such as the routine stay in the recovery room following surgery and preceding return to the ward, the expectation of some pain at the operative site for a time or the necessity of early ambulation. Some

---

* 32 *Journal of Medical Education* 703–707 (1957). Reprinted by permission.

patients presume that the total time off the ward was spent in the operating room in a lengthy, extensive and difficult procedure, misinterpret post-operative pain as surgical failure, and regard the effort of the nurse or aide to have them leave their bed a few days post-operatively as callousness if not sadism.

7. In amputation of the lower extremities due to peripheral vascular diseases, the patient seldom acquires a thorough understanding (to the limits of his individual ability to understand, of course) of the compelling necessity of this drastic procedure. His normal anxieties concerning the operation and his probable future adjustments do not usually undergo thorough discussion with the house staff physician. Few amputees who possess good rehabilitation potential acquire this hopeful information pre-operatively. Seldom are they made aware before operation, of the time, effort and services available to deal with re-ambulation, rehabilitation and prostheses.

8. In general, house staff physicians on the surgical service do not often conceive of the physician-patient relationship as an integral, important part of their role. There is little agreement among them concerning the communicative aspect of their relation to the surgical patient, and a tendency to view this as quite incidental and peripheral to their "real" concerns. Some house staff physicians believe that the teaching hospital does not provide the proper setting or amount of time for developing their relations with patients, but that once they enter private practice this phase of their work will develop naturally or spontaneously.

*   *   *

NOTE 4.

D. OGSTON AND G. M. MCANDREW
ATTITUDES OF PATIENTS TO
CLINICAL TEACHING*

Few clinical teachers would dispute the value of repeated personal contact with patients in the training of medical students. . . . In view of the paucity of objective information about the attitudes of patients to their use in clinical teaching, this study was undertaken to obtain the views of an unselected group of patients who had been used for teaching purposes in the general medical wards of a teaching hospital.

The hospital in which this study was carried

out (Aberdeen Royal Infirmary) belongs to a group serving a population of about 500,000. The wards are used for the clinical instruction of medical students attending the University of Aberdeen. There is no non-teaching hospital of comparable size in the region.

*   *   *

At the time of this survey no formal notification of the possibility of clinical teaching was given to patients before admission; this is now included in the admission booklet issued to patients.

The normal practice is the allocation of one or two students to a patient for one hour to obtain a history and carry out a physical examination followed by an hour in which one patient is selected for presentation and discussion with four to 10 students and a member of the teaching staff. This normally takes place at the bedside. Students attend the wards for such clinical instruction 5 days in the week.

The medical students were in the third to sixth year of the medical curriculum. Twenty-five of the 94 students who had spent time in the wards during the period of this study were women, and nine were coloured. The number of students by whom each patient was examined varied from one to 12 (mean 3.4).

*   *   *

Forty-three patients out of the 100 interviewed had not realized that they might be seen by students during their stay in hospital. Thirty-seven of the remaining 57 patients expected to be seen by students because of their experience in previous admissions to the same hospital. The remaining 20 patients had heard of the presence of students from relatives or friends. One patient had, in addition, heard a discussion about patients' attitudes to medical students on the radio.

With a single exception all the patients considered that it was reasonable that students be allowed to examine them during their stay in hospital; 40 specifically volunteered the comment that 'students must learn.' Qualifying comments included: 'if well enough' (four patients), 'not too often,' and 'if permission asked first.'

*   *   *

Seventy-three per cent of the patients interviewed did not know of their right to refuse to be examined by students, but only one patient said that he would have refused if he had known of this right on admission. Eleven of the patients who were unaware that they could refuse con-

* 1 *British Journal of Medical Education* 316–319 (1967). Reprinted by permission.

sidered that refusal would prejudice the medical staff against them.

Eight patients (five women and three men) declined to be seen by students on at least one occasion. The reason given by six patients was that they felt unwell, one patient did not like the manner of a student, and one patient finally refused after being seen by six students over the first 14 days of his admission. This patient indicated that he was unwilling to help medical students to complete their medical training because they would then emigrate. Six of the eight patients were unaware of their right to refuse and their refusal took the form of a request to their allocated student not to be examined on a particular day.

*   *   *

Although our findings indicate that patients accept the need for their participation in the clinical training of medical students and that the great majority cooperate willingly, there is a small minority who, while not refusing, find that examination by students is an unpleasant experience. While there is general recognition of the value of teaching devices such as closed-circuit television, these do not eliminate the need for the personal examination of patients by students, and in a period of increasing student numbers it is essential that as many patients as possible cooperate for this purpose. There is thus a conflict between the need for patients for clinical instruction and the personal feelings of a relatively small number of patients. The right of patients to refuse to be examined by students is beyond question; the problem concerns those who do not refuse but find examination distasteful—usually because of embarrassment at any exposure of the body or because of colour prejudice. Such attitudes are not readily changed; we consider, therefore, that the only reasonable course is to exclude such patients from clinical teaching.

*   *   *

e.

Andrew Watson
The Lawyer as Counselor*

*   *   *

[T]he role a person occupies is determined by the society in which it exists. The practitioner himself has little to do with its definition, nor

* 5 *Journal of Family Law* 7, 8–16 (1965). Copyright 1965 by the University of Louisville. Reprinted by permission.

can he freely modify it without running into serious difficulties. For example, lawyers have had considerable to do with shaping the physician's role through the laws of malpractice, contract, and assault and battery, which limit and define the ways in which a doctor may and must relate to a patient. Physicians may challenge and protest these definitions, but they have no freedom whatsoever to change them. While these more tangible aspects of role are also present for the lawyer, I wish to focus upon some aspects of his role which are not so frequently the subject of comment.

First of all, a lawyer as a professional, in contrast to an artist or artisan, has several characteristics which place upon him very specific role demands. First of all, he is the possessor and purveyor of highly technical knowledge and skill, which is the product of a long and involved educative process. Second, this technical information is so completely unintelligible and beyond the scope of judgment to laymen, that a client has no capacity to evaluate the professional skill or effectiveness of the lawyer and his work. Third, because of the two factors mentioned above, the client therefore places himself entirely in the hands of the lawyer and must *trust* that his best interest will be protected by him. This weighty obligation is the motive force for the development by all truly professional groups, of a code of ethics which is self-administered by the professional group and which is dedicated to the protection of those served. These ethical limitations set the standards of practice and are the principal method for controlling professional efficiency. It should be clear upon a moment's reflection, that it is virtually impossible to control professional standards from without, since non-professionals will always suffer the same incapacity to assay professional activity accurately, as do patients or clients.

Clearly this places lawyers as professionals, in a posture which shall cause them to be both revered and feared. Those who function in a manner which looks both omniscient and omnipotent, stand in close psychological proximity to the status of gods, and it is no accident that ancient civilizations inevitably deified both lawgivers and healers. All who have functioned in a professional role have no doubt experienced many occasions in which they fairly glowed under the worshipful attitudes of patients or clients. I do not suggest that we should deny ourselves this pleasure, but I would urge that we be aware of the other side of this emotional axis. Gods with power to produce reverence must also be feared, and wherever there is fear, there will be latent hatred. Just as the ancient gods suffered frequent assaults from mortals below, so professionals will be common targets for the irrational anger created and propagated by the helplessness of the client relationship. This fear and potential fury may be assumed omnipresent as a potent source of complication in the lawyer-client relationship. In fact, one can safely assert that there are *always* problems in professional relationships due to this normal, irrational force, but skillful and competent professionals know how to deal with it either intuitively or consciously. . . .

The lawyer's contribution to the professional relationship is not only composed of all the personal emotional factors present in the client, but he also provides the complication produced by his need to perform a highly technical task. Because he has selected his own professional activity, there will also be a series of emotional needs, some of which are largely unconscious, which caused him to choose the profession of law. Though we do not yet have well established information about these factors, it would appear that many select law as a vocation because it gives them opportunities to operate from a position of power and authority, as they organize, conceptualize, and manipulate the social forces known as law. To comment about this is not to criticize these impulses, for they are present in every human being in some degree. It is merely to emphasize that each of us, in selecting our vocation, responds to inner needs and desires by seeking out tasks which provide probabilities for such gratification. These tasks may be of enormous social value, but the professional role necessitates, or at least makes desirable, some awareness of the manner in which these internal forces may enter into professional activities.

Another emotional factor which will be present in many professionals, is a powerful desire to be helpful to others and thus secure a supply route to sources of approval, affection, or love. All human beings need such guarantees of attachment to the group, and professional activities are one of the surest sources of supply for this need. However, such emotional need may become of such overriding importance, that it can distort the professional relationship and produce inappropriate decisions and actions. One of the burdens of professionalism is to make occasional moves which by their nature are bound to

be unpopular, even when they are desirable and ultimately helpful. This is reflected in the oft repeated protest of punishing parents, that "this will hurt me more than you." No child nor any client can recognize this while suffering pain or frustration, and it is only by hindsight and mature reflection that the truth of the statement and the reason of its offering can become known.

Another important need which can be gratified in the law and which may be a well-forged portion of a lawyer's identity, is the wish to create orderliness in ideas, institutions, and relationships. While clearly of enormous social importance, if too urgent a pressure, it can result in premature limitation of hypothesis and result in constriction of viewpoint. No doubt all lawyers recall if their memory is jogged, early frustrations in their legal studies, when they first discovered that the "known certaintie of the law" even when stated by the venerable Coke, is chimerical at best. However, after overcoming initial panic, most learned how to be orderly about disorder, and thus restored a sense of well-being. I would suggest, parenthetically, that perhaps some of this need for order still rests latently in most, where it may occasionally cause problems through forcing premature decisions about clients, their needs, and their wishes.

Because of the psychological components of the lawyer's self-image described above, as well as other and perhaps more subtle ones, each lawyer has tended to select an area of professional activity which best suits the balance of his individual needs. This empirically and perhaps gropingly effected result has placed each lawyer in his position of best strength as well as greatest weakness. Strength, because it facilitates the use of the sharpest tools possessed; weakness, because it is closest to the built-in blindspots which emanate from the largely unconscious forces which led to the position from which each functions, and by which each is invisibly bound. To get behind this invisible net should be part of the lifetime educational goal of every professional. It is the road to both professional success as well as a sense of personal well-being.

*   *   *

[B]ecoming involved with clients produces high probability that even such concrete matters as choice of legal tactics, whether or not to take a client, whether to negotiate or go to trial, which witnesses to use and which to shelve, which jurors to empanel and which to avoid, and, in the last analysis, even which aspect of law to practice, will at least be partially determined by emotions of which the lawyer will be only vaguely aware or completely ignorant.

These omnipresent and disturbing emotional forces in the professional relationship will place the legal counselor under constant internal pressure to resolve questions in a way which will tend to make him more comfortable, with at least some semblance of control in the variables. In practice, this results in premature decisions with curtailment of fact gathering. Tactical and strategic decisions will be drawn from insufficient and sometimes less-than-optimal data. Decisions of this sort can only result in poor practice which is likely to be less than effective for clients and far from satisfying to the lawyer. Let me emphasize that these premature maneuvers are not the function of slovenliness, technical ineptitude, or lack of a conscientious interest in clients. Rather, they are due to the inner needs of a lawyer to alleviate anxiety by "settling matters." Also it should be emphasized, that many lawyers do not "feel" this anxiety since their training and experience has provided them with excellent means for avoiding this sensation and thus missing the more obvious clues to conflict in the situation. The desirable approach sounds paradoxical, since the optimal psychological posture for pursuing these professional problems is to be able to sustain comfortably, the discomfort of open-ended situations. . . .

At this point, let me enumerate and describe briefly, some of the built-in emotional difficulties in the practice of law. . . .

* * *

The legal counselor in his professional operations has from the offset a potentially difficult problem in that he must serve the best interest of his client, and at the same time maintain his responsibility to the bar. Thus he serves two masters who may have different goals and this places him in the psychologically difficult position of balancing and judging the merits and relationships between these competing claims. I do not suggest that this is inappropriate or undesirable, but merely wish to point out that if one were to contrive a psychological situation which would produce great stress and anxiety, this set of circumstances could hardly be improved upon. This is greatly augmented by the fact that law, ethics of practice, and the authority of judges on the bench, all have great psychological potential for being cloaked in [a] kind of blind and irrational authority, ... When this occurs, rational approaches tend to be immobilized and press one toward automatic submission to the authority. When this happens and is side by side with the ideal of serving the client, internal conflict may be stirred up sufficiently to produce paralysis.

It is my impression from observing the legal process, and most especially the relationship of lawyers to clients, that a great many decisions are made in response to these blind internal forces and are detrimental to clients, or are seriously questionable in relationship to responsibility to the bar. Many lawyers resist discussing some of the more difficult questions which involve potential conflict in this area. They reject them with what I would call pseudo-callousness in order to avoid this stress. For example, the problem of representing the unpopular client is often brushed aside with a rationalization. I do not personally believe that lawyers are less interested than most in the problems of other persons, and in many instances they are the most sensitive members of the community in regard to such questions. I merely put the notion that they appear to fall strikingly into two groups which represent both sides of this question. They may be too quick and too casual in their judgments in order to avoid the difficult problems involved. On the other hand, they may have suffered through such trial-by-fire, and through maturing will take the issues on rationally and with enormous social responsibility. At any rate, it behooves the laymen to appreciate the fantastic difficulty that such a professional responsibility carries with it.

Another operation of the legal counselor, which can provide difficulty, stems from ramifications of the adversary method of trial. The necessity for aggressive statement of position is one of the built-in and fundamental ethical demands of the method, and it is essential that the lawyer argue his client's position as aggressively as possible with the facts he has at hand. This must occur regardless of whether or not he agrees with the position or action of his client. There is much psychological difficulty in this situation since it may result in the active espousal of a question which is diametrically opposed to one's own inner value system. One must possess considerable emotional maturity to accomplish this goal without adopting some kind of psychological defense maneuver to deal with the anxiety created by holding a double position. . . .

Another source of potential difficulty for lawyers is that they always represent a partisan interest. While there are clear and cogent reasons for this, it also carries built-in difficulties for the lawyer who must often function as a negotiator. To do this successfully he must be able to identify himself emotionally with both sides of a question in order to understand it well, and to negotiate skillfully. . . .

The last example of difficulties which the lawyer-counselor needs to handle has to do with the kind of intimacy which is involved in professional relationships. Due to the psychological tendency on the part of the client to invest the counselor with all sorts of power, authority, and a nearly magical belief in their helpfulness, there will also be a powerful tendency to bestow affection. These feelings largely are unrelated to truly personal involvement and are mostly a function of the relationship itself. Therefore, for a lawyer to take advantage of them would be quite as unethical as making personal use of the client's money or property which had been entrusted to him in the course of carrying out the professional role. These powerful and yet irrational emotions can be disquieting to say the least. They are capable of producing a variety of defensive maneuvers which may range from callous advantage-taking, to total withdrawal carried out in blind, rationalized ways, or in the context of overt anger caused by the threat which such feelings may pose. One need not feel guilty about sensing internal responses to these emotional manifestations, nor indeed is it unlikely or inappropriate that one should gain some pleasure and satisfaction from the allegation of affection displayed by the client. It is only in the area of action that the professional obligation exists, and it is therefore a matter of professional concern that these feelings be handled in a way which will not interfere with professional obligations to the client.

*　　*　　*

NOTES

NOTE 1.

Douglas E. Rosenthal
Client Participation in Professional
Decision—The Lawyer-Client
Relationship in Personal Injury Cases*

*　　*　　*

I do not think it unfair to say that at the national, state and local levels, the "organized

* Yale University: Doctoral Dissertation 194–206 (1970). Reprinted by permission of the author who retains all rights.

bar" has been complacent about the problem of professional self-policing. The comprehensive review of lawyer performance commissioned by the American Bar Association shortly after World War II came to the conclusion that criticism of the profession is largely unfounded and that, while there is room for improvement, the primary fault of the profession is not performance but "public relations." Consistent with the traditional approach to professional performance, the bar has defined the problem as one best dealt with by screening out the untrained and the unfit, treating proficient performance as synonymous with a lawyer being a person of "integrity and good character." The law schools are encouraged to teach legal ethics. Bar associations are encouraged to develop and implement effective certification procedures for admitting new lawyers, and practicing attorneys are encouraged to cooperate in "purging the profession of the unworthy." However, these traditional principles are not implemented. While many law schools teach ethics courses, they are not designed to relate to the specific and real world pressures and dilemmas of practice. Students are taught almost nothing about how to deal with clients. Students end their law school careers more cynical than when they started and consistently report that their law school experience did not prepare them for the realities of law practice. . . . [I]nstead of reporting ethical violations and gross incompetence of colleagues (as mandated by Disciplinary Rule 1–103 of the Code of Professional Responsibility), lawyers ignore them. Even Henry Drinker, an approving friend of the legal profession, has remarked that

One of the principle features resulting in just public criticism of the bar is the unwillingness of lawyers to expose the abuses of which they know that certain of their brethren are guilty, as well as the reluctance of judges to disbar, suspend, or even publicly reprimand such lawyers. . . . [M]ost of the abuses of which lawyers are guilty could be eliminated if the bar and the courts were constantly alert and willing to do their full duty in this regard.

While the bar has been more active in establishing principles of professional responsibility than in enforcing them, the existing legal doctrine defining lawyer duties and client rights is neither clear nor extensive, nor especially protective of the client. Three overlapping standards have been used by different courts to define the performance owed a client by his attorney. A lawyer is responsible for any loss to his client which proximately results from a want to that degree of knowledge and skill (1) ordinarily possessed by others of his profession similarly situated, or (2) from the omission to use reasonable care and diligence, or (3) from the failure to exercise in good faith his best judgment in attending to the litigation committed to his care.[13]

The first standard has been incorrectly interpreted as setting as the norm the average conduct of general practice attorneys in the same community. Such an interpretation sets a lower standard of care for the attorney than the reasonable man standard of negligence applied to his client. A reasonable man is expected to perform prudently. The law says a person is not freed from liability for negligence on the mere showing that his conduct was average or normal. The third standard implies, among other things, that if a lawyer is specially trained in a specific area of the law, he may be held to a higher standard of care—the skill and knowledge reasonable for a specialist. Though widely approved, it has yet to be applied in a specific case.

The reasonable care standard is usually applied to the omissions of attorneys rather than to their affirmative acts. Attorneys have been held not to have exercised reasonable care for failing to push a claim diligently, for failing properly to arrange for witnesses at the trial, for incorrectly serving a summons and complaint, for defective pleadings and for not researching the relevant law of a foreign jurisdiction. An attorney may be liable for failing to follow with reasonable promptness and care the explicit instructions of his client—even in the honest belief that the instructions were not in the client's best interest. The attorney is clearly constrained from acting in his client's behalf without his permission only with respect to three issues: he may not settle the claim unilaterally; he may not farm out the case without the client's consent; and he may not unilaterally waive judgment and seek a new trial. More than 70 years ago, New York courts were divided on whether an attorney could stipulate not to appeal a decision without his client's permission. No more recent case has settled the matter.

These rulings may appear to constitute strong protection for the client's right to competent representation. In fact they fall far short of extensive protection. An important erosion of the due care standard has come with the application of the principle that an attorney is freed from

liability where the law is considered uncertain or unsettled. Judges and juries are invited to view a negligent act or judgment as an honest mistake. In a recent California case, for example, an attorney was not held liable for damages resulting from drafting a will which excluded an intended beneficiary from an inheritance. The court so held notwithstanding that the particular error had been the subject of prior authoritative California court decisions interpreting the relevant statute. The court felt that the area of law was sufficiently difficult, anyway, that the honest mistake was not negligence. Ironically, though "ignorance of the law will not excuse" the client, it will excuse the lawyer who is trained to learn the law. Further examples of lawyer omissions that have been judicially sanctioned include: failure to bring a timely appeal—where this was not specifically directed by the client,— failure to receive the client's permission to waive trial by jury and failure to get the client's approval for extending the adversary's permissible time to serve the complaint.

All of the principles promulgated by the organized bar which we have considered to this point are consistent with the traditional professional model. Active client participation is disfavored. As one judge put it, "clients should not be forced to act as hawklike inquisitors of their own counsel, suspicious of every step and quick to switch lawyers. The legal profession knows no worse headache than the client who mistrusts his attorney." Because clients are passive and dependent they deserve the bar's vigilance in weeding out the unscrupulous and incompetent and in establishing principles of lawyer responsibility to be enforced against specific cases of lawyer nonconduct and mis-conduct. Even if implementation is not as extensive and effective as it should be, the ideals are legitimate and consistent. One reason, however, why these principles are not better enforced is the fear that granting relief for every attorney error will tie up the courts with endless petitions from "overly litigious or chronically dissatisfied persons who refuse to accede to the sound judgment of their lawyers." The bar —especially the judiciary—is torn between the policies of putting an end to litigation and guaranteeing clients effective legal representation. To resolve this conflict, the Supreme Court has abandoned the traditional model. The Warren Court has held that the client must be presumed to control his lawyer's conduct. The lawyer is merely the client's passive agent. Therefore any errors of judgment or performance by the lawyer are presumed to be approved by the client. In

[13] *Hodges v. Carter*, 239 N.C. 517, 80 S.E.2d 144, 146 (1954).

the leading case of *Link v. Wabash Railraod Company,* the majority said,

> Petitioner voluntarily chose this attorney as his representative in the action, and he cannot now avoid the consequences of the acts or omissions of this freely selected agent. Any other notion would be wholly inconsistent with our system of representative litigation.[34]

In dissent, Justice Black (joined by Chief Justice Warren) reminded the Court that lawyers want and encourage clients to be passive and are therefore being unfair in punishing them for this trusting behavior.

> How could [the client] know or why should he be presumed to know that it was his duty to see that the many steps a lawyer needs to take to bring his case to trial had been taken by his lawyer. . . . [S]o far as this record shows [the client] was simply trusting his lawyer to take care of his case as clients generally do.[35]

In the *Link* case, the court's rule denied the plaintiff, an accident victim, any recovery in his claim. As frequently happens, more than three years had elapsed between the day of the accident and the day of the ruling. There is a three-year statute of limitations for bringing negligence actions.

The policy of the *Link* case can be partially defended on the theory that the client still had the possible remedy of a malpractice suit. "Malpractice" suits are brought by aggrieved clients—represented by a second lawyer—against the attorney representing them in a prior unsuccessful lawsuit. If successful, the client may recover from his lawyer the damages to which he was entitled had his prior claim been handled properly. In reality, there are serious hurdles impairing the client's chances for success. First of all, there is also a three-year statute of limitations on suits claiming attorney negligence. The three-year period begins to run from the time the negligent act is committed, not from the time that the client discovers it. Even if the lawyer conceals the negligence from his client until the statute has run, New York courts have held that the lawyer is not liable for fraudulent concealment (with its longer six-year statute of limitations). Thus in the *Link* case, the client would have been denied a malpractice remedy. More than three years had elapsed since his attorney failed to meet the initial trial date. The second hurdle for the client

is that in the malpractice action he must show not only that the first attorney was negligent but that the result would have been different *but for* that negligence. As has been noted, the client must win a "suit within a suit." Courts, so inclined, are given the "easy out" of finding that while, yes, the attorney was negligent, his negligence did not proximately cause the client's damages since the client might well have lost the first suit anyway. A third hurdle is that in many communities (though probably not in Manhattan) it is difficult to find attorneys who will represent clients in malpractice suits against colleagues. The fourth hurdle is the bias of the judges who hear malpractice cases. In the words of a *Columbia Law Review* comment,

> Although the overwhelming majority of decisions indicate that the question of negligence is one of fact, judicial reluctance actually to submit the issue to the jury is manifest. Allocating responsibility between judge and jury in attorney malpractice suits raises questions even more delicate and complex than those presented in ordinary negligence cases, which normally involve mixed questions of law and fact. The nature of the relationship between bench and bar inevitably influences judicial attitudes. . . . Notwithstanding their frequent statements that attorneys occupy a position with respect to those they serve similar if not identical to that of members of the medical profession, the courts have treated attorney malpractice suits as sui generis. The majority of decisions reflect a superficial analysis that is almost certainly colored by the fraternal concern of the judiciary for members of the practicing bar. . . . The defense that "errors of judgment" were made has generally been sustained uncritically. The defendant should be required to demonstrate that his choice of alternatives, though subsequently mistaken, was not unreasonable, for only then is the allegation of negligence rebutted.[38]

Even if the client overcomes these hurdles and wins the malpractice suit he may well find that the liable lawyer is not sufficiently covered by malpractice insurance to pay damages. The costs of malpractice insurance are steadily rising as more suits are undertaken. The one most likely to be underprotected—or not protected at all—is the general practice attorney who is also the one most likely to make a mistake in representation. Some local bar associations have established client security funds, with contributions provided by member attorneys, to pay defaulted claims brought against guilty attorneys. Unfortunately, for the victim of ordinary negligence, client security funds are only used to pay the

[34] 370 U.S. 626, at 633, 634, 8 L.Ed.2d 734, 82 S.Ct. 1386 (1962).
[35] *Ibid.,* at 643 (dissenting opinion).
[38] *Attorney Malpractice,* 63 COLUMBIA LAW REVIEW 1309, 1312 (1963).

victims of serious misconduct—misappropriation of trust funds, fraud, forgery, larceny and the like.

There is a third possible "remedy" for aggrieved clients who fail to recover damages. They may receive the moral satisfaction of seeing the attorney "disciplined" by the court. Judicial discipline for negligence rarely if ever exceeds the simple wrist-slap of "censure." The attorney is free to continue his practice otherwise unimpaired. It has been found that the effects of a malpractice suit on the practices of a sample of 58 Connecticut physicians were insignificant. The same is probably true for the practice of censured attorneys.

In sum, current legal doctrine is designed to frustrate the client seeking effective representation. If he behaves passively and trusts his lawyer, as encouraged under the traditional approach, he will be held liable for all but the most serious forms of misconduct by his attorney, thereby forfeiting his claim. If he behaves actively and tries to monitor the actions of his attorney he risks incurring the wrath of the lawyer and being branded a troublemaker. The legal profession departs from advocacy of the traditional model of client passivity only so far as to deny the client the very protection the profession claims to provide. Since laymen cannot rely upon the legal profession to insure that all practicing lawyers give good service, choosing a lawyer becomes a real problem.

*   *   *

NOTE 2.

LINK v. WABASH RAILROAD CO.
370 U.S. 626, 646–49 (1962)

MR. JUSTICE BLACK with whom THE CHIEF JUSTICE concurs, dissenting.

*   *   *

[T]o say that the sins or faults or delinquencies of a lawyer must always be visited upon his client so as to impose tremendous financial penalties upon him, as here, is to ignore the practicalities and realities of the lawyer-client relationship. Lawyers everywhere in this country are granted licenses presumably because of their skill, their integrity, their learning in the law and their dependability. While there may be some clients sophisticated enough in the affairs of the world to be able to select the good from the bad among this mass of lawyers throughout the country, this unfortunately cannot always be

the case. The average individual called upon, perhaps for the first time in his life, to select a lawyer to try a lawsuit may happen to choose the best lawyer or he may happen to choose one of the worst. He has a right to rely at least to some extent upon the fact that a lawyer has a license. From this he is also entitled to believe that the lawyer has the ability to look out for his case and that he should leave the lawyer free from constraint in doing so. Surely it cannot be said that there was a duty resting upon Link, a layman plaintiff, to try to supervise the daily professional services of the lawyer he had chosen to represent him. How could he know, even assuming that it is true, that his lawyer was a careless man or that he would have an adverse effect upon the trial judge by failing to appear when ordered? How could he know or why should he be presumed to know that it was his duty to see that the many steps a lawyer needs to take to bring his case to trial had been taken by his lawyer? Why should a client be awakened to his lawyer's incapacity for the first time by a sudden brutal pronouncement of the court: "Your lawyer has failed to perform his duty in prosecuting your case and we are therefore throwing you out of court on your heels"? So far as this record shows, the plaintiff never received one iota of information of any kind, character or type that should have put him on notice as an ordinary layman that his lawyer was not doing his duty.

Any general rule that clients must always suffer for the mistakes of their lawyers simply ignores all these problems. If a general rule is to be adopted, I think it would be far better in the interest of the administration of *justice,* and far more realistic in the light of what the relationship between a lawyer and his client actually is, to adopt the rule that no client is ever to be penalized, as this plaintiff has been, because of the conduct of his lawyer unless notice is given to the client himself that such a threat hangs over his head. Such a rule would do nothing more than incorporate basic constitutional requirements of fairness into the administration of justice in this country.

The Court seems to find some reason for holding that this plaintiff can be penalized without notice because of a program certain courts have adopted to end congestion on their dockets by setting down long-pending cases for trial. It is of course desirable that the congestion on court dockets be reduced in every way possible consistent with the fair administration of justice. But that laudable objective should not be sought in a way which undercuts the very purposes for which courts were created—that is, to try cases on their merits and render judgments in accordance with the substantial rights of the parties. Where a case has so little merit that it is not being prosecuted, a trial court can of course properly dispose of it under fair constitutional procedures. There is not one fact in this record, however, from which an inference can be drawn that the case of Link against the Wabash Railroad Company is such a case. When we allow the desire to reduce court congestion to justify the sacrifice of substantial rights of the litigants in cases like this, we attempt to promote speed in administration, which is desirable, at the expense of justice, which is indispensable to any court system worthy of its name.

*   *   *

3.

The Professional in Practice— Can Power Be Shared?

a.

Thomas S. Szasz and Marc H. Hollender A Contribution to the Philosophy of Medicine—The Basic Models of the Doctor-Patient Relationship*

*   *   *

The three basic models of the doctor-patient relationship, which we will describe, embrace modes of interaction ubiquitous in human relationships and in no way specific for the contact between physician and patient. The specificity of the medical situation probably derives from a combination of these modes of interaction with certain technical procedures and social settings.

1. *The Model of Activity-Passivity.*—Historically, this is the oldest conceptual model. Psychologically, it is not an interaction, because it is based on the effect of one person on another in such a way and under such circumstances that the person acted upon is unable to contribute actively, or is considered to be inanimate. This frame of reference (in which the physician does something to the patient) underlies the application of some of the outstanding advances of modern medicine (e.g., anesthesia and surgery, antibiotics, etc.). The physician is active; the pa-

---

* 97 *Archives of Internal Medicine* 585, 586–587 (1956). Reprinted by permission of the American Medical Association.

tient, passive. This orientation has originated in —and is entirely appropriate for—the treatment of emergencies (e.g., for the patient who is severely injured, bleeding, delirious, or in coma). "Treatment" takes place irrespective of the patient's contribution and regardless of the outcome. There is a similarity here between the patient and a helpless infant, on the one hand, and between the physician and a parent, on the other. It may be recalled that psychoanalysis, too, evolved from a procedure (hypnosis) which was based on this model. Various physical measures to which psychotics are subjected today are another example of the activity-passivity frame of reference.

2. *The Model of Guidance-Cooperation.* —This model underlies much of medical practice. It is employed in situations which are less desperate than those previously mentioned (e.g., acute infections). Although the patient is ill, he is conscious and has feelings and aspirations of his own. Since he suffers from pain, anxiety, and other distressing symptoms, he seeks help and is ready and willing to "cooperate." When he turns to a physician, he places the latter (even if only in some limited ways) in a position of power. This is due not only to a "transference reaction" (i.e., his regarding the physician as he did his father when he was a child) but also to the fact that the physician possesses knowledge of his bodily processes which he does not have. In some ways it may seem that this, like the first model, is an active-passive phenomenon. Actually, this is more apparent than real. Both persons are "active" in that they contribute to the relationship and what ensues from it. The main difference between the two participants pertains to power, and to its actual or potential use. The more powerful of the two (parent, physician, employer, etc.) will speak of guidance or leadership and will expect cooperation of the other member of the pair (child, patient, employee, etc.). The patient is expected to "look up to" and to "obey" his doctor. Moreover, he is neither to question nor to argue or disagree with the orders he receives. This model has its prototype in the relationship of the parent and his (adolescent) child. Often, threats and other undisguised weapons of force are employed, even though presumably these are for the patient's "own good." It should be added that the possibility of the exploitation of the situation—as in any relationship between persons of unequal power—for the sole benefit of the physician, albeit under the guise of altruism, is ever present.

3. *The Model of Mutual Participation.*— Philosophically, this model is predicated on the postulate that equality among human beings is desirable. It is fundamental to the social structure of democracy and has played a crucial role in occidental civilization for more than two hundred years. Psychologically, mutuality rests on complex processes of identification—which facilitate conceiving of others in terms of oneself—together with maintaining and tolerating the discrete individuality of the observer and the observed. It is crucial to this type of interaction that the participants (1) have approximately equal power, (2) be mutually interdependent (i.e., need each other), and (3) engage in activity that will be in some ways satisfying to both.

This model is favored by patients who, for various reasons, want to take care of themselves (at least in part). This may be an overcompensatory attempt at mastering anxieties associated with helplessness and passivity. It may also be "realistic" and necessary, as, for example, in the management of most chronic illnesses (e.g., diabetes mellitus, chronic heart disease, etc.). Here the patient's own experiences provide reliable and important clues for therapy. Moreover, the treatment program itself is principally carried out by the patient. Essentially, the physician helps the patient to help himself.

In an evolutionary sense, the pattern of mutual participation is more highly developed than the other two models of the doctor-patient relationship. It requires a more complex psychological and social organization on the part of both participants. Accordingly, it is rarely appropriate for children or for those persons who are mentally deficient, very poorly educated, or profoundly immature. On the other hand, the greater the intellectual, educational, and general experiential similarity between physician and patient the more appropriate and necessary this model of therapy becomes.

* * *

b.

Robert Rubenstein and Harold Lasswell
The Sharing of Power in a
Psychiatric Hospital*

* * *

The great social movements of our time concern the demand for full participation as equals in the affairs of the community by the

---

* New Haven: Yale University Press 2–6 (1966). Reprinted by permission.

disadvantaged. Sermons and speeches have long acknowledged the justice of this demand, but the insistence that we take the democratic ideology seriously and live by it is revolutionary. All of us may be viewed in some context as disadvantaged. Two prominent examples are Negroes and women; two groups less aware of being deprived are students and patients.

* * *

Patients are . . . among the disadvantaged. It is customary to view them as having to be taken care of because they are ill, incapacitated, or defective. Hospitalized psychiatric patients, the subgroup we shall focus upon, have been defeated in long, protracted, at times subtle, at times violent, power struggles within their families, and by friends and colleagues in school, work, and the other communities in which they have unsuccessfully sought to participate. Unable to find a way to share effectively in the decision-making processes of the family, they remain in unresolved conflict with those exercising power and at odds with their critical decisions, their perspectives, preferred outcomes, and strategies.

* * *

Conventional psychiatric institutions reinforce the self-image of the hospitalized as losers, sufferers, and victims. Decisions about fundamental and pressing issues in the lives of patients are decided by others; the individuals most concerned participate not at all. In an authoritarian hospital, the roles of doctors, nurses, and patients are clearly defined. The "good patient" is compliant, cooperative, accepting, unquestioning, the recipient of the good, established, known care from doctors, nurses, and other staff members. He is regarded as a troublemaker, uncooperative, and cantankerous if he questions procedures, seeks information about why this is being done and that isn't, or presumes to take a more active position by volunteering judgments about what is wrong with him and what should be done, or the nature of the difficulties and the treatment of other patients. One part of the hospital—the staff—does things to that other part of the hospital—the patients—"to get 'them' well." The patients comply with these implicit expectations by assuming the passive role of those to whom things are done by others.

Once more, society and the doctors, experts with extraordinary authority over the lives of others, justify such exemptions from democratic practices and drastic usurpation of rights by describing the mentally ill as fragile, childlike, irresponsible, and dangerous to themselves and others. Not protecting them, failing to administer their affairs as dependents, would be a breach of professional obligation. But now the possibility is being considered that the traditional medical model is not appropriate for reprocessing these defeated and disadvantaged, and new institutions specifically elaborated in response to their needs are developing. This shift was prompted both by convincing demonstrations of the beneficial effects of patients participating actively with staff in determining and assessing what happens in the hospital and by conflicts of conscience among those exercising power, the doctors who knew, but had not previously been forced to acknowledge, the necessity of extending throughout the patient's experience the dignity, respect, responsibility, autonomy, and self-determination long acknowledged as central to psychoanalytic treatment. [P]atients respond completely and responsibly to such opportunities and expectations; in such an atmosphere they assert their dissatisfaction with being the passive recipients of the ministrations of others. That fact renders the doctor's authoritarian position uncertain and conflictful. He cannot continue to violate the canons of shared power and fulfill his obligations as a physician, for these deviations from democratic practice are no longer justifiable on therapeutic grounds.

*　　*　　*

c.

Douglas E. Rosenthal
Client Participation in Professional Decision —The Lawyer-Client Relationship in Personal Injury Cases*

The traditional model proposes that the client who participates actively in problem-solving, who shares in controlling the decisions, will end up in a poorer position—and certainly no better off—than the client who passively delegates decision-making to the professional. The participatory model posits the opposite. . . . I will test the proposition that active clients get poorer results than passive clients. . . . The data about client participation and case worth is taken from extended personal interviews with 59 Manhattan residents who brought accident claims and who were represented by an attorney. These clients had their claims terminated during 1968 and

* Yale University: Doctoral Dissertation 48–64 (1970). Reprinted by permission of the author who retains all rights.

each received at least $2,000 in compensation for their accident. . . .

*　　*　　*

Inspection of the interview protocols points up six distinguishable types of client activity that tend to have an impact on decisions made in pursuing a case. The first is seeking out quality medical attention for recuperation and making sure that medical expenses and related non-medical expenses are included in provable claim damages. The second is impressing one's wishes and concerns about the claim upon the lawyer—having the client's wishes reflected in the handling of the claim, and having the lawyer's support in dealing with client anxieties. Third is the client persuading the lawyer to give special attention to his case. Fourth is helping the lawyer to marshal evidence to build a solid claim that will be worth his extra time and energy. Fifth is a client tactic of continually appraising his lawyer's performance according to criteria of responsiveness, thoroughness and consistency and, if dissatisfied, "comparison shopping" to support additional demands or for a replacement. Sixth is bargaining with the lawyer about the fee. Any client who took all six of these types of actions would have initiated the search for information bearing on his problem, would have alerted his attorney to his special interests, would have received some feedback on how well the attorney was responding to these concerns and would have had the opportunity for an informed intermediate review before a final settlement was irrevocably made. Any client who took none of these steps would exhibit a passive problem-solving strategy. Only one client sampled, Mr. Bates, a civil engineer, reported having taken all six types of action. Almost one third (19/59) of the client sample reported taking none of them. In Table II–1, we see how frequent are the various forms of client action as reported by the interviewees (listed in rank order of frequency).

*　　*　　*

Plaintiffs' trial lawyers share a consensus view that there is an objective value that can be placed, approximately, on various types of liability claims. This view facilitates compromise settlements. The going values are based on prior settlements, recent jury verdicts in similar types of cases and some rules-of-the-game, such as that a fair settlement in a strong case should not depart too greatly from a figure that reflects the victim's out-of-pocket expenses multiplied by 3. Recent jury awards within various jurisdic-

TABLE II–1
Frequencies of Types of Client Activity

activity type	number of clients reporting it	percentage of sample
1. expresses a special want or concern	25	42%
2. makes follow-up demands for attention	19	32%
3. marshals information to aid lawyer	14	24%
4. seeks quality medical attention	12	20%
5. seeks second legal opinion	10	15%
6. bargains about the fee	7	12%

tions are codified and reported by national research services. Thus it is possible to find value precedents for most types of injuries. Nonetheless, it remains an open question just how objective and consensual expert case evaluation can be.

One analytical way to make use of an "objective" consensus value on case result is to have a disinterested panel of experts make a case by case appraisal. This was done for each of the 59 cases in the sample. A fact sheet was prepared based upon the more important determinants of any case's worth. It was submitted to a panel of three experienced plaintiff's personal injury attorneys. They were asked to put an exact dollar value on each claim—based on the given facts—at three different time periods: one year after the accident, four years after the accident (approximately pre-trial), and what could be expected from a jury's trial judgment. . . .

. . . If client activity does influence case result, we should expect to find a statistically significant rank order correlation between the two variables [client participation and case result]. I have used Kendall's Tau to determine the rank order correlation for the 43 cases where the mean panel evaluation is acceptable, and find a moderately strong positive relationship: contrary to the expectation from the traditional professional model, active clients not only do not get worse results, but actually get better recoveries from their legal claims.

But this is only the first step in casting doubt on the traditional hypothesis. It may well be expected that client activity only masks some deeper more important explanation of good case outcome. In fact, there are three additional factors which might be thought to have a significant causal impact on case outcome. These factors are the social status of the client, the dollar worth of the claim, and the "perfection" of the liability issue in the claim.

. . . If social position significantly influences

case result we would expect to find a high positive rank order correlation between the status and case result scales. Surprisingly, the two factors are not significantly related. A client's high social standing does not noticeably improve his chances of receiving a good claim disposition. Therefore, even though client status is significantly related to active client participation . . . it is the client's activity rather than his status which better explains the success of his claim.

Though not intuitively obvious, the worth of a case and the perfection of the liability issue in it are significant rival explanations of why some clients get better case results than others. Ironically, the greater the dollar amount of recovery that can be anticipated in a claim (case worth), the smaller the chances of making a good recovery. Also, and more plausibly, the stronger the evidence that the one accused of causing the accident was negligent and that the accident victim was free from contributory negligence, the greater the chances of a successful recovery.

There is a statistical procedure for performing a partial correlation of client activity with case result, controlling for each of these three alternative variables one at a time. If client activity is not a valid independent causal variable, the correlation should "wash out." Computation of the partial Kendall correlation reveals that client activity is indeed a potent explanatory factor. At the level of aggregate analysis, active client participation definitely pays off. . . .

*   *   *

d.
Washington-Greene Legal Aid Society Application
45 D. & C. 2d 563 (Pa. 1968)

*   *   *

SWEET, P. J.—This matter comes before the court on the application of the O. E. O.

Legal Services for a nonprofit corporation charter. The Washington-Greene Legal Aid Society has asked us, pursuant to the Act of May 5, 1933, P. L. 289, 15 PS §7201 et seq., to grant them powers of a nonprofit corporation ". . . to make available legal aid to all residents in the Counties of Washington and Greene, Commonwealth of Pennsylvania, who, because of their financial inability are unable to procure such legal aid, and to undertake educational programs in which indigent residents may be instructed in and advised of their fundamental private legal rights and obligations, to the end that their performance, motivation and productivity as citizens may be improved and their respect for the law increased."

Because of the controversial nature of this application, the amount of money involved and the relatively novel nature of the proposal, we ordered a hearing, "as to the necessity, the legality, the propriety and the wisdom of the activities of the proposed corporation."

*   *   *

The application before us . . . has some non-lawyers representative of the poor in a position of control of policy, but it provides for a director of legal service employees who will exercise executive authority in the office. Probably this is the best compromise that could be planned.

It seems fairly clear that the Canon of Ethics does not prohibit such an organization as this. Canon 35 says that while a lawyer should not be controlled by any corporate lay agency which comes between him and his client that "charitable societies rendering aid to the indigent are not deemed such intermediaries."

Liberals favoring these offices may find some delicious irony in the fact that the American Bar Association once approved a plan by which attorneys associated with the Liberty League publicly advertised free legal services to those challenging the constitutionality of New Deal Legislation. A.B.A. Opinions of the Committee on Professional Ethics and Grievances #148 (1935) said in part the canon ". . . certainly was never aimed at a situation such as this, in which a group of lawyers announced that they are willing to devote some of their time and energy to the *interests of indigent citizens whose constitutional rights are believed to be infringed.*"

*   *   *

The most ambitious scholarly study of this field which we have been able to find is "Neighborhood Law Offices," 80 *Harv. L. Rev.* 805, February (1967). This characteristically documented article points out the inadequacy of existing charitable legal aid services. It suggests the importance of the neighborhood concept in the furnishing of legal services to the poor and makes a careful distinction between the service function and the nonservice function of the new legal services programs in their component role in the war on poverty. "While the service function—the representation by the neighborhood lawyer of individual clients without regard for broader reform—is the least novel aspect of the New Wave, it is nevertheless crucial to any neighborhood law office program. The service function occupies the great majority of the working hours of most of the lawyers and is the day-to-day means of building the community's trust and confidence in the program, so that the neighborhood concept may become a reality." A fairly large percentage of the article is devoted to the nonservice functions. These are categorized (A) law reform, (B) community action, and (C) community education. "In order to restore the overall integrity of the adversary system, OEO-funded legal services programs are required to list as one of their goals the reform of substantive law in the interest of the poor." This is squarely based on the guidelines which say, "that advocacy of appropriate reforms . . . should be among the services afforded by the program."

*   *   *

We also find in the *Harvard Law Review* article considerable stress laid on participation of the poor. It is critical of the technique, used by our applicant here, in placing responsibility for the poor on the Board of Trustees. While the N.Y.S. case, supra, was critical of any non-lawyer control over lawyers the *Harvard Law Review* article tends the other way. "But there are disadvantages in giving the poor full control of a legal services program. The attorneys have special responsibilities to their clients, and the poor on the board may not understand the lawyer-client relationship, expecting the attorney to be dedicated to the interest of the poor as a class or even to the more narrow interests of the representatives. Although the attorney should be able to resist pressures to sacrifice his client's interest, it would be preferable not to put him in such a position. *It seems undesirable, however, to attempt to avoid this pressure by giving the organized bar control of the program;* local bar associations tend to be critical of innovation and close to the established interests in society with whom the poor are often in conflict. The adverse effect that control by the organized bar might have on the nonservice functions outweighs the possible advantages of a professionally supervised program."

*   *   *

It seems to us that we should grant the application. There is little reason to question the legality of the plan nor are we convinced that it will be injurious to the community. At this point, however, a word of caution, precatory perhaps, but none the same strongly felt, seems in order. We are gravely disturbed by the implications of the "non-service" function referred to indirectly in the application as education, training and research activities. The business of a lawyer engaged by such a nonprofit corporation is to represent indigent persons one by one as they have a need for representation. It is not a class representation of the indigent, as such, nor a collective representation, nor are the poor a single and collective client. . . .

*   *   *

We take this occasion to remind the public generally that any person aggrieved by the operations of this society has recourse to the courts. It would be invidious indeed were O.E.O. Legal Services organized to prevent injustice to the poor only to become an instrument of malevolence and illegality toward any person, however affluent.

*   *   *

NOTES

NOTE 1.
THE NEW PUBLIC INTEREST LAWYERS*

*   *   *

Though there are a great variety of checks and controls the lawyer may adopt in his selection of cases, the issues are focused most clearly by comparing two models: "independence" and "community control." The "independent" lawyer relies solely on personal values and his own sense of what is important. Monroe Freedman, director of the Philip Stern Community Law Office in Washington, justified the independence model, arguing that lawyers totally released from external constraints serve a highly useful social

---

* 79 *Yale Law Journal* 1069, 1132–35 (1970). Reprinted by permission of The Yale Law Journal Company and Fred B. Rothman and Company.

purpose: they provide a perspective on the legal process and social change which cannot be achieved by those concerned with their own immediate problems.

I do not mean to say that people in the community, groups in the community, don't know what they want or are not entitled to have representation on what they want or think they want. I am saying that there is a place for lawyers who don't serve that function. It's in part a matter of expertise and values and of the public not knowing what they're going to need in the future. I'll use a dirty word. It's very elitist, and although I'm a very strong believer in participatory democracy, it doesn't prevent me from being an elitist.

Set against the "independence" model is the "community control" model, which subordinates the lawyer's decisions on cases to handle to control by those whose interests are at stake in his work. This model is usually implemented by a board composed of true representatives of the constituency—rather than lawyers or inveterate board sitters—who have effective power to control the lawyer's allocation decisions. The contemporary movement for decentralization and democratization of institutions urges that people are the best judges of their own best interests and ought to participate in decisions which affect their lives—and thus it supports the notion that the lawyer should be accountable to those he serves. Since lawyers for the underrepresented are by definition scarce, a lawyer's decision to handle one kind of case rather than another is also a decision setting priorities in the community's legal representation. The "community control" model asserts that those decisions are properly the people's.

The two models are true alternatives where —as in Neighborhood Legal Services—the question is how best to serve the interests of a poor community. Here there exists a group which is able, through representatives, to exercise control over the lawyer; yet the lawyer can also, while still claiming to serve the group's best interests, be independent of it in allocating his services among various types of cases. The dilemma is well focused: who should decide how to allocate the community's legal resources, the lawyer or the community?

The justification for independence in this situation is paternalistic; the lawyer is properly a social engineer, deciding what is really important for a community or constituency, because he is skilled, rational, and benevolent. Independence allows rational action and the use of expertise free from the need to spend energy and time dealing with people who may be uneducated, prone to irrationality, unaware of their best interests, and difficult to organize. But this notion of benevolent expertise is undercut by the community's conflicting claim of "expertise" in matters which concern it, and by the danger that, in following his own instincts, the lawyer may be misled by the limitations of his perspective, and mistake personal interests for those of the group on whose behalf he speaks. Thus the lawyer's personal interest in furthering his career or his organization, or in amusing himself, and the limitations of his perspective because of his class and racial background, may undermine the goals to which he professes devotion.

No one really knows which of these models will produce "better" decisions, nor is there agreement on what "better" means. Given what have been publicized as failures of expertise in the country's recent history, however, and given the demoralizing powerlessness so many citizens feel today, the arguments seem stronger in the direction of community control; where there is popular participation, decisions are at least likely to be perceived as more "legitimate," and, even should there be increased in-fighting among groups, community organization is likely to be furthered. This is not to say that lawyers whose selection of cases is not controlled by the community are somehow illegitimate advocates of the underrepresented. They may be handling matters affecting the community to which no other lawyer is giving consideration; and they may even be handling matters which *they* perceive are the *most* important for the community. But where a lawyer, a foundation, or a program administrator is faced with the choice between the independence and community control models of service, we can favor the latter, insisting that only it will offer the poor more than "expert"—though presumably benevolent—manipulation of their future.

*　　*　　*

NOTE 2.

STEPHEN WEXLER
PRACTICING LAW FOR POOR PEOPLE*

*　　*　　*

The dominant attitude in law school is that the client is a troublesome pain-in-the-neck. Occasionally, the law student hears hints that he should present his clients with the legal alternatives, among which the client should choose. Many lawyers are now aware that people should control their lawyer, and are beginning to present alternatives from which their clients can choose. But the control which poor people should exercise over their lawyer is much greater than that of merely selecting among his proposals. Because he does know more about the possibilities in the law, the lawyer should present new knowledge and options to his clients; but, because they know what is helpful to them and possible for them, they can and must structure their own alternatives and make their own choices. The lawyer should not push his clients toward or away from jail. "Jail" must, of course, be read as a metaphor for the whole range of possible consequences of possible actions, of which jail is only the worst.

The last portion of the preceding sentence makes clear why a lawyer must not lead his clients. For me, as for most lawyers, jail is the worst possible consequence of a political action. But it is clear that jail is not the worst consequence. Welfare recipients have lost the only money they have to live on because they protested the policies of welfare departments; people have lost their homes; children have been unable to obtain medical care; Fred Hampton was shot.

*　　*　　*

* 79 *Yale Law Journal* 1049, 1063–64 (1970). Reprinted by permission of the Yale Law Journal Company and Fred B. Rothman and Company.

CHAPTER FOUR

Perspectives on Decisionmaking

The case studies in the first two chapters revealed considerable confusion about the rights and duties of the various participants as well as the absence of a conceptual framework to guide the human experimentation process. Before turning to a detailed analysis of the authority of the participants at each stage—formulation, administration, and review—of the experimentation process, we pause briefly to examine some theories of decisionmaking. These theories raise fundamental questions for students of human experimentation about the extent of man's ability to plan rationally for human institutions.

At one extreme the pure market system of "free contract" suggests that all control over experimentation should be left to individual investigators and the subjects whom they persuade to join their projects. At the other extreme, some theorists maintain that decisions are better made collectively after a thorough analysis of all relevant values and a comparison of the extent to which alternative plans maximize these values. Under this system, for example, a central planning agency would decide which experiments to pursue and would prescribe in detail the rights and duties of all participants. Other analysts agree that some planning is needed, but believe that limitations on time, resources, and rationality preclude "comprehensive" planning. Their approach would lead to intervention directed at specific evils in the process or to marginal changes in regulations which are easily modified in the light of experience.

This chapter does not present a complete examination of competing decisionmaking theories. Rather, a sampling of the literature is offered to stimulate questions as the student turns to Parts Two, Three, and Four of this book and analyzes specific proposals for exercising control over human experimentation, especially by the professions and the state. Thus, the materials should facilitate consideration of the advantages and disadvantages of various decisionmaking models for each stage in the human experimentation process. Throughout the remaining chapters we return not only to the decisionmaking questions raised in this chapter but also to an examination of the values on which such decisions rest. For example, the discussion of individual liberty in Chapter Eight bears on both the value of freedom and the kinds of regulations society may wish to pursue to implement this value.

In studying these materials, on the basis of problems already raised about human experimentation, consider the following questions:

1. What are the limits of planning by man for man?

2. What values of man and society are reinforced or undermined by these theories of decisionmaking?

3. What impact would the adoption of the various decisionmaking theories have had on the resolution of the problems which surfaced in the Jewish Chronic Disease Hospital and Wichita Jury Recording cases?

A.
Planning by Individuals—The Market System

1.
Cooperation without Coercion?

a.
Milton Friedman
Capitalism and Freedom*

* * *

Fundamentally, there are only two ways of coordinating the economic activities of millions. One is central direction involving the use of coercion—the technique of the army and of the modern totalitarian state. The other is voluntary cooperation of individuals—the technique of the market place.

The possibility of coordination through voluntary cooperation rests on the elementary—yet frequently denied—proposition that both parties to an economic transaction benefit from it, *provided the transaction is bilaterally voluntary and informed.*

Exchange can therefore bring about coordination without coercion. A working model of a society organized through voluntary exchange is

a *free private enterprise exchange economy*—what we have been calling competitive capitalism.

In its simplest form, such a society consists of a number of independent households—a collection of Robinson Crusoes, as it were. Each household uses the resources it controls to produce goods and services that it exchanges for goods and services produced by other households, on terms mutually acceptable to the two parties to the bargain. It is thereby enabled to satisfy its wants indirectly by producing goods and services for others, rather than directly by producing goods for its own immediate use. The incentive for adopting this indirect route is, of course, the increased product made possible by division of labor and specialization of function. Since the household always has the alternative of producing directly for itself, it need not enter into any exchange unless it benefits from it. Hence, no exchange will take place unless both parties do benefit from it. Cooperation is thereby achieved without coercion.

Specialization of function and division of labor would not go far if the ultimate productive unit were the household. In a modern society, we have gone much farther. We have introduced enterprises which are intermediaries between in-

* Chicago: University of Chicago Press, 13–15, 23–24, 33–34 (1962). © 1962 by the University of Chicago. Reprinted by permission.

dividuals in their capacities as suppliers of service and as purchasers of goods. And similarly, specialization of function and division of labor could not go very far if we had to continue to rely on the barter of product for product. In consequence, money has been introduced as a means of facilitating exchange, and of enabling the acts of purchase and of sale to be separated into two parts.

Despite the important role of enterprises and of money in our actual economy, and despite the numerous and complex problems they raise, the central characteristic of the market technique of achieving coordination is fully displayed in the simple exchange economy that contains neither enterprises nor money. As in that simple model, so in the complex enterprise and money-exchange economy, cooperation is strictly individual and voluntary *provided:* (a) that enterprises are private, so that the ultimate contracting parties are individuals and (b) that individuals are effectively free to enter or not to enter into any particular exchange, so that every transaction is strictly voluntary.

It is far easier to state these provisos in general terms than to spell them out in detail, or to specify precisely the institutional arrangements most conducive to their maintenance. Indeed, much of technical economic literature is concerned with precisely these questions. The basic requisite is the maintenance of law and order to prevent physical coercion of one individual by another and to enforce contracts voluntarily entered into, thus giving substantive meaning to "private." Aside from this, perhaps the most difficult problems arise from monopoly—which inhibits effective freedom by denying individuals alternatives to the particular exchange—and from "neighborhood effects"—effects on third parties for which it is not feasible to charge or recompense them. . . .

So long as effective freedom of exchange is maintained, the central feature of the market organization of economic activity is that it prevents one person from interfering with another in respect of most of his activities. The consumer is protected from coercion by the seller because of the presence of other sellers with whom he can deal. The seller is protected from coercion by the consumer because of other consumers to whom he can sell. The employee is protected from coercion by the employer because of other employers for whom he can work, and so on. And the market does this impersonally and without centralized authority.

Indeed, a major source of objection to a free economy is precisely that it does this task so well. It gives people what they want instead of what a particular group thinks they ought to want. Underlying most arguments against the free market is a lack of belief in freedom itself.

The existence of a free market does not of course eliminate the need for government. On the contrary, government is essential both as a forum for determining the "rules of the game" and as an umpire to interpret and enforce the rules decided on. What the market does is to reduce greatly the range of issues that must be decided through political means, and thereby to minimize the extent to which government need participate directly in the game. The characteristic feature of action through political channels is that it tends to require or enforce substantial conformity. The great advantage of the market, on the other hand, is that it permits wide diversity. It is, in political terms, a system of proportional representation. Each man can vote, as it were, for the color of tie he wants and get it; he does not have to see what color the majority wants and then, if he is in the minority, submit.

It is this feature of the market that we refer to when we say that the market provides economic freedom. . . .

*   *   *

There are clearly some matters with respect to which effective proportional representation is impossible. I cannot get the amount of national defense I want and you, a different amount. With respect to such indivisible matters we can discuss, and argue, and vote. But having decided, we must conform. It is precisely the existence of such indivisible matters—protection of the individual and the nation from coercion are clearly the most basic—that prevents exclusive reliance on individual action through the market. If we are to use some of our resources for such indivisible items, we must employ political channels to reconcile differences.

The use of political channels, while inevitable, tends to strain the social cohesion essential for a stable society. The strain is least if agreement for joint action need be reached only on a limited range of issues on which people in any event have common views. Every extension of the range of issues for which explicit agreement is sought strains further the delicate threads that hold society together. If it goes so far as to touch an issue on which men feel deeply yet differently, it may well disrupt the society. Fundamental differences in basic values can seldom if ever be resolved at the ballot box; ultimately they can only be decided, though not resolved, by conflict. The religious and civil wars of history are a bloody testament to this judgment.

The widespread use of the market reduces the strain on the social fabric by rendering conformity unnecessary with respect to any activities it encompasses. The wider the range of activities covered by the market, the fewer are the issues on which explicitly political decisions are required and hence on which it is necessary to achieve agreement. In turn, the fewer the issues on which agreement is necessary, the greater is the likelihood of getting agreement while maintaining a free society.

*   *   *

Freedom is a tenable objective only for responsible individuals. We do not believe in freedom for madmen or children. The necessity of drawing a line between responsible individuals and others is inescapable, yet it means that there is an essential ambiguity in our ultimate objective of freedom. Paternalism is inescapable for those whom we designate as not responsible.

The clearest case, perhaps, is that of madmen. We are willing neither to permit them freedom nor to shoot them. It would be nice if we could rely on voluntary activities of individuals to house and care for the madmen. But I think we cannot rule out the possibility that such charitable activities will be inadequate, if only because of the neighborhood effect involved in the fact that I benefit if another man contributes to the care of the insane. For this reason, we may be willing to arrange for their care through government.

Children offer a more difficult case. The ultimate operative unit in our society is the family, not the individual. Yet the acceptance of the family as the unit rests in considerable part on expediency rather than principle. We believe that parents are generally best able to protect their children and to provide for their development into responsible individuals for whom freedom is appropriate. But we do not believe in the freedom of parents to do what they will with other people. The children are responsible individuals in embryo, and a believer in freedom believes in protecting their ultimate rights.

To put this in a different and what may seem a more callous way, children are at one and the same time consumer goods and potentially responsible members of society. The freedom of individuals to use their economic resources as they want includes the freedom to use them to have children—to buy, as it were, the services of children as a particular form of consumption. But once this choice is exercised, the children have a value in and of themselves and have a freedom of their own that is not simply an extension of the freedom of the parents.

The paternalistic ground for governmental activity is in many ways the most troublesome to a liberal [*]; for it involves the acceptance of a principle—that some shall decide for others—which he finds objectionable in most applications and which he rightly regards as a hallmark of his chief intellectual opponents, the proponents of collectivism in one or another of its guises, whether it be communism, socialism, or a welfare state. Yet there is no use pretending that problems are simpler than in fact they are. There is no avoiding the need for some measure of paternalism. As Dicey wrote in 1914 about an act for the protection of mental defectives, "The Mental Deficiency Act is the first step along a path on which no sane man can decline to enter, but which, if too far pursued, will bring statesmen across difficulties hard to meet without considerable interference with individual liberty." There is no formula that can tell us where to stop. We must rely on our fallible judgment and, having reached a judgment, on our ability to persuade our fellow men that it is a correct judgment, or on their ability to persuade us to modify our views. We must put our faith, here as elsewhere, in a consensus reached by imperfect and biased men through free discussion and trial and error.

*   *   *

b.

Sumner H. Slichter
Modern Economic Society†

*   *   *

The reasoning in support of the belief that freedom of enterprise is the maximum of satisfaction at the minimum of cost is very simple. Each individual, it is said, is better able than any one else to judge his own interests. If men are at liberty to spend their money as they choose,

---

[*] Friedman uses the term "liberal" in its classical nineteenth century meaning, not in the meaning it has come to have in the United States in recent decades.

† New York: Henry Holt & Co. 43–46, 49 (1928). Reprinted by permission.

they will naturally purchase those things that will yield them the most satisfaction. Consequently the very commodities which give consumers the greatest pleasure are the most profitable for business enterprises to produce. Likewise, if men are free to use such methods of production as they wish, they will select those which involve the least cost per unit of output. With the goods which give the greatest gratification being made by the methods which are least costly, it follows, according to the theory, that there will be the maximum surplus of satisfaction over sacrifice.

But if this result is to follow, two things would appear to be necessary: (1) goods must go to the consumers who will derive the greatest pleasure from them, and (2) the tasks of making goods must be assigned to the workers who can perform them with the least sacrifice for each unit of product. Does freedom of enterprise cause either goods or jobs to be distributed in this manner?

[U]nder a system of free enterprise goods tend to get into the hands of those who offer the best prices for them. But how then can they be consumed so as to yield the maximum of satisfaction? Are the people who are willing and able to pay most for goods also those who will derive the most satisfaction from using them? If they are not, it would appear possible to increase the surplus of satisfaction over sacrifice by causing goods to be distributed more in accordance with needs and less in accordance with ability to pay. We have no way of comparing the amount of pleasure which two persons derive from consuming an article. And yet it seems ridiculous to assert that ability to derive satisfaction from goods is proportionate to ability to pay for them. . . .

We are no better able to compare the pains suffered by different persons than we are the pleasures which they enjoy. Nevertheless it does not appear probable that freedom of enterprise necessarily causes jobs to be distributed so as to result in a minimum sacrifice for each unit of output—so that, for example, persons who can do heavy work with least fatigue will be given heavy work. Rather jobs tend to go to those who are willing to do the most work for the least money. . . .

In face of the fact that ability to derive pleasure from goods does not appear to correspond to capacity to pay for them and that jobs are not necessarily given to the men who can do them with the least sacrifice for each unit of product, how can it be asserted that industrial liberty results in a maximum of satisfaction over

sacrifice? But the exponents of free enterprise are not without a reply. To interfere with liberty in order to bring about a distribution of goods upon the basis of needs rather than ability to pay, or in order to cause jobs to be assigned to those who perform them with least sacrifice, might have the *immediate* effect of increasing the surplus of satisfaction over sacrifice. But this result, it is said, would be short lived. Men have the greatest incentive to improve their efficiency when they are free to compete for any jobs which they desire and to spend their income as they see fit. Were this incentive diminished by distributing jobs to those who could perform them with the least sacrifice and goods to those who would derive the most pleasure from them, output would inevitably decline. What would be gained by a different distribution of goods and jobs would be lost through smaller production.

* * *

The theory of free enterprise does not, it is important to emphasize, assert that restraints upon human selfishness are not needed. It simply assumes that they are provided by *competition*. This, according to the theory, is the great regulative force which establishes effective control over economic activities and gives each of us an incentive to observe the interests of others. Thus business establishments are deterred from furnishing adulterated or poorly made goods by the fear that customers may shift their patronage to rivals. Likewise the enterprises which fail to protect their men against accidents or industrial disease or which work them unusually hard are penalized by the refusal of laborers to work for them except at a higher wage than other employers pay.

The mere existence of competition, however, is not enough. For it to perform satisfactorily the protective function attributed to it, certain very definite conditions must be present.

To begin with, an appreciable proportion of buyers and sellers must be willing to discriminate against those sellers or buyers who ignore, and in favor of those who take account of, the welfare of others. Otherwise, of course, no one has an economic incentive to pay attention to the well-being of his fellows. Assume, for example, that an enterprise pollutes a stream by dumping refuse and chemicals into it. From the standpoint of the firm, this may be an economical method of production. But from the standpoint of the community it is an expensive one, because it kills the fish, spoils the stream for bathing, and makes it foul and ill-smelling. But competition will not stop the pollution unless an appreciable number of consumers, wage earners, or investors refuse to deal with the firm which is responsible—that is, unless a substantial number of consumers refuse to buy from it, or wage earners to work for it, or investors to put money into it. But if the enterprise charges no more than its rivals for goods of equal grade, offers equally attractive conditions of employment, and pays as high dividends, who has an interest in discriminating against it? Perhaps the very fact that the enterprise pollutes the stream enables it to offer better terms than its rivals. Or take the case of child labor—another method of production cheap in dollars and cents but expensive in terms of human cost. If the firms which employ children are able, *because of that very fact,* to sell for less or to pay higher wages to adults or higher profits to investors, who is going to discriminate against them? Under these circumstances, does not competition positively encourage the employment of children?

But willingness to discriminate between those who consider the interests of others and those who do not is insufficient. Competition protects consumers against inferior ware only when they know good quality from bad; it protects laborers from unguarded machines only when they know which employers have and which have not guarded their machines. In other words, competition is an efficient protective agency only when buyers or sellers have the information necessary to make intelligent choices. It fails, for example, to protect consumers against milk from tubercular cattle because the ordinary buyer of milk has no way of distinguishing the milk of healthy cows from that of diseased.

*　　*　　*

Perhaps the most striking aspect of the theory of free enterprise is its assertion that intervention of the government in economic activities is unnecessary. The theory, as we have said, does not deny that restraints on human selfishness are needed. It simply asserts that we can trust competition to provide them. But closer inquiry reveals that the defenders of free enterprise do not trust competition to do all things. However much they trust it to guard the lives and limbs of workmen against dangerous machinery or to protect consumers against injurious foods, they do not rely upon it to enforce contracts or to prevent fraud. But the same reasoning which is used to prove that the government need not intervene on behalf of wage earners and consumers can be employed to show that laws are not required to guard business men against fraud or breach of contractual obligations. Would not a customer who refused to pay his bills soon experience difficulty in getting dealers to sell to him, and would not an enterprise which violated its contracts find other concerns unwilling to deal with it? Is not the aid of the courts in these matters as superfluous as laws to protect workmen against dangerous machines or consumers against adulterated wares?

NOTE

W. J. M. MacKenzie
Politics and Social Science*

The invisible hand of perfect competition was deemed to maximize utility by making decisions which were in a sense not decisions at all. Part of the puzzle is that in common use the word "decision" has something to do with an individual choosing, according to criteria which he has chosen or at least accepted, between options present to his mind. A market in a sense sums individual decisions, and it is easy to slip into talking of market "decisions," as one slips into talking of computer "decisions." But one of the blessed characteristics of a market is that the outcome is no one's "decision": it is an "event." As has been said often, seriously or in sarcasm, it is a situation almost too good to be true, that nature should thus optimize and distribute for us, without human responsibility.

2.

Free Choice about Risktaking?

Guido Calabresi
The Costs of Accidents—A Legal and Economic Analysis†

*　　*　　*

[T]he primary way in which a society may seek to reduce accident costs is to discourage activities that are "accident prone" and substitute

---

* Baltimore: Penguin Books 139 (1967). © W. J. M. MacKenzie, 1967. Reprinted by permission.

† New Haven: Yale University Press 68–94 (1970). Reprinted by permission.

safer activities as well as safer ways of engaging in the same activities. But such a statement suggests neither the degree to which we wish to discourage such activities nor the means for doing so. [W]e certainly do not wish to avoid accident costs at all costs by forbidding all accident-prone activities. Most activities can be carried out safely enough or be sufficiently reduced in frequency so that there is a point at which their worth outweights the costs of the accidents they cause. Specific prohibition or deterrence of most activities would cost society more than it would save in accident costs prevented. We want the fact that activities cause accidents to influence our choices among activities and among ways of doing them. But we want to limit this influence to a degree that is justified by the cost of these accidents. The obvious question is, how do we do this?

There are two basic approaches to making these difficult "decisions for accidents," and our society has always used both, though not always to the same degree. The first, which I have termed the specific deterrence or collective approach . . . involves deciding collectively the degree to which we want any given activity, who should participate in it, and how we want it done. These decisions may or may not be made solely on the basis of the accident costs the activity causes. The collective decisions are enforced by penalties on those who violate them.

The other approach . . . involves attempting instead to decide what the accident costs of activities are and letting the *market* determine the degree to which, and the ways in which, activities are desired given such costs. Similarly, it involves giving people freedom to choose whether they would rather engage in the activity and pay the cost of doing so, including accident costs, or, given the accident costs, engage in safer activities that might otherwise have seemed less desirable. I call this approach general, or market, deterrence.

The crucial thing about the general deterrence approach to accidents is that it does not involve an a priori collective decision as to the correct number of accidents. General deterrence implies that accident costs would be treated as one of the many costs we face whenever we do anything. Since we cannot have everything we want, individually or as a society, whenever we choose one thing we give up others. General deterrence attempts to force individuals to consider accident costs in choosing among activities. The problem is getting the best combination of choices available. The general deterrence ap-

proach would let the free market or price system tally the choices.

* * *

The general deterrence approach treats accident costs as it does any other costs of goods and activities—such as the metal, or the time it takes, to make cars. If all activities reflect the accident costs they "cause," each individual will be able to choose for himself whether an activity is worth the accident costs it "causes." The sum of these choices is, *ex hypothesis,* the best combination available and will determine the degree to which accident-prone activities are engaged in (if at all), how they are engaged in, and who will engage in them. Failure to include accident costs in the prices of activities will, according to the theory, cause people to choose more accident-prone activities than they would if the prices of these activities made them pay for these accident costs, resulting in more accident costs than we want. Forbidding accident-prone activities *despite* the fact that they can "pay" their costs would, in theory, bring about an equally bad result from the resource allocation point of view. Either way, the postulate that individuals know best for themselves would be violated.

* * *

For the theory to make some sense there is no need to postulate a world made up of economic men who consciously consider the relative costs of each different good and the relative pleasure derived from each. If the cost of all automobile accidents were suddenly to be paid out of a general social insurance fund, the expense of owning a car would be a good deal lower than it is now since people would no longer need to worry about buying insurance. The result would be that some people would buy more cars. Perhaps they would be teen-agers who can afford $100 for an old jalopy but who cannot afford—or whose fathers cannot afford—the insurance. Or they might be people who could only afford a second car so long as no added insurance was involved. In any event, the demand for cars would increase, and so would the number of cars produced. Indeed, the effect on car purchases would be much the same as if the government suddenly chose to pay the cost of the steel used by automobile manufacturers and to raise the money out of general taxes. In each case the objection would be the same. In each, an economist would say, resources are mis-allocated in that goods are produced that the consumer would not want if he had to pay the full extent of their cost to society, whether in terms of the physical components of the product or in terms of the expense of accidents associated with its production and use.

*   *   *

To describe a world of perfect general deterrence is to refute its possibility. In the extreme, general deterrence would consider the problem of accident costs to be precisely one of market decisions to buy and sell goods, and accident costs would give rise to *no* collective decisions regarding whether activities were worthwhile. If an activity could pay for the accidents it caused and make a go of it, it would be considered worthwhile; if it could not pay such costs, it would be priced out of the market. But for this to work properly, activities would have to be able to "buy" willing victims. Just as the potential injurer would have to decide whether the accident was worth its costs to him, so the victim would have to decide whether the payment to be received in compensation made the accident worthwhile from his point of view. The costs of accidents would then be determined freely by the market, and there would be no need for collective intervention.

Obviously this is a highly improbable situation. In the extreme, it presupposes such perfect knowledge that all "accidents" would be come intentional killings, mayhems, or taking of property by the injurer; and suicides or sales of person or property by the victim. Short of the extreme, it presupposes at least a *statistical* intention to injure and a *statistical* willingness to be injured (for a price) that does not and cannot represent the attitudes of actual injurers and victims in our society. An examination of each of these "theoretical" worlds of general deterrence will disclose what an actual world of optimal general deterence would look like.

The first of these theoretical worlds requires perfect knowledge, so that both the victim and the injurer would know that a particular act performed at a particulra time in a particular way would result in a particular injury. Victim and injurer could then bargain without collective intervention for an appropriate price to be paid for the injury. But it is virtually inconceivable that with such perfect knowledge the parties would not find it cheaper to act in a slightly different way and avoid the injury. In other words, with such perfect knowledge there would be no "accidents" and virtually no injuries—general deter-

rence would work perfectly. The few injuries that would remain would be acts of madmen, and intolerable—or perfect martyrdoms, and divine.

It might be thought that even without perfect knowledge, pure general de_.rrence, requiring no collective determination of accident costs, could exist so long as we have statistically certain injurers and victims. People willing to take a risk for a price would form a supply of victims, and people willing to pay the price in order to undertake activities which injure would form a demand side for the victims.

*   *   *

It may appear that potential victims do undertake some risky enterprises in exchange for payments that compensate them for the risk of being injured. Thus it may seem that both the supply and the demand sides of an injury market exist, and that no collective decisions are necessary to the determination of the costs of accidents. Closer examination, however, casts severe doubt on the feasibility of this statistical world of pure general deterrence.

It depends on market bargains—establishing the value of accident costs—between *potential* injurers and *potential* victims *before the accident*. In practice this presupposes that the potential victims are already in a bargaining relationship with the potential injurers *before* the accident and can therefore ask for payment for being potential victims. Market determination of accident costs is not meaningful in any practical sense in situations where the injuring party has no bargaining relationship with the potential victims before the accident. For example, while it may appear that coal miners receive, and mine owners pay, wages that reflect the costs of mine accidents as estimated by both sides, it is hard to see how a similar bargain could be struck between drivers and pedestrians. In theory, drivers might seek out all the pedestrians whom they could conceivably injure, offer them an amount of money in exchange for taking the risk, receive counteroffers from them, and ultimately strike bargains establishing market values for the costs of car-pedestrian accidents. But such bargains are inconceivable in reality.

Even in the case where potential victims *are* in a bargaining relationship with potential injurers before the accident, it is usually unrealistic to treat market determination of the value of accident costs as adequate.

In the first place, adequate market determination of accident costs requires freedom on the part of victims to refuse the bargain and thus avoid the risk of injury. If the organization of our society is such that the only alternative work available to coal miners is the almost equally dangerous occupation of lumberjacking, it is hard to accept the valuation of accident costs arrived at through the "free" bargains between miners and mine owners as a satisfactory estimate of the accident costs involved.

In the second place, free market determination of the value of accident costs will lead to an acceptable result only if the potential injurers and victims are reasonably aware of and take account of the risks, i.e., only if they have adequate statistical knowledge of the risks involved and act on that knowledge. Injurers may often obtain and act on such knowledge, but as we have seen in our discussion of why private insurance is not likely to bring about adequate loss spreading, victims are unlikely to do either. Virtually all the arguments made there apply here: it may be very expensive for potential victims to obtain adequate knowledge of what the risk is; they may be psychologically incapable of viewing themselves as *actual* victims; they may suffer from the Faust complex and inevitably choose the good life now and regret it later; and they may not be the only ones to bear the costs when they occur.

In the third place, statistical willingness to take risks does not give an adequate value for what an accident costs if it actually occurs. This is because the value individuals give to a particular accident depends on the likelihood of its occurring. A man may take $1,000 for one chance in a thousand of being killed, thus seeming to value his life at $1,000,000, and still require much more than $10,000 for one chance in a hundred of being killed. And if he accepted $50,000 for one chance in a hundred, thus valuing his life at $5,000,000, this would be no indication that he would accept $2,500,000 for one chance in two of being killed, or $5,000,000 in exchange for the certainty of death. [T]his does not mean we should not try to give values to lives and limbs, but especially when coupled with the other factors I have just mentioned, it makes any purely market determination of the costs of accidents entirely inadequate.

For all these reasons, even a society that is basically committed to the general notion that individuals know best for themselves, and hence to general deterrence, will not leave valuations of accident costs to the free market. Some of the problems with free market determination of the value of accident costs will be mitigated in situations where the bargaining on the part of potential victims is carried out by representatives (such as unions) who presumably are aware of the risks and do not suffer from the same psychological disadvantages. But this mitigation will occur, at best, only in some of the bargaining situations, which themselves are only a part of the world of accident costs.

*   *   *

Of course, even if we thought that the problems with free market accident cost determination could all be overcome, we might still find a world of total general deterrence not to our liking. The allocation of losses necessary in such a world might result in intolerable concentrations of losses, the administrative costs of establishing and running this world might be too high, and our "moral" sense might be offended by activities that could pay their way under such a system. As a result, collective judgments would still be required. In other words, a world of total general deterrence might not be desirable because it does not allow room for our other goals.

*   *   *

NOTE

FRANK H. KNIGHT
FREEDOM AND REFORM*

*   *   *

Individual freedom of patients to select their doctors, and of men generally to be doctors, is exactly the meaning of what is called free competition or, more accurately, the open-market organization. Social planners usually misconceive these facts. There is no implication of competition in the psychological sense of a feeling of rivalry, or action motivated by this feeling; on the contrary, such feeling and action are definitely irrational, in the instrumental or means-and-end definition. Economic competition is one of the unfortunate accidents of terminology; what it means is simply the freedom of individuals to cooperate through exchange with the others who offer (or accept) the best terms. The idea of "bargaining" is likewise misleading. In an effective market there is no bargaining in the sense of higgling or discussion or influence, and in most real markets there is very little.

* New York: Harper and Brothers 360–364 (1947). Copyright, 1947, by Harper & Row, Publishers, Inc. Reprinted by permission.

To discuss market competition as a method of organized action would mean summarizing the science of economics. It may be viewed either as an alternative to collective rationality or as an alternative form of the latter or method of achieving the same general result. We can only assert "dogmatically" that the theoretically perfect, or "perfectly competitive" market has certain consequences for the given individuals involved. It leads to the "maximum" of efficiency consistent with individual freedom, in the only sense in which association can be free, i.e., based on rational mutual consent, and also results in "justice" in the sense of exchange of equal values. That is, the return to each participant is equal to his contribution to the total result of the joint activity; each takes out the equivalent of what he puts in, in the only possible meaning of quantitative equivalence.

This of course is "theory." On the other side we note two general facts, also without explanation or argument. The first is that real markets are more or less imperfect; the second, the far more important fact that the ethical quality of the result is limited by the consideration that the individuals are taken as given, specifically with respect to their desires and their possession and control of productive capacity in all forms. The main mechanical limitations are monopoly and the business cycle. Popular ideas about monopoly fantastically exaggerate both its amount and the evil of that which exists, particularly when society is not already demoralized by crisis conditions. A considerable amount of monopoly is inevitable and more is natural and useful in a free and progressive economy. In extreme cases, where conditions make reasonably effective competition impossible or grossly wasteful (such as public utilities, railways, etc.) public authority always steps in to "regulate" the industry or to operate it directly. As to cycle phenomena, the main fact is that depressions benefit virtually no one and accordingly do not arise out of conflicts of interest. Consequently, the remedy does not present an ethical problem but is purely a matter of science and political competence.

The major ethical problem of economic organization arises out of the grossly unequal distribution of economic capacity, and consequently of the product, among individuals, and the fact that distribution is determined for the most part by forces beyond the control of the disadvantaged individuals and classes, while the working of the free exchange system naturally tends toward increasing inequality. The simple and obvious remedy for inequality, insofar as it is unjust and is practically remediable, is not planning by a central authority, but progressive taxation, particularly of inheritances, with use of the proceeds to provide services for the poorer people. Particularly in point are relief of destitution, health measures, and educational opportunities for the young. This remedy has long been widely applied. . . .

. . . This points in a very different direction from central planning, which obviously means curing the root evil of excessively unequal distribution of economic power through an enormously greater concentration—in economic terms, a universal monopoly. And if any prediction is possible, this would not tend either to equalize the distribution of income itself, or to increase efficiency, while freedom, the greatest of the fundamental human values, would be largely sacrificed. Within wide limits, free government is to be preferred to good government (in any other meaning) or freer to better; and the reasonable inference from history, current experience, and reasoning in general terms is that planning by any central authority would sacrifice the one and mean a loss rather than a gain in terms of the other. Any government which had the task of managing the economic life of a modern nation, to say nothing of the world, would have to be a dictatorship and to repress the primary freedoms of thought, communication and association. This would be true even if it were staffed with people who personally abhorred power—and the contention that power would fall into the hands of such people will appeal only to the most romantic credulity.

However, the problem is complex, and certainly calls for a combination of practically all conceivable forms of solution. The positive values in what we call economic life itself are more aesthetic, social and cultural than really individual; and even where they seem to be individualistic, there are limits to the possibility of allowing each individual to be his own judge of what is good for him, or the means of achieving it. The real defects of the "competitive" economic order as revealed by objective analysis are largely due to limitations of the rationality of individuals and free groups, and a general replacement of free action and voluntary association with political compulsion would certainly mean a decrease and not an increase in rationality. Centralization of authority within any political unit would be achieved through the domination, by force, emotional appeal, or outright trickery, of some particular interest group, and under conditions which probably mean mobilization for war against opposed internal interests or externally against other units. . . .

Yet there is a place for centralized planning under authority, with some use of force, of innumerable activities and with an infinite variety in the scope of the units. All government is by nature central planning. But there is a vast difference in principle between general laws, of the nature of traffic regulations or rules of the game, and concrete prescription of where, when, and how to travel or what game to play. The main difficulty is that planning always means replanning, and the imposition of some particular plan out of an infinite number of possibilities, and under some particular authority, among innumerable claimants. Most of the possibilities under both heads have both merits and limitations, and the real question is how far to go at the same time in most of the possible directions.

* * *

B.
Collective Planning—The Rational-Comprehensive Approach

1.

Cooperation through Comprehensive Analysis?

a.

Harold D. Lasswell
The Political Science of Science*

* * *

[The] task is to construct a continuing institutional activity by which central theory is related continuously to events as they unfold. . . .

The limited degree of success achieved by the profession in perfecting or in encouraging the body politic to perfect such an institutional process had adverse consequences for our role in regard to nuclear weapons. Long before atomic weapons were introduced we were well aware of the importance of scientific knowledge for the technology of fighting. But we did not correctly anticipate the approximate timing of the impact of nuclear physics upon military technology. Although we were equipped to assess the political consequences of sudden and stupendous increases of fighting effectiveness we did not foresee that such an emergent was imminent. Since technical developments were not explicitly anticipated we did not clarify in advance the main policy alternatives open to decision makers in this country or elsewhere. We did not create a literature or a body of oral analysis that seriously anticipated these issues. As political scientists we should have anticipated fully both the bomb and the significant problems of policy that came with it.

I do not want to create the impression that all would have been well if we had been better political scientists, and that we must bear upon our puny shoulders the burden of culpability for the situation of the world today. We are not so grandiose as to magnify our role or our responsibility beyond all proportion. Yet I cannot refrain from acknowledging, as I look back, that we left the minds of our decision makers flagrantly unprepared to meet the crisis precipitated by the bomb. I have no desire to hold a kangaroo court on President Truman's momentous decision or upon his principal advisers; or to give credence to the insinuation that "results" had become necessary in the face of Congressional restiveness about the cost of research and development. In the light of hindsight (that should have been foresight) I want to underline the probability that the new weapon was introduced in a manner that contributed unnecessarily to world insecurity. Perhaps the critics are right who say that the bomb should have been demonstrated on an uninhabited island before the live drops were made on Hiroshima and Nagasaki. More important is the question of how formal and effective control might have been extended beyond the decision makers of a single power. At least some members of the winning coalition might wisely have been brought into a system that operated through a common agency of inspection and direction.

Plainly there were not enough political scientists trained in physics, or sufficiently aware of the implication of impending scientific developments, to do much forward thinking and planning. This points to a failure of professional recruitment and training, and calls in question the then-prevailing conception of the political

* 50 *The American Political Science Review* 961–979 (1956). Reprinted by permission.

scientist's role. . . . Part of our role, as the venerable metaphor has it, is scanning the horizon of the unfolding future with a view to defining in advance the probable import of what is foreseeable for the navigators of the Ship of State. It is our responsibility to flagellate our minds toward creativity, toward bringing into the stream of emerging events conceptions of future strategy that, if adopted, will increase the probability that ideal aspirations will be more approximately realized.

An implication for our future relation to science and armament is that we need to develop more political scientists who have the competence to infer the weapon implications of science and technology. It then becomes possible to anticipate the implications for collective policy.

Even a moderate degree of cross-disciplinary training or continuing contact should have enabled us to prepare for the advent of nuclear fission (and fusion). The *Review of Modern Physics* carried an article by Louis Turner of Princeton University in January 1940 in which 133 papers were appraised. They began with Fermi's original report of 1934 and came down to the Hahn-Strassman-Meitner researches which made explicit the import of Fermi's original experiment. In passing it may be noted that the contributions of a dozen nations were catalogued in Turner's review. Not more than half a dozen of the 133 papers were by American authors. Perhaps American political scientists may be partially absolved for lack of foresight under these circumstances. But the over-all record of the profession is not thereby improved, since I do not find that colleagues in other countries were any more in touch than we were. Incidentally, it is worth recording that a standard college textbook in physics included a chapter in which the implications of current research were clearly spelled out. Ernest Pollard of Yale University referred in 1940 to the possibility of nuclear reactors that might generate electrical power or detonate as immensely destructive bombs; or that might produce radioactive substances for research and industrial processes or for a new and frightful kind of chemical warfare. I note further that at the time of the Fermi-Dunning experiment at the Columbia University cyclotron in early 1939 some science writers (especially of the *New York Times*) were quite definite about what was at stake.

*   *   *

In many ways the most disturbing result of the laggard position of political scientists in comprehending science and technology is that we have displayed no intellectual initiative in furnishing guidance to those who are in command of modern knowledge and its instrumentalities. Alert businessmen have long been on the lookout for promising applications in the marketplace. The professional military man is now accustomed to take the initiative. The question for us as political scientists is whether we have given enough serious attention to the task of reducing the human cost of whatever violence we cannot dispense with.

As an exercise in this line of thought I invite you to use your imagination to ask what an instrument of coercion would look like that incapacitates without killing, mutilating or in any way imposing permanent incapacity. You and I will probably come up with the same answer: a gas or a drug or a beam that when applied will induce sleep or a similar state of suspension. We spent several billion dollars on A and H bombs; and it is commonly said, with some plausibility, that scientists and engineers give you what you pay for. Our suggestion (and I repeat an old proposal) is that we go down the alphabet to the P bomb, the "paralysis bomb." The technical difficulties in the way of paralyzing a city or a region are very great, given current means of delivering a concentrated gas. Possibly the instrument can be a "P beam," a paralyzing beam of sound or of some other kind capable of accomplishing the purpose.

Without being in the least committed to the specific devices referred to, I nevertheless assert that in the future we need not remain as passive as we have been in approaching the problem of harmonizing considerations of humanity with the use of whatever coercion cannot be avoided.

*   *   *

As clarifiers of the goals and alternatives implicit in a decision process and as advisers of the participants we have an opportunity to reduce the amount of unnecessary friction by establishing a frame of reference in advance of the facts. When factual details appear they will of course exhibit some novel elements; common goals and principles will not. The members of the world community have a long history of accommodating "exclusive" claims and "sharing" claims with one another (as new resources provide new base values for the participants in the world arena).

It is, or course, essential that in taking advantage of this opportunity we deal with the entire context of value goals and principles as they relate to potential facts. I have referred to sets of doctrines that in all probability will be invoked when claims are made. The chief function of these formulations is to guide the attention of decision makers to the context in which pertinent activities occur. Formulas assist in recognizing and evaluating the consequences for international public order of accepting the exclusive or the sharing claim in particular cases or categories of cases.

* * *

When we think configuratively about the problems raised in reference to the new resources it is clear that instead of relying on blanket principles (like "freedom of the seas" or "freedom of the air") the most fruitful policy alternatives are likely to emerge when we anticipate the appearance of characteristic factual contexts, and consider how the values chiefly at stake in them can be maximized. Hence we would not expect to apply the same prescription (1) to the sharing of air space for weather observation (where equipment is used that is expressly designed for the purpose and perhaps registered, and when the information obtained is made public) and (2) to the sharing of air space for projects of weather or climate control that may be deleterious to local values.

The contextual (or, synonymously, the configurative) approach is a challenge to imagine the full range of possible means of anticipating and resolving difficulties. On the most uncertain matters it is appropriate to call attention to the need of exploring the possibilities of agreement in advance of conflict. The inference is that no time should be lost, for instance, in putting into the hands of the UN the facilities for research, development and operation of satellites, "space platforms" and travel beyond the limits of the earth's atmospheric and gravitational fields. Doubtless the USA and the USSR will continue to compete with independent programs. Since the polar powers have a stake in moderating the conflict in which they are engaged in the hope of eventual harmony through agreement, not catastrophe, a practical method would appear to be to strengthen the "third factor," especially when both powers are also included within it.

The rapid introduction of new resources under present conditions calls for some degree of community and regional planning; and planning poses thorny questions about the structure and ideology of society. To an increasing extent questions of this kind need to be answered directly rather than by default. . . . For instance,

we have not explored the principles of proportion that are most likely to consolidate or to sustain at various stages of industrial growth the perspectives and operational technique of popular government. Shall we, for example, rely upon a 30–40–50 rule to guide public policy in regard to the permissible degree of market control permitted to private interests? (For example: When one interest has 30 per cent control of output, shall it be subject to special regulations designed to nullify the side-effects of power that go along with economic control? When one interest rises to 40 per cent shall we put governmentally appointed trustees on the Board of Directors? At 50 per cent shall government trustees predominate?)

Whatever the workable rules of proportion may be in representative contexts it is evident that we need to guide our studies of trend correlation and of comparative cases in order to improve the available bases of inference in such matters.

The same approach—the search for rules of proportion—applies to every institutional and personality pattern in a body politic. What are the optimum proportions of community resources to devote to elementary, intermediate, advanced and ultra-advanced education? To research and development in science and technology? To positive and negative sanctions for correctional and other purposes?

One way to jar "cakes of custom" out of the mind is to draft specifications for the first Mayflower expedition to establish continuing occupation outside the earth. (Possibly it could be "Noah's Jet"?) What proportion of men, women and children of which culture or combination of earth cultures shall we select? What ideological traditions, secular and sacred? What class backgrounds (elite, mid-elite, mass)? What individual and group interests? What personality structures?

By asking questions of this kind we are in a position to assess our present stock of knowledge concerning the interdependence of institutions specialized to power, and all other institutions in the social process of any community, together with the forms of personality involved. These, of course, are the recurring issues of political science and historical interpretation as well as policy.

. . . As political scientists we are perhaps even less well prepared to anticipate developments in genetics, experimental embryology and related disciplines. Taken together these fields signify that, as Julian Huxley has often put it, man is on the threshold of taking evolution into his own hands. By influencing the genes that constitute the key units in man's biological inheritance we affect the entire potential of future generations.

*   *   *

It has been pointed out that perhaps the most satisfactory index of genetic damage is the sum of tangible defects existing among living individuals. We are speaking of such stigmata as "mental defects, epilepsy, congenital malformations, neuromuscular defects, hematological and endocrine defects, defects in vision or hearing, cutaneous and skeletal defects, or defects in the gastrointestinal or genitourinary tracts." We are informed that about 2 per cent of the live births in the United States have defects that are of "simple genetic origin and appear prior to sexual maturity." If mankind were subjected to a "double dosing" of radiation the present level of genetic defects would rise, and would eventually be doubled.

Regulatory measures are obviously needed against wars and weapon tests; and they are essential to the disposition of nuclear waste from industrial plants. (It has been remarked that a nuclear power plant is to be viewed as a large-scale production of both highly poisonous gas and explosives under a single roof.)

The principal questions to which I desire to call attention pose issues of a relatively new and different order. Some of these questions have already come up in controversies over artificial insemination. They have embarrassed the champions of the orthodox prescriptions that prevail in several fields (theology, ethics, jurisprudence). Shall we call a child legitimate whose biological father is not identical with the sociological father? Even with the consent of the latter? With spermatozoa from a known or unknown source? (A possible international question is whether a nation state like the United States can claim the child as a citizen if the spermatozoa employed originated with an American mail order house and was sent by air mail for use abroad.)

Poignant as these issues are in specific cases they do not confront us with the consequences for public order that are to be anticipated if the progress of biology separates insemination and child-bearing from genital contact. The assumption is often made that the continuation of sexual rectitude and even civic order depends upon charging every genital contact with the blessings and perils of procreation. The impending improvement of oral contraceptives, joined with other recent advances, are factors that already suggest the wisdom of other norms and sanctions of public order.

Other developments are threatening current ratios of the influence and power of the sexes. Given the millions and millions of spermatozoa produced by one male and the technique of canning by refrigeration, any very large number of males becomes relatively redundant for purposes of procreation. Must the male rest his future upon other values such as the strictly aesthetic appeal of the male contour? Before the female of the species becomes too complacent in this context it may be worth recalling the significance of some current experiments for the removal of the primordial female function from the body and into other receptacles. (Women, too, may have to rely upon their charm, a role for which their experience has provided extensive preparation.)

Appparently we are closer than most of us like to think to the production of species that occupy an intermediate position between man and the lower animals (or even plants). It is sometimes said, even in august quarters, that "one has not yet succeeded in making a species from another species." Theodosius Dobzhansky notes, however, that "the feat of obtaining a new species was accomplished more than a quarter of a century ago." In recent decades a fair number of new species have been brought into being. It is also true that some species that exist in nature have been recreated experimentally. A garrison police regime fully cognizant of science and technology can, in all probability, eventually aspire to biologize the class and caste system by selective breeding and training. Such beings can, in effect, be sown and harvested for specialized garrison police services or for other chosen operations.

Great strides have been taken in brain design. Experimental models of robots have been built who solve problems of a rather complex order in a given environment. Some of these machines look after themselves to a degree, obtaining and using the raw materials required for energy and repairs. Already it is claimed that the function of reproducing its kind, and of interacting with others, can be in-built.

The question then rises: Given our concern for human dignity when do we wisely extend all or part of the Universal Declaration of Human Rights to these forms? When do we accept the humanoids—the species intermediate between lower species and man, and which may resemble us in physique as well as in the possession of an approximately equivalent central nervous and cortical system—as at least partial participants in the body politic? And at what point do we accept the incorporation of relatively self-perpetuating and mutually influencing "super-machines" or "ex-robots" as beings entitled to the policies expressed in the Universal Declaration?

It is obvious that we are not too well equipped by cultural tradition to cope with these problems. A trait of our civilization is the intense sentimentalization of superficial differences in the visible format of the groupings to be found even within the human species. Recall the theologians, ethicists and jurists who have devoted themselves to the elaboration of symbols to show that the white race alone is genuinely human and hence solely entitled to the dignity of freedom. Recall, too, the counter-assertions, nourished in the soil of humiliation, that have arisen among ethnic groups that seek to overcome their contempt for themselves by dragging down the pretensions of the white imperialist.

*   *   *

The most disturbing question, perhaps, arises when we reflect upon the possibility that super-gifted men, or even new species possessing superior talent, will emerge as a result of research and development by geneticists, embryologists or machine makers. In principle, it is not too difficult to imagine a superior form. For instance, our sensory equipment does not enable us to take note of dangerous radiation levels in the environment. We have no inborn chattering of a Geiger counter.

I spoke before of taking the intellectual initiative for the use of science and technology for the fuller realization of our value goals. It is plain that if we bring certain kinds of living forms into the world we may be introducing a biological elite capable of treating us in the manner in which imperial powers have so often treated the weak. A question is whether the cultivation of superior qualities ought to be limited to intellectual capability. The answer, I feel confident you will agree, is in the negative. We need to be sufficiently vigilant to prevent the turning loose on the world of a hyper-intelligent species driven by an instinctual system especially inclined toward predation. The blood-stained story of our own species is only too familiar (the

stories about succulent missionaries whose bodies were more readily incorporated than their messages are not wholly without foundation). Can we improve the prospects of developing a form of intelligent life copied not after our own image, but after the image of our nobler aspirations?

It is not to be overlooked that the problem of human capability can become acute if in the years ahead we escape from our present habitat on the earth, or are visited by other forms of intelligent life. There are, after all, untold millions of environments resembling our solar system, and it would be more remarkable to find that but one planet is inhabited by a complex living form than to encounter parallel developments. It would of course be embarrassing, at least, to discover that we are the savages or that we are put together on a markedly inferior biological plan.

The fact is that many of the problems to which I have been referring will be upon us long before we can make great changes in the ideological outlook or the socio-political patterns of life in this country or elsewhere. The same point applies to ourselves in our role as individuals and as members of the political science profession. Considering our present predispositions how can we improve the likelihood of contributing to the decision process at every level, from the neighborhood to the world as a whole?

It is abundantly clear that the impact of science and technology does not occur in a social vacuum, but in a context of human identifications, demands and expectations. I make the modest proposal that it is appropriate for political scientists, in company with other scientists and scholars dealing with human affairs, to improve our procedures of continuous deliberation upon the potential impacts of science and technology upon human affairs. No doubt the American Political Science Association and other professional societies constitute an appropriate network for the purpose. We can sustain continuing conferences devoted to the examination of emerging developments. As fellow professionals we have special responsibility for giving thought to the aggregate effects of any specific innovation.

Our first professional contribution, it appears, is to project a comprehensive image of the future for the purpose of indicating how our overriding goal values are likely to be affected if current policies continue.

A closely related contribution consists in clarifying the fundamental goal values of the body politic. We are accustomed to confront political ideologies with new factual contingencies and to suggest appropriate specific interpretations. We also confront political doctrines with rival doctrines, and with comprehensive theological and metaphysical systems. I have called attention to the point that the basic value systems of European civilization, in particular, are likely to be exposed to sweeping challenge as biology and engineering narrow the obvious differences between man and neighboring species, and between man and centrally operating machines. The crisis will be peculiarly sharp if we create or discover forms of life superior to man in intellect or instinctual predispositions. Our traditions have not been life-centered, but man-centered. We possess various paranoid-like traditions of being "chosen." Clearly a difficult task of modifying these egocentric perspectives lies ahead.

The third task is historical and scientific. It is historical in the sense that by mobilizing knowledge about the past we are enabled to recognize the appearance of new patterns and the diffusion or restriction of the old. It is scientific in the sense that we summarize the past in order to confirm (or disconfirm) propositions about the interplay of predisposition and environment. If we are to serve the aims of historic recognition and of scientific analysis, one of our professional responsibilities is to expedite the development of more perfect institutions specialized to continual self-observation on a global scale. Self-observation requires guidance by a system of theoretical models of the political process in which a continuing gradation is maintained between the most inclusive model and submodels adjusted to more limited contexts in time and space. Continual self-observation renders it necessary at each step through time to reevaluate the appropriateness of the operational indices for the variables and concepts employed at the most recent step. In this way all the concepts that figure in systematic, descriptive political science can be kept chronically pertinent to the ordering of political events as the future unfolds.

The fourth task is inventive and evaluative. It consists in originating policy alternatives by means of which goal values can be maximized. In estimating the likely occurrence of an event (or event category), it is essential to take into account the historical trends and the scientifically ascertained predispositions in the world arena or any pertinent part thereof.

* * *

NOTE

STUART CHASE
DEMOCRACY UNDER PRESSURE—
SPECIAL INTERESTS VS. THE PUBLIC WELFARE*

* * *

Sometimes I have a clear picture of the way the Agenda . . . could be presented to the people. I see perhaps a hundred leading Americans, men and women, meeting in some high, quiet place to prepare it. . . . They are scientists, judges, teachers, university people, philosophers of business, lovers of the land, statesmen; and they think in terms of the whole community.

I picture them as people without ideologies or dogmatic principles, aware of their own shortcomings and the general inadequacy of mankind, as Wells put it. They are accustomed to approach a question with the scientific attitude, and to look at all the major characteristics of a situation before leaping to a conclusion. They are aware of the pitfalls of language.

* * *

They ought, I think, to go up into the mountains somewhere.

* * *

They could hold general meetings in the big Lodge, while subcommittees, working on detail problems, could meet wherever they pleased.

* * *

It ought to clear the brain. The meeting should be held in summer rather than winter, with wild flowers, not snow. The delegates would do better to take their exercise on horseback, or fishing, rather than risk their tibias on the Canyon run.

I can see the Chairman getting to his feet in front of the big blue tapestry in the Lodge dining room to open the conference.

. . . I shall not quote him directly, but paraphrase his address, as I imagine it.

* * *

We who are meeting here, I take it, represent no economic interest except that of the consumer, which means everybody. We are not specifically for "labor," for "capital," for farmers,

---

* New York: Twentieth Century Fund. 133–142 (1945). © 1945 by The Twentieth Century Fund, New York. Reprinted by permission.

for organized medicine, for Wall Street, the West Coast, the export trade, the department stores, or for the manufacturers of Shocking Radiance perfume.

We are not in favor of "capitalism," "Socialism," "Fascism," "Communism," "individualism," or saving the world by the introduction of planned parenthood. We have gone through these vague ideologies and come out on the other side. We are in favor of keeping our minds open and the machines running. We want the community to go on, not to stop dead in its tracks as in 1929.

* * *

We must have first-rate men in government, and public service made an attractive career to keen youngsters. We need a more enlightened civil service, better rules for tenure, many more schools of public administration.

* * *

We want to offer reasoned suggestions as to which public activities should be centralized and handled from Washington, and which should be decentralized and handled regionally, like the TVA, or by the states, or by local governments. We want to know why we should tolerate 165,000 units of government at all levels.

We want to develop some pretty clear ideas about the three major forms of government control: regulation, control-without-ownership, and outright ownership. Which is best for a given activity?

* * *

These are some of the concrete matters we are going to take up, the Chairman went on. In order to handle them wisely, we must keep in mind some longer-range principles. We must remember that it is the era of abundance we are trying to adjust to.

* * *

Since 1929, the Chairman went on, any expectation of free, unmanaged economies is academic. We all know that, in our minds if not in our emotional nervous systems. Men cannot return to free, unmanaged economies so long as inanimate energy and mass production dominate human activity. Furthermore, I do not know how many of us, when we get right down to it, would like the London of Adam Smith. We have to cope with the age that is here. To run away from it is to become impotent. The parade back

to unlimited free enterprise is not an inspiring spectacle. It leaves young people confused and baffled. They want leaders, not retreaters.

Economic systems must now be managed. Have people in the democracies the brains to work out a kind of management which deals only with a few key functions and leaves most activities in private hands?

* * *

Americans, the Chairman continues, were not brought up to plan for, or even think about, their national survival. It was taken for granted.

* * *

Our forefathers set up an elaborate plan in 1787. They gave it a push and let it go. The expanding frontier carried it on for a hundred and fifty years. Lincoln had to do some managing, and so did Woodrow Wilson. But the New Deal marked the first time it was ever necessary to make over-all plans coordinating banks, farmers, and employment.

* * *

The Chairman paused again . . . My time is about up. This isn't a speech but some ideas thrown out to get us started. A preliminary draft prepared by the steering committee is now before you. Each delegate has his copy. Your task is to round out this preliminary draft; take it as far as you can, as deep as you can, while holding general agreement. We want to obtain maximum agreement among ourselves. None of us belongs to pressure groups, but some of us have pet ideas. I implore you to drop them if they stand in the way of agreement. It isn't you who must be vindicated, it is your country. Broader still, it is democracy which must be vindicated.

b.

Bertrand Russell
The Scientific Outlook*

. . . The scientific society, as I conceive it, is one which employs the best scientific technique in production, in education, and in propaganda. But in addition to this, it has a characteristic which distinguishes it from the societies of the past, which have grown up by natural causes,

* New York: W. W. Norton & Co., Inc. 203–205, 227–228, 233–235, 260–261, 268–269 (1931). Reprinted by permission of George Allen & Unwin, Ltd. and W. W. Norton & Co., Inc. Copyright 1931, renewed 1959 by Bertrand Russell.

without much conscious planning as regards their collective purpose and structure. No society can be regarded as fully scientific unless it has been created deliberately with a certain structure in order to fulfill certain purposes. . . .

[S]cientific technique has so enormously increased the power of governments that it has now become possible to produce . . . profound and intimate changes in social structure. . . . Science first taught us to create machines; it is now teaching us by Mendelian breeding and experimental embryology to create new plants and animals. There can be little doubt that similar methods will before long give us power, within wide limits, to create new human individuals differing in predetermined ways from the individuals produced by unaided nature. And by means of psychological and economic technique it is becoming possible to create societies as artificial as the steam engine, and as different from anything that would grow up of its own accord without deliberate intention on the part of human agents.

Such artificial societies will, of course, until social science is much more perfected than it is at present, have many unintended characteristics, even if their creators succeed in giving them all the characteristics that were intended. The unintended characteristics may easily prove more important than those that were foreseen, and may cause the artificially constructed societies to break down in one way or another. But I do not think it is open to doubt that the artificial creation of societies will continue and increase so long as scientific technique persists. The pleasure in planned construction is one of the most powerful motives in men who combine intelligence with energy; whatever can be constructed according to a plan, such men will endeavour to construct. So long as the technique for creating a new type of society exists there will be men seeking to employ this technique. They are likely to suppose themselves actuated by some idealistic motive, and it is possible that such motives may play a part in determining what sort of society they shall aim at creating. But the desire to create is not itself idealistic, since it is a form of the love of power, and while the power to create exists there will be men desirous of using this power even if unaided nature would produce a better result than any that can be brought about by deliberate intention.

* * *

When I speak of scientific government I ought, perhaps, to explain what I mean by the term. . . . I should define a government as in a greater or less degree scientific in proportion as it can produce intended results: the greater the number of results that it can both intend and produce, the more scientific it is. . . .

Owing to the increase of knowledge, it is possible for governments nowadays to achieve many more intended results than were possible in former times, and it is likely that before very long results which even now are impossible will become possible. The total abolition of poverty, for example, is at the present moment technically possible; that is to say, known methods of production, if wisely organized, would suffice to produce enough goods to keep the whole population of the globe in tolerable comfort. But although this is technically possible, it is not yet psychologically possible. International competition, class antagonisms, and the anarchic system of private enterprise stand in the way, and to remove these obstacles is no light task. The diminution of disease is a purpose which in Western nations encounters fewer obstacles and has therefore been more successfully pursued, but to this purpose also there are great obstacles throughout Asia. Eugenics, except in the form of sterilization of the feeble-minded, is not yet practical politics, but may become so within the next fifty years. [I]t may be superseded, when embryology is more advanced, by direct methods of operating upon the foetus.

* * *

The man who dreams of a scientifically organized world and wishes to translate his dream into practice finds himself faced with many obstacles. There is the opposition of inertia and habit: people wish to continue behaving as they always have behaved, and living as they always have lived. There is the opposition of vested interest: an economic system inherited from feudal times gives advantages to men who have done nothing to deserve them, and these men, being rich and powerful, are able to place formidable obstacles in the way of fundamental change. In addition to these forces, there are also hostile idealisms. Christian ethics is in certain fundamental respects opposed to the scientific ethic which is gradually growing up. Christianity emphasizes the importance of the individual soul, and is not prepared to sanction the sacrifice of an innocent man for the sake of some ulterior good to the majority. Christianity, in a word, is unpolitical, as is natural since it grew up among men devoid of political power. The new ethic which is gradually growing in connexion with scientific technique will have its eye upon society rather than upon the individual. It will have little use for the superstition of guilt and punishment, but will be prepared to make individuals suffer for the public good without inventing reasons purporting to show that they deserve to suffer. In this sense it will be ruthless, and according to traditional ideas immoral, but the change will have come about naturally through the habit of viewing society as a whole rather than as a collection of individuals. We view a human body as a whole, and if, for example, it is necessary to amputate a limb we do not consider it necessary to prove first that the limb is wicked. We consider the good of the whole body a quite sufficient argument. Similarly the man who thinks of society as a whole will sacrifice a member of society for the good of the whole, without much consideration for that individual's welfare. This has always been the practice in war, because war is a collective enterprise. Soldiers are exposed to the risk of death for the public good, although no one suggests that they deserve death. But men have not hitherto attached the same importance to social purposes other than war, and have therefore shrunk from inflicting sacrifices which were felt to be unjust. I think it probable that the scientific idealists of the future will be free from this scruple, not only in time of war, but in time of peace....

But, the reader will say, how is all this to come about? Is it not merely a phantasy of wish-fulfillment, utterly remote from practical politics? I do not think so. The future which I foresee is, to begin with, only very partially in agreement with my own wishes. I find pleasure in splendid individuals rather than in powerful organizations, and I fear that the place for splendid individuals will be much more restricted in the future than in the past....

* * *

... The impulse towards scientific construction is admirable when it does not thwart any of the major impulses that give value to human life, but when it is allowed to forbid all outlet to everything but itself it becomes a form of cruel tyranny. There is, I think, a real danger lest the world should become subject to a tyranny of this sort....

Science in the course of the few centuries of its history has undergone an internal development which appears to be not yet completed. One may sum up this development as the passage from contemplation to manipulation. The love of knowledge to which the growth of science is

due is itself the product of a twofold impulse. We may seek knowledge of an object because we love the object or because we wish to have power over it. The former impulse leads to the kind of knowledge that is contemplative, the latter to the kind that is practical. In the development of science the power impulse has increasingly prevailed over the love impulse. The power impulse is embodied in industrialism and in governmental technique. It is embodied also in the philosophies known as pragmatism and instrumentalism. Each of these philosophies holds, broadly speaking, that our beliefs about any object are true in so far as they enable us to manipulate it with advantage to ourselves. This is what may be called a governmental view of truth. Of truth so conceived science offers us a great deal; indeed there seems no limit to its possible triumphs. To the man who wishes to change his environment science offers astonishingly powerful tools, and if knowledge consists in the power to produce intended changes, then science gives knowledge in abundance.

* * *

... The new powers that science has given to man can only be wielded safely by those who, whether through the study of history or though their own experience of life, have acquired some reverence for human feelings and some tenderness towards the emotions that give colour to the daily existence of men and women. I do not mean to deny that scientific technique may in time build an artificial world in every way preferable to that in which men have hitherto lived, but I do say that if this is to be done it must be done tentatively and with a realization that the purpose of government is not merely to afford pleasure to those who govern, but to make life tolerable for those who are governed. Scientific technique must no longer be allowed to form the whole culture of the holders of power, and it must become an essential part of men's ethical outlook to realize that the will alone cannot make a good life. Knowing and feeling are equally essential ingredients both in the life of the individual and in that of the community. Knowledge, if it is wide and intimate, brings with it a realization of distant times and places, an awareness that the individual is not omnipotent or all-important, and a perspective in which values are seen more clearly than by those to whom a distant view is impossible. Even more important than knowledge is the life of the emotions. A world without delight and without affection is a world destitute of value. These things the scientific manipulator must remember, and if he does his manipulation may be wholly beneficial. All that is needed is that men should not be so intoxicated by new power as to forget the truths that were familiar to every previous generation. Not all wisdom is new, nor is all folly out of date.

Man has been disciplined hitherto by his subjection to nature. Having emancipated himself from this subjection, he is showing something of the defects of slave-turned-master. A new moral outlook is called for in which submission to the powers of nature is replaced by respect for what is best in man. It is where this respect is lacking that scientific technique is dangerous. So long as it is present, science, having delivered man from bondage to nature, can proceed to deliver him from bondage to the slavish part of himself. The dangers exist, but they are not inevitable, and hope for the future is at least as rational as fear.

2.

Rational Choice about Alternatives?

a.

Directive Committee on Regional Planning—Yale University
The Case for Regional Planning*

* * *

To the most general question: Why plan? the answer is that man is in some measure a rational animal and plans because it is by planning that he is able to insure the fullest achievement of his specific goals and basic values. By trial and error and success, he has learned that it is by clear vision of goals, careful calculation of probabilities, and intelligent appraisal of alternative courses of action that both individuals and human communities, of whatever size or purpose, most effectively achieve their goals, whether individual or communal. Experience has taught him that he plans, whether he knows it or not, and that the more conscious he is of his planning and the more systematically he appraises its results, the better he is able to adapt it to his purposes. The reason why contemporary people give so much conscious thought and effort to planning is, therefore, to make certain that all

———

* Myres S. McDougal and Maurice E. H. Rotival, Chairmen. New Haven: Yale University Press 7–18, 19–20 (1947). Reprinted by permission.

of their planning, whether for peace or general welfare or individual happiness, is as effective as contemporary science and knowledge will permit.

To the slightly less general question: Why plan through government? the answer is that government is the one general institution of society established and maintained for the very purpose of planning and acting for communal ends. It is the institution especially designed to marshal all the other institutions, to keep them from interfering with each other, and to promote their most efficient contribution to the values of the community. Government is the intelligence-receiving, communicating, directing, central nervous system of community life. By appropriate techniques of representation, government can, further, be made the most amenable of all society's institutions to democratic control, and hence can best be trusted with that power over people and resources which is necessarily involved in the shaping of a community's physical environment and in providing its public services, by whomsoever these tasks may be performed.

* * *

Planning is the rational adaptation of means to ends. It is a process of thought, a method of work, the way in which man makes use of his intelligence. People always act with some anticipations of the future—with some picture, however cloudy, of the ends they are seeking; with some notion, however inaccurate, of the conditions that determine the extent to which they can achieve their ends; and with some appraisal, however inadept, of what are appropriate means to attain their ends under such conditions. It is the function of planning to make such anticipations of the future—such prevision of goals, such calculation of probabilities, and such appraisal of alternative courses of action—as clear, as realistic, and as effective as possible.

This conscious application of intelligence to the task of creating appropriate means to attain defined ends, which we call planning, is a process that is characteristic of man—however irrational he may appear or be on occasion—in all of his activities. It extends from the shaping of individual careers to the conduct of all his communities or associations, public and private. It is a process which is applied, with varying degrees of success, from the small rural community, at one extreme, through the various levels of local, state, or national government and through the great private or public-private associations of business to, at the other extreme, world society. When planning is thus understood, there can be no question of a choice between planning and not planning. Planning in this sense is not a political philosophy which can be accepted or rejected. It is a mode of exercising foresight in action and is indispensable to effective action in any walk of life. Differences between political philosophies are to be found in the ends to which planning is put (as well as in, of course, the means by which such ends are effected) and not in the fact of planning. Planning can be used to implement any political philosophy. Under contemporary world conditions, it is especially needed to implement democracy.

In government, specifically, it is the function of planning to apply scientific knowledge and common sense to the creation and execution of programs, designed to achieve the general purposes and specific goals for which any particular institution of government exists.

*   *   *

The first task of the planner in any community or governmental institution is, therefore, to clarify and define objectives.

In a democratic society the basic values, with which planning for any community or institution must begin, are the more general values common to the individual citizens of such a society. In highest abstraction these values may be described in terms of a wider sharing of power, respect, knowledge, income, safety, health, and character and of all other values that contribute to the dignity of the individual and the possibilities of his maturing his latent talents, without discrimination, into socially valued expression.

*   *   *

It is obvious, however, that . . . specific goals for community action cannot be completely clarified without realistic knowledge of the conditions which determine or limit the possibilities of the community's achievement of basic values.

The second task of the planner, which must be carried out concomitantly with the first is, therefore, to study such determining conditions.

These conditions include many interdependent variables, such as the numbers and characteristics of the people, the structure and functioning of external political and economic power, the efficiency of the community's institutions and technology, and the resources, natural and manmade, that are available for development. The exact interrelation of these conditioning factors

varies from community to community and can seldom be precisely known, but the planner assumes that, given a certain stability in population and in the effects of power exercised from outside the area, the extent to which the people of any particular area achieve their values depends upon the efficiency with which they apply their institutions and technology to the development of their resources. Even common observation suggests that certain variations in a people's organizational practices and in their design and use of natural resources greatly affect the degree of their achievement of their values and that man has a very large capacity to adapt natural resources and forces to his ends. It is with these modifiable factors in organizational practice and in the design and use of resources that the planner must work.

One of the variables which most directly affects the extent to which a community can achieve its values in the future is the extent to which it has achieved them in the past. The degree to which any of the basic values of a community are achieved conditions in part the achievement of all the other values. Thus, the extent to which knowledge, respect, and character are shared affects the extent to which real income can be produced and shared, and vice versa. It is important, therefore, for the planner first to inquire to what extent the people of the area under study have hitherto realized their various major values.

*   *   *

In exploring adequately the extent to which any given community is achieving its basic values, the planner must of course study all of the major institutions and organizational practices of the community under observation. Since, however, the community's over-all achievement is so largely dependent upon the efficiency of its component institutions and the practices within them, these institutions and practices call for a more direct investigation, with attention focused squarely upon them and their functioning.

*   *   *

The third task of the planner, which must be kept constantly in mind while goals are being clarified and conditions determined, is to appraise or devise appropriate means for securing the goals that are finally established.

In a democratic society, people plan to achieve most of their values by voluntary, private, or civic undertakings and to preserve the widest possible zones of action for private decision. The function of government is to create the conditions—to supply the basic framework of efficient material environment and public services and regulation—under which voluntary, private activity and individual development can flourish. In a federal nation of interdependent regions such as the United States, however, the creation of such conditions calls for planning and action at all levels of government—national, regional, state, and local.

* * *

A fourth and final task is to assist in carrying recommendations into action.

His contribution to the implementation of plans is as indispensable as his contribution to their conception. . . .

[He must also] observe closely all day-to-day activities in the execution of programs, conducting what amounts to a continuous survey of the extent to which the action being taken is effective in securing the specific goals and basic values sought. This process of evaluation is indeed a part of his general function of determining the conditions which affect the achievement of specific goals and basic values and here leads directly to subsequent recommendations for action. It is exactly for this reason that the planning process is a continuing one and the role of the planner a permanent one. The purposes of planning cannot be achieved in one blow by a single exercise of the four separate steps involved in the process of planning. The continuing achievement of the major values of any community requires a continuous exercise of all its powers of foresight and rational decision.

* * *

It might, therefore, be helpful if a reasonably routinized order of work could be adopted.

* * *

The first chapter in a study of the order proposed would investigate the people and their values and aspirations. This would comprehend all the ascertainable facts about population, including numbers, births, deaths, biological traits, health, personality types, spatial distribution and migrations; about groups, classes, and skills and about movements and conflicts between groups; about the basic disciplines imposed by the family and other small in-groups for the conditioning of character; about the intellectual, spiritual, es-

thetic, moral, and philosophical concepts, attitudes, and aspirations of the people; and finally, about the details of the standard of living, the real income, achieved in the community.

A second chapter would study institutions and resources. To make these manageable, a seamless web of areal activities and resources must be broken up into specific types of component functional activities. Any classification of components of a community organism adequate to satisfy all of man's basic needs must be somewhat arbitrary. Each component must also consist, if it is to represent reality, of a complex of people pursuing values through organizational practices applied to specific resource bases.

* * *

A third chapter would single out design, as a most influential variable, for especial emphasis. . . . It would consider explicitly how norms and practices might be modified to secure a more efficient use of resources in promoting major purposes.

The fourth and final chapter would concentrate on government, potentially the most quickly responsive of all man's instruments of social change. This would survey institutions, rules, and practices at all levels of areal organization and seek to determine how these might be modified to implement any new moulding . . . to promote a fuller and richer achievement of major objectives.

* * *

The planning process follows also an order in time, representing degrees in the advancement of the work. Certain commonly accepted divisions are in terms of analysis, diagnosis, synthesis, and action.

Analysis represents the systematic study of conditions, following the sequence outlined above. Diagnosis is the careful appraisal of such conditions to determine which are most critical in effect and easiest of modification. Synthesis is an integration of all the relevant factors to achieve a final choice of means, a concrete vision of the kind of community desired and how to effect it—a vision so concrete that it can be embodied in plans, drawings, and programs for action. Action is what is required, in effective time sequence, at each level of government or by voluntary agencies to achieve ends sought.

* * *

b.

Harold Lasswell and Myres S. McDougal
Law, Science and Policy—
The Jurisprudence of a Free Society*

*   *   *

. . . A relevant jurisprudence must, in sum, seek a comprehensiveness and realism in focus which will encourage both a systematic, configurative examination of all the significant variables affecting decision and the rational appraisal of the aggregate value consequences of alternatives in decision.

*   *   *

. . . In any community, this process of authoritative and controlling decision, as an integral part of a more comprehensive process of effective power, can be seen to be composed of two different kinds of decisions: first, the decisions which establish and maintain the most comprehensive process of authoritative decision and, secondly, the flow of particular decisions which emerge from the process so established for the regulation of all the other community value processes. The first of these types of decision may be conveniently described as "constitutive," and the second as "public order."

For the comprehensive and economic description of a process of decision, as of other social processes, it is necessary to employ some systematic set of terms (the precise words do not matter if equivalences can be made clear) to refer to the participants in the process, their perspectives (demands, identifications, expectations), the situations of intersection, the base values at the disposal of participants, the strategies employed in management of base values, and the immediate outcomes and long-term effects achieved.

In the terms we find convenient, the "constitutive process" of a community may be described as the decisions which identify and characterize the different authoritative decisionmakers, specify and clarify basic community policies, establish appropriate structures of authority, allocate bases of power for sanctioning purposes, authorize procedures for making the different kinds of decisions, and secure the continuous performance of all the different kinds of decision functions (intelligence, promotion,

* Unpublished manuscript 23, 40–54 (1970). Printed by permission of the authors who retain all rights.

prescription, etc.) necessary to making and administering general community policy.

In complementary terms, the "public order" decisions of a community may be described as those, emerging in continuous flow from the constitutive process, which shape and maintain the protected features of the community's various value processes. These are the decisions which determine how resources are allocated and developed, and wealth produced and distributed; how human rights are promoted and protected or deprived; how enlightenment is encouraged or retarded; how health is fostered, or neglected; how rectitude and civic responsibility are matured; and so on through the whole gamut of demanded values.

It will be obvious in any community that an intimate relationship exists between constitutive process and public order. The economy and effectiveness of the constitutive process a community can achieve vitally affects the freedom, security, and abundance of its public order; while the quality of the public order a community attains, in turn, affects the viability of the constitutive process it can maintain. By distinguishing, however, between these two different types of decisions, and seeking systematic coverage of both, inquiry may avoid destructive fixation upon the mere application of allegedly given rules and vacuous controversies about the differences between "political" and "legal" decisions, and may appropriately extend its concern to all relevant features of the processes by which law is made and applied and to their consequences for preferred public order.

The conventional description of the different phases in authoritative decision which we describe as "authority functions" is in such terms as "legislative," "executive," "judicial," and "administrative" but these terms would appear to refer more to authority structures than functions. Inquiry seeking both greater precision and comprehensiveness in describing authority functions might distinguish the following (or their equivalents):

Intelligence:	Obtaining information about the past, making etimates of the future, planning.
Promoting:	Urging proposals.
Prescribing:	Projecting authoritative policies.
Invoking:	Confronting concrete situations with provisional char-

acterization in terms of a prescription to concrete circumstances.

Applying: Final characterization and execution of a prescription in a concrete situation.

Terminating: Ending a prescription or arrangement within the scope of a prescription.

Appraising: Comparison between goals and performance.

*   *   *

Every phase in the processes of authoritative decision is affected both by the past distribution of values and by the perspectives (demands, identifications, and expectations) of participants about future distribution. The outcomes of processes of authoritative decision, in turn, not only directly affect the future distribution of values among the claimants and others but, in total impact and in the long run, determine and secure a community's public order.

For comprehensive and precise description of the social process context of decision, any categorizations of values and institutional practices which can be given detailed operational indices in terms of specific, empirical relations between human beings can be made to serve the purposes of policy-oriented inquiry. The most general conceptualization we recommend is in terms of eight value-institution categories made familiar by contemporary social science:

Power: government, law, politics.
Wealth: production, distribution, consumption.
Respect: social class and caste.
Well-being: health, safety, comfort arrangements.
Affection: family, friendship circles, loyalty.
Skill: artistic, vocational, professional training and activity.
Rectitude: churches and related articulators and appliers of standards of responsible conduct.
Enlightenment: mass media, research.

When these or equivalent value-institutional categories are employed, in appropriately detailed phase analysis, to describe the events in social process which precipitate claims to authoritative decision, the claims which participants make about such precipitating events and relevant policies in their appeals to decision, and the choices which the established decision-makers actually make in their prescriptions and applications of policy, then effective comparisons can be made through time within single communities, and across the boundaries of communities, for study of the factors that affect decision and of the public order consequences of decision.

*   *   *

Every phase of decision process, whether of constitutive process or relating to public order, and every facet of conditioning context, will be examined for opportunities in innovation which may influence decision toward greater conformity with clarified goal. Assessment of particular alternatives will be made in terms of gains and losses with respect to all clarified goals and disciplined by the knowledge acquired of trends, conditioning factors, and future probabilities. All the other intellectual tasks will be synthesized and brought to bear upon search for integrative solutions characterized by maximum gains and minimum losses. Special procedures for encouraging creativity will be employed, including expansions and contractions of the focus of attention, alternation of periods of intensive concentration and inattention, free association, and experiment with random combinations.

c.

Gordon S. Fulcher
Common Sense Decision-Making*

[W]e shall devote most of our attention to thoughtful decision-making, especially to procedures useful for making very important, difficult, and complex decisions. Such procedures can readily be modified for use when making less important, less difficult, and less complex decisions. . . .

The *main factors* which may be involved in thoughtful decision-making are the following:

1. *Problem situation* with which the decision will deal: a situation which is unsatisfactory in some respect and is a problem because the proper action to take, if any, is not obvious.

2. *Purpose* to be achieved if practicable; the end to be aimed at.

3. *Available alternative decisions;* alternative means for dealing with the situation so as to

---

* Evanston: Northwestern University Press 7–12 (1965). Reprinted by permission.

achieve the desired purpose. Since each decision is a choice between alternative possible decisions, at least two such alternatives should be known, but one may be to take no action.

4. *Probable consequences* of each alternative. Since each alternative will have, if chosen, its natural consequences, a choice between the alternatives is, in effect, a choice between their consequences.

5. *Values* to the decision-maker of the probable consequences of the alternatives. A comparison of such values is necessary to determine which alternative is likly to have the most desirable consequences to him or, if the decision-maker is faced with a choice of evils, the least undesirable consequences.

. . . If one step is devoted to each of the five factors listed above and one step is added to check the evidence, assumptions, and reasoning on which a tentative decision, reached after taking the first five steps, is based, we arrive at the following list of steps which may be required in making a thoughtful decision:

To determine the available alternatives:
1. Investigation of the problem situation to determine the unsatisfactory features, the causes of these, and other pertinent facts.

2. Selection of the purpose to be achieved, the goal to have in mind, the end to be aimed at.

3. Determination of the courses of action or policies available to achieve the purpose selected, the means available to achieve the goal.

To make the best choice between the alternatives:
4. Prediction of the probable consequences of each of the alternatives or the probable differences in the consequences of the alternatives, so that the decision-maker may know what difference it is likely to make if he chooses one rather than the other.

5. Evaluation of these predictions by the decision-maker so as to determine which alternative, if chosen, is likely to have for him the most desirable results, or the least undesirable results if it is a choice of evils, and thus achieve the purpose most satisfactorily.

To check the tentative decision:
6. Checking of the evidence, the assumptions, and the reasoning on which the decision is based so as to make reasonably sure that the decision is the best decision available, a sound decision.

Each step may, of course, involve minor conclusions, judgments, and decisions. For example, step 1 may involve judgments as to which features of the problem situation are most unsatisfactory and conclusions as to the causes of the unsatisfactory features. Step 3 may involve decisions as to which alternatives should receive further consideration. Also, step 5 naturally involves judgments as to the relative desirability of various predicted consequences; and all the steps may involve decisions as to how to obtain needed facts, ideas, and predictions. Thus, making a sound decision to deal with an important personal or social problem may be very complex. For such problems the advantage to the decision-maker of training and practice in the art of decision-making should be obvious.

The numerical sequence of the steps indicates the order in which they are normally completed, since after each has been checked, there is usually no need for further consideration of any preceding steps.

The relative importance of the six steps varies greatly for different types of a problem situation as well as for different situations of the same general type. When the unsatisfactory features of the situation are not well enough known or the causes are not well enough understood, the first step may be the most important. When no satisfactory alternative is known, the third step may be the most important. When all available alternatives are clear or easily known from past experience, the first three steps are not needed, and either the fourth or the fifth step may be the most important.

Best decisions. From the point of view of the decision-maker, the best decision he can make to deal with a certain problem situation is, naturally, the decision he would make if he knew all the factors involved—including all available alternatives and their probable consequences—well enough to be sure which alternative would have the most desirable results according to his highest standards. . . .

Sound decisions. Even when a decision-maker cannot be sure which decision is the best to deal with the situation, he can arrive at a sound decision, as we shall use the term, by making a reasonable effort to determine the available alternatives, to predict the probable consequences, and to make a sound choice between them. In other words, a decision will be considered sound if after reasonable effort the decision-maker is reasonably sure that the decision is a logical decision based on sound premises, one for each of the factors involved, as listed below. The premises are:

1. That the pertinent facts and causal factors of the problem situation are sufficiently well known;

2. That the purpose selected is the best under the circumstances;

3. That the alternatives considered include the best available;

4. That the predicted probable consequences are sufficiently complete, accurate, and far-sighted; and

5. That the evaluation of the expected consequences is sufficiently objective, conscientious, and idealistic.

NOTES

NOTE 1.
DAVID BRAYBROOKE AND CHARLES E. LINDBLOM
A STRATEGY OF DECISION*

*   *   *

[The] more sophisticated lines of thought, which many social scientists have followed—and philosophers before them—find their fullest expression in what we shall call "the rational-deductive ideal" . . . Many people, social scientists among them, are inclined to think that the most rational and satisfactory procedure for evaluating policies would be something like that described in the following instructions, assuming that they could be carried out:

Let ultimate values be expressed in general principles satisfactory to everybody who is ready to attend to the arguments identifying them—or, if there is no hope of that, satisfactory at least to those who are now undertaking a specific job of evaluation. Let these principles, which may embody notions of happiness, welfare, justice, or intuitive notions of goodness, be stated so exactly that they may be arranged intelligibly in an order of priority that indicates precisely which principles govern the application of others and when. Then derive within the limits of such a system intermediate principles that are suitable for application in particular cases, and that—allowing for rare cases of equality in net benefits—will indicate unambiguously which of alternative policies is to be chosen, according to the values they would promote.

---

* New York: The Free Press of Glencoe 9–12 (1963). Reprinted by permission of The Macmillan Company. Copyright © 1963 by The Free Press of Glencoe, a Division of The Macmillan Company.

The intermediate principles of such a system would specify the sort of information that would be decisive for rating any policy above or below its alternatives. If these principles are formulated as hypothetical propositions (which is the most convenient way to formulate them), they take something like the following form:

In conditions C, D, E, etc. (themselves derived from the ultimate principles), if such-and-such are the facts about Policy P and such-and-such are the facts about Policy Q, then P is better than Q.

For example, given that due process is observed and compensation is paid and (perhaps certain other conditions), if Policy P would remove certain dangers to the health and safety of the community caused by an existing use of private property, while Policy Q, although it would improve certain recreational facilities, would leave those dangers (and the existing use of private property) untouched, then P is better than Q. Once we substitute, in this intermediate principle, "compelling the dye-works in the town center to shut down," for "Policy P" and explain that the dangers consist of fumes and excessive traffic, the way is open for us to move directly from these facts to recommending the policy of shutting down the dye-works rather than Policy Q ("spending the money on a new playground").

Ideally, the system would be complete, not necessarily in the sense that it mentioned every contingency but in the sense that its ultimate principles were rich enough to supply the intermediate principles or the sequence of intermediate principles that one would need to decide any case that might come up. With such a system, the uncertainties of evaluation would have been mastered on the values side. For, on the values side, determination of policy becomes simply a matter of calculation, a question of feeding in the observed facts and thinking consistently through a sequence of logical transformations. One discovers the facts, looks up (or derives) the relevant hypotheticals, and deduces by strict logic which policy is to be selected. Nowadays, the work does not even seem impossibly tedious; one imagines that a suitably programmed computer could do it.

The rational-deductive ideal, so conceived, represents an ideal of science transferred to the field of values. For on the facts side too, the traditional ideal of science, going back to Plato and Aristotle, is the ideal of a complete deductive system—as a way of organizing knowledge (not, of course, for empirical scientists, as the sole way of obtaining it). If it is fantastic to imagine having such a system for all phenomena, it has not necessarily been thought fantastic to have it for a specific range of phenomena. The triumph that men attributed to Newton was a triumph of this kind—invested with fantasy by Laplace's boast of being able to calculate the positions and velocities of all the particles in the universe at any time if he knew their positions and velocities at any other.

In ethics, all manner of philosophers have subscribed to this ideal, beginning with the man who first conceived it, Plato. Both Aristotle and St. Thomas had reservations about the precision with which what can be known of values determines what is to be done in particular cases. In Aristotle's case, at least, if these reservations are explored, they lead away from the rational-deductive ideal. But it is fair to say that the historical effect of both men's writings has been to promote the view that, insofar as there is genuine knowledge in ethics, it can be elaborated in the form of a deductive system. John Locke also held this ideal; in ethics, furthermore, he was no more of an empiricist than Plato, for he believed that the content of ethics could be established with absolute certainty by a priori reasoning. Kant thought that we can discover a priori a universally effective method of testing decisively every moral judgment. If it is made an axiom that one ought to do whatever the test of the Categorical Imperative requires, then this universal method furnishes a system containing every judgment that passes the test.

The ethical discussions of most philosophers, from the Middle Ages through modern times, have concentrated on ethics in the narrow sense, which is concerned with the actions that it is our duty to do, the policies that it is our duty to choose. One has to guess from this what they would say of ethics in the larger sense, which involves choices among actions and policies all of which are morally permissible, although they differ in benefits. In the case of one major philosopher—the doggedly fact-minded Bentham—we do not have to guess. Bentham thought that the way to discover moral principles was to consider what could be consistently and effectively recommended to people, taking people as they are. His manifold lexicographical investigations aside, the system that he championed was meant to be fundamentally very simple. At the same time, it was meant to be a complete system, which applied to every choice of policy; it not only went beyond ethics in the

"duty" sense, but it subordinated "duty" to the criteria laid down for the larger sphere. The principle of utility, accompanied by the felicific calculus, is offered as a way of determining every conceivable policy question.

The example of Bentham—and, in another way, the example of Kant—shows that the ethical system offered to satisfy the rational-deductive ideal need not be a complicated one. If the right key can be found, the whole plan of the system will open up immediately—or so it may seem before getting down to cases. Whether the complications appear in the basic formulation of the system or only in its applications, however, people who subscribe to the rational-deductive ideal are ready to confront them bravely. In an intrepid statement of the ideal, the sociologist Florian Znaniecki writes,

You cannot isolate . . . arbitrarily one practical cultural problem and its solution from the rest of the human cultural world; you must take into consideration all the other practical cultural problems which are connected with it now and may become connected with it as an actual consequence of your activity—your own problems, those of the individuals and groups whose cooperation you must enlist, and those of the wider society whom you wish to influence through those individuals or groups. Otherwise, divergent, perhaps conflicting, standards of valuation and norms of conduct will continually interfere with the planful realization of your cultural "end." This "end" as a value and the activity pursuing it must be incorporated into an axiological and normative system organizing conceptually all the values and activities which are or will be connected with it in the active experience of all the people who are or will be involved in the realization of your plan.

Znaniecki will not allow anything relevant to be excluded from consideration. He will not spare himself or other evaluators even the difficulties involved in obtaining agreement on the system from all the people who will be affected by its determinations.

* * *

NOTE 2.

ABRAHAM KAPLAN
SOME LIMITATIONS ON RATIONALITY*

Few would argue that the human animal has become more rational in the twentieth century, but there can be no doubt that more than

* Carl J. Friedrich, ed.: *Nomos VII—Rational Decision.* New York: Atherton Press 55–59 (1964). Copyright 1964 by Atherton Press. Reprinted by permission of Aldine-Atherton, Inc.

ever before we know what we're missing. Within our lifetimes the advances in the exact formulation and analysis of what constitutes rational behavior have been greater, I venture to say, than in the whole of history. The theory of games, of information, and of decision-making and associated techniques like linear programming, operations research, and data-processing all have provided us, not just with an impressive new vocabulary, but with new and profound insights into the nature of rational choice, incomparably richer and more subtle than those underlying the *mos geometricus* which defined rationality from Plato to Spinoza and beyond. At the same time a new technology has sprung up, whose electronic components and magnetic tapes allow an exploitation of the theoretical possibilities incomparably beyond the capacity of a brain of flesh and blood; and if machines do not think, whatever it is they do puts our thinking to shame, given the same data and problems. More and more areas of rational decision have been brought into the domain of such theory and practice, and its frontier is expanding. A brave new world of rationality is in the making.

*   *   *

Rationality, I should suppose, is more than a matter of acting so as to secure the values pursued. Would we not also want to say that the reason judges them to be worth pursuing? I need not rehearse here the decades of discussion of the mutuality of ends and means. What seems to me unexceptionable is that rationality is not limited to a choice among means. The paranoid who waits till dark before turning on his persecutors may be a master strategist; he is surely not a paragon of rationality. A theory which demands only consistency of preference scales (a stable transitivity of utilities) is grossly inadequate to the political process. Political theorists have recognized at least since Burke that the decision-maker has a responsibility beyond giving the people what they want; he owes them also his own best judgment of what they *should* want. It could be said, to be sure, that rationality is not the only desideratum for political decisions, and that what I see as a problem for rationality lies, in fact, beyond its limits. But that Satan has a fine mind and is lacking only in heart is more than I am willing to admit; I believe he is a fool from beginning to end.

In politics, above all, decision-making cannot escape the responsibility of judging the relative worth of disparate and perhaps conflicting values. Even decisions affecting only ourselves may involve this problem, for we are individuals only by courtesy; in truth the individual is a congress of selves, each pursuing values to which the other selves may be indifferent or hostile— if, indeed, they are even aware of the pursuit. . . .

*   *   *

Given determinate values as well as the probabilities of their attainment by alternative courses of action, there is still the question of the criterion by which a rational choice is to be made. Risks can vary though expectations remain constant; what is a rational valuation of the element of risk itself? Gambling has a positive utility for players of Russian roulette, a negative utility for the young man in de Maupassant's story who is so afraid he might die in a scheduled duel that he kills himself the night before. The political game of "Chicken!" is grossly irrational, Bertrand Russell has tirelessly argued; under the designation of "brinkmanship" it has been defended by others as rational indeed. Agreement on expected outcomes might still lead to different decisions. The mathematical expectation is the same whether we match pennies or hundred-dollar bills, it being zero in both cases; for my part, the smaller stake is the more rational. This example is complicated by uncertainties as to the utility of money, but the excitement of the gamble itself also plays a part.

A criterion must also make some assessment of the value of the future, that is, of how utilities are affected by the mere fact that they lie in the future. A miser saves all he can, spends only what he must; a child does just the reverse. We might all agree with Aristotle that the rational course lies somewhere between these extremes; but where? I am not raising the problem of hedging against inflation, for example; expected changes of this kind can be discounted. The question is how to allocate resources between consumption and capital goods—as it were, how to choose between consuming something now or more later, how to decide how much the generation of the revolution should sacrifice to ensure the great leap forward. For a democracy the formulation is that the welfare of the unborn must be taken into account even though they cast no vote. What is the basis of a rational assignment of such utilities or, for that matter, a rational assignment of the utilities for our own future selves? Is it rational to decide now in terms of what I may want then? Love's way never changes of promising never to change, but those unblinded by love know better.

NOTE 3.

FELIX E. OPPENHEIM
RATIONAL DECISIONS AND
INTRINSIC VALUATIONS*

I am an advocate of birth control. Moreover, I maintain that, in view of certain further goals, it is *rational* for people in overpopulated countries to practice contraception and for government to encourage the practice. I have then the burden of proving that birth control is *desirable* under those conditions. I may justify contraception by pointing out that such a policy is required to reduce the population to the point where the necessities of life become available to all and that this condition is in turn a necessary means to "the greatest happiness of the greatest number." Now, means-end statements can be translated without loss of meaning into cause-effect statements which can, in principle, be empirically tested. Accordingly, if my prediction of the causal chain (contraception = decrease of population = increase of the average living standard = general well-being and happiness) is empirically warranted and if I am committed to the principle of utility, then my advocacy of contraception is rational, and it will be rational for any government which aims at maximizing the general welfare and happiness to adopt a policy of contraception in case of actual or threatened overpopulation.

Now, suppose someone disagrees with me. Suppose, however, he does not challenge my factual allegations. He concedes that failure to check the threatened population explosion will with practical certainty lead to the greatest unhappiness of the greatest number. He realizes the ineffectiveness of the rhythm method and the futility of preaching continence. He nevertheless opposes contraception, and his sole argument is that such practices are contrary to God's will. Our disagreement then boils down to the question: Should everyone (including every government) aim at maximizing the general welfare, or at complying with allegedly divine commands, even if in conflict with the principle of utility?

* Carl J. Friedrich, ed.: *Nomos VII—Rational Decision.* New York: Atherton Press 217–219 (1964). Copyright 1964 by Atherton Press. Reprinted by permission of Aldine-Atherton, Inc.

Professor Kaplan points out the unsatisfactory state of the theory of rational choice even for the purpose "of acting so as to secure the values pursued." But, on the other hand, he is convinced "that rationality is not limited to the choice among means" but applies also to the determination of "the relative worth of disparate and perhaps conflicting values" in the sense of ultimate goals. He would presumably claim that it is either rational or irrational to adopt the principle of utility as an aim in itself. He thereby espouses the meta-ethical theory of value cognitivism, according to which not only extrinsic, but also intrinsic, value judgments have cognitive status. Accordingly, the intrinsic value judgment that the greatest happiness principle is worth implementing for its own sake would be either demonstrably true or demonstrably false. If true, it would follow that it is rational to pursue this goal and irrational to be guided by any conflicting value, for example, my opponent's.

I cannot think of any scientific argument by which either my opponent or I could justify our respective intrinsic valuations. He might contend that an action is demonstrably rational if and only if it does not deviate from the moral law ordained by God and that the practice of contraception violates this principle and is therefore irrational as well as immoral. This argument may be *persuasive,* but only to those who happen to believe in an anthropomorphic God issuing commands—commands incompatible with birth control. However, an argument which is in principle acceptable only to some is not *valid* in the intersubjective, scientific sense. But I deny just as categorically the possibility of validating the greatest happiness principle or any other intrinsic value judgment. I agree with the meta-ethical position of value noncognitivism. Intrinsic valuations are a matter of subjective commitment, not of objective truth. Neither my adoption of the utilitarian standard nor my opponent's adherence to a particular religious faith can be called *either* rational *or* irrational. Both are commitments and, as such, nonrational.

I nevertheless agree with Professor Kaplan that rationality is not limited to the choice of means, and value noncognitivism does not entail that it is. To arrive at a rational decision, one does not start with the arbitrary selection of some ultimate end and then proceed to the choice of whatever means are most conducive to its realization. Means have consequences other than the goal, and the negative utility of the former may outweigh the positive utility of the latter. A rational actor must therefore predict (with as high a degree of probability as possible) the *total* outcome of each alternative action open to him in the given situation. Then he must establish a preference rank order among these total outcomes. The preferred outcome may include elements which the actor would disvalue if he considered them in isolation, and it need not include his original, but tentative, ultimate goal. Intrinsic valuations in connection with rational choice do not pertain to separate goals but to total outcomes. I have thus oversimplified the previous example. I must ask the following, more complicated question. What do I prefer on the whole: government-sponsored birth control *and* a higher living standard *and* increased promiscuity *and* a disregarding of certain religious beliefs and so on; or the outlawing of information about contraception *and* increased misery *and* the upholding of a particular faith and the like? This is the type of question which the theory of rational choice cannot answer; it does cover all other steps of the decision-making process.

*   *   *

d.

Karl R. Popper
The Open Society and Its Enemies*

[Utopian engineering] may be described as follows. Any rational action must have a certain aim. It is rational in the same degree as it pursues its aim consciously and consistently, and as it determines its means according to this end. To choose the end is therefore the first thing we have to do if we wish to act rationally; and we must be careful to determine our real or ultimate ends, from which we must distinguish clearly those intermediate or partial ends which actually are only means, or steps on the way, to the ultimate end. If we neglect this distinction, then we must also neglect to ask whether these partial ends are likely to promote the ultimate end, and accordingly, we must fail to act rationally. These principles, if applied to the realm of political activity, demand that we must determine our ultimate political aim, or the Ideal State, before taking any practical action. Only when this ultimate aim is determined, in rough outlines at least, only when we are in the posses-

* Princeton: Princeton University Press, Vol. 1, 157–163 (5th rev. ed., 1966). Copyright © 1962, 1966 by Karl Raimund Popper. Reprinted by permission of the author, Princeton University Press, and Routledge & Kegan Paul, Ltd., London.

sion of something like a blueprint of the society at which we aim, only then can we begin to consider the best ways and means for its realization, and to draw up a plan for practical action. These are the necessary preliminaries of any practical political move that can be called rational, and especially of social engineering.

*   *   *

Before proceeding to criticize Utopian engineering in detail, I wish to outline another approach to social engineering, namely that of piecemeal engineering. It is an approach which I think to be methodologically sound. The politician who adopts this method may or may not have a blueprint of society before his mind, he may or may not hope that mankind will one day realize an ideal state, and achieve happiness and perfection on earth. But he will be aware that perfection, if at all attainable, is far distant, and that every generation of men, and therefore also the living, have a claim; perhaps not so much a claim to be made happy, for there are no institutional means of making a man happy, but a claim not to be made unhappy, where it can be avoided. They have a claim to be given all possible help, if they suffer. The piecemeal engineer will, accordingly, adopt the method of searching for, and fighting against, the greatest and most urgent evils of society, rather than searching for, and fighting for, its greatest ultimate good. This difference is far from being merely verbal. In fact, it is most important. It is the difference between a reasonable method of improving the lot of man, and a method which, if really tried, may easily lead to an intolerable increase in human suffering. It is the difference between a method which can be applied at any moment, and a method whose advocacy may easily become a means of continually postponing action until a later date, when conditions are more favourable. And it is also the difference between the only method of improving matters which has so far been really successful, at any time, and in any place . . . and a method which, wherever it has been tried, has led only to the use of violence in place of reason, and if not to its own abandonment, at any rate to that of its original blueprint.

In favour of his method, the piecemeal engineer can claim that a systematic fight against suffering and injustice and war is more likely to be supported by the approval and agreement of a great number of people than the fight for the establishment of some ideal. The existence of social evils, that is to say of social conditions under which many men were suffering, can be comparatively well established. Those who suffer can judge for themselves, and the others can hardly deny that they would not like to change places. It is infinitely more difficult to reason about an ideal society. Social life is so complicated that few men, or none at all, could judge a blueprint for social engineering on the grand scale; whether it be practicable; whether it would result in a real improvement; what kind of suffering it may involve; and what may be the means for its realization. As opposed to this, blueprints for piecemeal engineering are comparatively simple. They are blueprints for single institutions, for health and unemployed insurance, for instance, or arbitration courts, or antidepression budgeting or educational reform. If they go wrong, the damage is not very great, and a re-adjustment not very difficult. They are less risky, and for this very reason less controversial. But if it is easier to reach a reasonable agreement about existing evils and the means of combating them than it is about an ideal good and the means of its realization, then there is also more hope that by using the piecemeal method we may get over the very greatest practical difficulty of all reasonable political reform, namely, the use of reason, instead of passion and violence, in executing the programme. There will be a possibility of reaching a reasonable compromise and therefore of achieving the improvement by democratic methods. ("Compromise" is an ugly word, but it is important for us to learn its proper use. *Institutions* are inevitably the result of a compromise with circumstances, interests, etc., though as *persons* we should resist influences of this kind.)

[T]he Utopian attempt to realize an ideal state, using a blueprint of society as a whole, is one which demands a strong centralized rule of a few, which therefore is likely to lead to a dictatorship. . . . One of the difficulties faced by a benevolent dictator is to find whether the effects of his measures agree with his good intentions. . . . The difficulty arises out of the fact that authoritarianism must discourage criticism; accordingly, the benevolent dictator will not easily hear of complaints concerning the measures he has taken. But without some such check, he can hardly find whether his measures achieve the desired benevolent aim. The situation must become even worse for the Utopian engineer. The reconstruction of society is a big undertaking which must cause considerable inconvenience to many, and for a considerable span of time. Accordingly, the Utopian engineer will have to be deaf to many complaints; in fact, it will be part of his business to suppress unreasonable objections. . . . But with

it, he must invariably suppress reasonable criticism also. . . . The very sweep of . . . a Utopian undertaking makes it improbable that it will realize its ends during the lifetime of one social engineer, or group of engineers. And if the successors do not pursue the same ideal, then all the sufferings of the people for the sake of the ideal may have been in vain.

A generalization of this argument leads to a further criticism of the Utopian approach. This approach, it is clear, can be of practical value only if we assume that the original blueprint, perhaps with certain adjustments, remains the basis of the work until it is completed. But that will take some time. It will be a time of revolutions, both political and spiritual, and of new experiments and experience in the political field. It is therefore to be expected that ideas and ideals will change. What had appeared the ideal state to the people who made the original blueprint, may not appear so to their successors. If that is granted, then the whole approach breaks down. The method of first establishing an ultimate political aim and then beginning to move towards it is futile if we admit that the aim may be considerably changed during the process of its realization. It may at any moment turn out that the steps so far taken actually lead away from the realization of the new aim. And if we change our direction according to the new aim, then we expose ourselves to the same risk again. In spite of all the sacrifices made, we may never get anywhere at all. . . .

[T]he Utopian approach can be saved only by the Platonic belief in one absolute and unchanging ideal, together with two further assumptions, namely (a) that there are rational methods to determine once and for all what this ideal is, and (b) what the best means of its realization are. Only such far-reaching assumptions could prevent us from declaring the Utopian methodology to be utterly futile. But even Plato himself and the most ardent Platonists would admit that (a) is certainly not true; that there is no rational method for determining the ultimate aim, but, if anything, only some kind of intuition. Any difference of opinion between Utopian engineers must therefore lead, in the absence of rational methods, to the use of power instead of reason, i.e., to violence. If any progress in any definite direction is made at all, then it is made in spite of the method adopted, not because of it. The success may be due, for instance, to the excellence of the leaders; but we must never forget that excellent leaders cannot be produced by rational methods, but only by luck.

It is important to understand this criticism properly; I do not criticize the ideal by claiming that an ideal can never be realized, that it must always remain a Utopia. This would not be a valid criticism, for many things have been realized which have once been dogmatically declared to be unrealizable, for instance, the establishment of institutions for securing civil peace, i.e. for the prevention of crime *within* the state; and I think that, for instance, the establishment of corresponding institutions for the prevention of international crime, i.e. armed aggression or blackmail, though often branded as Utopian, is not even a very difficult problem. What I criticize under the name Utopian engineering recommends the reconstruction of society as a whole, i.e. very sweeping changes whose practical consequences are hard to calculate, owing to our limited experiences. It claims to plan rationally for the whole of society, although we do not possess anything like the factual knowledge which would be necessary to make good such an ambitious claim. We cannot possess such knowledge since we have insufficient practical experience in this kind of planning, and knowledge of facts must be based upon experience. At present, the sociological knowledge necessary for large-scale engineering is simply non-existent.

In view of this criticism, the Utopian engineer is likely to grant the need for practical experience, and for a social technology based upon practical experiences. But he will argue that we shall never know more about these matters if we recoil from making social experiments which alone can furnish us with the practical experience needed. And he might add that Utopian engineering is nothing but the application of the experimental method to society. Experiments cannot be carried out without involving sweeping changes. They must be on a large scale, owing to the peculiar character of modern society with its great masses of people. An experiment in socialism, for instance, if confined to a factory, or to a village, or even to a district, would never give us the kind of realistic information which we need so urgently.

[T]he Utopian engineer . . . is convinced that we must recast the whole structure of society, when we experiment with it; and he can therefore conceive a more *modest* experiment only as one that recasts the whole structure of a *small* society. But the kind of experiment from which we can learn most is the alteration of one social institution at a time. For only in this way can we learn how to fit institutions into the framework of other institutions, and how to adjust them so that they work according to our intentions. And only in this way can we make mistakes, and learn from our mistakes, without risking repercussions of a gravity that must endanger the will to future reforms. Furthermore, the Utopian method must lead to a dangerous dogmatic attachment to a blueprint for which countless sacrifices have been made. Powerful interests must become linked up with the success of the experiment. All this does not contribute to the rationality, or to the scientific value, of the experiment. But the piecemeal method permits repeated experiments and continuous readjustments. In fact, it might lead to the happy situation where politicians begin to look out for their own mistakes instead of trying to explain them away and to prove that they have always been right. This—and not Utopian planning or historical prophecy—would mean the introduction of scientific method into politics since the whole secret of scientific method is a readiness to learn from mistakes.

*　　*　　*

C.
Collective Planning—The Step-by-Step Approach

Choice by Mutual Adjustment?

a.

Charles E. Lindblom
The Science of "Muddling Through"*

Suppose an administrator is given responsibility for formulating policy with respect to in-

* 29 *Public Administration Review* 79–88 (Spring, 1959). Reprinted by permission.

flation. He might start by trying to list all related values in order of importance, e.g., full employment, reasonable business profit, protection of small savings, prevention of a stock market crash. Then all possible policy outcomes could be rated as more or less efficient in attaining a maximum of these values. This would of course require a prodigious inquiry into values held by members of society and an equally prodigious set of calculations on how much of each value is equal to how much of each other value. He could then proceed to outline all possible policy alternatives. In a third step, he would undertake systematic comparison of his multitude of alternatives to determine which attains the greatest amount of values.

In comparing policies, he would take advantage of any theory available that generalized about classes of policies. In considering inflation, for example, he would compare all policies in the light of the theory of prices. Since no alternatives are beyond his investigation, he would consider strict central control and the abolition of all prices and markets on the one hand and elimination of all public controls with reliance completely on the free market on the other, both in the light of whatever theoretical generalizations he could find on such hypothetical economies.

Finally, he would try to make the choice that would in fact maximize his values.

An alternative line of attack would be to set as his principal objective, either explicitly or without conscious thought, the relatively simple goal of keeping prices level. This objective might be compromised or complicated by only a few other goals, such as full employment. He would in fact disregard most other social values as beyond his present interest, and he would for the moment not even attempt to rank the few values that he regarded as immediately relevant. Were he pressed, he would quickly admit that he was ignoring many related values and many possible important consequences of his policies.

As a second step, he would outline those relatively few policy alternatives that occurred to him. He would then compare them. In comparing his limited number of alternatives, most of them familiar from past controversies, he would not ordinarily find a body of theory precise enough to carry him through a comparison of their respective consequences. Instead he would rely heavily on the record of past experience with small policy steps to predict the consequences of similar steps extended into the future.

Moreover, he would find that the policy alternatives combined objectives or values in different ways. For example, one policy might offer price level stability at the cost of some risk of unemployment; another might offer less price stability but also less risk of unemployment. Hence, the next step in his approach—the final selection would combine into one the choice among values and the choice among instruments for reaching values. It would not, as in the first method of policy-making, approximate a more mechanical process of choosing the means that best satisfied

goals that were previously clarified and ranked. Because practitioners of the second approach expect to achieve their goals only partially, they would expect to repeat endlessly the sequence just described, as conditions and aspirations changed and as accuracy of prediction improved.

For complex problems, the first of these two approaches is of course impossible. Although such an approach can be described, it cannot be practiced except for relatively simple problems and even then only in a somewhat modified form. It assumes intellectual capacities and sources of information that men simply do not possess, and it is even more absurd as an approach to policy when the time and money that can be allocated to a policy problem is limited as is always the case. . . . It is the second method that is practiced.

. . . This might be described as the method of *successive limited comparisons.* I will contrast it with the first approach, which might be called the rational-comprehensive method. More impressionistically and briefly—and therefore generally used in this article—they could be characterized as the branch method and root method, the former continually building out from the current situation, step-by-step and by small degrees; the latter starting from fundamentals anew each time, building on the past only as experience is embodied in a theory, and always prepared to start completely from the ground up.

* * *

*Intertwining Evaluation and
Empirical Analysis*

The quickest way to understand how values are handled in the method of successive limited comparisons is to see how the root method often breaks down in *its* handling of values or objectives. The idea that values should be clarified, and in advance of the examination of alternative policies, is appealing. But what happens when we attempt it for complex social problems? The first difficulty is that on many critical values or objectives, citizens disagree, congressmen disagree, and public administrators disagree. Even where a fairly specific objective is prescribed for the administrator, there remains considerable room for disagreement on sub-objectives. . . .

Administrators cannot escape these conflicts by ascertaining the majority's preference, for preferences have not been registered on most issues; indeed, there often *are* no preferences in the absence of public discussion sufficient to bring an issue to the attention of the electorate. Furthermore, there is a question of whether intensity of feeling should be considered as well as the number of persons preferring each alternative. By the impossibility of doing otherwise, administrators often are reduced to deciding policy without clarifying objectives first.

Even when an administrator resolves to follow his own values as a criterion for decisions, he often will not know how to rank them when they conflict with one another, as they usually do.

*   *   *

A more subtle third point underlies both the first two. Social objectives do not always have the same relative values. One objective may be highly prized in one circumstance, another in another circumstance. If, for example, an administrator values highly both the dispatch with which his agency can carry through its projects and good public relations, it matters little which of the two possibly conflicting values he favors in some abstract or general sense. Policy questions arise in forms which put to administrators such a question as: Given the degree to which we are or are not already achieving the values of dispatch and the values of good public relations, is it worth sacrificing a little speed for a happier clientele, or is it better to risk offending the clientele so that we can get on with our work? The answer to such a question varies with circumstances.

The value problem is, as the example shows, always a problem of adjustments at a margin. But there is no practicable way to state marginal objectives or values except in terms of particular policies. That one value is preferred to another in one decision situation does not mean that it will be preferred in another decision situation in which it can be had only at great sacrifice of another value. Attempts to rank or order values in general and abstract terms so that they do not shift from decision to decision end up by ignoring the relevant marginal preferences. The significance of this third point thus goes very far. Even if all administrators had at hand an agreed set of values, objectives, and constraints, and an agreed ranking of these values, objectives, and constraints, their marginal values in actual choice situations would be impossible to formulate.

*   *   *

In summary, two aspects of the process by which values are actually handled can be distinguished. The first is clear: evaluation and empirical analysis are intertwined; that is, one chooses among values and among policies at one and the same time. Put a little more elaborately, one simultaneously chooses a policy to attain certain objectives and chooses the objectives themselves. The second aspect is related but distinct: the administrator focuses his attention on marginal or incremental values. . . .

*   *   *

As to whether the attempt to clarify objectives in advance of policy selection is more or less rational than the close intertwining of marginal evaluation and empirical analysis, the principal difference established is that for complex problems the first is impossible and irrelevant, and the second is both possible and relevant. The second is possible because the administrator need not try to analyze any values except the values by which alternative policies differ and need not be concerned with them except as they differ marginally. His need for information on values or objectives is drastically reduced as compared with the root method; and his capacity for grasping, comprehending, and relating values to one another is not strained beyond the breaking point.

Relations between Means and Ends

Decision-making is ordinarily formalized as a means-ends relationship: means are conceived to be evaluated and chosen in the light of ends finally selected independently of and prior to the choice of means. This is the means-ends relationship of the root method. But it follows from all that has just been said that such a means-end relationship is possible only to the extent that values are agreed upon, are reconcilable, and are stable at the margin. Typically, therefore, such a means-ends relationship is absent from the branch method, where means and ends are simultaneously chosen.

Yet any departure from the means-ends relationship of the root method will strike some readers as inconceivable. For it will appear to them that only in such a relationship is it possible to determine whether one policy choice is better or worse than another. How can an administrator know whether he has made a wise or foolish decision if he is without prior values or objectives by which to judge his decisions? The answer to this question calls up the third distinctive difference between root and branch methods: how to decide the best policy.

The Test of "Good" Policy

In the root method, a decision is "correct," "good," or "rational" if it can be shown to attain some specified objective, where the objective can be specified without simply describing the decision itself. Where objectives are defined only through the marginal or incremental approach to values described above, it is still sometimes possible to test whether a policy does in fact attain the desired objectives; but a precise statement of the objectives takes the form of a description of the policy chosen or some alternative to it. To show that a policy is mistaken one cannot offer an abstract argument that important objectives are not achieved; one must instead argue that another policy is more to be preferred.

. . . But what of the situation in which administrators cannot agree on values or objectives, either abstractly or in marginal terms? What then is the test of "good" policy? For the root method, there is no test. Agreement on objectives failing, there is no standard of "correctness." For the method of successive limited comparisons, the test is agreement on policy itself, which remains possible even when agreement on values is not.

*   *   *

If agreement directly on policy as a test for "best" policy seems a poor substitute for testing the policy against its objectives, it ought to be remembered that objectives themselves have no ultimate validity other than they are agreed upon. Hence agreement is the test of "best" policy in both methods. But where the root method requires agreement on what elements in the decision constitute objectives and on which of these objectives should be sought, the branch method falls back on agreement wherever it can be found.

In an important sense, therefore, it is not irrational for an administrator to defend a policy as good without being able to specify what it is good for.

Non-Comprehensive Analysis

Ideally, rational-comprehensive analysis leaves out nothing important. But it is impossible to take everything important into consideration unless "important" is so narrowly defined that analysis is in fact quite limited. Limits on human intellectual capacities and on available information set definite limits to man's capacity to be comprehensive. . . .

In the method of successive limited comparisons, simplification is systematically achieved in two principal ways. First, it is achieved through limitation of policy comparisons to those policies that differ in relatively small degree from policies presently in effect. Such a limitation im-

mediately reduces the number of alternatives to be investigated and also drastically simplifies the character of the investigation of each. For it is not necessary to undertake fundamental inquiry into an alternative and its consequences; it is necessary only to study those respects in which the proposed alternative and its consequences differ from the status quo. . . .

*   *   *

Since the policies ignored by the administrator are politically impossible and so irrelevant, the simplification of analysis achieved by concentrating on policies that differ only incrementally is not a capricious kind of simplification. In addition, it can be argued that, given the limits on knowledge within which policy-makers are confined, simplifying by limiting the focus to small variations from present policy makes the most of available knowledge. Because policies being considered are like present and past policies, the administrator can obtain information and claim some insight. Non-incremental policy proposals are therefore typically not only politically irrelevant but also unpredictable in their consequences.

*   *   *

The second method of simplification of analysis is the practice of ignoring important possible consequences of possible policies, as well as the values attached to the neglected consequences. If this appears to disclose a shocking shortcoming of successive limited comparisons, it can be replied that, even if the exclusions are random, policies may nevertheless be more intelligently formulated than through futile attempts to achieve a comprehensiveness beyond human capacity. Actually, however, the exclusions, seeming arbitrary or random from one point of view, need be neither.

*   *   *

Suppose that each value neglected by one policy-making agency were a major concern of at least one other agency. In that case, a helpful division of labor would be achieved, and no agency need find its task beyond its capacities. The shortcomings of such a system would be that one agency might destroy a value either before another agency could be activated to safeguard it or in spite of another agency's efforts. But the possibility that important values may be lost is present in any form of organization, even where agencies attempt to comprehend in planning more than is humanly possible.

The virtue of such a hypothetical division of labor is that every important interest or value has its watchdog. And these watchdogs can protect the interests in their jurisdiction in two quite different ways: first, by redressing damages done by other agencies; and, second, by anticipating and heading off injury before it occurs.

*　　*　　*

Mutual adjustment is more pervasive than the explicit forms it takes in negotiation between groups; it persists through the mutual impacts of groups upon each other even where they are not in communication. For all the imperfections and latent dangers in this ubiquitous process of mutual adjustment, it will often accomplish an adaptation of policies to a wider range of interests than could be done by one group centrally.

Note, too, how the incremental pattern of policy-making fits with the multiple pressure pattern. For when decisions are only incremental—closely related to known policies, it is easier for one group to anticipate the kind of moves another might make and easier too for it to make correction for injury already accomplished. . . .

Succession of Comparisons

The final distinctive element in the branch method is that the comparisons, together with the policy choice, proceed in a chronological series. Policy is not made once and for all; it is made and re-made endlessly. Policy-making is a process of successive approximation to some desired objectives in which what is desired itself continues to change under reconsideration.

*　　*　　*

In the first place, past sequences of policy steps have given him knowledge about the probable consequences of further similar steps. Second, he need not attempt big jumps toward his goals that would require predictions beyond his or anyone else's knowledge, because he never expects his policy to be a final resolution of a problem. His decision is only one step, one that if successful can quickly be followed by another. Third, he is in effect able to test his previous predictions as he moves on to each further step. Lastly, he often can remedy a past error fairly quickly—more quickly than if policy proceeded through more distinct steps widely spaced in time.

*　　*　　*

Successive limited comparisons is, then, indeed a method or system; it is not a failure of method for which administrators ought to apologize. None the less, its imperfections, which have not been explored in this paper, are many. For example, the method is without a built-in safeguard for all relevant values, and it also may lead the decision-maker to overlook excellent policies for no other reason than that they are not suggested by the chain of successive policy steps leading up to the present. Hence, it ought to be said that under this method, as well as under some of the most sophisticated variants of the root method—operations research, for example—policies will continue to be as foolish as they are wise.

*　　*　　*

b.

Charles E. Lindblom
The Policy-Making Process*

*　　*　　*

The limits on analyses . . . are of a particular kind. They indicate how far man might go, *if he tried,* toward settling policy disputes by investigating their merits—that is, by studying and reasoning about policy instead of fighting over it. Often, however, he does not even try. Why?

Irrationality. Men turn an indifferent or hostile eye on policy analysis because they are not wholly rational. Because, specifically, it is easier to feel than to think. Because they cling to beliefs that serve the needs of their personalities. Because words or symbols with which they talk about politics come to be more dear to them than the things to which the symbols refer. Because sometimes it pains them to change their minds. Because they have picked up all kinds of beliefs from their families, friends, churches, and other groups—beliefs that give them a comforting orientation to the world about them and which they consequently dare not challenge. Because it may not have occurred to them that policy analysis is of potential great value.

*　　*　　*

Assaults on the mind. Moreover, man is forever assaulted by a barrage of communications from other men who want to manipulate him. If he wants to pursue analysis, or encourage those who do, he must fight off the seductive irrational and nonrational appeals of political parties, candidates for office, interest groups, and propagandists of other kinds. They everywhere tug at his

* Englewood Cliffs, N.J.: Prentice-Hall, Inc. 18–20, 24–29, 116–117 (1968). © 1968. Reprinted by permission.

attention and try to commit his mind before he has had time to think. They are always at his ear.

Men who "know" what they want. And those at his ear may not want to analyze policy either, for they may have decided that they already know what they want. Senator Joseph McCarthy wanted no analysis of the threat of internal communism in the U.S.; he wanted to proceed directly against a whole class of people he indiscriminately associated with communism, socialism, liberalism, and internationalism. Similarly, most taxpayers' councils scattered around the United States want only limited analysis of government fiscal policy; on their basic antagonism to government expenditures they have already made up their minds: on that issue, they feel, the less discussion and the less study, the better.

Reasoned grounds for rejection. Even those people most interested in analysis will know that analysis will always be influenced by the biases of the analysts and by their incompetences, and that hence it is not always to be trusted. And they will know that, since most analysis takes place in organizations, it will always be marred by organizational biases, rigidities, and other incompetence. Take for example the unhappy failure of organizations to define relevant problems. An organization like the Air Force is primarily established to exploit the usefulness of aircraft for national defense. Its policy problems therefore revolve around the question: How best to use aircraft for defense? As an organization, however, it is most unlikely ever to ask the question (which as time passes and new techniques of warfare are developed comes to be a critical question): Should aircraft give way to missiles? And the organization may even try to suppress the question elsewhere in the Department of Defense.

Organizational obstacles to satisfactory analysis constitute a subject in themselves. Differences of rank in organizations obstruct communication; the generalist's rivalry with the specialist sows distrust and becomes a source of bias; the organization's hiring policies may not attract competent personnel; promotion may be based on fitting in with the organization rather than on analytical skill; and so on. No few examples, however, can represent the luxuriant variety of organizational barriers to analysis.

*   *   *

It is not . . . man's use of language, of quantification, of other universal tools, or of ideology that changes the character of policy analysis in surprising ways. We begin to see a somewhat unexpected new face on policy analysis only when we look at certain strategies or dodges that man has developed for dealing with very complex problems—strategies that are especially well adapted to public policy analysis. Some of the most important are as follows:

Satisficing

In the conventional ideal of a rational decision, a decision maker maximizes something—utility or want satisfaction, income, national security, the general welfare, or some other such value. But, as we have already noted, an exhaustive search for the maximum, for the best of all possible policies, is not usually worth what it costs, and may in fact be impossible of accomplishment. An alternative strategy, therefore, is not to try too hard, to decide instead on some acceptable level of goal accomplishment short of maximization, and then pursue the search until a policy is found that attains that level. One "satisfices" instead of maximizes.

The Next Chance

Sometimes policy analysts deliberately make little mistakes to avoid big ones. One can deliberately choose a policy (knowing that it is not quite the right policy) that leaves open the possibility of doing better in a next step, instead of a policy designed to be on target but difficult to amend. While an Indian civil servant, for example is inclined to shoot for his target with little thought of a second chance, an American civil servant never expects to be wholly right and values a second chance. In as relatively simple a policy problem as routing New Haven traffic, to try out one-way traffic going south and stand ready, if that is unsuccessful, to try a northbound flow may be better than to gamble, through an *a priori* study of traffic flows, on a permanent installation of expensive controls to inaugurate southbound one-way movement.

Feedback

A policy analyst may want to deal inconclusively with a problem—that is, keep a next chance open because he thinks that with the passage of time he will come to know more. But if he can choose a policy that will, as in the traffic example, itself feed back information necessary to a better choice of policy, so much the better. Policy feedback is of course a commonplace phenomenon: it is hard to imagine a policy that feeds back no useful information at all. Monetary and fiscal policy is an example of especially quick and powerful feedback because of its immediate impact on business activity. But policy-making systems differ in sensitivity to feedback and in the skill with which they choose policies in order to induce feedback. A policy chosen because it is ideologically correct—like Soviet policy on collective farms—may persist for years in spite of failure, with its advocates blind to feedback.

Remediality

In the classical model of rational decision making a policy analyst concerned about American Negroes would be required to formulate in his mind an organized set of policy aspirations and to specify for various dates in the future the income, educational status, and other social and cultural goals at which policy should aim. In actual fact, some policy analysts greatly simplify this otherwise impossible goal-setting task by refusing to look very far ahead—focusing instead on the removal of all-too-observable disadvantages now suffered by the Negroes. That is, if they cannot decide with any precision the state of affairs they want to achieve, they can at least specify the state of affairs from which they want to escape. They deal more confidently with what is wrong than with what in the future may or may not be right.

Critics will say that policy would be more rational if it were guided by positive instead of negative objectives, but it is not at all certain that positive objectives could win assent, or that they would be as operational as negative objectives. . . . If in this sense policy analysts look backward instead of forward, they sometimes gain rather than lose competence.

Seriality

A policy analyst who appreciates a next chance, exploits feedback, and keeps his eye on ills to be remedied will come to take for granted that policy making is typically serial, or sequential. He will see that policy making is typically a never-ending process of successive steps in which continual nibbling is a substitute for a good bite. He will design policy not merely on the expectation of a second step but on the projection of a third, or a fourth—of an endless series. In this style of policy analysis, he sees possibilities for revising both policies and objectives, and he comes to treat policy making as open-ended in all its aspects. He and any political system of this style may therefore develop a high level of flexibility, resilience and pertinency that greatly raises his or its ability to make good policy in the face of complexity. In a system in which policy making is frankly recognized to be serial or sequential, the whole system may be tailored to rapid sequences so that, though no one policy move is great, the frequency of small moves makes rapid social change possible.

In the U.S., policy analysts nibble endlessly at taxation, social security, national defense, conservation, foreign aid and the like. Policy analysts assume that these problems are never solved, and hold themselves in readiness to return to them again and again. That kind of persistence in policy making has transformed the society. America, observers say, has gone through an industrial revolution, an organizational revolution, a revolution in economic organization (from *laissez faire* to a highly regulated economy) and a revolution in the role of the family—but all through policy sequences so undramatic as to obscure the magnitude of change.

Bottlenecks

Every policy analyst—and you and I in our personal problems—makes frequent use of the tactic of bottleneck breaking to simplify complex problems. On a superficial view of policy making, a bottleneck is nothing more than clear evidence of a breakdown in decision making. If something is running behind schedule, or something necessary to action is missing, or there is a congestion, we say a bottleneck exists. But since bottlenecks are inevitable for complex policy making, policy analysts have discovered how to use them to make the best of a less-than-ideal situation.

*   *   *

At an extreme, one can see the two contrasting possibilities for policy analysis: on the one hand, plan everything to fit with everything else; on the other hand, plan to break specific bottlenecks as they arise. The first is impossible; the second, though far from ideal, works.

Incrementalism

Usually—though not always—what is feasible politically is policy only incrementally, or marginally, different from existing policies. Drastically different policies fall beyond the pale. That aside, a preoccupation with no more than incremental or marginal changes in policy often serves for still other reasons to raise the level of competence of policy. Where applicable, such a strategy:

1. concentrates the policy maker's analysis on familiar, better-known experience;

2. sharply reduces the number of different alternative policies to be explored; and

3. sharply reduces the number and complexity of factors he has to analyze.

*   *   *

What is the ordinary interpretation put on these strategies or dodges? On superficial examination they are often dismissed as irrational. For they are seen as indecisiveness, patching up, timidity, triviality, narrowness of view, inclusiveness, caution, and procrastination. But we have seen them to be useful devices for stretching man's analytic capacities. Man has had to be devilishly inventive to cope with the staggering difficulties he faces. His analytical methods cannot be restricted to tidy scholarly procedures. The piecemealing, remedial incrementalist or satisficer may not look like an heroic figure. He is nevertheless a shrewd, resourceful problem-solver who is wrestling bravely with a universe that he is wise enough to know is too big for him.

*   *   *

We now come back to face up to the fact that, however extended, policy analysis is inadequate. If it is not possible through analysis to find policies that are everywhere accepted because proved to be correct, what can be done? Someone has to take on the task of deciding on policy for society. But because no one can perform the task of making a decision on policy without the "power" to do so, the more usual way to put the point is to say that, in the absence of universal agreement on what is to be done, someone has to either seize or be given "power" to decide.

In actual fact, of course, "power" is always held by a number of persons rather than by one; *hence policy is made through the complex processes by which these persons exert power or influence over each other.* What is the character of this play of power in policy making? And how is policy analysis incorporated into it?

*   *   *

"Power" to decide. . . . Some person or persons must simply make policy choices for the society, the rest of the population simply accepting the decisions. The policy-making task or function has to be seized or assigned.

Whoever takes on the task will of course employ analysis up to a point. He must, however,

come to a decision—by guess, considered judgment, or whim.

The task or responsibility cannot be laid upon one man or small group. Even an authoritarian ruler needs a structure of subordinate colleagues to assist him in policy making. In the democracies, almost every adult is offered a share of the task, and many accept. For example—though examples do not do justice to the complexities of task definition and assignment—some (President, Prime Minister, or Cabinet) accept the principal responsibility for initiating policy decisions; others the (legislative) task of amending, ratifying, or rejecting these policy decisions; others the (judicial) task of testing policy decisions for consistency with constitutional rules; and others, the task of deciding who will be a member, say, of the legislative group—a task they are able to discharge through voting.

Rules and authority. Such a process—both the relatively simpler one of authoritarian policy making and the intricate one of democratic policy making—works because somehow people perform the tasks they accept, and others accept the results. But why do people accept? They may be terrorized into so doing by someone or some group that can command a personal guard, police force, or army. In democratic societies, however, they do so for a variety of other reasons. Some people like the tasks that have been assigned, or the money, prestige, and sense of power that go with them. Others who like to be left free of responsibility are willing to accept what is decided upon. Some people simply believe that, since some assignment of tasks is necessary, they ought morally to perform their assigned task and go along with others who perform theirs. Others perform their tasks, or accept the results of those who do, because they fear the enmity of their neighbors and associates if they fail to do so, or because those who do accept their assignments have organized routines for fining, jailing, or otherwise punishing others.

Whatever the reasons, most people adopt a rule of performing an accepted task according to the task's specifications, and a *rule* of accepting the decisions of those to whom tasks have been assigned. They do not ask themselves at every opportunity: "Could I get away with defaulting?" Some of the rules they accept are those of obedience on specified matters to specified categories of persons, thus establishing the *authority* of those persons.

Specialization. A proliferation of specialized tasks in policy making arises both as a method of raising the competence of policy makers (since no one participant in the process can be competent in all areas and on all aspects of policy making) and as a method of limiting the power or influence of any one policy maker. In democratic societies, an especially intricate specialization of function—carried to an extreme in the American pattern of checks and balances—greatly constrains the power or influence of any one policy maker.

Cooperation. Hence in all policy-making systems, but especially in democratic systems, policies can be made only through the cooperation of many participants, each of whom performs a task that is necessary, but itself insufficient, to establish a policy decision. Policy making is a cooperative collective effort, and policy a joint output, beyond the capacity of any one person or any small group of those to whom policy-making tasks are assigned.

c.

Aaron Wildavsky
The Politics of the Budgetary Process*

Budgeting is incremental, not comprehensive. The beginning of wisdom about an agency budget is that it is almost never actively reviewed as a whole every year in the sense of reconsidering the value of all existing programs as compared to all possible alternatives. Instead, it is based on last year's budget with special attention given to a narrow range of increases or decreases. Thus the men who make the budget are concerned with relatively small increments to an existing base. Their attention is focused on a small number of items over which the budgetary battle is fought. As Representative Norrel declared in testifying before the House Rules Committee, "If you will read the hearings of the subcommittees you will find that most of our time is spent in talking about the changes in the bill which we will have next year from the one we had this year, the reductions made, and the increases made. That which is not changed has very little, if anything, said about it." Most appropriations committee members, like Senator Hayden in dismissing an item brought up by the Bureau of Indian Affairs, "do not think it is necessary to go into details of the estimate, as the committee has had this appropriation before it for many years." Asked to defend this procedure,

---

* Boston: Little, Brown & Co. 15, 128–138 (1964). Copyright © 1964 by Little, Brown & Company, Inc. Reprinted by permission.

a budget officer (or his counterparts in the Budget Bureau and Congress) will say that it is a waste of time to go back to the beginning as if every year was a blank slate. "No need to build the car over again."

*   *   *

If a normative theory of budgeting is to be more than an academic exercise, it must actually guide the making of governmental decisions. The items of expenditures that are passed by Congress, enacted into law, and spent must in large measure conform to the theory if it is to have any practical effect. This is tantamount to prescribing that virtually all the activities of government be carried on according to the theory. For whatever the government does must be paid for from public funds; it is difficult to think of any policy that can be carried out without money.

The budget is the lifeblood of the government, the financial reflection of what the government does or intends to do. A theory that contains criteria for determining what ought to be in the budget is nothing less than a theory stating what the government ought to do. If we substitute the words "what the government ought to do" for the words "ought to be in the budget," it becomes clear that a normative theory of budgeting would be a comprehensive and specific political theory detailing what the government's activities ought to be at a particular time. A normative theory of budgeting, therefore, is utopian in the fullest sense of that word: its accomplishment and acceptance would mean the end of conflict over the government's role in society.

By suppressing dissent, totalitarian regimes enforce their normative theories of budgeting on others. Presumably, we reject this solution to the problem of conflict in society and insist on democratic procedures. How then arrive at a theory of budgeting that is something more than one man's preferences?

The crucial aspect of budgeting is whose preferences are to prevail in disputes about which activities are to be carried on and to what degree, in the light of limited resources. The problem is not only "how shall budgetary benefits be maximized?" as if it made no difference who received them, but also "who shall receive budgetary benefits and how much?" One may purport to solve the problem of budgeting by proposing a normative theory (or a welfare function or a hierarchy of values) which specifies a method for maximizing returns for budgetary expendi-

THE STEP-BY-STEP APPROACH 277

tures. In the absence of ability to impose a set of preferred policies on others, however, this solution breaks down. It amounts to no more than saying that if you can persuade others to agree with you, then you will have achieved agreement. Or it begs the question of what kind of policies will be fed into the scheme by assuming that these are agreed upon. Yet we hardly need argue that a state of universal agreement has not yet arisen.

Another way of avoiding the problem of budgeting is to treat society as a single organism with a consistent set of desires and a life of its own, much as a single consumer might be assumed to have a stable demand and indifference schedule. Instead of revenue being raised and the budget being spent by and for many individuals who may have their own preferences and feelings, as is surely the case, these processes are treated, in effect, as if a single individual were the only one concerned. This approach avoids the central problems of social conflict, of somehow aggregating different preferences so that a decision may emerge. How can we compare the worth of expenditures for irrigation to certain farmers with the worth of widening a highway to motorists and the desirability of aiding old people to pay medical bills as against the degree of safety provided by an expanded defense program?

The process we have developed for dealing with interpersonal comparisons in government is not economic but political. Conflicts are resolved (under agreed-upon rules) by translating different preferences through the political system into units called votes or into types of authority like a veto power. There need not be (and there is not) full agreement on goals or the preferential weights to be accorded to different goals. Congressmen directly threaten, compromise, and trade favors in regard to policies in which values are implicitly weighted, and then agree to register the results according to the rules for tallying votes.

The burden of calculation is enormously reduced for three primary reasons: first, only the small number of alternatives politically feasible at any one time are considered; second, these policies in a democracy typically differ only in small increments from previous policies on which there is a store of relevant information; and, third, each participant may ordinarily assume that he need consider only his preferences and those of his powerful opponents since the American political system works to assure that every significant interest has representation at some key point.

*   *   *

The basic idea behind program budgeting is that instead of presenting budgetary requests in the usual line-item form, which focuses on categories like supplies, maintenance, and personnel, the presentation is made in terms of the end-products, of program packages like public health or limited war or strategic retaliatory forces. The virtues of the program budget are said to be its usefulness in relating ends to means in a comprehensive fashion, the emphasis it puts upon the policy implications of budgeting, and the ease with which it permits consideration of the budget as a whole as each program competes with every other for funds. Interestingly enough, the distinguishing characteristics of the program procedure are precisely the reverse of those of the traditional practice. Federal budgeting today is incremental rather than comprehensive, calculated in bits and pieces rather than as a whole, and veils policy implications rather than emphasizing them.

*   *   *

The incremental, fragmented, non-programmatic, and sequential procedures of the present budgetary process aid in securing agreement and reducing the burden of calculation. It is much easier to agree on an addition or reduction of a few thousand or a million than to agree on whether a program is good in the abstract. It is much easier to agree on a small addition or decrease than to compare the worth of one program to that of all others. Conflict is reduced by an incremental approach because the area open to dispute is reduced. In much the same way the burden of calculation is eased because no one has to make all the calculations that would be involved in a comprehensive evaluation of all expenditures.

*   *   *

Procedures that de-emphasize overt conflicts among competing programs also encourage secret deliberations, non-partisanship, and the recruitment of personnel who feel comfortable in sidestepping policy decisions most of the time.

*   *   *

Consider by contrast some likely consequences of program budgeting. The practice of focusing attention on programs means that policy implications can hardly be avoided. The gains and the losses for the interests involved become far more evident to all concerned. Conflict is heightened by the stress on policy differences and increased still further by an in-built tendency to an all-or-nothing, "yes" or "no" response to the policy in dispute. The very concept of program packages suggests that the policy in dispute is indivisible, that the appropriate response is to be for or against rather than bargaining for a little more or a little less. Logrolling and bargaining are hindered because it is much easier to trade increments conceived in monetary terms than it is to give in on basic policy differences. Problems of calculation are vastly increased by the necessity, if program budgeting is to have meaning, of evaluating the desirability of every program as compared to all others, instead of the traditional practice of considering budgets in relatively independent segments. Conflict would become much more prevalent as the specialist whose verdict was usually accepted in his limited sphere gave way to the generalist whose decisons were fought over by all his fellow legislators who could claim as much or (considering the staggering burden of calculation) as little competence as he. The Hobbesian war of all against all, though no doubt an exaggeration, is suggestive on this score.

I wish to make it clear that I am not saying that the traditional method of budgeting is good because it tends to reduce the amount of conflict. Many of us may well want more conflict in specific areas rather than less. What I am saying is that mitigation of conflict is a widely shared value in our society, and that we ought to realize that program budgeting is likely to affect that value.

NOTES

NOTE 1.

WILLIAM M. CAPRON
THE IMPACT OF ANALYSIS ON BARGAINING IN GOVERNMENT*

Does the current addition to Washington's alphabetic vocabulary—PPBS—signify that a real and important change is occurring in the Federal government's decision-making process? Or do the techniques, devices, and ground rules

* A. A. Altshuler, ed.: *The Politics of the Federal Bureaucracy* 196–207 (1968). New York: Dodd, Mead & Co. Reprinted by permission.

summed up in the terms for which those initials stand — Planning - Programming - Budgeting System—merely represent a systematic eruption which will leave unaffected the real elements—and the actual results of—the "bargaining," or decision-making process, in government?

*   *   *

[O]ne of the hallmarks of good systems analysis as it has come to be practiced is that simultaneously with a definition and testing of alternative means is the refinement and specification of objectives. Furthermore, the *comprehensiveness* of any given systems analysis will depend on the ingenuity of the analyst, the kind of data available to him, and the amount of resources that are at his command in undertaking the analysis. I would urge even if Lindblom's preferred approach—successive limited comparisons —is selected as appropriate to the case in hand that it should be undertaken *systematically* with assumptions clearly specified. This is particularly necessary since in this approach, as he points out, many of the interrelationships with other parts of the system are ignored. It is important that those who will use the results of the "analysis" have called to their attention the limited nature of the analysis so that the limited, partial and incomplete nature of the argument will be understood. I am not so concerned with "comprehensiveness" or the lack thereof, but rather with the use of a very casual and inarticulate "analysis" in place of a specific, "spelled-out" analysis. The "consumer" of the results should be in a position to judge whether or not the particular analysis is in fact useful to him—whether he wants to be guided, in whole or in part, by the results of that "analysis."

*   *   *

. . . I must refer to one other theme which is frequently emphasized by the skeptics, namely, the value in many areas of government activity in *not* being explicit about objectives. Representatives of this view have pointed out that at least in some instances agreement on specific programs is possible, even though the interests of various affected groups in the program may be not only quite different but, in terms of their overall value schemes, antithetical. From this one *might* draw the inference that an attempt at articulating an analysis which identifies objectives will actually make agreement on programs and on budgets *more* difficult than reliance on implicit reasoning and bargaining to arrive at the program's contours and level. It is, moreover, pointed out that the implicit "analysis" in a bargaining system with various interests and values "taken care of" by the representation of these interests and values by one or more players at the bargaining table is a good and workable system. I would agree that, by and large, the system has been pretty good and pretty workable and I further agree that one can undoubtedly identify specific cases (especially where feelings run high) which might be put back rather than forward by an attempt to subject the program to an explicit analysis—or at least to make that analysis public. (But the Executive Branch can develop its position based on analysis without injecting analysis into public debate.) However, I am not persuaded by this view as a regular and basic guide. For one thing, the fact that there are different interests and different values concerned with particular programs does not mean that systematic analysis will necessarily make agreement on specific program decisions and specific budget decisions impossible. It is possible, for example, to reflect explicitly the degree and extent to which different objectives or values will be realized under different alternative approaches and different levels in a given program area. Thus, the interested parties will be able to identify the extent to which *their* own particular interests—their own particular weighing of the outcomes—will be achieved.

*   *   *

. . . PPBS was designed and is being pushed as a technique or set of techniques which will improve the *Presidential* budget decision process. The President, having made his decisions, can forward his recommendations to the Congress in a variety of forms. It is worth emphasizing that in any case the *implementation* of the President's budget once the Congress has authorized and appropriated funds requires expression of these budgetary decisions in the familiar "object class," input-oriented, and organizational-unit oriented terms of the traditional budget. There is no special difficulty or extra burden placed on the Executive Branch in translating the results of the program budget and the decisions reflected therein to the Congress in the familiar terms which they seem, at least up until now, to prefer. Thus, I see no particular technical difficulty in acceding to the apparent will of Congress that the familiar budget structure be maintained with regard to their deliberations.

There is, however, one central and sensitive

point involved in the implications of PPB for Congressional-Executive relations: a key element in the new system is its emphasis on *multi-year* programming and budgeting. The standard pattern is that each program be developed in terms of a five-year program plan and that this be translated into a five-year financial plan.

. . . Even though the President decides not to submit formally the five-year program and financial plans to the Congress, there is little question, given the facts of life in Washington, that the existence of these plans will not only be well known but that they will, one way or another—above or below the table—come into the hands of the Congress. I recognize that there is a certain amount of risk for the President in this situation. Only by the repeated and steadfast reiteration of the fact that the plans for each program beyond the next budget year—the year for which he must make specific recommendations—are only tentative and do *not* represent any kind of Presidential determination or commitment, can he avoid creating the impression that he is committed for the future.

*   *   *

NOTE 2.

ALLEN SCHICK
SYSTEMS FOR ANALYSIS—
PPB AND ITS ALTERNATIVES*

*   *   *

. . . Despite all the talk about cost-benefit analysis, there are too many conceptual and operational difficulties to the implementation of useful benefit analysis at this time. Economists who have joined the analytic staffs have had to trim their sails and put a good deal of their methodological equipment into storage. It is not that the problems confronting Government are simple; they are too difficult to solve with the high-powered methods now at hand. Before benefits can be measured, they have to be identified. Some scale of values must be set. The question of values is especially troublesome, for each discipline and interest has its own way of seeing and evaluating things.

If policy analysis were focused on public benefits, it would be appropriate to have a system structured according to the purposes of Gov-

---

* *The Analysis and Evaluation of Public Expenditures—The PPB System,* Joint Economic Committee, Subcommittee on Economy in Government, 91st Congress, 1st Session 825–827, 832–833 (1969)

ernment. An end product program structure would facilitate the comparison of alternative program opportunities on some homogeneous value scale. Such is not the case, however. Most policy analysis deals not with benefits, but with program effectiveness. Only implicitly does the analyst put a value on the program he is studying. For example, a billion-dollar health care program might be adjudged the most cost effective if it yields a lower infant mortality rate than any alternative billion-dollar program. Unlike benefit analysis which begins with some social value, effectiveness analysis begins with a concrete set of objectives that are embodied in specific programs or with a problem that concerns policymakers. In appraising a health care program, one need not place some value on the life of an infant. One need only assume that more lives saved is preferable (i.e., more effective) to fewer lives saved.

*   *   *

. . . Unless the categories are designed with sensitive attention to problems as they are perceived by top officials and unless they are revised frequently to reflect changing perspectives, the program categories will hinder rather than abet useful policy analysis. It is very doubtful that this kind of categorization can be devised. The analyses undertaken in HEW ignored the boundaries imposed by the program categories. Problems don't come packaged according to some grand formulation of governmental ends. The analyst must pursue his problem in whatever format is appropriate, regardless of the constraints of the data system. Sometimes he will want to look at health from the viewpoint of target groups—expectant mothers, the needy, the elderly. Other times, he will want to study

health in terms of diseases—heart, kidney, cancer, and so on.

*   *   *

The attempt to link analysis to budgeting is a logical recognition of the place and potency of the budget process in public policymaking. . . . Yet it is appropriate to question the connection to budgeting and to raise the possibility of some alternative outlet for analysis.

[B]udgeting is nonanalytic and . . . a rigid integration of analysis and budgeting will not be successful.

[T]he cause of analysis would be better served if analytic work were addressed to the processes of program determination and legislative recommendation. These processes are not well formalized, but they are the processes which deal with the big issues, which mark departures from the status quo and changes in direction. The overwhelming weight of the budget process favors the continuation of what is already on the books. When a President wishes to launch new programs, he is impelled to rely on task forces, advisory staff, and ad hoc arrangement. All these are lacking sustained analytic focus, but perhaps they are more useful than the budget process. In the crowded months of the budget cycle, there just isn't enough time or inclination to consider the bigger issues, to look beyond the present and the certain to the future and the speculative.

While analysis can be channeled to both planning and budgeting, I would urge that attention be given to the neglected opportunities for planning. We tend to rely too heavily on an overburdened budget process and not enough on other decisional institutions.

*   *   *

PART TWO

The Authority of the Investigator as Guardian of Science, Subject and Society

This Part explores the role of the investigator in the human experimentation process. Unlike theoretical scientists whose freedom to pursue their studies, though sometimes challenged, is generally accepted in contemporary society, investigators involved in human research often find their freedom encumbered by the rights and interests of their subjects. Consequently, the student of human experimentation must confront issues which would be only remotely relevant, and perhaps even overreaching, to someone examining decisionmaking in theoretical science.

To familiarize the student with the range of activities investigators pursue with human subjects, research studies from a variety of disciplines are presented in this Part. Among the analytic tasks which emerge from an examination of these materials are: (1) to identify those decisions of investigators which conflict with the interests and values of subject and society; (2) to determine whether the investigator, once aware of these conflicts, can resolve them on his own initiative to the satisfaction of society and subject; (3) if not, to explore those consequences to subject and society which should affect his authority; and (4) to decide by what rules and procedures the extent of his authority should be established.

We begin this inquiry with a question: Can complete authority over experimentation be left to the investigator, placing trust in his professional conscience? Materials from settings in which investigators were permitted to work with considerable or even unlimited freedom are presented in Chapter Five, in order to explore the problems created by relying on an investigator's personal and professional conscience, ambition, and training, without providing him with rules and procedures to guide his personal choices. Abandoned to their scientific curiosity, some researchers are impelled to proceed in disregard of the consequences for themselves or mankind, while other researchers, abandoned to their ethical doubts, hold back on experiments of great potential value.

If investigators are to be responsive to the rights and interests of others, the nature and extent of their authority must be defined. This involves determining how to minimize intentional and unintentional harm to subject, science, and society. Thus, Chapters Six and Seven seek first to define categories of harm to which research may expose subjects and society and then to identify additional elements of experimental design and objectives (*e.g.*, the subject's awareness of participating in an experiment, the subject's understanding of its risks, or the benefits of an experiment to subject, science, and society) which may aggravate or mitigate an experiment's harmful consequences. Both the nature of harm and the conditions under which it may arise must be examined in any attempt to define the proper scope of an investigator's authority for the formulation, administration, and review of experimentation with human beings.

Throughout we ask:

1. What are the professional and personal goals of the investigator, and what consequences to subjects and society result from the pursuit of these goals as well as the means employed to pursue them?

2. What interests of investigator, subject, and society are affected by these consequences?

3. Which of these consequences and interests can be taken into account by the investigator alone, and how should they affect his decisions?

4. In what areas are investigators competent to make informed judgments, and what are the limits of their personal and professional competence?

5. What aspects of experimental design and objectives should either extend or limit the investigator's authority and who else, if anyone, should participate in his decisionmaking?

6. To what extent should the investigator's authority be affected by a coexisting intention to benefit subjects and society?

CHAPTER FIVE

Experimentation without Restriction

What consequences ensue for society and subjects if no external restraints are imposed on an investigator's utilization of human subjects for research purposes? Perhaps the most extreme example of experimentation without restrictions occurred in Nazi Germany. In the concentration camps "political," "racial," and "military" prisoners, considered unworthy of the protections ordinarily afforded to citizens of any society, were made available to physicians for research. This environment provided the investigators with an opportunity to carry out studies with unlimited freedom. In scrutinizing these materials from the vantage point of experimentation without restriction, we disregard their cultural origins and focus on those aspects which may offer insights relevant to our society.

The legal proceedings against the Nazi doctors at Nuremberg exposed in their starkest form the inherent conflicts between scientific interests and societal interests (seen as the interest of the world community). We do not suggest that other cases comparable to the concentration camp experiments in magnitude or cruelty can be found elsewhere in the literature. Yet examples from the pre- and post-World War II periods demonstrate that the actions of the Nazi physicians were not isolated instances of "crimes against humanity." Whenever subjects are too helpless or ignorant to resist participation, the investigator is in a position to pursue his scientific interests constrained only by his personal and professional conscience and values. Thus, similar transgressions occurred prior to the Nuremberg trials and continue to occur, though because they are less dramatic their existence is more likely to be denied.

In examining these materials consider the following questions:

Do investigators require external guides in order to make decisions about the limits of human experimentation? If so, what form should they take?

A.
Prologue—Experiments Prior to 1939

Vikenty Veressayev
The Memoirs of a Physician*

. . . I will now occupy myself with a question to which but one answer is possible, and that a perfectly straight one. It deals with gross and entirely conscious disregard for that consideration which is due to the human being. I approach the subject with regret, but it is impossible to pass it by.

"A certain Dr. Koch," we read in the Russian medical paper, *Physician,* "has published a pamphlet, entitled, . . . Medical Experiments on Living Man, than which nothing were better calculated to further undermine the respect for, and confidence of the laity in, our profession. The author essays to prove that 'vivisection has long crossed the thresholds of our hospitals'— in other words, that experiments similar to those conducted upon the lower animals in the laboratory, are practised on living man in our infirmaries. . . ."

[U]nfortunately there is much substantial truth even in the title of Dr. Koch's booklet alone. In proof of the above it would be easy enough to adduce a very long array of facts— facts of such a nature, too, that they could not be bracketed in inverted commas, for this simple reason—they are substantiated in black and white by the perpetrators themselves.

As we proceed, I shall point out the original sources of my information with every possible care, that the reader may verify my statements.

I shall restrict myself to the venereal diseases. . . . I was compelled in my choice to single out the above, because they furnish us with the greatest wealth of the facts I wish to draw public attention to. For venereal complaints are the exclusive lot of man, and not a single one of them can be transmitted to the lower animals.[1]

Owing to this, many questions which, in other branches of medicine, find their answer in experiments on animals, can, in venerology, only be decided through human inoculation, and venerologists have not hesitated to take the plunge. . . .

* * *

The specific micro-organism of gonorrhoea was discovered by Neisser in 1879. His experiments, conducted with exemplary care, tended to prove, with a considerable degree of probability, that the gonococcus he had discovered was the specific agent of that disease. But in bacteriology the proof positive of the specific quality of any micro-organism is only absolute when obtained through inoculation; if, on inoculating an animal with a pure culture of the micro-organism, we call forth a given disease, this fact proves that the above micro-organism is the specific agent of the latter. Unfortunately, not a single animal, as we already know, is liable to gonorrhoea. Either the discovery had to remain doubtful, or else it was necessary to inoculate man. For himself, Neisser chose the first alternative.

His followers were not so nicely conscientious. The first to inoculate man with gonococcus was Dr. Max Bockhart, assistant to Professor Rinecker.

"Geheimrath von Rinecker," writes Bockhart, "held the view, that the discovery of the causes of venereal disease was only possible through the inoculation of human beings."[2] Acting upon the suggestion of his patron, Bockhart inoculated a patient suffering from creeping paralysis in its last stages with a pure culture of gonococcus: a few months previously the patient had lost his sense of feeling and his death was awaited very shortly.

---

* Translated from Russian by Simeon Linden. New York: Alfred A. Knopf, 332–366 (1916). [Wherever possible the references in Dr. Veressayev's book were checked against the original sources; their accuracy was confirmed in every instance.]

[1] It has been possible to infect monkeys with syphilis.

[2] "Beitrag zur Aetiologie des Harnröhrentrippers": *Vierteljahrschr. für Dermatol. und Syphilis,* 1883, p. 7.

The inoculation proved successful, but the discharge was very insignificant. To increase it, the patient was given half a litre of beer. "The success was brilliant," writes Bockhart; "the discharge became very copious. . . . Ten days after inoculation the patient died of a paralytic fit. Autopsy showed acute gonorrhoeic inflammation of the urethra and bladder, with incipient kidney mortification, and a large number of abscesses in the left kidney; numerous gonococci were found in the pus taken from these abscesses."[3]

The methods of pure culture employed by Bockhart were very crude, and his experiment had but small scientific value. The first undoubtedly pure culture of gonococcus was obtained by Ernst Bumm.[4] To prove that it was the specific agent, Bumm, by means of a platinum wire, introduced the culture into a woman's urethra, which had been found perfectly healthy after repeated examinations. Typical urethritis developed which required six weeks for its cure (op. cit., p. 147). Studying the various peculiarities of his cultures, Bumm inoculated his gonococcus upon another woman in the same manner, obtaining an identical result (p. 150). Here we must note that, more than twenty years previously, Noeggerath proved how serious and painful were the effects—especially in the case of women, following so-called "innocent" gonorrhoea. . . . Bumm himself declares, in the preface to his work, that "gonorrhoeic infection is one of the most important causes of painful and serious affections of the sexual organs";[6] which knowledge did not, however, deter him from subjecting two of his patients to such a risk. It is true that, according to his accounts, "every measure of precaution (?) against infection of the sexual organs" was taken, but such precautions are extremely unreliable. We may further add that even gonorrhoeic affection of the urethra alone is sufficient to cause the most painful complications later.

The next step in the culture of the gonoccus was made by Dr. Ernst Wertheim,[7] who succeeded in obtaining a pure culture on plates. "To prove conclusively," writes Wertheim, "that the colonies growing on the plates were really those of Neisser's gonococci, it was naturally necessary to perform inoculation upon the urethra of man." Wertheim inoculated four paralytic patients with his culture and also a certain S. (an idiot of thirty-three). "Fairly abundant discharge was still noticeable in S. two months after inoculation."[8] Wertheim made no further experiments "owing to lack of suitable material."[9]

Wertheim's methods were verified by other investigators . . . Karl Menge . . . inoculated a woman suffering from a vesico-vaginal carcinomatous fistula, with gonococcus; it was he also, who inoculated a woman, suffering from tumour on the brain, with gonorrhoea, two days before her death.[11]

But especially comprehensive were the experiments of Finger, Ghon and Schlangenhaufen.[12] They inoculated fourteen patients, all of them hopeless cases, chiefly consumptives, who mostly died from three to eight days after inoculation. "Extremely valuable histological material was furnished by the patient F.D., 21, who died three days after inoculation. Taking into consideration," remarked the joint authors, "the short duration of the process, which lasted but three days, one is surprised at its intensity, which caused such deep histological changes."

Gonorrhoea is one of the commonest causes of inflammation of the eyes in newly born infants. Many investigators studied the relationship of gonococcus to eye-disease in newly born children. E. Fraenkel inoculated the eyes of infants, which could not have lived in any case, with the inflammatory secretions of gonorrhoeic patients. One of the infants lived for ten days after inoculation, developing typical purulent inflammation of the eyes.[13]

Tischendorff inoculated the eyes of atrophic

---

[3] "Beitrag zur Aetiologie des Harnröhrentrippers": *Vierteljahrschr. für Dermatol. und Syphilis,* 1883, pp. 7–10.

[4] E. Bumm, "Die Micro-organismus der gonorrhosichen Schleimhauterkrankheiten." 2. Ausg. Wiesbaden, 1887.

[6] *Op. cit.,* p. iv.

[7] Provisional report in the *Deutsche med. Wochenschrift,* 1891, No. 50 ("Reinzuchtung des Gonococcus Neisser mittels des Platenverfahrens"). Detailed description in *Archiv für Gynaecologie,* Bd. 42 (1892): "Die ascendirende Gonorrhoe beim Weibe."

[8] *Archiv,* pp. 17, 28, 33–34, 37, 39.

[9] I will here draw attention to the fact of Wertheim having injected pure culture of gonococcus into *his own* body—each time with positive results.

[11] "Ein Beitrag zur Kultur des Gonococcus": *Centralblatt für Gynaecologie,* 1893, No. 8.

[12] "Zur Biologie des Gonococcus": *Archiv für Dermatologie und Syphilis,* Bd. 28, 1894, pp. 304–306, 317–324.

[13] "Bericht über eine bei Kindern beobachtete Endemie infectiöser Kolpitis": *Virchow's Archiv* Bd. 99, Heft 2 (1885), pp. 263–264.

children with gonorrhoeic discharge of little girls suffering from that disease: purulent inflammation, with characteristic gonococci, was the result.[14] Kroner inoculated six adult blind persons with the muco-purulent discharge of pregnant and parturient women (with negative results).[15]

* * *

[W]e pass on to syphilis. Without going far back into antiquity, I shall give an account of the history of that disease dating from the times of the celebrated French syphilologist, Philippe Ricord.

Ricord cleared up many obscure problems of his specialty and entirely reconstructed the science of venerology. But, of course, he did not escape error. One of his most lamentable mistakes was the affirmation that syphilis was not contagious in its secondary stage. This mistake was due to the fact that while Ricord performed endless inoculations upon venereal *patients,* he never ventured to experiment upon the healthy.[17] Let us see how this fallacy was set right.

One of the first to express himself in favour of secondary syphilis being contagious was the Dublin physician, William Wallace, in his highly instructive "lectures on Cutaneous and Venereal Disease."[18] These lectures are remarkable for the classical shamelessness with which their author tells us of his criminal experiments in inoculating healthy people with syphilis.

* * *

In his . . . lectures, he gives a detailed account of his inoculations performed upon five healthy individuals from 19 to 35 years of age. All developed characteristic syphilis.[19]

In his twenty-second lecture Wallace declared that the facts above mentioned were "only a portion, yes, a very small portion of those of a similar kind which I could adduce."[20] In his twenty-third he again lays stress on the circumstance that the experiments described were only a small part of those he had conducted.[21]

"Is it permissible to expect more convincing proofs of the contagiousness of the secondary stage of syphilis?" queries Dr. Schnepf,[22] writing on the subject of these experiments. "No further experiments on the healthy are required. Wallace's make them entirely superfluous. The problem is solved, science desires no more victims; all the worse for those who close their eyes to this fact."

But the orgy was only about to commence. . . . In 1851 the "remarkable epoch-making" experiments of Waller were published. This is how he described them:—

"First experiment: Durst, a boy of 12, registration number 1396, suffered for a number of years from sores on the head. Otherwise quite healthy, never had rash or scrofula. As his disease required his detention in hospital for several months, and as he had not suffered from syphilis in the past, I found him to be very suitable for inoculation, which was performed on August 6th. The skin of the right thigh was incised and the pus taken from a syphilitic patient introduced into the fresh and slightly bleeding wounds. I rubbed the matter into the abrasions with a spatula, then I rubbed the scarified surface with lint soaked in the same matter, and having covered it with the same lint, applied a bandage." About the beginning of October the child developed a typical syphilitic rash.[23]

"Second experiment: Friedrich, 15, registration number 5676, suffered for the last seven years from lupus of the right cheek and the chin. Up to now the patient had not had syphilis and was therefore eligible for inoculation. This was performed on July 27th. I introduced the blood of a syphilitic woman into fresh incisions made on the left thigh and then dressed the wounds with lint soaked in the same blood." About the

[14] "Verhandlungen der 57 Versammlung deutscher Naturforscher u. Aerzte in Magdeburg, 1884": *Archiv fur Gynaecologie,* Bd. 25 (1885), p. 114.

[15] *Ibid.,* p. 113.

[17] Rinecker, referring to this fact, very justly remarks: "It is hard to understand why Ricord condemned the inoculation of the healthy so absolutely; taking into consideration the vast number of his experiments, he could not have remained in ignorance of the fact that the inoculation of the sick is not infrequently dangerous to the latter." The sum-total of Ricord's gonorrhoeic inoculations, as well as those of syphilis and soft ulcer, amounted to *seven hundred.*

[18] W. Wallace, "Lectures on Cutaneous and Venereal Diseases": *The Lancet* for 1835–36 vol. ii., p. 132.

[19] "Clinical Lectures on Venereal Diseases": *The Lancet* 1836–1837, vol. ii., pp. 535, 536, 538, 620, 621.

[20] *Ibid.,* p. 539.

[21] *Ibid.,* p. 615.

[22] "De la contagion des accidents consecutifs de la syphilis": *Annales des maladies de la peau et du syphilis.* Publ. par A. Cazenave. Vol. iv., 1851–52, p. 44.

[23] Waller, "Die Contagiosität der secondaren Syphilis": *Vierteljahrschr. für d. prakt. Heilkunde.* Prag. 1851, Bd. I. (xxix), pp. 124–126.

beginning of October the success of the inoculation was beyond a doubt.[24]

"I showed both patients expressly to the director of the hospital, Riedel," adds Waller, "to the head physicians of the hospital (Boehm and others), to many of the city physicians, to several professors (Jackisch, Kubik, Oppolzer, Dietrich and others), to almost all the hospital physicians of the city and to many foreigners. All unanimously substantiated the accuracy of my diagnosis of the syphilitic rash and declared themselves ready, if necessary, to step forward as witnesses of the reality of the results of my inoculations."

Is not this a complete and accurate . . . criminal report? All the details of the "case" are communicated, the victims are indicated and the witnesses cited name by name. . . . If the public prosecutor had peeped into this province, he would have found his task wonderfully simplified.

Waller's were the signal for general and universal experiments for the verification of the contagiousness of secondary syphilis.

In March, 1852, Professor Rinecker inoculated a boy of 12, suffering from incurable St. Vitus' dance, with the pus taken from a syphilitic patient. After the lapse of a month the inoculated part developed infiltration and induration. There were no constitutional symptoms in this case.[25]

In 1855, at a convocation of Pfalz doctors, while the contagiousness of secondary syphilis was under discussion (in connection with Waller's experiments), the assembly was acquainted by its secretary with the contents of a communication received from an absent colleague.

"A peculiar coincidence made it possible for the above-mentioned colleague to carry out experiments in connection with the contagiousness of secondary syphilis, without infringing the laws of humanity." These experiments consisted of the following.[26] The discharge of flat moist condylomata and the secretion of the fissures of a female syphilitic patient, were inoculated upon eleven persons—three women of 17,

20 and 25 years of age respectively, and eight men of ages varying from 18 to 28 years. All developed syphilis. The pus of syphilitic ulcers was used for inoculating three women of 24, 26 and 35 years of age respectively. All three developed syphilis. Sores on the feet of six patients were smeared with blood taken from a syphilitic patient; three of the above contracted syphilis. The blood of a syphilitic patient was introduced into the wounds left after wet cupping of three persons. There was no result.[27]

Thus *twenty-three persons* were inoculated; seventeen of these developed syphilis; and it was found possible to do all this "without infringing the laws of humanity!" Truly, a wonderful coincidence! As we proceed, we shall see that such "coincidences" are not rare in syphilology. . . . The identity of the author of these experiments never transpired; he found it best to keep his infamous name forever in the dark, and he is known in science to this day as the *"Anonimus of Pfalz."*

The same question of the contagiousness of secondary syphilis was the subject of the researches of Professor H. von Hubbenet. Among others, he made the following experiments:—

1. "F. Susikoff, medical orderly, 20 years of age, in February, 1852, underwent inoculation with mucous papulae of a syphilitic patient, while in blooming health. I blistered his left thigh, and, after thus removing the cuticle, transferred the matter of the mucous papule, by means of a spatula, to the raw surface, and applied lint dressing impregnated with the same secretion. . . . Roseolae appeared on his chest and abdomen in five weeks. From that moment the syphilitic affection made rapid progress. I kept the patient in this condition for a week longer, to enable me to demonstrate him before as large a number of physicians as possible, and thus allow them to assure themselves of the actuality of the fact. At last I applied the mercurial treatment, and the patient was cured in three months."

2. "Private Timothy Maximoff, 33, admitted to the surgical clinic on January 13th, 1858, suffering from an inveterate fistula of the urethra. As according to every calculation the patient was to remain in hospital for a considerable period, and there was thus sufficient time at our disposal to await results, this case struck me

[24] *Ibid.,* pp. 126–128.
[25] "Über die Ansteckungsfähigkeit der constitutionellen Syphilis": *Verhandlungen der phys. medic. Gesellschaft in Wurzburg,* Bd. III. (1852), p. 391. In the clinic of the same Prof. Rinecker two physicians, Drs. Warneri of Lausanne and W. P., consented to be inoculated and both developed syphilis.
[26] *Ibid.*
[27] "Auszüge aus den Protocollen des Vereins pfalzischer Aerzte vom Jahre 1855": *Aerztliche Intellegenzblatt,* 1856 No. 35, pp. 425, 426.

as being a suitable one for experiment. On March 14th, inoculation with the matter taken from the ulcerated tonsils of Private Nesteroff was performed. . . . By May 22nd characteristic roseolae. . . . Mercurial treatment started on June 2nd, and in six weeks the patient was cured."[28]

Commenting upon these descriptions, Professor V. A. Manassein expresses himself as follows: "We do not know what to be more amazed at: the cold-blooded way in which the experimenter allows syphilis to develop more acutely for the purposes of clearer illustration and 'so as to show the patient to a larger number of physicians;' or at that logic of the superior, which permits him to subject a subordinate to the dangers of a serious and, not infrequently, fatal disease, without so much as obtaining his consent thereto! I should very much like to know whether Professor Hubbenet would inoculate his own son with syphilis, even were he to acquiesce!"[29]

Professor von Hubbenet concludes his article with the following words: "I consider it necessary to remark that, having carried out a multitude of ineffective experiments on sick persons, I was perfectly convinced that, in the case of the healthy, I would meet with the same lack of success: this conviction alone made it possible for me to proceed with these dangerous experiments." Needless to say that a professor and specialist could not have been ignorant of Waller's successful inoculations. Besides, Prof. Hubbenet performed his first successful inoculation in 1852, while his last dates 1858. Are we to believe that in 1858 the professor proceeded with his incoulations full of the same "conviction"?

The publication of these observations, continues Hubbenet, "will perhaps restrain others, even with such a sceptical nature as my own, from making further experiments, often leading to the complete wrecking of the lives of the persons subjected to them. It would add considerably to my peace of mind in respect to the victims' fate, if these experiments were to spread the conviction that the secondary stage is contagious. If they lead to the establishing of such an important truth, the sufferings of a few individuals were not too high a price to be paid by mankind for the attainment of such a truly beneficial and practical result."

If that is the case, it is hard to understand why Professor Hubbenet did not inoculate *himself* with syphilis. Perhaps, after all, such a price would have been too high to pay even "in the cause of humanity."

In 1858 the French Government applied to the Parisian Medical Academy for elucidation on the still contested question of the contagiousness of secondary syphilis. A commission was nominated and Dr. Gibert was appointed as its referee. Among other things, he stated that with a view to clear this question up, Dr. Auzias-Turenne had inoculated two adult patients suffering from lupus, and that both developed syphilis.

The referee himself inoculated two patients, also suffering from lupus, and in both cases he obtained syphilis.[30]

Gibert's report gave rise to stormy and lengthy debates in the Academy; Ricord, who had hitherto obstinately denied the contagiousness of secondary syphilis, notwithstanding overwhelming confirmatory evidence, entered the lists with great heat, but was compelled, in the end, to confess his mistake, and went over to the opposite camp.

Thus the most powerful and authoritative opponent of the new view taken by science was vanquished. But, nevertheless, experiments, now absolutely unwarrantable, went on and on. . . . In 1859 Guyenot inoculated T.B.B., a boy of ten, suffering from sores of the head, with the secretions of syphilitic plaques, and obtained syphilis.[31]

In the same year Professor Baerensprung successfully inoculated Bertha B., a girl of eighteen, with syphilitic pus. It was also he who inoculated the prostitute Marie G. with the secretions of hard chancre.[32]

Prof. Lindwurm, in 1860–1861, inoculated five women lying in his hospital, aged 18, 19, 30, 45 and 71 years respectively, with syphilis.

[28] Prof. H. v. Hubbenet, "Observations and Experiments in Syphilis": *The Medical-Military Journal*, Part 77 (1860), pp. 423–427.

[29] "Lectures on General Therapeutics," Part I. St. P. 1879, p. 66.

[30] *Bulletin de l'Academie Imperiale de Médécine*, Tome xxiv. Paris. 1858–1859, pp. 888–890.

[31] "Nouveau fait d'inoculation d'accidents Syphil. Secondaires": *Gaz. hebdomad. de med. et de chirurgie*, 1859, No. 15. Guyenot was terribly punished for his experiment: the Tribunal of Correction of Lyons condemned him to a fine of *one hundred* francs!

[32] "Mitteilungen aus der Klinik für syphil. Kranke." *Annalen des Charite-Krankenhauses* Bd. IX. Heft I (1860), pp. 167, 168.

We quote the description of the last of these experiments: "Mary E., aged 71 years, suffering for many years from an extensive and deep ulcer in the forehead. Both *sinera frontalia,* thanks to the destruction of the front walls, are open; the bottom of the ulcer is covered deeply with granulations, through which the probe easily reaches the bone, and, in places, traverses the latter. . . . On May 27th, 1861, the blood of a syphilitic patient was injected subcutaneously between the shoulder blades." The patient developed syphilis.[33]

According to Zeissel, Dr. Rosnerom, acting under Prof. Hebra's directions, made the following experiments: "(1) The secretion of a flat condyloma, located on the breast of a certain wet-nurse, was inoculated upon a patient of 50, suffering from acute itch."—Syphilis. (2) A wet-nurse, suffering from innocuous syphilis, was inoculated in the forearm with chancrous pus. This woman, impregnated with syphilis, developed characteristic pustules. The pus of the latter was used to inoculate a certain leprous patient, who had not previously suffered from syphilis. . . . This inoculation also was successful."[34]

Dr. Puche inoculated a patient lying at the *Hôpital du Midi,* in the ventral regions, with the secretion of an indurated ulcer of a syphilitic patient, but without results. Three weeks later Puche inoculated his victim with the matter of another syphilitic. This time the experiment was crowned with success: the patient contracted syphilis.[35]

To settle the question once and for all whether a person who had once had syphilis could contract it again, Prof. Vidal de Cassi made the following experiments. "M., age 37." (Had been cured of syphilis, entered hospital with paralysis of the lower extremities, formerly employed in a tannery and afterwards as a watchman.) "The patient began to recover but wished to remain in hospital for a certain time longer, in expectation of a government post. In January, 1852, small blisters were applied to each thigh because of the inactivity of the bladder; when the skin was removed, *the wounds were dressed with lint soaked in matter taken from the mucous papules of another patient.* This inoculation was barren of results. Later I proposed that the experiment should be repeated. On April 12th, 1852, when the patient began to complain of difficulty in breathing, blisters were applied to the upper parts of his arms; these were dressed on April 13th with lint saturated in the pus of the mucous papules of another patient. April 15th, the wounds on each arm had become covered with a greyish membrane, suppuration very copious and of disgusting odour; lint saturated with the same pus as previously was freshly applied to the wounds," etc.[36] Vidal was very dissatisfied with the squeamishness of those savants who did not venture upon such experiments. "Unfortunately," he remarks, "the cleverest of syphilologists, who could be of the greatest service to science thanks to their logic and clinical observations, regard experiment as immoral, and neglect it accordingly."[37]

*   *   *

For the sake of ascertaining whether the milk of women suffering from syphilis was infectious. . . .

. . . Dr. R. Voss . . . inoculated three prostitutes, *"having obtained their consent,"* with the milk of a syphilitic patient.

First experiment: P.A., aged thirteen, a peasant from the Province of Novgorod; had had syphilis, but was cured. On September 25th, 1875, the milk of a syphilitic patient was injected into her back. The only result was an abscess the size of a "small fist."

Second experiment: Natalie K., age fifteen, had taken up prostitution but recently. Admitted with urethritis and vaginitis. Milk of a syphilitic patient injected. No result.

Third experiment: Lubov U., age sixteen, a prostitute; admitted into hospital suffering from urethritis; never had syphilis. September 27th, a full Pravaz syringe of milk from a syphilitic patient injected beneath the left shoulder blade. *The girl developed syphilis.*[48]

Dr. Voss, as also Prof. Gay, assures us that his victims gave their consent to these ex-

[33] "Über die Verschiedenheit der syphilischen Krankheiten": *Würzburger medicinische Zeitschrift* Bd. III., pp. 146–148, 174 (1862).

[34] Herrmann Zeissel, "Guide to the Study of General Syphilis." St. Petersburg, 1866, p. 29.

[35] Henry Lee, "Hunterian Lectures on Syphilis": *The Lancet* 1875, vol. ii, p. 122.

[36] Prof. A. Vidal, *"On Venereal Disease"* Transl. from the French, St. Petersburg, 1857, pp. 560–561.

[37] Prof. A. Vidal, *"On Venereal Disease"* Transl. from the French, St. Petersburg, 1857, p. 31.

[48] "Ist die Syphilis durch Milch übertragbar?" *St. Petersburger med. Wochenschrift,* 1876, No. 23. In the original all three girls were named in full.

periments. Is this mockery? The eldest of the girls was but sixteen years of age! Even if their consent had really been obtained, did these children know what they were agreeing to, could any importance have been attached to their acquiescence?

. . . In conclusion, I will only quote a few more experiments from other spheres of medicine. Although the latter are comparatively rarer (thanks to the possibility of experimenting upon animals), nevertheless their absolute number is more than sufficient.

While investigating the channels of human infection with worms, Professors Grassi and Calandruccio administered a pill, containing the germs of ascaris, to a boy of seven, who had not hitherto suffered from worms: in the course of three months the child evacuated 143 ascaris of lengths varying from 18 to 23 centimetres each.[50]

*   *   *

In March, 1887, a woman, suffering from cancer of the mammary gland, applied to the surgeon, Eugene Hahn, of Berlin. The performance of an operation was impossible. "Not wishing to divulge before the patient the hopelessness of her condition by declining to operate upon her, and so as to relieve and reassure her by the psychical illusion of having performed the operation," Dr. Hahn removed a portion of the tumour of the patient's diseased breast and . . . transplanted it into the other healthy one; the inoculation was successful.[55]

*   *   *

Dr. N. A. Finn studied the question of the infectiousness of typhoid fever in one of the military hospitals of the Caucasus. Following his instructions, assistant house-physician Artemovitch injected the blood of typhoid patients subcutaneously into the systems of seventeen healthy soldiers. Not one of those inoculated contracted the disease; "only ten of them developed ordinary abscesses at the places of puncture." In addition, twenty-eight young and healthy soldiers were placed by Dr. Finn in the same ward with typhoid patients. They lay in hospital in the vicinity of the sick, "for four or five days, the beds being moved close together,

and sometimes they were covered with the blankets of the typhoid patients."[56]

During December, 1887, Dr. Stickler read a paper before the Academy of Medicine of New York on preventive inoculation against scarlet fever. He had observed that persons who had contracted hoof and other kindred diseases from the lower animals became immune to scarlet fever. To verify his observations, Stickler inoculated children with the blood of sick horses and cows. After this he placed the children on bedding which had been in the use of scarlet fever patients and made them inhale the air exhaled by the latter; these children numbered twenty. Stickler also injected the blood of scarlet fever patients into the systems of the twenty children. Of their number several did not take the fever at all, the rest developed it in very mild form; there were no serious cases.[57]

Professor Roberts Bartholow of Ohio, U.S.A., attended a female patient, the posterior part of whose cerebrum had become exposed, owing to cancer of the cranial integuments. The professor took advantage of this rare case for the purpose of conducting a series of experiments of electric irritation of his patient's brain. Galvanic irritation of the *dura mater* proved to be painless, while faradic current caused muscular contraction throughout the opposite side of the body. After this he "passed an isolated needle into the left posterior lobe; the other isolated needle was placed in contact with the *dura mater*. When the circuit was closed, muscular contractions of the right upper and lower extremities ensued; faint but visible contractions of the left orbicularis palpebrarum and dilation of the pupils also ensued. Notwithstanding the very evident pain from which she suffered, she smiled as if amused."

The same experiment was repeated upon the right cerebral hemisphere. "When the needle entered the brain substance she complained of acute pain in the neck. In order to develop more decided reactions, the strength of the current was increased. When communication was made

---

[50] Prof. B. Grassi, "Trichocephalus u. Ascarisentwicklung": *Centralbl. für Bacteriol. u. Paras.,* 1887 Bd. I., p. 131.

[55] E. Hahn, "Über Transplantation der carcin. Haut." *Berlin. klin. Woch.* 1888 No. 21.

[56] The minutes of the meetings of the *Imperial Caucasian Medical Society* for 1878–1879, No. 8, p. 107. Drs. Finn and Artemovitch also injected the blood of typhoid patients *into their own systems.*

[57] Summary of Stickler's paper, as it appeared in one of the American medical journals. The *Centralblatt für Bacteriologie u. Parasitenkunde,* Bd. IV., 1888, p. 369, remarks: "The results obtained are, in any case, sufficiently important to encourage further research in the same direction."

with the needles, her countenance exhibited great distress, and she began to cry. Her eyes became fixed, with pupils widely dilated, lips blue, and she frothed at the mouth. She lost consciousness and was violently convulsed on the left side. The convulsion lasted five minutes, and was succeeded by coma. She returned to consciousness in twenty minutes from the beginning of the attack." After the lapse of a certain time the experiment was repeated once more with a weaker current, and three days later her condition was decidedly worse. In the evening she "had a convulsive seizure, lasting about five minutes. After this attack she relapsed into profound unconsciousness and was found to be completely paralysed on the right side."

The unfortunate woman died soon afterwards. According to Professor Bartholow's opinion her death was caused by the original disease.[58]

. . . The existence of a few hundred doctors, to whom the sick are merely so many objects for experiment, does not justify the branding of the entire profession. As a parallel, I might bring forward a no less array of facts, which would show that, in the past, doctors have conducted —and continue to do so now—no less dangerous experiments *upon their own persons.* Thus, Pettenkoffer's and Emerich's experiments are still fresh in the memory of all: both swallowed

---

[58] See *British Medical Journal,* 1874, vol. i. p. 687. In reviewing the above communication which appeared in an American contemporary, the *British Medical Journal* censured the author for his experiments. Bartholow wrote a letter to the editor, in which he sought to vindicate his action by remarking that his patient was bound to die very soon and that she had agreed to the experiments, which, according to his opinion, presented no danger. "Notwithstanding my sanguine expectation that small isolated needle electrodes could be introduced without injury into the cerebral substance," wrote the professor, "I now know that I was mistaken. To repeat such experiments with the knowledge we now have that injury will be done by them would be in the highest degree criminal. I can only now express my regret that facts which I hoped would further, in some slight degree, the progress of knowledge were obtained at the expense of some injury to the patient." According to the journal's opinion, this letter was "one which is likely to disarm further criticism," and the editor found it both sincere and worthy of the author's profession, and even . . . humane (p. 728). All this was said without a trace of irony. On the whole, however, Bartholow's experiments aroused the indignation of the entire medical press.

pure cultures of cholera bacilli, after having had the acids of the stomach neutralised with soda. This was repeated by Professor Metschnikoff, Drs. Hasterlick and Latapie. Drs. Borgioni, Warneri, and Lindemann, and many others, inoculated themselves with syphilis; young and healthy, in the name of Science, they faced experiments which crippled and ruined their entire lives. To conclude that the entire medical body is made up of heroes, because a few devoted men martyred themselves in the name of Science, was as erroneous as to write all doctors down brutes, callous of their patients' interest, in consequence of the comparative few having conducted criminal experiments as described. But the latter establish one thing beyond all vestige of a doubt—and that is the shameful indifference with which the medical world contemplates such atrocities. For this martyrology of the unhappy patients offered up as victims to science was not compiled by any underhand means—the culprits publicly blazoned their own infamy in black and white. One would suppose that the mere fact of publication of such experiments would make their repetition utterly impossible, the first to attempt anything of the kind being cast forever from the medical corporation! But, unfortunately, this is not so. With heads proudly erect, these bizarre disciples of science proceed upon their way without encountering any effective opposition, either from their colleagues or the medical press. . . .

*   *   *

[T]he moment has also arrived for society to take its own measures of self-protection against those zealots of science who have ceased to distinguish between their brothers and guinea-pigs, without waiting for the faculty to emerge from its lethargy.

NOTES

NOTE 1.

R. J. V. PULVERTAFT
THE INDIVIDUAL AND THE GROUP
IN MODERN MEDICINE*

*   *   *

. . . It is in fact remarkable how irresponsibly attempts were made at the end of the last century to produce venereal disease experimentally. Urethritis was produced with pure cul-

---

* 2 *The Lancet* 841 (1952). Reprinted by permission.

tures of the gonococcus in both men and women by at least five separate workers. It is hard to believe that they were not aware of the implications both to the human beings infected and to their children. . . .

. . . I once met a lawyer who held office during the prosecution of Germans for war crimes, and asked him how a nation so renowned for its humanitarian services could have perpetrated such horrors. "There is only one step to take," he answered. "You may not think it possible to take it; but I assure you that men I thought decent men did take it. You have only to decide that one group of human beings have lost human rights."

* * *

NOTE 2.
MYRON PRINZMETAL
ON THE HUMANE TREATMENT
OF CHARITY PATIENTS*

During my training in medical school, as well as during my residency in St. Louis, fellowships at Harvard, New York City, and London, and visits to Vienna, Budapest, and other European medical centers, I was always horrified by the inhumane manner in which charity patients were treated. Occasionally, private patients were similarly abused.

I distinctly remember the degradation of a poor man with a prolapsed rectum who was asked to defecate in a wastebasket before the class in the proctology clinic, which included women medical students. I remember the Ne-

groes—two in a bed—called only by their first names. I remember a poor young woman at the San Francisco County Hospital who was stripped from neck to knees in front of the entire class. Cringing with shame and embarrassment, she closed her eyes.

The most detailed histories, including terms such as cancer, cardiac murmurs, leukemia, were on occasions given while the patient was in the room. X-rays demonstrating cancers, enlarged hearts, and other serious diseases were described in great detail. This was followed by long discussions and arguments among the doctors, all within hearing distance of the terrified patient.

The doctors and medical students would then consult, palpate, listen to the heart, argue over electrocardiograms, before the patient was rolled out.

* * *

New drugs, new experimental surgical procedures were commonly tested on charity patients, who rarely understood what was being done to them. Often they were maimed or killed —experimental "animals" sacrificed in the interests of medical progress. In former years, American doctors would actually pay the authorities in certain European capitals for the privilege of doing completely unnecessary operations on peasants.

In a word—some patients were not treated like animals, but often worse than animals—for some of them understood.

* * *

B.
United States v. Karl Brandt†

1.

Indictment

The United States of America, by the undersigned Telford Taylor, Chief of Counsel for War Crimes, duly appointed to represent said Government in the prosecution of war criminals, charges that the defendants herein participated

in a common design or conspiracy to commit and did commit war crimes and crimes against humanity, as defined in Control Council Law No. 10, duly enacted by the Allied Control Council on 20 December 1945. . . .

* * *

Count Two [and Three]—War Crimes [and Crimes against Humanity]

Between September 1939 and April 1945 all of the defendants herein unlawfully, willfully, and knowingly committed war crimes [and crimes against humanity], as defined by Article II of Control Council Law No. 10, in that they

---

* 6 *Medical Tribune* 15 (September 22, 1965). Reprinted by permission.
† *Trials of War Criminals Before the Nuremberg Military Tribunals. Volumes I and II, The Medical Case.* Washington, D.C.: U.S. Government Printing Office (1948).

were principals in, accessories to, ordered, abetted, took a consenting part in, and were connected with plans and enterprises involving medical experiments without the subjects' consent, upon [German civilians and] civilians and members of the armed forces of nations then at war with the German Reich . . . in the course of which experiments the defendants committed murders, brutalities, cruelties, tortures, atrocities, and other inhuman acts. Such experiments included, but were not limited to the following:

High-Altitude Experiments. From about March 1942 to about August 1942 experiments were conducted at the Dachau concentration camp, for the benefit of the German Air Force, to investigate the limits of human endurance and existence at extremely high altitudes. The experiments were carried out in a low-pressure chamber in which the atmospheric conditions and pressures prevailing at high altitude (up to 68,000 feet) could be duplicated. The experimental subjects were placed in the low-pressure chamber and thereafter the simulated altitude therein was raised. Many victims died as a result of these experiments and others suffered grave injury, torture, and ill-treatment. . . .

Freezing Experiments. From about August 1942 to about May 1943 experiments were conducted at the Dachau concentration camp, primarily for the benefit of the German Air Force, to investigate the most effective means of treating persons who had been severely chilled or frozen. In one series of experiments the subjects were forced to remain in a tank of ice water for periods up to 3 hours. Extreme rigor developed in a short time. Numerous victims died in the course of these experiments. After the survivors were severely chilled, rewarming was attempted by various means. In another series of experiments, the subjects were kept naked outdoors for many hours at temperatures below freezing. The victims screamed with pain as parts of their bodies froze. . . .

Malaria Experiments. From about February 1942 to about April 1945 experiments were conducted at the Dachau concentration camp in order to investigate immunization for and treatment of malaria. Healthy concentration-camp inmates were infected by mosquitoes or by injections of extracts of the mucous glands of mosquitoes. After having contracted malaria the subjects were treated with various drugs to test their relative efficacy. Over 1,000 involuntary subjects were used in these experiments. Many of the victims died and others suffered severe pain and permanent disability. . . .

* * *

Sulfanilamide Experiments. From about July 1942 to about September 1943 experiments to investigate the effectiveness of sulfanilamide were conducted at the Ravensbrueck concentration camp for the benefit of the German Armed Forces. Wounds deliberately inflicted on the experimental subjects were infected with bacteria such as streptococcus, gas gangrene, and tentanus. Circulation of blood was interrupted by tying off blood vessels at both ends of the wound to create a condition similar to that of a battlefield wound. Infection was aggravated by forcing wood shavings and ground glass into the wounds. The infection was treated with sulfanilamide and other drugs to determine their effectiveness. Some subjects died as a result of these experiments and others suffered serious injury and intense agony. . . .

* * *

Epidemic Jaundice Experiments. From about June 1943 to about January 1945 experiments were conducted at the Sachsenhausen and Natzweiler concentration camps, for the benefit of the German Armed Forces, to investigate the causes of, and inoculations against, epidemic jaundice. Experimental subjects were deliberately infected with epidemic jaundice, some of whom died as a result, and others were caused great pain and suffering. . . .

* * *

Spotted Fever [Typhus] Experiments. From about December 1941 to about February 1945 experiments were conducted at the Buchenwald and Natzweiler concentration camps, for the benefit of the German Armed Forces, to investigate the effectiveness of spotted fever and other vaccines. At Buchenwald numerous healthy inmates were deliberately infected with spotted fever virus in order to keep the virus alive; over 90 percent of the victims died as a result. Other healthy inmates were used to determine the effectiveness of different spotted fever vaccines and of various chemical substances. In the course of these experiments 75 percent of the selected number of inmates were vaccinated with one of the vaccines or nourished with one of the chemical substances and, after a period of 3 to 4 weeks, were infected with spotted fever germs. The remaining 25 percent were infected without any previous protection in order to compare the effectiveness of the vaccines and the chemical substances. As a result, hundreds of the persons experimented upon died. . . .

Experiments with Poison. In or about December 1943, and in or about October 1944, experiments were conducted at the Buchenwald concentration camp to investigate the effect of various poisons upon human beings. The poisons were secretly administered to experimental subjects in their food. The victims died as a result of the poison or were killed immediately in order to permit autopsies. In or about September 1944 experimental subjects were shot with poison bullets and suffered torture and death. . . .

* * *

Between June 1943 and September 1944 the defendants Rudolf Brandt and Sievers . . . were principals in, accessories to, ordered, abetted, took a consenting part in, and were connected with plans and enterprises involving the murder of civilians and members of the armed forces of nations then at war with the German Reich and who were in the custody of the German Reich in exercise of belligerent control. One hundred twelve Jews were selected for the purpose of completing a skeleton collection for the Reich University of Strasbourg. Their photographs and anthropological measurements were taken. Then they were killed. Thereafter, comparison tests, anatomical research, studies regarding race, pathological features of the body, form and size of the brain, and other tests, were made. The bodies were sent to Strasbourg and defleshed.

* * *

The said war crimes [and crimes against humanity] constitute violations of international conventions, particularly . . . of the Hague Regulations, 1907 . . . the laws and customs of war, the general principles of criminal law as derived from the criminal laws of all civilized nations, the internal penal laws of the countries in which such crimes were committed. . . .

* * *

2.

Opening Statement of the Prosecution by Brigadier General Telford Taylor

The defendants in this case are charged with murders, tortures, and other atrocities committed in the name of medical science. The victims of these crimes are numbered in the hundreds of thousands. A handful only are still alive; a few of the survivors will appear in this courtroom. But most of these miserable victims were slaughtered outright or died in the course of the tortures to which they were subjected.

For the most part they are nameless dead. To their murderers, these wretched people were not individuals at all. They came in wholesale lots and were treated worse than animals. They were 200 Jews in good physical condition, 50 gypsies, 500 tubercular Poles, or 1,000 Russians. . . .

The charges against these defendants are brought in the name of the United States of America. They are being tried by a court of American judges. The responsibilities thus imposed upon the representatives of the United States, prosecutors and judges alike, are grave and unusual. It is owed, not only to the victims and to the parents and children of the victims, that just punishment be imposed on the guilty, but also to the defendants that they be accorded a fair hearing and decision. Such responsibilities are the ordinary burden of any tribunal. Far wider are the duties which we must fulfill here.

These larger obligations run to the peoples and races on whom the scourge of these crimes was laid. The mere punishment of the defendants, or even of thousands of others equally guilty, can never redress the terrible injuries which the Nazis visited on these unfortunate peoples. For them it is far more important that these incredible events be established by clear and public proof, so that no one can ever doubt that they were fact and not fable; and that this Court, as the agent of the United States and as the voice of humanity, stamp these acts, and the ideas which engendered them, as barbarous and criminal.

We have still other responsibilities here. The defendants in the dock are charged with murder, but this is no mere murder trial. We cannot rest content when we have shown that crimes were committed and that certain persons committed them. To kill, to maim, and to torture is criminal under all modern systems of law. These defendants did not kill in hot blood, nor for personal enrichment. Some of them may be sadists who killed and tortured for sport, but they are not all perverts. They are not ignorant men. Most of them are trained physicians and some of them are distinguished scientists. Yet these defendants, all of whom were fully able to comprehend the nature of their acts, and most of whom were exceptionally qualified to form a moral and professional judgment in this respect, are responsible for wholesale murder and unspeakably cruel tortures.

It is our deep obligation to all peoples of the world to show why and how these things happened. It is incumbent upon us to set forth with conspicuous clarity the ideas and motives which moved these defendants to treat their fellow men as less than beasts. The perverse thoughts and distorted concepts which brought about these savageries are not dead. They cannot be killed by force of arms. They must not become a spreading cancer in the breast of humanity. They must be cut out and exposed, for the reason so well stated by Mr. Justice Jackson in this courtroom a year ago—

> The wrongs which we seek to condemn and punish have been so calculated, so malignant, and so devastating, that civilization cannot tolerate their being ignored because it cannot survive their being repeated.

*   *   *

I pass now to the facts of the case in hand. There are 23 defendants in the box. All but three of them—Rudolf Brandt, Sievers, and Brack—are doctors. Of the 20 doctors, all but one—Pokorny—held positions in the medical services of the Third Reich. . . .

*   *   *

I turn now to the main part of the indictment and will outline at this point the prosecution's case relating to those crimes alleged to have been committed in the name of medical or scientific research. . . . What I will cover now comprehends all in the experiments charged as war crimes . . . and as crimes against humanity in . . . the indictment. . . .

*   *   *

A sort of rough pattern is apparent on the face of the indictment. Experiments concerning high altitude, the effect of cold, and the potability of processed sea water have an obvious relation to aeronautical and naval combat and rescue problems. The mustard gas and phosphorous burn experiments, as well as those relating to the healing value of sulfanilamide for wounds, can be related to air-raid and battlefield medical problems. It is well known that malaria, epidemic jaundice, and typhus were among the principal diseases which had to be combated by the German Armed Forces and by German authorities in occupied territories.

To some degree, the therapeutic pattern outlined above is undoubtedly a valid one, and explains why the Wehrmacht, and especially the German Air Force, participated in these experiments. Fanatically bent upon conquest, utterly ruthless as to the means or instruments to be used in achieving victory, and callous to the sufferings of people whom they regarded as inferior, the German militarists were willing to gather whatever scientific fruit these experiments might yield.

But our proof will show that a quite different and even more sinister objective runs like a red thread through these hideous researches. We will show that in some instances the true object of these experiments was not how to rescue or to cure, but how to destroy and kill. The sterilization experiments were, it is clear, purely destructive in purpose. The prisoners at Buchenwald who were shot with poisoned bullets were not guinea pigs to test an antidote for the poison; their murderers really wanted to know how quickly the poison would kill. This destructive objective is not superficially as apparent in the other experiments, but we will show that it was often there.

Mankind has not heretofore felt the need of a word to denominate the science of how to kill prisoners most rapidly and subjugated people in large numbers. This case and these defendants have created this gruesome question for the lexicographer. For the moment we will christen this macabre science "thanatology," the science of producing death. The thanatological knowledge, derived in part from these experiments, supplied the techniques for genocide, a policy of the Third Reich, exemplified in the "euthanasia" program and in the widespread slaughter of Jews, gypsies, Poles, and Russians. This policy of mass extermination could not have been so effectively carried out without the active participation of German medical scientists.

*   *   *

The experiments known as "high-altitude" or "low-pressure" experiments were carried out at the Dachau concentration camp in 1942. According to the proof, the original proposal that such experiments be carried out on human beings originated in the spring of 1941 with a Dr. Sigmund Rascher. Rascher was at that time a captain in the medical service of the German Air Force, and also held officer rank in the SS. He is believed now to be dead.

The origin of the idea is revealed in a letter which Rascher wrote to Himmler in May 1941 at which time Rascher was taking a course in aviation medicine at a German Air Force headquarters in Munich. According to the letter, this course included researches into high-altitude flying and

> considerable regret was expressed at the fact that no tests with human material had yet been possible for us, as such experiments are very dangerous and nobody volunteers for them. (1602-PS.)

Rascher, in this letter, went on to ask Himmler to put human subjects at his disposal and baldly stated that the experiments might result in death to the subjects but that the tests theretofore made with monkeys had not been satisfactory.

Rascher's letter was answered by Himmler's adjutant, the defendant, Rudolf Brandt, who informed Rascher that—". . . Prisoners will, of course, gladly be made available for the high-flight researches."

. . . The tests themselves were carried out in the spring and summer of 1942, using the pressure chamber which the German Air Force had provided. The victims were locked in the low-pressure chamber, which was an airtight ball-like compartment, and then the pressure in the chamber was altered to simulate the atmospheric conditions prevailing at extremely high altitudes. The pressure in the chamber could be varied with great rapidity, which permitted the defendants to duplicate the atmospheric conditions which an aviator might encounter in falling great distances through space without a parachute and without oxygen.

. . . The first report by Rascher was made in April 1942, and contains a description of the effect of the low-pressure chamber on a 37-year-old Jew. (1971-A-PS.) I quote:

> The third experiment of this type took such an extraordinary course that I called an SS physician of the camp as witness, since I had worked on these experiments all by myself. It was a continuous experiment without oxygen at a height of 12 kilometers conducted on a 37-year-old Jew in good general condition. Breathing continued up to 30 minutes. After 4 minutes the experimental subject began to perspire and wiggle his head, after 5 minutes cramps occurred, between 6 and 10 minutes breathing increased in speed and the experimental subject became unconscious; from 11 to 30 minutes breathing slowed down to three breaths per minute, finally stopping altogether.
>
> Severest cyanosis developed in between and foam appeared at the mouth.
>
> At 5 minute intervals electrocardiograms from three leads were written. After breathing

had stopped Ekg (electrocardiogram) was continuously written until the action of the heart had come to a complete standstill. About ½ hour after breathing had stopped, dissection was started.

*   *   *

Another series of experiments carried out at the Dachau concentration camp concerned immunization for and treatment of malaria. Over 1,200 inmates of practically every nationality were experimented upon. Many persons who participated in these experiments have already been tried before a general military court held at Dachau, and the findings of that court will be laid before this Tribunal. The malaria experiments were carried out under the general supervision of a Dr. Schilling, with whom the defendant Sievers and others in the box collaborated. The evidence will show that healthy persons were infected by mosquitoes or by injections from the glands of mosquitoes. Catholic priests were among the subjects. The defendant Gebhardt kept Himmler informed of the progress of these experiments. Rose furnished Schilling with fly eggs for them, and others of the defendants participated in various ways which the evidence will demonstrate.

After the victims had been infected they were variously treated with quinine, neosalvarsan, pyramidon, antipyrin, and several combinations of these drugs. Many deaths occurred from excessive doses of neosalvarsan and pyramidon. According to the findings of the Dachau court, malaria was the direct cause of 30 deaths and 300 to 400 others died as the result of subsequent complications.

*   *   *

From December 1941, until near the end of the war, a large program of medical experimentation was carried out upon concentration camp inmates at Buchenwald and Natzweiler to investigate the value of various vaccines. This research involved a variety of diseases—typhus, yellow fever, smallpox, paratyphoid A and B, cholera, and diphtheria. . . .

*   *   *

The general pattern of these typhus experiments was as follows. A group of concentration camp inmates, selected from the healthier ones who had some resistance to disease, were injected with an anti-typhus vaccine, the efficacy of which was to be tested. Thereafter, all the persons in the group would be infected with typhus. At the same time, other inmates who had not been vaccinated were also infected for purposes of comparison—these unvaccinated victims were called the "control" group. But perhaps the most wicked and murderous circumstance in this whole case is that still other inmates were deliberately infected with typhus with the sole purpose of keeping the typhus virus alive and generally available in the bloodstream of the inmates.

*   *   *

The 20 physicians in the dock range from leaders of German scientific medicine, with excellent international reputations, down to the dregs of the German medical profession. All of them have in common a callous lack of consideration and human regard for, and an unprincipled willingness to abuse their power over the poor, unfortunate, defenseless creatures who had been deprived of their rights by a ruthless and criminal government. All of them violated the Hippocratic commandments which they had solemnly sworn to uphold and abide by, including the fundamental principles never to do harm —"primum non nocere."

Outstanding men of science, distinguished for their scientific ability in Germany and abroad, are the defendants Rostock and Rose. Both exemplify, in their training and practice alike, the highest traditions of German medicine. Rostock headed the Department of Surgery at the University of Berlin and served as dean of its medical school. Rose studied under the famous surgeon, Enderlen, at Heidelberg and then became a distinguished specialist in the fields of public health and tropical diseases. Handloser and Schroeder are outstanding medical administrators. Both of them made their careers in military medicine and reached the peak of their profession. Five more defendants are much younger men who are nevertheless already known as the possessors of considerable scientific ability, or capacity in medical administration. These include the defendants Karl Brandt, Ruff, Beiglboeck, Schaefer, and Becker-Freyseng.

A number of the others such as Romberg and Fischer are well trained, and several of them attained high professional position. But among the remainder few were known as outstanding scientific men. Among them at the foot of the list is Blome who has published his autobiography entitled "Embattled Doctor" in which he sets forth that he eventually decided to become a doctor because a medical career would enable him to become "master over life and death."

*   *   *

I intend to pass very briefly over matters of medical ethics, such as the conditions under which a physician may lawfully perform a medical experiment upon a person who has voluntarily subjected himself to it, or whether experiments may lawfully be performed upon criminals who have been condemned to death. This case does not present such problems. No refined questions confront us here.

None of the victims of the atrocities perpetrated by these defendants were volunteers, and this is true regardless of what these unfortunate people may have said or signed before their tortures began. Most of the victims had not been condemned to death, and those who had been were not criminals, unless it be a crime to be a Jew, or a Pole, or a gypsy, or a Russian prisoner of war.

*   *   *

Were it necessary, one could make a long list of the respects in which the experiments which these defendants performed departed from every known standard of medical ethics. But the gulf between these atrocities and serious research in the healing art is so patent that such a tabulation would be cynical.

*   *   *

These experiments revealed nothing which civilized medicine can use. It was, indeed, ascertained that phenol or gasoline injected intravenously will kill a man inexpensively and within 60 seconds. This and a few other "advances" are all in the field of thanatology. . . .

Apart from these deadly fruits, the experiments were not only criminal but a scientific failure. It is indeed as if a just deity had shrouded the solutions which they attempted to reach with murderous means. The moral shortcomings of the defendants and the precipitous ease with which they decided to commit murder in quest of "scientific results," dulled also that scientific hesitancy, that thorough thinking-through, that responsible weighing of every single step which alone can insure scientifically valid results. Even if they had merely been forced to pay as little as two dollars for human experimental subjects, such as American investigators may have to pay for a cat, they might have thought twice before wasting unnecessary numbers, and thought of simpler and better ways to solve their problems. The fact that these investigators had free and unrestricted access to human beings to be experimented upon misled them to the dangerous and fallacious conclusion that the results would thus be better and more quickly obtainable than if they had gone through the labor of preparation, thinking, and meticulous preinvestigation.

A particularly striking example is the sea-water experiment. I believe that three of the accused . . . will today admit that this problem could have been solved simply and definitively within the space of one afternoon. On 20 May 1944 when these accused convened to discuss the problem, a thinking chemist could have solved it right in the presence of the assembly within the space of a few hours by the use of nothing more gruesome than a piece of jelly, a semipermeable membrane and a salt solution, and the German Armed Forces would have had the answer on 21 May 1944. But what happened instead? The vast armies of the disenfranchised slaves were at the beck and call of this sinister assembly; and instead of thinking, they simply relied on their power over human beings rendered rightless by a criminal state and government. . . .

*　*　*

. . . Who could German medicine look to to keep the profession true to its traditions and protect it from the ravaging inroads of Nazi pseudo-science? This was the supreme responsibility of the leaders of German medicine—men like Rostock and Rose and Schroeder and Handloser. That is why their guilt is greater than that of any of the other defendants in the dock. They are the men who utterly failed their country and their profession, who showed neither courage nor wisdom nor the vestiges of moral character. . . .

*　*　*

3.

Extracts from Argumentation and Evidence of Prosecution and Defense

a.

Testimony of Defense Expert Witness Dr. Franz Vollhardt

Direct Examination.

*　*　*

DR. MARX: Please, would you briefly tell the Tribunal what your scientific activities have been and in what special field you have taken a particularly great interest, and since when?

WITNESS VOLLHARDT: I am Professor of Internal Medicine at Frankfurt and predominantly I have dealt with the questions of circulation, metabolism, blood pressure, and kidney diseases.

*　*　*

Q: Which foreign academies and foreign societies have you been a member of? . . .

A: I am Honorary Doctor of the Sorbonne, Paris, of Goettingen and Freiburg; and, as far as societies are concerned, there are a lot of them, Medical Society at Edinburgh, at Geneva, at Luxembourg. I am an Honorary Member of the University at Santiago, and so on and so forth.

*　*　*

Q: Now, Professor, have you sufficient insight into the planning and carrying out of the so-called sea-water experiments to give an expert opinion on that subject?

*　*　*

A: I think that scientifically speaking the planning was excellent and I have no objection to the entire plan. It was good to add a hunger-and-thirst group because we know by experience that thirst can be borne less well than hunger, and if people are suffering from hunger and thirst too, they do not suffer from hunger, but do suffer from thirst; and that resembles what shipwrecked persons would be subjected to because they only suffer from thirst. It was excellent that Wofatit was to be introduced into the experiments too, although it was expected from the beginning that this wonderful discovery would show its value. . . .

*　*　*

Q: Could the aim of these experiments have been achieved with a semipermeable membrane?

A: I don't understand how one can imagine this. What we are concerned with is the question of how long the human body can survive without water and under the excess quantity of salt. Now, that is subject to the water content of the body and it depends first of all, upon whether water is only used by the intermediary tissues or whether the cell liquid too is being used up. In the latter case, there is a danger which becomes apparent through excess potassium quantitites, and this was also continuously observed and checked during such experiments, and there were no excess potassium quantities such as can be expected after 6 days.

Q: Nor would it be right to say that these experiments were not planned scientifically and medically, is that correct?

A: Absolutely not.

Q: Could they have been planned differently?

A: I couldn't imagine how.

Q: Were these experiments in the interests of active warfare, or in the interests of the care of shipwrecked sailors or soldiers?

A: The latter.

Q: In other words, for aviators and sailors who were shipwrecked or might be shipwrecked?

A: Towards the end of the war there was an increase in the number of pilots shot down as well as of shipwrecked personnel, and it was, therefore, the duty of the hygiene department concerned to consider the question of how one could best deal with such cases of shipwrecked personnel. . . .

* * *

Q: Now, Professor, the experiments we were talking about; did they have a practical valuable aim and did they show a corresponding result?

A: Yes, that is correct. For instance an important observation was made which Eppinger had expected; he wanted to see if the kidneys did concentrate salt under such extreme conditions to an even higher extent than one expectedly previously. One thought that it would be something like 2.0 percent but 2.6 or 2.7 percent and record figures of 3.0, 3.5, 3.6, and 4 percent are shown, so that the fortunate man who is in a position to concentrate 3.6 percent or 4 percent of salt would be able to live on sea water for quite a long period.

* * *

Finally, one unsuspected fact was shown which may be connected with this, and that is that the drinking of small quantities of sea water up to 500 cc. given over a lengthy period turned out to be better than unalleviated thirst.

* * *

Q: So, you think that the result of these experiments is not only of importance in wartime, but is also of importance for the problems of seafaring nations?

A: Quite right, it is a wonderful thing for all seafaring nations.

* * *

b.

Final Plea for Defendant Joachim Mrugowsky

* * *

The case with the typhus experiments is different. No order was given to kill a man in order to obtain knowledge. But the typhus experiments were dangerous experiments. Out of 724 experimental persons, 154 died. But these 154 deaths from the typhus experiments have to be compared with the 15,000 who died of typhus every day in the camps for Soviet prisoners of war, and the innumerable deaths from typhus among the civilian population of the occupied eastern territories and the German troops. This enormous number of deaths led to the absolute necessity of having effective vaccines against typhus in sufficient quantity. The newly developed vaccines had been tested in the animal experiments as to their compatibility.

* * *

The Tribunal will have to decide whether, in view of the enormous extent of epidemic typhus, in view of the 15,000 deaths it was causing daily in the camps for Russian prisoners of war alone, the order given by the government authorities to test the typhus vaccines was justified or not. If the answer is in the affirmative, then the typhus experiments at Buchenwald were not criminal, since the prosecution did not contest that they were carried out according to the rules of medical science.

* * *

c.

Testimony of Defendant Gerhard Rose

Direct Examination.

* * *

DR. FRITZ: What do you know about the reasons for this protest (against experiments) being ignored and the typhus experiments being carried out in spite of it?

* * *

DEFENDANT ROSE: The Buchenwald experiments (with typhus vaccine) had four main results. First of all, they showed that belief in the protective effect of Weigl vaccine was a mistake, although this belief seemed to be based on long observation. Secondly, they showed that the useful vaccines did not protect against infection, but almost certainly prevented death, under the conditions of the Buchenwald experiments. Thirdly, they showed that the objections of the biological experts to the vitelline membrane vaccines and to the lice vaccines were unjustified, and that vitelline membrane, rabbit lungs, and lice intestines were of equal value. We learned this only through the Buchenwald experiments. This left the way open to mass production of typhus vaccines.

The Buchenwald experiments showed in time that several vaccines were useless: First, the process according to Otto and Wohlrab, the process according to Cox, the process of Rickettsia Prowazeki and Rickettsia murina, that is, vaccine from egg cultures; secondly, the vaccines of the Behring works which were produced according to the Otto process, but with other concentrations; finally the Ipsen vaccines from mouse liver. The vaccines of the Behring works were in actual use at that time in thousands of doses. They always represented a danger to health. Without these experiments the vaccines, which were recognized as useless, would have been produced in large quantities because they all had one thing in common: their technical production was much simpler and cheaper than that of the useful vaccines. In any case, one thing is certain, that the victims of this Buchenwald typhus test did not suffer in vain and did not die in vain. There was only one choice, the sacrifice of human lives, of persons determined for that purpose, or to let things run their course, to endanger the lives of innumerable human beings who would be selected not by the Reich Criminal Police Office but by blind fate.

*   *   *

d.
Testimony of Prosecution Expert Witness Dr. Andrew C. Ivy

Direct Examination.

*   *   *

Mr. Hardy: It is your opinion, then, that the state cannot assume the moral responsibility of a physician to his patient or experimental subject?

Witness Dr. Ivy: That is my opinion.

Q: On what do you base your opinion? What is the reason for that opinion?

A: I base that opinion on the principles of ethics and morals contained in the oath of Hippocrates. I think it should be obvious that a state cannot follow a physician around in his daily administration to see that the moral responsibility inherent therein is properly carried out. This moral responsibility that controls or should control the conduct of a physician should be inculcated into the minds of physicians just as moral responsibility of other sorts, and those principles are clearly depicted or enunciated in the oath of Hippocrates with which every physician should be acquainted.

Q: Is the oath of Hippocrates the Golden Rule in the United States and to your knowledge throughout the world?

A: According to my knowledge it represents the Golden Rule of the medical profession. It states how one doctor would like to be treated by another doctor in case he were ill. And in that way how a doctor should treat his patients or experimental subjects. He should treat them as though he were serving as a subject.

Q: Several of the defendants have pointed out in this case that the oath of Hippocrates is obsolete today. Do you follow that opinion?

A: I do not. The moral imperative of the oath of Hippocrates I believe is necessary for the survival of the scientific and technical philosophy of medicine.

*   *   *

e.
Closing Brief for Defendant Siegfried Ruff

*   *   *

Experiments which time and again have been described in international literature without meeting any opposition do not constitute a crime from the medical point of view. For nowhere did a plaintiff arise from the side of the responsible professional organization, or from that of the administration of justice, to denounce as criminal the experiments described in literature. On the contrary, the authors of those reports on their human experiments gained general recognition and fame; they were awarded the highest honors; they gained historical importance. And in spite of all this, are they supposed to have been criminals? No! In view of the complete lack of written legal norms, the physician, who generally knows only little about the law, has to rely on and refer to the admissibility of what is generally recognized to be admissible all over the world.

The defense is convinced that the Tribunal, when deciding this problem without prejudice, will first study the many experiments performed all over the world on healthy and sick persons, on prisoners and free people, on criminals and on the poor, even on children and mentally ill persons, in order to see how the medical profession in its international totality answers the question of the admissibility of human experiments, not only in theory but also in practice.

It is psychologically understandable that German research workers today will, if possible, have nothing to do with human experiments and will try to avoid them, or would like to describe them as inadmissible even if before 1933 they were perhaps of the opposite opinion. However, experiments performed in 1905–1912 by a highly respected American in Asia for the fight against the plague, which made him famous all over the world, cannot and ought not to be labelled as criminal because a Blome is supposed to have performed the same experiments during the Hitler period (which, in fact, however, were not performed at all); and experiments for which, before 1933, a foreign research worker, the Englishman Ross, was awarded the Nobel Prize for his malaria experiments, do not deserve to be condemned only because a German physician performed similar experiments during the Hitler regime. . . .

*   *   *

f.
Testimony of Prosecution Expert Witness Dr. Andrew C. Ivy

*   *   *

Cross-Examination.

DR. SAUTER: Witness, you spoke yesterday of a number of experiments carried out in the United States and in other countries outside of Germany. For example, pellagra, swamp fever, beri-beri, plague, etc. Now, I should like to have a very clear answer from you to the following question. In these experiments which you heard of partly from persons involved in them and partly from international literature, did deaths occur during the experiments and as a result of the experiments or not? Professor, I ask you this question because you said yesterday that you examined all international literature concerning this question and, therefore, have a certain specialized knowledge on this question.

WITNESS DR. IVY: I also said that when one reviews the literature, he cannot be sure that he has done a complete or perfect job.

So far as the reports I have read and pre-

sented yesterday are concerned, there were no deaths in trench fever. There were no deaths mentioned, to my knowledge, in the article on pellagra. There were no deaths mentioned, to my knowledge, in the article on beri-beri, and there were no deaths in the article, according to my knowledge, in Colonel Strong's article on plague. I would not testify that I have read all the articles in the medical literature involving the use of human beings as subjects in medical experiments.

Q: And, in the literature which you have read, Witness, there was not a single case where deaths occurred? Did I understand you correctly?

A: Yes, in the yellow fever experiments I indicated that Dr. Carroll and Dr. Lazare died.

Q: That is the only case you know of?

A: That's all that I know of.

*   *   *

g.
Testimony of Defendant Gerhard Rose

Cross-Examination.

*   *   *

MR. MCHANEY: Now, would the extreme necessity for the large-scale production of typhus vaccines and the resultant experiments on human beings in concentration camps have arisen had not Germany been engaged in a war?

DEFENDANT ROSE: That question cannot simply be answered with "yes" or "no." It is, on the whole, not very probable that without the war typhus would have broken out in the German camps, but it is not altogether beyond the bounds of possibility because in times of peace too typhus has broken out in individual cases from time to time. The primary danger in the camps is the louse danger, and infection by lice also occurs in times of peace. If typhus breaks out in a camp that is infected with lice, a typhus epidemic can arise in peacetime too, of course.

Q: But Germany had never experienced any difficulty with typhus before the war. Isn't that right?

A: Not for many decades, no.

Q: You stated that nine hundred persons were used in Dr. Strong's plague experiments?

A: Yes, I know that number from the literature on the subject.

Q: What is the usual mortality in plague?

A: That depends on whether it is bubonic

plague or lung pest. In one, namely, bubonic plague, the mortality can be as high as sixty or seventy percent. It also can be lower. In lung pest, the mortality is just about one hundred.

Q: How many people died in Dr. Strong's plague experiments?

A: According to what his reports say, none of them died, but this result could not have been anticipated because this was the first time that anyone had attempted to inoculate living plague virus into human beings, and Strong said in his first publication in 1905 that he himself was surprised that no unpleasant incidents occurred and that there was only severe fever reaction. That despite this unexpectedly favorable outcome of Strong's experiments the specialists had considerable misgivings about this procedure can be seen first of all from publications where that is explicitly stated; for example, two Englishmen say that, contrary to expectations, these experiments went off well but nevertheless this process cannot be used for general vaccination because there is always the danger that, through some unexpected event, this strain again becomes virulent. Moreover, from other works that Strong later published it can be seen that guinea pigs and monkeys that he vaccinated with this vaccine died not of the plague, but of the toxic affects of the vaccine. All these difficulties are the reason why this enormously important discovery, which Koller and Otto made in 1903, and Strong in 1905, has only been generally applied, for all practical purposes, since 1926. That is an indication of the care and fear with which this whole matter was first approached, and Strong could not know ahead of time that his experiments would turn out well. I described here the enormous concern that Strong felt during all these months regarding the fact that that might happen which every specialist feared, viz., that the virus would become virulent again.That is an enormous responsibility.

Q: Be that as it may, nobody died. That is a fact, isn't it?

A: If anyone did die, the publications say nothing about it. There were deaths only among the monkeys and guinea pigs that are mentioned in the publication. If human beings died, there is no mention in the publication. It is generally known that if there are serious accidents in such experiments as this, they are only most reluctantly made public.

*   *   *

NOTE

Leo Alexander
Medical Science under Dictatorship*

*   *   *

[A] series of experiments gave results that might have been an important medical contribution if an important lead had not been ignored. The efficacy of various vaccines and drugs against typhus was tested at the Buchenwald and Natzweiler concentration camps. Prevaccinated persons and non-vaccinated controls were injected with live typhus rickettsias, and the death rates of the two series compared. After a certain number of passages, the Matelska strain of typhus rickettsia proved to become avirulent for man. Instead of seizing upon this as a possibility to develop a live vaccine, the experimenters, including the chief consultant, Professor Gerhard Rose, who should have known better, were merely annoyed at the fact that the controls did not die either, discarded this strain and continued testing their relatively ineffective dead vaccines against a new virulent strain. This incident shows that the basic unconscious motivation and attitude has a great influence in determining the scientists's awareness of the phenomena that pass through his vision.

*   *   *

4.

Final Plea for Defendant Karl Brandt by Dr. Robert Servatius

*   *   *

It is contended that the state finds its limits in the eternal basic elements of law, which are said to be so clear that anyone could discern their violation as a crime, and that loyalty to the state beyond these limits is therefore a crime. One forgets that eternal law, the law of nature, is but a guiding principle for the state and the legislator and not a counter-code of law which the subject might use as a support against the state. It is emphasized that no other state had made such decisions up to now. This is true only to a certain extent. It is no proof, however,

* 241 *New England Journal of Medicine* 39, 43 (1949). Reprinted by permission.

that such decisions were not necessary and admissible now. There is no prohibition against daring to progress.

The progress of medical science opened up the problem of experiments on human beings already in the past century, and eventually made it ripe for decision. It is not the first time that a state has adopted a certain attitude with regard to euthanasia with a change of ideology.

Only the statesmen decide what is to be done in the interests of the community, and they have never hesitated to issue such a decision whenever they deemed it necessary in the interest of their people. Thereupon their rules and orders were carried through under the authority of the state, which is the basis of society.

Inquisition, witch trials, and revolutionary tribunals have existed in the name of the state and eternal justice, and the executive participants did not consider themselves criminals but servants of their community. They would have been killed if they had stood up against what was believed to be newly discovered eternal justice. What is the subject to do if the orders of the state exceed the customary limits which the individual himself took for inviolable according to tradition.

What did the airman think who dropped the first atomic bomb on Hiroshima? Did he consider himself a criminal? What did the statesmen think who ordered this atomic bomb to be used. We know from the history of this event that the motive was patriotism, based on the harsh necessity of sacrificing hundreds of thousands to save their own soldiers' lives. This motive was stronger than the prohibition of the Hague Convention, under which belligerents have no unlimited right in the choice of methods for inflicting damage on the enemy.

"My cause is just and my quarrel honorable," says the king. And Shakespeare's soldier answers him: "That's more than we know." Another soldier adds: "Ay, or more than we should seek after; for we know enough if we know we are the king's subjects; if his cause be wrong, our obedience to the king wipes the crime out of us."

It is the hard necessity of the state on which the defense for Karl Brandt is based against the charge of having performed criminal experiments on human beings.

Here also—in addition to the care for the population—the lives of soldiers were at stake, soldiers who had to be protected from death

and epidemics. In Professor Bickenbach's experiment, the issue was the lives of women and children who without 45 million gas masks would have been as unprotected against the expected gas attack as the Japanese were against the atomic bomb. Biological warfare was imminent, even praised abroad as cheaper and more effective than the atomic bomb.

The prosecution opposes to this necessity the condition of absolute voluntariness.

It was a surprise to hear from the expert Professor Ivy that in the penitentiaries many hundreds of volunteers were pressing for admission to experiments, and that more volunteered than could be used. I do not want to dispose of this phenomenon with irony and sarcasm. There may be people who realize that the community has the right to ask them for a sacrifice. Their feeling of justice may tell them that insistence on humanity has its limits. If humanity means the appeal to the strong not to forget the weak in the abundance of might and wealth, the weak should also make their contribution when all are in need.

But what if in the emergency of war the convicts, and those declared to be unworthy to serve in the armed forces, refuse to accept such a sacrifice voluntarily, and only prove an asocial burden to state and community and bring about the downfall of the community? Is not compulsion by the state then admissible as an additional expiation?

The prosecution says "No." According to this, human rights demand the downfall of human beings.

But there is a mixture of voluntariness and compulsory expiation, "purchased voluntariness." Here the experimental subject does not make a sacrifice out of conviction for the good of the community but for his own good. The subject gives his consent because he is to receive money, cigarettes, a mitigation of punishment, etc. There may be isolated cases of this nature where the person is really a volunteer, but as a rule it is not so.

If one compares the actual risk with the advantage granted, one cannot admit the consent of these "voluntary prisoners" as legal, in spite of all the protective forms they have to sign, for these can only have been obtained by taking advantage of inexperience, imprudence, or distress.

Looking through medical literature, one cannot escape the growing conviction that the word "volunteer," where it appears at all, is used only as a word of protection and camouflage; it is hardly ever missing since the struggle over this problem became acute.

I will touch only briefly on what I have explained in detail in my closing brief. No one will contend that human beings really allowed themselves to be infected voluntarily with venereal disease; this has nowhere been stated explicitly in literature. Cholera and plague are also not minor inconveniences one is likely to undergo voluntarily for a trifle in the interest of science. Above all, it is not customary to hand over children for experimental purposes, and I cannot believe that in the 13 experiments carried out on a total of 223 children, as stated in Document Karl Brandt 117, . . . the mothers gave their consent. Would not the mothers have deserved the praise of the scientist for the sacrifice they trustfully made in the interest of science, praise which is otherwise liberally granted to real volunteers in reports on experiments?

Is it not likely to have been similar to the experiments carried out by Professor McCance? The German authorities who condemn the defendants in a particularly violent form have no objection to raise here against the order to hand over weakling children to a research commission for experimental purposes. The questionnaires which the Tribunal approved for me in order to get further information about this matter have not been answered as the higher authorities did not give permission for such statements to be made. This silence says enough; it is proof of what is supposed to be legal today in the line of "voluntariness."

It is repeatedly shown that the experiments for which no consent was given were permitted with the full knowledge of the government authorities. It is further shown that these experiments were published in professional literature without meeting any objection, and that they were even accepted by the public without concern as a normal phenomenon when reports about them appeared in popular magazines.

This happens at a time when the same press is stigmatizing as crimes against humanity the German experiments which were necessary in the interests of the state. Voluntariness is a fiction; the emergency of the state hard reality.

In all countries experiments on human beings have been performed by doctors, certainly not because they took pleasure in killing or tormenting, but only at the instigation and under the protection of their state, and in accordance with their own conviction of the necessity for these experiments in the struggle for the existence of the people.

* * *

5.

Final Statements of the Defendants

* * *

a.

Final Statement of Defendant Siegfried Handloser

* * *

More than 150 years ago, the motto and guiding principle created for German military doctors and their successors was "Scientiae, Humanitati, Patriae" (For Science, Humanity, and Fatherland). Like the medical officers in their entirety I also have remained true to that guiding principle in thought and in deed. Realizing the outcome of the events of these recent times, may the joint endeavors of all the nations succeed in avoiding in future the immeasurable misfortune of war, the dreadful side of which nobody knows better than the military doctor.

b.

Final Statement of Defendant Gerhard Rose

* * *

. . . Everyone who, as a scientist, has an insight into the history of dangerous medical experiments, knows with certainty the following fact. Aside from the self-experiments of doctors, which represent a very small minority of such experiments, the extent to which subjects are volunteers is often deceptive. At the very best they amount to self-deceit on the part of the physician who conducts the experiment, but very frequently to a deliberate misleading of the public. In the majority of such cases, if we ethically examine facts, we find an exploitation of the ignorance, the frivolity, the economic distress, or other emergency on the part of the experimental subjects. I may only refer to the example which was presented to the Tribunal by Dr. Ivy when he presented the forms for the American malaria experiments.

You yourselves, gentlemen of the Tribunal, are in a position to examine whether, on the basis of the information contained in these forms, individuals of the average education of an inmate of a prison can form a sufficiently clear opinion of the risks of an experiment made with pernicious malaria. These facts will be confirmed by any sincere and decent scientist in a personal conversation, though he would not like to make such a statement in public. . . .

*   *   *

6.

Judgment

*   *   *

BEALS, SEBRING, CRAWFORD, J.J.: . . . Judged by any standard of proof the record clearly shows the commission of war crimes and crimes against humanity substantially as alleged in counts two and three of the indictment. Beginning with the outbreak of World War II criminal medical experiments on non-German nationals, both prisoners of war and civilians, including Jews and "asocial" persons, were carried out on a large scale in Germany and the occupied countries. These experiments were not the isolated and casual acts of individual doctors and scientists working solely on their own responsibility, but were the product of coordinated policy-making and planning at high governmental, military, and Nazi Party levels, conducted as an integral part of the total war effort. They were ordered, sanctioned, permitted, or approved by persons in positions of authority who under all principles of law were under the duty to know about these things and to take steps to terminate or prevent them.

The great weight of the evidence before us is to the effect that certain types of medical experiments on human beings, when kept within reasonably well-defined bounds, conform to the ethics of the medical profession generally. The protagonists of the practice of human experimentation justify their views on the basis that such experiments yield results for the good of society that are unprocurable by other methods or means of study. All agree, however, that certain basic principles[*] must be observed in order to satisfy moral, ethical, and legal concepts:

1. The voluntary consent of the human subject is absolutely essential.

This means that the person involved should have legal capacity to give consent; should be so situated as to be able to exercise free power of choice, without the intervention of any element of force, fraud, deceit, duress, over-reaching, or other ulterior form of constraint or coercion; and should have sufficient knowledge and comprehension of the elements of the subject matter involved as to enable him to make an understanding and enlightened decision. This latter element requires that before the acceptance of an affirmative decision by the experimental subject there should be made known to him the nature, duration, and purpose of the experiment; the method and means by which it is to be conducted; all inconveniences and hazards reasonably to be expected; and the effects upon his health or person which may possibly come from his participation in the experiment.

The duty and responsibility for ascertaining the quality of the consent rests upon each individual who initiates, directs, or engages in the experiment. It is a personal duty and responsibility which may not be delegated to another with impunity.

2. The experiment should be such as to yield fruitful results for the good of society, unprocurable by other methods or means of study, and not random and unnecessary in nature.

3. The experiment should be so designed and based on the results of animal experimentation and a knowledge of the natural history of the disease or other problem under study that the anticipated results will justify the performance of the experiment.

4. The experiment should be so conducted as to avoid all unnecessary physical and mental suffering and injury.

5. No experiment should be conducted where there is an *a priori* reason to believe that death or disabling injury will occur; except, perhaps, in those experiments where the experimental physicians also serve as subjects.

6. The degree of risk to be taken should never exceed that determined by the humanitarian importance of the problem to be solved by the experiment.

Proper preparations should be made and adequate facilities provided to protect the experimental subject against even remote possibilities of injury, disability, or death.

8. The experiment should be conducted only by scientifically qualified persons. The highest degree of skill and care should be required through all stages of the experiment of those who conduct or engage in the experiment.

---

[*] These ten principles are now known as the Nuremberg Code.

9. During the course of the experiment the human subject should be at liberty to bring the experiment to an end if he has reached the physical or mental state where continuation of the experiment seems to him to be impossible.

10. During the course of the experiment the scientist in charge must be prepared to terminate the experiment at any stage, if he has probable cause to believe, in the exercise of the good faith, superior skill, and careful judgment required of him that a continuation of the experiment is likely to result in injury, disability, or death to the experimental subject.

Of the ten principles which have been enumerated our judicial concern, of course, is with those requirements which are purely legal in nature—or which at least are so clearly related to matters legal that they assist us in determining criminal culpability and punishment. To go beyond that point would lead us into a field that would be beyond our sphere of competence. However, the point need not be labored. We find from the evidence that in the medical experiments which have been proved, these ten principles were much more frequently honored in their breach than in their observance. Many of the concentration camp inmates who were the victims of these atrocities were citizens of countries other than the German Reich. They were non-German nationals, including Jews and "asocial persons," both prisoners of war and civilians, who had been imprisoned and forced to submit to these tortures and barbarities without so much as a semblance of trial. In every single instance appearing in the record, subjects were used who did not consent to the experiments; indeed, as to some of the experiments, it is not even contended by the defendants that the subjects occupied the status of volunteers. In no case was the experimental subject at liberty of his own free choice to withdraw from any experiment. In many cases experiments were performed by unqualified persons; were conducted at random for no adequate scientific reason, and under revolting physical conditions. All of the experiments were conducted with unnecessary suffering and injury, and but very

little, if any, precautions were taken to protect or safeguard the human subjects from the possibilities of injury, disability, or death. In every one of the experiments the subjects experienced extreme pain or torture, and in most of them they suffered permanent injury, mutilation, or death, either as a direct result of the experiments or because of lack of adequate follow-up care.

Obviously all of these experiments involving brutalities, tortures, disabling injury, and death were performed in complete disregard of international conventions, the laws and customs of war [and] the general principles of criminal law as derived from the criminal laws of all civilized nations. . . . Manifestly human experiments under such conditions are contrary to "the principles of the law of nations as they result from the usages established among civilized peoples, from the laws of humanity, and from the dictates of public conscience."

*　　*　　*

There is some evidence to the effect that the camp inmates used as subjects in the first series submitted to being used as experimental subjects after being told that the experiments were harmless and that additional food would be given to volunteers. But these victims were not informed that they would be artificially infected with a highly virulent virus nor that they might die as a result. Certainly no one would seriously suggest that under the circumstances these men gave their legal consent to act as subjects. One does not ordinarily consent to be the special object of a murder, and if one did, such consent would not absolve his slayer.

*　　*　　*

[Sixteen of the twenty-three defendants were found guilty of war crimes and crimes against humanity. Seven, including Karl Brandt, Rudolf Brandt, and Joachim Mrugowsky, were sentenced to death by hanging; the other nine, including Siegfried Handloser and Gerhard Rose, to imprisonment varying from ten years to life.]

C.

Epilogue—Experiments Subsequent to 1945

In 1966 Dr. Henry K. Beecher, Dorr Professor of Research in Anesthesia at the Harvard Medical School, surveyed the tremendous postwar increase in research involving human subjects and charged that "many of the patients [who were used in these experiments] never had the risk satisfactorily explained to them, and . . . further hundreds have not known that they were the subjects of an experiment although grave consequences have been suffered as the direct result. . . ."* We have selected excerpts from his article, which was checked for accuracy by the editors of one of the most prestigious American medical journals, as illustrative of "the ease with which the admonition first of all to do no harm is allowed . . . to slip from the investigator's consciousness."† Despite his "troubling charges," Dr. Beecher concluded that in addition to informed consent, a "more reliable safeguard [for an ethical approach to experimentation is] provided by the presence of an intelligent, informed, conscientious, compassionate, responsible investigator."‡

Dr. Beecher's conclusion in turn raises further questions: Does or can science produce such ideal investigators? And, if not, how can professional training be reformed to provide "reliable safeguards" for human subjects? Before turning to an analysis of the extent and limits of the investigator's authority, we examine a few of the major documents on medical ethics as well as selected commentaries on research responsibility. In studying these documents we ask:

1. How adequately do codes of ethics guide the investigator in formulating specific rules of conduct for himself?

2. How adequate are these documents in themselves as rules of conduct?

3. To what extent are these documents counterproductive as guides or as rules of conduct for investigators?

1.

The Experiments

Henry K. Beecher
Ethics and Clinical Research**

*   *   *

Nearly everyone agrees that ethical violations do occur. The practical question is, how often? A preliminary examination of the matter was based on 17 examples, which were easily increased to 50. These 50 studies†† contained references to 186 further likely examples, on the average 3.7 leads per study; they at times overlapped from paper to paper, but this figure indicates how conveniently one can proceed in a search for such material. The data are suggestive of widespread problems, but there is need for another kind of information, which was obtained by examination of 100 consecutive human studies published in 1964, in an excellent journal; 12 of these seemed to be unethical. If only one quarter of them is truly unethical, this still indicates the existence of a serious situation. Pappworth, in England, has collected, he says, more than 500 papers based upon unethical experimentation. It is evident from such observations that unethical or questionably ethical procedures are not uncommon.

*   *   *

Known Effective Treatment Withheld

Example 1. It is known that rheumatic fever can usually be prevented by adequate treatment of streptococcal respiratory infections by the parenteral administration of penicillin. Nevertheless, definitive treatment was withheld, and placebos were given to a group of 109 men in service, while benzathine penicillin G was given to others.

The therapy that each patient received was determined automatically by his military serial number arranged so that more men received penicillin than received placebo. In the small

---

* Henry K. Beecher: "Ethics and Clinical Research," 274 *New England Journal of Medicine* 1354 (1966).

† "Experimentation on Man" (Editorial), 274 *New England Journal of Medicine* 1383 (1966).

‡ Beecher, at 1360.

** 274 *New England Journal of Medicine* 1354–1360 (1966). Reprinted by permission.

†† [The editors of the *Journal,* "for reasons of space," published only twenty-two studies.]

group of patients studied 2 cases of acute rheumatic fever and 1 of acute nephritis developed in the control patients, whereas these complications did not occur among those who received benzathine penicillin G.

Example 2. The sulfonamides were for many years the only antibacterial drugs effective in shortening the duration of acute streptococcal pharyngitis and in reducing its suppurative complications. The investigators in this study undertook to determine if the occurence of the serious nonsuppurative complications, rheumatic fever and acute glomerulonephritis, would be reduced by this treatment. This study was made despite the general experience that certain antibiotics, including penicillin, will prevent the development of rheumatic fever.

The subjects were a large group of hospital patients; a control group of approximately the same size, also with exudative Group A streptococcus, was included. The latter group received only non-specific therapy (no sulfadiazine). The total group denied the effective penicillin comprised over 500 men.

Rheumatic fever was diagnosed in 5.4 per cent of those treated with sulfadiazine. In the control group rheumatic fever developed in 4.2 per cent.

In reference to this study a medical officer stated in writing that the subjects were not informed, did not consent and were not aware that they had been involved in an experiment, and yet admittedly 25 acquired rheumatic fever. According to this same medical officer *more than 70* who had had known definitive treatment withheld were on the wards with rheumatic fever when he was there.

Example 3. This involved a study of the relapse rate in typhoid fever treated in two ways. In an earlier study by the present investigators chloramphenicol had been recognized as an effective treatment for typhoid fever, being attended by half the mortality that was experienced when this agent was not used. Others had made the same observations, indicating that to withhold this effective remedy can be a life-or-death decision. The present study was carried out to determine the relapse rate under the two methods of treatment; of 408 charity patients 251 were treated with chloramphenicol, of whom 20, or 7.97 per cent, died. Symptomatic treatment was given, but chloramphenicol was withheld in 157, of whom 36, or 22.9 per cent died. According to the data presented, 23 patients died in the course of this study who would

not have been expected to succumb if they had received specific therapy.

* * *

Physiologic Studies

Example 5. In this controlled, double-blind study of the hematologic toxicity of chloramphenicol, it was recognized that chloramphenicol is "well known as a cause of aplastic anemia" and that there is a "prolonged morbidity and high mortality of aplastic anemia" and that ". . . chloramphenicol-induced aplastic anemia can be related to dose. . . ." The aim of the study was "further definition of the toxicology of the drug. . . ."

Forty-one randomly chosen patients were given either 2 or 6 gm. of chloramphenicol per day; 12 control patients were used. "Toxic bone-marrow depression, predominantly affecting erythropoiesis, developed in 2 of 20 patients given 2.0 gm. and in 18 of 21 given 6 gm. of chloramphenicol daily." The smaller dose is recommended for routine use.

Example 6. In a study of the effect of thymectomy on the survival of skin homografts 18 children, three and a half months to eighteen years of age, about to undergo surgery for congenital heart disease, were selected. Eleven were to have total thymectomy as part of the operation, and 7 were to serve as controls. As part of the experiment, full-thickness skin homografts from an unrelated adult donor were sutured to the chest wall in each case. (Total thymectomy is occasionally, although not usually part of the primary cardiovascular surgery involved, and whereas it may not greatly add to the hazards of the necessary operation, its eventual effects in children are not known.) This work was proposed as part of a long-range study of "the growth and development of these children over the years." No difference in the survival of the skin homograft was observed in the 2 groups.

* * *

Example 8. Since the minimum blood-flow requirements of the cerebral circulation are not accurately known, this study was carried out to determine "cerebral hemodynamic and metabolic changes . . . before and during acute reductions in arterial pressure induced by drug administration and/or postural adjustments." Forty-four patients whose ages varied from the second to the tenth decade were involved. They included normotensive subjects, those with essential hypertension and finally a group with malignant hypertension. Fifteen had abnormal electrocardiograms. Few details about the reasons for hospitalization are given.

Signs of cerebral circulatory insufficiency, which were easily recognized, included confusion and in some cases a nonresponsive state. By alteration in the tilt of the patient "the clinical state of the subject could be changed in a matter of seconds from one of alertness to confusion, and for the remainder of the flow, the subject was maintained in the latter state." The femoral arteries were cannulated in all subjects, and the internal jugular veins in 14.

The mean arterial pressure fell in 37 subjects from 109 to 48 mm. of mercury, with signs of cerebral ischemia. "With the onset of collapse, cardiac output and right ventricular pressures decreased sharply."

Since signs of cerebral insufficiency developed without evidence of coronary insufficiency the authors concluded that "the brain may be more sensitive to acute hypotension than is the heart."

*   *   *

Studies to Improve the Understanding of Disease

Example 14. In this study of the syndrome of impending hepatic coma in patients with cirrhosis of the liver certain nitrogenous substances were administered to 9 patients with chronic alcoholism and advanced cirrhosis: ammonium chloride, di-ammonium citrate, urea or dietary protein. In all patients a reaction that included mental disturbances, a "flapping tremor," and electroencephalographic changes developed. Similar signs had occurred in only 1 of the patients before these substances were administered:

> The first sign noted was usually clouding of the consciousness. Three patients had a second or a third course of administration of a nitrogenous substance with the same results. It was concluded that marked resemblance between this reaction and impending hepatic coma implied that the administration of these [nitrogenous] substances to patients with cirrhosis may be hazardous.

Example 18. Melanoma was transplanted from a daughter to her volunteering and informed mother, "in the hope of gaining a little better understanding of cancer immunity and in the hope that the production of tumor antibodies might be helpful in the treatment of the cancer patient." Since the daughter died on the day after the transplantation of the tumor into her mother, the hope expressed seems to have

been more theoretical than practical, and the daughter's condition was described as "terminal" at the time the mother volunteered to be a recipient. The primary implant was widely excised on the twenty-fourth day after it had been placed in the mother. She died from metastatic melanoma on the four hundred and fifty-first day after transplantation. The evidence that this patient died of diffuse melanoma that metastasized from a small piece of transplanted tumor was considered conclusive.

Technical Study of Disease

Example 19. During bronchoscopy a special needle was inserted through a bronchus into the left atrium of the heart. This was done in an unspecified number of subjects, both with cardiac disease and with normal hearts.

The technic was a new approach whose hazards were at the beginning quite unknown. The subjects with normal hearts were used, not for their possible benefit but for that of patients in general.

*   *   *

Example 21. This was a study of the effect of exercise on cardiac output and pulmonary-artery pressure in 8 "normal" persons (that is, patients whose diseases were not related to the cardiovascular system), in 8 with congestive heart failure severe enough to have recently required complete bed rest, in 6 with hypertension, in 2 with aortic insufficiency, in 7 with mitral stenosis, and in 5 with pulmonary emphysema.

Intracardiac catheterization was carried out, and the catheter then inserted into the right or left main branch of the pulmonary artery. The brachial artery was usually catheterized; sometimes, the radial or femoral arteries were catheterized. The subjects exercised in a supine position by pushing their feet against weighted pedals. "The ability of these patients to carry on sustained work was severely limited by weakness and dyspnea." Several were in severe failure. This was not a therapeutic attempt but rather a physiologic study.

Bizarre Study

Example 22. There is a question whether ureteral reflux can occur in the normal bladder. With this in mind, vesicourethrography was carried out on 26 normal babies less than forty-eight hours old. The infants were exposed to x-rays while the bladder was filling and during voiding. Multiple spot films were made to record the presence or absence of ureteral reflux. None was found in this group, and fortunately no infection followed the catheterization. What the results of the extensive x-ray exposure may be, no one can yet say.

Comment on Death Rates

In the foregoing examples a number of procedures, some with their own demonstrated death rates, were carried out. The following data were provided by 3 distinguished investigators in the field and represent widely held views.

Cardiac catheterization: right side of the heart, about 1 death per 1000 cases; left side, 5 death per 1000 cases. "Probably considerably higher in some places, depending on the portal of entry." (One investigator had 15 deaths in his first 150 cases.) It is possible that catheterization of a hepatic vein or the renal vein would have a lower death rate than that of catheterization of the right side of the heart, for if it is properly carried out, only the atrium is entered en route to the liver or the kidney, not the right ventricle, which can lead to serious cardiac irregularities. There is always the possibility, however, that the ventricle will be entered inadvertently. This occurs in at least half the cases, according to 1 expert—"but if properly done is too transient to be of importance."

Liver biopsy: the death rate here is estimated at 2 to 3 per 1000, depending in considerable part on the condition of the subject.

Anesthesia: the anesthesia death rate can be placed in general at about 1 death per 2000 cases. The hazard is doubtless higher when certain practices such as deliberate evocation of ventricular extrasystoles under cyclopropane are involved.

*   *   *

NOTES

NOTE 1.

LETTER FROM OWEN H. WANGENSTEEN
TO SENATOR WALTER F. MONDALE—
JANUARY 28, 1968*

Your letter of January 10, 1968, has crossed my desk together with a memorandum relative to a proposal you intend bringing before the

---

* *Hearings on S.J. Res. 145 before the Subcommittee on Government Research of the Senate Committee on Government Operations,* 90th Congress, 2d Session 98–99 (1968).

Congress with the intent of creating a commission to adjudicate the Social and Ethical Implications of Health Science Research and Development.

Senator, I would urge you with all the strength I can muster to leave this subject to the conscionable people in the profession who are struggling valiantly to advance medicine. We are living through an era in which the innovator is often under suspicion, being second-guessed by self-appointed arbiters more versed in the art of criticism than in the subject under scrutiny. We need to take great care lest the wells of creativity and the spring of the mind of those who break with tradition are not manacled by well-intentioned but meddlesome intruders. I will only recount three items here:

First, when the Minnesota group under the leadership of Drs. C. Walton Lillehei, Richard Varco, and Richard De Wall gave intracardiac surgery its first real impetus, they and I too found it necessary to defend ourselves and our position. At meetings my colleagues were viciously attacked by the keenest exponents of cardiac surgery in America. I too became a target of these assaults. I remember well Walt Lillehei saying very patiently but firmly in reply to these charges: "Your procedure is palliative; mine is corrective. Time will dispel the difference in surgical mortality." As we all know, it has. . . .

In Paris for generations it was customary to adjudicate scientific matters by assigning them for arbitration to a commission—a thumbs-up or Pollicis Versus Phenomenon which determined the life or the death of the proposal. How progress was stifled by such structures! Antiseptic surgery might have come much earlier if a few enterprising and knowledgeable surgeons of those days had not been influenced too much by the unfavorable verdict of committees that expressed firm judgments upon proposals of which they had little or no orientation.

When anesthesia, an American invention of 1846 came it found generally warm acceptance because the world had been waiting patiently for centuries for a lenitive to pain. Even so there were those who raised the question of the morality of making a patient unconscious when he was undergoing an operative procedure.

I would urge you to leave these matters in the hands of their proponents, the persons who are actually doing the work. They know more about all this than any of us possibly could. They have wrestled with the problem day and night, almost invariably over many years. Theirs are not overnight judgments or convictions. In the academic community in which I have worked and spent my entire professional life of almost 50 years, you will find as warm, sympathetic human beings as are to be found on this earth. . . .

It is important that we look back as well as forward. To have no concern for history is tantamount to having a physician with total amnesia. If we leave this matter alone, it will simmer down. Discussion should not be restrained, but legislative action, never!

NOTE 2.

EDWARD A. SHILS
SOCIAL INQUIRY AND THE AUTONOMY
OF THE INDIVIDUAL*

*   *   *

More serious experimentation by social psychologists and sociologists in the present state of the subject must be viewed very cautiously. Many restraints should accompany its recommendation or execution. In medicine, where knowledge is admittedly fragmentary, although undoubtedly less fragmentary than in the social sciences, experimentation is guided by a strongly rooted therapeutic tradition and is almost always a link in a continuing sequence of scientific activity. One of the chief features of social psychological and sociological research today is the absence of both therapeutic intent and a tradition of cumulative scientific growth. This renders more doubtful the scientific value of the results attained by experimentation which would deal with the more vital features of individual or corporate life.

Furthermore, because the therapeutic tradition of medicine is lacking, the probability that sociological and psychological experimentation on more important variables might have harmful consequences is greater. The professional ethos formed by the weight of a powerful tradition and inculcated in medical schools, where ethical responsibility is one of the best precipitates of a course of study which includes much that is not technically necessary for the medical practitioner, is still lacking in the social and psychological sciences. This *ethos* is not by any means just a product of scientific maturity, al-

though the latter does not make a positive difference. It flows from a deeper attitude that is still lacking in the scientific study of man.

*   *   *

2.

Professional Guidelines

a.

Oath of Hippocrates (5th century B.C.)

I swear by Apollo the physician, and Aesculapius and Health, and All-heal, and all the gods and goddesses, that, according to my ability and judgment, I will keep this Oath and this stipulation—to reckon him who taught me this Art equally dear to me as my parents, to share my substance with him, and relieve his necessities if required; to look upon his offspring in the same footing as my own brothers, and to teach them this art, if they shall wish to learn it, without fee or stipulation; and that by precept, lecture, and every other mode of instruction, I will impart a knowledge of the Art to my own sons, and those of my teachers, and to disciples bound by a stipulation and oath according to the law of medicine, but to none others. I will follow that system of regimen which, according to my ability and judgment, I consider for the benefit of my patients, and abstain from whatever is deleterious and mischievous. I will give no deadly medicine to anyone if asked, nor suggest any such counsel: and in like manner I will not give to a woman a pessary to produce abortion. With purity and with holiness I will pass my life and practise my Art. I will not cut persons labouring under the stone, but will leave this to be done by men who are practitioners of this work. Into whatever houses I enter, I will go into them for the benefit of the sick, and will abstain from every voluntary act of mischief and corruption; and, further, from the seduction of females or males, or freemen or slaves. Whatever, in connection with my professional practice, or not in connection with it, I see or hear, in the life of men, which ought not to be spoken of abroad, I will not divulge, as reckoning that all such should be kept secret. While I continue to keep this Oath unviolated, may it be granted to me to enjoy life and the practice of the Art, respected by all men, in all times. But should I trespass and violate this Oath, may the reverse be my lot.

---

* Daniel Lerner, ed.: *The Human Meaning of the Social Sciences.* New York: Meridian Books, Inc. 114, 146 (1959). © 1959 by the World Publishing Co. Reprinted by permission.

NOTE

WORLD MEDICAL ASSOCIATION
THE HIPPOCRATIC OATH
FORMULATED AT GENEVA (SEPTEMBER 1948)

Now being admitted to the profession of medicine I solemnly pledge to consecrate my life to the service of humanity. I will give respect and gratitude to my deserving teachers. I will practice medicine with conscience and dignity. The health and life of my patient will be my first consideration. I will hold in confidence all that my patient confides in me. I will maintain the honor and the noble traditions of the medical profession. My colleagues will be as my brothers. I will not permit consideration of race, religion, nationality, party politics or social standing to intervene between my duty and my patient. I will maintain the utmost respect for human life from the time of its conception. Even under threat I will not use my knowledge contrary to the laws of humanity. These promises I make freely and upon my honor.

b.

World Medical Association Declaration of Helsinki*

It is the mission of the doctor to safeguard the health of the people. His knowledge and conscience are dedicated to the fulfillment of this mission.

The Declaration of Geneva of the World Medical Association binds the doctor with the words, "The health of my patient will be my first consideration"; and the International Code of Medical Ethics which declares that "Any act or advice which could weaken physical or mental resistance of a human being may be used only in his interest."

Because it is essential that the results of laboratory experiments be applied to human beings to further scientific knowledge and to help suffering humanity, the World Medical Association has prepared the following recommendations as a guide to each doctor in clinical research. It must be stressed that the standards as drafted are only a guide to physicians all over the world. Doctors are not relieved from criminal, civil, and ethical responsibilities under the laws of their own countries.

In the field of clinical research a funda-

mental distinction must be recognized between clinical research in which the aim is essentially therapeutic for a patient, and clinical research the essential object of which is purely scientific and without therapeutic value to the person subjected to the research.

I. Basic Principles

1. Clinical research must conform to the moral and scientific principles that justify medical research, and should be based on laboratory and animal experiments or other scientifically established facts.

2. Clinical research should be conducted only by scientifically qualified persons and under the supervision of a qualified medical man.

3. Clinical research cannot legitimately be carried out unless the importance of the objective is in proportion to the inherent risk to the subject.

4. Every clinical research project should be preceded by careful assessment of inherent risks in comparison to foreseeable benefits to the subject or to others.

5. Special caution should be exercised by the doctor in performing clinical research in which the personality of the subject is liable to be altered by drugs or experimental procedure.

II. Clinical Research Combined with Professional Care

1. In the treatment of the sick person the doctor must be free to use a new therapeutic measure if in his judgment it offers hope of saving life, re-establishing health, or alleviating suffering.

If at all possible, consistent with patient psychology, the doctor should obtain the patient's freely given consent after the patient has been given a full explanation. In case of legal incapacity consent should also be procured from the legal guardian; in case of physical incapacity the permission of the legal guardian replaces that of the patient.

2. The doctor can combine clinical research with professional care, the objective being the acquisition of new medical knowledge, only to the extent that clinical research is justified by its therapeutic value for the patient.

III. Non-therapeutic Clinical Research

1. In the purely scientific application of clinical research carried out on a human being it is the duty of the doctor to remain the protector of the life and health of that person on whom clinical research is being carried out.

---

* 271 New England Journal of Medicine 473 (1964). Reprinted by permission.

2. The nature, the purpose, and the risk of clinical research must be explained to the subject by the doctor.

3a. Clinical research on a human being cannot be undertaken without his free consent, after he has been fully informed; if he is legally incompetent the consent of the legal guardian should be procured.

3b. The subject of clinical research should be in such a mental, physical, and legal state as to be able to exercise fully his power of choice.

3c. Consent should as a rule be obtained in writing. However, the responsibility for clinical research always remains with the research worker; it never falls on the subject, even after consent is obtained.

4a. The investigator must respect the right of each individual to safeguard his personal integrity, especially if the subject is in a dependent relationship to the investigator.

4b. At any time during the course of clinical research the subject or his guardian should be free to withdraw permission for research to be continued. The investigator or the investigating team should discontinue the research if in his or their judgment it may, if continued, be harmful to the individual.

c.

American Medical Association Principles of Medical Ethics*

Introduction

*   *   *

Ethical principles are basic and fundamental. Men of good conscience inherently know what is right or wrong, and what is to be done or to be avoided. Written documents attempt to express for the guidance of all what each knows to be true. Thus the Principles of Medical Ethics are truly guides to good conduct.

*   *   *

Principles of Medical Ethics
Preamble
These principles are intended to aid physicians individually and collectively in maintaining a high level of ethical conduct. They are not laws but standards by which a physician may determine the propriety of his conduct in his relationship with patients, with colleagues, with members of allied professions, and with the public.

Section 1
The principal objective of the medical profession is to render service to humanity with full respect for the dignity of man. Physicians should merit the confidence of patients entrusted to their care, rendering to each a full measure of service and devotion.

Section 2
Physicians should strive continually to improve medical knowledge and skill, and should make available to their patients and colleagues the benefits of their professional attainments.

Section 3
A physician should practice a method of healing founded on a scientific basis; and he should not voluntarily associate professionally with anyone who violates this principle.

Section 4
The medical profession should safeguard the public and itself against physicians deficient in moral character or professional competence. Physicians should observe all laws, uphold the dignity and honor of the profession and accept its self-imposed disciplines. They should expose, without hesitation, illegal or unethical conduct of fellow members of the profession.

Section 5
A physician may choose whom he will serve. In an emergency, however, he should render service to the best of his ability. Having undertaken the care of a patient, he may not neglect him; and unless he has been discharged he may discontinue his services only after giving adequate notice. He should not solicit patients.

Section 6
A physician should not dispose of his services under terms or conditions which tend to interfere with or impair the free and complete exercise of his medical judgment and skill or tend to cause a deterioration of the quality of medical care.

Section 7
In the practice of medicine a physician should limit the source of his professional income to medical services actually rendered by him, or under his supervision, to his patients. His fee should be commensurate with the services rendered and the patient's ability to pay. He should neither pay nor receive a commission for referral

* *Opinions and Reports of the Judicial Council.* Chicago: American Medical Association iii–vii (1969). Reprinted by permission.

of patients. Drugs, remedies or appliances may be dispensed or supplied by the physician provided it is in the best interests of the patient.

Section 8
A physician should seek consultation upon request; in doubtful or difficult cases; or whenever it appears that the quality of medical service may be enhanced thereby.

Section 9
A physician may not reveal the confidences entrusted to him in the course of medical attendance, or the deficiencies he may observe in the character of patients, unless he is required to do so by law or unless it becomes necessary in order to protect the welfare of the individual or of the community.

Section 10
The honored ideals of the medical profession imply that the responsibilities of the physician extend not only to the individual, but also to society where these responsibilities deserve his interest and participation in activities which have the purpose of improving both the health and the well-being of the individual and the community.

NOTE

AMERICAN MEDICAL ASSOCIATION
OPINIONS OF THE JUDICIAL COUNCIL RELATING
TO THE PRINCIPLES OF MEDICAL ETHICS*

*   *   *

Section 1—Opinion 5. Substitution of Surgeon without Patient's Knowledge or Consent

*   *   *

The surgeon's obligation to the patient requires him to perform the surgical operation: (1) within the scope of authority granted him by the consent to the operation; (2) in accordance with the terms of the contractual relationship; (3) with complete disclosure of all facts relevant to the need and the performance of the operation; and (4) to utilize his best skill in performing the operation.

*   *   *

---

* *Opinions and Reports of the Judicial Council.* Chicago: American Medical Association 5, 9, 55 (1969). Reprinted by permission.

Section 2—Opinion 2. Experimentation: New Drugs or Procedures [1946][†]

In order to conform to the ethics of the American Medical Association, three requirements must be satisfied in connection with the use of experimental drugs or procedures:
(1) the voluntary consent of the person on whom the experiment is to be performed should be obtained;
(2) the danger of each experiment must be previously investigated by animal experimentation; and
(3) the experiment must be performed under proper medical protection and management.

*   *   *

Section 9—Opinion 2. Prognosis

The physician should neither exaggerate nor minimize the gravity of a patient's condition. He should assure himself that the patient, his relatives or his responsible friends have such knowledge of the patient's condition as will serve the best interests of the patient and the family.

d.
American Psychological Association Ethical Standards of Psychologists*

The psychologist believes in the dignity and worth of the individual human being. He is committed to increasing man's understanding of himself and others. While pursuing this endeavor, he protects the welfare of any person who may seek his service or of any subject, human or animal, that may be the object of his study. He does not use his professional position or relationships, nor does he knowingly permit his own services to be used by others, for purposes inconsistent with these values. While demanding for himself freedom of inquiry and communication, he accepts the responsibility this freedom confers: for competence where he claims it, for objectivity in the report of his findings, and for consideration of the best interests of his colleagues and of society.

[†] The opinion of the Judicial Council on the "Ethical Guidelines for Clinical Investigation" (1966) appears at pp. 845–846 *infra.*

* 18 *American Psychologist* 56–60 (1963). Reprinted by permission.

Specific Principles

Principle 1. Responsibility. The psychologist,[2] committed to increasing man's understanding of man, places high value on objectivity and integrity, and maintains the highest standards in the services he offers.

a. As a scientist, the psychologist believes that society will be best served when he investigates where his judgment indicates investigation is needed; he plans his research in such a way as to minimize the possibility that his findings will be misleading; and he publishes full reports of his work, never discarding without explanation data which may modify the interpretation of results.

* * *

Principle 6. Confidentiality. Safeguarding information about an individual that has been obtained by the psychologist in the course of his teaching, practice, or investigation is a primary obligation of the psychologist. Such information is not communicated to others unless certain important conditions are met.

a. Information received in confidence is revealed only after most careful deliberation and when there is clear and imminent danger to an individual or to society, and then only to appropriate professional workers or public authorities.

* * *

e. Only after explicit permission has been granted is the identity of research subjects published. When data have been published without permission for identification, the psychologist assumes responsibility for adequately disguising their sources.

f. The psychologist makes provisions for the maintenance of confidentiality in the preservation and ultimate disposition of confidential records.

* * *

Principle 16. Research Precautions. The psychologist assumes obligations for the welfare of his research subjects, both animal and human.

a. Only when a problem is of scientific significance and it is not practicable to investigate it in any other way is the psychologist justi-

fied in exposing research subjects, whether children or adults, to physical or emotional stress as part of an investigation.

b. When a reasonable possibility of injurious aftereffects exists, research is conducted only when the subjects or their responsible agents are fully informed of this possibility and agree to participate nevertheless.

c. The psychologist seriously considers the possibility of harmful aftereffects and avoids them, or removes them as soon as permitted by the design of the experiment.

d. A psychologist using animals in research adheres to the provisions of the Rules Regarding Animals, drawn up by the Committee on Precautions and Standards in Animal Experimentation, and adopted by the American Psychological Association.

e. Investigations of human subjects using experimental drugs (for example: hallucinogenic, psychotomimetic, psychedelic, or similar substances) should be conducted only in such settings as clinics, hospitals, or research facilities maintaining appropriate safeguards for the subjects.

* * *

NOTES

NOTE 1.

HENRY K. BEECHER
TENTATIVE STATEMENT OUTLINING THE
PHILOSOPHY AND ETHICAL PRINCIPLES
GOVERNING THE CONDUCT OF RESEARCH ON
HUMAN BEINGS AT THE HARVARD
MEDICAL SCHOOL*

* * *

The breaches of ethical conduct which have come to the personal attention of the writer are owing to ignorance or thoughtlessness. They were not of willful or unscrupulous origin. Basic considerations in human experimentation at Harvard are the same as they are everywhere: protection of the subject, protection of the investigator and protection of research and the institutions involved, and the sound development of medicine. These all require a levelheaded approach to experimentation in man. It is everywhere recognized that man is the final essential test site—the animal of necessity, so to speak, when it comes to the evaluation of new drugs and new procedures.

* * *

[2] A student of psychology who assumes the role of psychologist shall be considered a psychologist for the purpose of this code of ethics.

* Unpublished manuscript (undated). Printed by permission of the author who retains all rights.

The inescapable responsibility for determining what investigations may be done on a particular patient must rest with the investigator or physician concerned, bearing in mind that present-day specialization in medicine and complexity of procedures proposed or undertaken are frequently beyond the grasp of the subjects involved.

All of the so-called codes as guides to human experimentation emphasize the necessity that the experimenter be well trained and adequate as a scientist to undertake the study proposed. Medical research, when it involves treatment of any physical procedures beyond the simplest, requires that the investigator or his close associate be a qualified physician. No other profession gives such prerogatives and no other profession, probably, presents such a generally high level of unselfishness and compassion in directly caring for the sick or in planning procedures for the future. Of the qualities of the investigators, unselfishness is the most important for subject and project alike. Imagination, objectivity, and the power to generalize soundly are all essential. In the forefront of the qualities which lead to protection of subject and patient in investigation is a deep sense of responsibility on the part of the investigator, coupled with unselfishness and a keen and well-trained intelligence.

NOTE 2.

WALTER MODELL
COMMENT ON "SOME FALLACIES AND ERRORS"*

*   *   *

. . . I suspect that every species of ostrich selects its own kind of sand to stick its head into. Here is how I do it. I bury my head in my notions of the status of medicine in modern Western culture and of the nature of the license given the physician by society (and as you will recall, medicine has a place close to religion in virtually all cultures). I then choose to believe this covers both categories of consent, the straightforward as well as for the experiment which does not benefit the subject.

It is my feeling that Western civilization accepts medicine as an experimental discipline and that, in expecting it to continue to grow, to be a progressive science, as against the attitudes of the medicine man whose incantations and medicaments were not expected to nor designed for change, an acceptance of the trial of the new and the search for the better is implicit. I also think that when society confers the degree of physician on a man it instructs him to experiment on his fellow. I think that when a patient goes to a modern physician for treatment, regardless of whether he consciously consents to it, he is also unconsciously presenting himself for the purpose of experimentation.

There is really nothing new in this. Modern society accepts this all the time. It is the nature of life in our time. When you become a passenger on a new airplane, you automatically become the subject of an experiment in modern travel. When you purchase your ticket you give consent; when society licenses the pilot, it instructs him to experiment with your life at stake. In this case, no one seems to worry about the ethical or philosophic implications. Nor do I see much difference in the ethics of experimentation between an old doctor trying a new drug on a patient or a new doctor trying an old one.

It is this kind of thinking that makes me feel that there is nothing that I, as an ostrich, can do to shelter or protect the end of me that is so openly exposed to attack. I am fully conscious of my responsibilities as well as the apparent arrogance of my attitude, but I also wonder whether I am not much more honest and even more humble about what I do than a practitioner who prescribes pills all day long thinking that he is not doing experiments and that he is not taking risks with his patients' lives without their explicit instruction. . . .

NOTE 3.

WALSH MCDERMOTT
OPENING COMMENTS ON THE CHANGING
MORES OF BIOMEDICAL RESEARCH*

When the needs of society come in head-on conflict with the rights of an individual, someone has to play God. We can avoid this responsibility so long as the power to decide the particular case-in-point is clearly vested in someone else, for example, a duly elected governmental official. But in clinical investigation, the power to determine this issue of "the individual versus society" is clearly vested in the physician. Both the power itself and, above all, *our awareness that we are wielding it* are increasing every day and can be expected to increase much further.

* 3 *Clinical Pharmacology and Therapeutics* 145, 146 (1962). Reprinted by permission.

* 67 *Annals of Internal Medicine,* Supplement 7: 39–42 (1967). Reprinted by permission.

It is this inescapable *awareness* that we are wielding power that has us so deeply troubled, for we are a generation nurtured on the slogan "the end does not justify the means" in matters concerning the individual and his society. Yet as a society we enforce the social good over the individual good across a whole spectrum of non-medical activities every day, and many of these activities ultimately affect the health or the life of an individual.

Traditionally in our Judeo-Christian culture we have handled this issue by one of two mechanisms. When, as in our racial problem for example, the conflict contains no built-in contradiction, we publicly and officially subscribe to a set of ideals. We can work privately and publicly toward the attainment of these ideals, and with their attainment would come the solution of the problem. This mechanism works when the forces in conflict are intrinsically reconcilable even though the reconciliation might take many decades or a century. But we use another mechanism when the conflict is head on, when the group interest and the individual interest are basically irreconcilable.

In circumstances like these, such as the decision to impose capital punishment or the selection of only a minority of our young men to become soldiers, the issue is decided by a judgment that is arbitrary as it affects the individual. In short, we play God. When we take away an individual's life or liberty by one of these arbitrary judgments we try to depersonalize the process by spreading responsibility for the decision throughout a framework of legal institutions. Thus, it is usually a jury, not a judge, that determines the death penalty; a local draft board, not a bureaucrat, that decides who goes to Vietnam. This second type of mechanism works only because there is widespread public acceptance that society has rights too, and that it is preferable that the power to enforce these rights over the rights of the individual be institutionalized.

I submit that the core of this ethical issue as it arises in clinical investigation lies in this second category—the one wherein, to ensure the rights of society, an arbitrary judgment must be made against an individual.

This is not to say that all ethical problems in clinical investigation fall into the irreconcilable category. On the contrary, in numerical terms most of them probably do not.

Without question, a considerable portion of the lapses in fully protecting individual rights in clinical investigation can be avoided by more careful and open attention to the subject and by our ingenuity in developing new practices to attain some of the same old ends. This will prove quite costly in financial terms, but what is being accomplished in this way is very much to the good and is to be strongly encouraged. But there remains that hard core of the problem: the kind of situation in which it clearly seems to be in the best interests of society that the information be obtained. It can be obtained only from studies on certain already unlucky individuals, and no convincing case can be made that they can expect much in the way of benefits except those accruing to them as members of society.

Clearly there are three questions here: (1) From where does society get its rights or interest that makes it imperative to perform biomedical studies on an individual? (2) how is the individual subject selected? and (3) how are the social priorities decided?

The social priorities are easy; any small group of certified medical statesmen can settle them in an afternoon. As we all know, however, it is the other two questions that are so thorny.

Without too deep reflection it seems to me that society's actually having a right here is a relatively new phenomenon that is chiefly derived from the demonstration that knowledge gained by studies in a few humans can show us how to operate programs of great practical benefit to the group. Until the late nineteenth century, as I understand it, most human experimentation expanded knowledge but did not increase the power to control disease. The physicians of that day thus had no problem in maintaining the double ethical charge still preserved in the Helsinki Declaration: to "safeguard the health of the people," on the one hand, and to make the health of "my patient" the first consideration, on the other hand. But starting, I suppose, with the yellow fever studies in Havana, we have seen large social payoffs from certain experiments in humans, and there is no reason to doubt that the process could continue. It is by this demonstration, analogous to the great "invention of invention" of Newton's era, that medicine has given to society the case for its rights in the continuation of clinical investigation. Once this demonstration was made, we could no longer maintain, in strict honesty, that in the study of disease the interests of the individual are invariably paramount.

Yet we are temperamentally incapable of

leaving it at that. Our reflex action here is to try to imitate what we do when the same conflict arises in irreconcilable form elsewhere in our society. That is to say, we are willing to concede that some judgments must be arbitrary, but we attempt to clothe them with institutional forms so that at least the judgments are not made solely by one person. We will play God, but we would like to do it by group effort.

I am deeply convinced that such efforts provide no real solution because our culture has not yet faced up to the irreconcilable nature of the conflict at the heart of this particular issue. And until it does so, there exists no recognized consensus or article in the "social contract," if you will, to provide that base on which any law or regulation must rest if it is to be viable.

Conventional juridical procedures including the traditional jury system are too slow to fit the urgent nature of many clinical decisions. [B]y the terms of our culture, as may be seen in the Declaration of Helsinki, no matter who the investigator takes into partnership when he acts, he acts alone.

What can we do to solve this agonizing dilemma? Obviously we cannot convene a constitutional convention of the Judeo-Christian culture and add a few amendments to it. Yet, in a figurative sense, until we can do something very much like that, I believe deeply that the problem, at its roots, is unsolvable and that we must continue to live with it.

To be sure, by careful attention we can cut down the number of instances in which the problem presents itself to us in its starkest form. But there is no escape from the fact that, if the future good of society is to be served, there will be times when the clinical investigator must make an arbitrary judgment with respect to an individual. The necessity for such arbitrary judgments has had *tacit* social recognition and approval for some time. Because the approval *was* tacit, however, there was an imbalance of actions and words, in effect, a hypocrisy, that marvelous human invention by which we are enabled to adapt to problems judged to be not yet ripe for solution. By this hypocrisy society had its future medical interests fully protected. At the same time the attitude could be maintained that in medical matters, *as contrasted with those in many other walks of life,* the sole public interest was in the inviolability of the individual.

Now, most unfortunately, these essentially harmless hypocrisies of our culture have been codified. For the Helsinki Declaration . . . if

. . . followed to the letter . . . would produce the curious situation in which the only stated public interest is that of the individual. The future interest of society and its sometime conflict with the interest of the individual, in effect, are ignored. I believe it has been most unwise to try to extend the principle of "a government of laws and not men" into areas of such great ethical subtlety as clinical investigation.

When in our cultural evolution it has not yet been possible to develop an institutional framework for a particular kind of arbitrary decision that may affect an individual, there is only one basis on which to proceed, and that is on the basis of trust. My position may sound paternalistic, as indeed it is. Making arbitrary decisions concerning an individual in conflicts as yet unsolved by our society is one of the major responsibilities of a parent.

Society may not have given us a clear blueprint for clinical investigation, but it has long since given us immense trust to handle moral dilemmas of other sorts, including many in which, in effect, we have to play God. Thus, the moral dilemma of clinical investigation is not something new; what is new about the problem is its rapid increase in size. This rapid increase in size is no help to us now, but it may hasten the day, still far off, when in medical investigations we can institutionalize this making of arbitrary decisions between an individual and his society.

In the meantime we can do no more than carry on under the mantle of the trust we now possess. To continue to receive that trust we must be ever conscious that the issue of the individual vis-à-vis society is always *there,* and we can try our best to create an environment of awareness of it on our clinical services. For once a moral dilemma has become clearly recognized; whenever each person acts within that dilemma, his act can be seen for what it is, and the extent to which he has seemed to act with acceptable propriety can be judged.

But the hard core of our moral dilemma will not yield to the approaches of "Declarations" or "Regulations"; for as things stand today such statements must completely ignore the fact that society, too, has rights in human experimentation. Somehow, somewhere, in this question of human experimentation, as in so many other aspects of our society, we will have to learn how to institutionalize "playing God" while still maintaining the key elements of a free society.

*   *   *

NOTE 4.

HOWARD S. BECKER
AGAINST THE CODE OF ETHICS*

Sociologists face moral problems in every sphere of their lives. Most of these problems are shared with all men, many only with those who teach and do research, and relatively few with social scientists alone. To be of any use, a Code of Ethics for the American Sociological Association must deal successfully with the moral problems generic to social science. But these are precisely the problems dealt with least adequately by the draft code of ethics.

In dealing with general academic problems, the draft code can, for example, assert without equivocation that a professor should not appear as principal author of an article based on his student's dissertation. But in areas most characteristic of social science, the draft code cannot be as forthright. It cannot, for example, say that undercover research roles are not justified: it must equivocate by adding "unless they are clearly the only feasible means for reaching important scientific goals." Such equivocation only moves the problem back to a consideration of whether the scientific goals are important enough or truly cannot be reached in any other way, and helps us little.

The code is equivocal or unenlighteningly vague in dealing with most of the problems distinct to social science. This is so in spite of the intelligence and energy of the Committee on Ethics. It is so because there is no consensus about such problems; many sociologists would disagree with any more forthright statement in either direction.

The moral issues of our work, however, are important and deserve attention. I believe that they should be debated freely and fully rather than be obscured behind over-general "principles." I therefore wish to recommend that instead of adopting a code of ethics, the Association officially sponsor a symposium on the ethical problems characteristic of sociology.

Subsequently, the Association should undertake to publish the symposium, not as official doctrine, but as official recognition that ethical problems exist and that there are a number of ways of interpreting and coping with them. This would substantially advance our understanding of the complex moral issues of our craft.

*   *   *

* 29 American Sociological Review 409–410 (1964). Reprinted by permission.

NOTE 5.

JAY KATZ
THE EDUCATION OF
THE PHYSICIAN-INVESTIGATOR*

. . . The problems confronting modern medicine are the result not so much of the increase in research activities, but of the awareness that research and therapy, pursuit of knowledge and treatment, are not separate but intertwined. Therefore, the focus on experimentation and the concomitant emphasis on "informed consent" created new difficulties not merely because of the requirement to inform patient-subjects about proposed research, but also because consent raised troublesome questions about what all patients should be told about medical interventions.

It is a task of medical education to teach students how to deal with these emerging problems. Yet we have not explored in a systematic fashion whether education can serve medicine well as a method of control. I have often wondered how and by whom the Nazi concentration-camp experiments would have been conducted had the physician's responsibilities toward his patient-subject been exposed to careful scrutiny in the medical education of the nineteenth and early-twentieth centuries. The Nazi studies, despite opinions to the contrary, had their antecedents. There are, for example, reports of French and German experiments in which cancer tissue surgically removed from one diseased breast was transplanted into the apparently healthy other breast or experiments with variola vaccine performed on children in Sweden about which the experimenter commented that "perhaps I should have first experimented upon animals, but calves—most suitable for these purposes—were difficult to obtain because of their cost and their keep."

In my own medical education I have never forgotten Conrad Wesselhoeft's brilliant lecture on "The Care of the Patient." I turned over in my mind again and again one story he told— probably because its "lesson" did not satisfy me, though I was not aware of it then. He related one of his first experiences as a house officer. A patient with appendicitis had come to the emergency room and Dr. Wesselhoeft, once having made the diagnosis, recommended immedi-

* 98 Daedalus 480, 484–487 (1969). Reprinted by permission of Daedalus, Journal of the American Academy of Arts and Sciences, Boston, Massachusetts.

ate surgery. The patient pleaded an important business engagement and asked that the operation be postponed for a few hours. Dr. Wesselhoeft reluctantly agreed and eventually the operation was successfully performed by him. That evening, at dinner, he related the story and noticed that his father, an eminent physician of his day, looked increasingly disturbed and did not say a word beyond sternly telling him: "Conrad, I want to see you in my study after dinner." There he chided his son severely for having taken too lightly his medical responsibilities by giving his patient leave for a few hours. Young Dr. Wesselhoeft felt that he had learned an important lesson that he wished to communicate to us. But what was the lesson? As I remember, he did not answer this question because it seemed so obvious.

I believe that I now know what troubled me then. Traditionally the concept of medical responsibility has been defined as responsibility for the patient's well-being. While such a definition could encompass, within the context of a medical relationship, concern for the patient's total functioning—physical, psychological, social, economic, spiritual—it is often limited to physical aspects. In order to exercise this more limited responsibility, patients must be carefully diagnosed, given the best treatment for their condition, and not be abandoned. Many students learn well to fulfill these obligations.[20] But there are other aspects to medical responsibility, and the controversy about what to disclose to patient-subjects in investigative settings has put one of them into sharper perspective—namely, the dialogue that should be pursued with the patient about treatment or no treatment or available alternative treatments in light of the risks, benefits, and prognosis as well as the totality of the

patient's life situation. Put another way, so long as medical responsibility primarily addressed itself to dispensing physical benefits, it was easier to view the physician as the sole decision-maker. Once physical benefits are placed in the web of the patient's total situation, the patient may have to be given a greater role in the decision-making process.

Not only does modern medicine command extensive therapeutic options—each with its known and unknown risks and benefits—but almost daily new therapeutic possibilities are introduced that have not yet met the test of time. Moreover, physicians are much more critical than they used to be about the efficacy of their therapeutic interventions. These considerations raise questions about the extent to which patients should participate in decisions affecting their health. To return briefly to Dr. Wesselhoeft's father, why did he seem so convinced that his son had not behaved with the utmost sense of professional responsibility?

Since medical experimentation is generally conducted with patients, the emphasis on "informed consent" raises questions about the nature of the dialogue between physicians and patients with respect to all interventions. This component of professional responsibility has not received the systematic attention it deserves. In medical commentary on professional responsibility, considerable agreement exists on the extent and limits of permissible physical interventions, but there is less consensus on or little systematic exploration into the dialogue that should take place between physicians and their patients. The Hippocratic Oath is silent on this point; it merely states that "I will follow that system of regimen which according to my ability and judgment, I consider for the benefit of my patients, and abstain from whatever is deleteri-

<hr>

[20] Becker and his associates, on the basis of detailed observations of an entire medical school class, have described the development of the "responsibility perspective." They state that "basically the term [responsibility] refers to the archetypal feature of medical practice: the physician who holds his patient's fate in his hands and on whom the patient's life and death may depend." While concern with his "fate" could include the patient's entire functioning, the authors note that "two areas of activity seem most involved with questions of medical responsibility. The first consists . . . of arriving at a correct diagnosis on the basis of a thorough and accurate examination. . . . The second activity consists of performing diagnostic and therapeutic procedures containing some element of danger to the patient." The accompanying interview material sug-

gests that in these two activities concern for physical well-being is of primary or exclusive importance and that this aspect of medical responsibility is presented well and in great detail. In contrast, other aspects seem to be neglected. I found only one reference to the problem of disclosure. A student asked what to tell patients "who would die very shortly of an inoperable tumor. . . . The staff member gave a long and complex answer, pointing out that frequently patients figure it out for themselves, or on the other hand, didn't want to know anything about it. In either case the physician had no decision to make about whether to tell or not." See H. S. Becker, B. Geer, E. C. Hughes, and A. L. Strauss, *Boys in White* (Chicago: University of Chicago Press, 1961).

ous and mischievous." Dr. Thomas Percival, whose book *Medical Ethics* influenced profoundly the subsequent codifications of medical ethics in England and the United States, only commented once and in a very restricted fashion on the discourse between physicians and patients:

> A physician should not be forward to make gloomy prognostications, because they savor of empiricism, by magnifying the importance of his services in the treatment or care of disease. But he should not fail, on proper occasions, to give to the friends of the patient, timely notice of danger, when it really occurs, and *even* to the patient himself, *if absolutely necessary* [emphasis supplied].

Nowhere in his detailed book, which carries the subtitle "A Code of Institutes and Precepts, Adapted to the Professional Conduct of Physicians and Surgeons," does Percival discuss the obligations of physicians to inform patients about the nature, purposes, and risks of therapeutic interventions. Nor does he comment on when a patient's consent should be obtained prior to a therapeutic intervention. Such omissions suggest

that Percival did not consider this issue important. And subsequent codes and commentaries by the American Medical Association have similarly treated this problem, if at all, briefly and without any elaboration.

These considerations put in question statements by commentators that experimental subjects are best safeguarded by the ethical training which investigators have received in their prior education as physicians. If disclosure and consent are posited as important problems for medical research, these commentators forgot to realize that physicians could not draw on systematic prior training. In an article on "Ethics and Clinical Research," Henry Beecher concluded that while "it is absolutely essential to strive" for informed consent, a "more reliable safeguard [in experimentation is] provided by the presence of an intelligent, informed, conscientious, compassionate, responsible investigator." One cannot quarrel with such a prescription, but has medicine trained physicians to analyze the complex and conflicting issues that medical decisionmaking often entails?

*   *   *

CHAPTER SIX

What Consequences to Subjects Should Affect the Authority of the Investigator?

This chapter examines those research conditions which give rise to tension between the actions of the investigator and the rights and interests of the subject. Since a primary concern in research is the protection of subjects against harm, our first analytic task is to specify the categories of harm which can result from experimental interventions. We have identified three major interests of the subject which, if interfered with, may cause him harm: (1) self-determination and privacy, (2) psychological integrity, and (3) physical integrity.

Though the categories of harm overlap, we treat them separately to highlight the distinctive problems which arise from each. For example, interferences with a subject's psychological or physical integrity may also violate his primary right to privacy and self-determination. Thus, experiments which employ deception may not only cause psychological harm but may also invade the subject's right to privacy and self-determination if he suffers unanticipated psychological exposure. Furthermore, we give special attention to interferences with self-determination because they are frequently overlooked in analyses of harm which have emphasized actual physical or psychological injury and neglected the impact of undisclosed manipulation. Accordingly, we include in the section on interferences with self-determination and privacy those interactions in which the subjects remain partially or completely uninformed about the nature, the impact, or even the existence of the investigation.

The remaining studies emphasize interferences with the subjects' psychological and physical integrity. Though in most of these instances the subjects were also unaware of some or all of the conditions inherent in the investigation, this is not an inevitable concomitant of these categories.

Clearly, a central task is to determine what actually constitutes harm. It has been argued that the minor risks or inconveniences to which some subjects are exposed do not rise to the level of harm and that in the absence of "direct personal injury" to subjects an investigator should be permitted to proceed on his own initiative. Alternatively it has been suggested that even if an experiment involves substantial risks, the investigator is still best situated to weigh those risks against the benefits which the research may provide. In any event, whatever the authority of the investigator, criteria for identifying the nature and extent of harm need to be articulated.

Once categories of harm have been identified, we turn to other elements of experimental objectives and design which may bear on extending or limiting the investigator's authority. We present ten such factors. Some focus on the investigator, such as his values, his attitude toward and method of selecting subjects, and the limitations on his ability to predict the consequences of his work. Others are addressed to the subject's role in the process: whether he is made aware of his participation in an experiment and of the risks and manipulation involved, as well as whether the experiment benefits him. Finally, we consider the impact of the pursuit of knowledge and other professional and societal interests on the investigator's authority. The relevance of these factors must be appraised separately for each category of harm and evaluated in terms of their bearing on the decisions that have to be made at each stage—formulation, administration, and review—in the human experimentation process.

Commentators on research with human beings disagree about the extent to which decisions about experimentation can be left to the discretion of investigators. The materials in this and the succeeding chapter delineate the investigator's values and specify those factors which he is best, and least, able to evaluate alone. Accordingly, they provide a basis for deciding when others, besides the investigator, ought to make decisions about human experimentation.

In examining these materials consider the following questions:

1. Do the categories of harm—interferences with self-determination, privacy, psychological integrity, and physical integrity—draw meaningful distinctions, and do they suggest different consequences for the authority of the investigator?

2. For each category of harm, whenever relevant, how should the authority of the investigator be affected by:

(a) The degree of harm—*e.g.*, slight, moderate or severe; reversible or irreversible?

(b) The type of harm—*e.g.*, to body, emotions, conduct, character, personal and societal values, dignity, anonymity, or reputation?

(c) The explanation of harm—*e.g.*, disclosure or nondisclosure about being a participant or about specific aspects of the design?

(d) The balancing of harm—*e.g.*, against benefits to subject, science, or society?

(e) The recipients of harm—*e.g.,* subjects who are considered worthy, inferior, normal, or deviant?

(f) The awareness of harm—*e.g.,* the ability to know, predict, and comprehend consequences?

3. For each element in the previous question, what difference does it make if the subject accepts the harm?

A.
What Constitutes Harm?

1.

Interferences with Self-Determination and Privacy

a.

Unawareness about Being a Participant in Research*

[i]
*Laud Humphreys
Tearoom Trade—
Impersonal Sex in Public Places†*

The methods employed in this study of men who engage in restroom sex are the outgrowth of three ethical assumptions: First, I do not believe the social scientist should ever ignore or avoid an area of research simply because it is difficult or socially sensitive. Second, he should approach any aspect of human behavior with those means that least distort the observed phenomena. Third, he must protect respondents from harm—regardless of what such protection may cost the researcher.

Because the majority of arrests on homosexual charges in the United States result from encounters in public restrooms, I felt this form of sexual behavior to provide a legitimate, even essential, topic for sociological investigation. In our society the social control forces, not the criminologist, determine what the latter shall study.

Following this decision, the question is one of choosing research methods which permit the

investigator to achieve maximum fidelity to the world he is studying. I believe ethnographic methods are the only truly empirical ones for the social scientist. When human behavior is being examined, systematic observation is essential; so I had to become a participant-observer of furtive, felonious acts.

Fortunately, the very fear and suspicion of tearoom participants produces a mechanism that makes such observation possible: a third man (generally one who obtains voyeuristic pleasure from his duties) serves as a lookout, moving back and forth from door to windows. Such a "watchqueen," as he is labeled in the homosexual argot, coughs when a police car stops nearby or when a stranger approaches. He nods affirmatively when he recognizes a man entering as being a "regular." Having been taught the watchqueen role by a cooperating respondent, I played that part faithfully while observing hundreds of acts of fellatio.

* * *

Although primarily interested in the stigmatized behavior, I also wanted to know about the men who take such risks for a few moments of impersonal sex. . . .

* * *

How could I approach these covert deviants for interviews? By passing as deviant, I had observed their sexual behavior without disturbing it. Now, I was faced with interviewing these men (often in the presence of their wives) without destroying them.

* * *

To overcome the danger of having a subject recognize me as a watchqueen, I changed my hair style, attire and automobile. At the risk of losing more transient respondents, I waited a

---
* For examples from medicine, see The Jewish Chronic Disease Hospital Case, pp. 9–65 *supra* and H. K. Beecher: Ethics and Clinical Research, pp. 307–310 *supra.*
† 7 *Trans-action* 15 (January 1970). Reprinted by permission.

year between the sample gathering and the interviews, during which time I took notes on their homes and neighborhoods and acquired data on them from the city and county directories.

* * *

This study, then, results from a confluence of strategies: systematic, first-hand observation, in-depth interviews with available respondents, the use of archival data, and structured interviews of a representative sample and a matched control group. At each level of research, I applied those measures which provided maximum protection for research subjects and the truest measurement of persons and behavior observed.

NOTES

NOTE 1.

NICHOLAS VON HOFFMAN
SOCIOLOGICAL SNOOPERS*

We're so preoccupied with defending our privacy against insurance investigators, dope sleuths, counterespionage men, divorce detectives and credit checkers, that we overlook the social scientists behind the hunting blinds who're also peeping into what we thought were our most private and secret lives. But they are there, studying us, taking notes, getting to know us, as indifferent as everybody else to the feeling that to be a complete human involves having an aspect of ourselves that's unknown.

If there was any doubt about there being somebody who wants to know about anything any other human being might be doing it is cancelled out in the latest issue of *Trans-action,* a popular but respected sociological monthly. The lead article, entitled "Impersonal Sex in Public Places," is a resumé of a study done about the nature and pattern of homosexual activities in men's rooms. Laud Humphreys, the author, is an Episcopal priest, a duly pee-aich-deed sociologist, holding the rank of assistant professor at Southern Illinois University.

* * *

Most of the people Humphreys observed and took notes on had no idea what he was doing or that they, in disguised form, would be showing up in print at some time in the future. Of

* *The Washington Post* B1, col. 1; B9, col. 5 (January 30, 1970). Reprinted by permission. © 1970, The Washington Post.

all the men he studied only a dozen were ever told what his real purpose was, yet as a sociologist he had to learn about the backgrounds and vital facts of the other tearoom visitors he'd seen. To do this Humphreys noted their license numbers and by tracing their cars learned their identities. He then allowed time to pass, disguised himself and visited these men under the color of doing a different, more innocuous door-to-door survey.

* * *

Humphreys said that he did everything possible to make sure the names of the men whose secrets he knew would never get out: "I kept only one copy of the master list of names and that was in a safe deposit box. I did all the transcribing of taped interviews myself and changed all identifying marks and signs. In one instance, I allowed myself to be arrested rather than let the police know what I was doing and the kind of information I had."

Even so, it remains true that he collected information that could be used for blackmail, extortion, and the worst kind of mischief without the knowledge of the people involved. *Trans-action* defends the ethics of Humphreys' methodology on the basis of purity of motive and the argument that he was doing it for a good cause, that is getting needed, reliable information about a difficult and painful social problem.

Everybody who goes snooping around and spying on people can be said to have good motives. The people whom Sen. Sam Ervin is fighting, the ones who want to give the police the right to smash down your door without announcing who they are if they think you have pot in your house, believe they are well motivated. They think they are preventing young people from destroying themselves. J. Edgar Hoover unquestionably believes he's protecting the country against subversion when he orders your telephone tapped. Those who may want to overthrow the government are just as well motivated by their lights. Since everybody can be said to be equally well motivated, it's impossible to form a judgment on what people do by assessing their intentions.

To this Laud Humphreys replies that his methods were less objectionable than getting his data by working through the police: "You do walk a really perilous tightrope in regard to ethical matters in studies like this, but, unless someone will walk it, the only source of information will be the police department, and that's dangerous for a society. The methods I used were the least intrusive possible. Oh, I could have hidden in the ceiling as the police do, but then I would have been an accomplice in what they were doing."

*   *   *

Incontestably such information is useful to parents, teen-agers themselves, to policemen, legislators and many others, but it was done by invading some people's privacy. This newspaper could probably learn a lot of things that the public has a right and need to know if its reporters were to use disguises and the gimmickry of modern, transistorized, domestic espionage, but there is a policy against it. No information is valuable enough to obtain by nipping away at personal liberty, and that is true no matter who's doing the gnawing, John Mitchell and the conservatives over at the Justice Department or Laud Humphreys and the liberals over at the Sociology Department.

NOTE 2.
IRVING LOUIS HOROWITZ AND LEE RAINWATER
JOURNALISTIC MORALIZERS*

Columnist Nicholas Von Hoffman's quarrel with Laud Humphreys' "Impersonal Sex in Public Places" starkly raises an issue that has grown almost imperceptibly over the last few years, and now threatens to create in the next decade a tame sociology to replace the fairly robust one that developed during the sixties. . . .

*   *   *

Sociologists have tended to assume that well-intentioned people fully accept the desirability of demystification of human life and culture. In the age of Aquarius, however, perhaps such a view will be recognized as naive.

"They are there, studying us, taking notes, getting to know us, as indifferent as everybody else to the feeling that to be a complete human involves having an aspect of ourselves that's unknown." Von Hoffman seems to mean this to be a statement about the right to privacy in a legal sense, but it really represents a denial of the ability of people to understand themselves and each other in an existential sense. This denial masks a fear, not that intimate details of our lives will be revealed to *others,* but rather that

we may get to know *ourselves* better and have to confront what up to now we did not know about ourselves. Just as psychoanalysis was a scientific revolution as threatening to traditional conceptions as those of Galileo and Kepler had been, it may well be that the sociologist's budding ability to say something about the how's and why's of men's relationships to each other is deeply threatening not only to the established institutions in society, but also in a more personal way to all members of society.

*   *   *

Von Hoffman recognizes that his most appealing charge has to do with privacy, and so he makes much of the fact that Humphreys' collected information that could be used for "blackmail, extortion, and the worst kind of mischief without the knowledge of the people involved."

Here his double standard is most glaringly apparent. Journalists routinely, day in, day out, collect information that could be used for "blackmail, extortion, and the worst kind of mischief without the knowledge of the people involved." But von Hoffman knows that the purpose of their work is none of those things, and so long as their information is collected from public sources, I assume he wouldn't attack them. Yet he nowhere compares the things sociologists do with the things his fellow journalists do. Instead, he couples Humphreys' "snooping around," "spying on people" with similarly "well-motivated" invaders of privacy as J. Edgar Hoover and John Mitchell.

To say the least, the comparison is invidious; the two kinds of enterprises are fundamentally different. No police group seeks to acquire information about people with any other goal than that of, in some way, prosecuting them. Policemen collect data, openly or under cover, in order to put someone in jail. Whatever it is, the sociological enterprise is not that. Sociologists are not interested in directly affecting the lives of the particular people they study. They are interested in those individuals only as representatives of some larger aggregate—in Humphreys' case, all participants in the tearoom action. Therefore, in almost all sociological research, the necessity to preserve the anonymity of the respondent is not an onerous one, because no purpose at all would be served by identifying the respondents.

*   *   *

* 7 *Trans-action* 5–8 (May 1970). Reprinted by permission.

Von Hoffman's points are: that in studying the sexual behavior of men in restrooms, Humphreys violated their rights to intimacy and privacy; that the homosexuals were and remain unaware of the true purpose of Humphreys' presence as a lookout; and that in the follow-up questionnaire the researcher further disguised himself and the true nature of his inquiry. For von Hoffman the point of principle is this: that although Humphreys' intent may have been above reproach and that in point of fact his purposes are antithetical to those of the police and other public officials, he nonetheless in his own way chipped away at the essential rights of individuals in conducting his investigations. Therefore, the ends, the goals, however noble and favorable to the plight of sexual deviants, do not justify the use of any means that further undermine personal liberties. Let us respond to these propositions as directly as possible.

First, the question of the invasion of privacy has several dimensions. We have already noted the public rather than the private nature of park restrooms. It further has to be appreciated that all participants in sexual activities in restrooms run the constant risk that they have among them people who have ulterior purposes. The vocabulary of motives is surely not limited or circumscribed by one man doing research but is as rich and as varied as the number of participants themselves. The fact that in this instance there was a scientific rather than a sexual or criminal "ulterior motive" does not necessarily make it more hideous or more subject to criticism, but perhaps less so.

Second, the question of disguising "the true nature" and purpose of this piece of research has to be put into some perspective. To begin with, let us assume that the research was worth doing in the first place. We know almost nothing about impersonal sex in public places, and the fact that we know so little has in no small way contributed to the fact that the cops feel that *they* know all that needs to be known about the matter. Who, then, is going to gather this countervailing knowledge? . . . Moreover, to assume that the investigator must share all of his knowledge with those being investigated also assumes a common universe of discourse very rarely found in any kind of research, much less the kind involving sexual deviance. Furthermore, the conduct of Humphreys' follow-up inquiries had to be performed with tact and with skill precisely because he discovered that so many of the people in his survey were married men

and family men. Indeed, one of the great merits of Humphreys' research is that it reveals clearly etched class, ethnic, political and occupational characteristics of sexual participants never before properly understood. Had he not conducted the follow-up interviews, we would once again be thrown back on simpleminded, psychological explanations that are truly more voyeuristic than analytic, or on the policeman's kind of knowledge. It is the sociological dimensions of sexuality in public places that make this a truly scientific breakthrough.

To take on the ethic of full disclosure at the point of follow-up interviews was impossible given the purposes of the research. If Humphreys had told his respondents that he knew they were tearoom participants, most of them would have cooperated. But in gaining their cooperation in this way he would have had to reveal that he knew of their behavior. This he could not responsibly do, because he could not control the potentially destructive impact of that knowledge. . . . Therefore, the posture of Humphreys toward those interviewed must be viewed as humane and considerate.

But what von Hoffman is arguing is that this research ought not to have been done, that Humphreys should have laid aside his obligation to society as a sociologist and taken more seriously his obligation to society as a citizen. Von Hoffman maintains that the researcher's intentions—the pursuit of truth, the creation of countervailing knowledge, the demystification of shadowy areas of human experience—are immaterial.

*   *   *

The only interesting issue raised by von Hoffman is one that he cannot, being a moralizer, do justice to. It is whether the work one does is good, and whether the good it does outweighs the bad. "No information," he writes, "is valuable enough to obtain by nipping away at personal liberty. . . ." It remains to be proven that Humphreys did in fact nip away at anyone's liberty; so far we have only von Hoffman's assertions that he did and Humphreys' assurance that he did not. But no amount of self-righteous dogmatizing can still the uneasy and troublesome thought that what we have here is not a conflict between nasty snoopers and the right to privacy, but a conflict between two goods: the right to privacy and the right to know.

What is required is a distinction between the responsibilities of social scientists to seek and to obtain greater knowledge and the responsibilities of the legal system to seek and obtain maximum security for the private rights of private citizens. . . .

It is certainly not that sociologists should deliberately violate any laws of the land, only that they should leave to the courtrooms and to the legislatures just what interpretation of these laws governing the protection of private citizens is to be made. . . . The really tough moral problem is that the idea of an inviolable right of privacy may move counter to the belief that society is obligated to secure the other rights and welfare of its citizenry. Indeed one might say that this is a key contradiction in the contemporary position of the liberal: he wants to protect the rights of private citizens, but at the same time he wants to develop a welfare system that could hardly function without at least some knowledge about these citizens.

* * *

NOTE 3.

PAVESICH V. NEW ENGLAND LIFE INSURANCE CO. 122 GA. 190, 193–198, 50 S.E. 68, 69–71 (1905)

COBB. J. . . . The question . . . to be determined is whether an individual has a right of privacy which he can enforce, and which the courts will protect against invasion. It is to be conceded that prior to 1890 every adjudicated case, both in this country and in England, which might be said to have involved a right of privacy, was not based upon the existence of such right, but was founded upon a supposed right of property, or a breach of trust or confidence, or the like, and that therefore a claim to a right of privacy, independent of a property or contractual right, or some right of a similar nature, had, up to that time, never been recognized in terms in any decision. . . . The individual surrenders to society many rights and privileges which he would be free to exercise in a state of nature, in exchange for the benefits which he receives as a member of society. But he is not presumed to surrender all those rights, and the public has no more right, without his consent, to invade the domain of those rights which it is necessarily to be presumed he has reserved, than he has to violate the valid regulations of the organized government under which he lives. The right of privacy has its foundation in the instincts of nature. It is recognized intuitively, consciousness being the witness that can be called to establish its existence. Any person whose intellect is in a normal condition recognizes at once that as to each individual member of society there are matters private, and there are matters public so far as the individual is concerned. Each individual as instinctively resents any encroachment by the public upon his rights which are of a private nature as he does the withdrawal of those of his rights which are of a public nature. A right of privacy in matters purely private is therefore derived from the natural law. . . . It is one of those rights referred to by some law writers as "absolute"—"such as would belong to their persons merely in a state of nature, and which every man is entitled to enjoy, whether out of society or in it."—Blackstone 123.

. . . An individual has a right to enjoy life in any way that may be most agreeable and pleasant to him, according to his temperament and nature, provided that in such enjoyment he does not invade the rights of his neighbor, or violate public law or policy. The right of personal security is not fully accorded by allowing an individual to go through life in possession of all of his members, and his body unmarred; nor is his right to personal liberty fully accorded by merely allowing him to remain out of jail, or free from other physical restraints. The liberty which he derives from natural law, and which is recognized by municipal law, embraces far more than freedom from physical restraint. The term *liberty* is not to be so dwarfed, "but is deemed to embrace the right of a man to be free in the enjoyment of the faculties with which he has been endowed by his Creator, subject only to such restraints as are necessary for the common welfare. . . ."

* * *

[A]ncient law recognized that a person had a legal right "to be let alone," so long as he was not interfering with the rights of other individuals or of the public. This idea has been carried into the common law, and appears from time to time in various places. . . . "Eavesdroppers, or such as listen under walls or windows or the eaves of a house to hearken after discourse, and thereupon to frame slanderous and mischievous tales," were a nuisance at common law, and indictable, and were required, in the discretion of the court, to find sureties for their good behavior. (4 Blackstone 168.) The offense consisted in lingering about dwelling houses and other places where persons meet for private intercourse, and listening to what is said, and then tattling it abroad. . . . Instances might be multiplied where the common law has both tacitly and expressly recognized the right of an individual to repose and privacy. . . .

*   *   *

NOTE 4.

EDWARD A. SHILS
SOCIAL INQUIRY AND THE AUTONOMY
OF THE INDIVIDUAL*

*   *   *

The respect for privacy rests on the appreciation of human dignity, with its high evaluation of individual self-determination, free from the bonds of prejudice, passion, and superstition. In this, the respect for human dignity and individuality shares an historical comradeship with the freedom of scientific inquiry, which is equally precious to modern liberalism. The tension between these values, so essential to each other in so many profoundly important ways, is one of the antimonies of modern liberalism. The ethical problems with which we are dealing . . . arise from the confrontation of autonomy and privacy by a free intellectual curiosity, enriched by a modern awareness of the depth and complexity of the forces that work in us and implemented by the devices of a passionate effort to transform this awareness into scientific knowledge.

*   *   *

[ii]
*Mortimer A. Sullivan, Jr., Stuart A. Queen,
and Ralph C. Patrick, Jr.
Participant Observation as Employed in the
Study of a Military Training Program*†

Until recently the Air Force included in its research and development planning an extensive social science program. This program, itself part of a larger and more elaborate organization devoted to the Air Force's personnel and training requirements, utilized in its studies classical experimental design, polling, the interview, and, occasionally, observation and the ethnographic or survey approach. There existed, however, certain aspects of the Air Force training situation which apparently could not adequately be understood through the use of these techniques. In particular, certain officers wished to gain a better notion of how basic and technical training were lived, understood, and felt by new airmen. Hence, after a year of preliminary study, a plan was drawn up and approved for the utilization of a participant observer.[1]

The general purpose of the study was to gain insight into the motivations and attitudes of personnel (in training) as reflected in both their military and social behavior. Through such insight into airmen's own views and feelings it was hoped to find leads to new ways of reducing disciplinary problems (particularly AWOL), failures in the course of training, poor performance thereafter, and non-re-enlistment. . . .

To accomplish this purpose it was decided that a research officer should "enlist" as a basic trainee. He would be a fullfledged member of the group under study, his identity, mission, and role as a researcher unknown to every one (except the investigators), even to his own commanding officer. This then became one of the few cases of real participant observation.

There were literally thousands of problems to overcome, not only in deciding how the study would be conducted, but also in determining how the participant-observer would be guided in his work, the things to be looked for or recorded if observed, the form reports should take, and how the data would be used after the study was completed. . . .

*   *   *

The preliminary arrangements for the "enlistment" of the observer and the recording and transporting of data were well taken care of by high-ranking Air Force personnel. The provost marshal of the command for which the study was undertaken worked closely with those primarily concerned in providing the needed support and information, and the Air Force's so-

* Daniel Lerner, ed.: *The Human Meaning of the Social Science.* New York: Meridian Books, Inc. 114, 120–121 (1959). © 1959 by the World Publishing Company. Reprinted by permission.

† 23 *American Sociological Review* 660–667 (1958). Reprinted by permission.

[1] Participant observation is defined by Florence R. Kluckhohn as ". . . conscious and systematic sharing, insofar as circumstances permit, in the life-activities and, on occasion, in the interests and affects of a group of persons. Its purpose is to obtain data about behavior through direct contact and in terms of specific situations in which the distortion that results from the investigator's being an outside agent is reduced to a minimum." "The Participant-Observer Technique in Small Communities," 46 *American Journal of Sociology* (November 1940), p. 331.

cial science agency which guided the study made available a capable member of its organization, a civilian sociologist, to oversee and coordinate the research.

* * *

In addition to the other team members, the provost marshal, and the Air Force's civilian sociologist, there were many individuals who contributed to the study. After the participant-observer left the South and arrived at the technical training base, he was told that an additional person had been informed of his presence and of his mission, a young chaplain who had had enlisted service in World War II and whose primary duty, in addition to ministerial responsibilities, was counseling newly arrived trainees. The chaplain contributed to the investigation not only through his familiarity with the training situation, but also by his personal interest in the problems of the observer. While the observer came to rely heavily upon the team for professional guidance whenever they met, he also depended upon the chaplain as his sole contact between meetings with the other team members.

The creation of a "new personality" for the observer was of some importance to the study. It would have been entirely possible for him to have "enlisted" and undergone training without disguising his name, age, or education. On the other hand, it appeared advantageous to provide the observer with an identity through which he might achieve a maximum of rapport with other trainees—most of whom, it was known, were under twenty years old and few of whom had any college education. . . .

For nine months before the beginning of the field study itself, the observer was coached in the ways of the adolescent subculture. A young airman was told the requirements of the study and given the job of creating a "new personality" for the observer. Dress, speech, and mannerism, as well as interests, attitudes, and general appearance were "corrected" by the observer's enthusiastic coach. . . . So successful was the airman's tutoring that when the time for "enlistment" arrived, the recruiting sergeant (who did not know of the study) suggested that the observer not be accepted by the Air Force because by all appearances he was a juvenile delinquent. . . .

* * *

In deliberately cultivating a second self the research observer was engaged in something su-

perficially like intelligence work or espionage. But there was a very important difference in goal for, in this case, it was a general understanding of a significant subculture, the processes of its development and transmission to new recruits, and its effect on the official training program. It was not the indictment of anybody or the immediate change of anyone's behavior. In fact, the data were so safeguarded that they could not lead to disciplinary action against any of the men under study. Neither was the objective a general indictment or defense of the Air Force. It was simply to gather a body of previously unavailable information and to interpret in it a way that might be helpful both to the military and to social scientists.

* * *

[T]he most interesting phenomenon to the participant-observer was the ease with which he was able to carry out his role with the other trainees. The men not only accepted him and his cover story, but identified many aspects of his past as being similar to their own lives. The observer shared the sorrows and hopes of the other trainees and felt compelled to do his best out of loyalty to them. When the others learned of "tricks" by which to pass inspections or to give the appearance of doing a job which they had actually not done, the observer joined in and suffered no guilt for doing what he, as an officer, knew was "wrong." The observer is convinced that his complete integration into the trainees' subculture was essential for understanding and conveying the attitudes and problems which he reported. However, he also attaches importance to the professional guidance given by the other team members and the counsel and reassurance which they and the chaplain offered.

* * *

. . . The method of participant observation was adopted in this case only after responsible Air Force personnel believed they had obtained about all they could from general observation, questionnaires, and formal interviews. In addition, they suspected that airmen, like other human beings, could and did maintain "false fronts," often deceiving officers, researchers, and perhaps themselves. Here seemed to be a new approach that might probe beneath the surface in a revealing way. . . .

* * *

NOTES

NOTE 1.

JULIUS A. ROTH
DANGEROUS AND DIFFICULT ENTERPRISE?*

The article on participant observation in a military program is remarkable to me in a number of respects.

For one thing, the authors make it sound as if the undercover type of participant observation is extremely rare. Yet, without any careful search, I can think of a number of studies of this type in recent years. There is Mann's article on the marine radioman, Caudill's study of the psychiatric patient's role, the book *Why Prophecy Fails* by Festinger, Riecken, and Schachter. A number of dissertations on occupational groups at the University of Chicago are based entirely or largely on information collected by students who worked at the job they studied without revealing their professional interest in their fellow workers. . . . Some of these people took their jobs mainly to make money to pay tuition and living expenses, and *then* decided to use the opportunity to collect data for a study of an occupation. But the priority of their other motives does not detract from the value of their observations. In my own current study of the social psychology of the treatment of tuberculosis, I have collected my most valuable data while a tuberculosis hospital patient and later as a tuberculosis hospital attendant, in each case keeping daily notes on my observations and experience without the knowledge of the persons [being observed].

In the second place, Sullivan, Queen, and Patrick make such secret observation sound extraordinarily difficult. Note the elaborate nine-month preparation of their observer. To cite again my own experience, I made no preparation and took no training for the observational roles I played. For example, my vocabulary and English usage were much better than those of my fellow patients and, later on, of my fellow attendants and even of the nurses who supervised us. Yet I made no attempt to disguise my speech or modify my vocabulary and I had no difficulty mixing comfortably with my temporary colleagues. The several University of Chicago sociologists I know who have engaged in such "undercover research" never mentioned making any special preparation for their participant role

and, with one exception, had no difficulty carrying out their study.

I am quite sure that the observer airman could readily have stepped into his role despite some deviations from the "average" without any noticeable effect on his observations. I believe these researchers have entirely too narrow a conception of people's tolerance of somewhat deviant behavior.

It is my opinion that for studying the dynamics of complex social interaction there is no substitute for participation in the activities of the group (or groups) in which one is interested. I am afraid that the . . . article is more likely to scare off social scientists who have had no experience with this approach than it is to win more recruits. I want to say to such people: It's not nearly as difficult as they make it sound. Give it a try yourself.

NOTE 2.

HENRY W. RIECKEN
THE UNIDENTIFIED INTERVIEWER*

[A] major problem for the participant-observers in this study† was to . . . avoid exerting influence on the beliefs and actions of the members. We wished especially to avoid doing or saying anything that would affect the extent of proselyting; but we also wanted to avoid increasing or decreasing the conviction and the commitment of the members.

From our very first contact with the chief figures it was apparent that a study could not be conducted openly. The leaders had not yet adopted a policy of secrecy and exclusion, but they were at that time neither seeking publicity nor recruiting converts. Rather, their attitude can be best described as one of passive accept-

---

* 24 *American Sociological Review* 398 (1959). Reprinted by permission.

* 62 *American Journal of Sociology* 210–212 (1956). Reprinted by permission.

† This study concerned an apocalyptic group which "had gathered around a middle-aged housewife in a suburb of an American city. She believed that, through 'automatic writing,' she had received a number of messages from beings dwelling in outer space, forecasting the destruction of the earth by flood on a certain date. She made known this prediction among her acquaintances, and a number of people began calling on her regularly to be instructed in the 'lessons' from outer space and to discuss the possibilities of salvation. Most 'members' were adult men and women, of between about twenty to about fifty-five years of age, of middle socio-economic status and well educated, all but two having at least attended college." *Ibid.* at 210.

ance of individuals who came to call and seemed to be interested in the messages from outer space. Our observers were welcomed politely, and their questions were answered, for the most part, fully, but they were not proselyted vigorously or enlisted to spread the word. . . .

. . . In gathering the data . . . the observers tried to be non-directive, sympathetic listeners —passive participants who were inquisitive and eager to learn whatever others might want to tell them. But such a role was not without its difficulties.

In the first place, the passive-member role greatly hampered inquiry. . . . Second, while the attitude we strove for was easy enough for an observer to take during his first few contacts, it became increasingly difficult to maintain as he began to be seen as a "regular." Non-directive inquiry about others, while revealing little about one's own feelings or actions, is appropriate enough behavior for a newcomer, but, if prolonged, it tends to cast doubt on either the intelligence or the motives of interrogator. . . . Nearly every conversation he had with a member about his conviction, commitment, or proselyting presented the observer with an unsought opportunity to influence the other; for it is difficult, outside the interviewer's role, to inquire of an individual how he feels about a matter without having him return the question. . . . The pressure on observers to take part in the process of mutual support and confirmation was ever present and often strong.

. . . The observers were forced . . . to present the appearance of agreement with the major beliefs of the group. While they avoided taking strong stands on these issues and never voluntarily or spontaneously spoke up to reinforce conviction, their general air of acceptance as well as their mere presence and interest in the affairs of the group undoubtedly had some strengthening effect on the conviction of the others. The goal of avoiding influence completely, proved unrealistic, for, in order to remain members and yet gather the necessary data, the observers had to offer some support to the members' convictions. And this, while indeed minimal, must have had some effect.

*   *   *

It is hard to estimate the effect of this apparent commitment by the observers. On the one hand, it probably reinforced members' convictions and confidence that they had been right in making whatever commitments they had made;

on the other hand, the observers' commitments may have made those of other members seem either more or less important. The perceived amount of the observers' commitment probably ranged from moderate to slight: there were at least two members whose commitment was less than that of any observer and at least four or five who exceeded that of any observer. For the latter, the lesser commitment of the observers probably made their own seem greater and more binding, whereas the former probably perceived their commitment to be even slighter in contrast to the observers'. In short, for most of the group the observers' investment in group activity was supportive, but the amount of support varied.

*   *   *

[F]rom our experience, it seems likely that observers cannot avoid exercising *some* influence on behavior and beliefs. The conflict in roles and its attendant consequences seem to be inherent in the process of doing a study such as this, although it may be possible to devise better ways of handling the conflict and of further reducing observer effect. . . .

[iii]
Norman Lefstein
Experimental Research in the Law—Ethical and Practical Considerations*

*   *   *

In the juvenile courts of two metropolitan communities a study of attorneys and their effects on the attitudes and behavior of boys accused of delinquency is being made. Initially, plans for this program—termed the lawyer project—were limited primarily to the opening of special legal aid offices to serve the two juvenile courts involved. Before the project commenced, however, an extensive program to evaluate counsel's effects—not originally planned—was developed.

An experimental method with random assignment to groups, specifically the "Solomon Four-Group Design," is employed in the study. Accordingly, in one of two treatment (lawyer) groups, boys are interviewed prior to an attorney's entry into the case; in one of two control (no lawyer) groups, boys are interviewed prior to their appearance in court. In all four groups the boys are interviewed at a designated interval

---

* Unpublished manuscript 1–3, 6–13 (1967). Printed by permission of the author who retains all rights.

after their court appearance. The interviews, which are based upon a structured questionnaire, are administered by a trained staff of field workers. The major content areas of the questionnaire include a boy's knowledge and attitude toward the law and legal process, his readiness to accept or reject court imposed sanctions, and his attitudes toward various court participants. Representation for boys in the treatment (lawyer) group is provided by one of the three full-time staff attorneys associated with the project's legal office.

The research activities are totally separated from operation of the lawyer project office. For example, the interviewers who operate out of their own headquarters have never been informed of the relationship between the lawyer project and their interviewing, thus minimizing the risk of their communicating to the boys that the questions asked are related directly to attorney representation in juvenile court. The lawyers do not know, nor will they be informed until the project's completion, of the precise content of the interview. Also, the lawyers are not told which of the boys they represent have been interviewed prior to the court hearing.

The families of boys in the lawyer group are specifically offered the services of a project attorney. They may, however, refuse the representation tendered and appear in juvenile court without an attorney or with an attorney of their choosing. The lawyer project, therefore, is experimental insofar as it "offers" to a randomly selected group of juveniles the opportunity to be represented by the project's attorneys. The control group consists of an equal number of randomly designated youths who are not offered the services of a project attorney, but who are free to obtain representation through the normal legal services available in the project cities. While these procedures detract from the project's experimental rigor, they tend to obviate a critical objection which otherwise certainly would be leveled, i.e., that the program forces some boys, who may not want an attorney, to accept representation, and deprives of counsel others who may wish to have a lawyer's services.

Implementation of the research design required a series of difficult administrative decisions, each of which was deemed essential to insure validity of the controlled experiment. Moreover, several of the decisions, much like the original choice of an experimental method, raised practical as well as ethical questions. . . .

*   *   *

Representation Limited to Experimental Cases. In order to insure external validity, the project lawyer offices have been made to resemble those of typical legal aid programs. The project lawyers, just like other attorneys furnishing legal aid in juvenile courts, become involved in delinquency cases after a court complaint has been filed. In one important respect, however, the lawyer project had to differ from typical legal services programs. This difference, though not affecting external validity, further serves to illustrate how the experimental design has influenced the action program. Normally legal aid attorneys will accept appointments to cases assigned by the court and will provide representation at the request of indigent persons referred for legal services. This practice could not be allowed with the lawyer project, for it would seriously have threatened operation of the research by requiring the attorneys to spend too much of their time working on non-experimental cases. Accordingly, the juvenile courts agreed not to appoint the project's lawyers to indigent cases in which counsel was requested. Similarly, referral cases are not accepted; persons seeking legal representation are directed to other legal services in the community or to the juvenile court.

Form Letter and Field Representative. Implementation of the research design required permission from the juvenile courts to allow daily inspection of all new delinquency filings, for random assignment to treatment and control groups is made possible with this information. Permission also was obtained for a form letter to be mailed to the parents of boys assigned to the treatment group informing them that they might have a project lawyer represent their son. The letter states that the project is authorized to provide representation without cost, and encourages parents to phone the project office to arrange an appointment with one of the staff attorneys. When the form letter fails to bring a response, a field representative employed by the project, whose function also was approved by the juvenile courts, visits the parents to determine whether they will accept legal representation for their child. . . .

Beyond complexities of administering experimental research programs in legal areas, there are broader, more difficult questions, such as the ethical propriety of doling out different treatment to random subjects without their consent, and failing to furnish complete information about the experiment to persons connected with it. In the lawyer project, there are several instances during the processing of cases in which information is concealed from subjects of the experiment—indeed must not be revealed if the study is to have validity. For example, when the field representative contacts the child and his parents, he informs them that they may be represented by a project attorney; no mention is made of how the boy's name was obtained from juvenile court, that the effects of lawyer representation on the youth will be studied, and that a comparable control group of boys also is being studied. Similarly, when the lawyer speaks with the youth and his parents, the overall purposes of the project are not revealed. Although the attorneys know of the interviewing and its relationship to their representation, they are instructed, as is the field representative, not to reveal the existence of this relationship to their clients. Finally, the parents and child are never apprised of the various hypotheses which the research is designed to test. In light of these circumstances, it may be argued that subjects of this experiment are unable to make an informed, intelligent decision on whether they wish representation by a project attorney.

Incomplete disclosure of information during administration of a research study obviously is not peculiar to the experimental method; on the other hand, only an experimental design involves random assignment to groups without the knowledge and consent of those being studied. In articles dealing with use of this research method in the law, various justifications and principles have been advanced in support of random assignment, which, although persuasive for some experiments, are not altogether satisfactory when applied to others.

It is argued, for example, that with random assignment each person, "before the lot is drawn, has an initial, equal chance to become a member of either group." Consequently, random assignment is less arbitrary, therefore presumably fairer, than any other conceivable dividing line. Theoretically this appears to be unassailable. But is the proposition necessarily true in practice for all experiments? Are there not legal innovations for which some persons would readily qualify absent an experimental design, but, with an experimental design imposed, their chances of qualifying for the innovation are severely reduced? Professor Norval Morris, writing about programs to test the effects of early release from prison, pointed out this potential occurrence. Without an experimental design, a particular in-

mate's chances of qualifying for an early release from prison project, based upon his record and ability to impress the parole board, might have been excellent, perhaps even an 80 percent to 90 percent chance. As a member of the sample population for the experiment, his chances of release would be reduced to 50 percent.

Another argument by which random assignment is justified goes like this: given the presence of a legal innovation, an experimental design involves not the basic issue of differential treatment itself but merely a shift in an existing and tolerated line of differentiation so that it is of use in evaluation; in other words, since any innovation in the law involves discrimination, it might as well be planned in such a way as to maximize our knowledge of its effects. But this argument, besides overlooking that the differential treatment may not correspond with the desires of those in the experiment, disregards the fact that the demands of the research design may contribute to altering the *degree* of differential treatment. To illustrate, with the lawyer project it would be possible for the lawyers to handle substantially more cases than just those which can be randomly assigned. As noted earlier, however, cases of persons referred to the project office are not taken, due to the potential interference of this practice with the research design. Although persons seeking representation by a project attorney are referred to other legal aid or to the juvenile court, it is not certain that they always obtain a lawyer. In both of the juvenile courts in which the project operates, requests for the appointment of counsel are discouraged, and occasionally indigent persons seeking counsel are pressured into proceeding without a lawyer, despite a constitutional right to have counsel appointed. In light of these circumstances, it is conceivable that the lawyer project directly alters, because of its experimental design, the extent of differential treatment; that is to say, absent the lawyer project's experimental design, greater numbers of persons probably would receive "lawyer treatment."

The Manhattan Bail Study conducted in New York City several years ago, which was designed to test the effects of releasing defendants prior to trial on their personal recognizance, provides a clearer illustration of how an experimental design may alter the degree of differential treatment. During its first year, random assignment to treatment and control groups was maintained. Prisoners were interviewed shortly after arrest and their references in the community screened; eligibility for release on recognizance was determined according to certain established criteria. Then, based upon random assignment, from among those found to be eligible, a treatment group was recommended to the court for release, whereas those in a control group, despite their eligibility, were not recommended. The results were significant: 60 percent of those in the treatment group were released by the court on their recognizance in contrast to only 14 percent in the control group. Clearly the extent of differential treatment was heightened as a direct consequence of the experimental research design, for one can reasonably infer that if the legal innovation—recommendation for release on personal recognizance—had been applied to those in the control group, a larger number of persons would have obtained their liberty.

To minimize possible discrimination with experimental designs, Professor Morris urges that a principle of "less severity" be adopted, i.e., no person in an experiment should receive more severe treatment than would commonly be accorded—some simply should receive "less severe" treatment. [I]n the lawyer project, the hypothesis has been that having an attorney will lead to a more favorable result and hence "less severe" treatment. But what if the boys represented by project attorneys receive substantially harsher sentences than those without counsel? Or suppose that the youths represented by the project's lawyers do receive more lenient dispositions than those without counsel, but, as a group, those who have had attorneys consistently get into additional difficulty, and ultimately are incarcerated far longer than those in the control group. In circumstances such as these, the principle of "less severe" treatment appears to lose much of its meaning.

*   *   *

[iv]
Philip R. A. May and A. H. Tuma
The Effect of Psychotherapy and Stelazine
on Length of Hospital Stay, Release Rate,
and Supplemental Treatment of
*Schizophrenic Patients**

It is unlikely that any one treatment by itself will be universally effective—in every way, for all types of patients, in everyone's hands, in every type of setting. Since large numbers of patients are treated in public mental hospitals, it was believed important to study the relative effectiveness of treatment modalities in common use for schizophrenic patients under the sort of conditions that might be expected in such hospitals within the reasonably foreseeable future.

There is some difference of opinion about the effectiveness of individual psychotherapy, either alone or in combination with ataraxic drugs, in the treatment of schizophrenic patients: this has particular significance since a large part of public hospital time and effort is devoted to the treatment of such patients. It is important to the therapist and to the administrator to have knowledge of the outcome of psychotherapeutic treatment in a hospital setting, for this will have a direct bearing on the selection of patients for psychotherapy and on the assignment of skilled professional time to a variety of functions in the total treatment program. There is still considerable controversy as to whether tranquilizing drugs facilitate or inhibit the therapeutic process when given as an adjunct to psychotherapy. Other arguments center around the "sufficiency" of a chemical treatment for an illness that is thought to have its etiology, at least in part, in psychosocial processes. It is the writers' belief that such controversies will undoubtedly continue until scientific evidence can replace the process of self-fulfilling and wish-fulfilling prophecy.

Selected first-admission schizophrenic patients with no previous treatment were assigned by a random method to four treatment groups in a factorial design—individual psychotherapy; individual psychotherapy plus tranquilizing drugs; tranquilizing drugs alone; and a control group that did not receive any of the specific treatments stated above. Evaluation was carried out before and after treatment, using multiple independent criteria.

The patient sample consists of 40 male and 40 female first-admission schizophrenic patients between 18 and 40 years of age, selected from consecutive admissions to Camarillo State Hospital. . . .

*   *   *

All patients, regardless of their specific treatment, were housed in one male and one female research ward with similar staffing pattern, ward program and general milieu. The latter included routine nursing care, sedation, hydrotherapy, occupational, industrial and recre-

---

* 139 *Journal of Nervous and Mental Disease* 362–369 (1964). © 1964, The Williams & Wilkins Co., Baltimore, Maryland. Reprinted by permission.

ational therapies, ward meetings and social case work.

The patients were treated by physicians who had had less than five years psychiatric experience and who were in residency training or had completed it. This corresponds with the level of experience of physicians who may reasonably be expected to be found to treat patients in state hospitals. Each patient's treatment was supervised by a psychiatric consultant who believed in the particular treatment to which the patient was assigned and who was responsible for discussing with the patient's doctor the timing, management, dosage, process and duration of treatment as well as tactics and operational details.

Patients had psychotherapy for an average of not less than two hours a week, supervised by a psychoanalyst experienced in the treatment of schizophrenic patients, with one hour of supervision for each patient every two weeks.

With ataraxic drugs, the aim was to give whatever type or dose the experienced supervisor judged most likely to be effective for a particular patient—to study treatment under "battlefield conditions," and not to conduct a study of one particular drug. . . .

Treatment was given up to a maximum of one year, until *either* the patient was released *or* had been in the hospital for at least six months and the supervisor and the therapist agreed that treatment had been given a good trial and that further treatment with that particular method was unlikely to succeed. A six- to twelve-month treatment period would seem to be more realistic than the shorter periods often reported in many research studies. It is more congruent with the natural history of the disease and therefore may increase the possibility of differentiating clinically significant differences in response to treatment. It also permits meaningful use and interpretation of two ultimate objective criteria of outcome—length of hospital stay and release rate.

*   *   *

This report presents the outcome of treatment in terms of the following four measures: release rate, length of stay in hospital for those successfully released, amount of supplemental treatment required, and estimated change on the Menninger Health-sickness Scale. Ratings for this latter measure were provided by a team of two psychoanalysts who had no direct connection with the patients' treatment.

An important criterion of treatment effectiveness is the release rate. [M]ore patients were released when treated with "Drugs plus psychotherapy" or with "Drugs" than "Psychotherapy" or "Controls" (release rates—95 and 90 per cent vs. 70 and 65 per cent respectively), the overall difference being statistically significant at the .05 level.

The combined "Control" and "Psychotherapy" groups were compared with the combined "Drug" and "Psychotherapy plus drug" groups to test the difference in release rates between the groups receiving drug and those not receiving it, regardless of any other considerations. For this comparison the difference is significant at the .01 level. . . .

Another criterion of the usefulness of a treatment is the length of hospital stay for patients released. The mean stay (in days) for each of the four groups is as follows: Psychotherapy, 191.00; Control, 187.15; Drug, 151.00; Drug plus psychotherapy, 126.32. . . . [D]rug treatment has the only significant effect in reducing length of stay. Neither psychotherapy alone nor its interaction with drug treatment had significant influence on the variation in length of stay.

In considering the effectiveness of a treatment, it is reasonable to consider how much supplemental care the patient has to be given in addition to the experimental treatment. Since sedatives and hydrotherapy were available for all patients on all treatments, the frequency and duration of their use were recorded and the groups were compared on this basis. . . . [T]he most supplemental treatment was given to patients in the control group, the least to those who received drugs alone. Psychotherapy, with or without drugs, falls between the extremes.

*   *   *

Perhaps one of the most critical considerations from the viewpoint of the clinician is the amount of improvement in clinical status. . . . The greatest differences lie between the "Control" group on the one hand and the "Drug," "Psychotherapy plus drug" and "Psychotherapy" groups in this descending order. There seems to be virtually no difference between "Drug alone" and "Psychotherapy plus drug." Again, when we look for the source of this variation in the amount of clinical change we find it to be the drug treatment. Psychotherapy had virtually no effect on the amount of change, while the interaction between psychotherapy and drug was significant at the .20 level, suggesting a possible advantage in the combination of these two therapeutic agents.

Discussion

*   *   *

It is not a simple matter to carry out a controlled experimental study of seriously ill schizophrenic patients treated for six to twelve months, and particularly to maintain a control group with no specific treatment for this length of time. This particular study of 80 patients took some three years to complete, not including the design and pilot stages. Under the circumstances, a study of 80 patients is a formidable affair—yet from a statistical point of view, the numbers are small: for example, they are sufficient only to be 50 per cent certain of detecting a shift from 70 per cent to 95 per cent improvement rate, with statistical tests at the .05 level. The reporting of relatively high percentage levels of significance seems appropriate in clinical research and especially in preliminary reports dealing with small numbers, where it is important to be sure of uncovering a true difference when it *does* exist. For example, use of a .20 level of significance gives odds of one in five that spurious differences or relationships will be reported as true: however, in severe and potentially ruinous disorders such as schizophrenia, the physician, the patient and his family may willingly take the risk that there is one chance in five that a given treatment will lead to results that are in reality no different than "milieu" treatment alone.

The figures for psychotherapy and drugs illustrate particularly well one of the difficulties of research in this area. If "Drug alone" produces a release rate of 90 per cent, and if the addition of psychotherapy produces a real increase of release rate to 95 per cent, it would be necessary to have 188 cases in each group to be even 50 per cent certain of detecting the above difference as significant at the .05 level.

In the present study, with a small sample size, none of the differences between the "Drug alone" and "Drug plus psychotherapy" groups were statistically significant although, for improvement on the Menninger Health-sickness Rating Scale, there was an interaction effect significant at the .20 level. Clearly, definitive answers in this particular area must await replication with a larger sample at some future time.

However, the figures do not support the contention that psychotherapy keeps patients hospitalized longer. It may be that a particular treatment has an effect on the doctor who gives it, so that, for example, hospital stay *seems* longer to the psychotherapist; or it may be that psychotherapists keep some patients in longer and release others earlier.

On the other hand, the use of drugs, with or without psychotherapy, seems to reduce hospital stay; in the present study, the shortest mean stay was associated with the use of Stelazine and individual psychotherapy combined.

*   *   *

[P]rolongation of hospital stay is seldom advisable. From the point of view of psychotherapy, the patient who is not psychologically minded is unlikely to benefit psychotherapeutically from a prolonged hospital stay. If more prolonged therapy is indicated, the therapist will usually wish to change to outpatient care as soon as possible. A prolonged regressive experience may promote chronicity; for patients with little financial reserve, it may be ruinous.

*   *   *

b.

Threats to Anonymity and Reputation

[i]
Lee Rainwater and David J. Pittman
Ethical Problems in Studying a Politically
Sensitive and Deviant Community*

*   *   *

The Pruitt-Igoe Housing projects were planned in the early 1950's and first occupied in 1954. Originally the plan was to build two segregated projects, Pruitt for Negroes, and Igoe, across the street, for whites. This plan was ruled unconstitutional, however, and after a short period of integration the project became all-Negro. . . .

By 1959 the project had become a community scandal both because of certain unattractive design features (for example, the elevators stop only on the fourth, seventh and tenth floors) and as a result of the wide publicity given to crimes (rape, murder, robbery) and accidents (people fell down elevator shafts and children fell out of windows in the project). In response to the steady unfavorable publicity and a grand jury investigation of the project, former Mayor Tucker of St. Louis appointed in 1960 a committee on public housing and social services that

* 14 *Social Problems* 357–366 (1967). Reprinted by permission.

WHAT CONSTITUTES HARM? 339

included representatives of business, labor, and the general public as well as the various private and public agencies whose services and facilities were available to public housing residents. The committee directed its primary attention to Pruitt-Igoe, "because it had been much in the public eye and because the tangle of needs and services, present and potential, could be grappled with in the smaller area first." By February, 1961, the committee had presented both its findings of fact and its recommendations.

About the same time in Washington the Federal government's concern with urban problems was quickening. The President's Committee on Juvenile Delinquency and Youth Crime, which had been the main instrumentality of Federal interest, had been supplemented by a Joint Task Force of the Public Housing Administration and the Department of Health, Education, and Welfare, which came to be most centrally concerned with "Community Planning for Concerted Services in Public Housing." Concerted services meant that special efforts would be made in selected demonstration areas to maximize the input of social services and to maximize the coordination of these services. . . .

It was planned that accompanying the concerted services program would be a research project to study the community and to evaluate the effectiveness of the concerted services. . . .

*　　*　　*

[A]n ethical aspect of the public interest in our study arose not in relations with outsiders but within our own group. Some of the fifteen faculty and graduate student researchers expressed concern early in the study over the effect a really penetrating analysis of the style of life of poor Negroes might have on the public dialogue about race relations and poverty. That is, if one describes in full and honest detail behavior which the public will regard as immoral, degraded, deviant, and criminal, will not the effect be to damage the very people we hope our study will eventually help? We have heard such views offered by others, by eminent social scientists in universities and in government. The question is generally phrased something along the following line, "How do you know that the constructive effect of our research will outweigh the damage to the reputations of the people we study? Our science isn't that good yet. Maybe all that will happen is that we will strengthen prejudices and provide rationalizations for bigotry."

This is a knotty issue, and one which per-

haps can only be resolved by an act of faith. If you believe that in the long run truth makes men freer and more autonomous, then you are willing to run the risk that some people will use the facts you turn up and the interpretations you make to fight a rear guard action. If you don't believe this, if you believe instead that truth may or may not free men depending on the situation, even in the long run, then perhaps it is better to avoid these kinds of research subjects. We say perhaps it is better, because it seems to us that a watered-down set of findings would violate other ethical standards, and would have little chance of providing practical guides to action; thus it would hardly be worth the expenditure of one's time and someone else's money.

At the level of strategy, however, this concern for the effect of findings on public issues sensitizes one to the question of how research results will be interpreted by others, and to his responsibility to anticipate probable misuses, and from this anticipation attempt to counteract the possibility of misuse. That is, though we do not feel a researcher must avoid telling the truth because it may hurt a group (problems of confidentiality aside) we do believe that he must take this possibility into account in presenting his findings and make every reasonable effort to deny weapons to potential misusers.

For example, several years ago one of us published a study analyzing the problems of motivation and marital role difficulty that lead lower-class women to be poor family planners.[3] The study was commissioned by the Planned Parenthood Federation of America in hope of learning how to operate their clinics more effectively. The findings indicated that most lower-class women could not sustain the kinds of habits required to practice contraception effectively with the then existing methods (this was before the introduction of the "pill" and the intrauterine device). During the two years after the study appeared, there was considerable agitation in several cities and states to establish family planning services in public health and welfare facilities. In the course of the controversy that ensued several officials who opposed the establishment of family planning services in this way quoted the study to support their contention that lower-class women really did not want help in

---

[3] Lee Rainwater, *And the Poor Get Children: Sex, Contraception, and Family Planning in the Working Class*, Chicago: Quadrangle Books, Inc. 1960.

limiting their families. In examining what he had written, the author realized that he had not taken this possibility into account at all, although knowing the strong feelings people have about family planning and contraception he should have known better. He had not made crystal clear that there was no question but that these lower-class women wanted fewer children, even though they needed a good deal of help in realizing that desire. In his desire to get at the problems that created difficulties in Planned Parenthood's clinic organization, he had not sufficiently emphasized the wishes that lower-class women have for some kind of really effective help in family limitation.

Another example of the misuse of social science findings can be found in controversies dealing with problems of integration and segregation. Much recent research on the problems of slums and ghettos has emphasized the destructive effects of lower-class family and neighborhood systems. The authors of these studies clearly hope that by understanding the dynamics of slum living it will be possible to develop programs that do not fail as present housing, welfare, and retraining programs seem to be failing. However, since these researchers deal with the internal dynamics of the ghetto, their findings can prove quite attractive to individuals and institutions that seek to perpetuate containment of Negroes in segregated areas. Recently Rainwater testified for the National Association for the Advancement of Colored People in a de facto segregation suit against the Cincinnati School Board. In direct testimony he said some very elementary things about the destructive effects of going to a ghetto school and thus contributed to the plaintiff's case that de facto segregation, as much as legal segregation, affects negatively the "hearts and minds" of Negro children and therefore violates the due process clause of the Fourteenth Amendment. However, on cross-examination he found himself exposed to a fairly sophisticated line of questioning that sought to have him "admit" that the low achievement scores and high drop-out rate of Negro children in ghetto schools have nothing to do with the fact that these schools are "racially imbalanced" but rather is due to the home and neighborhood environment. The Board of Education obviously felt that it had a defense against the plaintiff's charges which was validated by social science research on Negro slum family and neighborhood behavior. This is apparently a popular defense by boards of education in several parts

of the country. They seek to substantiate the view that ghetto schools do not damage Negro children but that the damage is instead done by the family and the neighborhood over which the schools have no control. Indeed, we have heard of one other social scientist expert witness in a de facto segregation case who was cross-examined for five days along exactly this line. In that case the court was not impressed and found for the plaintiffs, but given the jaundiced eyes with which courts view social science testimony anyway, it seems likely that more often the effect of such "conflicting" findings will be beneficial to the case of those who wish to maintain a segregated school system.

It probably would have been difficult to anticipate such a sophisticated misuse of research findings before the fact. After all, that families may damage their children says nothing about whether schools do or do not also damage the same children. But once we know that such misuse is being made of the products of our discipline, perhaps we have a responsibility to try to do something about it, much as psychologists have done with the misuses of intelligence test data on racial groups. Perhaps we need some kind of "intelligence service" which appraises us of this kind of misuse so that in our subsequent writings we can make it less easy for people to misuse the findings and also so that as a group we can make efforts to counteract this kind of misinterpretation.

More generally, it seems evident that as sociology is more and more accepted as of relevance to the important issues the country must cope with, what sociologists have to say will be increasingly fateful in the lives of individuals and groups. It behooves us then, not only to study significant problems and report our findings accurately, but also to be sensitive to the way these findings are used, particularly to whether or not they are used in ways that seem illegitimate, given the findings. In this respect sociologists will come increasingly to have the same kinds of problems that historians, political scientists, economists, and psychologists have had for some time.

*   *   *

The traditions of our field emphasize anonymity as necessary and desirable in research. We generally think of ourselves as studying social behavior about which our informants are protective. They may be protective because their deepest interests are involved, or for reasons that are less vital, but it is traditional to honor our subjects' wish that what we learn about them not be communicated to a larger public in any way that will affect their interests or identify them. Confidentiality is deemed technically necessary, and once it is offered we are ethically bound to honor our promise.

However, there are some situations for which the offer of confidentiality may be both unnecessary and technically a bad choice. In some situations the applicability of research findings to applied goals will be rendered almost impossible if true confidentiality is maintained. And in some other situations it may be impossible to communicate the findings once the informants have been told that what we see and hear will be kept confidential.

It seems to us that we should rethink our automatic assumption that we offer to maintain the privacy of our informants. The question of whether or not to make such an offer demands a conscious and thoughtful decision that is made in the light of needs and goals of a particular research. Let us offer a couple of examples of situations in which confidentiality has not been offered and then suggest a principle which underlies these examples.

In our Pruitt-Igoe research, we have not made promises of confidentiality to anyone in the Housing Authority management. We have not done so since we feel that were the information we collect from them regarded as confidential it would not be possible to publish a sensible report of our findings. This applies both to individual functionaries in the Housing Authority and to the Authority as an organization. We cannot possibly conceal the identity of this particular project when we publish our results. We must be free to identify the organization and its various constituent units. Similarly we could not possibly discuss the role of the executive director of the Housing Authority or of the project managers without their being identified as particular persons. While in the end we might adopt some cover of pseudonyms it would be more to avoid becoming enmeshed in questions of personality than to prevent the identification of the actual persons involved. Thus, while we feel that no useful purpose would be served by not concealing the identities of the tenants in the project and of the low-level employees, at the higher reaches of the organization our presumably useful purpose can be served only by openness about the identities of the organization and the top level executives involved.

These persons know that it is possible that our study will have unpleasant repercussions on them, but they also are used to being exposed to the light of publicity.

*   *   *

The decision not to promise confidentiality makes explicit our claim to a *right* to study social behavior in certain situations. Obviously we do not claim the right to study all kinds of behavior in non-confidential ways and to make public our findings, but we do and should study certain kinds of behavior in this way. As an initial formulation, we suggest that sociologists have the right (and perhaps also the obligation) to study publicly accountable behavior. By publicly accountable behavior we do not simply mean the behavior of public officials (though there the case is clearest) but also the behavior of any individual as he goes about performing public or secondary roles for which he is socially accountable—this would include businessmen, college teachers, physicians, etc.; in short, all people as they carry out jobs for which they are in some sense publicly accountable. One of the functions of our discipline, along with those of political science, history, economics, journalism, and intellectual pursuits generally, is to further public accountability in a society whose complexity makes it easier for people to avoid their responsibilities.

We would suggest that, in principle, anyone is publicly accountable for the actions which it is his duty to perform. Most of the time, however, since sociologists are not muckrakers, it is not necessary or desirable to single out individuals or even clearly identifiable small groups. In such situations one may reasonably use confidentiality as an inducement to cooperation. In other situations, however, this is clearly unwarranted. If one wishes to study the functioning of courts, or of a mayor's office, or of General Motors, or of unions, it is perhaps better to put up with the difficulties of only doing what one can do without promising to keep information confidential. Since publicly accountable individuals often recognize the fact of their accountability and the useful purposes that might be served by sociologists studying them, one can often gain a good deal of cooperation without the promise of confidentiality.

We are suggesting that sociologists in this respect have the same rights that journalists have. Our understanding of the social process may be such that we do not use this right in the same way as journalists, because we are not interested in momentary sensations but in developing an understanding of the persisting tendencies of social systems, large or small.

[ii]
Diane Bauer
*Maryland Tests for Criminal Potential**

With the approval of both state and Federal agencies, some 15,000 Maryland boys are being submitted to blood tests at the risk of being labeled for life as potential criminals. The testing, to be administered in a majority of cases without legal consent of parents, has been attacked by lawyers, doctors and civil liberties groups.

The search for boys with an XYY chromosome pattern, which some scientists theorize may be linked with violent criminal behavior, is being conducted by Johns Hopkins University with Federal funds. The study will include two main test groups over the next three years—6,000 boys confined to Maryland's juvenile jails . . . and 7,500 from a group of largely underprivileged Negro families enrolled in a free Johns Hopkins medical program.

*   *   *

Both Maryland Children's Center and Waxter [Children's Center], court officials acknowledge, detain some children who are not accused of crimes, but are "dependent and neglected."

*   *   *

Results of the tests on the 6,000 boys in state institutions will be turned over to juvenile correctional agencies by the staff conducting the study.

Dr. Digamber Borgaonkar, who heads the three-year project under a $300,000 grant from the National Institutes of Health's Center of Crime and Delinquency, said he plans to give the parents test results only if requested and then only "as much as they can understand."

*   *   *

Parents of 7,500 East Baltimore boys, 95 per cent from underprivileged Negro families enrolled in a free child care program at Johns Hopkins, are not being asked for a signed legal consent for their childrens' participation in the study, Dr. James Hudson said.

Dr. Hudson, project director of the Com-

prehensive Child Care Program, said Johns Hopkins does not have a "blanket permission" from the parents for test studies. He said blood is "drawn routinely to check for anemia," and by using the same samples for the chromosome test the problem of asking parents for legal permission to look for the XYY factor in the youngsters' blood is avoided.

*   *   *

The results of the blood tests—which lawyers say would "label boys for life with the criminal stigma of a yet unproven scientific theory," according to Robert C. Hilson, director of Juvenile Services, "will probably be passed on to the courts for whatever use they can make of it."

Maryland juvenile court probation officers will be used to persuade resisting parents to sign a permission to take a blood sample, Dr. Borgaonkar said, with the single explanation on the document "for examination by the staff of the Division of Medical Genetics" of Johns Hopkins.

*   *   *

Neither the [preliminary] letter nor the permission form [see NOTE 1.] tell parents anything about the theories relating XYY chromosome patterns to criminal violence which sparked the study, the ACLU complains.

Lawyers originally saw the XYY defect as a basis for a plea of insanity for clients charged with violent crimes.

Maryland courts have twice in the past year rejected the XYY diagnosis as a basis for an insanity plea. Both a local circuit court and the state Court of Special Appeals refused Ray Millard, convicted of armed robbery in Prince Georges County, permission to use his XYY chromosome pattern to prove his legal insanity.

[I]n Australia a murder suspect diagnosed as XYY was last year found not guilty by reason of insanity.

"What can be used by the defense can also be used for the prosecution," said a leading Montgomery County lawyer who represents juveniles in Maryland courts.

"With the state co-operating in such a study, a juvenile could be sent away for life to a state hospital or Patuxent," he warned, "not because he did anything serious, but just because some guy in a laboratory thinks he has one chromosome too many."

Timothy Crofton, assistant director of Edgemeade, a private psychiatric treatment center,

---

* *Washington Daily News* 7, cols. 1–3 (January 22, 1970). Reprinted by permission.

said he assisted Dr. Borgaonkar in obtaining the NIH grant and will act as "administrative co-ordinator" for the project, which will include the 500 emotionally disturbed boys under his care during the next three years.

Parents of these boys will not be asked for signed legal permissions for this specific test because a blanket permission is signed when each child is admitted. Mr. Crofton said, however, that he is "sure all parents are aware of the study."

Mr. Crofton, a former Montgomery County probation officer, said "my assignment is to try to get the co-operation of various probation officers to get parents to sign up when their child is committed to an institution."

*   *   *

A baby's sex is determined by whether it receives an X or a Y chromosome from its father. Normal men receive an X from their mothers and a Y from their fathers. Women get one X from each parent. The usual number of chromosomes is 46.

This study is chiefly concerned with who receives an extra Y. Some geneticists believe that boys born with XYY chromosomes get a double dose of masculinity that makes them prone to violent, aggressive behavior.

Genetic scientists don't agree on the significance of chromosome abnormalities. A California doctor believes an abnormal number of chromosomes may result in a high potential for committing rape or other sex crimes. Other scientists say chromosome abnormalities are not as uncommon as previously believed and are of concern only in unusual cases.

Dr. Borgaonkar believes XYY males are more impulsive than aggressive, but may react more violently than others under certain stresses. He says earlier studies reported that the majority of XYY's have low IQs and are tall, acned and aggressive, but only the height factor has been proven so far.

NOTES

NOTE 1.

JOHNS HOPKINS HOSPITAL
CONSENT FORM AND COVER LETTER (1969)*

Your son, who is presently at _____, has been included in a special diagnostic genetic

(chromosome) study. This test is being conducted with the administrative approval of the Director, Department of Juvenile Services, State of Maryland, Baltimore, Maryland. We plan to test 6,000 boys, in a period of three years, from all the state institutions.

Please sign the enclosed form and mail it in the enclosed stamped, addressed envelope at your earliest convenience.

*   *   *

Date:

BOY'S NAME: _____

As his parents and/or legal guardian, I give permission for a blood sample to be drawn from the above named youngster for examination by the staff of the Division of Medical Genetics of this institution.

It is understood that no drugs or medication will be administered; that the results of the examination will be made known to me upon request; and that there will be no charge for this service.

_____
Signature of parent(s) or legal guardian

NOTE 2.

DIANE BAUER
XYY TESTS STOP*

Dr. Saleem Shah, chief of the National Institute of Mental Health's Center for Studies of Crime and Delinquency, said yesterday that as a result of articles in *The Washington Daily News* he has suspended a blood test search for the rare XYY chromosome pattern among some 14,000 Maryland juveniles.

*   *   *

A law suit, which names Dr. Shah as one of nine defendants, filed in Montgomery County Circuit Court last week charged that the study violates the civil liberties of the youths.

It accuses NIMH and Johns Hopkins of neglecting to obtain proper legal consent to the testing from parents, failing to inform parents of the legal consequences of the testing and destroying the confidentiality of the doctor-patient relationship by turning over the results to state juvenile courts.

"It is clear," said Dr. Shah, "that the procedures for getting informed consent (for the blood tests) have to be revised and made stricter.

---

* Reprinted by permission of Dr. Digamber S. Borgaonkar, The Johns Hopkins University School of Medicine, Baltimore, Maryland.

* *Washington Daily News* 5, cols. 1–3 (Feb. 13, 1970). Reprinted by permission.

Until that is clarified the taking of blood samples has been stopped."

Dr. Shah said that he could not say whether or not the study had violated the constitutional rights of the boys as charged by civil liberties groups and some experts in medical and legal ethics, because Johns Hopkins has not completed a review of the procedures which are being used by the project director, Dr. Digamber Borgaonkar.

Dr. Shah refused to show reporters the written procedures outlining the methods the researchers agreed to use in order to safeguard the boys' rights and which Johns Hopkins is required by law to file with NIMH.

A spokesman for Dr. Shah, James Helsing, said that NIMH is not required to provide the information to the public even under the new federal public information law because it "constitutes trade secrets."

* * *

NOTE 3.

DIANE BAUER

CRIMINAL-PRONE TESTS RESUMED*

The Government has quietly resumed testing the blood of underprivileged Maryland boys in an effort to find and label potential troublemakers by the make-up of their chromosomes. . . .

The Health, Education and Welfare Department is permitting the blood testing to be touted to impoverished black parents as a free $100 medical bargain, apparently in order to obtain parents' signatures on a new consent form that was revised after it had been sharply criticized.

Rep. Cornelius E. Gallagher, D-N.J., who recently scheduled hearings on a similar—and abortive—proposal by a Dr. Arnold Hutschnecker to psychologically test the nation's 6-year olds for incipient anti-social behavior, now plans a full-scale investigation of the XYY chromosome blood testing being funded by HEW's National Institute of Mental Health (NIMH). . . .

* * *

Project director Borgaonkar refused to reveal the percentage of Negroes included in the testing, but the population of Maryland juvenile institutions is about 75 percent black. Of the non-incarcerated children in the project, 95 percent are boys fron black ghettos.

---

* *Washington Daily News* 1, col. 4 (May 4, 1970). Reprinted by permission.

A new consent form was drafted by the ACLU after *The Daily News* revealed that Johns Hopkins could produce no written record that it had either sought or received permission from the parents of the underprivileged boys included in the study. The ACLU also charged that the consent form being used for institutionalized youths was inadequate and misleading.

HEW standards require that "informed consent" be obtained before any project funded by tax money can use humans as research subjects. In a letter to Sen. Ervin, Dr. Roger Egeberg, assistant HEW secretary for health and scientific affairs, said that, as required by law, "this project had been reviewed by the committee on clinical investigation of the Johns Hopkins University school of medicine."

But Dr. Gordon Walker, chairman of the university's committee on clinical investigation, said his committee had never held a meeting to discuss the original XYY proposal funded by NIMH. However, the proposal was circulated to the members individually for approval.

* * *

The form does not point out that Maryland has no confidentiality law for doctors and that therefore the test results could be introduced in court. . . .

The consent form does assure parents that test results will be confidential, but unlike some standard consent forms used in Maryland jails, no official signs the XYY form to bind the state or the Baltimore hospital to observe the agreement.

* * *

While Johns Hopkins and NIMH acknowledged that they suspended XYY testing in view of complaints about failure to inform the boys and their families of its nature and possible legal consequences, project officials said they had no plans to inform boys already tested that their rights may have been violated or that a new consent form is now in use.

Blood from the institutionalized boys is being drawn by students—"psychology majors"—without medical supervision, Mr. Ventura [legal counsel for Johns Hopkins] said. He refused to say if they had any other qualifications for taking blood by hypodermic needles from the boys. Project director Borgaonkar is not a physician.

"We feel the detailed information of the type you're looking for has no legitimate public interest," Mr. Ventura told *The News*.

* * *

NOTE 4.

JOHNS HOPKINS HOSPITAL
CONSENT FORM FOR CHROMOSOME STUDY OF
INSTITUTIONALIZED JUVENILE DELINQUENTS
(1970)*

This is to ask your permission to include your son (name) in a research study of chromosomes. Chromosomes are things in a person's body that determine such factors as sex and color of eyes. The purpose of the study is to locate and compare boys with unusual chromosome patterns and to learn whether unusual chromosome patterns are related to such factors as a person's physical and mental development and behavior problems (including a tendency to violate the law).

Over a period of approximately three years, we hope to study all of the State's 6,000 institutionalized juvenile delinquents, all of the 500 boys at the Edgemeade Center, as well as 7,500 other boys.

If you elect to permit your son to participate, a member of the Johns Hopkins Hospital staff will draw about 2 cc's (about a thimbleful) of blood from him. *No drugs or medication will be given.* Further studies will be done in certain cases, but your son will be included only after we have obtained your further consent.

The chromosome study ordinarily costs about $100 and, once performed in a lifetime, need ordinarily never be done again. However, no fees will be charged to you. You, and only you, will be told of the medically useful results of the study and we will explain the significance of this information to you.

This study has been cleared by the Maryland Departments of Health and Juvenile Services. However, the results will be used only by our medical researchers for scientific study and *will not be disclosed to any other person or agency.*

Because this program involves important medical research, we would very much appreciate your cooperation. However, *this program is purely voluntary; you are not required to sign this authorization.* If you do not, no tests will be run on your son. If you desire to authorize your son's participation, please sign below and mail this letter in the enclosed, stamped, addressed envelope at your earliest convenience. If your son is over 14, we will request him to sign this voluntary consent form at the institution. A copy is enclosed for your records. If you have any questions, please call us collect at the above number—or call Mr. Timothy Crofton at Adelphi, Md.—Area Code 301-434-3206, evenings and weekends.

☐ I agree

to permit my son to participate
in this study.

☐ I do not agree

_____ Date _____
Signature of parent(s)/legal guardian

NOTE 5.

ROBERT C. COWEN
BIOLOGISTS DEBUNK CRIMINAL GENE*

London.—Geneticists feel embarrased by the so-called "criminal" chromosome.

It is a human genetic factor that recently, and falsely, was thought to make its possessor criminally inclined.

This notion was introduced in American courts as an indication of criminal "insanity." It has been used, in Britain at least, as reason for abortion of unborn children.

All of this was the result of an erroneous conclusion drawn from bad statistics.

Now geneticists are concerned lest people again be improperly stigmatized as "abnormal" on equally hazy genetic grounds as medical centers build up files on the genetic background of adults and children.

This is one of the dangers cited at a meeting here on the social implications of biology, a meeting convened by the British Society for Social Responsibility in Science.

* * *

Studies made over the past five years at certain penal and mental institutions indicated what seemed an abnormally high percentage of males with the XYY chromosome set among inmates. This was taken as evidence that the extra Y inclined its possessors toward aggressive criminality.

As experts pointed out at the meeting, geneticists now consider such a conclusion scientific rubbish. It was drawn without any knowledge of or reference to the proportion of XYY males in

---

* Reprinted by permission of Dr. Digamber S. Borgaonkar, The Johns Hopkins University School of Medicine, Baltimore, Maryland.

the "normal" population. It was drawn with no knowledge whatsoever of how the extra Y chromosome actually does manifest itself in bodily structure or human behavior. Finding this out would take massive research, which has scarcely begun to be tackled.

Yet invalid as the concept of the "criminal" chromosome may have been, it had begun to be used publicly as a criterion for judging people. This, said Prof. Geoffrey Beale of Edinburgh University, has shocked geneticists. They just had not been aware of what the social consequences could be when they released socially sensitive research information.

While valid as research, the XYY studies were no basis for social decisions. Scientists, he said, must exercise more control over how much information is released to the public.

* * *

[iii]
William Foote Whyte
Freedom and Responsibility in Research—
The "Springdale" Case*

A small upstate New York village has now been immortalized in anthropological literature under the name of "Springdale". . . .

* * *

[Prof. Arthur] Vidich spent two and a half years living in "Springdale" as field director of a Cornell project carried out in the Department of Child Development and Family Relations. The project was directed by Urie Bronfenbrenner, a social psychologist. As a result of this research experience, Vidich published several articles, but the official report in book form regarding the project did not materialize during his tenure at Cornell and is only getting into print at this writing. Some time after he left Cornell, Vidich began work on a book of his own, in collaboration with Joseph Bensman, who had had no previous association with the project.

The Vidich manuscript gave rise to considerable controversy between the author and the Springdale project director. . . .

The points of controversy were essentially these:

1. Should individuals be identified in the book?
2. If individuals were identified, what—if

anything—should be done to avoid damage to them?

* * *

Before Vidich came onto the scene, Springdale people had been assured, when their collaboration was sought, that no individuals would be identified in printed reports. While all of the Vidich characters are given fictitious names, they can easily be identified within Springdale. The author argues that, when there is only one mayor and a small number of village and town officials and school board members, it is impossible to discuss the dynamics of the community without identifying individuals. He further argues that what he has reported in the book is "public knowledge" within Springdale. Even if this be true, is there a different between "public knowledge" which circulates from mouth to mouth in the village and the same stories which appear in print?

In addition to his objections regarding the anonymity pledge, Bronfenbrenner claimed that certain individuals were described in ways which could be damaging to them. On this he submitted a long bill of particulars. One example:

One member of invisible government, in agreement with the principal's educational policy, has remarked that "He's a little too inhuman—has never got into anything in the town. He's good for Springdale until he gets things straightened out. Then we'll have to get rid of him."

* * *

The Springdale experience also raises a general problem regarding the relations of a staff member to the project director in a team project, especially when there is a long period between the initiation of the study and the publication of major research reports. The junior member of such a staff must naturally think about establishing his own professional reputation, which he can do primarily through publication. An article or two will help, but a book would help even more. Is he to be a co-author on a book which represents a major report of the study? In that case, he may have to wait some time for the appearance of the book, and, in the meantime, he has little in the way of credentials to offer as he seeks new teaching and research jobs. . . .

* * *

We will let the author have the next-to-last word on the controversy. Replying in the *Ithaca*

* 17 *Human Organization* 1–2 (Summer 1958). Reprinted by permission.

Journal to a statement made by Bronfenbrenner, Vidich writes:

Strictly speaking, I take the position that in the interests of the pursuit of scientific truth, no one, including research organizations, has a right to lay claims of ownership of research data.

That is a violation of the entire spirit of disinterested research.

Asked whether he was aware that there would be a reaction in Springdale, Vidich replied:

I was aware that there would be a reaction in the town when the book was published. While writing the book, however, it did not occur to us to anticipate what these reactions might be, nor did it occur to us to use such anticipations of reactions as a basis for selecting the data or carrying out the analysis.

One can't gear social science writing to the expected reactions of any audience, and, if one does, the writing quickly degenerates into dishonesty, all objectivity in the sense that one can speak of objectivity in the social sciences is lost.

We do not have any firm answers to the various problems raised by this case, but we are quite convinced that the Vidich answer will not serve. He seems to take the position that he has a responsibility only to science. Has the researcher no responsibility to the people whom he studies? We are not prepared to state what the nature of this responsibility should be, but we find it strange indeed to hear a researcher argue that he assumes no responsibility at all.

* * *

NOTES

NOTE 1.

ARTHUR VIDICH AND JOSEPH BENSMAN
FREEDOM AND RESPONSIBILITY IN RESEARCH*

We are pleased to be invited to join in the discussion of the issues which the Editor opened up in the editorial. . . .

* * *

We feel, however, that his phrasing of the issues was too narrow, in that it was limited to the social and public relations problems of social science investigation. It failed to consider any of the problems related to the purposes of inquiry and to the scientific problems which social in-

* 17 *Human Organization* 2–5 (Winter 1958–59). Reprinted by permission.

quiry presumes to state and solve. For example, his editorial gave attention exclusively to the social scientist's responsibilities to the community and the research organization, and to his personal problems, such as career aspirations, rewards, publications, and the gaining of publicity. While all of these things are important as far as the organization of the discipline is concerned, they are irrelevant; progress in a science is somehow related to important substantive problems and issues and the activities which lead to progress in the solution of the problems posed. This he altogether failed to bring up in his discussion.

* * *

The particular fates of Vidich, Bensman, the project, the department, Cornell University, Springdale, etc. are of much less significance than the problems which the editorial raises for the future of scientific investigation in western society. Not that the Springdale example presents a new problem; on the contrary, negative reactions by organizations, individuals, and interest groups have been characteristic for the Lynds' study of Middletown, West's study of Plainville, Warner's study of Yankee City, Selznick's study of the T.V.A., Hunter's study of Community Power, and Whyte's study of Street Corner Society. In the latter case, Doc still suffers from the recognition he received in the book.

Historically, this problem has not appeared, or has appeared to a much lesser extent, in the anthropology of non-western society. This is because primitive populations have been less concerned, aware, and vocal in their response to the anthropological description of their societies. The life history, studies of native politics and organizations, etc., all invade the native's "privacy," subject his inner life to exposure, and strip him of the magic on which his existence rests. Because it was possible to do this with native society, sociologists and anthropologists have learned a great deal about social life which they could apply to western society. Now that so many primitives have become westernized and are aware of the implications of anthropological research, they, too, resent the invasion of privacy and descriptions of the inner structure of their society.

There is an interesting parallel between the license taken by anthropologists and that taken by sociologists who have studied crime, minority groups, caste groups, factory workers, prostitutes, psychopathic personalities, hoboes, taxidancers, beggars, marginal workers, slum dwellers, and other voiceless, powerless, unrespected, and disreputable groups. Negative reaction to community and organizational research is only heard when results describe articulate, powerful, and respected individuals and organizations. We believe there would have been no objection to our study if it had been limited solely to the shack people.

We think all of the community and organizational studies mentioned above made important contributions. The problem is: *At what price should a contribution be made?*

One of the principal ideas of our book is that the public atmosphere of an organization or a community tends to be optimistic, positive, and geared to the public relations image of the community or the organization. The public mentality veils the dynamics and functional determinants of the group being studied. Any attempt in social analysis at presenting other than public relations rends the veil and must necessarily cause resentment. Moreover, any organization tends to represent a balance of divergent interests held in some kind of equilibrium by the power status of the parties involved. A simple description of these factors, no matter how stated, will offend some of the groups in question.

The only way to avoid such problems is not to deal with articulate groups who will publicly resist the attention which research gives to them, or to deal with the problems in such a way that they are inoffensive. Research of this type becomes banal, irrespective of its technical and methodological virtuosity. We think this has always been the case and that the Springdale example presents nothing new.

* * *

If, however, as in our work, fundamental issues which are related to the basic problems of social science are raised, one cannot predict in advance the embarrassment which research may cause, including the embarrassment to oneself. If the social scientist wants to raise these kinds of issues, he has to risk the possibility of getting into these kinds of troubles. We foresaw this, as the research progressed, and there is no easy solution to the problem.

We think the social scientist can only answer the problem for himself, by asking himself what kind of research he wants to do. If he wants to do practical research which is important to some sponsoring body, he must accept the ethic of responsibility and give up the illusion of independent inquiry. If he wishes to do serious re-

search on problems which are not practical (as practicality is now defined in modern society) he must almost certainly conclude that he must work outside the framework of large research organizations, large institutional grants, or research-servicing organizations. The choice he makes must then be a personal one and, in each case, he can preserve the ethical system he has selected.

* * *

NOTE 2.

ARTHUR J. VIDICH AND JOSEPH BENSMAN
THE SPRINGDALE CASE—ACADEMIC
BUREAUCRATS AND SENSITIVE TOWNSPEOPLE*

* * *

After three years of contact with the community, the members of the project and "The Project" as an official organization had established many personal and official contacts, commitments, friendships, and confidences. This was inevitable simply because of the duration and closeness of the contact. The problem was how these personal and official relations relate to scientific reporting. In the Springdale case the project director took the position that certain materials were questionable from the point of view of ethics and possible injury to persons.

I have just finished reading the manuscript of you and Bensman and, in response to your request, am giving concrete examples of material which, though it may represent public knowledge, is, in our judgment, highly questionable from the point of view of professional ethics and possible injury to the person involved. Since there are many instances of this kind, I shall confine myself to a few outstanding examples.

1. There are many references to the enmity between Flint and Lee. . . . Since, as you yourself have emphasized, these two persons will be immediately recognizable to anyone familiar with the community, assertions that Flint "has been excluded from town politics by Lee" who harbors "resentment" against him are fairly strong accusations. Moreover, the discussion of their personal antagonism is not really central to your analysis of the way in which the community operates and hence you would not lose much by omitting mention of the matter.

2. The whole discussion of Peabody, the school principal, and his relation to the community could,

* Arthur J. Vidich, Joseph Bensman, and Maurice Stein, eds.: *Reflections on Community Studies.* New York: John Wiley and Sons, Inc. 313, 331–335, 338–341, 347–349 (1964). Reprinted by permission.

if it remained in its present form, do a good deal of harm and arouse justifiable resentment. For example, consider the possible impact on him and others of reading the following direct quotation attributed "to a prominent member of invisible government": "He's a little too inhuman—has never gone into anything in the town. He's good for Springdale until he gets things straightened out. Then we will have to get rid of him." Potentially equally damaging are the statements quoted from the observers' report, but these, along with all excerpts from the project files, would of course no longer appear in the manuscript.

3. In pointing out that the Polish community is controlled by political leaders through intermediaries who are willing to do their bidding in exchange for acceptance, is it necessary to point the finger so visibly at Kinserna? You do this very pointedly . . . you go so far as to assert that the upshot of his activities is "to get the Poles to accept measures and policies which are disadvantageous to them."

4. Personality descriptions of the ministers are likewise conspicuously on the *ad hominem* side. For example, you refer to one as "awkward, condescending, and not of the people" and to another as a "cantankerous troublemaker." Also, I wonder whether the description of the Episcopalian minister as trained in "one of the 'radical' Eastern seminaries" is not subject to misinterpretation by Springdale readers despite your use of quotations around the word radical. Given upstate New York's climate of opinion, such a statement may have some unfortunate consequences for the man concerned.

5. The clearly uncomplimentary remarks about Grainger . . . have especial importance for not only is he likely to read them himself, even though he is no longer living in the community, but they are also likely to be read by his colleagues and superiors in the Extension Service. It would be particularly unfair and unfortunate, especially in view of Grainger's whole-hearted cooperation with the project, if any statement made by you jeopardized Grainger's professional future. As the manuscript now stands, such a possibility is by no means out of the question. . . .[16]

The issue here is not the specific items of censorship, but rather the assumption of protective attitudes toward specific community members on the basis of personal attractiveness, entangling commitments, respondent's earlier cooperativeness, and other nonresearch considerations. As a result of personal, social, and organizational commitments, the project finds itself in the position of writing its findings with an eye to other than research or theoretical interests and issues.

As a final step in viewing the community as a reference group, the project decided that:

. . . Before any manuscripts are shown to outside representatives, such as publishers or their agents, we will ask one or two persons within the college and possibly in Springdale to read the manuscripts from the point of view of public relations. Although the final responsibility for deciding what we publish will rest with the project staff, the reactions of such readers would receive serious consideration and we would probably rewrite and omit in accordance with their recommendations. . . .[17]

In this instance, to avoid personal responsibility for the project's research reporting, selected nonresearch respondents would be invited to pass on manuscripts purely as a way of avoiding bad public relations, so that aspects of community life that may be theoretically relevant can be censored by local individuals on nonresearch grounds. Moreover, the local individuals to be selected would be specifically those who constituted the project's dominant reference group in the town, namely, the town's official leaders and spokesmen who represented most forcefully the stereotyped image of the positive-minded community which the project has absorbed as its own image of the town.

The identification of the project and its personnel with the town's interests and with the feelings and sentiments of individuals and groups being studied leads to a subtle adaptation of the research to the problems of the community even though those problems are not the problems of the research. In an extreme instance this policy would lead to no point of view except the point of view of the community. . . .

* * *

At certain stages the community may become a more important reference group for the project than is the scientific community to which the research is ostensibly addressed. In Springdale, for example, the study of constructive activities in the community gradually came to include the ideology that the project and its members assume constructive attitudes toward Springdale in all phases of work including community relations, field work, participation, analysis of data, and reporting of scientific results.

* * *

The town itself came to its own defense in

[16] Personal communication from project director, July 1956.

[17] Personal letter from project director, January 1956.

reviews of the book which appeared in Springdale and neighboring towns. For example, the *Times* in the county seat:[24]

The Small Town in Mass Society—[Springdale]
Says It Isn't So

Small Town in Mass Society, by Arthur J. Vidich and Joseph Bensam (Princeton University Press, $6.00)

An accurate review of this book should be from the viewpoint of a professional sociologist since it is intended as a textbook for the social sciences.

Lacking that point of view, our interest in the book stems from the fact that it is written by a former resident of [Springdale] and concerns itself with "class, power and religion" in [Springdale], called Springdale in the book.

Mr. Vidich is currently about as popular in [Springdale] as the author of *Peyton Place* is in her small town and for the same reason—both authors violate what Vidich calls the etiquette of gossip.

During the three years he lived here, Vidich was engaged in a research project, "Cornell Studies in Social Growth" sponsored by the New York State College of Home Economics and with the aid of funds from the National Institute of Mental Health, United States Public Health Service and the Social Science Research Council.

He then proceeded to use portions of the survey material, making Cornell very unhappy, added a considerable amount of misinformation and gossip and drew certain conclusions based on the three sources.

The Cornell survey material is fairly accurate and pertains to economics and population trends. The misinformation indicates that Vidich is something less than a scientist and has either deliberately distorted facts to prove his personal conclusions or has failed to inquire into basic facts. For example, he states that the railroad running through the village has not made a stop there in years: this misstatement seems immaterial except that he uses it to bolster his conclusion that local business is at a standstill.

He discusses the failure of ecumenicalism in [Springdale], stating that Episcopal and Congregational churches failed to merge because of the opposition of powerful members of the older generation who were fearful of losing the traditions of their churches. Actually, no merger was ever contemplated

and the temporary arrangement of sharing one minister ceased when his superior decided he was being overworked.

The inference is that [Springdale] is living in the past, unable to accept new ideas of mass society, and, further, that it is run by certain individuals.

The theme of control runs throughout the book. [Springdale] citizens will be amazed to discover that practically every phase of daily living is subject to the whims of one man and his cohorts. They run local government, including the school, decide church policies and influence the economic life of the community.

No attempt is made to disguise the individuals who may be readily identified by anyone having any knowledge of [Springdale]. In this field, Vidich seems to have resorted to pure gossip as his source of material.

The author is shocked by the fact people settle their differences in private rather than resorting to public argument; economy in government becomes "the psychology of scarcity"; he arrives at the conclusion people work fantastically hard to avoid coming to terms with themselves.

He finally sums up the whole picture by proclaiming that the entire population is disenchanted, has surrendered all aspirations and illusions. But, says he, [Springdalers] are too stupid to realize they are frustrated. To a certain extent (they) live a full and not wholly unenjoyable life. "Because they do not recognize their defeat, they are not defeated."

"Life consists in making an adjustment that is as satisfactory as possible within a world which is not often tractable to basic wishes and desires."

It should not have taken 314 pages of repetition and technical language to discover that life, as so defined, is not a problem peculiar to a small town.—CC[25]

The reactions of some of the people in the community were recorded in one part of a three-part feature story about the book which was carried by the *Ithaca Journal.* The varied reactions indicate that the town's response was not monolithic, and, moreover, that not all persons had equally absorbed the public relations.

Book's Sales Spiral in Subject Village

Here is the last of three articles about a book and its effect on the town about which it was written.
By Donald Greet

For a book that costs $6 and is "slow" to read, *Small Town* proved to be a best-seller in [Springdale].

Elmer G. Kilpatric, proprietor of a main street store, sold more than two dozen copies. He says only *Peyton Place* in a half-dollar paperback did better.

---

[24] We were not able to secure a copy of the issue of the Springdale *Courier* which carried the review of the book. Though we wrote to the publishers asking for copies and enclosed funds to cover costs, no one ever replied to our request. Our relations with Cornell have been so strained that we have not asked to see their files on the matter. Reviews appeared in other regional papers like the *Ithaca Journal,* but we have made no effort to collect these.

[25] *Oswego Times,* January 31, 1958.

Mrs. Mary Lou Van Scoy, librarian at the village library (which does not have *Peyton Place*), says two copies "have been on the move since we got it."

One copy, she says, "got bitten up by a dog."

There is evidence, then, that a good many people in [Springdale] have read the book and a good many more have been treated to certain salient passages by their friends.

Ask a waitress in the local restaurant if she is acquainted with *Small Town* and she will say, "Oh, yes, that book."

The three persons who felt the chief impact of the book are called in its pages Sam Lee, Howard Jones and John Flint.

Villagers know these men respectively as C. Arthur Beebe, C. Paul Ward and Winston S. Ives. Beebe is the retired head of the [Springdale] *Courier*, Ward is a partner in Ward & Van Scoy Feed Mills and Ives is an attorney.

All three have been and are active in local politics. The book refers to the threesome as the "invisible government," a term that has provoked both merriment and anger in [Springdale].

All three proved real enough to give their impression of *Small Town*. Says Beebe: "People have talked over every situation in the book. They have not felt generally that the book was fair.

"It was not as objective as it was supposed to have been. It was only one man's opinion. He (author Vidich) was judging a small community by big city standards. We felt it was sneaky."

Ward comments: "The whole thing is based on gossip and is not a true study. He (Vidich) didn't find it out by any bona fide investigation.

"The book could just as well have been written from New York (City). It was not a scientific study, which is what it purports to be."

Attorney Ives is somewhat more generous:

"Two-thirds of the book is probably alright but he (Vidich) got into his biggest difficulty with personalities and in dealing with certain recent events.

"My principal objection to the book is that there are unfortunately a number of factual inaccuracies which in some cases create a distinctly misleading impression.

"Another objection is that the book suggests 'invisible government' had no motive but control. In my experience and to my knowledge leaders have been motivated to do what they thought best for the community."

Others in town added their comments. The Rev. V. F. Cline, minister of the Baptist Church for 14 years, said: "It (the book) has caused a suspicion between individuals and groups."

Funeral director Myron Miller puts it succinctly: "Much ado about nothing."

Off-the-cuff statements, not intended for quoted publication, indicate that some portions of the book struck pretty close to home and gave [Springdalers] the chance to see themselves as others see them.

Said one observer: "The book did more to allay apathy in [Springdale] than anything in a long time."

Perhaps it is just coincidence, but interest in a village election this spring shot up from the usual two dozen voters to 178.

The village's two fire companies, needled in the book for pursuing their separate ways over the years, recently joined forces.

One thing is certain: Walk into [Springdale] and mention *Small Town* and you won't get away without a reaction. Those reactions range from horselaughs, to polite smiles to the angry bristle of a porcupine.[26]

*   *   *

[T]here are at least three different criteria by which the fundamental values in research can be evaluated:

1. By the ethic of scientific inquiry—the pursuit of knowledge for the sake of knowledge regardless of its consequences.

2. By the ethic of bureaucratic inquiry. . . .

3. And by the ethic of Christian human relations—for the sake of helping or at least not hurting others.

Every organizational structure imposes its own set of ethics on the individuals who work in it. This is largely because ethics have largely come to be work rules. Knowing that bureaucratic research is here to stay means also that bureaucratic ethics are here to stay, and that, furthermore, they will be elaborated in formal codes as part of the bureaucratic rules. All current trends in bureaucratic research point in the direction of ethical and professional codes which try to specify codes of research conduct that will be consistent with the exigencies of the bureaucratic method of research.

*   *   *

However, the ethic of independent and disinterested research with regard only for the creation of new theories and the discovery of new facts is much older than the modern bureaucratic ethic. At some point almost everyone is willing to accept the ancient Greek ideal of personal integrity, especially after an individual scholar produces valuable and useful results.

*   *   *

The work of the individual scholar, no matter where he is located, and no matter how he is financed, organized, constrained, or aided, is perhaps the sole source of creativity. The successful placing of limitations on individual schol-

---

[26] *Ithaca Journal* June 13, 1958.

arship under the guise of "ethics," work rules, institutional responsibility, or higher considerations forces a society to live off the intellectual capital of its independent thinkers.

2.

Interferences with Psychological Integrity

a.

M. M. Berkun, H. M. Bialek, R. P. Kern, and K. Yagi
Experimental Studies of Psychological Stress in Man*

Degradation of behavior in combat has always occupied the attention of commanders. Behavior in battle may also maintain the prebattle level of proficiency, or surpass it even to the point of heroism; but this does not present a problem as does behavior that has visibly deteriorated under the stress of combat.

This apparently well-documented degradation of behavior in combat was one of the principal problems presented for research when the United States Army first entered into contract with the George Washington University for the establishment of the Human Resources Research Office (HumRRO). Research Task FIGHTER was organized within HumRRO to study the causes of behavioral degradation under psychological stress and to recommend personnel management and training procedures to the Army for reducing the severity of this problem.

*   *   *

The stratagem of inducing a threat by communicating information, rather than by presenting only the stimuli for primitive fears, can be used to create for S a situation in which he is expected or required to do something which is measurable and which is relevant to the threat he perceives.

As an illustration, consider a hypothetical experiment in which S is told to drive an ambulance to an isolated site to bring a critically injured man to the hospital. The ambulance stalls on the way out and the driver must get it going again without assistance. Now, the ambulance and its "gimmicked" motor are perceptual supports—merely props. The essential element in the stress is information given the driver verbally.

---

* 76 *Psychological Monographs* (No. 15) 1–8 (1962). Reprinted by permission.

There is a specific task: to trouble-shoot the engine and correct the defect which has been planted in it by the experimenter. This task is meaningful in terms of the emergency with which S must deal—and the emergency dominates his motivation. By being thus "embedded" in the situation, the task does not expose the deception to S, nor does his performance of it depend exclusively upon his motivation to please himself or to please his examiner with a high test score. Further, the measure is taken during the existence of the emergency, so that performance can be observed during as well as after the stress.

*   *   *

Five proposed stressor situations have been tested and compared with appropriate control situations on each of the above measures. . . .

*   *   *

Ss and Equipment

Ss were simply passengers aboard an apparently stricken plane which was being forced to "ditch" or crash-land, and the performance required of them consisted of filling out two forms which appeared reasonable for the situation. The first, called the Emergency Data Form, was a description of, and instructions for, disposition of the individual's personal possessions in case of death. It was an example of deliberately bad human engineering, consisting of complicated directions on 23 categories of items. The second form, Official Data on Emergency Instructions, was an achievement test with 12 multiple-choice items testing retention of airborne-emergency instructions which all Ss had been required to read, ostensibly as standard operating procedure before the flight. All materials developed for this purpose were pretested with a group of Ss comparable to those for whom they were intended.

A twin-engine DC-3 military aircraft, capable of carrying 12 passengers plus crew, was used. It was equipped with an earphone intercom and a reading table for each passenger. Sixty-six men, aged 18–24, in their first 8 weeks of Army Basic Training, who had demonstrated ordinary reading knowledge of English, were randomly selected and assigned to one of three groups—an Experimental group, a Flying Control group, and a Grounded Control group. The Flying Control group was taken up for a flight but was not exposed to a simulated emergency. The Grounded Controls were given the same measures as were the other Ss, but did not fly at all.

Procedure

The experiment was conducted on 2 successive days. On the morning of the first day half of the Controls flew, and in the afternoon half of the Experimentals flew. On the second day the sequence was reversed for the remaining flying Ss. The Grounded Control group was split into four subgroups, one tested each morning and one each afternoon. The time schedule for administration of the various tests was kept constant for all groups.

One group of 10 Ss at a time was taken to the airport, purportedly to participate in a study of the effects of altitude on psychomotor performance. One experimenter supposedly conducting this study, and another experimenter disguised as a steward accompanied Ss. Ss were informed that their urine was to be collected after the flight; its chemical analysis to be "correlated" with their psychological test performance. To permit collection of only the urine secreted during and immediately after the flight, these Ss were required to void their bladders ½ hour before take-off.

Prior to boarding, an airport representative gave all personnel, including the experimenters, a folder containing the emergency instructions to be studied for 10 minutes. As standard operating procedure aboard military aircraft, all personnel, including the plane crew, donned life preservers and parachute harnesses under supervision of the aircraft commander.

Once aloft, at 5,000 feet Ss completed one irrelevant test and then waited for the plane to reach a higher altitude. In the case of the Experimental group flights, the aircraft lurched while changing altitude. Ss saw that one propeller had stopped turning and heard about other malfunctions over the intercom; they were then informed directly that there was an emergency. A simulated pilot-to-tower conversation was provided to the Ss over their earphones to support the deception. As the aircraft passed within sight of the airfield, Ss could see fire trucks and ambulances on the airstrip in apparent expectation of a crash landing.

After several minutes the pilot ordered the plane steward to prepare for ditching in the nearby ocean, since the landing gear would not function properly. This was a prearranged signal for the "steward" to administer the questionnaires both to Ss and to the overt experimenter, to make it appear to Ss that this experimenter was in the same emergency situation in which they found themselves. The Emergency Data

Form was given first, on a straightforward basis, because requesting information of this sort would seem plausible under the circumstances. The Emergency Instructions test was given under the pretext that this would furnish proof to insurance companies that emergency precautions had been properly followed. These papers were supposedly to be put in a waterproof container and jettisoned before the aircraft came down on the ocean.

While Ss worked on both of these pencil-and-paper tests, the pilot-to-tower communication was cut out from their earphones to permit them to work without distraction. At no time was there any intercommunication among Ss since both the aircraft noise and the seating arrangement made any contact impossible. After a specified time period, the aircraft made a safe landing at the airport. Ss were taken to a nearby classroom where, after individually responding to the SSS (Table 1), they were thoroughly informed as to the true nature and purpose of the experiment.

About 1 hour later, a group interview was arranged to further probe the Ss for their reaction to the situation, to determine if any had seen through the deception, and to calm any fears which might remain about the seriousness of the situation. Urines were collected at 3 hours after landing.

The Flying Control group was exposed to the same flight procedure, except that no emergency was simulated. At the proper time, both the overt experimenter and Ss were given the measures by the steward, ostensibly as routine operating procedure aboard military aircraft.

The Grounded Control Ss did not fly at all; they were told that the purpose of the experiment was to develop forms and questionnaires for use by the military. Ss in this group were to fill out what they thought were trial versions of these forms as part of the developmental process.

Before any of the data were processed, five experimental Ss were eliminated because it was determined that they had not been deceived. During the interviews one S reported that he saw figures written on an airsickness bag used as scratch paper by a previous S. Another accidentally overheard a genuine conversation on the intercom between the pilot and the flight engineer of the aircraft. The other three had had considerable flight experience and were able, cognitively, to determine that the emergency was not authentic.

The group interview with the Experimental

Ss served generally to confirm the expectations of the experimenters that the situation was perceived as real, that various degrees of anxiety had been aroused in Ss about the possibility of death or injury, and that there were various degrees of self-confidence about ability to survive a possible ditching. The anxiety was determined to have disappeared by the time of the interview.

*   *   *

Three Cognitive Stresses Embedded into a Military Exercise

*   *   *

The three situations comprising this experiment have this in common: S is led to believe that he is in immediate danger of losing his life or of being seriously injured, and the task required of all Ss relevant to the predicament is the same. The situations differ only in the events contrived to cause the "emergency": accidental nuclear radiation in the area, a sudden forest fire in the area, or misdirected incoming artillery shells. These three events can be ordered along the dimension of amount of *perceptual support* (this term refers to the saliency and/or intensity of environmental cues confirming the cognitive elements of the stressor).

The situation with the least perceptual support is identified as Chemical, Biological, and Radiological (CBR) warfare. S is stationed alone at an isolated outpost and is told to report to the Command Post by radio the presence of any aircraft overhead. He later hears over his radio that an accident with radioactive material has resulted in dangerous fallout over his area. He is led to believe that the accident occurred during the exercise but is definitely not an intentional part of it. Immediate rescue is possible for him only if he can report his location over his radio transmitter, which has quite suddenly failed. The failure of his transmitter is, to his knowledge, coincidental with the accidental radiation hazard. The maneuver in which he was participating is canceled because of the accident and all activity now is concerned solely with the evacuation of personnel from the affected area. The only perceptual confirmation available at the position is an instrument which presumably (but not actually) measures the amount of nuclear radiation in the area.

The setting for the second situation is the same, except that the "accident" is a forest fire surrounding S's outpost. For perceptual support, S is enveloped in artificial smoke generated about

300 yards away. This cue is more obvious than the radiation dosimeter in the CBR situation. Again, his failing radio thwarts his rescue.

In the third situation a series of explosions simulates a barrage of artillery shells coming in and bursting near S. These explosions substantiate reports which S hears on his radio to the effect that some artillery shells appear to be hitting outside the designated target area. The explosions constitute the most salient of the perceptual supports used in these three situations. As in the other situations, S's transmitter—his key to rapid rescue—inexplicably fails, though he continues to receive messages.

The Control group, to be contrasted with each of the above three Experimental groups, needs radio communication in order to request future rations and water. This was an important incentive for their radio repair work but since their immediate needs had been met, it clearly was not at the same level of intensity as were those of the Experimental treatments.

*   *   *

b.

W. E. Glover, A. D. M. Greenfield, and R. G. Shanks
The Contribution Made by Adrenaline to the Vasodilation in the Human Forearm during Emotional Stress*

*   *   *

. . . In the present experiments DCI [dichloroisopropylnor-adrenaline] has been used to define the contribution of adrenaline to the changes in blood flow in the forearm in response to emotional stress.

The experiments were carried out on six healthy young men. The subject, wearing normal indoor clothing, lay on a couch in a laboratory, the temperature in which was maintained constant in the range 20–22°C. . . . A needle was inserted in the left brachial artery, and through it saline was infused at a rate of 4 ml./min by means of a mechanically driven syringe. In three experiments adrenaline hydrochloride was infused intra-arterially for 3–4 min., and in four experiments was infused into an antecubital vein for 5 min. Ascorbic acid was added to the perfusates as a preservative. DCI was infused intra-arterially for periods up to 30 min.

"Emotional stress" was produced by lead-

---

* 164 *Journal of Physiology* 422, 423, 428 (1962). Reprinted by permission.

ing the subject to believe that the wrong dose of a drug had been infused into his arm and that he was in considerable peril.* After 3–10 min. the subject was reassured and the purpose of the experiment was explained. Such observations can be made only once on each subject, and this limited the number of experiments we could make.

* * *

. . . The results . . . agree with the conclusion of Blair *et al.* that the humoral contribution to the increase in forearm blood flow during emotional stress may vary from subject to subject, and the conclusion of Barcroft *et al.* that both humoral and nervous factors are concerned. It would be interesting to know whether the same subject always produced the same type of response to varying emotional stimuli. Unfortunately, it is possible to hoax the subject on only one occasion.

c.

Allen E. Bergin
The Effect of Dissonant Persuasive Communications upon Changes in a Self-Referring Attitude†

* * *

The purposes of the present study were (*a*) to test whether conclusions regarding the role of credibility and discrepancy in attitude change research remain valid when "interpretations" about self-referring attitudes are involved, and (*b*) to test predictions derived from dissonance theory‡ concerning the effects of extremely dis-

crepant communications upon attitude change under conditions of high issue involvement and under varying levels of communicator credibility.

Specifically, it was predicted that (*a*) Ss receiving a communication from a source of high credibility would change their self-ratings in the direction of the communication significantly more than would Ss receiving a similar communication from a low-credibility source, (*b*) the amount of change in the high-credibility condition would increase monotonically as discrepancy increased, and (*c*) that the difference in amount of change between the low- and high-credibility conditions would increase as discrepancy increased.

Method

To test the hypotheses attempts were made to change the Ss' conceptions of their own masculinity or femininity by manipulating the discrepancy and credibility of a communication about those characteristics. Ss first rated themselves on masculinity-femininity following which they received a communication on this subject at one of three discrepancy levels from either a high- or low-credibility source. Ss subsequently made a second self-rating of masculinity-femininity and the difference between the two ratings was taken as the index of attitude change.

Ss were 60 freshmen and sophomores enrolled in an introductory psychology course at Stanford. They were distributed randomly among the six experimental conditions provided by the

---

* "[T]he words 'considerable peril' were perhaps wrongly chosen, and have caused some people to form an opinion of the experiments which differs from what actually happened. The aim of the experiments was physiological, not pathological, and was to reproduce in the laboratory a state of alarm of a quality that is frequently experienced in normal life—for example when driving, and a pedestrian emerges from behind a parked vehicle, or on missing an important connection for a vital appointment. One of my colleagues who was present on all occasions makes the important point that in the 'acting,' subjects were not led to think, for example, that there was any danger to life. We should obviously have taken more space to describe the methods more clearly." [Letter from A.D.M. Greenfield, May 1, 1971.]

† 30 *Journal of Personality* 423, 425–427, 434, 436 (1962). Reprinted by permission.

‡ Festinger's theory of cognitive dissonance (1957) provides a theoretical basis for organizing

the attitude-change variables with which we are principally concerned. The theory assumes that individuals strive to maintain consistency among their cognitions and that the existence of nonfitting cognitive elements produces tension which a person tries to reduce. A dissonance-producing situation common to both persuasion and interpretation is one in which a communicator presents a view contrary to the one held by the communicatee. In this event, the person is confronted with a need to reduce the dissonance produced by the presence of two contrary cognitions. A prediction of how he will choose to reduce the resultant state of dissonance will be in part a function of the credibility of the communicator, in part of the degree of discrepancy between the communicator and communicatee's positions, and in part of personal involvement with the communication content. Although these factors have been manipulated experimentally in studies of communication and persuasion, they have not been applied to the problem of changing attitudes about oneself which is a major purpose of interpretation.

three degrees of communication discrepancy and the two levels of communicator credibility. Males and females were distributed approximately evenly among the conditions in order to equalize any effects of sex differences in responses to the communication.

In the high-credibility condition Ss reported individually to the Psychiatry Department of the Stanford Medical Center where the E assumed the role of director of a personality assessment project. To further establish his credibility, Ss were sent to E by a receptionist, and the experimental room was furnished with elaborate equipment, a couch, an impressive array of medical and psychological volumes, and a large portrait of Freud. In the first session Ss were informed that the study was concerned with peoples' accuracy in evaluating their own personalities. The procedure was described as one in which S would rate himself on some scales after which he would take a battery of diagnostic tests. The degree of agreement between his self-description and that yielded by the objective measures would then be determined.

After rating himself, S was administered an elaborate battery of tests including cards from the Rorschach and TAT, the Fe scale from the California Personality Inventory (CPI), the Draw-A-Person test, a word-association test, and a specially devised figures-perception test concerning descriptions of male, female, and neutral figures. During this portion of the procedure Ss were hooked up to two disguised electroshock-therapy sets which were connected by means of false wiring to the S's chest and the palm of the right hand and in turn to a kymograph which reeled off (previously recorded) readings of S's responses to the test stimuli. Ss were informed that these instruments yielded physiological measures of their underlying emotional reactions which were extremely valid indicators of a person's underlying personality predispositions. The session was also tape recorded to further impress the Ss with the rigor of the procedures.

In a second session within the same week Ss were shown a Rorschach Psychogram and a set of Leary Interpersonal Diagrams which were purported to represent an analysis of their test responses. It was indicated that these diagrams summarized all of the test material and provided a set of discrepancy scores that could be translated back to the self-rating forms. After emphasizing the validity of the psychological evaluation, E described to S the (predetermined) discrepancy (moderate, high, or extreme) be-

tween the S's self-rating on masculinity-femininity and the rating supposedly derived from the test analysis.

*   *   *

In the low-credibility conditions Ss reported for the first session to a decrepit room in the basement of the Education Building where they simply filled out a set of self-ratings.

At the beginning of the second session Ss were introduced to another person, purportedly another subject with whom S would participate in the experiment. The "other" subject was actually E's confederate, a high school freshman. The Ss were told that the experiment was concerned with two different problems. The first, a study of interpersonal perception, required each of them to rate their partner on the personality dimensions they had rated themselves on several days earlier. The confederate then pretended to rate S on the dimensions; however, the actual ratings had been made by E in advance of the session according to the discrepancy condition to which S was assigned. When the confederate finished he was asked to transfer these ratings onto S's original self-ratings so that a direct comparison could be made. During this time S was kept busy answering the CPI. S was then shown his own self-rating in comparison to that made of him by the confederate. The discrepancy was discussed in the course of which E implied that high school students may not be the best judges of the traits of others.

*   *   *

Four rating scales were devised covering personality traits of concern to college students. These were: dominance-submission, masculinity-femininity, hostility, and independence-dependence. The masculinity-femininity scale was chosen as the dimension on which the discrepant communication was to be made, since the Ss were assumed to have special concern for their masculine or feminine image and, therefore, high involvement with communications on this topic. The masculinity-femininity scale consisted of seven defined points and six intermediate points, making a 13-point scale ranging from "completely feminine" to "slightly more masculine than feminine" for females and from "completely masculine" to "slightly more feminine than masculine" for males. The other three scales were used to provide a context for the critical scale and thus to disguise the persuasive intent of the relevant communication.

The three discrepancy levels (moderate, high, extreme) used were defined in terms of latitudes of acceptance and rejection. . . . In this experiment, a communication of moderate discrepancy was one within S's latitude of acceptance and at least two points away from his most acceptable rating. A high discrepancy was within S's latitude of rejection and at least four points away from his most acceptable rating. An extreme discrepancy was at the point S had rated as most contrary to his own view of himself and was at least six points away from his most acceptable rating. The communication of these ratings was accomplished by marking S's self-rating in red at the predetermined discrepancy level so that the comparison was obvious. . . .

*   *   *

To prevent distorted perceptions of the message in the direction of one's previous beliefs the communications were made as unambiguous as possible. The communicator's rating was shown as a distinct red mark on the self-rating scale with the distance away from Ss own rating clearly shown. His attention was explicitly focused on this difference by E's instructions. . . .

*   *   *

Discussion

The results are consistent with the predictions derived from cognitive dissonance theory. They suggest that amount of dissonance increases monotonically with amount of discrepancy and when attitude change is the primary means available to the S for reducing dissonance, attitude change will also increase monotonically. On the other hand, when involvement and dissonance are high and credibility is low, other means—such as discrediting the communicator—become the primary dissonance-reducing response and amount of change is minimized.

*   *   *

It could be argued that the changes in self-ratings simply represent compliance with the wishes of a prestigeful figure rather than a reorientation in the way Ss view themselves. It appears that such compliance effects were minimized as is evidenced by the following: (a) the emotional reactions of Ss (grasping, turning redfaced, poring over the rating scale) in the high-credibility condition indicated that they were more serious about the discrepancies and what they implied than if they intended merely

to comply, (b) the avoidance by the E of giving the impression that he wanted Ss to change their self-ratings, and (c) the fact that in the post-experimental interview when Ss were asked whether they had changed their self-ratings, a sizable proportion (35 per cent) had changed significantly without being aware of it. They reported that the second rating was their own view and that it had not changed since the time of the original ratings. This was quite startling in light of the fact that many of these people had shifted several points in the direction of the communication. Apparently they were committed to the new rating, not simply publicly espousing it while privately rejecting it.

*   *   *

NOTES

NOTE 1.

HERBERT C. KELMAN
HUMAN USE OF HUMAN SUBJECTS—THE PROBLEM OF DECEPTION IN SOCIAL PSYCHOLOGICAL EXPERIMENTS*

*   *   *

Ethical problems of a rather obvious nature arise in the experiments in which deception has potentially harmful consequences for the subject. Take, for example, the brilliant experiment by Mulder and Stemerding on the effects of threat on attraction to the group and need for strong leadership. In this study—one of the very rare examples of an experiment conducted in a natural setting—independent food merchants in a number of Dutch towns were brought together for group meetings in the course of which they were informed that a large organization was planning to open up a series of supermarkets in the Netherlands. In the High Threat condition, subjects were told that there was a high probability that their town would be selected as a site for such markets and that the advent of these markets would cause a considerable drop in their business. On the advice of the executives of the shopkeepers' organizations, who had helped to arrange the group meetings, the investigators did not reveal the experimental manipulations to their subjects. I have been worried about these Dutch merchants ever since I heard about this study for the first time. Did some of them go out of business in anticipation of the heavy competition? Do some of them have an

* 67 *Psychological Bulletin* 1, 3–4 (1967). © 1967, American Psychological Association. Reprinted by permission.

anxiety reaction every time they see a bulldozer? Chances are that they soon forgot about this threat (unless, of course, supermarkets actually did move into town) and that it became just one of the many little moments of anxiety that must occur in every shopkeeper's life. Do we have a right, however, to add to life's little anxieties and to risk the possibility of more extensive anxiety purely for the purposes of our experiments, particularly since deception deprives the subject of the opportunity to choose whether or not he wishes to expose himself to the risks that might be entailed?

*   *   *

NOTE 2.

JULIUS SEEMAN
DECEPTION IN PSYCHOLOGICAL RESEARCH*

*   *   *

With respect to the incidence of deception, it may be useful to note the frequency with which deception appears in the published literature and to determine whether any long-term trends are evident. For this purpose, the total published literature in several journals was analyzed for the years 1948 and 1963. Journals were chosen to reflect different fields within psychology.

[J]ournals emphasizing "experimental" and "clinical" areas had a relatively low incidence of deception studies in comparison with "personality and social" areas. The latter areas also showed a distinct rise in the use of deception. When the figures for the *Journal of Personality* and the *Journal of Abnormal and Social Psychology* are combined, the mean for 1948 is 18.47 percent and the mean for 1963 is 38.17 percent. It seems safe to conclude that to some degree deception has come to be the method of choice in this area of research.

*   *   *

d.

Stanley Milgram
Some Conditions of Obedience and
Disobedience to Authority†

The situation in which one agent commands another to hurt a third turns up time and again as a significant theme in human relations. . . .
. . . We describe an experimental program,

recently concluded at Yale University, in which a particular expression of this conflict is studied by experimental means.

In its most general form the problem may be defined thus: if X tells Y to hurt Z, under what conditions will Y carry out the command of X and under what conditions will he refuse. In the more limited form possible in laboratory research, the question becomes: if an experimenter tells a subject to hurt another person, under what conditions will the subject go along with this instruction, and under what conditions will he refuse to obey. The laboratory problem is not so much a dilution of the general statement as one concrete expression of the many particular forms this question may assume.

One aim of the research was to study behavior in a strong situation of deep consequence to the participants, for the psychological forces operative in powerful and lifelike forms of the conflict may not be brought into play under diluted conditions.

This approach meant, first, that we had a special obligation to protect the welfare and dignity of the persons who took part in the study; subjects were, of necessity, placed in a difficult predicament, and steps had to be taken to ensure their well-being before they were discharged from the laboratory. Toward this end, a careful, post-experimental treatment was devised and has been carried through for subjects in all conditions.[3]

---

[3] It consisted of an extended discussion with the experimenter and, of equal importance, a friendly reconciliation with the victim. It is made clear that the victim did not receive painful electric shocks. After the completion of the experimental series, subjects were sent a detailed report of the results and full purposes of the experimental program. A formal assessment of this procedure points to its overall effectiveness. Of the subjects, 83.7 per cent indicated that they were glad to have taken part in the study; 15.1 per cent reported neutral feelings; and 1.3 per cent stated that they were sorry to have participated. A large number of subjects spontaneously requested that they be used in further experimentation. Four-fifths of the subjects felt that more experiments of this sort should be carried out, and 74 per cent indicated that they had learned something of personal importance as a result of being in the study. Furthermore, a university psychiatrist, experienced in outpatient treatment, interviewed a sample of experimental subjects with the aim of uncovering possible injurious effects resulting from participation. No such effects were in evidence. Indeed, subjects typically felt that their participation was instructive and enriching. . . .

---

* 24 *American Psychologist* 1025 (1969). Reprinted by permission.
† 18 *Human Relations* 57–75 (1965). Reprinted by permission.

Terminology. If Y follows the command of X we shall say that he has obeyed X; if he fails to carry out the command of X, we shall say that he has disobeyed X. The terms *to obey* and *to disobey,* as used here, refer to the subject's overt action only, and carry no implication for the motive or experiential states accompanying the action.

* * *

A subject who complies with the entire series of experimental commands will be termed an *obedient* subject; one who at any point in the command series defies the experimenter will be called a *disobedient* or *defiant* subject. As used in this report, the terms refer only to the subject's performance in the experiment, and do not necessarily imply a general personality disposition to submit to or reject authority.

Subject Population. The subjects used in all experimental conditions were male adults, residing in the greater New Haven and Bridgeport areas, aged 20 to 50 years, and engaged in a wide variety of occupations. Each experimental condition described in this report employed 40 fresh subjects and was carefully balanced for age and occupational types. The occupational composition for each experiment was: workers, skilled and unskilled: 40 per cent; white collar, sales, business: 40 per cent; professionals: 20 per cent. . . .

The General Laboratory Procedure. The focus of the study concerns the amount of electric shock a subject is willing to administer to another person when ordered by an experimenter to give the "victim" increasingly more severe punishment. The act of administering shock is set in the context of a learning experiment, ostensibly designed to study the effect of punishment on memory. Aside from the experimenter, one naive subject and one accomplice perform in each session. On arrival each subject is paid $4.50. After a general talk by the experimenter, telling how little scientists know about the effect of punishment on memory, subjects are informed that one member of the pair will serve as teacher and one as learner. A rigged drawing is held so that the naive subject is always the teacher, and the accomplice becomes the learner. The learner is taken to an adjacent room and strapped into an "electric chair."

The naive subject is told that it is his task to teach the learner a list of paired associates, to test him on the list, and to administer punishment whenever the learner errs in the test. Punishment takes the form of electric shock, delivered to the learner by means of a shock generator controlled by the naive subject. The teacher is instructed to increase the intensity of electric shock one step on the generator on each error. The learner, according to plan, provides many wrong answers, so that before long the naive subject must give him the strongest shock on the generator. Increases in shock level are met by increasingly insistent demands from the learner that the experiment be stopped because of the growing discomfort to him. However, in clear terms the experimenter orders the teacher to continue with the procedure in disregard of the learner's protests. *Thus, the naive subject must resolve a conflict between two mutually incompatible demands from the social field. He may continue to follow the orders of the experimenter and shock the learner with increasing severity, or he may refuse to follow the orders of the experimenter and heed the learner's pleas. The experimenter's authority operates not in a free field, but against ever-mounting countervailing pressures from the person being punished.*

A few technical points need to be considered before the findings of the study are described. For the purpose of delivering shock, a simulated shock generator is used, with 30 clearly marked voltage levels that range from 15 to 450 volts (and each activated by one of 30 individual lever switches set in a horizontal line). The naive subject is given a sample shock of 45 volts to convince him of the authenticity of the instrument. The generator bears verbal designations that range from "Slight Shock" to "Danger: Severe Shock."

The responses of the victim are standardized on tape, and each protest is coordinated to a particular voltage level on the shock generator. Starting with 75 volts the learner begins to grunt and moan. At 150 volts he demands to be let out of the experiment. At 180 volts he cries out that he can no longer stand the pain. At 300 volts he refuses to provide any more answers to the memory test, insisting that he is no longer a participant in the experiment and must be freed. In response to this last tactic, the experimenter instructs the naive subject to treat the absence of an answer as equivalent to a wrong answer, and to follow the usual shock procedure. The experimenter reinforces his demand with the statement: "You have no other choice, you must go on!" (This imperative is used whenever the naive subject tries to break off the experiment.) If the subject refuses to give the next higher level of shock, the experiment is considered at an end. A quantitative value is assigned to the subject's performance based on the maximum intensity shock he administered before breaking off. Thus any subject's score may range from zero (for a subject unwilling to administer the first shock level) to 30 (for a subject who proceeds to the highest voltage level on the board). For any particular subject and for any particular experimental condition the degree to which participants have followed the experimenter's orders may be specified with a numerical value, corresponding to the metric on the shock generator.

*　　*　　*

Pilot Studies. Pilot studies for the present research were completed in the winter of 1960; they differed from the regular experiments in a few details: for one, the victim was placed behind a silvered glass, with the light balance on the glass such that the victim could be dimly perceived by the subject.

Though essentially qualitative in treatment, these studies pointed to several significant features of the experimental situation. At first no vocal feedback was used from the victim. It was thought that the verbal and voltage designations on the control panel would create sufficient pressure to curtail the subject's obedience. However, this was not the case. In the absence of protests from the learner, virtually all subjects, once commanded, went blithely to the end of the board, seemingly indifferent to the verbal designations ("Extreme Shock" and "Danger, Severe Shock"). This deprived us of an adequate basis for scaling obedient tendencies. A force had to be introduced that would strengthen the subject's resistance to the experimenter's commands, and reveal individual differences in terms of a distribution of break-off points.

This force took the form of protests from the victim. Initially, mild protests were used, but proved inadequate. Subsequently, more vehement protests were inserted into the experimental procedure. To our consternation, even the strongest protests from the victim did not prevent all subjects from administering the harshest punishment ordered by the experimenter; but the protests did lower the mean maximum shock somewhat and created some spread in the subject's performance; therefore, the victim's cries were standardized on tape and incorporated into the regular experimental procedure.

The situation did more than highlight the technical difficulties of finding a workable experimental procedure: it indicated that subjects would obey authority to a greater extent than we had supposed. It also pointed to the importance of feedback from the victim in controlling the subject's behavior.

One further aspect of the pilot study was that subjects frequently averted their eyes from the person they were shocking, often turning their heads in an awkward and conspicuous manner. One subject explained: "I didn't want to see the consequences of what I had done." Observers wrote:

. . . subjects showed a reluctance to look at the victim, whom they could see through the glass in front of them. When this fact was brought to their attention they indicated that it caused them discomfort to see the victim in agony. We note, however, that although the subject refuses to look at the victim, he continues to administer shocks.

This suggested that the salience of the victim may have, in some degree, regulated the subject's performance. If, in obeying the experimenter, the subject found it necessary to avoid scrutiny of the victim, would the converse be true? If the victim were rendered increasingly more salient to the subject, would obedience diminish? The first set of regular experiments was designed to answer this question.

Immediacy of the Victim. This series consisted of four experimental conditions. In each condition the victim was brought "psychologically" closer to the subject giving him shocks.

In the first condition (Remote Feedback) the victim was placed in another room and could not be heard or seen by the subject, except that, at 300 volts, he pounded on the wall in protest. After 315 volts he no longer answered or was heard from.

The second condition (Voice Feedback) was identical to the first except that voice protests were introduced. As in the first condition the victim was placed in an adjacent room, but his complaints could be heard clearly through a door left slightly ajar, and through the walls of the laboratory.[6]

---

[6] It is difficult to convey on the printed page the full tenor of the victim's responses, for we have no adequate notation for vocal intensity, timing, and general qualities of delivery. Yet these features are crucial to producing the effect of an increasingly severe reaction to mounting voltage levels. (They can be communicated fully only by sending interested parties the recorded tapes.) In general terms,

The third experimental condition (Proximity) was similar to the second, except that the victim was now placed in the same room as the subject, and 1½ feet from him. Thus he was visible as well as audible, and voice cues were provided.

The fourth, and final, condition of this series (Touch-Proximity) was identical to the third, with this exception: the victim received a shock only when his hand rested on a shockplate. At the 150-volt level the victim again demanded to be let free and, in this condition, refused to place his hand on the shockplate. The experimenter ordered the naive subject to force the victim's hand onto the plate. Thus obedience in this condition required that the subject have physical contact with the victim in order to give him punishment beyond the 150-volt level.

Forty adult subjects were studied in each condition. The data revealed that obedience was significantly reduced as the victim was rendered more immediate to the subject. . . .

Expressed in terms of the proportion of obedient to defiant subjects, the findings are that 34 per cent of the subjects defied the experimenter in the Remote condition, 37.5 per cent in Voice Feedback, 60 per cent in Proximity, and 70 per cent in Touch-Proximity.

How are we to account for this effect? A first conjecture might be that as the victim was brought closer the subject became more aware of the intensity of his suffering and regulated his behavior accordingly. This makes sense, but

---

however, the victim indicates no discomfort until the 75-volt shock is administered, at which time there is a light grunt in response to the punishment. Similar reactions follow the 90- and 105-volt shocks, and at 120 volts the victim shouts to the experimenter that the shocks are becoming painful. Painful groans are heard on administration of the 135-volt shock, and at 150 volts the victim cries out, "Experimenter, get me out of here! I won't be in the experiment any more! I refuse to go on!" Cries of this type continue with generally rising intensity, so that at 180 volts the victim cries out, "I can't stand the pain," and by 270 volts his response to the shock is definitely an agonized scream. Throughout, he insists that he be let out of the experiment. At 300 volts the victim shouts in desperation that he will no longer provide answers to the memory test; and at 315 volts, after a violent scream, he reaffirms with vehemence that he is no longer a participant. From this point on, he provides no answers, but shrieks in agony whenever a shock is administered; this continues through 450 volts. Of course, many subjects will have broken off before this point.

our evidence does not support the interpretation. There are no consistent differences in the attributed level of pain across the four conditions (i.e. the amount of pain experienced by the victime as estimated by the subject and expressed on a 14-point scale). But it is easy to speculate about alternative mechanisms:

Empathic cues. In the Remote and to a lesser extent the Voice Feedback condition, the victim's suffering possesses an abstract, remote quality for the subject. He is aware, but only in a conceptual sense, that his actions cause pain to another person; the fact is apprehended, but not felt. The phenomenon is common enough. The bombardier can reasonably suppose that his weapons will inflict suffering and death, yet this knowledge is divested of affect, and does not move him to a felt, emotional response to the suffering resulting from his actions. . . .

Denial and narrowing of the cognitive field. The Remote condition allows a narrowing of the cognitive field so that the victim is put out of mind. The subject no longer considers the act of depressing a lever relevant to moral judgment, for it is no longer associated with the victim's suffering. When the victim is close it is more difficult to exclude him phenomenologically. He necessarily intrudes on the subject's awareness since he is continuously visible. . . .

Reciprocal fields. If in the Proximity condition the subject is in an improved position to observe the victim, the reverse is also true. The actions of the subject now come under proximal scrutiny by the victim. Possibly, it is easier to harm a person when he is unable to observe our actions than when he can see what we are doing. His surveillance of the action directed against him may give rise to shame, or guilt, which may then serve to curtail the action. . . .

*   *   *

Closeness of Authority. If the spatial relationship of the subject and victim is relevant to the degree of obedience, would not the relationship of subject to experimenter also play a part?

There are reasons to feel that, on arrival, the subject is oriented primarily to the experimenter rather than to the victim. He has come to the laboratory to fit into the structure that the experimenter—not the victim—would provide. He has come less to understand his behavior than to *reveal* that behavior to a competent scientist, and he is willing to display himself as the scientist's purposes require. Most subjects seem quite concerned about the appearance they are making before the experimenter, and one could argue that this preoccupation in a relatively new and strange setting makes the subject somewhat insensitive to the triadic nature of the social situation. In other words, the subject is so concerned about the show he is putting on for the experimenter that influences from other parts of the social field do not receive as much weight as they ordinarily would. This overdetermined orientation to the experimenter would account for the relative insensitivity of the subject to the victim, and would also lead us to believe that alterations in the relationship between subject and experimenter would have important consequences for obedience.

In a series of experiments we varied the physical closeness and degree of surveillance of the experimenter. In one condition the experimenter sat just a few feet away from the subject. In a second condition, after giving initial instructions, the experimenter left the laboratory and gave his orders by telephone; in still a third condition the experimenter was never seen, providing instructions by means of a tape recording activated when the subjects entered the laboratory.

Obedience dropped sharply as the experimenter was physically removed from the laboratory. The number of obedient subjects in the first condition (Experimenter Present) was almost three times as great as in the second, where the experimenter gave his orders by telephone. Twenty-six subjects were fully obedient in the first condition, and only 9 in the second. . . .

Moreover, when the experimenter was absent, subjects displayed an interesting form of behavior that had not occurred under his surveillance. Though continuing with the experiment, several subjects administered lower shocks than were required and never informed the experimenter of their deviation from the correct procedure. (Unknown to the subjects, shock levels were automatically recorded by an Esterline-Angus event recorder wired directly into the shock generator; the instrument provided us with an objective record of the subjects' performance.) Indeed, in telephone conversations some subjects specifically assured the experimenter that they were raising the shock level according to instruction, whereas in fact they were repeatedly using the lowest shock on the board. This form of behavior is particularly interesting: although these subjects acted in a way that clearly undermined the avowed purposes of the experiment, they found it easier to handle the conflict in this manner than to precipitate an open break with authority.

* * *

Tensions. The description of final scores does not fully convey the character of the subjects' performance, and it would be useful to interrupt our reporting of quantitative relationships to remark on the subjects' general reaction to the situation.

One might suppose that a subject would simply break off or continue as his conscience and temperament dictated. Yet this is very far from what happened. There were powerful reactions of tension and emotional strain in a substantial proportion of the participants. Persons were observed to sweat, tremble, stutter, bite their lips, and groan as they found themselves increasingly implicated in the experimental conflict. Some sense of the subjects' mood can be gotten from a transcript of their remarks at break-off point. Here are the remarks of two defiant subjects:

Is he banging? . . . Is he hurt out there? Well, I don't want to be responsible for anything that happens to him. No, I can't go on with it. I don't know whether he's alright or not. I mean he may have a heart condition or something; I wouldn't feel right doing it. He's banging for help. He's evidently in trouble or he wouldn't bang. . . . I don't see any sense to this—to knocking him out or something. I just can't see it.

(Subject refuses to administer shocks.)

The man is banging. He wants to get out. . . . I'm sorry. If the man wants to get out I'd just as soon stop. . . . I don't want to administer any more [extremely excited]. . . I will gladly refund the check, but I will not harm this man. . . . I'm sorry, I will not give him any more if he obviously wants to get out. There is no money in the world that will make me hurt another individual.

And here is a transcript from an obedient subject. He began the experiment calmly, but became increasingly tense as the experiment proceded. After administering the 150-volt shock, he began to address the experimenter in agitated tones:

(150 *volts delivered.*) You want me to keep going?
(165 *volts delivered.*) That guy is hollering in there. There's a lot of them here. He's liable to have a heart condition. You want me to go?
(180 *volts delivered.*) He can't stand it! I'm not going to kill that man in there! You hear him hollering? He's hollering. He can't stand it. What if something happens to him? . . . I'm not going to get that man sick in there. He's hollering in there. You know what I mean? I mean I refuse to take responsibility. He's getting hurt in there. He's in there hollering. Too many left here. Geez, if he gets them wrong.

There's too many of them left. I mean who is going to take responsibility if anything happens to that gentleman?
[*The experimenter accepts responsibility.*]
All right.
(195 *volts delivered.*) You see he's hollering. Hear that. Gee, I don't know. [*The experimenter says: "The experiment requires that you go on."*]—I know it does, sir, but I mean—huh—he don't know what he's in for. He's up to 195 volts.
(210 *volts delivered.*)
(225 *volts delivered.*)
(240 *volts delivered.*) Aw, no! You mean I've got to keep going up with the scale? No sir. I'm not going to kill that man! I'm not going to give him 450 volts! [*The experimenter says: "The experiment requires that you go on."*]—I know it does, but that man is hollering in there, sir. . . .

Despite his numerous, agitated objections, which were constant accompaniments to his actions, the subject unfailingly obeyed the experimenter, proceeding to the highest shock level on the generator. He displayed a curious dissociation between word and action. Although at the verbal level he had resolved not to go on, his actions were fully in accord with the experimenter's commands. This subject did not want to shock the victim, and he found it an extremely disagreeable task, but he was unable to invent a response that would free him from *E*'s authority. Many subjects cannot find the specific verbal formula that would enable them to reject the role assigned to them by the experimenter. Perhaps our culture does not provide adequate models for disobedience.

One puzzling sign of tension was the regular occurrence of nervous laughing fits. In the first four conditions 71 of the 160 subjects showed definite signs of nervous laughter and smiling. The laughter seemed entirely out of place, even bizarre. Full-blown, uncontrollable seizures were observed for 15 of these subjects. On one occasion we observed a seizure so violently convulsive that it was necessary to call a halt to the experiment. In the post-experimental interviews subjects took pains to point out that they were not sadistic types and that the laughter did not mean they enjoyed shocking the victim.

In the interview following the experiment subjects were asked to indicate on a 14-point scale just how nervous or tense they felt at the point of maximum tension. The scale ranged from "Not at all tense and nervous" to "Extremely tense and nervous." Self-reports of this sort are of limited precision, and at best provide only a rough indication of the subject's emo-

tional response. Still, taking the reports for what they are worth, it can be seen that the distribution of responses spans the entire range of the scale, with the majority of subjects concentrated at the center and upper extreme. A further breakdown showed that obedient subjects reported themselves as having been slightly more tense and nervous than the defiant subjects at the point of maximum tension.

* * *

Background authority. . . . The effectiveness of the experimenter's commands may depend in an important way on the larger institutional context in which they are issued. The experiments described thus far were conducted at Yale University, an organization which most subjects regarded with respect and sometimes awe. In post-experimental interviews several participants remarked that the locale and sponsorship of the study gave them confidence in the integrity, competence, and benign purposes of the personnel; many indicated that they would not have shocked the learner if the experiments had been done elsewhere.

This issue of background authority seemed to us important for an interpretation of the results that had been obtained thus far; moreover it is highly relevant to any comprehensive theory of human obedience. Consider, for example, how closely our compliance with the imperatives of others is tied to particular institutions and locales in our day-to-day activities. On request, we expose our throats to a man with a razor blade in the barber shop, but would not do so in a shoe store; in the latter setting we willingly follow the clerk's request to stand in our stockinged feet, but resist the command in a bank. In the laboratory of a great university, subjects may comply with a set of commands that would be resisted if given elsewhere. *One must always question the relationship of obedience to a person's sense of the context in which he is operating.*

To explore the problem we moved our apparatus to an office building in industrial Bridgeport and replicated experimental conditions, without any visible tie to the university.

Bridgeport subjects were invited to the experiment through a mail circular similar to the one used in the Yale study, with appropriate changes in letterhead, etc. As in the earlier study, subjects were paid $4.50 for coming to the laboratory. The same age and occupational distributions used at Yale, and the identical personnel, were employed.

The purpose in relocating in Bridgeport was to assure a complete dissociation from Yale, and in this regard we were fully successful. On the surface, the study appeared to be conducted by RESEARCH ASSOCIATES OF BRIDGEPORT, an organization of unknown character (the title had been concocted exclusively for use in this study).

The experiments were conducted in a three-room office suite in a somewhat run-down commercial building located in the downtown shopping area. The laboratory was sparsely furnished, though clean, and marginally respectable in appearance. When subjects inquired about professional affiliations, they were informed only that we were a private firm conducting research for industry.

Some subjects displayed skepticism concerning the motives of the Bridgeport experimenter. One gentleman gave us a written account of the thoughts he experienced at the control board:

. . . Should I quit this damn test? Maybe he passed out? What dopes we were not to check up on this deal. How do we know that these guys are legit? No furniture, bare walls, no telephone. We could of called the police up or the Better Business Bureau. I learned a lesson tonight. How do I know that Mr. Williams [the experimenter] is telling the truth. . . . I wish I knew how many volts a person could take before lapsing into unconsciousness. . . .

Another subject stated:

I questioned on my arrival my own judgment [about coming]. I had doubts as to the legitimacy of the operation and the consequences of participation. I felt it was a heartless way to conduct memory or learning processes on human beings and certainly dangerous without the presence of a medical doctor.

There was no noticeable reduction in tension for the Bridgeport subjects. And the subjects' estimation of the amount of pain felt by the victim was slightly, though not significantly, higher than in the Yale study.

A failure to obtain complete obedience in Bridgeport would indicate that the extreme compliance found in New Haven subjects was tied closely to the background authority of Yale University; if a large proportion of the subjects remained fully obedient, very different conclusions would be called for.

As it turned out, the level of obedience in Bridgeport, although somewhat reduced, was not significantly lower than that obtained at Yale. A large proportion of the Bridgeport subjects were fully obedient to the experimenter's commands (48 per cent of the Bridgeport subjects delivered the maximum shock *vs.* 65 per cent in the corresponding conditions at Yale).

*   *   *

Levels of Obedience and Defiance. One general finding that merits attention is the high level of obedience manifested in the experimental situation. Subjects often expressed deep disapproval of shocking a man in the face of his objections, and others denounced it as senseless and stupid. Yet many subjects complied even while they protested. The proportion of obedient subjects greatly exceeded the expectations of the experimenter and his colleagues. At the outset, we had conjectured that subjects would not, in general, go above the level of "Strong Shock." In practice, many subjects were willing to administer the most extreme shocks available when commanded by the experimenter. For some subjects the experiment provides an occasion for aggressive release. And for others it demonstrates the extent to which obedient dispositions are deeply ingrained, and are engaged irrespective of their consequences for others. Yet this is not the whole story. Somehow, the subject becomes implicated in a situation from which he cannot disengage himself.

The departure of the experimental results from intelligent expectation, to some extent, has been formalized. The procedure was to describe the experimental situations in concrete detail to a group of competent persons, and to ask them to predict the performance of 100 hypothetical subjects. For purposes of indicating the distribution of break-off points judges were provided with a diagram of the shock generator, and recorded their predictions before being informed of the actual results. Judges typically underestimated the amount of obedience demonstrated by subjects.

. . . The psychiatrists predicted that most subjects would not go beyond the tenth shock level (150 volts; at this point the victim makes his first explicit demand to be freed). They further predicted that by the twentieth shock level (300 volts; the victim refuses to answer) 3.73 per cent of the subjects would still be obedient; and that only a little over one-tenth of one per cent of the subjects would administer the highest shock on the board. But, as the graph indicates, the obtained behavior was very different. Sixty-two per cent of the subjects obeyed the experimenter's commands fully. Between expectation and occurrence there is a whopping discrepancy.

Many people, not knowing much about the experiment, claim that subjects who go to the end of the board are sadistic. Nothing could be more foolish as an overall characterization of these persons. It is like saying that a person thrown into a swift-flowing stream is necessarily a fast swimmer, or that he has great stamina because he moves so rapidly relative to the bank. The context of action must always be considered. The individual, upon entering the laboratory, becomes integrated into a situation that carries its own momentum. The subject's problem then is how to become disengaged from a situation which is moving in an altogether ugly direction.

The fact that disengagement is so difficult testifies to the potency of the forces that keep the subject at the control board. Are these forces to be conceptualized as individual motives and expressed in the language of personality dynamics, or are they to be seen as the effects of social structure and pressures arising from the situational field?

A full understanding of the subject's action will, I feel, require that both perspectives be adopted. The person brings to the laboratory enduring dispositions toward authority and aggression, and at the same time he becomes enmeshed in a social structure that is no less an objective fact of the case. From the standpoint of personality theory one may ask: What mechanisms of personality enable a person to transfer responsibility to authority? What are the motives underlying obedient and disobedient performance? Does orientation to authority lead to a short-circuiting of the shame-guilt system? What cognitive and emotional defenses are brought into play in the case of obedient and defiant subjects?

* * *

Postscript. Almost a thousand adults were individually studied in the obedience research, and there were many specific conclusions regarding the variables that control obedience and disobedience to authority. . . .

* * *

What is the limit of such obedience? At many points we attempted to establish a boundary. Cries from the victim were inserted; not good enough. The victim claimed heart trouble; subjects still shocked him on command. The victim pleaded that he be let free, and his answers no longer registered on the signal box; subjects continued to shock him. At the outset we had not conceived that such drastic procedures would be needed to generate disobedience, and each step was added only as the ineffectiveness of the earlier techniques became clear. The final effort to establish a limit was the Touch-Proximity condition. But the very first subject in this condition subdued the victim on command, and proceeded to the highest shock level. A quarter of the subjects in this condition performed similarly.

The results, as seen and felt in the laboratory, are to this author disturbing. They raise the possibility that human nature, or—more specifically—the kind of character produced in American democratic society, cannot be counted on to insulate its citizens from brutality and inhumane treatment at the direction of malevolent authority. A substantial proportion of people do what they are told to do, irrespective of the content of the act and without limitations of conscience, so long as they perceive that the command comes from a legitimate authority. If in this study an anonymous experimenter could successfully command adults to subdue a fifty-year-old man, and force on him painful electric shocks against his protests, one can only wonder what government, with its vastly greater authority and prestige, can command of its subjects. There is, of course, the extremely important question of whether malevolent political institutions could or would arise in American society. The present research contributes nothing to this issue.

* * *

e.

Bernard Bressler, Albert J. Silverman, Sanford I. Cohen, and Barry Shmavonian Research in Human Subjects and the Artificial Traumatic Neurosis— Where Does Our Responsibility Lie?*

The authors are engaged in a research project at Duke University dealing with isolation and sensory deprivation which uses human subjects selected at random. These subjects evidenced no gross psychopathology. The experiment is, on the surface, a comparatively simple one. Without previous instruction the subject is placed in a small, soundproof, completely darkened chamber for a period of two hours, at the end of which he is interviewed in the chamber to obtain his immediate impressions and reactions.

* 116 *American Journal of Psychiatry* 522–526 (1959). Copyright 1959, the American Psychiatric Association. Reprinted by permission.

Following this, he is seen outside the chamber by another interviewer, who questions him further on the cues picked up in the initial interview (which is taped). Then the subject fills out a comparatively simple written questionnaire regarding his impression of the experiment. On the day following the experiment he meets with a third interviewer for evaluation of his memory of his reaction to the experiment and also, generally, to determine how he has handled the total experience.

Reviewing our experience with one subject, a seemingly well adjusted, bright young woman obtaining her Ph.D. in psychology, we were confronted with an important problem which deserves considerable discussion and sober thought. A brief description of her progress during and following the experiment will indicate the exact nature of our concern.

It was quite apparent from the initial interview inside the chamber that the subject was experiencing a great deal of anxiety, and as she described it,

"My heart is beating quite fast." She described the feeling of "trying to get some kind of anchor; some kind of bearing," since all of her visual cues were gone. She reported periods of uneasiness, reassuring herself that she didn't have claustrophobia, and a headache which lasted for a short time. It was readily apparent (as is typical for almost all subjects) that she had no idea of the time elapsed despite her intellectual realization that she hadn't been in the chamber very long. When asked for a specific time estimate of her isolation she replied "Oh, hours." Her initial appearance was that of a perplexed, frightened, uncomfortable and anxious person. Her thinking process was quite slowed, and there was a great change in her verbalization and general speech patterns. As the interviewer entered the chamber her first impression was that he looked much larger than his actual size, and it was at this moment that she began to feel anxiety. Also she produced several bizarre fantasies: one about a submarine and another, derived from a science fiction story, about people locked in a room where they were slowly frozen to death. She required roughly an hour and a half to recover her normal intellectual functioning since, as she stated, "I was bewildered."

Following the isolation experience the subject described her feelings as "being shaken up inside." She said that she had a tremendous impulse to find someone she could trust and tell him "all about it." On her arrival home she was very hungry, something quite unusual for her, since she rarely eats at night. She played a few records and fixed something to eat although "it wasn't real hunger, just something to do." Finally, after great difficulty she went to sleep, awakening in the morning to find that the sheets had all been kicked away from the bed.

In the interview the next day she further elaborated some of her isolation fantasies. For example, she had the thought that "Maybe there was only two or three hours' worth of oxygen in the room." She identified herself with sailors in a submarine, a submarine which was obviously in danger. She recalled skipping from one dangerous situation to another and stated that she had concentrated on such situations. One of the dangers was "that the experimenter walked into the room, and an enemy closed the door behind him. Of course, there were no locks. He couldn't get out, and the fellow froze to death." At times she had some near paranoid ideas, i.e., thinking that the room was deliberately overheated, that her headache was due to deliberate oxygen deprivation, etc. At one point she became very threatened and thought "Well, I'll play a trick on you. If I go to sleep, you'll get me out." She said she had tried sleeping, and actually it was at this moment that the experiment was interrupted, and an interviewer entered.

At first, "You know I couldn't answer properly. I had a feeling I had nothing to say. I felt slowed down. Then there was that tremendous thumping of my heart." She said that at one point she reviewed her past and present life but had no thoughts about the future. Although she had a lot of love fantasies, she was unable to describe them to the interviewer who had teased her in the past. She thought about the opera "Aida," in which Radames was put into a vault to die. Her reaction to the total isolation experiment was: "There was something fascinating about it. It's not entertaining like going to a movie, but it's something fascinating, it's like having gone through the war. I'll never regret having gone through the war and having had my experiences despite the fact that they were pretty uncomfortable. There is something about it that just fascinates me."

Some time elapsed during which we had no further contact with the subject. However, it was subsequently decided to retest this subject (and others) in order to further evaluate the material under different circumstances. The experiment was repeated exactly as before, except that this time she was told in detail exactly what would happen.

One of the most remarkable effects of this second isolation experience on the subject was:

"I said to myself now I can really get my fantasies going. In other words I didn't start thinking of the present as I did before; this time I tended to wander more towards the past and towards the future, towards trying to solve problems. You know it seemed a lot longer this time, it was much harder for me to stay awake, and I was much less alert."

Later she indicated that she was sure she fell asleep, despite her intention to stay awake and watch her fantasies, and although she had taken a nap earlier to avoid being sleepy during the experiment. She also noticed a difference in her thought processes. "Well, they were sort of level, then going up and down, up and down, like a slow wave. This is unlike before when there were lots of things which kept me alert." Further, she essentially described a tremendous amount of passivity and massive denial, which she grudgingly admitted were related to "having to avoid something." The subject indicated that she was quite surprised at her total reaction.

Her previous experiences in the chamber had been so vivid that she assumed that by "letting herself go" they would be even more vivid, yet actually they weren't. Another important factor of the isolation experience was that many of her thoughts were directly concerned with or immediately related to her childhood, particularly of a period of summer vacation. At one time she referred to the underwater submarine scene which she described earlier; note this was associated with a story she read at age 9 or 10 in which a heroic diver died after a very exciting episode.

Throughout the second experiment the subject experienced periods of boredom which puzzled her since they seemed to be completely out of control. Usually associated with the boredom were feelings of wanting to get out and a return to some of her projective thinking, for example, "I thought that the boys were holding me in here longer than they did before," (despite the fact that she had been carefully reassured that she would remain in the chamber only two hours).

She had many feelings of being in a dangerous situation, despite the reassurance that she had been through this before and that "nothing had happened." As this material was elaborated her ninth and tenth years of childhood became most important. During this time she had spent a vacation in the country, following which she had left her home in Europe to come to the United States. Associated with this move was much unhappiness since "I was perfectly happy. I mean I couldn't see why . . . the fact that . . . my friends were doing this. They said the United States was a place where we could live much freer than we were, yet I felt perfectly free."

It is to be noted that this woman was in a period of transition; she was leaving her present position, a very protective training program, to go on her own. This leaving was directly reminiscent by association of leaving her homeland in childhood.

One other interesting incident occurred during the second interview. At one time the subject suddenly felt as if the room were tilted and noticed that her head was tilted, too. Try as she might she could not right herself. Not until she forcefully "straightened" her head with her hands did the room resume its normal position.

In the interview on the day following the experiment the subject greatly elaborated the material reported in the previous interview. She described her experience as "a kind of numbness. In a sense all my feelings were sort of on even keel." This is a sec-

ondary distortion. Despite her massive denial, she did experience moments of anxiety. She said in reply to a question that it was "as if I weren't responding to anything." This statement again exposes her attempted repression and—when this was unsuccessful—massive denial.

She reported an interesting dream in which "people were bunched together, people from my high school days and people that I knew (in her home country) as a little girl, and the people I knew here. . . . I was sort of surprised. I thought to myself what on earth are all these people doing here, I haven't seen them for years."

The dream and her subsequent elaborations were associated to her memory of the vacation in the country before she came to the United States. Her feelings about the separation trauma were very much like her feelings about being separated from Duke. She said further about the experience in the chamber "I said I'd come back again. I didn't enjoy the experience but it was so weird; it was fascinating." (We never explained her excessive use of the word fascination.")

Following this interview it was necessary to have another session because of a very peculiar symptom she developed.

She seemed to have lost sense of direction and was confused whether to take a left or right turn as she was leaving a room. This symptom was clearly related to her tremendous indecision over "where to go," *i.e.,* the separation in the present was, in turn, related to the feelings of separation from her country as a child which had been stirred up by the isolation experiment.

Another subject reported immediately following the experiment that he had directed his thinking during the period of isolation. He said that thinking of specific events made him more comfortable and that he found these thoughts reassuring since the darkness and silence were disquieting.

The subject, a medical student, mentioned that one of the things he had reviewed was an interview with a young patient the day before, and he implied that thinking of this kept his mind from other thoughts. The initial interviewer believed the subject to be more upset by the experience than he described, but there was no direct evidence thereof. Associations during the interview were only followed in terms of the immediate experimental situation for fear that allowing the subject to associate to past events might either (a) enhance any disorganization which the subject already felt or (b) allow the subject to escape into the past and "forget" the present provocative events. Furthermore it had been decided that extensive exploration should not be attempted during the first interview if the subject appeared to be confused, disoriented or extremely uncomfortable. When the subject was interviewed on the following day, he was considerably more comfortable although he still expressed much embarrassment and discomfort in regard to the previous day's experience. To reassure him the interviewer spoke of the many unusual thoughts subjects had during this experiment and pointed out that sometimes discussing these feelings and ideas allowed the subject to look at them realistically and feel more comfortable about them. At this point the subject remarked that not only had he been thinking about his young male patient, but that there were some sexual connotations. Furthermore, the previous interview conducted in the chamber just after the completion of the experiment was associated with sexual feelings he experienced in regard to the interviewer. He described feeling panic at this time and feeling panic at the previous thoughts about the patient but he had felt unable to report it. Certainly the experience acted as a traumatic event for this subject by bringing to the conscious level latent homosexual feelings and thoughts.

There is some evidence that these feelings have remained conscious. For several days thereafter and indeed, until the present time, this subject is unable to look directly at the interviewer and apparently is embarrassed when they chance to meet.

A female subject requested release from the chamber, and, when this was not done rapidly enough, she located the emergency door and walked out of the chamber a half hour before the official termination of the experiment.

In the interview which followed, the subject stated that she was beginning to feel restless, and described a certain amount of anxiety and fear although she did not consider the experience overwhelming. All of the interviewers noted that the subject's usual vivaciousness was replaced by an affective state which varied from flatness to irritability and petulance. She seemed extremely suspicious, exhibited poor judgment in the things she had expressed and the manner in which she expressed them. When she was first seen, she appeared quite confused and had the appearance of sleepwalking. This state lasted for several days, and a full month passed before she was her usual vivacious self.

During the interview on the following day the subject related that she had always been afraid of darkness and that this was particularly true for the past year since the death of her father; she insists that each night one or two lights be left on in the house, because she and her mother "are alone and some prowler might enter the house." She then described how she had attempted to resist this thought by thinking of pleasant things while she was in isolation. As the thought that someone might be "prowling on the outside" and that *he* might break into the chamber came closer to awareness, the subject's anxiety and restlessness increased until she had to leave the chamber despite strong inhibitions based on her desire to help and to please the experimenters.

Discussion

It seems reasonably clear that the processing of these subjects in an experiment which was, on the surface, comparatively innocuous, acted as a traumatic event. This result is even more significant in view of the fact that the subjects were carefully chosen as individuals with "strong egos." Although intelligence and education are not necessarily the attributes of a strong ego, these factors plus our knowledge of the subjects had made us reasonably secure in our evaluations of them.

By definition the amount of psychic energy which one's ego is unable to master within a reasonable span of time is designated as a trauma; ordinarily there are protective barriers (*i.e.,* the defenses) against the outcropping of such stimuli (*i.e.,* id impulses). It is also known that there are numerous instances in which the ability of the defenses erected by the ego to maintain usual or normal functioning is diminished. We believe this to be particularly true in the sensory deprivation experiment we have conducted in which we have introduced a *temporary abrogation of usual ego functioning.* In other words we deliberately (or artificially) deprive the ego of many of the usual activities and resources which help to keep its defenses intact. In our experiment the paralysis of voluntary motion and withdrawal of many of the usual sensory stimuli which guide the ego produce a strange, potentially dangerous situation for the ego. Under these circumstances, if the protective defense barriers break down, the ego loses its ability to react with purposeful reactions, and anxiety, in one form or another, will appear. Although the ego opposes the emergence of an id impulse that is equated with some dangerous situation by producing anxiety, it is equally possible, as indicated above, that the ego, unaware, is helpless or temporarily overwhelmed in the face of some conflict and this, in turn, produces anxiety. Thus we believe that the artificial abrogation of ego functioning markedly weakens the ability of the ego to utilize countercathexis so that repressed and conflictual material tends to emerge into consciousness. This is particularly true for those conflicts which might otherwise be handled slowly or more realistically but which can no longer be put off by a paralyzed and weakened ego.

Subsequently it is our feeling that the experiment produced a temporary artificial traumatic neurosis. Although the problems indicated were naturally latent, we believe they would not have emerged with the same intensity in ordinary circumstances.

*   *   *

3.

Interferences with Physical Integrity

Renée C. Fox
Experiment Perilous*

*   *   *

All physicians are confronted with problems of uncertainty. Some of these result from their own incomplete or imperfect mastery of available medical knowledge and skills; others derive from limitations in current medical knowledge; and still others grow out of difficulties in distinguishing between personal ignorance or ineptitude and the limitations of medical science.

In a sense, the physicians of the Metabolic Group can be thought of as specialists in problems of uncertainty—particularly those uncertainties related to limits of present medical knowledge. As clinical investigators, it was their special role to work on the periphery of what is medically known: to concern themselves with ill-understood basic mechanisms underlying the normal and abnormal functioning of the human body, and with unresolved problems in the diagnosis, treatment, and prognosis of human disease. Chiefly by means of experimentation, their task was to devise, explore, and appraise new ideas, methods, procedures, and drugs that might possibly contribute to medical knowledge, skill, and clinical prowess.

Because they worked "close to the growing edge of things" in the capacity of researchers, the physicians of the Metabolic Group were confronted with uncertainties of the medically unknown in a variety of forms. These included uncertainties regarding fundamental biochemical and physiological mechanisms underlying the phenomena and conditions they studied; uncertainties connected with the experimental compounds and procedures with which they worked —their basic properties and potential clinical effects; methodological uncertainties, related to the laboratory techniques they were developing;

* Glencoe, Ill.: The Free Press 28–33, 43–60 (1959). © The Free Press, Inc., 1959. Reprinted by permission of The Macmillan Company.

and finally, clinical uncertainties that were non-experimental in nature, which had to do with the diagnosis, treatment, and prognosis of their patients' illnesses.

As research pioneers or trail-blazers, who often worked outside the terrain of well-established medical knowledge, the physicians of the Metabolic Group were perhaps more continuously and immediately exposed to problems of uncertainty that result from limits of the field than were many of their nonresearch colleagues. The advances in knowledge and skill which their work effected helped to clarify and occasionally even dispel some of these uncertainties. But at the same time, as in all research, these gains in knowledge frequently uncovered new problems of uncertainty to be explored.

Things multiply. You solve one problem, and you're faced with two others. Things you didn't know once become obvious. But then other things you didn't even know existed arise. . . .

As we shall see, "chance" factors, which the physicians of the Metabolic Group did not necessarily plan or anticipate, played a considerable role in bringing various uncertainties to the attention of these physicians, and in determining the direction of their experimental work. The greater part of their research, of course, consisted of rationally-organized experimental attempts to learn more about various problems of uncertainty, or, hopefully, to resolve them. For the purpose of experimentation, one might say that the physicians of the Metabolic Group intentionally sought out problems of uncertainty, and, to some extent, deliberately induced them. In this sense, they were actively responsible for creating some of the uncertainties with which they worked. As we shall see, this affected the way that they felt about the consequences of these uncertainties for their research subjects, who were also their patients.

*   *   *

[T]he major share of the Metabolic Group's investigative and clinical activities centered around problems related to the normal and abnormal functioning of the adrenal glands. A considerable number of their studies involved estimating the metabolic activity of newly synthesized adrenal steroids and related compounds that had been tested on animals and had shown promising evidence of being useful as therapeutic agents. . . . The Group "hoped that through long-term studies extensive correlations might be made between modifications of steroid structures and modifications of their biological activity in man." However, in spite of the intensive investigative work they devoted to this problem and some empirical success in the treatment of various clinical syndromes with these adrenocortical hormones, the physicians of the Metabolic Group were "still largely in the dark as to their exact nature and basic mechanisms of action."

The Metabolic Group received the steroid preparations which they assayed directly from the laboratories of the pharmaceutical firms that manufactured them. Since methods for synthesizing steroid compounds are still "far from foolproof," these preparations sometimes contained impurities that could adversely affect patients who received them. However, the Group had no sure way of detecting these impurities before administering the steroids to patients; nor could they always explain the reactions that such impure compounds evoked. "We have had five reactions of the type you had to Lot No. 2179," a member of the Group wrote to a patient,

but we must admit that we are not certain why this particular lot has caused these reactions. It is essentially no different from previous lots in any way we have so far been able to determine, except for the obvious important fact that no reactions have occurred with other batches. . . .

The laboratory methods which the group had developed for investigating the nature and quantities of steroids secreted by the adrenal cortex were still characterized by a considerable degree of error, and were not yet refined enough to separate steroids originating from the adrenal cortex from those originating from other tissues. . . .

*   *   *

The fact that the medical sciences have not yet developed a "broad, over-all theory of drug action" also contributed to the many elements of uncertainty which characterized the Group's investigative work with steroids.

*   *   *

Partly as a consequence, many of the experiments conceived by the Group were highly empirical in nature: "trial-and-error shots in the dark" of which the outcome was very uncertain and unpredictable. . . .

*   *   *

The fact that the Group conducted most of its research on patients—individuals who were af-

flicted with some form of illness—rather than on healthy subjects, added to the elements of uncertainty which so often complicated the course of their experiments, or "clouded" their interpretation. . . .

*   *   *

Gradually, out of experimental "casting in the dark," the Metabolic Group (and other research units like it) have been able to advance understanding of the adrenal gland and its secretions, develop programs for the treatment of patients suffering from disorder of adrenal function, and modify certain generalized disease processes of nonadrenal origin by manipulation of the type and quantity of adrenal steroid secretion, or by surgical removal of adrenal tissue. But "the problem is never finally solved; the last word is never said." For, as we have indicated, the advance in knowledge and clinical efficacy which the Group's research brought about led to the detection of and, in a sense, to the creation of problems of uncertainty not previously encountered, recognized, or explored:

Before cortisone, the treatment of diabetes and Addison's disease combined was frightful—just hopeless. Jim Hayes, for example, was in the hospital fifty-five times—most of those admissions because he was hypoglycemic. But cortisone has really changed this whole disease picture. In the last two or three years, he hasn't had to come in at all. . . . *Now* the trouble is that when Addisonians *do* arrive, they come in with "crisis *sine* crisis." According to the textbook definitions, they're not actually in crisis. It's a different sort of picture. How would you classify Ed Murray's symptoms, for example? And how do you treat them? Well, in the past three or four years, we've had only one case come in with the classic symptoms. All the rest arrive they way he did. . . . What's more, Addisonians live longer now. So they are developing neoplastic and degenerative diseases. Last year, for instance, we had three hypertensive Addisonians; and we can expect to have more diabetic Addisonians as time goes on. . . .

[I]n collaboration with the surgical service, the Metabolic Group was also engaged in studying the effects of several types of experimental surgery on patients: the effects of bilateral complete adrenalectomy on patients with severe advanced hypertensive vascular disease, reactivated cancer of the prostate, and hyperadrenalism; the effects of transplanting a healthy kidney into the bodies of patients with terminal renal disease; and to a lesser extent, the effects of cardiac surgery on patients with serious heart disease.

Were such procedures "justified as an experimental approach in man"? Could they be "carried out with reasonable safety" in patients? How should patients be prepared for such surgery? What kind of anesthesia ought to be chosen? What kind of surgical approach ought to be used? How should patients be maintained postoperatively? What kinds of operative complications would be forthcoming? What therapeutic benefits, if any, could be derived from these procedures?

In the words of the Surgeon-in-Chief of the hospital, this kind of research "could not have been undertaken by the faint of heart." For the only way that such questions could be answered and problems resolved was by actually performing these procedures on a certain number of patients and studying their results. Medical ethics required the Group to try this radical experimental surgery on patients who were beyond help by conventional means, before attempting to carry it out on patients less gravely ill. The magnitude of the uncertainties with which the Group was faced in undertaking these procedures on patients this seriously ill is very great.

* * *

The fact that these physicians were frequently limited in the extent to which they could improve their patients' clinical status had implications for another constellation of problems with which the Metabolic Group was faced. These were the problems of meeting both their responsibilities as clinicians and their commitments to medical research to the fullest extent possible; ascertaining the limits of each set of obligations; and preventing or reconciling some of the conflicts that existed between them.

In many cases, the clinical and research activities of the Metabolic Group implemented one another. Some of the tests and procedures the Group asked patients to undergo, or the drugs they gave them primarily in order to diagnose or treat their diseases, also provided the Group with basic or general information about such conditions which was relevant to research in which they were engaged. In such instances (providing that things went well), the members of the Group simultaneously fulfilled their obligations as clinicians to further their patients' welfare and their responsibilities as investigators to advance medical knowledge.

* * *

However, there were also many occasions on which the procedures or drugs which the Group administered to patients did not benefit the persons subjected to them, or proved to have negative consequences for them. Situations of this sort were attributable to a number of factors. To begin with, as we know, the patients under the care of the Metabolic Group were likely to have serious, relatively ill-understood, or complicated diseases. Partly as a consequence, subjecting them to some of the procedures and agents that were used to diagnose or treat their disorders entailed a considerable amount of risk, some of which the Metabolic Group could calculate in advance, and some of which they could not. . . .

* * *

The Metabolic Group was also engaged in a considerable amount of research which they undertook primarily to advance general medical knowledge, and only secondarily or incidentally because they thought it might be helpful to patients who consented to act as their subjects. The members of the Group "hoped" that the patients who participated in these experiments might gain some clinical benefit from doing so, and they were pleased when this happened. But to the limited extent that medical ethics allowed them to do so, they subordinated their clinical desire to serve the immediate interests of the particular patients involved in such experiments, and gave priority to the more long-range, impersonal research task of acquiring information that might be of general value to medical science.

* * *

The physicians of the Metabolic Group were deeply committed to . . . [the principles of the Nuremberg Code] and conscientiously tried to live up to them in the research they carried out on patients. However, like most norms, the "basic principles of human experimentation" are formulated on such an abstract level that they only provide general guides to actual behavior. Partly as a consequence, the physicians of the Metabolic Group often found it difficult to judge whether or not a particular experiment in which they were engaged "kept within the bounds" delineated by these principles.

This was especially true of the experiments they conducted primarily to advance medical knowledge. The justification for this kind of research did not lie in its potential immediate value for the patients who acted as subjects. Rather, it was premised on the more remote, general, uncertain probability that its "anticipated results . . . their humanitarian importance . . . for the good of society" and the chance of achieving them—would exceed the immediate amount of "suffering" and "risk" the experiment might entail. The criteria on which physicians ought to form such a calculus are not specified by the rules of conduct for clinical research. Thus, without many established or "clean-cut" bases of judgment to guide them, the physicians of the Metabolic Group were constantly faced with the problem of trying to decide whether the particular experiments they were conducting fell within the limits of their rights as investigators, or whether they were overstepping those rights by subjecting the patients involved to more inconvenience and danger than the possible significance of those experiments for the "advancement of health, science, and human welfare" seemed to warrant.

In addition, as we know, the many uncertainties connected with experimentation and the clinical status of the patients who served as subjects made it hard to predict what the actual results of carrying out a procedure or administering a drug would prove to be. For this reason, the physicians of the Metabolic Group sometimes found themselves in situations where their experiments resulted in more inconvenience or suffering for their patient-subjects than they anticipated, intended, or desired.

Accounts of . . . experiments conducted by the Metabolic Group follow. The primary purpose of these experiments was to obtain scientific information. In this respect, and a number of other ways, they are characteristic of many studies conducted by the Group. Therefore, they suggest or illustrate some of the concrete problems the Metabolic Group faced in trying to determine the boundaries of their responsibilities as physicians to protect and further the welfare of their patients, and their rights as investigators to subject them to a certain amount of discomfort and risk, so as to strike a "proper balance" between these two potentially incompatible aspects of the role of clinical investigator.

*　　*　　*

Another characteristic these experiments had in common is that they all involved the use of a number of procedures which imposed varying degrees of risk upon the patients who underwent them. Most of these procedures were accepted clinical methods for establishing a diagnosis. In this context, risks that accompany these procedures are generally established as "tolerable"—that is, within the confines of ethical medical practice. However, in the research cases we are considering, these methods were not being used to diagnose patients' conditions in order to help them more effectively. Rather, they were being employed for general investigative purposes. . . . These were inquiries from which the patients acting as subjects could not expect to receive immediate clinical benefit, if any at all. Before they undertook such experiments the Group had to decide whether procedures which had "acquired respectability . . . in a diagnostic setting" could also be justifiably used "in an investigative setting" where the interests of patients were not being directly or immediately served. In these cases, the physicians of the Metabolic Group felt that they were. It was their considered judgment that given the cogency of the research problems they wished to explore, and the fact that the patients who acted as subjects for these experiments were ill with diseases which they could only help symptomatically, the discomforts and risks involved were not excessive.

The problems that the Group sometimes faced in deciding whether it was clinically wise and morally just to subject patients to this kind of investigation are well demonstrated by another experiment they conducted. This is one which had undesirable consequences for the patient, despite the fact that before they initiated the experiment the Group had carefully discussed the risks it might entail, and decided that they were not too great.

Mr. Max Gold, the patient involved, was afflicted with a rarely seen combination of disorders: Addison's disease and mitral stenosis. For the physicians of the Metabolic Group his condition was a "significant experiment of nature." It offered them an extraordinary opportunity to study the metabolic processes underlying a concurrence of disorders which they themselves had neither the moral right nor technical ability to induce. Mr. Gold was also the first patient with both these conditions to have undergone the procedure for surgical correction of mitral stenosis known as mitral valvuloplasty. This enhanced his potential importance as a research subject and the Metabolic Group's interest in studying the patterns of his metabolic processes.

It is a well-established fact that patients with Addison's disease generally have a defect in their ability to excrete administered water. For this reason, one of the phenomena the Group wished to observe was whether this would be equally characteristic of Mr. Gold, or whether because of his heart condition and the surgery he had recently undergone to correct it, his pattern of excretion would be different. For this purpose, the Group considered using what is known as the Robinson-Kepler-Power "water test." This is a simple screening examination; one of the clinical procedures which helps physicians to rule in the possibility that a patient has Addison's disease, or to rule it out. The test lasts for eighteen-and-a-half hours, during which time the patient is not allowed to eat any food or drink any fluids. He is then given a large amount of water to drink over a short period of time. Throughout the test all his urine is collected and its volume and specific gravity are measured. Whereas in normal subjects a prompt diuresis follows ingestion of the water, in patients with Addison's disease the diuresis is greatly delayed. The test is regarded as safe for patients with possible Addison's disease, as well as those who prove not to have it.

Before they finally decided to subject Mr. Gold to the water test, the Group tried to estimate the degree of stress the procedure might impose on him, and discussed the question of whether it was greater than what he ought to be asked to undergo for investigative rather than diagnostic purposes. The major reason for which various members of the Group felt some hesitancy about conducting the test was that it would entail witholding, while the test was in progress, the desoxycorticosterone acetate (DOCA) and cortisone therapy the patient was receiving daily. The possibility was raised that in his postoperative state the patient might "react more radically" than is usually the case to the withdrawal of medication, fasting, and the administration of a large volume of water under these circumstances. However, the members of the Group were somewhat more inclined to believe that because of the therapy he had received Mr. Gold was "well enough stocked" with DOCA and cortisone to sustain the stress of having them withheld for eighteen hours and undergoing the procedure. On the strength of this conviction and because they felt that Mr. Gold "might be the last case of Addison's disease and mitral stenosis that [they] would ever see," the Group decided to proceed with the experiment.

As already indicated, the optimism of the Group regarding the ability of Mr. Gold to withstand the procedure was not upheld. Due to factors they did not anticipate, could not control, and even in retrospect did not understand very well, the patient reacted to the test in a seriously adverse way. Thus, despite the caution with

which they proceeded, the effect of the experiment on the patient's clinical status conflicted sharply with what the Group had predicted, and with their desire as his personal physicians to protect him from harm. At the Group's Evening Rounds at the end of the day on which Mr. Gold underwent this test, his untoward reaction to it was described by one physician in the following way:

Well, I guess just about everybody knows that Mickey had a water test today. And out of the blue, he got very hot and dizzy. The room started to spin around, he said. His eyes began to twitch and his vision got blurred. . . . His pressure was still 100 over 80 when I took it; but his pulse was feeble and thready. Those symptoms lasted for about a half hour. Right now he's getting saline, desoxy, and Compound F. That should be enough. . . . And, of course, it's no longer possible to consider keeping him on a constant diet. We've got no choice but to treat this man. So our experiment ends right here. We might just as well put him on an all-therapeutic program.

The experiments described contain at least two other practices, at once characteristic of the Group's research and essential to it, that produced many of the situations in which they experienced conflict between their obligations to advance knowledge and their responsibility to promote the welfare of their patient-subjects. These were the practices of administering new drugs to patients and of witholding drugs from them, primarily for investigative purposes.

*   *   *

In their experiment with Mr. Ray Woodham, on the other hand, what the Group did to implement research interfered with the welfare of a patient in another characteristic way. For the purposes of metabolic study, the Group temporarily deprived the patient of cortisone: a drug which they had good reason to believe would help him excrete the many pounds of excessive water with which his body was swollen as a result of kidney disease. In fact, some of the Group's experiments were conducted primarily for the purpose of determining how long a patient could tolerate not receiving a needed drug, and exactly what the nature of his reaction would be to having it withheld. For example, the Group carried out the following experiment on Mr. Michael Terhune, a patient who had undergone total bilateral adrenalectomy for carcinoma of the prostate, and thus was not capable of producing his own cortisone:

1/7: Mike is at present undergoing DOCA withdrawal for the purpose of demonstrating sodium chloride diuresis. No attempt will be made to prolong this withdrawal; adequate demonstration of the electrolyte defect is all that is desired. Following this, he will resume DOCA therapy, and will then be gradually tapered off cortisone for the purpose of following 17-ketosteroids, FS, and androgenic excretions. In view of the fact that we were never able to withdraw Mr. Carr's cortisone longer than 2½ days without impending crisis, it will be important to determine the length of time Mike can tolerate this procedure. . . .

1/26: On 1/14 we began the slow tapering of Mr. Terhune's cortisone dose from 50 mgms. daily p.o. to 0. This is the fourth day off cortisone. The dose of DOCA has been maintained at 5 mgms. I.M. daily throughout this period. On or about 1/14 he began to complain that the pain in his back and legs was more severe. This has not been particularly progressive. There is no doubt that he has been frightened during the four days off cortisone. On several occasions he has raised the spectre of death. It has been difficult to reassure him that he is in no danger. This evening he complained of more marked weakness and excessive perspiration. He has noted some stuffiness in his nose for two days, and since last night, a dry cough. T 99 degrees (M), BP, 130/80, Pulse 72 min., strong. He is perspiring excessively about the forehead and neck. No sign of respiratory infection. We will however, watch him carefully. If there is any rise in temperature, we will have to restart his cortisone.

1/28: 100 mgms. cortisone p.o. at 11:25 A.M.

As this experiment, and also the studies conducted on Ray Woodham and Max Gold demonstrate, the conflict between their responsibilities as clinicians and as investigators which the physicians of the Metabolic Group faced was a "true dilemma." On the one hand, their using or withholding a procedure or drug for the purpose of experimentation often put them in the position where they were not serving the welfare of the patients who were subjects, or might even be jeopardizing it. On the other hand, what they did to benefit these patients or to protect them from harm often curtailed or impaired their research. Thus, when Mr. Gold reacted adversely to the water test, for example, in the words of one physician, the Group had "no choice but to treat this man," which in turn, meant the "end of the experiment." Similarly, the negative clinical effects of . . . withdrawing cortisone from Mr. Terhune made it necessary to terminate these experiments despite the research value that the Group could have derived from prolonging them. "No matter which way you slice it," a member of the Group explained,

being a clinical investigator has its problems. A lot of the research you do is of no benefit to patients, and there's a real possibility that you can do them harm. So, in order to do research you've got to close your eyes to some extent, or at least, take calculated risks with the patients on whom you run the experiments. . . . Still, you almost never attain the ideal research. . . . You rarely get to the basis of the problem you're investigating, because it's touch and go all along the way with these patients. Their care and welfare have to be taken into consideration. . . . So, you usually end up by compromising your research goals and standards. . . .

These conflicts between experimenting on patients and caring for them with which the physicians of the Metabolic Group were confronted were in some ways closely connected with another of their problems as clinical investigators: that of finding patients who would make appropriate subjects for their research, and of motivating them to serve in this capacity.

From the point of view of the Metabolic Group, the ideal research patient would have had the following characteristics. His medical condition would either be directly relevant to the research interests of the Group, or so unusual that it represented an opportunity to study phenomena rarely seen. He would be healthy enough to withstand the inconvenience and stresses of experimentation for long enough periods of time in order to enable the Group to realize high standards of accuracy and evidence in their research, and also to benefit him clinically through the procedures or drugs to which they subjected him. On the other hand, his condition would be sufficiently serious to justify asking him to undergo the degree of discomfort and risk that their experiments entailed, and to accept other than established methods of diagnosis and treatment. Furthermore, such an ideal research patient would not only be willing to submit to the conditions of the experiment, but he would be highly enough motivated to do so for a relatively long time. In short, the ideal research patient would have been one whose physical condition and attitudes allowed the physicians of the Metabolic Group to fulfill both their responsibilities as clinicians and investigators to an optimal degree.

Needless to say, the physicians of the Metabolic Group rarely, if ever, encountered a patient who met all these requirements. For example, the patients whose conditions were severe enough to justify subjecting them to an experimental procedure as radical as a total adrenalectomy, and to motivate them to consent to undergo it, were too ill to endure certain procedures that would have enabled the Metabolic Group to realize high standards of experimental precision, or to derive very much therapeutic value from it. On the other hand, because patients with Addison's disease had received so much clinical benefit from advances in the diagnosis and treatment of their condition which the research of the Group had helped to make possible, they did not present as many "interesting" possibilities for study as they once had, it was no longer justifiable to expose them to the stresses of experimentation on the grounds that there were no effective established means for helping them, and the patients themselves were not as willing as they formerly were to undergo the tedium and rigors of experimentation.

* * *

In sum, the problem for the Group was to find a sufficient number of patients with physical conditions which were suited to their research needs and interests and on whom it seemed morally justifiable to conduct the experiments they had in mind—and, if possible, to motivate those patients to serve as research subjects without violating their ethical responsibility to make known to the prospective subject all inconveniences and hazards the experiment might entail, or imposing any element of force, fraud, deceit, duress, overreaching, or other ulterior form of constraint or coercion upon them in order to obtain their consent to act as subjects.

Listening in on what the physicians of the Metabolic Group had to say one evening about the total bilateral adrenalectomy and the patients with hypertensive cardiovascular disease on whom they had carried out this experimental procedure, we hear many of the problems with which they were faced reviewed in this connection, and learn something about the way they were affected by them. The discussion that follows took place during the meeting which the Group customarily held at the end of each day. "Evening Rounds," as these meetings were called, were held in the Group's conference room, which rather appropriately was located half-way between the laboratory and the Metabolic Ward. The Group gathered around the long table in this room to discuss the clinical and research status of various patients for whom they were jointly responsible, and to make any decisions regarding them that were currently necessary. At this particular meeting, the Group were having a difficult time trying to decide what they ought to do for a seventeen-year-old patient with severe hypertension of unknown origin.

Dr. D.: There's one thing I want to do before Bob Baum is discharged, if he can tolerate it, and that's a histamine test. . . . The thing we ought to consider in following him is doing another retrogram on his left kidney some time in the future. Because if we definitely find bilateral kidney disease that way, then at least we've taken care of one specter. . . . He doesn't seem to be a good candidate for an exploratory now. So, what I'd do is send him out, plan to follow him closely, and have him come back in a few months. . . . I think our enthusiasm for doing an exploratory on this boy has waned considerably. . . .

Dr. R.: Actually, I'm not quite sure why we've changed.

Dr. D.: I'm not either.

Dr. R.: Because we really haven't found out a helluva lot that would make us change our minds. . . .

Dr. P.: I think there will be a great deal of feeling over exploring this boy, because he's young, and because we can't be sure that he doesn't have a pheo[chromocytoma]. . . . Then there'll probably be a great beating of the drums over sympathectomy and adrenalectomy. . . .

Dr. D.: As I see it, the only reason for discharging him now is for psychological reasons. . . .

Dr. P.: I agree. The real reason we're sending him out is because he needs more diagnostic tests of a traumatic nature.

Dr. G.: It's also a matter, too, of not having any definitive treatment to offer him, isn't it?

Dr. D.: We don't want to adrenalectomize him.

Dr. G.: Why not?

Dr. D.: I'm interested in doing some adrenalectomies, but not on him. . . . Do you mean to tell me we're going to start taking every young hypertensive case we find and do an adrenalectomy on them? Let me go on record right here and now, once and for all, about my position on adrenalectomies. I think now— and I've thought from the very first—that the adrenalectomy is a hopeless procedure—not one bit justifiable. There is no evidence whatsover so far as I'm concerned that it is a bona fide therapeutic procedure. However, once committed to a program, there is the necessity for doing adrenalectomies on a few carefully selected cases for evaluative purposes. If we're going to make a definitive evaluation of the role of the adrenal cortex in hypertension, we've got to select a group of patients who don't have such serious complications as the patients we've done adrenalectomy on up till now. . . . But I don't want to do it on this patient.

Dr., G.: It's just about time you went back to clinical medicine, Jim.

Dr. D.: You're perfectly right. Because this group has been puttering around with adrenalectomy for two years now. It seems to me that once and for all the technique deserves some sort of real trial. This is the one place where that can and should be done. So, I'm willing to try it on ten carefully selected cases.

Dr. G.: Quite apart from therapeutic considerations, then.

Dr. D.: Right.

DR. R.: I think the patients who have survived adrenalectomy are doing very well. (*Group laughter*) No, I mean it. I'm serious. Howard Beech, for instance, was just about as bad as this patient is. . . .

DR. D.: Oh, was he? Well, the fact of the matter is, he was much, much better than he is. He was far and away the earliest case of hypertension we did. . . . You can list Will as a good result— I'll take that. You can list Mr. Hemming, but he falls in a different category entirely. . . . Mr. Ardsley's pressure is 230 over 160. . . . So, it's been a tremendous triumph!

DR. C.: Well, I'm not enthusiastic about the procedure at all. But in Abe Samuelson's case, I really think it's done something for him.

DR. D.: Sure, it's done something for him. But he's become a real invalid as a result.

DR. H.: A vegetable. . . .

DR. D.: He's been sitting in the house for 400 consecutive days now, not moving a muscle, having his family wait on him hand and foot, and doing nothing but listening to the radio and watching TV all day. Even without the operation, on *that* regime his pressure would have come down!

DR. R.: So it's been a therapeutic success, but not a psychological one. (*Laughter*)

DR. D.: What you're doing, Bob, is evaluating these people as good merely on the basis of their not being dead, because so many of the others have died.

DR. C.: Bill Pappas is a good result.

DR. R.: And Walter Cousins was. . . .

DR. D.: Except he's now dead.

DR. R.: Well, you can't live forever! (*Group laughter*)

DR. P.: Well, we took a gamble, and maybe we lost.

DR. D.: I don't know. . . .

DR. C.: Now that we've gotten off *that* depressing subject, let's talk about the Cushing's disease cases. . . .

*   *   *

B.
In Determining the Investigator's Authority, What Is the Relevance of:

1.

Choice of and Attitude toward Subjects?

a.
Lawrence W. Shaw and Thomas C. Chalmers
Ethics in Cooperative Clinical Trials*

*   *   *

A well-designed scientific trial of a new therapeutic agent provides for the careful comparison of the new agent with some prior therapy, or with no specific therapy if such comparison is ethically warranted. The setting up of a valid comparison between the two modes of therapy involves, in the usual case, the random assignment of the eligible patients to the two modes of therapy. Our thesis is that the use of this sound scientific approach in the search for knowledge has been, and remains, at a low level because of unfortunate and unfounded prejudices concerning the ethical propriety of randomization as a technique of the decision-making process in the practice of medicine. In our view, the random allocation of patients in a scientific clinical trial is more ethical than the customary procedure, that of trying out a new therapy in an unscientific manner by relying on clinical impression and comparison with past ex-

perience. This conclusion follows from application of the fundamental principle that the physician-investigator's primary responsibility is to his patient. The sequence of thought is:

1. If the clinician knows, or he has good reason to believe, that a new therapy (A) is better than another therapy (B), he cannot participate in a comparative trial of Therapy A versus Therapy B. Ethically, the clinician is obligated to give Therapy A to each new patient with a need for one of these therapies.
2. If the physician (or his peers) has genuine doubt as to which therapy is better, he should give each patient an equal chance to receive one or the other therapy. The physician must fully recognize that the new therapy might be worse than the old. Each new patient must have a fair chance of receiving either the new and, hopefully, better therapy or the limited benefits of the old therapy.

If these principles are accepted, the physician must follow the course that if he *knows* which therapy is better, he does not conduct a trial in the human domain. If the physician does not know which therapy is better, he should randomize, and thus he can readily participate in a scientific trial. In fact, this latter methodology might be a more ethical way of practicing medicine than the routine prescription of a medication that has never been established as more beneficial than harmful. If this point of view were more widely appreciated, the literature would carry more reports of sound scientific trials and

* 169 *Annals of the New York Academy of Sciences* 487–488 (1970). Reprinted by permission.

fewer reports of inconclusive trials of new therapies.

* * *

NOTES

NOTE 1.

THOMAS C. CHALMERS
THE ETHICS OF RANDOMIZATION AS A DECISION
MAKING TECHNIQUE AND THE PROBLEM OF
INFORMED CONSENT*

* * *

Let me illustrate the value of randomization by presenting the data in some detail on a surgical operation for a vascular disorder in a serious disease, namely portacaval shunt surgery in patients with cirrhosis. It is now almost 20 years since the operation was introduced as a means of preventing fatal hemorrhage from esophageal varices, and 51 papers have been written in the English literature on the experiences of physicians who have treated more than 10 patients. Forty-five of these have concluded that the operation is effective, and only six have called it ineffective. Only four of the 51 studies were well controlled, and three of these found the operation ineffective, and one showed only slight enthusiasm. Yet, the operation is assumed to be effective by almost every physician in America and Britain.

Widespread performance of portacaval shunt surgery in patients with cirrhosis and esophageal varices has been primarily based on two observations—that patients who have survived the operation rarely bleed again from their varices, and they seem to live longer than a group of cirrhotics compiled as an example of the best so-called natural history of the disease. There have been a few dissenters to the view that all patients who have bled from varices should be shunted if they seem to be in good enough shape to survive surgery. However, opinions have been about equally divided with regard to the efficacy of shunts in patients whose varices have not yet bled. This equal division of opinion among both surgeons and internists made it seem to be entirely ethical to conduct a controlled trial of shunt surgery as a prophylactic

procedure. Three groups have now conducted reasonably well-controlled trials: The Boston Inter-Hospital Liver Group, Dr. H. O. Conn of New Haven, and a group of collaborating Veterans Administration Hospitals under the chairmanship of Dr. F. C. Jackson. Combined survival data from all three of these groups indicate that the operation actually shortens rather than prolongs life. This is true when the decision whether to operate or not is made at random, rather than according to the clinical condition of the patient. The explanation for the discrepancy between the data gathered in the controlled studies and those of other series lies in a comparison of the survival of patients selected for surgery in the Boston Inter-Hospital Liver Group studies, and those with esophageal varices who had not bled but who were not selected for surgery. The 50 percent survival time of the selected patients is five years and of the unselected patients with the same criteria for the diagnosis of esophageal varices is less than one year. But the operation had no significant influence on survival in the selected group. Even if one subtracts from the so-called control group all of the patients who died within three months after the diagnosis of their varices, because it was unlikely that they might have been candidates for surgery in that time, the difference still is striking after one year. In other words, the best way to survive if you have cirrhosis of the liver and esophageal varices that have not yet bled is to be selected for a portacaval shunt, and not have the operation performed.

Because of the negative findings in the controlled studies of prophylactic shunt surgery and the lack of any controlled trial of surgery in patients who have already bled, it is now considered entirely ethical to carry out the study in the latter group, and this is being done by the Boston Inter-Hospital Liver Group and by the Veterans Administration Group.

These data have been presented in some detail to illustrate the tremendous importance of the selection factor in the evaluation of therapies which are inherently dangerous themselves and for which patients in good condition are likely to be selected, i.e., the selected patients might very well live a long time because of their good condition and not because of the treatment, and it is even conceivable that the treatment might shorten their lives. This information can only be obtained by a controlled trial in which the decision as to whether to operate or not is made solely at random, and the patients are followed

---

* Report of Fourteenth Conference of Cardiovascular Training Grant Program Directors, National Heart Institute. Bethesda, Md.: U.S. Department of Health, Education, and Welfare 89–90 (1967). Reprinted by permission.

in such a way that the major therapy is the main variable.

*   *   *

NOTE 2.

THOMAS C. CHALMERS
WHEN SHOULD RANDOMISATION BEGIN?*

*   *   *

The series of articles on the anticoagulant effect of purified fraction of Malayan pit viper venom may be a milestone in the development of successful therapy for patients with thromboembolic disease, but it also raises a critical question as to the scientific and ethical requirements of new-drug trials in man. How early in the development of new drugs should the process of randomisation be introduced into the therapeutic trial? I am firmly convinced that the first patient to receive a new agent should be randomised. . . .

*   *   *

The standard argument against early randomisation is that an improper trial would result if the drug has not previously been explored in selected patients to determine the proper dose and to decide whether or not a randomised trial is ethical. Is it proper for patients to be selected arbitrarily for earliest trials of a new agent when it is even more likely at that time that they might do better if they received standard therapy?

*   *   *

NOTE 3.

PAUL FREUND
ETHICAL PROBLEMS IN HUMAN
EXPERIMENTATION†

*   *   *

. . . A juvenile court judge of rather progressive and scientific mind decided to try an experiment regarding sentencing. There were two institutions available: one an ordinary prison; and the other a minimum-security institution where the offenders would return in the evening after being allowed to go out into the town and work during the day. In sentencing to one or the other place of detention, this judge was not in-

clined to weigh the merits of the individual offenders or appraise the likelihood of their benefiting from one rather than the other form of treatment. What he did was to pair off the offenders coming before him in the best way he could, in point of age, ethnic grouping, intelligence quotient, family background and so on; one of the pair would be sent to one place of correction and the other to the other, and the plan was that at intervals careful observations would be made so that in the future there would be some basis for judging the kind of offender who can be expected to profit or not to profit from one or another type of treatment. Perhaps I should not be disturbed by this, but I am troubled because it seems to be an unprincipled way of taking liberties with the liberty of young offenders—unprincipled, that is, except from the standpoint of experimental design. I would be a little easier in my mind if this experiment were thought to be of benefit to the particular offenders who are being sentenced rather than to their successors or their children. If, for example, the risk of recidivism were such that these very offenders might be back before the court, and the data drawn from the experiments might be helpful in their own subsequent cases, a stronger argument could be made for this kind of randomized procedure. . . .

*   *   *

NOTE 4.

DONALD T. CAMPBELL AND
ALBERT ERLEBACHER
HOW REGRESSION ARTIFACTS IN QUASI-
EXPERIMENTAL EVALUATIONS CAN MISTAKENLY
MAKE COMPENSATORY EDUCATION LOOK
HARMFUL*

There are problems . . . with randomization experiments. Randomization at the invitational level avoids the disappointment problem generated by randomly allocating eager applicants to the control condition. But it exaggerates the always present problem of experimental mortality inasmuch as not all those randomly invited accept the treatment. Using only those invited who accept as the experimental group produces a selection bias with favorable pseudo-effects. . . .

*   *   *

---

* 1 *The Lancet* 858 (1968). Reprinted by permission.

† 273 *New England Journal of Medicine* 687, 689 (1965). Reprinted by permission.

* J. Hellmuth, ed.: *Compensatory Education: A National Debate,* Vol. III of *The Disadvantaged Child.* New York: Brunner-Mazel 22–25 (1970). Reprinted by permission.

Social ameliorative changes which are applied or made available to everyone do not readily permit the creation of control groups. . . . But those expensive remediations which are in short supply and which cannot be given everyone provide settings in which true experiments are readily possible. Once the decision makers in government and applied research are educated to their importance, they can become the standard evaluational procedure.

On the one hand, we must not create a political climate which demands that no ameliorative efforts be made unless they can be evaluated. There will be many things obviously worth doing which cannot be experimentally evaluated, and which should still be done. The shift to new math is an example. By making math achievement tests inappropriate it undermined the only convenient benchmark for its own evaluation. College education is another example, a boon for which we have almost no interpretable experimental or quasi-experimental evidence. (Since college education is given to those who need it least, the regression artifacts are biased to make it look effective.) We applied social methodologists should be alert to recognize such cases and not assume that every new program must be and can be evaluated.

On the other hand, where we can experiment and where the social costs of such experimentation are outweighed by the social value of reality testing, we should hold out for the least biased, most informative procedures.

There exist in administrators, researchers, legislators, and the general public "ethical" reluctances to random assignment. These center around a feeling that the control group is being deprived of a precious medicine it badly needs. But if it be recognized that the supposed boon is in fact in short supply, then it can be seen that the experiment has not increased the number so deprived, but has instead reassigned some of that deprivation so that the ethical value of knowing may be realized. Is randomization as the mode of such reassignment ethically defensible? It might represent an ethical cost (one nonetheless probably worth paying) if all the children in the nation had been rank ordered on need, and those most needy given the compensatory education up to the budgetary and staff limits of the program. But instead, the contrast is with a very haphazard and partially arbitrary process which contains unjust inversions of order of need far more extensive than a randomization experiment involving a few thousand children would entail. These unjust deprivations are normally not forced to our attention, and so do not trouble our ethical sensitivities as does the deprivation of the control group. But there is no genuine ethical contrast here.

Within randomization, there are some designs and stances that may ease any residual ethical burden. For example, the randomization could be limited to the boundary zone, at the least needy edge of those to be treated, the most needy edge of the untreated. For this narrow band of children, all considered as essentially tied at the cutting point on a coarse grained eligibility score, random assignment to treatment and nontreatment could be justified as a tie-breaking process. We would learn about the effects of the program only for a narrow band of talent. We would wonder about its effectiveness for the most disadvantaged. But this would be better than nothing, and better than quasi-experimental information.

The funds set aside for evaluation are funds taken away from treatment. This cost-benefit trade-off decision has already been made when quasi-experimental evaluation has been budgeted, or when funds are committed to any form of budgeting and accounting. Taking these evaluational funds, one could use nine tenths of them for providing experimental expansions of compensatory instruction, one tenth for measurement of effects on the small experimental and control samples thus created. Here the ethical focus could be on the lucky boon given to the experimentals. Since evaluation money would be used to expand treatment, the controls would not be deprived. . . .

b.

William A. Nolen
The Making of a Surgeon*

*   *   *

We weren't very "long" on research at Bellevue. Most city hospitals don't have the money that it takes to do basic, or laboratory, surgical research. The taxpayers, who foot the bill for municipal hospitals, would be up in arms if someone slipped in a request for an extra million

* New York: Random House 140, 143–146 (1970). Copyright © 1968, 1970 by William A. Nolen, M.D. Reprinted by permission of Random House, Inc.

for a complete dog lab with all the personnel and equipment needed.

On our division we didn't do any basic research at all, and that was fine with me. Some of my friends had chosen to train in research-oriented hospital centers without realizing what they were getting into, and most of them hated what they were doing.

*   *   *

I was glad that we weren't forced to do research, unless we were so inclined, but there was one drawback to this attitude. When we finished our training there were certain hospitals, like those under Dr. Ramsey's direction, where it was virtually impossible to obtain an appointment to the staff unless you had a bibliography as long as your arm. I had no desire to practice in that sort of institution but Al Johnson did. . . .

Al was determined to get the appointment and asked Dr. Stevens to intervene in his behalf. "What it boils down to, Al, is this," Dr. Stevens told him after talking with Dr. Ramsey. "If you're willing to spend some time doing research, and if you can come up with two or three papers that are publishable, Dr. Ramsey will reconsider your application. It's another year or so out of your life, but if you want the job you'll have to make the sacrifice. I'll try to arrange a grant from some foundation, and you can do your work here at Bellevue if you can find a suitable project."

My reaction to this proposition would have been an immediate and emphatic "No"; there were plenty of other hospitals as good as the one Dr. Ramsey headed. The appointment certainly wouldn't have been worth a year of my life. But Al felt differently. He accepted the deal, and after a few weeks of mulling it over, decided he'd devote his research time to solving the problem of leg ulcers. He couldn't have chosen a problem better suited to investigation at Bellevue, since there were always half a dozen such patients in the ward.

Al went to work. Healing was the problem. Leg ulcers are a result of poor circulation, infection and injury. They may, and frequently do, extend from the ankle halfway up the leg. In our patients, with their poor hygiene and substandard living conditions, it was virtually impossible to get these sores to heal without several weeks in bed and, eventually, a skin graft. Even when we finally did get them healed, it was 2 to 1 that within six months the patient would be back with a recurrence.

At the time when Al embarked on his research project there were reports in the surgical journals of an enzyme, a chemical substance, that had been used successfully to expedite healing in dogs, but the work hadn't yet been done on humans. After reading all the literature on the subject, Al decided to try the drug on some of our patients.

Jack Lesperance agreed to admit six leg-ulcer patients from the outpatient department for Al's purposes. We brought them in on a Monday morning. There was no problem from the legal point of view. These gentlemen would have sold their mothers into slavery just to spend two nights in a warm hospital away from the Bowery. They signed the releases authorizing Al's research without a moment's hesitation.

All day long Al could be seen running back and forth from the intern's lab to the small room into which we had jammed the six beds for his vagrants. He had to complete some base-line (preliminary) blood studies before he could give them the intravenous solutions which he hoped would hasten the healing of their leg ulcers. It was five-thirty in the evening before he really had things under way and all six of his patients had fluids running into their arms.

Everything went smoothly for the first fifteen minutes. He might as well have been giving them sugar water for all the effect it had. Then one of them, Russ Peters, an old friend of ours, called Al over. "Say, Doc," he said, "I feel kind of hot. Could I be getting a fever?"

"I wouldn't think so," Al answered, "but let me check."

Russ's temperature was 103; by the time Al had finished checking the others, all five of them were perspiring profusely and shouting for help. Al was beside himself. He ran out onto the ward looking for an intern and bumped into our entire house staff. We were just escorting Dr. Stevens onto the ward for his Monday-night rounds.

"Can we help you, Al?" Dr. Stevens asked.

Al couldn't stand still. "I'd just like to borrow an intern or two, if I may, Dr. Stevens," he answered. "I need a little help."

"Certainly, Al. Who would you like to send, Jack?"

Jack gave him two interns. Al all but ran off with them down the hall. He wrapped the patients in alcohol-soaked sheets, threw ice water on them, turned fans on each one. All during rounds, each time Dr. Stevens looked up he could see Al or one of his co-workers running through the hall with ice or some other cooling medium. "Al's certainly taking a vigorous approach to his research project, isn't he?" Dr. Stevens commented.

It was a near disaster. Even though he had shut off the I.V.'s as soon as temperatures started to climb, every patient hit 106 and five of them went temporarily off their rocker from the fever. The new chemical just wasn't ready for human use. . . .

NOTES

NOTE 1.

EDWARD A. SHILS
SOCIAL INQUIRY AND THE AUTONOMY
OF THE INDIVIDUAL*

* * *

Where, as in the United Kingdom, the direct approach of modern social science was developed in the study of living aborigines or of the lower social and economic classes of one's own society, serious issues did not arise. In the first place, these inquiries did not enter very deeply into the private sphere of their subjects; they confined themselves largely to external economic matters and to publicly observable actions. There was a restraint on curiosity, deriving from the puritanical ethos of the culture from whence the investigators came. There was, furthermore, no obvious problem in intruding on the privacy of savages or workingmen, particularly those at or near the poverty level, because, at bottom, the investigators did not feel that they shared membership in a common moral community with the persons investigated. They possessed no secrets which were sacred to the investigators; they possessed no secrets whose penetration could be expected to arouse discomfiture among the investigators or the circles in which they moved. The situation was little different in the United States. The first large-scale inquiries based on interviewing dealt with slum dwellers, Negroes, immigrants, juveniles on the margin of delinquency, persons with dubious moral standards, et al.—people regarded as not possessing the sensibilities which demand privacy or the moral dignity which requires its respect. Moreover, the investigators were inhibited in their curiosity by the wider culture and by the traditions of their discipline.

* * *

* Daniel Lerner, ed.: *The Human Meaning of the Social Sciences.* New York: Meridian Books, Inc. 114, 116–117 (1959). © 1959 by the World Publishing Company. Reprinted by permission.

NOTE 2.

LOUIS LASAGNA
SPECIAL SUBJECTS IN
HUMAN EXPERIMENTATION*

* * *

I am concerned . . . about the use of students as volunteers in experiments conducted by their academic superiors. If a student is of age to give consent, there would seem to be no special ethical problem about volunteering in *general*. But if a student in a classroom is asked to volunteer by his instructor, there is at least the implied threat of loss of affection (and decreased academic grade) if the student fails to volunteer, which takes the situation into a nasty area of restricted choice. Furthermore, it has been the practice in some institutions actually to give extra credits for such participation, a procedure that raises the issue of infringement of the rights of those who do not volunteer or are not chosen after volunteering. Should the non-volunteers at least be allowed another means (non-experimental) of earning extra credits equal in amount to those earned by the volunteers, so as not to be academically disadvantaged? Perhaps, but the problems involved in being "fair" to all parties concerned suggest that it may be simpler, as well as more ethical, for professors to avoid soliciting volunteers from student groups whose academic standing or future employment may be in their hands. It is not enough to say that a professor will not be swayed in his marking or writing of reference letters by whether a student has volunteered; the *belief* that he will do so is enough to act as a troublesome influence on both the volunteer and the non-volunteer.

* * *

c.

Joseph H. Fichter and William L. Kolb
Ethical Limitations on
Sociological Reporting†

* * *

Within the area of contemporary material a distinction can be drawn between studies of primitive societies and civilized communities. It is to be supposed that the details of social life

* 98 *Daedalus* 449, 456–457 (1969). Reprinted by permission of Daedalus, Journal of the American Academy of Arts and Sciences, Boston, Massachusetts.

† 18 *American Sociological Review* 544, 546–550 (1953). Reprinted by permission.

among the Samoans were not reported to these people, and if any reputations suffered from such study it was only among non-Samoans. There have been instances, however, of anthropologists' reports getting back to American Indian tribes, causing some dissension and suspicion among the members of the tribe. In either case the sociologist must consider these people as the subjects of human rights, even though the prospect of moral damage may not be great.

In studying contemporary communities the problem of reporting varies according to whether the data concerned are sacred or non-sacred. The analysis of behavior patterns which involve high traditional values (like religion, family and sex, ethnic and group loyalties) should, of course, be as objective as possible, but an effort should be made to avoid needless and callous affront to the people who hold such values and such an effort requires special attention and care. In non-sacred areas (such as economic and political activities, housing and recreational problems) there can be greater freedom of reporting.

* * *

. . . At the core of the Western value system is a belief in the basic dignity and worth of the human being. This belief is based on different assumptions according to the particular stream of tradition in which one locates it: the Fatherhood of God, natural law, universal human needs and aspirations, or human reason. Whatever the base, the belief implies that men are bound to one another in a moral community. Membership in this community requires that the individual's rights to privacy, secrecy, and reputation be respected, even though the human beings studied may not be members of the sociologist's own society.

The belief also implies that a man or group can renounce membership in the moral community by choosing modes of action which violate these basic values of dignity and worth. In mid-century it seems probable that men like Hitler and Stalin, organized groups like "Murder Incorporated," the Ku Klux Klan, and some others, have placed themselves outside the moral community and have surrendered the protection of its norms. Thus the social scientist need have no qualms about reporting in full detail the activities of such groups and people. Although this norm has never been explicitly formulated, it has guided a great deal of the research and reporting in social science.

Yet the decision of the sociologist to place particular persons or groups outside the moral community involves great responsibility, and he must be careful that his criteria of judgment permit tolerance, compassion, and wisdom. This is especially the case when he studies "unpopular" racial, religious and political groups, prostitutes, homosexuals, drug addicts, and the psychologically ill, the poor and powerless. It is hardly questionable that these people remain members of the moral community and hence retain their rights of privacy, respect, and secrecy. The needs of the society may require a limitation of their rights by the courts or by the social scientist in his reporting, but basic rights can be limited only to the extent that they *must* be limited. Beyond that point such people must be treated in the same way as other members of the moral community.

The recognition of basic human rights which accompany membership in the moral community is an important means by which social scientists can avoid the dangers of the use of purely subjective criteria. Within the consensus of the Western tradition it is objectively true that there are moral evils and modes of action which place the perpetrator outside this community. We must know as much as possible about such people and the scientist need have little inhibition in the report he provides about them. All other persons and groups, no matter how personally distasteful to the scientists, seem to require the respect of their fellow-members in the moral community.

NOTE

HOWARD S. BECKER
PROBLEMS IN THE PUBLICATION OF FIELD STUDIES*

* * *

Fichter and Kolb seem to assume that, except for Hitler, Stalin, and others who are not members of our moral community, there is no irreconcilable conflict between the researcher and those he studies. In some cases he will clearly harm people and will refrain from publication; in others no harm can be done and publication is not problematic. The vast majority of cases will fall between and, as men of good will,

* Arthur J. Vidich, Joseph Bensman, and Maurice R. Stein, eds.: *Reflections on Community Studies.* New York: John Wiley and Sons, Inc. 267, 272–274 (1964). Reprinted by permission.

the researcher and those he studies will be able to find some common ground for decision.

But this analysis can be true only when there is some consensus about norms and some community of interest between the two parties. In my view that consensus and community of interest do not exist for the sociologist and those he studies.

The impossibility of achieving consensus, and hence the necessity of conflict, stems in part from the difference between the characteristic approach of the social scientist and that of the layman to the analysis of social life. Everett Hughes has often pointed out that the sociological view of the world—abstract, relativistic, generalizing—necessarily deflates people's view of themselves and their organizations. Sociological analysis has this effect whether it consists of a detailed description of informal behavior or an abstract discussion of theoretical categories. The members of a church, for instance, may be no happier to learn that their behavior exhibits the influence of "pattern variables" than to read a description of their everyday behavior which shows that it differs radically from what they profess on Sunday morning in church. In either case something precious to them is treated as merely an instance of a class.

Consensus cannot be achieved also because organizations and communities are internally differentiated and the interests of subgroups differ. The scientific report that pleases one faction and serves its interests will offend another faction by attacking its interests. Even to say that factions exist may upset the faction in control. What upsets management may be welcomed by the lower ranks, who hope the report will improve their position. Since one cannot achieve consensus with all factions simultaneously, the problem is not to avoid harming people but rather to decide which people to harm.

* * *

d.

David McK. Rioch
Concluding Remarks*

* * *

It is not inconceivable that as our methods improve and as with increased information we

* E. R. Ramey and D. O'Doherty, eds.: *Electrical Studies of the Unanesthetized Brain.* New York: Paul B. Hoeber 411–412 (1960). Reprinted by permission of Harper & Row, Publishers.

can more precisely select relevant problems, certain patients with incurable diseases and short life expectancy might be willing to volunteer as subjects for collaborative studies utilizing implanted electrodes. Considering these problems I have necessarily done some thinking about my own attitudes. . . . It has seemed to me that when I come to retire and, as it were, only have use for my brain in getting around the yard, but will not be responsible for decisions significantly affecting other people's lives, I might quite reasonably approach an experimental neurosurgeon in whose work and scientific orientation I had confidence and say, "Let us do an experiment together, as there are a number of things both you and I would like to find out." Now, I find myself hesitating in discussing this subject as it has many nuances and conflicting factors. I am aware that there is a good deal of psychiatric opinion to the effect that people who volunteer as subjects for experiments are conceivably more crazy than people who don't. However, I also recognize that within the next few years I might want to ask a patient to volunteer for certain observations, and I would not want to be in the position of asking another person to do something which I would not do. It is clear that I could not be certain as to what cultural role I would be assuming, what my "motivation" would be, in becoming an experimental subject. . . .

. . . Although many people are "horrified" by experiments on human subjects, I find myself not infrequently somewhat more concerned about the effect of these experiments on the experimenters. The doing of experiments tends to shut out from the awareness of the experimenter most of those aspects of relationship with the patient that are really valuable in human interchange. That is, when one begins to look at the patient or the subject as part of an experimental operation one ceases to respond; the patient can no longer evoke from the observer those involved and intimate behaviors by which as *humans* we live. Such attitudes tend to feed upon themselves and become more general, and the experimenter becomes shut off from his subject and is no longer a physician. I sometimes think that much of our study of patients is directed toward coming closer to them as human beings, but we find it dangerous and shield our need with scientific methods.

* * *

NOTE

HERBERT C. KELMAN
HUMAN USE OF HUMAN SUBJECTS—
THE PROBLEM OF DECEPTION IN SOCIAL
PSYCHOLOGICAL EXPERIMENTS*

*   *   *

In our other interhuman relationships, most of us would never think of doing the kinds of things that we do to our subjects—exposing others to lies and tricks, deliberately misleading them about the purposes of the interaction or witholding pertinent information, making promises or giving assurances that we intend to disregard. We would view such behavior as a violation of the respect to which all fellow humans are entitled and of the whole basis of our relationship with them. Yet we seem to forget that the experimenter-subject relationship—whatever else it is—is a *real* interhuman relationship, in which we have responsibility toward the subject as another human being whose dignity we must preserve. The discontinuity between the experimenter's behavior in everyday life and his behavior in the laboratory is so marked that one wonders why there has been so little concern with this problem, and what mechanisms have allowed us to ignore it to such an extent. I am reminded, in this connection, of the intriguing phenomenon of the "holiness of sin," which characterizes certain messianic movements as well as other movements of the true-believer variety. Behavior that would normally be unacceptable actually takes on an aura of virtue in such movements through a redefinition of the situation in which the behavior takes place and thus of the context for evaluating it. A similar mechanism seems to be involved in our attitude toward the psychological experiment. We tend to regard it as a situation that is not quite real, that can be isolated from the rest of life like a play performed on stage, and to which, therefore, the usual criteria for ethical interpersonal conduct become irrelevant. Behavior is judged entirely in the context of the experiment's scientific contribution and, in this context, deception—which is normally unacceptable—can indeed be seen as a positive good.

*   *   *

* 67 *Psychological Bulletin* 1, 5 (1967). © 1967, American Psychological Association. Reprinted by permission.

2.

Awareness of Participation?

a.

Kai T. Erikson
**A Comment on Disguised Observation
in Sociology***

*   *   *

"[P]ersonal morality" and "professional ethics" are not the same thing. Personal morality has something to do with the way an individual conducts himself across the range of his human contacts; it is not local to a particular group of persons or to a particular set of occupational interests. Professional ethics, on the other hand, refer to the way a group of associates define their special responsibility to one another and to the rest of the social order in which they work. In this sense, professional ethics often deal with issues that are practical in their application and limited in their scope: they are the terms of a covenant among people gathered together into a given occupational group. For instance, it may or may not be ethical for an espionage agent or a journalist to represent himself as someone he is not in the course of gathering information, but it certainly does not follow that the conduct of a sociologist should be judged in the same terms; for the sociologist has a different relationship to the rest of the community, operates under a different warrant, and has a different set of professional and scientific interests to protect. In this sense, the ethics governing a particular discipline are in many ways local to the transactions that discipline has with the larger world.

*   *   *

. . . It may seem a little cranky to insist that disguised observation constitutes an ugly invasion of privacy and is, on that ground alone, objectionable. But it is a matter of cold calculation to point out that this particular research strategy can injure people in ways we can neither anticipate in advance nor compensate for afterward. For one thing, the sheer act of entering a human transaction on the basis of deliberate fraud may be painful to the people who are thereby misled; and even if that were not the case, there are countless ways in which a stranger who pretends to be something else can disturb

* 14 *Social Problems* 366, 367–373 (1967). Reprinted by permission.

others by failing to understand the conditions of intimacy that prevail in the group he has tried to invade. Nor does it matter very much how sympathetic the observer is toward the persons whose lives he is studying: the fact of the matter is that he does not *know* which of his actions are apt to hurt other people, and it is highly presumptuous of him to act as if he does—particularly when, as is ordinarily the case, he has elected to wear a disguise exactly because he is entering a social sphere so far from his own experience.

So the sheer act of wearing disguises in someone else's world may cause discomfort, no matter what we later write in our reports; and this possibility raises two questions. The first, of course, is whether we have the right to inflict pain at all when we are aware of these risks and the subjects of the study are not. The second, however, is perhaps more important from the narrow point of view of the profession itself: so long as we suspect that a method we use has at least *some* potential for harming others, we are in the extremely awkward position of having to weigh the scientific and social benefits of that procedure against its possible cost in human discomfort, and this is a difficult business under the best of circumstances. If we happen to harm people who have agreed to act as subjects, we can at least argue that they knew something of the risks involved and were willing to contribute to that vague program called the "advance of knowledge." But when we do so with people who have expressed no readiness to participate in our researches (indeed, people who would presumably have refused if asked directly), we are in very much the same ethical position as a physician who carries out medical experiments on human subjects without their consent. The only conceivable argument in favor of such experimentation is that the knowledge derived from it is worth the discomfort it may cause. And the difficulties here are that we do not know how to measure the value of the work we do or the methods we employ in this way, and, moreover, that we might be doing an extraordinary disservice to the idea of detached scholarship if we tried. Sociologists cannot protect their freedom of inquiry if they owe the rest of the community (not to mention themselves) an accounting for the distress they may have inadvertently imposed on people who have not volunteered to take that risk.

* * *

In one of the most sensible pieces written on the subject, Julius Roth has reminded us that all social research is disguised in one respect or another and that the range of ethical questions which bear on the issue must be visualized as falling on a continuum. Thus, it is all very well for someone to argue that deliberate disguises are improper for sociologists, but it is quite another matter for him to specify what varieties of research activity fall within the range of that principle. Every ethical statement seems to lose its crisp authority the moment it is carried over into marginal situations where the conditions governing research are not so clearly stipulated. For instance, some of the richest material in the social sciences has been gathered by sociologists who were true participants in the group under study but who did not announce to other members that they were employing this opportunity to collect research data. Sociologists live careers in which they occasionally become patients, occasionally take jobs as steel workers or taxi drivers, and frequently find themselves in social settings where their trained eye begins to look for data even though their presence in the situation was not engineered for that purpose. It would be absurd, then, to insist as a point of ethics that sociologists should always introduce themselves as investigators everywhere they go and should inform every person who figures in their thinking exactly what their research is all about.

But I do think we can find a place to begin. If disguised observation sits somewhere on a continuum and is not easily defined, this only suggests that we will have to seek further for a relevant ethic and recognize that any line we draw on that continuum will be a little artificial. What I propose, then, at least as a beginning, is the following: first, that it is unethical for a sociologist to *deliberately misrepresent* his identity for the purpose of entering a private domain *to which he is not otherwise eligible;* and second, that it is unethical for a sociologist to *deliberately misrepresent* the character of the research in which he is engaged. . . .

* * *

NOTE

Laud Humphreys
Tearoom Trade—Impersonal Sex
in Public Places*

* * *

At the conclusion of his article, Erikson proposes two rules regarding misrepresentation of the researcher's identity and purposes:

It is unethical for a sociologist to *deliberately misrepresent* his identity for the purpose of entering a private domain *to which he is not otherwise eligible.*

It is unethical for a sociologist to *deliberately misrepresent* the character of the research in which he is engaged.

Since one's identity within the interaction membrane of the tearoom is represented only in terms of the participant role he assumes, there was no misrepresentation of my part as an observer: I was indeed a "voyeur," though in the sociological and not the sexual sense. My role was primarily that of watchqueen, and that role I played well and faithfully. In that setting, then, I misrepresented my identity no more than anyone else. Furthermore, my activities were intended to gain entrance not to "a private domain" but to a public restroom. The only sign on its door said "Men," which makes me quite eligible for entering. It should be clear, then, that I have not violated Erikson's first canon. Although passing as deviant to avoid disrupting the behavior I wished to observe, I did not do so to achieve copresence in a private domain.

The second rule may be applied to the reactive part of my research, when I interviewed persons I had observed in the tearooms under the pretext of a social health survey. Here it should be noted that all interviews were in fact made as part of a larger social health survey, and abstracted data from my interviews are already in use in that study. The problem then may be viewed in two ways: First, I gave less than full representation of what I was doing, though without giving false representation. I wore only one of two possible hats, rather than going in disguise. Second, I made multiple use of my data. Is it unethical to use data that someone has gathered for purposes one of which is unknown to the respondent? With the employment of proper security precautions, I think such multiple use is quite ethical; it is frequently employed by

* Chicago: Aldine Publishing Co. 172 (1970). Reprinted by permission.

anyone using such data banks as the records of the Bureau of Census.

* * *

b.

Fred Davis
Comment on "Initial Interaction of Newcomers in Alcoholics Anonymous"*

* * *

In their article "Initial Interaction of Newcomers in Alcoholics Anonymous," John Lofland and Robert Lejeune report on an "experiment [which] consisted in sending six male agents (*sic*; graduate students in sociology) to A.A. open meetings where they posed as alcoholic newcomers"....

There is little need to dwell on the more narrowly professional issues occasioned by research strategies of this genre (i.e., those political ones having to do with the power and repute of sociologists to command access to persons and organizations in furtherance of scholarly objectives). Suffice it to say that the leaders and members of no corporate group, especially one imbued with a reformistic spirit of mission, can be reasonably expected to view such acts of premeditated deception with, to understate the case, indifference....

Beyond these . . . considerations however, there looms the more cogent issue of the character and extent of the sociologist's license to exempt himself from the expectations, common reciprocities and *modus operandi* of the persons and organizations to which he attaches himself in his role of participant-observer. I can only raise again the same kinds of disturbing, yet ever relevant, questions that many have raised before me. Is such license complete or partial? Enduring on all occasions, or terminal according to time, place and circumstances? Contingent when studying "good" causes and institutions, but uninhibited when studying "bad" ones? Equally applicable in whatever degree to the powerful and powerless alike or, as a matter of expedience, of differential applicability? (A colleague has ventured the disquieting allegation that while sociologists are as a rule scrupulous in setting forth their research auspices and purposes when making first-hand studies of such powerful groups as the military, labor unions and liberal professions, they tend to be a good deal less conscientious on

* 8 *Social Problems* 364–365 (1961). Reprinted by permission.

this score when studying such powerless groups and aggregates as isolated religious cults, deviants of various kinds and anonymous respondents at every twenty-third household.) ...

* * *

Last, there is what some may treat as only a sentimental objection, but one which despite its elusiveness, I feel, comes closest to the heart of the matter. That is, in field situations in which the sociologist (or anthropologist) openly represents himself to his subjects for what he is (i.e., a person whose interest in them is professional rather than personal) he unavoidably, and properly I would hold, invites unto himself the classic dilemma of compromising involvement in the lives of others. Filling him with gossip, advice, invitations to dinner and solicitations of opinion, they devilishly make it evident that whereas he may regard himself as the *tabula rasa* incarnate upon whom the mysteries of the group are to be writ, they can only see him as someone less detached and less sublime. There then follows for many a fieldworker the unsettling recognition that, within very broad limits, it is precisely when his subjects palpably relate to him in his "out-of-research role" self (or "presentation," depending on one's disassociative bent) that the *raison d'être* for his "in-role" self is most nearly realized; they are more themselves, they tell and "give away" more, they supply connections and insights which he would otherwise have never grasped. (One is tempted to conceive of this moral paradox as the sociologist's original sin, although happily the benign interpositions of area sampling, pre-coded questionnaires and paid interviewers now spare more and more of us from suffering its pangs.)

It is in large measure due to this ineluctable transmutation of role postures in field situations that, when he later reports, the sociologist often experiences a certain guilt, a sense of having betrayed, a stench of disreputability about himself; these, despite the covers, pseudonyms and deletions with which he clothes his subjects. (Or, have I alone heard such "confessions" from fellow sociologists?) In an almost Durkheimian sense, I would hold that it is just and fitting that he be made to squirm so, because in having exploited his non-scientific self (either deliberately or unwittingly) for ends other than those immediately apprehended by his subjects he has in some significant sense violated the collective conscience of the community, if not that of the profession.

Now, the resort to calculated and wholecloth deception of the type discussed here does not of course escape the final terms of this dilemma which may unalterably be our lot. It does, however, escape the intermediate ones: the discovery that *in vivo* the participant research role becomes something, both, more and less than itself; the conscious opening up of self to the possibility of rebuttal, disaffection, divided loyalties, compromising attachments and difficult disclosures; the price of engagement as opposed to that of mere doing. And, it is ultimately in this sense that such actions strike me as less than human, and hence unworthy of a discipline which, whatever else it represents itself as, also calls itself by that name.

* * *

NOTE

Julius A. Roth
Comments on "Secret Observation"*

* * *

All research is secret in some ways and to some degree—we never tell the subjects "everything." We can escape secrecy more or less completely only by making the subjects participants in the research effort, and this process, if carried far enough, means that there would be no more "subjects." So long as there exists a separation of role between the researchers and those researched upon, the gathering of information will inevitably have some hidden aspects even if one is an openly declared observer. The following are at least some of the reasons for this:

1. The researcher usually does not know everything he is looking for himself when he first starts out and structures his study to some extent as he goes along. Some of the things he finds of interest to study as the research goes on are things which the subjects might have objected to if they had been told about it in the beginning.

2. In many types of study of social behavior, the researcher does not want the subjects' behavior influenced by his knowledge of what the observer is interested in.

3. Even if the subjects of a study are given as precise and detailed an explanation of the purpose and procedure of the study as the investigator is able to give them, the subjects will not understand all the terms of the research in the same way that the investigator does. The terms

* 9 *Social Problems* 283–284 (1961). Reprinted by permission.

used have different connotations to them, their experiential contexts differ, and their conceptions of the goals of the study are likely to be different. Therefore, even in those cases where the researcher has made a deliberate effort to explain to his subjects just what he is going to do, he will frequently find them acting surprised when he actually goes ahead and does it.

When a psychologist gives a subject a TAT and tells the subject that he is simply telling stories, is this "secret research"? Or still further removed, when you give a prospective employee what looks like an application form and then do a personality analysis of his responses, is this or is this not equivalent to posing as a fake participant?

When we are observing a crowd welcoming a hero, it is obviously absurd to say that we should warn everybody in the crowd that a sociologist is interpreting their behavior. The same can probably be said if we observe the behavior of the passengers we ride on the bus with every day. But suppose we are systematically observing the behavior of fellow workers in a shop or an office? Or the members of one's own family?

Does the manner in which one comes to be a secret observer affect the morality of the situation? Is it moral if one gets a job in a factory to earn tuition and then takes advantage of the opportunity to carry out a sociological study, but immoral to deliberately plant oneself in the factory for the express purpose of observing one's fellow workers? If the outcome is the same— e.g., if the manner in which the observations are used are the same—I, for one, see no moral difference in these two situations, but I find some of my colleagues do not agree with this position.

If the possibility of disrespect for an organization or group is at issue, we are faced with the question of just when a collection of people becomes a self-identifiable group that may have considered itself being researched on. Would this mean that groups which are consciously organized deserve more consideration than those which are not? As observers must we be careful of how we deal with hospital nurses, but be more free in how we deal with patients who are unorganized and are not likely to read our reports? Might it perhaps be considered proper to keep secret notes on the behavior of truck drivers with whom one hitches a ride or with whom one works, but not upon the members of the Teamsters Union as an organization?

*   *   *

The point of all these illustrations is that social science research cannot be divided into the "secret" and the "non-secret." The question is rather how much secrecy shall there be with which people in which circumstances? Or, to state the question in a more positive (in more researchable) manner: When we are carrying out a piece of social science research involving the behavior of other people, what do we tell whom under what circumstances? Posing the question in this manner puts us in the same boat with physicians, social workers, prostitutes, policemen, and others who must deal with information which is sometimes delicate, threatening, and highly confidential. We are then in a position to draw upon our own knowledge of these other groups and the way in which they handle information to carry out their work and to draw analogies between those professions and our own.

*   *   *

c.

Edward A. Shils
Social Inquiry and the Autonomy
of the Individual*

*   *   *

Experimentation often involves manipulation, although it need not always do so. Manipulative experimentation involves the exercise of influence for an end which is not fully shared between experimenter and the experimental subject. Such experimentation is not a relation between equals; it is a relationship in which power is exercised, at best within a framework of consent and mutual good will.

Now authority is exercised throughout society, and most of us regard it as reasonable to accept within its proper limits. It is exercised by legislators, physicians, priests, teachers, and civil servants. In all these relationships, the end striven for by the person exercising authority is not perceived as clearly or shared equally by the person over whom it is exercised. That is in the nature of authority, and its inevitability renders it acceptable, even though it should be recognized that it often falls very far short of the highest ethical standards of liberal individualism. But apart from its inevitability, we regard it as proper by virtue of the common commitment to membership in the civil community. Even within

* Daniel Lerner, ed.: *The Human Meaning of the Social Sciences*. New York: Meridian Books, Inc. 114, 142–144 (1959). © 1959 by the World Publishing Company. Reprinted by permission.

this commitment, however, which is by no means entirely voluntary, there are limitations. When the exercise of civil authority shades off into manipulation, i.e., when the ends of the instigated action become more and more opaque to the person over whom it is exercised, and the opacity is a deliberate creation of the ruler, the bonds of obligation loosen. The authority of the experimenter has none of the claims of the civil authority; it is more like a contractual relationship, with the limitation on the right to contract away one's will or dignity or to serve unforeseen purposes of the experimenter. The less the experimental subject appreciates or desires the ends sought by the experimenter and the less intelligible to him are the means used for eliciting his obedience, the more problematic it becomes ethically. As consensus becomes attenuated, manipulation increases. This is the kind of power exercised in the operation of a sociological experiment.

The subject of an experiment will practically never know as much about the experiment and its meaning as the designer of the experiment, and if he did, it might prejudice the desired outcome. The problem that remains, therefore, given this irreducible trace of the ethically problematic in social and psychological experimentation, is whether it is kept down to a minimum in its pernicious effects. Here, on the whole, I think the record of social science experimentation is quite unblemished. Its purity, however, can be partly associated with its scientific inconsequentiality. If it studied more important variables which touch more deeply and lastingly on the life, conduct, and outlook of the subjects, it might perhaps have acquired more scientific substance, but it would have done so at a much greater ethical risk.

Recently, a group of Cornell University anthropologists came into control over a Peruvian *hacienda* of two thousand persons on whom they are using their authority to institute large-scale and long-range changes. They are undertaking to rule the lives of men and women without the legitimacy that any government, even a tyranny, possesses, but with the legitimacy of a large landowner. If we assume that they introduce no measures except what they think beneficial for their subjects, then they are a benevolent despotism. If, as seems to be the case, they attempt to establish democracy there, to raise the standard of living, to increase education and civic responsibility, their position is little different from that of the conventional liberal reforming land-

lord, except that they are also trying to observe precisely the results of their efforts. They have two claims to justification—one, the enhancement of welfare, and the other, the increase in their knowledge of how the changes came about —but as far as I can gather, no measure is instituted for exclusively cognitive purposes. Although I have not seen any detailed reports on this unprecedented undertaking in which the Peruvian government has rented two thousand of its citizens to a foreign landlord, the dominant impression I receive is that the Cornell group is trying to apply its already available knowledge to the practical task of improving the life of a hitherto impoverished and suppressed group, increasing their self-respect, their desire and capacity for self-government, their productivity, their understanding and skill. It should also be noted that in a formal sense, there is apparently no experimentation.

In trying to arrive at an assessment of sociological experimentation, the Cornell-Peru project is important because it reminds us that, whatever their attitude toward the larger social order and the institutions of authority which play important parts in regulating it, social scientists do not seek the gratifications of aggression in their relations with their experimental subjects. Unlike the experiments of the physicians who worked on Jews, Poles, and other "inferior races" in the German concentration camps, no deprivations are being knowingly inflicted on the Peruvian peasants. Social scientists, whatever their other imperfections, are usually not sadists.

3.

Disclosure of Risks?

a.

Authorization and Release of Responsibility for the Investigational Use of LSD-25 and Psilocybin (1964)*

I, the undersigned, hereby authorize [the] chief investigator, to administer to me the drugs LSD-25 and psilocybin, as well as concentration procedures, psychological examinations and tests. I hereby consent to the administration of the aforesaid drugs and to all psychological tests, examinations, procedures, and experiments involving their use as Doctor [A] deems neces-

---

* Reprinted by permission of the investigator.

sary or advisable. I hereby authorize Doctor [A] to make use of all records, tests and personal data derived from these experiments and previous experiments for the purposes of his research and to quote, summarize or otherwise incorporate in research reports or publication all records, tests and personal data derived from these experiments and previous experiments providing that there is no disclosure of the identity of the undersigned. I fully understand that the safety and usefulness of examinations, tests, treatments or therapies involving the use of LSD-25 and psilocybin are now being investigated and that the manufacturers and distributors of said agents have supplied them for research and investigational purposes. I have read and understood and signed the attached description of the potential risks and consequences of undergoing these experiments, examinations and tests involving the use of LSD-25 and psilocybin, and of concentration procedures. I hereby personally assume all risks known and unknown and agree to hold Doctor [A] and his agents and employees free and harmless from any claims, demands or suits for damages for any injuries or complications whatsoever which may result from or arrive out of these experiments, examinations, tests and procedures involving the use of LSD-25, psilocybin and concentration procedures.

It is understood that no charge is being made for LSD-25 and psilocybin used in the course of the experiments, examinations or tests.

This release is freely given, and I affirm that I am not acting under fraud, duress or menace of any person whomsoever.

DATED: _____

SIGNED: _____

WITNESS: _____

WITNESS: _____

NOTES

NOTE 1.

SUMMARY OF RISKS FROM EXPERIMENTAL ADMINISTRATION OF LSD-25 AND PSILOCYBIN (1964)*

LSD-25 and psilocybin are now classified by the Federal Food and Drug Administration as experimental. This summary describing risks attendant upon the use of such agents in investigational examinations, tests, treatments and thera-

------
* Reprinted by permission of the investigator.

pies has been prepared in compliance with legislation requiring that prospective patients or experimental subjects be acquainted with these risks.

The primary risks from use of psychedelic agents arise from the possibility of emotional upset leading either to suicide or a psychotic reaction (nervous breakdown). The most extensive summary of these risks is contained in an article by Dr. Sidney Cohen, written in 1960 in the *Journal of Nervous and Mental Disease* (Vol. 130, pp. 30–40). The data presented was obtained from questionnaires sent to various investigators who had experience in administering these agents. Of the almost 5,000 cases reported involving over 25,000 ingestions, psychotic reactions lasting more than 48 hours were reported in 0.8 cases per 1,000 among experimental subjects, and 1.8 cases per 1,000 among patients undergoing therapy. No attempted suicides were reported among the experimental subjects and 1.2 cases per 1,000 of attempted suicides, and 0.4 cases per 1,000 of completed suicides were reported among patients undergoing therapy.

Safeguards have been instituted in order to eliminate these major types of reactions. However, the risk of suicide or psychotic reaction is present and must, therefore, be recognized.

There are no known deleterious physical effects from use of psychedelic agents in the dosage range which the subject will undergo in these experiments. Physical injuries which might occur include tongue biting and bruises and result from a patient's inability to handle the emotional effects of uncovering his own mind.

Some anxiety and emotional turmoil is to be expected from the administration of these agents. These effects are typical of those which occur whenever exploration of a person's psyche is undertaken.

Concentration procedure, as performed in the experiment, may evoke anxiety and emotional turmoil but there are otherwise no known deleterious physical or psychological effects to be expected from them. Aside from the individual effects of the drugs and concentration exercises, there are no known deleterious effects from the combining of LSD-25 and/or psilocybin with concentration procedures.

DATED: _____

SIGNED: _____

WITNESS: _____

WITNESS: _____

NOTE 2.
J. KENNETH BENSON AND JAMES O. SMITH
THE HARVARD DRUG CONTROVERSY—
A CASE STUDY OF SUBJECT MANIPULATION
AND SOCIAL STRUCTURE*

*   *   *

. . . Perhaps the most frequent complaint lodged against the Leary-Alpert psilocybin research project concerns the alleged failure of the researchers to provide adequate safeguards for the health of their research subjects. Such a complaint was voiced by behavioral scientists at a meeting of the faculty and students of Harvard's Center for Research in Personality. Some public reactions to the research by individual members of the medical profession have included expressions of concern for the welfare of research subjects. During the controversy, some editorials (one written by Harvard's Farnsworth) appearing in medical journals warned of possible harm from hallucinogenic materials without naming the Harvard research project specifically.

The concern of critics seems to have been based on the following presumed dangers of exposure to psilocybin and other hallucinogenic drugs:

(1) short-term psychosis-like experiences are reported by some subjects;
(2) long-term mental disorders are precipitated in some cases;
(3) suicide attempts occur in a few instances;
(4) psychological dependence sometimes develops, even though physiological addiction apparently does not;
(5) the use of other, more dangerous, drugs may be encouraged;
(6) long-term changes in the personality of the subject may take place.

For their part, Leary and Alpert denied that the health of their research subjects was in jeopardy. They argued that the deleterious effects of the hallucinogens reported in earlier studies were accounted for by the variables of "set" and "setting." If research subjects expect a psychosis-mimicking experience and are exposed to the drugs in a clinic-like setting appropriate to psychosis, then a terrifying, potentially harmful experience will ensue, they contended. By contrast, exposure to the drugs in a friendly, relaxed, supportive atmosphere in which subjects have been

led to expect beneficial, insightful, educational experiences is productive of such experiences. In Leary's words,

Set and suggestive contexts account for ninety-nine per cent of the specific response to the drug. Thus, you cannot sensibly talk about the effects of psilocybin. It's always the set and suggestive context triggered off by the drug. A fascinating tension between these two factors—set and context—inevitably develops. If both are positive and holy, then a shatteringly sacred experience results. If both are negative then a hellish encounter ensues.

There is considerable agreement among psychopharmacologists that the suggestive context of the drug experience largely determines the psychological effects of the hallucinogens.

Leary and Alpert did not deny that personality changes were occurring among their research subjects. They argued, however, that the changes were for the better, providing the subject with a better understanding of himself and of others and enhancing his capacity for self-improvement, for creativity, and for love of others.

*   *   *

NOTE 3.
WILLIAM MCGLOTHLIN, SIDNEY COHEN,
AND MARCELLA S. MCGLOTHLIN
LONG-LASTING EFFECTS OF LSD ON NORMALS*

This is a report of a study designed to measure personality, attitude, value, interest, and performance changes resulting from the administration of LSD to normals. Several investigators using LSD with humans in nontherapy experiments have observed that some of their subjects report various lasting effects attributable to the drug experience. In addition, the recent controversy over the nonmedical use of LSD has given rise to numerous claims and counterclaims in this regard. We have previously reported on a pilot study in which tests of anxiety, attitudes, and creativity were given to 15 subjects prior to, and one week following, a single 200µg LSD session. Some significant changes in the anxiety and attitude tests were observed, but none were found for the creativity measures.

The assessment of lasting effects of hallucinogens involves extradrug variables to a greater extent than do most drug studies. We are asking, in effect, whether a dramatic drug-induced experience—one which temporarily dissolves the primacy of habitual perceptions of self-image, environment, beliefs, and values—

* G. Sjoberg, ed.: *Ethics, Politics and Social Research.* Cambridge, Mass.: Schenkman Publishing Co. 115, 119–120 (1967). Reprinted by permission.

* 17 *Archives of General Psychiatry* 521–532 (1967). Reprinted by permission.

will have a lasting impact on the individual's personality. We would expect any such impact to be influenced by the person's prior personality, motivation, and expectation, and by the presence of suggestion and reinforcement prior, during, and after the drug experience. In the present study, the subjects volunteered for a paid experiment without prior knowledge of its nature. A large battery of psychological tests was administered prior to a series of three, 200 μg LSD sessions, and again at intervals of two weeks and six months following the third session. The hypothesized postdrug personality changes include those most commonly reported in questionnaire evaluations: (1) lower anxiety; (2) attitude and value changes, primarily characterized by greater introspection, less defensiveness, aggression and rigidity, less materialism and competitiveness, and greater tolerance towards others; (3) increased creativity; and (4) enhanced interest and appreciation of music and art.

The subjects were US-born male graduate students who responded to an advertisement for experimental subjects to be paid at the rate of $2 per hour. The Minnesota Multiphasic Inventory (MMPI) was administered for screening . . . A subsequent interview dealt, in part, with the subject's experience, knowledge, and attitude on LSD and other hallucinogens. During this interview, the subjects were told that the experiment involved the use of drugs and they might or might not receive LSD.

Of the 155 subjects tested and interviewed in December 1964, 12 per cent knew a considerable amount about LSD, 15 per cent had never heard of it and the remainder had only casual knowledge. . . .

*   *   *

. . . Following the initial administration of the main test battery, each subject received a one-hour interview with the clinical psychologist who attended the drug session. The psychologist attempted to establish rapport with the subject, allay anxiety, assure him that he would be well cared for, and that no surprises, tests, or other demands would be introduced during the drug session. Special effort was made to convey the notion that, for maximum comfort, he should adopt an attitude of relaxing and "going with" the drug effect, i.e., to passively observe the effect without trying to control or direct its course. Questions pertaining to safety of LSD were answered, but no mention was made of possible personality or other changes resulting from the experience. The experiment was double blind during the preparation and until that point in the drug session at which there were sufficient symptoms to identify the drug given.

. . . Seventy-two subjects participated in the main experiment (mean age 24, range 21 to 35). There were three treatment groups, each with 24 subjects. The experimental group received 200 μg LSD, one control group received 20 mg amphetamine (5 mg immediate, and 15 mg sustained release), and the other control group received 25 μg LSD. . . .

*   *   *

After the six-month follow-up testing was completed, a questionnaire was administered which dealt with the subject's own evaluation of the drug experiences and any lasting effects. In a summary evaluation, 14 of the 24 experimental subjects indicated that the drug sessions had produced some lasting effects. . . .

. . . At the six-month testing, 33 per cent of the 200 μg LSD group subjectively reported lower anxiety and tension which they attributed to the drug experiences. The comparable percentages for the amphetamine and 25 μg LSD groups were 13 and 9. . . .

*   *   *

. . . The most frequently reported change in the experimental group on the six-month questionnaire was "a greater appreciation of music" (62 per cent). Forty-six per cent responded similarly with respect to art. These subjective evaluations were supported by certain behavioral changes. . . .

*   *   *

. . . At the six-month testing, 25 per cent of the 200 μg LSD group felt that the drug experience had resulted in enhanced creativity in their work, as compared to 9 per cent and 0 per cent for the amphetamine and 25 μg LSD groups respectively. . . .

*   *   *

. . . Of the 24 experimental subjects, the number reporting no effects, moderate, and pronounced lasting effects were 10, 10, and 4. The comparable results for the amphetamine and 25 μg LSD groups were 20, 3, 0, and 23, 0, 0 respectively.

*   *   *

The postdrug results for the personality, attitude, and value tests are generally consistent with the hypothesis, as well as the subjective reports of change, although the amounts of change are typically quite small. There is some evidence of a more introspective and passive orientation accompanied by a less defensive attitude in the experimental group. The subjective reports of increase in aesthetic appreciation were supported by behavioral activities, but there was no evidence of enhanced performance on the art tests. Similarly, there was no tendency for improvement in the postdrug measures of creativity.

The findings relating personality variables to attitude toward, and response to, the taking of LSD are much more definite. As would be expected, persons who place strong emphasis on structure and control generally have no taste for the experience and tend to respond minimally if exposed. Those who respond intensely tend to prefer a more unstructured, spontaneous, inward-turning (though not socially introverted) life, and score somewhat higher on tests of aesthetic sensitivity and imaginativeness. They also tend to be less aggressive, less competitive, and less conforming.

The above results should be interpreted in the context of the population from which the subjects were drawn. They were graduate students committed to a well-defined goal, and were typically not motivated to take LSD, nor to alter their values or aspirations. They received the drug in a secure aesthetically pleasing setting, but without suggestions of possible lasting effect. Under these conditions, 58 percent of the experimental group subjectively reported some lasting effect after six months. However, attempts to measure these changes via psychological tests provided only minimal supportive evidence.

b.

William P. Irvin
"Now, Mrs. Blare, About the Complications . . ."*

Mrs. Blare entered, sat down and lit a cigarette. Then she said calmly: "Well, here I am, Doctor. My husband was a little upset until I told him you said it was just a fibroid tumor, just a simple hysterectomy, and there really wasn't much to it."

Dr. Jones winced. What his lawyer had told him made him sorry he'd used those words. "Now, Mrs. Blare. I didn't exactly mean it that way. You see. . . ."

"Doctor, what is it? Do I have cancer?"

---

* 40 *Medical Economics* 102–108 (July 29, 1963). Reprinted by permission. © 1963 by Medical Economics, Inc., a subsidiary of Litton Publications, Inc., Division of Litton Industries, Inc., Oradell, N.J.

"No, still fibroids, Mrs. Blare. But a hysterectomy—well, frankly, there are some things that can go wrong. Not often, of course. But I should tell you of the possibilities."

"Oh, I'm not worried, Doctor. But if it'll make you feel better, go ahead and tell me."

"Well, after you're admitted to the hospital, they'll shave you. And occasionally they may nick the skin a little. . . . No, I realize that's not so bad. . . . Yes, I realize you're not the type to get upset over little things. . . . Well, then they'll draw your water. Sometimes this can cause a little inflammation of the bladder. . . . That's right —like you had with your last pregnancy. . . . Well, I know, it took four months, but usually we can cure it much faster. We'd use some of the newer drugs because they don't cause as many reactions. . . . A reaction? Well, you break out in a rash and itch and . . . That's right—like your cousin, John, after he got penicillin. . . . He died? Oh, I didn't know. Mrs. Blare, you're shaking ashes all over my rug.

"Next they'll draw some blood from your arm for tests. . . . Yes, I know you've had it done before. But sometimes you can get a virus infection that causes a little liver reaction. . . . Your friend's husband died, too? Well, most people get better. Of course, it takes years sometimes, and—well, anyway, it doesn't happen often. Mrs. Blare, you look pale. Here, take this pill. That's better.

"Now, at bedtime, they'll give you some drugs to help you rest. . . . Yes, I guess you could get a drug reaction from them, but usually. . . . No, I don't mean that would be your second drug reaction. I mean, you probably wouldn't have any reaction. . . . Yes, I know what I said about the bladder.

"You'll also get a little enema at bedtime. . . . Mrs. Blare what happened to your cousin in Omaha has nothing to do with this case. They won't punch a hole in *your* intestine. . . . Of course, I don't guarantee it. . . . Peritonitis? Well, yes, a hole in the intestine can cause it, but nobody will punch a hole in your intestine. . . . No, I wasn't aware that your brother is a lawyer.

"Well, let's see. Early the next day they'll take you to the operating room, which brings us to the anesthetic. Occasionally, it can cause a little problem. . . . Well, the heart might stop working. . . . Oh, yes, we can start it again. Usually. If we can get it going, it usually keeps on working O.K. Of course, if the brain has been damaged, the patient might not be too bright after surgery. . . . Yes, an idiot, you might say—but really, that doesn't happen often.

"Next we open the abdomen and remove the uterus. Of course, once in a while—not often, you understand—but sometimes. . . . Mrs. Blare, just because your grandmother said you were born under an unlucky star. . . . Now stop shaking. Here, take another pill. . . . No, it won't cause a drug reaction. . . . I don't think.

"Now, in removing the uterus, we might—on very rare occasions, you understand—get into the bowel. . . . I mean we might cut a small hole in the bowel. Sort of like the enema thing, yes. . . . Well, what we do is just sew it up. . . . Yes, peritonitis is possible.

"If all goes well, and we haven't nicked the ureter. . . . Oh, the tube that goes to the Bladder. . . . Well, it might cause a fistula and— let's talk about that later. . . . Yes, your insurance would cover it.

"Now the uterus is out, and the incision is closed. . . . No, we won't sew the bowel up too tight. I mean, we won't touch the bowel. . . . Yes, I know what I said before. . . . No, I'm not contradicting myself. Now please relax. . . . After the surgery you'll be given some fluids through a needle in your vein. . . . Well, yes, I guess so. That old virus and the liver again. . . . Yes, you mentioned that he died.

"If the wound doesn't break open. . . . Well, all your intestines would spill out. . . . Oh sure, we'd put them back. . . . No, that wouldn't cause idiocy.

"There's only one more thing. Of course, it doesn't happen often. We call it a staph infection. . . . Oh, you've read about it in the papers? . . . They all died? But that was in a nursery. . . . Well, yes, grownups can die from it, but we have drugs, and. . . . Well, a drug reaction isn't usually as bad as a staph infection.

"To sum it all up, Mrs. Blare, a hysterectomy really isn't so simple. Now if you'll just sign this paper that says I've informed you of these little complica—Mrs. Blare! We're not through. Where are you going? Come back, Mrs. Blare!"

NOTE

PAUL B. BEESON
MORAL ISSUES IN CLINICAL RESEARCH*

*   *   *

. . . I think in regard to the conscience of the physician, etc., one of the eroding things that

* 36 *Yale Journal of Biology and Medicine* 455, 465 (1964). Reprinted by permission.

does affect us is that physicians are accustomed to the fact that everything they do has a risk; every treatment has a potentiality for harming the patient; consequently the physician is constantly making a judgement whether a thing is more likely to help than to hinder. As a matter of fact we simply could not treat patients if we told them in advance every toxic effect of the treatment or diagnostic procedure we contemplated using in their case. We have to make that decision and we rely on the patient's trust and the fact that he cannot put himself in our place, and we make this decision. So we come to the business of clinical investigation and measure the risk; and the risk may be in our minds small, yet if we were to tell a person of all the possible things that could go wrong in the course of the experiment he probably would not wish to submit to it. This despite the fact, and I think this ought to be pointed out, that it is surprising how willing people are to submit to clinical experiments, to having tests made upon themselves, even when they realize these are tests which are made purely for knowledge and not with the idea of benefiting them directly.

*   *   *

c.

Ernst Prelinger
Safeguarding the Subject's Emotional Well-Being in the Context of Personality Research*

Consider the case of Dr. X who conducts research on the personality patterns and background factors of college students who have become political activists. Methodologically this research depends heavily on detailed, intensive, and fairly frequent interviews aimed at the subjects' past lives, family relations, ideologies, current experiences and activities, etc. The subject sample is obtained by approaching students who have become quite prominent and well-known activists on the campus and inviting their participation in the study. They are advised that they will be interviewed intensively and warned that the interviews may become upsetting to them. They are instructed, furthermore, that at any time they may terminate their participation in the research. They are also advised that psychotherapeutic referrals will be arranged in case of upset resulting from being in the study or in case that issues raised concerning their personality functioning stimulate their curiosity or interest

* Unpublished Manuscript (1970). Printed by permission of the author who retains all rights.

in further, personal self-exploration. As far as is known, no potential subject initially refused participation in the study as a result of these warnings; this fact may at least be partly the result of difficulties in anticipating the future impact of intensive interviews. Some subjects seem to have experienced some anxiety upon being thus warned but in at least some instances such anxiety in itself was perceived by them as a challenge to be mastered.

As the study progressed, a substantial proportion of the subjects became sufficiently upset to require referral to a psychotherapist. In most instances their participation in the research was diluted, in some instances terminated at that point. Reasons for this turn of events seem to be several: (1) The subjects, being late adolescents, activist, and also having been sufficiently interested in themselves to have volunteered for research of this kind, may be partly self-selected from a pool of rapidly developing, little settled or consolidated personalities. (2) The interview procedure, which by its very nature was directed toward investigation and probing, may have been lacking in providing supports available in the usual psychotherapeutic situation. (3) There is some evidence that the researcher, despite his own technical qualifications, may have had insufficient awareness of the transferences and transference expectations which are aroused within the subjects while they are being studied. (In a number of instances the subjects became quite demanding of the investigator, asked to live in his household, requested substantial financial loans, etc., and they apparently were indulged in these respects to some extent).

A number of issues, quite aside from the quality of the research project in itself, may be raised: (1) Are there definable conditions and safeguards which justify the conduct of such research altogether? (2) How can one assess the subjects' degree of understanding of the risks they assume by participating in the research? (3) What are the implications of interruptions of the subjects' participation in the research, with the resulting lack of closure of issues raised, whether the interruption is brought about by the investigator or by the subject? (4) What should be the relations between participation in the research and the undertaking of psychotherapy? Relevant here are questions of whether simultaneous participation in both enterprises limits or distorts participation in each one of them. There are issues of the relation between the researcher and the therapist (a special issue concerns the proba-

bly necessary scrutiny, in the therapy, of the subjects' relation with the investigator). (5) Is it necessary to make the subject's willingness possibly to enter psychotherapy part of the initial agreement between researcher and subjects?

4.

Disclosure of Manipulation?

a.

Kenneth Ring, Kenneth Wallston, and Michael Corey
Mode of Debriefing as a Factor Affecting Subjective Reaction to a Milgram-Type Obedience Experiment—An Ethical Inquiry*

*   *   *

This study represents an attempt to assess some effects of the Milgram-type experiment in order to provide a substantive basis for evaluating it and other experiments that pose ethical problems. . . .

*   *   *

[W]e have chosen to vary information that either clearly provides or fails to provide a subject with justification for her performance in the experiment. If, as we expect, offering a subject justification does significantly lower the level of emotional upset induced by participation in Milgram-type experiments, it would seem mandatory to exploit this device as long as we continue to carry out such experiments. . . .

Subjects. Fifty-seven female undergraduates enrolled in the introductory psychology course at the University of Connecticut served as subjects in this study. Most had not previously participated in a psychological experiment. All had volunteered, since participation in psychological experiments was not a requirement of the course; however, subjects did receive two points credit toward their final grade for having taken part.

Procedure. Although not an exact replication, the procedure followed in this study was designed to duplicate many of the features present in a Milgram-type obedience experiment.

*   *   *

First Debriefing. In the debriefing of experimental subjects, the experimenter explained that the

* 1 *Representative Research in Social Psychology* 67, 68–85 (1970). Reprinted by permission.

experiment involved a number of deceptions and proceeded to indicate them: (1) the experimenter was not really interested in the problem of how reinforcement works; (2) the other girl was actually an accomplice who (3) did not really receive any auditory stimulation; and (4) what the subject heard was in fact a prerecorded performance made by a drama student. The experimenter apologized for having had to so blatantly deceive the subject and hastened to justify the disguise of the experiment by giving a false though plausible account of its purposes.

The experimenter represented the experiment as a Milgram-type obedience study; specifically, he described it as an experiment dealing with "factors affecting conformity to an authority." After briefly elaborating this notion, he explained that not enough subjects had been run yet to enable him to give an account of how the results of the experiment were turning out; instead he offered to summarize some findings from (fictitious) related research concerned with personality differences between people who persist in the task and those who refuse to continue. Fortunately, subjects always expressed interest in hearing about them.

Subjects assigned to the *obedience justification (OJ)* condition were then told: In general, we find some rather clear-cut personality differences between what we call persistent subjects and those who quit before the experiment is over. Persistent subjects—those who continue in spite of the supposed reaction of the confederate—usually show higher ego-strength on personality inventories and seem better adjusted than those who quit. In other words, persistence in this experiment is usually, though of course not always, indicative of psychological well-being. We also have found that persisters more often seem to act in terms of long-range goals and are less often diverted from them by the pressures of the moment—of course, that's exactly how they behave in the experiment, so perhaps that's not so surprising a finding. Altogether then, persistence in this experiment may be considered a more desirable response than quitting before the experiment is over, though, obviously, we always get both kinds of people in these experiments.

Subjects in the *defiance justification (DJ)* condition, on the other hand, heard the experimenter say:

In general, we find some rather clear-cut personality differences between what we call defiant subjects and those who are fully obedient to the experimenter's instructions. Defiant subjects—those who before the experiment is officially over refuse to continue in spite of the experimenter's urging to do so—usually show higher ego-strength on personality inventories

and seem better adjusted than those who remain obedient. In other words, defiance in this experiment is usually, though of course not always, indicative of psychological well-being. We have also found that defiant subjects are in general less submissive to authority—of course, that's exactly how they behave in the experiment, so perhaps that's not so surprising a finding. Altogether, then, defiance in this experiment may be considered psychologically a more desirable response than complete obedience, though, obviously, we always get both kinds of people in these experiments.

It should be clear that we were attempting, through the use of these descriptions, to provide subjects with a basis for evaluating their behavior during the experiment: obedient subjects hearing the first account and defiant subjects hearing the second should feel, if they didn't already, that they behaved in a socially desirable fashion during the experiment and that their behavior is indicative of psychological well-being; defiant S's receiving the first description and obedient S's receiving the second, however, ought to feel they did not behave as they now wish they had and that they are less well-adjusted than people who performed in the opposite fashion during the experiment. It should perhaps be noted that providing a defiance justification evaluational set for obedient subjects represents an explicit effort to induce that cognitive state of affairs claimed by Baumrind and Kelman to characterize subjects after the experiment is over.

*　　*　　*

In the debriefing session for the control group, subjects were led to believe that the experiment was "on the level"—that everything really was as it appeared to be. The experimenter terminated subjects in this *no debriefing (ND)* condition by saying:

Well, that's the experiment, Miss ———. Miss (confederate's name), unfortunately, didn't learn the concept, but of course not all our subjects do. She did seem to find some of the latter stimulation painful, but that does happen occasionally. Since I explained the purpose of this experiment at the outset, I don't have much to add here. I wonder whether I could answer any questions you might have?

All questions were answered to uphold the initial cover story given for the experiment. If the subject inquired after the welfare of the learner, the experimenter responded, somewhat blandly, "I'm sure she's all right."

The purpose of this condition was to permit a comparison of the emotional state of subjects who believed that they had actually inflicted painful stimulation on the learner with that of subjects who had been disabused of that notion by the time an assessment of their emotional state was undertaken. In this way, we could determine the effects of a subjectively real performance in the experiment, uncontaminated by post-performance, experimenter-induced bases of evaluation.

Once this stage in the debriefing session had been reached for all subjects, the experimenter introduced a questionnaire designed to elicit the subject's reactions to the experiment. . . .

*   *   *

Once the subject had finished the questionnaire and sealed it in the envelope given to her, the experimenter (who had been sitting in the opposite corner of the room to encourage freedom of response) asked the subject to get her things and accompany him upstairs. After giving her envelope to a departmental secretary, she was escorted to the office of the senior author, who gave her a full and truthful debriefing.

Second Debriefing. Following Milgram's procedure, the second debriefing was varied depending on the subject's reaction to the experiment (all subjects had been observed through the one-way glass by the senior author) and whether she had been assigned to an experimental or control condition. Whenever a subject appeared quite upset, the experimenter's initial efforts were directed toward calming her down by whatever means seemed most appropriate and likely to be effective.

*   *   *

After the deceptions of the first debriefing had been indicated to the experimental subjects, the experimenter was able once again to follow a fairly standard sequence, description in varying detail depending on a subject's interest and mood, the background of the experiment, related research, and questions the present experiment was intended to answer. Subjects were encouraged to interrupt at any time to ask questions or comment.

Next (if they hadn't already been indicated) subjects were asked to express their reactions to the experiment and given a chance to "air their feelings."

The experimenter then endeavored to enlist the subject's cooperation in agreeing not to talk about the experiment with anyone until it was completed. He promised to (and did) send to each subject a written report of the major find-

ings of the experiment and, after thanking them again for their participation, mentioned that if they had any second thoughts about the experiment they should please return to his office to discuss them. (None ever did.)

Throughout this debriefing session, the experimenter sought to encourage subjects to feel they could speak freely and attempted to give a considerate and complete response to all comments and questions. The sessions themselves were of variable length, running from about 20 minutes to nearly an hour. No formal duration records were kept, but an approximate average for these debriefings would be 25 to 30 minutes.

Experimental Design and Hypothesis. . . . Of the 57 subjects in the experiment, 15 were eliminated from the analyses for the following reasons: five subjects defied the experimenter; six were suspicious in varying degrees concerning one or more aspects of the procedure; three indicated by their responses to the post-experimental form that they either did not grasp, believe, or remember the gist of what the first experimenter had told them concerning the desirability of obedience or defiance, and one subject was randomly eliminated from the *ND* condition to equilize *n*'s. Of the 42 subjects who remained, 14 were allocated to each condition; and in each condition, two experimenters ran exactly half the subjects.

Although in itself of only secondary interest, our hypothesis was that subjects in the *ND* condition would rate themselves as most upset, those in the *OJ* condition least upset, while *DJ* subjects would fall somewhere in between. The rationale underlying this hypothesis was simply that it would be somewhat comforting to know one was not really causing the learner to suffer pain and more comforting still to be given justification for one's experimentally demonstrated willingness to inflict what one thought was pain-eliciting stimuli. . . .

Followup interviews. Two to five weeks after they had participated in the experiment, 20 S's were selected (by a procedure neither random nor systematic) for followup interviews. The interviewer, who contacted subjects by phone, explained both over the phone and in the interview room that she was conducting an opinion survey concerning psychological experiments as part of the department's research assessment program. Subjects were told they had been chosen randomly and they should feel free to express their real opinions. They were told that the interview would be recorded but that they would be identified by a number that would protect their anonymity.

* * *

The subject was first asked to give a brief description of each experiment she had served in during the semester. If she had been only in the debriefing experiment, there was, of course, no problem in directing her attention to that experiment. If she had taken part in more than one, however, the interviewer, as if she herself had no preference, asked the subject to respond to the questions with the debriefing experiment in mind ("Suppose we start with, oh say, that concept-learning experiment you mentioned.").

Results

Behavior in the Experimental Setting. [O]f the 57 subjects taking part in the experiment, 52 (91 percent) were fully obedient. . . .

While there was nearly complete ultimate conformity to the experimenter's authority, the manner of obedient subjects' response was more variable. Some subjects persevered in their task with little overt show of emotion; others appeared extremely distressed. . . .

* * *

Of the five subjects classified as defiant, four simply refused to continue while one was so visibly upset that the experiment had to be halted.

* * *

On the basis of subjects' self-assessments of their emotional states, it is clear that the experimental procedure did generate substantial negative affect. Although there was some variation among the first ten items, the usual pattern was that subjects in the OJ condition tended to be somewhat less bothered by their experiences than were subjects in the DJ and ND conditions. These data suggest that the mode of debriefing received by a subject does make a difference: a significant reduction in emotional tension can be achieved by providing a subject with justification for her behavior; if she is (explicitly) led to think badly of her actions, however, the residual emotional tension is as great as if she believes she has actually harmed someone.

These general trends should not obscure differential treatment effects on specific emotional states. For example, the direction as well as the strength of a subject's anger is a function of her experimental treatment: OJ subjects tended not to be very angry either at themselves or at the experimenter; DJ subjects were angrier, but almost all their anger was focused on themselves; ND subjects were angrier still, but both at themselves *and* at the experimenter.

In view of these findings, perhaps the most intriguing data . . . deal with subjects' evaluations of the experiment as distinguished from their emotional reactions to it. As long as they were informed of the deceptions involved, their evaluation of the experiment was prevailingly and unmistakably positive. For the most part, these subjects indicated that they enjoyed the experiment, would be willing to participate in others like it, and found it an instructive and rewarding experience. Most notable of all, in our judgment, is that virtually none of these subjects resented being deceived, regretted being in the experiment, or thought that it involved anything unethical or should be discontinued.

It appears that even a cursory debriefing is sufficient to induce a marked discrepancy between how a subject reacts to an experiment and how she later comes to evaluate it. This discontinuity of affect and evaluation accords perfectly with Milgram's accounts which make clear that while many subjects are upset by the experimental procedure itself, they value the experiment and their participation. We fail to observe this pattern only for ND subjects whose evaluation of the experiment was consistently more negative; this is not surprising, of course, since at the time of their evaluation they still believe they had inflicted considerable pain on the learner.

Behavior during the Second Debriefing. Although many experimental subjects were greatly relieved by what they had learned from their first, partially false debriefing, some of them and most of the control group subjects were still quite agitated at the time they were given their second, truthful debriefing. Most of the subjects who arrived still feeling a little shaken were visibly calmer as soon as the real purposes of the experiment had been disclosed and usually evinced strong and sincere interest in learning more about the experiment. Most subjects responded remarkably well and with considerable good-humor on being informed of the deception-within-a-deception design of the experiment, and many displayed a lively sympathy with the objectives of the research. By the end of the debriefing, almost all subjects seemed emotionally intact and left with a clear understanding of what they had undergone that day and why.

Nevertheless, two cautionary remarks should be inserted here. The description given above is based entirely on the senior author's global impressions which may well be distorted both by the passage of time and his particular biases. No attempt was made to assess in any objective way a subject's emotional state after the second debriefing. In addition, as the foregoing account implied, there were a few who, even though they fully understood the purposes of the experiment and said that they were not resentful over what had happened, left the second debriefing still apparently somewhat upset, or at least not entirely free of their emotional tension. To determine the accuracy of the impressionistic observations made of the subjects during their second debriefing as well as to evaluate possible long-term negative aftereffects, we need to draw on the findings from the followup interviews.

Results of Followup Interviews. Subjects' responses to the interviewer's questions—many of which were the same as or similar to those that appeared on the post-experimental questionnaire—were in the main consistent with those they had expressed earlier: by and large, they regarded their experimental experience positively.

The modal subject indicated that (1) while she did not enjoy participating in the experiment at the time, (2) she did feel a lot better about it once it had been explained to her; (3) she was satisfied with the explanation she had received and (4) was grateful for it; (5) she felt she had learned something from the experiment, (6) did not regret being in it or (7) feel angry that she had been deceived; (8) she did not think any ethical standards were violated, or (9) that she was required to do anything she should not have been asked to do. . . .

Although the interview data that we collected are obviously not conclusive, we can say that they afford no evidence to indicate that there were any serious long-term aftereffects from this experiment. To affirm this, however, is not to deny that there were some significant negative consequences for varying numbers of subjects.

The most common of them was the view expressed by approximately half the interviewed subjects that they would now be more suspicious of psychological experiments and more wary about being deceived. In a number of instances, however, these subjects had subsequently been in other deception experiments which apparently served to reinforce their mistrust. Several subjects stated that they did not like the idea of deception per se, especially the deception that was foisted during the first debriefing and implied that the deception was more disturbing than the requirements of the experimental task itself.

Seven subjects approximately one-third of those interviewed, did indicate that they had been bothered by what they had done during the experiment. Some of these subjects commented that they had been disappointed or angry with themselves afterward for their behavior—a residual emotional state that was not entirely dissipated by the second debriefing. Others mentioned self-doubts. Several suggested that while they themselves were not that deeply affected by their experimental experience, they knew certain other people who would be and that "they wouldn't have been able to take it." One subject had clearly the most negative reaction to the experiment; when asked whether she regretted having been in the study, she replied:

It made me rather upset . . . for at least the rest of the day, if not the rest of the week. I felt very sick. I mean, I knew I hadn't done anything really, you know, to involve anyone getting pain, but the fact that, you know, I thought at the very beginning that I might have caused somebody pain and this was just getting me sick and even if they told me at the end that I wasn't doing anything to any other person, it still, you know, I had gotten past the point of being able to rationalize giving someone else pain.

*   *   *

Discussion

Taken as a whole, the data from this study fail to substantiate the charge that there are likely to be widespread and persistent negative aftereffects from Milgram-type obedience experiments. . . .

There was, however, one objection to Milgram-type experiments on which we were able to collect some supporting evidence. It will be recalled that Baumrind claimed that such experiments were potentially harmful because they might affect a subject's ability to trust adult authorities in the future. Our followup interview data suggested that, in fact, many subjects were experiencing such difficulties, even though there was no necessary concomitant decrease in their interest in serving as subjects in psychological experiments.

*   *   *

Although the findings of this experiment demonstrate that one kind of allegation against the Milgram-type obedience experiment—that based on its effects on subjects—is almost entirely without empirical foundation, they do not of course rule out other criticisms of this variety of experimentation. Indeed, it would be possible to utilize some of the data from the present experiment to argue against such research. For example, one could contend that:

1. Since a substantial number of subjects are upset during the experiment (18 of the 42 subjects retained for the principal analyses rated themselves 75 or higher on the "upset" scale), that in itself should give us pause, regardless of the effects of subsequent debriefings.
2. It is beside the point that only a small minority of subjects seem to be adversely, even if not severely, affected by the experiment; we should not conduct any experiments giving rise to such effects, however slight they may be and regardless of the number of people involved.
3. Whatever the ethical implications of such experiments, they raise serious methodological problems; for example, increasing subjects' suspicions about other experiments they might later be in.
4. Even though subjects themselves may not regret having taken part in such experiments or think that they entail any ethical violations, it is clear that they have in fact been made to act in a degrading way and that we should not conduct experiments that induce this kind of behavior, whatever subjects' own interpretation of it may be.

* * *

NOTE

PAUL ERRERA
STATEMENT BASED ON INTERVIEWS WITH
FORTY "WORST CASES" IN THE MILGRAM
OBEDIENCE EXPERIMENTS*

An attempt was made to evaluate whether subjects involved in Dr. Milgram's "Obedience to Authority" experiment had any harmful reactions as a result of their experience. Single 50 minute interviews were held with a selected sample of the population—individual and group sessions, some twelve months after the termination of the study.

Not enclosed in this report is a description of the selection process, a description of the population seen as compared to the overall sample, and an accounting of those who did not keep their return appointments.

The subjects seen responded to our invitation with obvious interest. Most of them participated actively in the discussions. None were

found by this interviewer to show signs of having been harmed by their experience.

The largest number claimed to have enjoyed participating in the project. Some reported marked anxiety and 3 described extreme stress at the time of the experiment. The reported distress was mostly relieved within a few days and completely dispelled after receiving the letter Dr. Milgram sent to each participant describing the purpose of the project and some preliminary findings.

The subjects seem to have handled their experience in a variety of ways. Some presented the task as a routine one void of any stress. They were asked to do something; they did it to the best of their ability. Others described the concerns they had in proceeding with the experiment. They expressed anger at the professor or at the institution responsible for the experiment; they became annoyed at the student for not learning and held him responsible for what happened—a few offered to switch roles with him.

Each subject seemed to handle his task in a manner consistent with well-established patterns of behavior. No evidence was found of any traumatic reactions. Those who had been the angriest appeared to be chronically angry at their environment—ever ready to attack available authority figures.

A few accepted responsibility for their actions and described their distress when faced with their willingness to inflict pain on another human being. They felt that as a result of the experiment they had learned something valuable about themselves.

b.

**Elaine Walster, Ellen Bersheid,
Darcy Abrahams, and Vera Aronson
Effectiveness of Debriefing
Following Deception Experiments***

* * *

Deception experiments differ so greatly from one another in the nature and degree of deception used that even the harshest critic of this technique would be hard pressed to state unequivocally that all deception has potentially harmful effects. There are, however, two frequently mentioned dangers of deception experiments, to which some experiments are more liable than others. First, some critics have voiced

* Unpublished manuscript (1963). Reprinted by permission of the author who retains all rights.

* 6 *Journal of Personality and Social Psychology* 371, 372–380 (1967). Reprinted by permission.

their concern that lying to people may lead them to lose faith in their fellow human beings. Because scientists are ordinarily highly respected, the discovery that a scientist will lie might upset subjects even more than lies told by others. Secondly, and perhaps more importantly, it has been pointed out that some deception manipulations are emotionally disturbing to a subject, and that some disturbances might not be entirely amendable by debriefing. . . .

Under what conditions might we expect debriefing to fail? Suppose that a subject is told that his test results indicate that he is not very creative. In fact, the experimenter reports, few people tested have ever scored so low on creativity. Further suppose that this subject happened to be a budding poet who picked up his mail on his way to the experimental session and discovered the fourteenth publisher's rejection slip for his first serious effort. While pursuing his way to the experiment, the subject might quite naturally wonder if the series or rejections should be attributed to his lack of talent or to the possibility that the uncultured masses are not clamoring for sonnets about the Crimean War.

It seems quite possible that the experimenter's authoritative evaluation of the subject's creative talents would initiate in this particular subject some independent thinking during the course of the experiment. It is quite likely, for example, that this subject would try to reach some consistency between the content of the experimenter's report and his own original ideas about his level of creativity. To do this, he might well reexamine his self-concept and selectively recall past incidents, most notably the 14 rejection slips, which would agree with the experimenter's information. Memories of criticisms from friends and family, the recollection of some low grades in English composition, would, when interpreted in the light of the test results, strengthen his belief in his supposed low creativity. Consequently, at some point in the course of the experiment, the subject might decide that since his own cognitions augment the experimental evidence, what the experimenter said was true. He might even come to the conclusion that he himself had been imperceptive not to realize his lack of creativity before.

At the completion of the experiment, of course, the subject-poet would be informed that the negative evaluation he received was chosen at random, and it would be explained that it was just as likely that he could have received a neutral or favorable evaluation of his creative tal-

ents. As previously mentioned, there is ordinarily little reason for the subject not to accept completely the notion that he has been deceived, that he is not the unimaginative dullard he thought he was, and be none the worse for wear. It even seems quite probable that the subject might believe the debriefing message in its entirety, that is, that the creativity test was not genuine. In this case, however, his own supporting and freshly organized cognitions might remain. It is still true that he *has* gotten 14 consecutive rejection slips and that he *did* receive those low grades. Consequently, it is possible that, though the specific anxieties produced by the deception might be completely removed by the debriefing, his general opinion about himself might well be lowered, and his life turned upon a new course, because of the extra thinking the manipulation initiated.

When the deception happens to strike an area of deep concern and worry to the individual, when it is likely to initiate a train of thought which would not be altered by the revelation of the deception, it is possible that the damage done to a subject by the deception might be irreversible.

The authors will report in this paper an experiment which tests the hypothesis that it will be more difficult to successfully debrief (i.e., return to his preexperimental state) a subject who has received false information on some aspect of himself about which he is currently concerned, than it will be to debrief a subject who has received information which is irrelevant to his current concerns. While the preceding discussion focussed on the possible residual effects of receiving negative information, a parallel result could be expected to occur when the subject has received positive information. That is, it might also be more difficult to debrief someone who receives positive information in an area of current concern. This experiment, then, was designed to test for the existence of both positive and negative residual effects after debriefing.

* * *

The 80 subjects who participated in this study were freshmen and sophomore women enrolled at the University of Minnesota. Subjects were recruited from an introductory psychology course and from the university library. All subjects had taken the MMPI as part of the freshman testing program.

In an initial contact, subjects agreed to participate in two separate experiments. They were told that the first experiment would have an hour delay between the first and second part. Thus, a second experiment had been scheduled during this hour for their convenience. They were told they could either participate in this experiment or not as they chose. In fact, all subjects chose to participate in both experiments. In reality, of course, the two experiments were both parts of the same experiment.

The purpose of Experiment 1 was twofold: (a) to *measure* the subject's preexperimental concern about the kind of social impression she makes, and (b) to randomly assign the subject to an experimental group and *manipulate* her concern about the kind of social impression she makes. We wanted half of our subjects to be highly concerned and curious about their social abilities and the other half to be little concerned about these abilities.

* * *

The purpose of Experiment 2 was to lead one-half of the unconcerned and one-half of the concerned subjects to believe for the duration of Experiment 2 that they possessed good social skills, and the remainder of the subjects to believe that they possessed poor social skills. . . .

* * *

Subjects were debriefed at great length after all of these measures were collected. Since subjects viewed this experiment as an effort to find out the extent to which deception might or might not be harmful to them, virtually all of them indicated that they were happy to have participated.

* * *

It was hypothesized that it would be more difficult to debrief the high-concern subjects than low-concern subjects. Thus, we expected high-concern subjects who were told they possessed good skills in Experiment 2 to overestimate their performance, even after debriefing, to a greater extent than would those low-concern subjects who were also told they possessed good social skills. Similarly, we expected high-concern subjects who were told they possessed poor social skills to underestimate their social skills, even after debriefing, to a greater extent than low-concern subjects.

* * *

From [our data] it is clear that regardless of whether we deal with manipulated concern or selected concern, and regardless of whether we consider self-estimates on the sociability index or on the interview performance index, high-concern subjects do *not* seem to be more difficult to debrief than low-concern subjects. Selected concern and type of deception do not interact in affecting subjects' estimates of their sociability . . . or of their interview performance . . . as we predicted they would. . . .

The data obtained from this experiment lead us to believe that our hypothesis is incorrect. This belief is further strengthened by . . . a very lengthy pilot study conducted by Abrahams (1967); the hypothesis of this paper was tested with only minor variations. (Ostensibly the Abrahams study was concerned with "problem solving ability" and "creativity" rather than with "interview performance" and "sociability.") The data from Abrahams' experiment also failed to provide any evidence that highly concerned subjects are more difficult to debrief than unconcerned subjects.

* * *

Although we feel that our hypothesis is incorrect, this does not mean that we have concluded that debriefing is uniformly effective with all subjects. Our data indicate that subjects in the various conditions do exhibit lingering aftereffects of the deception, although they are not the effects we predicted.

Let us first consider the estimates subjects made of their own sociability immediately after having been debriefed. For all subjects, it appears that the personality report had an impact which lasted at least for a few moments beyond the occurrence of debriefing. Regardless of whether concern was manipulated or selected, and regardless of level of concern, subjects who were given favorable sociability reports rated themselves significantly higher on the sociability index than did those subjects who received an unfavorable personality report. . . . Since the type of sociability report a girl received was determined by chance, we must assume these differences are due to the fact that the subjects were not entirely disabused of the information they received in Experiment 2.

* * *

In addition to the aftereffects previously discussed, there is one additional finding that seems worth commenting upon; though our manipulated-concern measure seemed to have little impact upon the success or failure of debriefing, there is some evidence that selected concern may be of importance.

From [our data] it is clear that a subject's initial degree of concern (with her social abilities) has a marked effect on her post-debriefing estimate of her interview performance.

When we consider only the data from *selected high-concern* subjects, we see that even after the passage of time, debriefing does not seem to be totally effective. Selected high-concern subjects who received good sociability reports in Experiment 2, even after being told these reports were false, estimated that they did better in the interview situation than did subjects who received poor sociability reports. *Selected low-concern* subjects who received good sociability reports estimated their interview performance very much as did high-concern subjects who received the good report. However, the interview performance estimates of the low-concern subjects who received a poor sociability report are markedly different from the estimates of comparable high-concern subjects. These low-concern subjects guessed they did *better* in the interview situation than did subjects in any other group. This finding is peculiar.

*   *   *

If low concern does in fact reflect high self-esteem, perhaps we can find an explanation for these findings. The apparent failure of debriefing for high-concern subjects is disturbing, but comprehensible. What is peculiar is the high performance estimates made by low-concern subjects who were given low personality results. Perhaps this simply demonstrates that high self-esteem individuals are especially likely to reject unpleasant information about themselves. . . .

*   *   *

We conclude two things from the preceding study:

1. The question of whether or not it is more difficult to successfully debrief concerned subjects than unconcerned subjects of information relevant to their current concerns remains unanswered. We can only say that two lengthy attempts to demonstrate this effect have been unsuccessful. Whether or not a stronger concern manipulation would produce the effect is, of course, a moot question, but we have been unable to produce evidence of even a slight tendency for subjects to behave in the predicted manner.

2. We have presented evidence that debriefing might not be as immediately effective as experimenters have hoped and assumed. This evidence is distressing for a number of reasons. First of all, it is disturbing that in the present experi-

ment and in the Abrahams experiment, even after a very lengthy and thorough debriefing (probably atypical in thoroughness), subjects still behaved to some extent as though the debriefing had not taken place. Subjects behaved in this manner even though they had voiced to the experimenter their understanding that the manipulation was false, their understanding of the true purpose of the experiment, and even though, by their manner and replies, the experimenter had been satisfied that they did indeed understand the nature of the deception.

Even more disturbing is the evidence that the aftereffects of debriefing might be complex, unpredictable, and may depend in part upon the personality traits of the subjects. The nature of the effect of personality traits in the present experiment was not totally explicable to us. Aftereffects in the Abrahams experiment were also present and somewhat inexplicable. The success of debriefing in that experiment was influenced by several significant interactions between sex of subject, sex of experimenter, and treatments. At the time the Abrahams experiment was run, we were willing to conclude that the significant interactions obtained were perhaps due to chance, to experimental error, to measurement error, and so on. The results of the present experiment, however, combined with the results of the Abrahams experiment, have aroused our suspicions and anxiety that there are often residual effects of debriefing, and that these effects appear to be complex and not easily interpreted. . . .

NOTE

Diana Baumrind
Principles of Ethical Conduct
in the Treatment of Subjects*

*   *   *

My own belief . . . is that subjects are less adversely affected by physical pain or psychological stress than they are by experiences which result in loss of trust in themselves and the investigator, and by extension in the meaningfulness of life itself. College students, who are the most frequently used subject pool, are particularly susceptible to conditions which produce an experience of anomie. My secretary, when typing an earlier version of this paper, described to me an incident which illustrates the way in which

* 26 *American Psychologist* 887, 888–889 (1971). © 1971, American Psychological Association. Reprinted by permission.

deception can contribute to the feeling of anomie in young people. She recounts the incident, which she remembers vividly although it occurred 8 years ago, as follows:

When I was 18, a sophomore in college, a psychologist from a nearby clinic came to my dormitory one evening and explained that he was looking for subjects for an experiment which involved simply telling stories about pictures which would be shown us. This sounded interesting, so I signed up. At the interview the same psychologist introduced me to a girl a few years my senior, who stayed bland and noncommittal throughout the time she interviewed me. She showed me a few pictures, and since they were extremely uninteresting I felt that the stories I was making up must be very poor. But she stopped at that point and told me that I was doing very well. I was gratified and said something to that effect before we went on to the rest of the pictures. Then I filled out a form about my reactions to the interview, the experimenter, etc., and she took it and left. After being alone for a few minutes I looked around the office and noticed a list of the last names of subjects, with "favorable" and "unfavorable" written alternately after each one. Shortly thereafter the male psychologist returned and said that, as I had guessed, what the interviewer had said had nothing to do with my performance. They were testing the effects of praise and disprraise on creative production, and he said so far they had discovered that disprraise had negative effects and praise seemed to have none at all. Since I expressed interest, he promised that the subjects would be given full results when they were tabulated (but we never heard from him).

My reaction to the experiment at the time was mixed. I assumed that the deception was necessary to get the proper reaction from me, and that since I had behaved unsuspiciously the results of the experiment were valid. However, I was embarrassed at having been manipulated into feeling pride at a nonachievement and gratification at praise I didn't deserve. Nevertheless, I felt that it was "right" that I was embarrassed, since I had always been taught a "pride goeth before a fall" philosophy of achievement. I had been an underachiever in school until just a few years previous to this experiment. Since in my early years in school I had alternated between being praised for doing well and being damned for doing too well, I had always been a poor judge of my own achievements and had no internal standards for evaluating my performance—although I knew I was very intelligent and felt that some sort of moral flaw kept me from doing as well as I might. At the time I was attending a very inferior college and felt (rightly) that my grades had nothing to do with how well I was really doing relative to my ability. This experiment confirmed my conviction that standards were completely arbitrary. Furthermore, for several years I had followed a pattern of achievement which it took me another 5 years to get free of: I would go along for quite a while doing well in classes, in-

terpersonal relations, etc. Then I would have a moment of hubris in which I was more self-confident or egotistical than it behooved me to be in that situation. At this point someone would cut me down to size; I would be totally devastated, and it would take me a long time to work myself up to my previous level of performance. The experiment had, in a lesser degree, the same effect upon me, and it may have served to confirm me in this pattern because the devastating blow was struck by a psychologist, whose competence to judge behavior I had never doubted before.

* * *

5.

Benefits to Subjects?

a.

Stanley Milgram
Issues in the Study of Obedience—
A Reply to Baumrind*

* * *

[T]here can be . . . an important positive side to participation [in experimentation]. Baumrind suggests that subjects derived no benefit from being in the obedience study, but this is false. By their statements and actions, subjects indicated that they had learned a good deal, and many felt gratified to have taken part in scientific research they considered to be of significance. A year after his participation one subject wrote:

This experiment has strengthened my belief that man should avoid harm to his fellow man even at the risk of violating authority.

Another stated:

To me, the experiment pointed up . . . the extent to which each individual should have or discover firm ground on which to base his decisions, no matter how trivial they appear to be. I think people should think more deeply about themselves and their relation to their world and to other people. If this experiment serves to jar people out of complacency, it will have served its end.

* * *

A concern with human dignity is based on a respect for a man's potential to act morally. Baumrind feels that the experimenter *made* the subject shock the victim. This conception is alien to my view. The experimenter tells the subject to

* 19 *American Psychologist* 848, 850–852 (1964). © 1964, American Psychological Association. Reprinted by permission.

do something. But between the command and the outcome there is a paramount force, the acting person who may obey or disobey. I started with the belief that every person who came to the laboratory was free to accept or to reject the dictates of authority. This view sustains a conception of human dignity insofar as it sees in each man a capacity for *choosing* his own behavior. And as it turned out, many subjects did, indeed, choose to reject the experimenter's commands, providing a powerful affirmation of human ideals.

*　　*　　*

If there is a moral to be learned from the obedience study, it is that every man must be responsible for his own actions. This author accepts full responsibility for the design and execution of the study. Some people may feel it should not have been done. I disagree and accept the burden of their judgment.

Baumrind's judgment, someone has said, not only represents a personal conviction, but also reflects a cleavage in American psychology between those whose primary concern is with *helping* people and those who are interested mainly in *learning* about people. I see little value in perpetuating diverse forces in psychology when there is so much to learn from every side. A schism may exist, but it does not correspond to the true ideals of the discipline. The psychologist intent on healing knows that his power to help rests on knowledge; he is aware that a scientific grasp of all aspects of life is essential for his work, and is in itself a worthy human aspiration. At the same time, the laboratory psychologist senses his work will lead to human betterment, not only because enlightenment is more dignified than ignorance, but because new knowledge is pregnant with humane consequences.

NOTES

NOTE 1.

ALAN C. ELMS
SOCIAL PSYCHOLOGY AND SOCIAL
RELEVANCE*

*　　*　　*

Not only can one justify imposing certain unpleasant experiences on psychological research participants; one might even argue that the experience these people undergo can sometimes be a moral good in itself. As I've noted, Milgram

* Brown: Little, Brown and Co., Inc. 271–272 (1972). Copyright © 1972 by Little, Brown and Co. Reprinted by permission.

did not falsely attribute any despicable qualities to his volunteers, as has occurred in a few studies; it happens to be quite true that the obedient volunteers were willing to shock innocent human beings upon command and each volunteer proved this to himself. Should we instead leave people to their moral inertia, or their grave moral laxity, so as not to disturb their privacy? Who is willing to justify privacy on this basis? Who would have done so, with foreknowledge of the results, in pre-Nazi Germany? Do we not try to wake our friends, our students, our followers or leaders from moral sloth when it becomes apparent, and are we bound to use our weakest appeals when we do so? Who now condemns the Old Testament prophets for having tried to arouse people to the evil within themselves? Milgram doesn't claim prophetic stature, but his experiments may similarly awaken some of the people involved. It's true that these people didn't *ask* to be shown their sinful tendencies; but people rarely do. That's why ministers lure people with church social functions, why writers clothe their hard moral lessons in pretty words and stories, why concerned artists . . . blend morality and estheticism: because people prefer not to face the truth about themselves if they can avoid it. I have heard the other side of this argument, come to think of it: the argument that a certain group of people doesn't want to be educated, that maybe they'd prefer to remain in happy ignorance, and therefore should be left to their familiar pattern of life. Yassuh, massa.

The thrust of such arguments in Milgram's case is that he was simply too effective in bringing volunteers into dramatic confrontation with their own conflicting moral trends and their own weaknesses. We don't hear the same complaints about other psychological studies, or about most public speakers or writers or teachers or preachers, because they seldom move their audiences enough to make complaints worthwhile. Plenty of ministers, I am sure, would be ecstatic over the possibility of giving their congregations such a harrowing contact with their own immoral inclinations as Milgram has done, and would feel the process producing this experience to be truly heaven-sent. (In fact, one doctor of divinity who was a research volunteer asked Milgram afterwards whether he would put some of the good reverend's divinity students through the procedure, and let the good reverend in on the results. Milgram, feeling a bit of doubt as to the ethics of such a procedure, said no.)

*　　*　　*

NOTE 2.

HERBERT C. KELMAN
HUMAN USE OF HUMAN SUBJECTS—
THE PROBLEM OF DECEPTION IN SOCIAL
PSYCHOLOGICAL EXPERIMENTS*

. . . If we do use deception, it is essential
that we find ways of counteracting and minimizing its negative effects. Sensitizing the apprentice
researcher to this necessity is at least as fundamental as any other part of research training.

In those experiments in which deception
carries the potential of harmful effects (in the
more usual sense of the term), there is an obvious requirement to build protections into every
phase of the process. Subjects must be selected
in a way that will exclude individuals who are
especially vulnerable; the potentially harmful
manipulation (such as the induction of stress)
must be kept at a moderate level of intensity;
the experimenter must be sensitive to danger signals in the reactions of his subjects and be prepared to deal with crises when they arise; and,
at the conclusion of the session, the experimenter
must take time not only to reassure the subject,
but also to help him work through his feelings
about the experience to whatever degree may be
required. In general, the principle that a subject
ought not to leave the laboratory with greater
anxiety or lower self-esteem than he came with
is a good one to follow. I would go beyond it to
argue that the subject should in some positive
way be enriched by the experience, that is, he
should come away from it with the feeling that
he has learned something, understood something,
or grown in some way. This, of course, adds special importance to the kind of feedback that is
given to the subject at the end of the experimental session.

*   *   *

b.

**Commonwealth v. Wiseman
350 Mass. 251, 249 N.E.2d 610 (1969)**

CUTTER, Justice.

This bill seeks, among other relief, to enjoin
all showings of a film entitled "Titicut Fol-
lies," containing scenes at Massachusetts Correctional Institution at Bridgewater (Bridgewater), to which insane persons charged with

* 67 *Psychological Bulletin* 1, 8 (1967). ©
1967, American Psychological Association. Reprinted
by permission.

crime and defective delinquents may be committed. . . . Mr. Wiseman and Bridgewater Film
Company, Inc. (BFC) appeal from an inter-
locutory decree, an order for a decree, and the
final decree which enjoins showing the film "to
any audience" and requires Mr. Wiseman and
BFC to deliver up for destruction specified films,
negatives, and sound tapes. The plaintiffs appeal
from the final de-
cree. . . .

*   *   *

The film shows many inmates in situations
which would be degrading to a person of normal
mentality and sensitivity. Although to a casual
observer most of the inmates portrayed make
little or no specific individual impression, others
are shown in close-up pictures. These inmates
are sufficiently clearly exhibited (in some instances naked) to enable acquaintances to identify them. Many display distressing mental symptoms. There is a collective, indecent intrusion
into the most private aspects of the lives of these
unfortunate persons in the Commonwealth's custody.

*   *   *

These considerations, taken with the failure
of Mr. Wiseman to comply with the contractual
condition that he obtain valid releases from all
persons portrayed in the film, amply justify
granting injunctive relief to the Commonwealth.
The impracticality of affording relief to the inmates individually also supports granting this collective relief to the Commonwealth as parens
patriae, in the interest of all the affected inmates. . . .

The defendants contend that no asserted interest of privacy may be protected from the publication of this film because the conditions at
Bridgewater are matters of continuing public
concern, as this court has recognized. . . .

Even an adequate presentation to the public
of conditions at Bridgewater, however, would
not necessitate the inclusion of some episodes
shown in the film, nor would it justify . . . the
depiction of identifiable inmates, who had not
given valid written consents and releases, naked
or in other embarrassing situations. We agree
with the trial judge that Mr. Wiseman's wide
ranging photography amounted to "abuse of the
privilege he was given to make a film" and a serious failure to comply with conditions reasonably
imposed upon him. Mr. Wiseman could hardly
have fairly believed that officials, solicitous about

obtaining consent and releases from all inmates portrayed, could have been expected to approve this type of film for general distribution.

*   *   *

That injunctive relief may be granted against showing the film to the general public on a commercial basis does not mean that all showings of the film must be prevented. . . . [T]he film gives a striking picture of life at Bridgewater and of the problems affecting treatment at that or any similar institution. It is a film which would be instructive to legislators, judges, lawyers, sociologists, social workers, doctors, psychiatrists, students in these or related fields, and organizations dealing with the social problems of custodial care and mental infirmity. The public interest in having such persons informed about Bridgewater, in our opinion, outweighs any countervailing interests of the inmates and of the Commonwealth (as parens patriae) in anonymity and privacy.

The effect upon inmates of showing the film to persons with a serious interest in rehabilitation, and with potential capacity to be helpful, is likely to be very different from the effect of its exhibition merely to satisfy general public curiosity. There is possibility that showings to specialized audiences may be of benefit to the public interest, to the inmates themselves, and to the conduct of an important state institution. Because of the character of such audiences, the likelihood of humiliation, even of identifiable inmates, is greatly reduced. In any event the likelihood of harm seems to us less than the probability of benefits.

*   *   *

c.

Jane E. Brody
Daring Is Urged in Cancer Cases*

The president of the American Cancer Society urged here today that scientists take more chances in applying experimental techniques to the treatment of human cancer.

Dr. Leonard W. Larson, noted that "when some of the present laboratory practices become clinical routine," the cancer death rate, now 800 Americans a day—can be expected to decline considerably.

*   *   *

* The New York Times 18, col. 3 (March 26, 1966). © 1966 by The New York Times Company. Reprinted by permission.

Dr. Larson emphasized that "we cannot be satisfied with the status quo in cancer therapy, which is saving one patient in three with the most obvious and easily cured cancers."

He expressed considerable impatience with the slow rate at which laboratory research methods were becoming clinically useful.

In an interview following his speech, Dr. Larson explained that the main reason for this time lag was scientists' fear of being accused of experimenting on humans.

Also contributing to the lag, he said, "is the reluctance of experimenters to take a chance. I realize there are dangers, I realize there are laws. But I think scientists should be permitted to try —say, a drug—which they feel has some chance of being effective and has a minimum of risk."

"Of course," he added, "this should only be done with the full knowledge and consent of the patient."

Dr. Larson, who is a former president of the American Medical Association, pointed out that taking "calculated risks" has characterized many of the greatest medical advances.

"In eradicating polio, we had to gamble that vaccines would not cause polio or cancer."

Early batches of polio vaccine were found to contain a virus that produced cancer in hamsters. The virus has since been eliminated from the vaccine.

"In removing greatly dreaded plagues from the list of lethal diseases, we had to take chances that sulfa drugs and antibiotics would not subject patients to deadly allergies and other diseases."

"Now," he noted, "important new knowledge has come from basic studies in the fields of hormones and immunity, and we should lose no time in applying it to human diseases like cancer."

An early effort along this line has resulted in spectacular disappearances of hopelessly advanced human skin cancer in a few patients at Roswell Park Memorial Institute in Buffalo, N.Y.

"There is reason for extreme caution in experimental medicine," Dr. Larson told the 50-odd science writers attending the seminar.

"But," he went on, "with the cure rates for leukemia at zero and for breast cancer at a complete standstill during recent decades, and with death rates for colon cancer rising and for lung cancer soaring, there is also reason for haste."

"We have a choice of living dangerously or dying early."

6.

Pursuit of Knowledge?

a.

Theodore Roszak
The Making of a Counter-Culture*

* * *

[T]here exists no way whatever, on strictly scientific grounds, to invalidate *any* objective quest for knowledge, regardless of where it may lead or how it may proceed. The particular project may be unpalatable to the more squeamish among us—for "purely personal reasons"; but it does not thereby cease to be a legitimate exercise of objectivity. After all, knowledge is knowledge; and the more of it, the better. Just as Leigh-Mallory set out to climb Everest simply because it was *there,* so the scientific mind sets out to solve puzzles and unravel mysteries because it perceives them as being *there*. What further justification need there be?

Once an area of experience has been identified as an object of study or experimental interference, there is no rational way in which to deny the inquiring mind its right to know, without calling into question the entire scientific enterprise. In order to do so, one would have to invoke some notion of the "sacred" or "sacrosanct" to designate an area of life that must be closed to inquiry and manipulation. But since the entire career of the objective consciousness has been one long running battle against such suspiciously nebulous ideas, these concepts survive in our society only as part of an atavistic vocabulary. They are withered roses we come upon, crushed in the diaries of a prescientific age.

We are sadly deceived by the old cliché which mournfully tells us that morality has failed to "keep up with" technical progress (as if indeed morality were a "field of knowledge" in the charge of unidentified, but presumably rather incompetent, experts). The expansion of objective consciousness must, of necessity, be undertaken at the expense of moral sensibility. Science deracinates the experience of sacredness wherever it abides, and does so unapologetically, if not with fanatic fervor. And lacking a warm and lively sense of the sacred, there can be no ethical commitment that is anything more than superficial humanist rhetoric. We are left with, at best,

good intentions and well-meaning gestures that have no relationship to authoritative experience, and which therefore collapse into embarrassed confusion as soon as a more hard-headed, more objective inquirer comes along and asks, "But why not?" Having used the keen blade of scientific skepticism to clear our cultural ground of all irrational barriers to inquiry and manipulation, the objective consciousness is free to range in all directions. And it so does.

* * *

b.

Sigmund Freud
Fragment of an Analysis of a Case of Hysteria (1905)*

* * *

[T]he presentation of my case histories remains a problem which is hard for me to solve. . . . If it is true that the causes of hysterical disorders are to be found in the intimacies of the patients' psychosexual life, and that hysterical symptoms are the expression of their most secret and repressed wishes, then the complete elucidation of a case of hysteria is bound to involve the revelation of those intimacies and the betrayal of those secrets. It is certain that the patients would never have spoken if it had occurred to them that their admissions might possibly be put to scientific uses; and it is equally certain that to ask them themselves for leave to publish their case would be quite unavailing. In such circumstances persons of delicacy, as well as those who were merely timid, would give first place to the duty of medical discretion and would declare with regret that the matter was one upon which they could offer science no enlightenment. But in my opinion the physician has taken upon himself duties not only towards the individual patient but towards science as well; and his duties toward science mean ultimately nothing else than his duties towards the many other patients who are suffering or will some day suffer from the same disorder. Thus it becomes the physician's duty to publish what he believes he knows of the causes and structure of hysteria, and it becomes a disgraceful piece of cowardice on his part to neglect doing so, as long as he can avoid causing direct personal injury to the single patient concerned. I think I have taken every precaution to prevent my patient from suffering any such injury. I have picked out a person the scenes of whose life were laid not in Vienna but in a remote provincial town, and whose personal circumstances must therefore be practically unknown in Vienna. I have from the very beginning kept the fact of her being under my treatment such a careful secret that only one other physician—and one in whose discretion I have complete confidence—can be aware that the girl was a patient of mine. I have waited for four whole years since the end of the treatment and have postponed publication till hearing that a change has taken place in the patient's life of such a character as allows me to suppose that her own interest in the occurrences and psychological events which are to be related here may now have grown faint. Needless to say, I have allowed no name to stand which could put a non-medical reader upon the scent; and the publication of the case in a purely scientific and technical periodical should, further, afford a guarantee against unauthorized readers of this sort. I naturally cannot prevent the patient herself from being pained if her own case history should accidentally fall into her hands. But she will learn nothing from it that she does not already know; and she may ask herself who besides her could discover from it that she is the subject of this paper.

* * *

NOTES

NOTE 1.

E. J. BLOUSTEIN
PRIVACY AS AN ASPECT OF HUMAN DIGNITY*

* * *

An intrusion on our privacy threatens our liberty as individuals to do as we will, just as an assault, a battery or imprisonment of our person does. And just as we may regard these latter torts as offenses "to the reasonable sense of personal dignity," as offensive to our concept of individualism and the liberty it entails, so too should we regard privacy as a dignitary tort. Unlike many other torts, the harm caused is not one which may be repaired and the loss suffered is not one which may be made good by an award of damages. The injury is to our individuality, to our

* 39 *New York University Law Review* 962, 1002–1004 (1964). Reprinted by permission.

dignity as individuals, and the legal remedy represents a social vindication of the human spirit thus threatened rather than a recompense for the loss suffered.

* * *

To be sure, this identification of the interest served by the law of privacy does not of itself "solve" any privacy problems; it does not furnish a ready-made solution to any particular case of a claimed invasion of privacy. In the first place, not every threat to privacy is of sufficient moment to warrant the imposition of civil liability or to evoke any other form of legal redress. We all are, and of necessity must be, subject to some minimum scrutiny of our neighbors as a very condition of life in a civilized community. Thus, even having identified the interest invaded, we are left with the problem whether, in the particular instance, the intrusion was of such outrageous and unreasonable character as to be made actionable.

Secondly, even where a clear violation of privacy is made out, one must still face the question whether it is not privileged or excused by some countervailing public policy or social interest. The most obvious such conflicting value is the public interest in news and information which, of necessity, must sometimes run counter to the individual's interest in privacy. Again, identification of the nature of the privacy interest does not resolve the conflict of values, except insofar as it makes clear at least one of the elements which is to be weighed in the balance.

* * *

NOTE 2.

RESTATEMENT OF THE LAW, SECOND
TORTS*

§ 652B.   *Intrusion upon Seclusion*

One who intentionally intrudes, physically or otherwise, upon the solitude or seclusion of another, or his private affairs or concerns, is subject to liability to the other for invasion of his privacy, if the intrusion would be highly offensive to a reasonable man.

Comment:

a. The form of invasion of privacy covered by this Section does not depend upon any pub-

* Tentative Draft No. 13. Philadelphia: The American Law Institute 103–132 (1967). Copyright 1967. Reprinted by permission of the American Law Institute.

licity given to the person whose interest is invaded, or to his affairs. It consists solely of an intentional interference with his interest in solitude or seclusion, either as to his person or as to his private affairs or concerns, of a kind that would be highly offensive to a reasonable man.

b. The invasion may be by physical intrusion into a place in which the plaintiff has secluded himself, as where the defendant forces his way into the plaintiff's room in a hotel, or insists over the plaintiff's objection in entering his home. It may also be by the use of the defendant's senses, with or without mechanical aids, to oversee or overhear the plaintiff's private affairs, as by looking into his upstairs windows with binoculars, or tapping his telephone wires. It may be by some other form of investigation or examination into his private concerns, as by opening his private and personal mail, searching his safe or his wallet, examining his private bank account, or compelling him by a forged court order to permit an inspection of his personal documents.

* * *

c. The defendant is subject to liability under the rule stated in this Section only when he has intruded into a private place, or has otherwise invaded a private seclusion which the plaintiff has thrown about his person or affairs. Thus there is no liability for the examination of a public record concerning the plaintiff, or of documents which the plaintiff is required to keep and make available for public inspection. Nor is there liability for observing him, or even taking his photograph while he is walking on the public highway, since he is not then in seclusion, and his appearance is public, and open to the public eye. Even in a public place, however, there may be some matters about the plaintiff, such as his underwear or lack of it, which are not exhibited to the public gaze; and there may still be invasion of privacy when there is intrusion upon such matters.

* * *

d. There is likewise no liability unless the interference with the plaintiff's seclusion is a substantial one, of a kind which would be highly offensive to the ordinary reasonable man, as the result of conduct to which the reasonable man would strongly object. . . .

* * *

§ 652D.   *Publicity Given to Private Life*

One who gives publicity to matters concerning the private life of another, of a kind highly offensive to a reasonable man, is subject to liability to the other for invasion of his privacy.

Comment:

* * *

c. Private life. The rule stated in this Section applies only to publicity given to matters concerning the private, as distinguished from the public, life of the individual. There is no liability when the defendant merely gives further publicity to information about the plaintiff which is already public. Thus there is no liability for giving publicity to facts about the plaintiff's life which are matters of public record, such as the date of his birth, the fact of his marriage, his military record, the fact that he is admitted to the practice of medicine or is licensed to drive a taxicab, or the pleadings which he has filed in a lawsuit. On the other hand, if the record is one not open to public inspection, as in the case of income tax returns, it is not public, and there is an invasion of privacy when it is made so.

* * *

Every individual has some phases of his life and his activities, and some facts about himself, which he does not expose to the public eye, but keeps entirely to himself, or at most reveals only to his family or to close personal friends. Sexual relations, for example, are normally entirely private matters, as are family quarrels, many unpleasant or disgraceful or humiliating illnesses, most intimate personal letters, most details of a man's life in his home, and some of his past history which he would rather forget. When these intimate details of his life are spread before the public gzae, in a manner highly offensive to the ordinary reasonable man, there is an actionable invasion of his privacy, unless, as stated in § 652F, there is a privilege to make the matter public because it is one of legitimate public interest.

* * *

§ 652F.   *Privilege to Give Publicity to Matters of Public Interest*

(1) One is privileged to give publicity to facts concerning another which would otherwise constitute an invasion of his privacy, to the extent that such publicity is given to [news or other] matters in which the public has a legitimate interest.

(2) The privilege stated in subsection (1) extends to false statements of such facts, unless they are made with knowledge of their falsity, or in reckless disregard whether they are true.

*   *   *

Comment:

a. The privilege stated in this Section rests primarily upon the traditional freedom of speech and of the press. . . .

*   *   *

h. Education and information. The privilege to give publicity to matters of public interest is not limited to "news," in the sense of reports of current events. It extends also to the use of names, likenesses or facts in giving information to the public for purposes of education, amusement or enlightenment, where the public may reasonably be expected to have a legitimate interest in what is published.

*   *   *

c.

Joseph H. Fichter and William L. Kolb
Ethical Limitations on Sociological Reporting*

*   *   *

As soon as the sociologist leaves the field of quantitative analysis and attempts to describe in conceptual terms the social relations in a small group or community, the problem of what to report becomes much greater. Even when the community is cloaked in anonymity, indirect identification is almost always possible, and there is likely to be a subtle and unintended violation of human rights. The threat becomes even greater when the sociologist adds to his description of the social relations in the group or community an interpretation of the motivation which supports these relations and other social behavior. Thus, where systematic sociological description and interpretation of motivation combine, the sociologist faces the gravest moral challenge, and particularly so where this mode of description and analysis is applied to a leading member of the group. The likelihood that such a person will be identified and his social behavior and personal reputation placed under scrutiny by his fellows on the basis of the research report is very great. Here, more than anywhere else, the sociologist

* 18 *American Sociological Review* 544, 547–548 (1953). Reprinted by permission.

must take care not to needlessly injure another human being.

The problem of truth telling thus becomes a circumstantial one. This means that while telling the truth cannot *per se* be wrong or harmful, the ethical question of whether or not to include a certain objective fact always arises in relation to person and circumstances. Thus complete objectivity, or telling all the truth in all circumstances, is not necessarily a morally good act.

This is true for several reasons. The researcher is, of course, bound to secrecy where information has been given in confidence or where he has made promises of secrecy. At the same time, as a scientist, he will discover natural secrets, which by their seriousness demand silence on the part of the reporter. There is also the problem of detraction—the injury of another's reputation by revealing what is detrimental but true about him. If the harmful fact is already widely disseminated or if the subject is mistaken in the belief that the fact will result in the impairment of his reputation, the sociologist may not have any obligation to conceal the fact. Otherwise its revelation is a serious matter.

*   *   *

. . . Some positivists seem to regard science only as a fascinating game played according to a set of rules. It is doubtful that the sociologist using this conception of science may ever legitimately overrule the rights of the people studied. The simple wish of the people to conceal certain aspects of their behavior must then be considered sufficient to bar the report of that behavior.

If one regards science as a search for truth as an end in itself, the demands of the objectivity of science will carry much weight in the decision to publish all pertinent data. Except in history, however, the truth for which the social scientist searches is nomothetic, not idiographic, truth. It may be necessary to base generalizations on certain idiographic items, but man has the entire span of his career on earth to discover and disclose such items. Certainly a particular item of current behavior turned up in a community study need not be used to support a generalization if such use inflicts injury on the people being investigated.

There is a third conception of pure science. Social scientists may believe that science is both a rigidly ruled game and a search for truth which is valuable for itself, but they usually also believe that science well developed and used by experts or disseminated among the people can make for a better life. There is a sense of urgency about accomplishing this mission of pure science in the modern world. Thus, within this perspective, considerable pressure arises to ignore the rights of people who are scientifically studied. Despite this pressure it remains true that a willful disregard for the rights of persons and groups to their privacy, reputations, and secrets, will tend to destroy the very values which the scientist hopes his basic research can render more achievable.

Frequently the scientist makes a community or small group study not as a pure scientist but in one sense or another as an applied scientist. He may carry on the research for what he himself consideres desirable practical ends; he may be employed by officials of the community or group or by those of the larger society; or he may be employed by some private group with a specific selfish or altruistic interest. In all three of these instances there is pressure to report all the significant findings even though injury may be done to the objects of the study. Nevertheless the sociologist must abide by the rule that he exercise every effort to determine whether or not the values to be implemented by the study, and the probability of being able to achieve them through the use of its findings, justify the harm done to the members of the community or group.

Preoccupation with applied science is frequently accompanied by the temptation to look for and publish data which will further the realization of what the researcher himself regards as the good society or community. He is likely to believe that all of his data must be revealed in all circumstances. It appears to us that a scientist of this persuasion is most in need of the virtues of tolerance, compassion, and love, because he is in danger of placing the considerations of the "good" society above all consideration of individual rights and injuries.

The hired scientist, moreover, cannot avoid responsibility for revealing data injurious to individuals and groups by pleading loyalty to community or nation or by indicating his contractural responsibilities to a private group. Loyalty to community or nation may require injury to individuals and groups, but in such cases the scientist shares whatever guilt is incurred with all other responsible agencies. In instances of purely contractual research the scientist must accept full responsibility, because loyalty to nation or community is not involved. He is free to refuse the job, and if the values of the employing group are wrong or do not justify the amount of injury done the scientist must accept the moral responsibility.

*   *   *

d.

Howard S. Becker
Problems in the Publication of Field Studies*

Unless the scientist deliberately restricts himself to research on the ideologies and beliefs of the people studied and does not touch on the behavior of the members of the community or organization, he must in some way deal with the disparity between reality and ideal, with the discrepancy between the number of crimes committed and the number of criminals apprehended. A study that purports to deal with social structure thus inevitably will reveal that the organization or community is not all it claims to be, not all it would like to be able to feel itself to be. A good study, therefore, will make somebody angry.

[A] good study of a community or organization must reflect the irreconcilable conflict between the interests of science and the interests of those studied, and thereby provoke a hostile reaction. Yet many studies conducted by competent scientists do not have this consequence. Under what circumstances will the report of a study fail to provoke conflict? Can such a failure be justified?

In the simplest case, the social scientist may be taken in by those he studies and be kept from seeing the things that would cause conflict were he to report them. . . .

*   *   *

This is probably an uncommon occurrence. Few people social scientists study are sophisticated enough to anticipate or control what the researcher will see. More frequently, the social scientist takes himself in, "goes native," becomes identified with the ideology of the dominant faction in the organization or community and frames the questions to which his research provides answers so that no one will be hurt. He does not do this deliberately or with the intent to suppress scientific knowledge. Rather, he unwittingly chooses problems that are not likely to cause trouble or inconvenience to those he has found to be such pleasant associates. . . .

* Arthur J. Vidich, Joseph Bensman, and Maurice R. Stein, eds.: *Reflections on Community Studies.* New York: John Wiley and Sons, Inc. 267, 275–276, 278–279, 283–284 (1964). Reprinted by permission.

* * *

[E]ven if he is not deceived . . . the social scientist may deliberately decide to suppress conflict-provoking findings. He may suppress his findings because publication will violate a bargain he has made with those studied. If, for example, he has given the subjects of his study the right to excise offensive portions of his manuscript prior to publication in return for the privilege of making the study, he will feel bound to honor that agreement. Because of the far-reaching consequences such an agreement could have, most social scientists take care to specify, when reaching an agreement with an organization they want to study, that they have the final say as to what will be published, though they often grant representatives of the organization the right to review the manuscript and suggest changes.

The social scientist may also suppress his findings because of an ideological commitment to the maintenance of society as it is now constituted. Shils makes the following case.

Good arguments can be made against continuous publicity about public institutions. It could be claimed that extreme publicity not only breaks the confidentiality which enhances the imaginativeness and reflectiveness necessary for the effective working of institutions but also destroys the respect in which they should, at least tentatively, be held by the citizenry.

He believes that the first of these considerations is probably correct and thus constitutes a legitimate restriction on scientific inquiry, whereas the second, although not entirely groundless ethically, is so unlikely to occur as not to constitute a clear danger.

* * *

Shils rests his case on the possibility that the publicity generated by research may interfere with the "effective working of institutions." When this occurs the scientist should restrict his inquiry. We can accept this argument only if we agree that the effective working of institutions as they are presently constituted is an overriding good. Shils, in his disdain for the "populistic" frame of mind that has informed much of American sociology (his way of characterizing the "easy-going irreverence toward authority" and the consequent tendency to social criticism among social scientists), is probably more ready to accept such a proposition than the majority of working social scientists. Furthermore, and I do not know that he would carry his argument so far, the right of public institutions to delude

themselves about the character of their actions and the consequences of those actions does not seem to me easily defended.

* * *

In discussing the several facets of the problem, I have avoided stating any ethical canons. I have relied on those canons implicit in the scientific enterprise in suggesting that the scientist must strive for the freest possible conditions of reporting. Beyond that I have said only that it is a matter of individual conscience. In so restricting my remarks and in discussing the problem largely in technical terms, I have not meant to indicate that one need have no conscience at all, but only that it must remain a matter of individual judgment.

I ought properly, therefore, to express my own judgment. Briefly, it is that one should refrain from publishing items of fact or conclusions that are not necessary to one's argument or that would cause suffering out of proportion to the scientific gain of making them public. This judgment is of course ambiguous. When is something "necessary" to an argument? What is "suffering"? When is an amount of suffering "out of proportion"? Even though the statement as it stands cannot determine a clear line of action for any given situation, I think it does suggest a viable vantage point, an appropriate mood, from which decisions can be approached. In particular, it suggests on the one hand that the scientist must be able to give himself good reasons for including potentially harmful material, rather than including it simply because it is "interesting." On the other hand, it guards him against either an overly formal or an overly sentimental view of the harm those he studies may suffer, requiring that it be serious and substantial enough to warrant calling it "suffering." Finally, it insists that he know enough about the situation he has studied to know whether the suffering will in any sense be proportional to gains science may expect from publication of his findings.

* * *

NOTE

EARL H. BELL
FREEDOM AND RESPONSIBILITY IN RESEARCH*

I read with great interest the editorial, "Freedom and Responsibility in Research: The

---

* 18 *Human Organization* 49 (1959). Reprinted by permission.

Springdale Case." The problem relative to responsibility of authors to the community is one which always pushes itself into focus when I start writing a report. Personally, I have come to the conclusion that responsibility to the community does *not* conflict with responsibility to science. As a matter of fact, I have found frequently that attempting to state material cooly and objectively, rather than in terms of personalities and anecdotes, sharpens my understanding of sociological processes.

After writing the first draft of the Haskell County, Kansas Study, I took the manuscript to the community and went over it with my major informants. In many ways, this was the most productive part of the field work. It enabled the informants, for the first time, to understand what I was attempting to accomplish. This broader understanding brought to mind many things which they had not told me, largely because I did not have the knowledge of the culture and social system to formulate some significant questions. They also pointed out numerous errors of both fact and interpretation and thus saved me personal embarrassment and scientific error.

* * *

e.
**Oscar M. Ruebhausen and Orville G. Brim, Jr.
Privacy and Behavioral Research***

* * *

[An] important safeguard for confidentiality can be provided through control techniques. For example, the identity of the respondent may be coded and separated from his response except for the code number. The code, in turn, may be made accessible only to a few of the most responsible officials, or perhaps, only on two signatures or by the use of double keys. Even as elementary a safeguard as a locked file can make for substantial improvement. Penalties within the profession may also be devised for any breach of the confidentiality which should be of the very essence of professionalism.

Another readily available step is the destruction of research data. At the very least, that part of the data which would identify any individual with any portion of it should be destroyed, and destroyed at the earliest moment it is possible to do so. . . . [B]ehavioral scientists have strong incentives to retain all original research data. Such data can provide information of a

* 65 *Columbia Law Review* 1184, 1205–1208 (1965). Reprinted by permission.

longitudinal nature about the development of personality or organizations over time, the early childhood antecedents of career success, the degree of change in interest and attitude from one age to another, the effects of marriage upon personality characteristics and other fascinating problems. There are now great repositories of such data in the United States collected about individuals in schools, both secondary and college, and other institutional settings, which have been maintained because of this natural resistance of the research scientist to discard anything of such potential value. Nevertheless, the maintenance and use of this information for purposes other than that originally agreed to, and the threat to confidentiality inherent in its continued maintenance, strongly suggest that the proper course of the person or institution possessing such data is either to obtain the consent of the individual involved to its continued preservation, or to destroy the data, painful as the latter prospect may be.

It should be emphasized that neither the integrity of the scientist nor the technical safeguards of locks and codes can protect research data against a valid subpoena; such data are at present quite clearly subject to subpoena. In the last analysis, therefore . . . confidentiality can be assured only by destruction of the data. . . .

* * *

Assuredly, one can visualize situations in which the release of research data for a use not initially contemplated would, because of the great public interest involved, be socially tolerable. . . .

* * *

7.

Values of Investigator?

a.

**Howard S. Becker
Whose Side Are We On?***

To have values or not to have values: the question is always with us. When sociologists undertake to study problems that have relevance to the world we live in, they find themselves caught in a crossfire. Some urge them not to take sides,

* 14 *Social Problems* 239, 245–247 (1967). Presidential Address, delivered at the annual meeting of the Society for the Study of Social Problems. Reprinted by permission.

to be neutral and do research that is technically correct and value free. Others tell them their work is shallow and useless if it does not express a deep commitment to a value position.

This dilemma, which seems so painful to so many, actually does not exist, for one of its horns is imaginary. For it to exist, one would have to assume, as some apparently do, that it is indeed possible to do research that is uncontaminated by personal and political sympathies. I propose to argue that it is not possible and, therefore, that the question is not whether we should take sides, since we inevitably will, but rather whose side we are on.

*   *   *

We must always look at the matter from someone's point of view. The scientist who proposes to understand society must, as Mead long ago pointed out, get into the situation enough to have a perspective on it. And it is likely that his perspective will be greatly affected by whatever positions are taken by any or all of the other participants in that varied situation. Even if his participation is limited to reading in the field, he will necessarily read the arguments of partisans of one or another side to a relationship and will thus be affected, at least, by having suggested to him what the relevant arguments and issues are. A student of medical sociology may decide that he will take neither the perspective of the patient nor the perspective of the physician, but he will necessarily take a perspective that impinges on the many questions that arise between physicians and patients; no matter what perspective he takes, his work either will take into account the attitude of subordinates, or it will not. If he fails to consider the questions they raise, he will be working on the side of the officials. If he does raise those questions seriously and does find, as he may, that there is some merit in them, he will then expose himself to the outrage of the officials and of all those sociologists who award them the top spot in the hierarchy of credibility. Almost all the topics that sociologists study, at least those that have some relation to the real world around us, are seen by society as morality plays and we shall find ourselves, willy-nilly, taking part in those plays on one side or the other.

*   *   *

We can never avoid taking sides. So we are left with the question of whether taking sides means that some distortion is introduced into our work so great as to make it useless. Or, less drastically, whether some distortion is introduced

that must be taken into account before the results of our work can be used. I do not refer here to feeling that the picture given by the research is not "balanced," the indignation aroused by having a conventionally discredited definition of reality given priority or equality with what "everyone knows," for it is clear that we cannot avoid that. That is the problem of officials, spokesmen and interested parties, not ours. Our problem is to make sure that, whatever point of view we take, our research meets the standards of good scientific work, that our unavoidable sympathies do not render our results invalid.

We might distort our findings, because of our sympathy with one of the parties in the relationship we are studying, by misusing the tools and techniques of our discipline. We might introduce loaded questions into a questionnaire, or act in some way in a field situation such that people would be constrained to tell us only the kind of thing we are already in sympathy with. All of our research techniques are hedged about with precautionary measures designed to guard against these errors. Similarly, though more abstractly, everyone of our theories presumably contains a set of directives which exhaustively covers the field we are to study, specifying all the things we are to look at and take into account in our research. By using our theories and techniques impartially, we ought to be able to study all the things that need to be studied in such a way as to get all the facts we require, even though some of the questions that will be raised and some of the facts that will be produced run counter to our biases.

But the question may be precisely this. Given all our techniques of theoretical and technical control, how can we be sure that we will apply them impartially and across the board as they need to be applied? Our textbooks in methodology are no help here. They tell us how to guard against error, but they do not tell us how to make sure that we will use all the safeguards available to us. We can, for a start, try to avoid sentimentality. We are sentimental when we refuse, for whatever reason, to investigate some matter that should properly be regarded as problematic. We are sentimental, especially, when our reason is that we would prefer not to know what is going on, if to know would be to violate some sympathy whose existence we may not even be aware of. Whatever side we are on, we must use our techniques impartially enough that a belief to which we are especially sympathetic could be proved untrue. We must always inspect our work carefully enough to know whether our techniques and theories are open enough to allow that possibility.

Let us consider, finally, what might seem a simple solution to the problems posed. If the difficulty is that we gain sympathy with underdogs by studying them, is it not also true that the superordinates in a hierarchical relationship usually have their own superordinates with whom they must contend? Is it not true that we might study those superordinates or subordinates, presenting their point of view on their relations with their superiors and thus gaining a deeper sympathy with them and avoiding the bias of one-sided identification with those below them? This is appealing, but deceptively so. For it only means that we will get into the same trouble with a new set of officials.

It is true, for instance, that the administrators of a prison are not free to do as they wish, not free to be responsive of the desires of inmates, for instance. If one talks to such an official, he will commonly tell us, in private, that of course the subordinates in the relationship have some right on their side, but that they fail to understand that his desire to do better is frustrated by his superiors or by the regulations they have established. Thus, if a prison administrator is angered because we take the complaints of his inmates seriously, we may feel that we can get around that and get a more balanced picture by interviewing him and his associates. If we do, we may then write a report which *his* superiors will respond to with cries of "bias." They, in their turn, will say that we have not presented a balanced picture, because we have not looked at *their* side of it. And we may worry that what they say is true.

The point is obvious. By pursuing this seemingly simple solution, we arrive at a problem of infinite regress. For everyone has someone standing above him who prevents him from doing things just as he likes. If we question the superiors of the prison administrator, a state department of corrections or prisons, they will complain of the governor and the legislature. And if we go to the governor and the legislature, they will complain of lobbyists, party machines, the public and the newspapers. There is no end to it and we can never have a "balanced picture" until we have studied all of society simultaneously. I do not propose to hold my breath until that happy day.

We can, I think, satisfy the demands of our science by always making clear the limits of what we have studied, marking the boundaries beyond which our findings cannot be safely applied. Not just the conventional disclaimer, in which we warn that we have only studied a prison in New York or California and the findings may not hold in the other forty-nine states—which is not a useful procedure anyway, since the findings may very well hold if the conditions are the same elsewhere. I refer to a more sociological disclaimer in which we say, for instance, that we have studied the prison through the eyes of the inmates and not through the eyes of the guards or other involved parties. We warn people, thus, that our study tells us only how things look from that vantage point—what kinds of objects guards are in the prisoners' world—and does not attempt to explain why guards do what they do or to absolve the guards of what may seem, from the prisoners' side, morally unacceptable behavior. This will not protect us from accusations of bias, however, for the guards will still be outraged by the unbalanced picture. If we implicitly accept the conventional hierarchy of credibility, we will feel the sting in that accusation.

It is something of a solution to say that over the years each "one-sided" study will provoke further studies that gradually enlarge our grasp of all the relevant facets of an institution's operation. But that is a long-term solution, and not much help to the individual researcher who has to contend with the anger of officials who feel he has done them wrong, the criticism of those of his colleagues who think he is presenting a one-sided view, and his own worries.

What do we do in the meantime? I suppose the answers are more or less obvious. We take sides as our personal and political commitments dictate, use our theoretical and technical resources to avoid the distortions that might introduce into our work, limit our conclusions carefully, recognize the hierarchy of credibility for what it is, and field as best we can the accusations and doubts that will surely be our fate.

b.

Alvin W. Gouldner
The Sociologist as Partisan—
Sociology and the Welfare State*

*   *   *

. . . I fear that the myth of a value-free social science is about to be supplanted by still another myth, and that the once glib acceptance of the value-free doctrine is about to be superseded by a new but no less glib rejection of it. . . .

*   *   *

* 3 *The American Sociologist* 103, 113 (1968). Reprinted by permission.

[W]hen we talk about the bias or impartiality of a sociologist we are, in effect, talking about the sociologist as if he were a "judge." Now, rendering a judgment premises the existence of conflicting or contending parties; but it does not imply an intention to *mediate* the difficulties between them. The function of a judge is not to bring parties together but is, quite simply, to do justice. Doing justice does not mean, as does mediation or arbitration, that both the parties must each be given or denied a bit of what they sought. Justice does not mean logrolling or "splitting the difference." For the doing of justice may, indeed, give all the benefits to one party and impose all the costs upon another.

What makes a judgment possessed of justice is not the fact that it distributes costs and benefits equally between the parties but, rather, that the allocation of benefits and costs is made in conformity with some stated normative standard. Justice, in short, is that which is justified in terms of some value. The "impartiality" or objectivity of the judge is an imputation made when it is believed that he had made his decision primarily or solely in terms of some moral value. In one part, then, the objectivity of the judge requires his explication of the moral value in terms of which his judgment has been rendered. One reason why Becker's analysis founders on the problem of objectivity is precisely because it regards the sociolgists' value commitment merely as an inescapable fact of nature, rather than viewing it as a necessary condition of his objectivity.

Insofar as the problem is seen as one of choosing up sides, rather than a working one's way through to a value commitment, I cannot see how it is ever possible for men to recognize that the side to which they are attached can be wrong. But men do not and need not always say, "my country right or wrong." Insofar as they are capable of distinguishing the side to which they are attached, from the *grounds* on which they are attached to it, they are, to that extent, capable of a significant objectivity.

It should again be clear, then, that I do not regard partisanship as incompatible with objectivity. The physician, after all, is not necessarily less objective because he has made a partisan commitment to his patient and against the germ. The physician's objectivity is in some measure vouchsafed because he has committed himself to a specific value: health. It is this commitment that constrains him to see and to say things about the patient's condition that neither may want to know.

But in saying that the explication of the so-

ciologist's value commitment is a necessary condition for his objectivity, we are saying little unless we recognize at the same time the grinding difficulties involved in this. For one, it is no easy thing to know what our own value commitments are. In an effort to seem frank and open, we all too easily pawn off a merely glib statement about our values without making any effort to be sure that these are the values to which we are actually committed. This is much of what happens when scientists conventionally assert that they believe only in "the truth." Secondly, a mere assertion of a value commitment is vainly ritualistic to the extent that the sociologist has no awareness of the way in which one of his commitments may conflict with or exclude another. For example, there is commonly some tension between a commitment to truth and a commitment to welfare. Third, we also have to recognize that the values in terms of which we may make our judgments may not necessarily be shared by the participants in the situations we have studied. Our objectivity, however, does not require us to share values with those we study, but only to apply the values that we claim are our own, however unpopular these may be. In other words, this form of objectivity requires that we be on guard against our own hypocrisy and our need to be loved. This creates a problem because the values we may actually hold may differ from those we feel that we must display in order to gain or maintain access to research sites.

* * *

8.

Limits of Prediction?

a.

Margaret Mead
The Problem of an Unpredictable Future Position of an Individual Identified in a Research Project—1953–1968 A Melanesian Leader in Papua, New Guinea*

In 1953, Theodore Schwartz and I made an extensvie study of a political movement in the Admiralty Islands, I as part of a restudy and Dr. Schwartz as a specific study of the movement and its native leader Paliau. At that time, Paliau

* 98 *Daedalus* 382–384 (1969). Reprinted by permission of Daedalus, Journal of the American Academy of Arts and Sciences, Boston, Massachusetts.

had become known in many parts of the world, especially in Australia and in Roman Catholic circles, as a leader who had transformed a cargo cult into a successful political movement. He was well known as a sergeant in the police force of the Mandated Territory of New Guinea. During World War II, he found himself behind the Japanese lines and took the responsibility for organizing the food and living arrangements for indentured laborers from other islands who had been left on New Britain when Rabaul fell to the Japanese. After the war, it was impossible to try as traitors Melanesians from the Mandated Territory of New Guinea who had worked under the Japanese administration: members of the Trust Territory that owed no allegiance to Australia. An attempt, however, was made to punish them as war criminals. Paliau maintained that he and others arraigned with him had been instructed by the Australians, when they evacuated Rabaul, to obey the Japanese. He successfully refuted the charges of being a war criminal, but his career in the police force was over. He returned to his own island of Balowan, and with many vicissitudes—a cargo cult, imprisonment for involvement in the cult under the heading of "spreading false rumors," an attack on his life by the insane former husband of a new wife, a trip to Port Moresby for "indoctrination"— he maintained a hold on some five thousand people whom he had succeeded in uniting in his new movement. He was first permitted to become chairman of half of this population, a local Council compound. While we were there in 1953, the local government Council authority was extended to the entire five thousand people, out of an estimated twenty thousand Admiralty Island inhabitants. It seemed unlikely at that time that he would increase his political importance further. Many local government officials were hostile; his original dream of operating in a larger sphere, including the entire Bismarck Archipelago, seemed completely incapable of realization.

In 1954, I wrote *New Lives for Old,* and in 1958, Theodore Schwartz completed the manuscript of *The Paliau Movement in the Admiralty Islands, 1946–1954.* In 1957, I discussed Paliau in one of the Terry Lectures at Yale as a man of unusual ability, comparable in quality to Churchill or Roosevelt, astonishing in a man who came from a small island group of only six hundred preliterate people. The Terry lectures were published in 1964 under the title of *Continuities in Cultural Evolution.*

In 1964, in the wake of the newly estab-

lished electoral proceedings in New Guinea, Paliau was elected a member to the new House of Assembly for the Admiralty Islands, in spite of active opposition. In September of that year, on my way back to the Admiralties, I was interviewed in Sydney, Australia, by a reporter for the *Pacific Island Monthly,* who had taken the trouble to look up *Continuities in Cultural Evolution,* a book of a type not usually presented in the popular and highly politicized periodical. As a consequence, *Pacific Island Monthly* published Paliau's picture with a full-page article entitled, "Paliau Compared to Roosevelt." This article might have been a hazard to a man who continued to be the target of much local mission attack. But Dr. Schwartz and I had written our descriptions so that they could be read by anyone interested in the Paliau movement, and because Dr. Schwartz had painstakingly gone over the text with Paliau (who was now operating on a wider, much more politically important stage than when we had done our original writing), he could be proud of, rather than hurt by, the discussions that had been published.

In 1967, National Education Television made a film of anthropological work in Manus from 1928 to the present and included Paliau as a prominent figure. The filming ended in the autumn of 1967, and it was clear then that it would take approximately a year to complete the editing. The next election for the General Assembly was coming up in May–June of 1968. Had Paliau lost, it might have been said, then or later, by commentators on the responsibilities of social scientists working among emerging peoples, that the film had lost him the election and his chance to be a significant molder of the future of Papua-New Guinea. However he was re-elected!

This case is presented in illustration of the vicissitudes of social research on living persons whose future roles cannot, in the nature of the case, be predicted.

NOTE

Joseph H. Fichter and William L. Kolb
Ethical Limitations on Sociological Reporting*

*   *   *

. . . Those instances in which the scientist can foretell with certitude that serious injury will be done to the objects of his study seem to be very few in number. It is also likely that the lar-

* 18 *American Sociological Review* 544, 548–549 (1953). Reprinted by permission.

gest proportion of his data will be free of possibly injurious materials. It is the in-between area of probable injury that is most difficult to determine and yet which must be determined.

To know what the effect of exposing a group's secrets will be, to realize how seriously a person's reputation may be damaged, and to visualize the effects of violation of privacy presupposes knowledge on the part of the scientist which he may not have. This knowledge can be approached to the extent to which the scientist saturates himself in the social relations of the group which he studies. It probably cannot be achieved by the aloof scientist who simply culls the reports of those who have done the actual and basic data collecting.

Since there is a great difference between imaginary and objective derogation of reputation, the sociologist may tend to brush off the former as relevant and uncontrollable. Human decency, however, would seem to require that the scientist make an effort to inquire even into this possibility of psychological and subjective injury. The scientist cannot guard against all such contingencies and against the unexpected and unwarranted complaints of people, but he should do his human best to avoid them ahead of time and to be sympathetic to them if they come.

If the sociologist attempts to interpret the social behavior of the people he studies, he must assess the responsibility of the people for their own actions. False sentimentality must not result in the denial of the fact that a person must accept the consequences of the acts for which he is responsible. The scientist cannot erase the responsibilities, duties, and obligations, of the objects of his study. Yet, at the same time, he must recognize that the human being is never completely responsible for his actions, and that in many cases factors over which the person or group has no control may come close to completely determining certain acts. Since the assessment of responsibility will be contained in the research report, injury can be done if the assessment is not carefully made.

b.

Diana Baumrind
Some Thoughts on Ethics of Research—After Reading Milgram's "Behavioral Study of Obedience"*

[I] regard the emotional disturbance described by Milgram as potentially harmful be-

cause it could easily effect an alteration in the subject's self-image or ability to trust adult authorities in the future. It is potentially harmful to a subject to commit, in the course of an experiment, acts which he himself considers unworthy, particularly when he has been entrapped into committing such acts by an individual he has reason to trust. The subject's personal responsibility for his actions is not erased because the experimenter reveals to him the means which he used to stimulate these actions. The subject realizes that he would have hurt the victim if the current were on. The realization that he also made a fool of himself by accepting the experimental set results in additional loss of self-esteem. Moreover, the subject finds it difficult to express his anger outwardly after the experimenter in a self-acceptant but friendly manner reveals the hoax.

A fairly intense corrective interpersonal experience is indicated wherein the subject admits and accepts his responsibility for his own actions, and at the same time gives vent to his hurt and anger at being fooled. Perhaps an experience as distressing as the one described by Milgram can be integrated by the subject, provided that careful thought is given to the matter. The propriety of such experimentation is still in question even if such a reparational experience were forthcoming. Without it I would expect a naive, sensitive subject to remain deeply hurt and anxious for some time, and a sophisticated, cynical subject to become even more alienated and distrustful.

* * *

NOTE

STANLEY MILGRAM
ISSUES IN THE STUDY OF OBEDIENCE—
A REPLY TO BAUMRIND†

* * *

. . . Baumrind confuses the unanticipated outcome of an experiment with its basic procedure. She writes, for example, as if the production of stress in our subjects was an intended and deliberate effect of the experimental manipulation. There are many laboratory procedures specifically designed to create stress . . . , but the obedience paradigm was not one of them. The extreme tension induced in some subjects was unexpected. Before conducting the experiment, the procedures were discussed with many colleagues, and none anticipated the reactions that subsequently took place. Foreknowledge of results can

* 19 *American Psychologist* 421–423 (1964). Reprinted by permission.

† 19 *American Psychologist* 848–849 (1964). Reprinted by permission.

never be the invariable accompaniment of an experimental probe. Understanding grows because we examine situations in which the end is unknown. An investigator unwilling to accept this degree of risk must give up the idea of scientific inquiry.

Moreover, there was every reason to expect, prior to actual experimentation, that subjects would refuse to follow the experimenter's instructions beyond the point where the victim protested; many colleagues and psychiatrists were questioned on this point, and they virtually all felt this would be the case. Indeed, to initiate an experiment in which the critical measure hangs on disobedience, one must start with a belief in certain spontaneous resources in men that enable them to overcome pressure from authority.

It is true that after a reasonable number of subjects had been exposed to the procedures, it became evident that some would go to the end of the shock board, and some would experience stress. That point, it seems to me, is the first legitimate juncture at which one could even start to wonder whether or not to abandon the study. But momentary excitement is not the same as harm. As the experiment progressed there was no indication of injurious effects in the subjects; and as the subjects themselves strongly endorsed the experiment, the judgment I made was to continue the investigation.

Is not Baumrind's criticism based as much on the unanticipated findings as on the method? The findings were that some subjects performed in what appeared to be a shockingly immoral way. If, instead, every one of the subjects had broken off at "slight shock," or at the first sign of the learner's discomfort, the results would have been pleasant, and reassuring, and who would protest?

A most important aspect of the procedure occurred at the end of the experimental session. A careful post-experimental treatment was administered to all subjects. The exact content of the dehoax varied from condition to condition and with increasing experience on our part. At the very least all subjects were told that the victim had not received dangerous electric shocks. Each subject had a friendly reconciliation with the unharmed victim, and an extended discussion with the experimenter. The experiment was explained to the defiant subjects in a way that supported their decision to disobey the experimenter. Obedient subjects were assured of the fact that their behavior was entirely normal and that their feelings of conflict or tension were shared by other participants. Subjects were told that they would receive a comprehensive report at the conclusion of the experimental series. In some instances, additional detailed and lengthy discussions of the experiments were also carried out with individual subjects.

When the experimental series was complete, subjects received a written report which presented details of the experimental procedure and results. Again their own part in the experiments was treated in a dignified way and their behavior in the experiment respected. All subjects received a follow-up questionnaire regarding their participation in the research, which again allowed expression of thoughts and feelings about their behavior.

The replies to the questionnaire confirmed my impression that participants felt positively toward the experiment. In its quantitative aspect . . . 84 percent of the subjects stated that they were glad to have been in the experiment; 15 percent indicated neutral feelings, and 1.3 percent indicated negative feelings. To be sure, such findings are to be interpreted cautiously, but they cannot be disregarded.

Further, four-fifths of the subjects felt that more experiments of this sort should be carried out, and 74 percent indicated that they had learned something of personal importance as a result of being in the study. . . .

c.

Alexander D. Langmuir
New Environmental Factor in
Congenital Disease*

This issue contains an original communication of great scientific importance and serious social implications. The highly significant correlation between the appearance of adenocarcinoma of the vagina in teen-age girls and young women, a very rare disease, and the ingestion of diethylstilbestrol by their mothers during the first trimester of pregnancy points to a new mechanism in the pathogenesis of congenital neoplastic disease and adds a new dimension to the whole matter of what drugs are safe or unsafe to administer to pregnant women.

The first indication of the existence of this effect was reported a year ago. A cluster of seven cases of adenocarcinoma of the vagina in young

* 284 New England Journal of Medicine 912–913 (1971). Reprinted by permission.

females, 15 to 22 years of age, was recognized in the New England area during the period 1966 to 1969. This report created interest within gynecologic and oncologic circles, but was largely overlooked by epidemiologists. Such a concentration of such a rare disease in such a young age group points vividly to the existence of a specific causative factor somewhere in the immediate environment of these patients.

Now the original discoverers of the cluster have pointed to the most likely factor—namely, the administration of stilbestrol to the mothers of these patients early in pregnancy. They had been treated between 1946 and 1951, a period when stilbestrol was being used for the therapy of repeated or threatened abortion. A confirmed history of this association has been elicited in seven of the eight patients so far studied, but in none of 32 carefully matched controls.

*   *   *

Although the authors have been conservative in reporting their observations as merely "an association," the epidemiologic evidence indicates a direct etiologic relation similar to other known congenital effects, such as maternal German measles as a cause of congenital rubella syndrome and thalidomide as a cause of phocomelia. The relation will be confirmed if additional cases associating this rare disease with maternal stilbestrol administration are reported.

The scientific implications of this discovery are evident. Presumably, the mechanism involves some derangement in the early development of the female urogenital tract at some critical phase, as yet unknown. The rare condition, vaginal adenosis, was present in five of the seven stilbestrol-associated cases and may well be an important stage in the evolution of the malignant process.

*   *   *

If the findings of this one group of workers is confirmed by others, it will become evident that the use of stilbestrol in pregnancy or even in suspected pregnancy will be contraindicated. Furthermore, until the pathogenesis of the effect has been established, it seems prudent for physicians to use caution in prescribing estrogenic substances during pregnancy. Indeed, physicians must think more seriously before administering any drug to a pregnant woman.

*   *   *

As the authors take care to point out, the extent and seriousness of the problem cannot

now be defined. The occurrence of the disease may not be limited to adolescence. Early lesions may be developing in prepubertal girls. Additional cases may continue to appear as the main cohort of exposed women, now in their early maturity, continue to experience normal cyclic endocrine stimuli through the menstrual cycle and pregnancy. Only when the data on the frequency of vaginal adenocarcinoma and adenosis in relation to maternal stilbestrol and other estrogenic therapy become available throughout the country, and, indeed, throughout the world, can the scope of the problem be measured.

In the meantime, physicians may be besieged by patients worried about the welfare of their daughters. At present writing they may be assured that the risk is extremely low. Although accurate data are not available on the number of women who received stilbestrol during pregnancy, reasonable estimates put the figure in the many thousands. Thus, the indicated risk to any individual girl is slight as has been emphasized by the authors. Nevertheless, it seems clear that all women, particularly girls entering menarche, who have persistent irregular bleeding should receive a careful intravaginal inspection to rule out possible neoplastic disease, not only of the uterus but also of the vagina.

NOTE

JUDAH FOLKMAN
TRANSPLACENTAL CARCINOGENESIS BY
STILBESTROL*

*   *   *

The fact that in mothers exposed to stilbestrol, neoplasms of the breast or genital tract did not develop after the same latent period when tumors appeared in their daughters may be explained by the exquisite sensitivity of fetal and neonatal tissues to carcinogens. For example, in mice fed griseofulvin, hepatomas develop. On a total dosage basis, tumors will appear in the infant mouse with only 1/4000th of the dose required to produce the same tumor in the adult mouse.

*   *   *

By avoidance of the prescription of stilbestrol to pregnant women, this unusual cancer may be prevented in the future. But more worrisome is stilbestrol residue in meat. Of 40,000,000

* 285 *New England Journal of Medicine* 404–405 (1971). Reprinted by permission.

cattle slaughtered in this country each year, 30,000,000 have been fed stilbestrol to increase their weight. This practice began about 1954. The surveillance program of the Department of Agriculture reveals that the finding of residue is infrequent. Since the fetus is so much more vulnerable to minute doses of carcinogen, there is no way of judging the risk of stilbestrol residue that remains undetected by the current government assay method. Advocates of the federal agricultural policy who believe that the present surveillance system is satisfactory might argue that stilbestrol ingestion is not any more dangerous than the contraceptive pill or the high levels of estrogens appearing in maternal blood during pregnancy. The argument is weak; there is an essential difference. Stilbestrol is a synthetic nonsteroidal estrogen known to be carcinogenic. Both maternal estrogen and the synthetic estrogens used in contraceptive pills are steroidal. Sweden and other countries have already banned the feeding of stilbestrol to cattle.

* * *

d.
A. Bradford Hill, John Marshall, and David A. Shaw
A Controlled Clinical Trial of Long-Term Anticoagulant Therapy in Cerebrovascular Disease*

* * *

In cerebrovascular disease the effect of anticoagulant therapy upon a recently established lesion is not entirely predictable. Thus it has been suggested that anaemic infarcts may become haemorrhagic under the influence of anticoagulants, and experimentally induced infarction in animals has been shown to behave in this way. On the other hand [some investigators] have failed to observe this effect in their experiments, nor can we be certain that experimentally induced infarction necessarily parallels naturally occurring thrombotic occlusion. Apart from the particular case of cerebrovascular disease, the precise mode of action of anticoagulant drugs, and their influence on the course of occlusive vascular disease generally, are not fully understood, and consequently the definition of "effective anticoagulation" is debatable. Furthermore, the treatment carries a risk of haemorrhagic complications; the frequency of these varies in

* 29 *Quarterly Journal of Medicine* 597–609 (1960). Reprinted by permission of the Clarendon Press, Oxford.

different reported series, but their occurrence has always to be weighed against the possible benefit which the treatment may confer. The history of the use of anticoagulants in disease of the coronary arteries, which constitute a vascular system less complex than the cerebral arteries, bears out the reluctance of these drugs to yield to clinical appraisal.

In spite of all these foreseeable difficulties, there is a need in cerebrovascular disease for a trial of a form of therapy which theoretically might improve the outlook for the immense number of patients for whom, at present, we have so little to offer. In the presence of so many unpredictable factors the only satisfactory approach is by a strictly controlled clinical trial, in which the progress of patients receiving the treatment is compared with that of a similar group not so treated, but managed in the same way in all other respects over the same period of time. This we have endeavoured to do in our present study of the place of long-term anticoagulant therapy in the treatment of cerebrovascular disease.

* * *

In 1958 Millikan, Siekert, and Whisnant reported their experience in a much larger group of patients, totalling 317, all of whom received anticoagulants. . . . Treatment appeared to confer striking benefit in stopping ischaemic episodes in the "insufficiency" groups and in reducing, in the "thrombotic" groups, the mortality anticipated on the basis of the authors' observations of untreated patients. . . .

* * *

There is thus a considerable weight of evidence to support the use of anticoagulants in chronic cerebrovascular disease, yet none of the studies referred to fulfill the criteria required in a strictly controlled trial. In particular, the use of the patient as his own "control" is regarded as unsatisfactory in a disease in which we have so little knowledge of the natural history, and in which the course is so variable and unpredictable. Furthermore, most authors have confined their attention to certain sharply defined diagnostic categories of cerebrovascular disease, though the issue that confronts the general physician, to whom the vast majority of patients with cerebrovascular disease is referred, is a broader one.

* * *

. . . For these reasons we have based our study on a broader plan, by including a wide range of cerebrovascular cases commonly encountered in general medical practice. We have attempted to answer the questions as to whether or not long-term anticoagulant therapy (1) increases the expectation of life, or (2) decreases the incidence of further cerebrovascular accidents, or (3) influences the functional capacity of patients with cerebrovascular disease in general, or in specific sub-groups thereof. In the present paper only the first two considerations will be discussed.

* * *

The trial was stopped in its present form earlier than had been anticipated, because of the emergence of a disturbing picture. Non-fatal cerebrovascular accidents were distributed about equally to the two groups (5 to 4), and so were deaths due to unrelated causes (3 to 2). On the other hand, the haemorrhagic fatalities that might be due to the treatment were very unevenly divided (5 to 0). While this difference does not quite reach the 0.05 level of significance, it so closely approaches it as to pose a serious ethical problem. It may well be that long-term anticoagulant therapy in patients with cerebrovascular disease carries a significant hazard of cerebral haemorrhage.

* * *

On the basis of some of the results already reported from the United States, when this trial was set up it might perhaps have been argued that it was unethical to withhold the treatment from half the patients. The wheel has turned so far that we feel it is unethical to proceed with the treated group without making the modification described. Although this result has emerged from the mortality figures, no conclusion can be drawn from the comparison of the non-fatal recurrence rates in the two groups. The low incidence of further non-fatal cerebrovascular accidents in the high-dosage group regarded in isolation might well give rise to the clinical impression that treatment had been beneficial. Yet comparison of the results with those in the low-dosage group clearly shows that this is not so. Indeed, the recurrence rate in the latter group is so low over the period of follow-up that any form of treatment would require to be almost one hundred per cent effective, and devoid of serious hazard, before it could claim to be of definite value. A longer period of follow-up, however, will be required before this point can be settled.

In conclusion, the present study strongly indicates that the general use of anticoagulant therapy in patients with cerebrovascular disease, who are selected and managed along the lines adopted in this trial, is hazardous, because of the risk of cerebral haemorrhage. This risk is present even when the anticoagulant therapy is carefully controlled, and the prothrombin time maintained at a level which is generally accepted to be safe. It may be that certain restricted types of cerebrovascular disease gain benefit from anticoagulant therapy, but, in view of the many variable factors present in the condition, this can be ascertained only in by properly designed and strictly controlled clinical trials.

* * *

9.

Interests of Profession?

a.

Herbert C. Kelman
Human Use of Human Subjects—
The Problem of Deception in Social
Psychological Experiments*

* * *

The use of deception has become more and more extensive, and it is now a commonplace and almost standard feature of social psychological experiments. Deception has been turned into a game, often played with great skill and virtuosity. A considerable amount of the creativity and ingenuity of social psychologists is invested in the development of increasingly elaborate deception situations. . . .

* * *

It is easy to view this problem with alarm, but it is much more difficult to formulate an unambiguous position on the problem. As a working experimental social psychologist, I cannot conceive the issue in absolutist terms. I am too well aware of the fact that there are good reasons for using deception in many experiments. There are many significant problems that probably cannot be investigated without the use of deception, at least not at the present level of development of our experimental methodology. Thus, we are always confronted with a conflict

* 67 *Psychological Bulletin* 1–9 (1967). © 1967, American Psychological Association. Reprinted by permission.

of values. If we regard the acquisition of scientific knowledge about human behavior as a positive value, and if an experiment using deception constitutes a significant contribution to such knowledge which could not very well be achieved by other means, then we cannot unequivocally rule out this experiment. The question for us is not simply whether it does or does not use deception, but whether the amount and type of deception are justified by the significance of the study and the unavailability of alternative (that is, deception-free) procedures.

I have . . . special concern about second-order deceptions, for example, the procedure of letting a person believe that he is acting as experimenter or as the experimenter's accomplice when he is in fact serving as the subject. Such a procedure undermines the relationship between experimenter and subject even further than simple misinformation about the purposes of the experiment; deception does not merely take place *within* the experiment, but encompasses the whole definition of the relationship between the parties involved. Deception that takes place while the person is within the role of subject for which he has contracted can, to some degree, be isolated, but deception about the very nature of the contract itself is more likely to suffuse the experimenter-subject relationship as a whole and to remove the possibility of mutual trust. Thus, I would be inclined to take a more absolutist stand with regard to such second-order deceptions—but even here the issue turns out to be more complicated. I am stopped short when I think, for example, of the ingenious studies on experimenter bias by Rosenthal and his associates. These experiments employed second-order deception in that subjects were led to believe that they were the experimenters. Since these were experiments about experiments, however, it is very hard to conceive of any alternative procedures that the investigators might have used. There is no question in my mind that these are significant studies; they provide fundamental inputs to present efforts at reexamining the social psychology of the experiment. These studies, then, help to underline even further the point that we are confronted with a conflict of values that cannot be resolved by fiat.

* * *

What concerns me most is not so much that deception is used, but precisely that it is used without question. It has now become standard operating procedure in the social psychologist's laboratory. I sometimes feel that we are training a generation of students who do not know that there is any other way of doing experiments in our field. . . .

* * *

A basic assumption in the use of deception is that a subject's awareness of the conditions that we are trying to create and of the phenomena that we wish to study would affect his behavior in such a way that we could not draw valid conclusions from it. For example, if we are interested in studying the effects of failure on conformity, we must create a situation in which the subjects actually feel that they have failed, and in which they can be kept unaware of our interest in observing conformity. In short, it is important to keep our subjects naive about the purposes of the experiment so that they can respond to the experimental inductions spontaneously.

How long, however, will it be possible for us to find naive subjects? Among college students, it is already very difficult. They may not know the exact purpose of the particular experiment in which they are participating, but at least they know, typically, that it is *not* what the experimenter says it is. Orne . . . pointed out that the use of deception "on the part of psychologists is so widely known in the college population that even if a psychologist is honest with the subject, more often than not he will be distrusted." As one subject pithily put it, " 'Psychologists always lie!' " Orne added that "This bit of paranoia has some support in reality." There are, of course, other sources of human subjects that have not been tapped, and we could turn to them in our quest for naiveté. But even there it is only a matter of time. As word about psychological experiments gets around in whatever network we happen to be using, sophistication is bound to increase. I wonder, therefore, whether there is any future in the use of deception.

* * *

For several reasons, however, the use of deception especially encourages the subject to dismiss the stated purposes of the experiment and to search for alternative interpretations of his own. First, the continued use of deception establishes the reputation of psychologists as people who cannot be believed. Thus, the desire "to penetrate the experimenter's inscrutability and discover the rationale of the experiment" . . . becomes especially strong. Generally, these efforts are motivated by the subject's desire to meet the expectations of the experimenter and of the situation. They may also be motivated, however, as I have already mentioned, by a desire to outwit the experimenter and to beat him at his own game, in a spirit of genuine hostility or playful one-upmanship. Second, a situation involving the use of deception is inevitably highly ambiguous since a great deal of information relevant to understanding the structure of the situation must be withheld from the subject. Thus, the subject is especially motivated to try to figure things out and likely to develop idiosyncratic interpretations. Third, the use of deception, by its very nature, causes the experimenter to transmit contradictory messages to the subject. In his verbal instructions and explanations he says one thing about the purposes of the experiment; but in the experimental situation that he has created, in the manipulations that he has introduced, and probably in covert cues that he emits, he says another thing. This again makes it imperative for the subject to seek his own interpretation of the situation.

*   *   *

. . . I have already stressed that I would not propose the complete elimination of deception under all circumstances, in view of the genuine conflict of values with which the experimenter is confronted. What is crucial, however, is that we always ask ourselves the question whether deception, in the given case, is necessary and justified. . . .

*   *   *

[My] final suggestion is that we invest some of the creativity and ingenuity, now devoted to the construction of elaborate deceptions, in the search for alternative experimental techniques that do not rely on the use of deception. . . .

NOTES

NOTE 1.

JOHN LOFLAND
REPLY TO DAVIS*

*   *   *

. . . Mr. Davis [in response to an experiment reported by Mr. Lejeune and myself]

_____

* 8 _Social Problems_ 365–367 (1961). Reprinted by permission. [The author no longer adheres to the views expressed in this NOTE. His present position is reflected in the following NOTE.]

writes that A.A. members will possibly be unhappy with our experiment and as a result make it difficult to get their cooperation in future research. This is a conceivable outcome in any field research, and one upon which we always take a chance. Mr. Davis' statement, in this case, assumes two things, both of which are unlikely. First, that A.A. members will read the report and, second, that they will be unhappy about what is reported. Concerning the former, the article was not written or reported to facilitate viewing by A.A. members; it is presented in scientific writing and appears in a professional journal, both of which very effectively limit its audience. As to the latter, if some members do read it, it is not evident that the reaction will be "indifferent," or as Mr. Davis means, hostile. In fact, personally, quite contrary to Mr. Davis' personal feelings, I judge the experiment to be favorable to A.A., and do not think that members will necessarily judge it any differently. . . .

*   *   *

It is generally agreed that our obligation to science is the objective, full and unbiased execution and reporting of observation. It is also generally agreed that our obligation to the profession is to conduct research in ways that will not injure the general repute of the profession or thwart subsequent access to research settings and thus hinder the development of the discipline. In his letter, Mr. Davis does not confine himself to his duty of upholding _these_ obligations. He almost exclusively devotes his attention to extra-scientific and extraprofessional standards because they appear to be different than his own. We all recognize that such statements are not, and cannot, be made as a scientist or professional; they are simply not part of the legitimate criteria for judging research. Therefore, _as_ scientists and professionals, we have no reason to be concerned with Mr. Davis' opinions of our personal moral standards; but this is not to say that personal standards are unimportant, quite the reverse as I will indicate below.

Beyond the fact that protestations like this are not relevant, except to one's self, and that they are rather presumptuous, there is, for those who would persist, the important problem of ever generalizing a personal standard and holding it nonviolate for the profession or, indeed, for one's self.

The difficulties involved in asserting immutable professional standards of conduct are clearly illustrated in Mr. Davis' personal standard that one should not study groups unless they know about it and give their permission. A professional rule to this effect would not only make for great past, present and future loss to the discipline, but would be an active violation of many people's moral standards who think that there are some groups, such as professional crime and fascist groups, that should be studied whether they are asked and give permission or not. In other words, in accepting this rule, we could not study "bad" groups, which, as it happens, are also especially likely to be "groups that do not want to be studied." Furthermore, conceivably, it might be important enough to the discipline to justify studying a group even though the particular group refuses. I suspect that Mr. Davis, in taking a second look, would agree.

*   *   *

[O]ur personal moral obligations and conflict of roles should not, and probably could not, be determined and/or solved by the intervention of the profession at large or other professionals speaking personally. It is probably an inescapable and insoluble part of the attempt to be both a scientist and a person in human groups that one must suffer the pains so eloquently portrayed by Mr. Davis, and that he must make his personal moral decisions alone, based on the situation. In addition, it is also doubtful that any amount of pleading for others to adopt one's own standards or prolonged demands to the profession for an edict of relief alters one's own, or others', personal dilemmas. The most legitimate and workable solution for the profession would appear to be the one we already have: each man works out, as best he can, his own, as Mr. Davis has so aptly captured it, "moral integration."

NOTE 2.

JOHN LOFLAND
DEVIANCE AND IDENTITY*

*   *   *

[T]here are . . . difficulties involved in the very character of the empirical materials classified under the topic of deviance. Deviance, by definition, is disapproved, and it therefore occurs in secret or at least is carried on in a very circumspect manner. Moreover, the study of episodic or isolated deviant acts is seriously ham-

------

* Englewood Cliffs: Prentice-Hall, Inc. 300–301 (1969). © 1969. Reprinted by permission of Prentice-Hall, Inc., Englewood Cliffs, N.J.

pered by their unpredictability. How, for example, would one arrange to study interaction scenes of homicide? There is little doubt that sound and film records of the interaction in the hours before the occurrence of acts of assault, rape, robbery, embezzlement or homicide would be of enormous value in understanding the constraining character of immediate space-time-bound locales. But it is less than clear how one is to know where and when to be in order to make such observations. Even if the "who, where and when" were foreknown, it is less than clear how one would arrange to be present without changing the entire situation and conducing some different outcome. . . .

*   *   *

[T]he moral implications of the methodological requirements of full, precise, systematic knowledge of deviance convince me that the moral price we would have to pay for full knowledge is much higher than the value of that knowledge. I, for one, would not be willing to condone—in fact, would actively oppose—the initiation of a series of precise experimental manipulations aimed at sorting out the exact effects of the various factors involved in the reconstitution of personal identity. Nor could I countenance the invasion of privacy that would be required for the natural-setting study of homicide, embezzlement or other deviant acts. The "research" activities of Nazi Germany taught us (or should have) very well that there are definite moral limits on what can be done in the name of science. In matters as fundamental as identity change and deviance, we must, as moral men who happen also to be social scientists, make what we can of the variations that occur in the natural world and that we can discover without undue invasions of privacy. We must hold in check our impulse to implement our research technology in ways that violate our beliefs about the essential dignity and inviolate character of human beings. And too, a variety of episodes in the 20th century occurring under totalitarian (and not so totalitarian) regimes have made quite clear the untenable character of arguments which justify some present condition of human debasement, degradation, suffering and even death for the sake of "enormous" benefits that will accrue to future generations—whether these benefits are to derive from knowledge gained or from something else. Ironically, of course, some such claims of future good based on present evil are probably true. But their truth or falsity is quite beside the point.

The point is, rather, that, with few exceptions (as perhaps when the future ends are quite concrete and immediate and as when the present suffering is voluntarily undertaken), the sacrifice of human beings for laudable ends is not morally acceptable.

b.

Margaret Mead
Research with Human Beings—A Model
Derived from Anthropological Field Practice*

In recent years there have been a great many experiments and investigations reported in which deliberate falsification has been introduced. Instructed stooges have been directed to deny sensory evidence, or to mimic pain that they did not feel, or to obstruct situations planned by their peers. Investigators have posed as possible converts to flying-saucer cults. Under the guise of "participant observation," various forms of "cover" have been developed for social investigators, which have later been revealed to the public in the reports on the experiments. These are, I believe, all deeply unsatisfactory in several ways:

*   *   *

[P]erhaps even more serious than the effect upon the subject or object or unwarned collaborator, which in most cases is brief and transitory, is the effect upon the investigator himself. Ethically, it means that he becomes accustomed to tricking, deceiving, and manipulating other human beings and, to that extent, to denigrating their humanity. Besides the ethical consequences that flow from contempt for other human beings, there are other consequences—such as increased selective insensitivity or delusions of grandeur and omnipotence—that may in time seriously interfere with the very thing which he has been attempting to protect: the integrity of his own scientific work. Encouraging styles of research and intervention that involve lying to other human beings therefore tends to establish a corps of progressively calloused individuals, insulated from self-criticism and increasingly available for clients who can become outspokenly cynical in their manipulating of other human beings, individually and in the mass.†

---

* 98 *Daedalus* 361, 374–377 (1969). Reprinted by permission of Daedalus, Journal of the American Academy of Arts and Sciences, Boston, Massachusetts.

† Here again, we should mention the other effect. Instead of being cynical about his manipula-

Both of these undesirable consequences are prevented to some extent by the honest belief that the deception is absolutely necessary to the conduct of an experiment and that the experiment itself must be performed. Arguments of this sort can be advanced for both laboratory and field tests of new drugs: Elimination of other factors of suggestion and belief must be made by the use of placebos, and so forth. When astronauts are being selected, it is vital to know their ability to withstand various kinds of strain, and this can only be found out by tests involving deception of various sorts, such as simulation, secret observation by long-distance TV, concealed indicators, and so forth. The ethical difficulties involved in even these situations are attested to by the number of cases where the experimenter with a new drug, for example, will insist on trying it on himself first.

Many of the situations where concealment is genuinely necessary and the experiment cannot be performed in some other way can be handled by general assent from the subjects, who know that they are agreeing to being deceived for the purposes of the experiment itself. Individuals who have particular diseases, conscientious objectors who wish to make a contribution to human welfare, candidates for dangerous secret activities or especially exacting forms of warfare or exploration, and students of psychology may volunteer to participate in activities where they consciously abrogate some of the dignities and freedoms that are associated with the status of a fully healthy, free citizen of a free society. The medical profession demands this of many patients, lawyers demand it of clients—"just put yourself in my hands and trust my judgment"— priests demand it of penitents, and parents demand it of their children. Such a status is not ennobling; it may be necessary; and it can be defined so that consent is given in such a general way that the particularities of placebos, stooges,

---

tions, the experimenter or interventionist who deceives may also take refuge behind the great good that he is doing to the subject as a patient or to other men who will benefit from his activities—in developing a new drug or writing advertising copy that will induce people to spend their money more wisely. Here the need to justify demeaning other human beings, in particular respects, is compensated for by another kind of delusion of grandeur: that of becoming someone who benefits mankind on a large scale, the omnipotent theorist, the all-knowing teacher, the scientist working for the intelligence agency of a particular government or conspiring with some secret plot to save the world.

and fabricated situations are left intact to test the physiological or psychological behavior of the subject. But the crucial question must be whether the deception is absolutely necessary in order to perform an experiment which is itself necessary. By the automatic inclusion of deception in a research or treatment plan, many research workers are simply relieved of any obligation to make new research designs which would not involve any deception at all.

c.

Kai T. Erikson
A Comment on Disguised Observation in Sociology*

* * *

[Another] problem with disguised observation . . . has to do with the sociologist's responsibilities to his colleagues. It probably goes without saying that research of this sort is liable to damage the reputation of sociology in the larger society and close off promising areas of research for future investigators. . . . And it is also true in the wider sense that any research tactic which attracts unfavorable notice may help diminish the general climate of trust toward sociology in the community as a whole. So long as this remains a serious possibility, the practice of disguised observation becomes a problem for everyone in the profession; and to this extent, it is wholly within the bounds of professional etiquette for one sociologist to challenge the work of another on this score.

This objection has been raised several times before, and the answer most often given to it is that the people who are studied in this fashion—alcoholics or spiritualists or mental patients, for example—are not likely to read what we say about them anyway. Now this argument has the advantage of being correct a good deal of the time, but this fact does not prevent it from being altogether irrelevant. To begin with, the experience of the past few years should surely have informed us that the press is more than ready to translate our technical reports into news copy, and this means that we can no longer provide shelter for other people behind the walls of our own anonymity. But even if that were not the case, it is a little absurd for us to claim that we derive some measure of protection from the narrowness of our audience when we devote so much time trying to broaden it. The fact is that

we are increasingly reaching audiences whose confidence we cannot afford to jeopardize, and we have every right to be afraid that such people may close their doors to sociological research if they learn to become too suspicious of our methods and intentions.

The [next] objection to be raised here, if only as a note in passing, concerns the responsibilities the profession should accept toward its students. The division of labor in contemporary sociology is such that a considerable proportion of the data we use in our work is gathered by graduate students or other apprentices, and this proportion is even higher for research procedures that require the amount of energy and time necessary for participant observation. Of the dozen or more observers who took part in the studies I have cited, for example, all but one was a graduate student. Now a number of sociologists who have engaged in disguised observation have reported that it is apt to pose serious moral problems and a good deal of personal discomfort, and I think one might well argue that this is a heavy burden to place on any person who is, by our own explicit standards, not yet ready for professional life. I am not suggesting here that students are too immature to make a seasoned choice in the matter. I am suggesting that they should not be asked to make what one defender of the method has called "real and excruciating moral decisions" while they are still students and presumably protected from the various dilemmas and contentions which occupy us in meetings like this—particularly since they are so likely to be academically, economically, and even psychologically dependent upon those elders who ask them to choose.

The [last] objection I would like to raise here about the use of undercover observation is probably the most important—and yet the most remote from what is usually meant by the term "ethics." It seems to me that any attempt to use masquerades in social research betrays an extraordinary disrespect for the complexities of human interaction, and for this reason can only lead to bad science. Perhaps the most important responsibility of any sociologist is to appreciate how little he really knows about his intricate and elusive subject matter. We have at best a poor understanding of the human mind, of the communication signals that link one mind to another, or the social structures that emerge from those linkages—and it is the most arrant kind of over-simplification for us to think that we can assess the effect which a clever costume or a few

* 14 *Social Problems* 366, 368–371 (1967). Reprinted by permission.

studied gestures have on the social setting. The pose might "work" in the sense that the observer is admitted into the situation; but once this passage has been accomplished, how is he to judge his own influence on the lives of the people he is studying? ...

* * *

... It may be possible for a trained person to rearrange the slant of his body and re-set his facial muscles to approximate the bearing of someone else, but his performance will never be anything more than a rough imposture. Now we know that these various physiological, linguistic, and kinetic cues play an important part in the context of human interaction, but we have no idea how to simulate them—and what is probably more to the point, we never will. For one thing, we cannot expect to learn in a matter of hours what others have been practicing throughout a lifetime. For another, to imitate always means to parody, to caricature, to exaggerate certain details of behavior at the expense of others, and to that extent any person who selects a disguise will naturally emphasize those details which *he* assumes are most important to the character he is portraying. In doing so, of course, he is really only portraying a piece of himself. It is interesting to speculate, for example, why the Air Force lieutenant mentioned earlier thought he needed to present himself as a near-delinquent youth with a visible layer of personal problems in order to pose as an enlisted man. Whatever the reasoning behind this particular charade, it would certainly be reasonable for someone to suspect that it tells us more about the investigators' impression of enlisted men than it does about the men themselves—and since we have no way of learning whether this is true or not, we have lost rather than gained an edge of control over the situation we are hoping to understand. What the investigators had introduced into the situation was a creature of their own invention, and it would be hardly surprising if the results of their inquiry corresponded to some image they had in advance of the enlisted man's condition. (It is perhaps worth noting here that impersonation always seems easier for people looking down rather than up the status ladder. We find it reasonable to assume that officers "know how" to portray enlisted men or that sociologists have the technical capacity to pose as drunks or religious mystics, but it is not at all clear that the reverse would be equally true.)

* * *

NOTE

MARGARET MEAD
THE CASE OF JOHN HOWARD GRIFFIN,
AUTHOR OF *Black Like Me**

During [a] discussion ... the question was raised as to whether John Howard Griffin's darkening his skin by a biochemical method so that he would be taken for a Negro and be able to explore the treatment of Negroes in the Southeast was an inadmissible type of deception. ... It is an interesting, perhaps crucial, case in many ways.

John Howard Griffin is a novelist, who became blind during the early days of World War II, when he had to abandon a medical career and became actively involved in helping Jewish children escape from the Nazis. He returned, completely blind, to Texas with his family and lived on a small farm for twelve years, where he wrote six successful novels. In 1957, he regained his sight and was horrified, when he could *see,* to realize how close the caste relationships in the South were to the racial attitudes that he had abhorred when practiced by the Nazis. His attention became fixed on the question of color and the responses which white and black people made to color. In order to explore this more thoroughly, he took a treatment that darkened his skin, was highly dangerous, and, in the form in which he took it, did him some irrevocable harm although the skin coloration was reversible. He then traveled through the South, finding out not what it was like to be a Negro, but how the indignities heaped on anyone suspected of being a Negro, and the help freely given by Negroes to others with a black skin, looked to a white man reared as he had been, protected from this knowledge.

As a commentary on this case I would say: (1) he was not a scientist but a writer with an ethical mission searching for material, as writers do search for material; (2) he took tremendous risks both with his personal safety, his sanity, and ultimately, after the book was published, with the life and the safety of his family—far out of proportion to any risk to which he exposed any of the people whom he met; (3) as his goal was to probe a situation—as a white man taken

* 98 *Daedalus* 381–382 (1969). Reprinted by permission of Daedalus, Journal of the American Academy of Arts and Sciences, Boston, Massachusetts.

for a black man—his means were completely appropriate to his ends. Individuals whom he deceived in passing were not experimental subjects or part of any experimental situation, nor were they identified in a way through which they could even recognize themselves again.

I believe this case falls quite outside the range of those scientific explorations which I have condemned, in which (1) the deception is unnecessary, (2) is damaging to subject and experimenter, and (3) when revealed is damaging to the trust of the public in scientists as such.

10.
Interests of Society?

a.
Julius Seeman
Deception in Psychological Research*

* * *

[T]he central dilemma posed by the use of deception . . . is the conflict between the rights of the individual and the needs of society. Those who justify the use of deception argue that the accumulation of scientifically derived knowledge sometimes exacts a price from individuals, and that this knowledge is worth the price. What does our society have to say on this point? The democratic ethic reflects continuing tensions generated by conflicts between individual and collective good. These conflicts rarely fail to take account of the central position that the rights of the individual hold in our social system. Even where there is collective danger, individual rights have a pivotal position. For example, our laws provide that even in time of war a person conscientiously opposed to military service may undertake civilian service.

* * *

. . . It is possible that the most correct position with regard to the use of deception may turn out to be an absolutist position. Such a position would advance the ends-means argument; namely, that the outcome of any process is inexorably embedded in the means used. Thus, a process that used deceptive means could not lead to a "good" end.

There is much to be said for such a view, both ethically and pragmatically. In learning ex-

___
* 24 *American Psychologist* 1025, 1026–1028 (1969). Reprinted by permission.

periments, for instance, it is clear that the end point of a learning curve is lawfully related to antecedent properties. In psychotherapy, the outcome is simply the end point of a process continuum. In an analogous way, the end point of an experience in which deception is embedded is functionally related to the deception process.

The ends-means view happens to be the view I hold. But one does not need to take an absolutist position in order to have reservations about the ethics of deception. One could argue that there are instances of innocuous deception that have no adverse consequences. This still leaves the question open with regard to other studies. The ethical issue is drawn most sharply in those studies that use noxious deception. . . .

* * *

There is one final consideration with respect to the use of deception. It is a difficult point to make because it requires a reexamination of the psychologist's most basic assumptions about his discipline. An empirical discipline takes for granted that the primary goal of its efforts is the accumulation of knowledge. Psychologists have been trained to a finely honed position with regard to empirical processes and they have learned to value knowledge above all else. Thus it is scarcely possible to argue for the importance of a nonempirical process. Yet that is what I propose. I suggest that the ultimate goal of the scientific enterprise ought to be not knowledge but wisdom. Knowledge alone has a neutrality that can be deadly in our time. It can destroy as well as create. The existence of a Hiroshima in man's history demonstrates that knowledge alone is not enough, and that the old question of "knowledge for what?" must still be asked. If knowledge in psychology is won at the cost of some essential humanness in one person's relationship to another, perhaps the price is too high.

NOTE

Diana Baumrind
Principles of Ethical Conduct in the
Treatment of Subjects*

* * *

There are no absolute principles of good and evil, and this all major systems of morality and mythic representations acknowledge. More-

___
* 26 *American Psychologist* 887, 890 (1971). © 1971, American Psychological Association. Reprinted by permission.

over, there is no human activity that under certain circumstances, settings, times, and places could not be viewed as good and under other circumstances as evil. But a given action under a given set of circumstances can be judged as good or evil; else what is the significant sphere of a code of ethics? It is my judgement that the research laboratory is the wrong place for Machiavellian encounters, and that this is the wrong time. I would judge many of [the experimenter's] actions as evil, for the precise reason that they are committed by a professional or scientist in the conduct of his work against an individual who has accepted an invitation to be a research subject. There is a time and place for deceit, inflicting pain, and putting other people down. But the psychologist's laboratory is not the place, and this is certainly not the time. . . . I am among those who believe that by such practices "behavioral research is contributing to the moral ills of society and that the influence is a direct one". . . . The influence of the research psychologist, such as it is, great or small, should be used as a positive moral vector and not a negative one. The research psychologist has many privileges not possessed by other people with whom the subject deals, and these privileges are granted to him on the assumption that he will be responsible, trustworthy, and altruistic in the conduct of his professional life. Fundamental moral principles of reciprocity and justice are violated when the research psychologist, using his position of trust, acts to deceive or degrade those whose extension of trust is granted on the basis of a contrary role expectation. It is unjust to use naïve, that is, trusting subjects, and then exploit their naïveté, no matter if the directly resulting harm is small. The harm is cumulative to the individual and society. At this time and in this place it is "evil" for research psychologists in pursuit of professional objectives to contribute an iota to "the attrition of human relationships in depersonalization and distrust," and the research enterprise does not intrinsically require that they do so.

*   *   *

b.

Joseph H. Fichter and William L. Kolb
Ethical Limitations on Sociological Reporting*

. . . Real urgency must be defined in terms of the pressing needs of a group, community, or society, or in terms of some impending problem of which the scientist but not the group or community being studied is aware. Rights and duties are never unqualified in society and one of the qualifications seems to be that the society sometimes has a prior right to information which is necessary and useful for itself even though it may be harmful to an individual or sub-group.

The social scientist may find himself in one of several moral situations when he is trying to determine whether or not the social need is greater than the individual or group right. If the duly appointed authorities of a community or of the larger society believe certain information to be vitally needed, there is a *prima facie* case for the scientist to reveal such information. However, these authorities must show to the scientist the ground for the need. If he does not know and cannot find out from the authorities whether there is an urgent need for certain data which will be harmful to individuals and sub-groups, he is free of moral obligation to reveal it. If he is certain that the information is not necessary, he may in good conscience refuse to reveal it even though the authorities demand to know it. It must be recognized that this freedom in such instances is moral and not legal, and he may have to pay a price for his refusal.

In a similar manner the obligations which the scientist has to the group studied may require the revelation of information damaging to individuals or sub-groups. In this instance the scientist himself is likely to be the best judge of the need for his data. If he understands and accepts the basic values of the group and takes his obligation to the group seriously, he may find it imperative to disclose such information. Since he cannot plead ignorance, and since there is no demand from competent higher authority, the responsibility for the assessment of urgency rests squarely on the scientist.

Finally, even though neither the higher authority nor the representatives of the group studied place any demands upon him, he may become aware of facts which are vitally needed by the social group studied or by the society. In such cases he must not only accept the responsibility for violating the rights of individuals and groups, but also must arrive at his decision with very little outside aid. In clear-cut instances where the comparison and balancing of the rights of the various claimants can be easily accomplished, the decision may be easily reached. But it is certainly in this area that the researcher will be forced to consider most thoroughly the im-

* 18 *American Sociological Review* 544, 550 (1953). Reprinted by permission.

portance which he, himself, has placed on the value of the information in its relation to the needs of the group.

*   *   *

NOTES

NOTE 1.

Ross Stagner
Problems Concerning Federal Support of Social Science Research*

*   *   *

No one has ever reported that an atom protested invasion of its privacy when bombarded by a particle accelerator. This type of research handicap is unique to investigations focused on the behavior of human beings. A man may plausibly object to questions about the violence of his temper, his impulses to attack and destroy others, his hostility toward minority groups, and so on. Yet the real hazard to society, and indeed to our civilization, rests not in the atom bombs but in the violence and aggression within human beings who can trigger these bombs.

Social scientists, of course, have a genuine obligation to devise protections for the right of privacy, and to avoid mere psychic voyeurism. At the same time they have a compelling obligation to accumulate data—and meaningful generalizations—about the powerful impulses of loyalty, hostility, fear, and ambition which shape human history. It seems to me that, on the whole, the record of the social scientists in this area of protecting privacy has been quite good. Ethical standards have been codified and students in these fields have been trained, as in medical and legal training, to observe these standards. Psychologists, have, I think, done a very good job in this regard. Renewed attention to this matter in recent years guarantees, according to most scholars, that researchers will exercise extreme caution in this respect.

*   *   *

There is an obvious conflict between the need of society to know and the right of the individual to dignity and privacy. The familiar analogy is that of medicine. For a thousand years or more, religious taboos forbade dissection of a

* *National Foundation for Social Sciences— Hearings on S.836 before the Subcommittee on Government Research of the Senate Committee on Government Operations,* 90th Congress, 1st Session 757– 760 (1967).

dead body. This prohibition was based on an appeal to the dignity of the individual, and the right of his relatives to know that his body was not violated. The consequence was that medical research and medical practice were blocked. It was only when a few brave souls defied the taboo and began such research that modern medicine began its remarkable advances. Clearly the scientists are under heavy obligation to avoid research techniques which endanger the health of their subjects; but there is also some need to consider the potential lifesaving and health-bringing developments in this equation. The medical profession has only recently been compelled to take a new look at this question. The social sciences must also consider it carefully.

My point in raising the medical analogy is that great social dangers cry for investigations which may be blocked by excessive emphasis on the right of privacy. Consider the case of the rapist, the violent criminal. As a youth he may certainly object to "prying questions" which might reveal his explosive, destructive, antisocial tendencies. Yet society is clearly entitled to look for measures to protect women from his hostile sexuality. A loaded way to phrase this question is to ask how we balance the right of the young man to privacy against the right of the young woman to walk safely in the streets. A more defensible question is: How can social scientists gather the data which we so desperately need, the basic information for the prevention and correction of violent behavior, with proper consideration for the right to privacy?

*   *   *

My purpose in elaborating on this point about the privacy is also to suggest that people in general, and the Congress in particular, must become aware of the possible conflicts between values, all of which are respected in our society: the value of knowledge and the value of privacy, the value of the individual and the value of society as a whole. When belief in an earth-centered universe was enforced by religious and civil punishment, no progress was made in astronomy. When similar taboos forbade anatomical dissection, no progress was made in medicine. The Congress should, in my opinion, recognize that no one of these is absolute; that the welfare of large numbers of individuals needs to be weighed against the privacy of a few. Obviously I am not suggesting that the proposed National Social Science Foundation should be authorized to underwrite unrestrained and frivolous prying into people's private lives. What must be said is that it will be futile to appropriate large sums of money for social science research if the investigators are forbidden to use psychological procedures which penetrate deeply into the thoughts and emotions of the person studied.

There has been, for example, some concern expressed on the floor of Congress in recent years about the use of personality tests. I hear that they have actually been banned for certain purposes within the Federal Government. This is probably a minor matter, because the validity of most such tests for employment purposes has not been adequately demonstrated. On the other hand, if agencies supporting basic social research should ban such tests, much important work will simply be impossible. Let me mention again the problem of rape and other violent assaults on persons. Our only rational hope is to try to identify the potential criminal and reeducate him before he begins these kinds of activities. Now I do not know how you put a dollar value on the trauma to a young woman who is raped, nor do I know how to put a dollar value on the invasion of privacy of the young men who might be studied in such a research program. But I do believe that, if the Congress is sincere in its desire that advances be made in the prevention of crime, legislation must be drafted in such a way that the research use of personality tests is permissible within the code of ethics of the American Psychological Association.

* * *

NOTE 2.

DIANA BAUMRIND
SOME THOUGHTS ON ETHICS OF RESEARCH—
AFTER READING MILGRAM'S "BEHAVIORAL
STUDY OF OBEDIENCE"*

* * *

[T]he subject is not always treated with the respect he deserves. It has become more commonplace in sociopsychological laboratory studies to manipulate, embarrass, and discomfort subjects. At times the insult to the subject's sensibilities extends to the journal reader when the results are reported. Milgram's study is a case in point. . . .

* * *

Milgram . . . partially explains the subject's destructive obedience as follows, "Thus they as-

---

* 19 *American Psychologist* 421–422 (1964). Reprinted by permission.

sume that the discomfort caused the victim is momentary, while the scientific gains resulting from the experiment are enduring. . . ." Indeed such a rationale might suffice to justify the means used to achieve his end if that end were of inestimable value to humanity or were not itself transformed by the means by which it was attained.

The behavioral psychologist is not in as good a position to objectify his faith in the significance of his work as medical colleagues at points of breakthrough. His experimental situations are not sufficiently accurate models of real-life experience; his sampling techniques are seldom of a scope which would justify the meaning with which he would like to endow his results; and these results are hard to reproduce by colleagues with opposing theoretical views. Unlike the Sabin vaccine, for example, the concrete benefit to humanity of his particular piece of work, no matter how competently handled, cannot justify the risk that real harm will be done to the subject. I am not speaking of physical discomfort, inconvenience, or experimental deception per se, but of permanent harm, however slight. . . .

c.

Henry K. Beecher
Research and the Individual—
Human Studies*

* * *

When the wonders of penicillin were new, but recognized, and the supply heartbreakingly meager, a small shipment finally arrived in North Africa during World War II. The hospital beds were overflowing with wounded men. Many had been wounded in battles; many had also been wounded in brothels. Which group would get the penicillin? By all that is just, it would go to the heroes who had risked their lives, who were still in jeopardy, and some of whom were dying. They did not receive it, nor should they have; it was given to those infected in brothels. Before indignation takes over, let us examine the situation. First, there were desperate shortages of manpower at the front. Second, those with broken bodies and broken bones would not be swiftly restored to the battle line even with penicillin, whereas those with venereal disease, on being treated with penicillin, would in a matter of

---

* Boston: Little, Brown and Co. 209–210 (1970). Reprinted by permission.

days free the beds they were occupying and return to the front. Third, no one will catch osteomyelitis from his neighbor; the man with venereal disease remains, until he is cured, a reservoir of infection and a constant threat. In terms of customary morality, a great injustice was done; in view of the circumstances, I believe that the course chosen was the proper one.

*   *   *

CHAPTER SEVEN

What Consequences to Society Should Affect the Authority of the Investigator?

In the previous chapter we explored the nature and extent of the investigator's authority in his interactions with individual subjects. Whenever these interactions interfere with the rights and well-being of research subjects, they also threaten the community as a whole. Thus, the problems presented for analysis in Chapter Six merge with those selected for this chapter. In some situations, however, the predictable and unpredictable risks for society go beyond the harm done to individual subjects. Accordingly, this chapter focuses on those situations in which the investigator's actions bring him into conflict with the rights and interests of the community. We have selected three categories of actual or potential harm to society, arising from interferences with: (1) human behavior, (2) human biology, and (3) mores and laws.

Since these investigations also expose individual subjects to harm, the questions set forth in Chapter Six should be asked once again. One question comes into sharper focus: When and to what extent should the scientist's freedom of inquiry be curtailed "in the interests of society"? Clearly, some experiments already performed and some now being contemplated may ultimately have far-reaching consequences for society. Investigations into ways of radically altering the psychology and biology of man have already proceeded to a considerable extent in the laboratory or in "therapeutic" settings. Once the means are at hand, the impetus to employ them more extensively may be irresistible unless prior thought has been given to the limits of their employment. In addition, some of these studies may have been carried out in violation of existing laws, while others may have been shelved in deference to legal barriers. Thus, decisions to experiment or not experiment which involve the interests of society have perhaps too often been made unilaterally by investigators.

Our continuing objectives remain (1) to identify those consequences to society which should be labeled harmful and (2) to determine whether the decision to permit or preclude these consequences should be left to the discretion of the investigator alone or whether it requires approval from other participants in the human experimentation process. In examining these materials the following specific questions should also be considered:

1. When, if ever, in the development of a new procedure, should society make judgments about research activities?

2. What persons or institutions should have the authority to establish guides and criteria for conducting investigations with human beings, either in "therapeutic" settings, limited human trials, or mass applications?

3. What persons or institutions should be given authority to decide which investigations violate existing laws and which are exempt from criminal or civil liability because of their significance to science and society?

A.
What Constitutes Harm?

1.
Interferences with Human Behavior

a.
José M. R. Delgado
Evolution of Physical Control of the Brain*

During the last decade we have reached an historical turning point because of the development of methods which permit the coordination and synthesis of physical, physiological, pharmacological, and psychological research. . . . [S]cience has developed a new electrical methodology for the study and control of cerebral functions in animals and humans. Learning, emotions, drives, memory, consciousness, and other phenomena which in the past belonged only in the realm of philosophy are now the subjects of neurophysiological experimentation. In the last few years, the scalpel of the brain surgeon has modified psychological reactions and a wealth of wonder drugs has liberated many patients from mental institutions.

I am not so naive as to think that cerebral

research holds all the answers to mankind's present problems, but I do believe that an understanding of the biological bases of social and antisocial behavior and of mental activities, which for the first time in history can now be explored in the conscious brain, may be of decisive importance in the search for intelligent solutions to some of our present anxieties, frustrations, and conflicts. Also, it is essential to introduce a balance into the future development of the human mind, and I think that we now have the means to investigate and to influence our own intellect.

* * *

The social interaction of animals requires continuous mutual adaptation, and activities depend on a variety of factors, including sensory inputs, problem-solving capacity, emotional background, previous experience, conditioning, drives, instincts, and intelligent integration of all these processes. In spite of the extraordinary complexity of these supporting mechanisms, there is experimental evidence that electrical stimulation of specific areas of the brain may influence social interaction such as contactual relations, hierarchical situations, submissive manifestations, sexual activity, aggressive behavior, and social fear. . . .

* James Arthur Lecture. New York: The American Museum of Natural History 2–3, 27–28, 30, 32, 41–42, 45–46, 48–51 (1965). Reprinted by permission.

... The fact that one animal can be electrically driven to fight against another has been established. In [an] experiment, stimulation of the tectal area in a male cat evoked the well-known pattern of offensive-defensive reactions. When this animal was placed on a testing stage in the company of a larger cat, they enjoyed friendly relations, lying close to each other and purring happily until the smaller cat was stimulated in the tectal area. At this moment, it started growling, unsheathed its claws, and launched a fierce attack against the larger animal which flattened its ears, withdrew a few steps, and retaliated with powerful blows. The fight continued as long as the stimulation was applied. The effect could be repeated, and the stimulated cat always took the initiative in spite of the fact that it was smaller and was always overpowered in the battle. After several stimulations, a state of mistrust was created between the two animals, and they watched each other with hostility.

* * *

Rhesus monkeys are destructive and dangerous creatures which do not hesitate to bite anything within reach, including leads, instrumentation, and occasionally the experimenter's hands. Would it be possible to tame these ferocious animals by means of electrical stimulation? To investigate this question, a monkey was strapped to a chair where it made faces and threatened the investigator until the rostral part of the caudate nucleus was electrically stimulated. At this moment, the monkey lost its aggressive expression and did not try to grab or bite the experimenter, who could safely put a finger into its mouth! As soon as stimulation was discontinued, the monkey was as aggressive as before. Later, similar experiments were repeated with the monkeys free inside the colony, and it was evident that their autocratic social structure could be manipulated by radio stimulation. In one case in which the boss monkey was excited in the caudate nucleus with 1.5 mA for five seconds every minute, after several minutes the other monkeys started to circulate more freely around the cage, often in proximity to the boss, and from time to time they crowded him without fear. The intermittent stimulation continued for one hour, and during this time the territoriality of the boss dropped to zero, his walking time was diminished, and he performed no aggressive acts against the other members of the colony. About 12 minutes after the stimulation hour ended, the boss had reasserted his authority, and

his territoriality seemed to be as well established as during the control period. ...

* * *

Elemental psychic phenomena such as hunger and fear can be analyzed in both animal and man, but processes like ideation and imagery that are expressed verbally can be studied only in human beings. ...

* * *

In three different patients, thoughts and expressions with sexual content were induced by electrical stimulation of the temporal lobe. The first case, S.S., was an intelligent and attractive woman, 32 years old, who had suffered from uncontrollable epileptic attacks for several years. During the interviews she was usually reserved, but the first time that point A in the second temporal convulsion was excited with 6 volts, she became visibly affected, holding the hands of the therapist to express her fondness for him and to thank him for all his efforts. Several minutes later, after another stimulation of the same point, she started to say how much she would like to be cured so that she might marry, and other stimulations of point A were also followed by flirtatious conversation. The provocative play and ideas expressed under stimulation of point A did not appear following stimulation of other cerebral points and contrasted with this woman's usually reserved spontaneous behavior.

The second patient, V.P., was a woman 36 years old who had suffered from epilepsy since childhood. Point C in the temporal lobe was excited five times at intervals of from five to 10 minutes, and after each stimulation the patient's mood became friendlier; she smiled, questioned the therapist directly about his nationality, background, and friends, and declared that he "was nice," that his country (Spain) "must be very beautiful," that "Spaniards are very attractive," and she ended with the statement "I would like to marry a Spaniard." This particular train of thought and manner of speaking seemed completely spontaneous, but it appeared only after stimulation of point C in the temporal lobe, and no such shift to a flirtatious mood was noted in her spontaneous conversations following stimulations of other cerebral points.

The third case of evoked change in sexual ideology was a young epileptic boy, A.F., who, following stimulation of point LP 5–6 in the left temporal cortex, suddenly began to discuss his desire to get married. After subsequent stimulations of the point, he elaborated on this subject, revealed doubts about his sexual identity, and voiced a thinly veiled wish to marry the male interviewer.

*   *   *

Probably the most significant conclusion derived from electrical stimulation of the awake brain is that functions traditionally related to the psyche such as friendliness, pleasure, and verbal expression can be induced, modified, and inhibited by direct stimulation of cerebral structures. This discovery may be compared with the revolutionary finding almost two centuries ago that contraction of frog muscle may be induced by electricity without need of the soul's "animal spirits," because experimental analysis of mental functions can now proceed without implicating metaphysical entities. Research concerning the electrical driving of emotions, anatomical correlates of memory, or electrical signals related to learning does not interfere with personal ideas about the natural or supernatural destiny of man and does not involve theological questions, which should be disassociated from neurophysiological inquiry. . . . The task that we are facing is the correlation of neuro-anatomy and physiology with mental functions; the investigation of cerebral areas involved in psychic manifestations; the analysis of their electrical and chemical background; and the development of methods to induce or inhibit specific activities of the mind.

. . . Human behavior, happiness, good, and evil are, after all, products of cerebral physiology. In my opinion, it is necessary to shift the center of scientific research from the study and control of natural elements to the analysis and patterning of mental activities. There is a sense of urgency in this redirection because the most important problem of our present age is the reorganization of man's social relations. While the mind of future generations will be formed by pedagogic, cultural, political, and philosophical factors, it is also true that education is based on the transmission of behavioral, emotional, and intellectual patterns related to still unknown neuro-physiological mechanisms. Investigators will not be able to prevent the clash of conflicting desires or ideologies, but they can discover the neuronal mechanisms of anger, hate, aggressiveness, or territoriality, providing clues for the direction of emotions and for the education of more sociable and less cruel human beings. The precarious race between intelligent brains and unchained atoms must be won if the human race is going to survive, and learning the biological mechanisms of social relations will favor the cerebral victory.

*   *   *

From its beginning, wiring of the human brain aroused emotional opposition even among scientists, while similar wiring of the heart or of the bladder has been received enthusiastically. The difference in attitude was no doubt related to a more or less conscious personal fear that our identity could be attacked and that our mind could be controlled. Personal traits such as friendliness, sexual inclination, or hostility have already been modified during cerebral stimulation, and we can foresee other influences on emotional tone and behavioral reactions. Electricity is only a trigger of pre-existing mechanisms which could not, for example, teach a person to speak Spanish, although it could arouse memories expressed in Spanish if they were already stored in the brain.

Entering into the field of speculation, I would like to comment on one question which has already caused widespread concern. Would it be feasible to control the behavior of a population by electrical stimulation of the brain? From the times of slavery and galleys up to the present forced-labor camps, man has certainly tried to control the behavior of other human beings. In civilized life, the intervention of governments in our private biology has become so deeply rooted that in general we are not aware of it. Many countries, including the United States, do not allow a bride and groom to marry until blood has been drawn from their veins to prove the absence of syphilis. To cross international borders, it is necessary to certify that a scarification has been made on the skin and inoculated with smallpox. In many cities, the drinking water contains fluoride to strengthen our teeth, and table salt is fortified with iodine to prevent thyroid misfunction. These intrusions into our private blood, teeth, and glands are accepted, practised, and enforced. Naturally, they have been legally introduced, are useful for the prevention of illness, and do generally benefit society and individuals, but they have established a precedent of official manipulation of our personal biology, introducing the possibility that governments could try to control general behavior or to increase the happiness of citizens by electrically influencing their brains. Fortunately, this prospect is remote, if not impossible, not only for obvious ethical reasons, but also because of its impracticability. Theoretically it would be possible to regulate aggressiveness, productivity, or sleep by means of electrodes implanted in the brain, but this technique requires specialized knowledge, refined skills, and a detailed and complex exploration in each individual, because of the existence of anatomical and physiological variability. The feasibility of mass control of behavior by brain stimulation is very unlikely, and the application of intracerebral electrodes in man will probably remain highly individualized and restricted to medical practice. Clinical usefulness of electrode implantation in epilepsy and involuntary movements has already been proved, and its therapeutical extension to behavioral disorders, anxiety, depression, and other illness is at present being explored. The increasing capacity to understand and manipulate mental functions of patients will certainly increase man's ability to influence the behavior of man.

If we discover the cerebral basis of anxiety, pleasure, aggression, and other mental functions, we shall be in a much better position to influence their development and manifestations through electrical stimulation, drugs, surgery, and especially by means of more scientifically programmed education.

These possibilities pose tremendous problems. As Skinner asked recently, "Is the deliberate manipulation of a culture a threat to the very essence of man or, at the other extreme, an unfathomed source of strength for the culture which encourages it?" Scientific discoveries and technology cannot be shelved because of real or imaginary dangers, and it may certainly be predicted that the evolution of physical control of the brain and the acquisition of knowledge derived from it will continue at an accelerated pace, pointing hopefully toward the development of a more intelligent and peaceful mind of the species without loss of individual identity, and toward the exploitation of the most suitable kind of feedback mechanism: the human brain studying the human brain.

b.

Hudson Hoagland
Potentialities in the Control of Behavior*

*   *   *

The idea of the control of one person by another usually elicits strong adverse reactions in people. We treasure our convictions of freedom,

* Gordon Wolstenholme, ed.: *Man and His Future.* Boston: Little, Brown and Co. 299, 303–310, 312–313 (1963). Reprinted by permission of J. & A. Churchill, London.

and know either at first hand or vicariously the misery produced by coercion and tyranny. But we often fail to recognize that we are continually controlled in a variety of ways. Sanctions are derived from parents and other representatives of society, by laws and customs, and by the impact of irrational persuasion through myths and symbols that appeal to our subconscious drives, and may have little to do with the reason and logic we believe we use in making choices. A huckster or political propagandist may make us wish to have things we would be better off without. We are none the less controlled because we wish to do the things we do.

The great problem of control of behaviour resides in the question of who controls whom and for what purposes. It is clear that control by a Hitler or a Stalin is bad; but control is real and pervasive. How can it be used to advance human welfare?

We control each other in a great variety of ways. Force and the threat of force, which are clearly objectionable, may not be used but education, persuasion and moral pressure have the same effects. Cajolery, seduction, incitement and a variety of other techniques are used. B. F. Skinner has pointed out that ethical counter-controls in most countries prevent exploitation by the use of force and deception. But he emphasizes that there is real danger that the rapid development of new techniques of control will outstrip counter-control. Despite objections, science will increasingly facilitate control of human behaviour and it must be used wisely if we are to avoid disaster.

The behavioral sciences have developed new methods to modify and direct conduct. Examples are Pavlovian conditioning and the conditioning methods developed by Skinner, which have become widely used in studies of animal and human behaviour. By the use of appropriate reinforcing stimuli, behaviour may be modified and directed. The techniques involve carefully programmed rewards, reinforcing the subject's known hierarchies of values. Operant conditioning is the basis of the programming of teaching machines which are increasingly being used in education. The use by advertisers and others of subliminal messages in television has caused alarm and been made illegal in some countries. The effectiveness of this clandestine form of subconscious communication is, however, questionable.

C. H. Waddington, in his book *The Ethical Animal,* has considered that the long range objectives of the control of behaviour are ethical systems, the values of which may be judged in relation to their ability to further a desirable evolutionary direction, unique for mankind, and he discusses the nature of this evolutionary progress. Human culture, he points out, is based on a mechanism that requires people to be brought up in such a way that they accept beliefs given them by others such as parents and other influential persons in authority. Of course such beliefs are subject to later testing and rejection or retention, but before this can happen ideas must be transmitted as a form of social heredity. Ideas thus function in cultural evolution in a way analogous to genes in biological evolution, and Henry A. Murray has referred to germinal ideas as idenes.

The moulding of the newborn human individual into a being ready to believe what it is told seems to involve many very peculiar processes, which at present may be explained as the formation of the superego and the repression of the id, to use Freudian terminology. A frequent result of the process seems to be that people believe too much and too strongly. The process that evolution has provided us with seems often to lead to considerable exaggeration of the ability to believe.

Waddington argues that many of the world's evils and social ills stem from over-activity of the superego, leading to the acceptance of socially regressive beliefs with undesirable impact upon politics, religion and group identifications. Intense and irrational loyalties stemming from early authoritarian acceptance of communication have repeatedly led to fanaticism, bigotry and wars. One has but to recall pictures in the American press of squawking New Orleans women with children in their arms, hurling imprecations at a white father taking his small daughter to a desegregated school, to see pathological ethics in action. As Brock Chisholm has pointed out, most of the ethical beliefs we hold so strongly are established by accidents of birth and what we learn, hit or miss, before we are seven years old. Emotionally charged prejudices are propagated from generation to generation by parental and adult prestige. The strongest beliefs may bear little relation to the common good. The world has continually been sundered by the hates of rival groups and these could, in the nuclear age, soon render man an extinct species.

The rate of increase of scientific information is said now to be doubling every ten years, and its technological applications are changing society in ways for which there are no precedents. The fate of man has become the prize in a gruelling race between education and disaster. Traditional methods of education and ethical transmission appear to be inadequate, and the behavioural sciences so far have not been effective in meeting major challenges of the twentieth century. Fear that the behavioural and social sciences may be used for evil purposes has slowed their development and blocked their use for constructive purposes. We need a larger investment of talent in these fields, commensurate with their importance. As someone has said, understanding the atom is child's play compared to understanding child's play.

* * *

Psychopharmacology is a new empirical field that has developed rapidly over the last decade, and the use of drugs for the treatment of psychiatric disorders has furnished its major thrust. The pharmaceutical industry has produced hundreds of compounds faster than they can be tested in the clinic. These substances fall roughly into five groups. There are the stimulant drugs, such as ephedrine and its derivatives, which increase wakefulness and decrease fatigue under some conditions but also have some undesirable side effects on the central nervous system. The anti-depressant drugs include iproniazid (Marsilid) and a number of other monoamine oxidase inhibitors, together with some anti-depressants of other chemical types. These agents may produce euphoria, increase verbal productivity, speed reaction times and otherwise act as stimulants, but their principal value is in combating severe depressions of mental patients. The tranquillizers are a third group extensively employed in the treatment of disturbed mental patients, including schizophrenics. These drugs include chlorpromazine and a variety of other phenothiazine derivatives, as well as reserpine and a few related *Rauwolfia* alkaloids. A fourth category consists of substances that act as mild tranquillizers and sedatives. One of these, meprobamate, is sold under a number of trade names of which Miltown is perhaps the best known, and another is methaminodiazepoxide (Librium). These drugs may relieve neurotic anxiety without producing the sedative effects of barbiturates and bromides.

A fifth group of psychoactive drugs produce transient psychotic states. Their primary value is for research purposes in producing model psychoses in normal persons. Some effects of some of this group have been known for a long time. In crude form, as they occur in native plants, they have been used to produce mystical states during primitive religious rites. They include mescaline, psilocybin, the powerful synthetic psychologen LSD-25 (lysergic acid diethylamide) and other synthetic products.

All these drugs except those of the fifth group primarily affect mood. None of them acts upon the information content of the brain. The tranquillizers and psychic energizers are primarily responsible for the large increase in discharge rates of mental patients from hospitals in recent years.

The promiscuous use of the milder tranquillizers has given cause for alarm. These substances can inhibit initiative, vigour and drive, and may have deleterious side effects. They constitute the largest item of sale in American drug stores today. Barbiturate sleeping pills, bootlegged from druggists, are being used as a substitute for alcohol by some juvenile groups. A drink called a "goof ball" is made from sleeping pills dissolved in Coca Cola, and barbiturate addiction has become a serious problem among some teen-agers.

At present there seems to be little likelihood of the deliberate use of any of the known psychoactive drugs for the control of the behaviour of normal people. Even in the hands of a dictator, it is hard to see how any of these compounds could be used effectively to manipulate the actions of a population towards directed ends. Although these drugs may relieve depression and reduce anxiety in neurotic and psychotic patients, they can only disturb normal persons and make them miserable. Ephedrine and its derivatives may briefly spur a fatigued individual to greater output of activity but the subsequent hangover can negate such transient benefit. The functions of normal healthy organs, including the brain, have not so far been improved significantly by the use of drugs. . . .

There are historical examples of the use of drugs to control populations. Alcohol was used deliberately by some of our American forebears to debilitate and destroy the will to resist of some Indian tribes, and oriental despots have promoted the use of opium by subject populations for similar purposes. The consumption of tobacco and alcoholic beverages is promoted by commercial interests for their own profit—a control, in general, approved by the public. But people tend to resent the use of chemical agents when urged upon them for their own good. Irrational opposition to vaccination in the past and to the fluoridation of water supplies today are cases in point. Despite the magnitude of the population problem, many most in need of birth control refuse the use of oral contraceptives even in the absence of religious taboos.

It has been popularly believed that drugs have been employed extensively in brain-washing procedures in Communist-controlled countries. However, from the evidence available, this has not been the case. According to reliable reports, coercion of persons for the purpose of extracting confessions has involved methods similar to police state practices used since the time of Napoleon. Neither scientifically directed Pavlovian conditioned reflex procedure nor pharmacology appear to have been used in any significant way in breaking the morale of political prisoners.

Extensive work by neurophysiologists, using operations on the brains of animals, has shown that it is possible markedly to modify emotional and aggressive behaviour. When experimental lesions in monkeys are carefully restricted to the pyriform lobe of the amygdaloid complex and hippocampus without interference with neocortical regions, most fear and anger responses disappear, without gross motor or sensory deficiencies. Although these animals can express anger and rage in response to appropriate stimuli, they are rendered remarkably docile and fearless, and their behaviour is accompanied by a reduction in sexual activity. Studies of cats, including the lynx, show there is marked docility following bilateral lesions of the pyriform lobe. But the amygdalectomized cat can be turned into a vicious and rageful animal by additional superimposed lesions in the ventro-medial nucleus of the hypothalamus. Changes have been reported in the hierarchical position of individual rhesus monkeys from dominant to submissive positions in the pecking order following amygdalectomy, and clinical observations indicate that some amygdala lesions in man are followed by diminished social aggressiveness.

It thus appears that surgical operations on the brain's limbic system can markedly change emotional behaviour. Presumably chemical agents may ultimately be found which will act selectively on specific brain centres and have similar effects. It has been reported that cats exposed to certain agents of potential use in chemical warfare are terrified at the sight of mice.

Despite the values of the neurosurgical findings to medicine, it is difficult to see any practical application of psycho-surgery in the future, to enable men deliberately to control each other's behaviour in any socially significant way.

There is however one field which may hold promise for constructive purposes. It is possible that agents may be found to facilitate learning, memory and recall. It would clearly be desirable to find chemical and pharmacological procedures to facilitate processes of education, even at the risk of their perversion for political purposes.

* * *

Holger Hydén and his collaborators have developed elegant microchemical methods to study individual neurones in different parts of the nervous system. . . . Of special interest in this connexion was the finding that tricyano-amino-propine administered to human subjects is followed by an increase in suggestibility. Hyden considers that this substance or others might affect mental states in such a way that a police-controlled government, by putting such agents in drinking water, could make propaganda more palatable. . . .

* * *

NOTES

NOTE 1.

DAVID KRECH
PSYCHOCHEMICAL MANIPULATION AND
SOCIAL POLICY*

* * *

It is my considered judgment—well, fairly well considered—that within 5 to 10 years there will be available a regimen combining psychological and chemical measures that will significantly increase the intelligence of man. This troubles me, and should trouble you, for reasons that may soon become clear. To give some substance to these predictions and forebodings, let me cite first some supporting experimental chapter and verse.

I start with Prof. James McGaugh's demonstration that certain central nervous system stimulants can improve an animal's ability to learn. . . . The experimental mice were presented with the task of learning to choose a white alley leading to food over a black alley. Note that the

saline control animals averaged about 20 errors before they learned always to choose the white alley, but the Metrazol (pentylenetetrazol)-dosed animals improved with increasing strengths of the drug until, at the dose level of 10mg/kg of body weight, the mice solved the problem after but 5 errors; beyond that dosage there was no appreciable improvement. There seems to be a limit to the intellectual power of even a hopped-up California supermouse. In another experiment two different strains of mice were trained to solve a simple maze. Note first that we had here hereditary differences in learning ability: a relatively bright strain and a relatively stupid one. Secondly, note that the stupid treated with 10 mg/kg of pentylenetetrazol did as well as their untreated but hereditarily superior colleagues. Chemotherapy here compensated for the stupid parents. In another series of experiments McGaugh found that different drugs worked differentially for different strains, individuals, and intellectual tasks. Thus, for some problems picrotoxin helped the dull animal but not the bright, while for other problems pentylenetetrazol seemed to help everyone.

Does all of this mean that we will soon be able to substitute an inexpensive get-smart pill for our expensive school enrichment programs? The answer is no, as our Berkeley experiments on the effects of experience on the brain suggest. Let me describe a typical experiment. At weaning age, 12 rats are put into a psychologically enriched living group while their twin brothers are placed in a psychologically impoverished group. They all have the same food, of course. All 12 enriched pups live in 1 large cage equipped with inviting rat toys in a well-lighted, noisy, and busy laboratory. As the rats grow older, they are given various little learning tasks to master for which they are rewarded with bits of sugar. While these animals are enjoying the richest intellectual environment that Berkeley can provide for rats (but they are not on drugs!), their brothers lead quite different lives. Each impoverished animal lives out his solitary confinement in a small cage situated in a dimly lit and quiet room. It is rarely handled by its keeper and never invited to solve problems or join in fun and games with fellow rats or graduate students. At the age of 105 days all the rats are sacrificed, and their brains are analyzed morphologically and chemically.

This standard experiment that I have just described has been repeated dozens of times and has yielded the [following] results. . . . As the

* 67 *Annals of Internal Medicine,* Supplement 7: 19–24 (1967). Reprinted by permission. © 1967, American College of Physicians.

more fortunate litter mate lives out his life in the enriched condition, the bulk of his cortex expands and grows deeper and heavier than that of his culturally deprived brother. Part of this increase in cortical mass is accounted for by an increase in the number of cortical glia cells, part by an increase in the size of the neuronal cell bodies and their nuclei, and part by an increase in the diameter of the cortical blood vessels. Biochemical changes also occur. The enriched brain shows both more acetylcholinesterase and more cholinesterase activity.

Now, what does all this mean? Let me return to McGaugh's results for a moment. Whether a drug will improve an animal's learning ability will depend, of course, upon how the drug changes the chemistry of the animal's brain. And it is now clear from our own work that the chemical status of the brain, *before the introduction of any drug,* is partly dependent upon the psychological milieu in which the animal has been living. Therefore, putting McGaugh's results and our results together, it seems clear that *how* a drug, introduced from the outside, will change the brain chemistry and, thus, affect learning will depend upon the organism's psychological environment. I am not talking about some sort of mysterious interaction between "psychological forces" and "chemical compounds." I am talking about interactions between chemical factors in the brain induced by environment and chemical factors introduced into the brain by injections or pills. This is what lay behind my opening conclusion that within a few years psychology and chemistry will be able to raise the intelligence of man significantly.

Why does this worry me? To answer this question, I shall ask you to take a very brief look at some human data and then join me in an old parlor game. [In] the theoretical IQ distribution for our population . . . the mental retardates are separated into the so-called "organics"— comprising those retardates whose difficulties can be traced to clearly identifiable physical defects such as phenylketonuria or serious head injuries—and the "familial retardates"—made up of children with IQ's between 40 and 70 in whom there has been found no clear physiological defect. The causes cited for familial retardation include defects in brain biochemistry, hereditary factors, and cultural factors; indeed, this group is often labeled "the cultural familial retardates."

Now the most likely development from the research that I have been discussing will undoubtedly produce effective treatment for many

of the cultural familial retardates. But if we will be able to raise the IQs of the cultural familial retardates, how about the "cultural familial geniuses"? And what about the many millions of men, women, and children in the largest group of all—the "cultural familial mediocrities"? Let me suggest three possible answers.

The first possibility I will label "Brave New World, Mark I." Here . . . we assume that our psychological chemical procedures will raise the intelligence of all men and women so that the distribution curve would shift in the direction of higher IQ levels. Now, let us play the old parlor game of "what if?". Remember how it goes? You say, "What if through a genetic mutation induced by radioactive fallout from our liberty-loving anticommunist, democratic, nuclear-testing program, all babies were born with three arms? What changes do you foresee?" And your guests begin to speculate. Someone suggests that the whole clothing industry would have to be retooled—three sleeves instead of two; the deodorant industry would boom; speakers would have to revise their "on-the-one-hand and on-the-other-hand" clichés; handholding under the dinner table would be facilitated, leading to an increase in off-the-reservation dalliance, divorce, and eventual total moral decay. Very well. What would happen if, through psychochemistry, we raise the IQ level of most people by 20 points? What new demands would this place on our educational facilities and practices? What political changes might such a population bring about? What moral changes? How about religious practices and institutions?

Let me propose another possibility and another set of questions. You will remember that McGaugh found that some drugs can help only the duller strains and individuals of his experimental animal populations. Perhaps we shall find that with the human being we can raise only the lower IQs, the higher IQs being resistant to further improvement. . . . In "Brave New World, Mark II" we would have relatively little spread from the brightest to the dullest. Who now will be the hewers of wood and the drawers of water and the inhabitants of the slums and the wastelands—and who, the WASPS and the gentry? What changes will all of this induce when we are all pretty much alike intellectually? How long can we remain segregated into different political, economic, and social groups?

Let me end with the "Mark III" model. You will also remember that different drugs may be effective for different kinds of problems. On the human level this means that we may be able, through psychochemistry, to raise verbal abilities in some, arithmetic reasoning in others, artistic abilities in still others. Now, who gets what raised and who decides for whom? The parent? The family pediatrician? The family physician? The school board? And on what basis do they decide? On the effectiveness of the pharmaceutical industry's advertising? On the effectiveness or the persuasiveness of detail men? On the ability to pay for the more expensive abilities? These problems—surpassingly strange in their novelty, bafflingly complex, and of serious import—are problems with which you will inevitably become intimately involved. Yet it seems clear to me that the physician alone does not have the wisdom and the knowledge to handle these matters. Here, most certainly, the physician cannot be allowed to write social policy on his prescription pad. And here, most certainly, the physician should be prepared to welcome guidance from the laity and even accede gracefully to social control.

NOTE 2.

PERRY LONDON
BEHAVIOR CONTROL*

The first true technology of individual behavior control through verbal information was probably psychotherapy, especially the multitude of systems and subsystems called insight therapy, which aims to help people solve personal problems primarily by special ways of talking to them and listening to them talk. . . .

Psychotherapy is a technologically primitive means of behavior control compared to what will come after it, but it is significant in its own right because of the breadth of its applications, if not their power, and because it embodies virtually all the ethical problems which conscientious students of behavior control must encounter. . . .

*   *   *

Even were its scope less broad, psychotherapy would still be an important prototype of informational behavior-control technology because of its noncoercive character. All psychotherapies are merely special cases of the many kinds of situations in which some rational, persuasive, and nonviolent means are needed for controlling individual behavior or for teaching responsible agents of society how to do so. Part of its value

------

* New York: Harper & Row 39–41 (1969). Reprinted by permission of Harper & Row, Publishers.

as an area of study is that it involves the development of controls under conditions of maximum disadvantage to any controlling agency. "The therapist," as Neal Miller of Rockefeller University puts it, "does not have direct control over the important rewards and punishments in the patient's environment." Neither coercion by police power nor continuous charge over rewards and punishments, such as parents have, are ordinarily available to a psychotherapist; this turns his operations into relatively pure attempts to influence with only limited resources, the chief of which is language. It is not cynical, therefore, to say that the systematic persuasion methods which are psychotherapy are salesmanship elevated to the level of technology.

Because it relies on this most complex medium—the "higher processes" of language and symbol (sometimes considered the only uniquely human attributes)—psychotherapy is also a straightforward extension of education which, in the ethical perspective of our age, is regarded as the antithesis of control through coercion. And because it addresses individuals directly, it may be the closest thing extant to an agency for individual control that also satisfies the modern morality of freedom and individual choice.

*   *   *

All forms of psychotherapy aim to control behavior which, by one standard or another, is considered mentally deranged, diseased, disturbed, or otherwise disordered. For this reason, psychotherapists commonly refer to their methods as techniques of treatment rather than control. Such terminology makes no difference to their operations.

*   *   *

c.

Arnold M. Ludwig, Arnold J. Mary, Phillip A. Hill, and Robert M. Browning
The Control of Violent Behavior through Faradic Shock*

This study concerns an evaluation of the use of faradic shock as punishment for the purpose of suppressing the violent, potentially homicidal behavior of a hospitalized, chronic paranoid schizophrenic patient. The uniqueness of the study lies in four general areas: a) the type of

------

* 148 *Journal of Nervous and Mental Disease* 624–627, 633–637 (1969). © 1969, The Williams & Wilkins Co., Baltimore, Maryland. Reprinted by permission.

patient treated, b) the particular kinds of behaviors chosen for modification, c) the fact that this procedure was administered against the expressed will of the patient and d) the clinical-experimental format employed.

* * *

[P]ertinent to the present study is the previous use of electric shock as an aversive conditioning agent. In most of these clinical studies, the investigators have used a special apparatus, capable of delivering about 70 to 100 volts (the actual voltage can be adjusted by a rheostat) through electrodes on a cuff applied to the patient's forearm, wrist or calf. The procedure involves shocking the patient immediately after the repeated visual presentation (actual object, picture, slide) of his deviant interest. The conditions treated by this means include cases of compulsive gambling, homosexuality, compulsive eating, fetishism, transvestism, car stealing, obsessional ruminations, smoking, writer's cramp, alcoholism, and even habitual blushing, compulsive copulation with sheep and marital infidelity. It is important to emphasize that in all these cases the "voluntary" consent and active cooperation of the patients were required as a precondition for treatment.

Of a somewhat different nature are the studies concerned with autistic and severely retarded children. Lovaas and co-workers, pioneers in this field, have used slapping, electrified grills and the cattle prod (the "shock stick") as a means of controlling and modifying self-mutilative, aggressive and other forms of maladaptive behavior in these children. Employing similar techniques, other investigators have extended this work and reported equally impressive therapeutic results in otherwise hopeless, self-destructive children. In these cases, of course, the consent and active cooperation of the children were not necessarily sought.

Three factors contributed to our choice of a punishment treatment paradigm: a) the dangerousness to self and others of the patient's behavior, b) the inability of previously employed treatment methods to modify this behavior and c) the far more drastic nature of other possible treatment alternatives.

The patient was a 31-year-old female with an established diagnosis of chronic paranoid schizophrenia. She had been hospitalized for the better part of 9 years. Her intelligence and verbal facility were normal, but the content of her ideation and speech was predominantly vindictive

and accusatory with marked delusions of persecution. Although she manifested agitation and depression on occasion, this symptomatology would usually undergo a rapid paranoid transformation whereby she would begin to blame others for her predicament. She showed poor socialization, resisting most efforts of both patients and staff to engage her in conversations or activities, and responded poorly to praise or other positive social reinforcers. The most serious feature of her behavior was her frequent, vicious physical assaultiveness toward staff and fellow patients. Less frequently, she had been known to set fire to herself or apply lit cigarettes to her skin. This self-destructive behavior, however, had not been observed during the last 2 years of her hospitalization.

Housed on various locked wards over the years, she had succeeded in terrorizing patients and staff alike. She would bully and threaten patients into giving her cigarettes, money and other articles. In regard to staff, she would threaten to kill them or their families if they did not accede to her wishes or did not leave her alone. Often these threats would be translated into physical assaults. The predictable result was that patients and staff treated her gingerly and tended to keep a "safe distance."

Although many of her physical attacks upon staff were in response to limit-setting attempts, there were other instances where there were no discernible antecedents for this violence. These latter situations were especially frightening because of their lightening suddenness and unexpected quality. For example, she would walk up to staff members or patients and without warning punch them in the face. In other instances, she would lie in wait for her intended "victims" in the bathroom or some other unsupervised ward area and attack them mercilessly once they entered.

Over the long period of her hospitalization, the patient had been exposed to almost every variety of psychiatric therapy. Massive doses of tranquilizers and sedatives, electroconvulsive therapy, intensive milieu, group and individual psychotherapy, and a variety of special psychosocial techniques had been tried—all to no avail in curbing her assaultive behavior. There were, to be sure, brief periods of quiescence of her symptomatology, but these seemed relatively independent of her treatment at those times.

Clearly, the management of this patient represented a serious medical-psychiatric problem and something had to be done before she killed

someone or was seriously injured or killed herself through the retaliation of another patient. Faced with the ineffectiveness of prior treatment approaches, we were forced to consider other more extreme procedures such as prefrontal lobotomy, shackling her in physical restraints, or isolating her through prolonged seclusion. We were naturally reluctant to resort to these procedures and believed it would be far more humane and potentially therapeutic to try to modify her behavior through aversive conditioning. After securing the support of a group of board-certified psychiatrists and obtaining the necessary administrative clearance, we initiated the treatment program.

The aims of the treatment program were essentially two-fold: a) the elimination of serious aggressive-assaultive behavior and b) the stimulation of appropriate, socialized, responsible behavior. In order to realize the first goal, we felt it would be important not only to apply punishment (i.e., faradic shock) systematically upon the appearance of behaviors defined as physical aggression but also to suppress certain antecedent, related behaviors. It was our plan to establish a hierarchy of responses associated with aggression and then proceed to modify each successive level in this hierarchy in a stepwise manner through the aversive therapy paradigm. . . .

To achieve the second goal, namely the fostering of prosocial responses in this patient, we planned to provide copious positive reinforcement in terms of praise, compliments and other more material rewards for all desirable and adaptive behavior. This intensive program of positive social reinforcement was to accompany the aversive conditioning aspects of treatment throughout the entire program.

There were a number of reasons for choosing the cattle prod as the means of delivering the aversive stimulus or punishment. From a technical standpoint, this instrument (Sabre-Six model, Hot Shot Products Co.) seemed to represent an excellent device for providing a potent, noxious stimulus. It was capable of producing a faradic shock spike of approximately 1400 volts at 0.5 milli-amperes, the resulting pain lasting only as long as the current was permitted to flow. From the standpoint of safety, the shock caused no tissue damage or other adverse physical effects. In comparing the treatment to such standard psychiatric procedures as electro-convulsive therapy or even psychotropic medication, the possibility of serious physical side effects was regarded as far more remote. Moreover, when compared to the dangers and relative unpredictability of onset and duration of action of other aversive agents, such as emetic and muscle-paralyzing drugs, this instrument was far safer and could be applied in a more specific manner with a minimal time lag between the appearance of the undesirable behavior and the aversive stimulus. Also, from a practical standpoint, the instrument was portable, inexpensive and easy to use.

*   *   *

General Clinical Observations

It seems reasonable to presume that if a stimulus is to be defined as aversive or punishment, it should elicit a reaction indicative of displeasure, discomfort or pain. The more profound the reaction, the greater should be the individual's efforts to avoid behavior associated with the application of the aversive stimulus. There were a number of clinical observations that indicated that the faradic shock possessed all the properties of a punishing stimulus for our patient. After being shocked, the patient would let out a cry, stiffen all over and then begin whimpering.

We had anecdotal confirmation from the patient herself that the faradic shock was specifically instrumental in making her cautious about striking out. For example, in the early stages of the therapy program it was common to hear her exclaim "The only thing holding me back is the faradic stimulator," "If it wasn't for the faradic shock, you'd be on your ass," "You are doing this to me, getting away with everything because of the faradic stimulator," "I wouldn't hit you . . . I don't want that faradic thing," "Maybe I better not say that . . . it might be blaming. It's better to be safe than sorry."

Of incidental interest was the anticipated finding that the patient was quite capable of making the mental connection between the performance of a punishable act and the subsequent punishment, regardless of the time lag between these events. Pertinent to this matter was the patient's response to one instance of delayed punishment when she chided a staff member by saying "You're supposed to do this right after I say it (referring to level III behavior)."

In contrast to our impressions about the potency of faradic shock as an aversive stimulus are our observations on the relative impotence of primary rewards (goodies, cigarettes) or social rewards (praise) to shape or reinforce constructive, adaptive behavior. For the most part, the patient typically had responded to praise, emotional warmth and rewards in an antagonistic and surly manner. Although we continued to provide intensive and copious positive reinforcements for appropriate behavior throughout the entire treatment program, including the several base line periods, it was not until the spontaneous appearance of the approach behavior following the start of the level III program that positive reinforcement (particularly social) seemed to take on increasingly appropriate emotional valence.

Concluding Comments

Although we were able to establish "effective" control over the intensity, duration and frequency of aggression and its antecedents, these behaviors were never eliminated completely and, therefore, control over them could not be regarded as absolute. Throughout the entire treatment program, there were occasional flareups of each of the three levels of punishable behaviors. . . .

Of great clinical interest was the spontaneous appearance of relatively new behaviors following the suppression of the patient's dominant aggressive responses. Generally, these outlets proved to be milder, less destructive and more innocuous than the deviant behaviors they substituted for, and they were relatively short-lived. We suspected that the reason for their transiency was that they did not serve as satisfactory outlets for her feelings.

Aside from a reduction in aggressive behaviors, we also noted a concomitant increase in more socialized behaviors following the punishment of each successive level in the hierarchy of aggressive and antecedent behaviors. It was not simply that the patient became more tractable, compliant or automaton-like in response to these punishment procedures: rather, the patient gradually began to show tentative warmth to others (i.e., "I like you . . . no I don't"), engaged in occasional humorous interchanges and showed some diminution in her general hating and surliness. . . .

One possible mechanism for the shift from antagonistic to approach behaviors, as well as for her general clinical improvement, involves the concept of "functional incompatibility." . . . For . . . new behaviors to become established, the stereotyped behaviors must first be reduced or eliminated. With our patient, an even clearer incompatibility between her prior aggressive and hating mode and any prosocial responses could be demonstrated.

From several of the patient's statements, such as "If I can't fight you guys, I'll join you.

. . . Nothing else works," we might also invoke the mechanism of "identification with the aggressor." With such a view, we would expect that the patient, feeling impotent and frightened when having her habitual sources of displaying power over others blocked, would attempt to regain strength and security through her identification with the staff. . . .

Perhaps the most straightforward explanation for the increase in the patient's social approach behavior related to the obvious change in attitudes and behavior of the staff and fellow patients toward her once her aggressive tendencies were reduced. Before this reduction took place, the staff might have felt that they were being warm and accepting much of the time with the patient, but it was difficult to relate with unconditional positive regard to someone who punched them in the jaw just 1 week ago. With this threat of harm diminished, the staff could be more genuinely affectionate, thereby increasing the possibility that the patient could respond in kind. . . .

* * *

Another factor contributing to the relative success of the aversive therapy program seemed related to the subjective meaning of punishment for the patient. From clinical observations, we had become convinced that the patient, at some level of consciousness or volition, wanted to be effectively controlled and have limits set and enforced. In the course of our therapy program, we collected much anecdotal "evidence" that seemed to support this view. For example, shortly after the initiation of the punishment program for level I behaviors, the patient eloped from the hospital. Following previous elopements, she was always picked up by the community authorities and escorted involuntarily back to the hospital. On this particular occasion, she returned on her own, claiming "They're trying to kill me out there . . . at least in here you'll protect me!" Also, during the course of the program, she made the following revealing statement: "I know what you're trying to do. . . . You're trying to make a human being out of me."

From a therapeutic standpoint, we must regard the aversive conditioning program as a qualified success. Although the patient remains far from "cured," she nevertheless has progressed considerably from the primitiveness, violence and malignant paranoia which characterized her pretherapy behavior. Most important, she has begun to display many positive attributes which make her more approachable by others and more responsive to social reinforcers. However, even with these gains, we anticipate having to deal with periodic flare ups of aggressive and antecedent behaviors. We are not so naive as to expect the aversive program alone to be sufficient to eliminate the patient's core psychopathology and completely reverse the effects of the superimposed psychopathology acquired, and inadvertently reinforced by others, over long years of institutionalization. We also have no way of predicting just how lasting even her current gains will be. It is quite possible that if and when the patient becomes inured to faradic shock, she may lapse to former behavior patterns rather than continue to show improvement. Nevertheless, with the threat of violence reduced and with the beginning responsiveness to social reinforcers, we now at least have a therapeutic foothold for exploring less drastic psychosocial procedures.

In conclusion, we wish to state that we are well aware of the many sensitive ethical issues associated with the use of punishment as therapy. No responsible clinicians can embark on this type of treatment program without first asking and answering for themselves the crucial questions dealing with the use of coercion for the modification of human behavior, the rights of patients and the time-worn ends-means controversy. Since we have dealt with many of these issues elsewhere, we feel that there is little to be gained from repeating our views. Suffice it to say that given the dangerousness of the patient's behavior, the ineffectiveness of prior treatment approaches and the safety of faradic shock as compared to the possible consequences of more drastic therapies, we were able to conduct this program with few ethical qualms. Even if the program had not proved successful, we would have felt that the exploration of this therapeutic modality was ethically justified.

NOTES

NOTE 1.

ROBERT G. HEATH
ELECTRICAL SELF-STIMULATION OF THE
BRAIN IN MAN*

Two patients were used in the study. Patient No. B-7, age 28, with a diagnosis of narcolepsy and cataplexy, had failed to respond to conventional treatments. He had electrodes implanted

* 120 *American Journal of Psychiatry* 571–576 (1963). Copyright 1963, the American Psychiatric Association. Reprinted by permission.

by the method developed in our laboratory into 14 predetermined brain regions and fixed to remain in exact position for prolonged study.

Patient No. B-10, age 25, a psychomotor epileptic with episodic brief periods of impulsive behavior uncontrolled with the usual treatments, had 51 leads implanted into 17 brain sites.

*   *   *

Stimuli were delivered from a specially constructed transistorized self-contained unit which was worn on the patient's belt. The unit generated a pre-set train of bi-directional stimulus pulses each time that one of the 3 control buttons was depressed. Each button directed the pulse train to a different electrode pair permitting the operator a possible selection of cerebral sites. . . .

*   *   *

Patient No. B-7. After randomly exploring the effects of stimulation with presses of each of the 3 buttons, Patient No. B-7 almost exclusively pressed the septal button.

Stimulation to the mesencephalic tegmentum resulted in a prompt alerting, but was quite aversive. The patient, complaining of intense discomfort and looking fearful, requested that the stimulus not be repeated. To make certain that the region was not stimulated, he ingeniously modified a hair pin to fit under the button which directed a pulse train to the mesencephalic tegmentum so it could not be depressed.

Hippocampal stimulation was mildly rewarding.

Stimulation to the septal region was the most rewarding of the stimulations and, additionally, it alerted the patient, thereby combatting the narcolepsy. By virtue of his ability to control symptoms with the stimulator, he was employed part-time, while wearing the unit, as an entertainer in a night club.

The patient's narcolepsy was severe. He would move from an alert state into a deep sleep in the matter of a second. Recognizing that button pressing promptly awakened him, fellow patients and friends occasionally resorted to pushing the button if he fell asleep so rapidly that he was unable to stimulate himself.

The patient, in explaining why he pressed the septal button with such frequency, stated that the feeling was "good"; it was as if he were building up to a sexual orgasm. He reported that he was unable to achieve the orgastic end point, however, explaining that his frequent, sometimes frantic, pushing of the button was an attempt to reach the end point. This futile effort was frustrating at times and described by him on these occasions as a "nervous feeling."

Patient No. B-10. Studies conducted on the psychomotor epileptic patient were more varied and provided more information concerning subjective responses. . . .

The button most frequently pushed provided a stimulus to the centromedian thalamus. This stimulus did not, however, induce the most pleasurable response; in fact, it induced irritability. The subject reported that he was almost able to recall a memory during this stimulation, but he could not quite grasp it. The frequent self-stimulations were an endeavor to bring this elusive memory into clear focus.

The patient most consistently reported pleasurable feelings with stimulation to two electrodes in the septal region and one in the mesencephalic tegmentum. With the pleasurable response to septal stimuli, he frequently produced associations in the sexual area. Actual content varied considerably, but regardless of his baseline emotional state and the subject under discussion in the room, the stimulation was accompanied by the patient's introduction of a sexual subject, usually with a broad grin. When questioned about this, he would say, "I don't know why that came to mind—I just happened to think of it."[*] The "happy feelings" with mesencephalic stimulation were not accompanied by sexual thought.

* * *

Changes in parameters of stimuli to a given region of the brain, including current intensity, wave form, pulse width, and frequency, in many

_____

[*] . . . Patient No. B-10, the psychomotor epileptic, was stimulated in the septal region during a period when he was exhibiting agitated, violent psychotic behavior. The stimulus was introduced without his knowledge. Almost instantly his behavioral state changed from one of disorganization, rage, and persecution to one of happiness and mild euphoria. He described the beginning of a sexual motive state. He was unable, when questioned directly, to explain the sudden shift in his feelings and thoughts. This case demonstrates a phenomenon which appears to be consistent and which has been repeated in a large number of patients in our laboratories. This phenomenon is the ability to obliterate immediately painful emergency emotional feelings in a human subject through introduction of a pleasurable state by physical or chemical techniques.

instances altered the patients' responses. This has similarly been reported with animal ICSS [Intracranial Self-Stimulation].

Information acquired from the patients' reporting of their reasons for button pressing indicates that all ICSS is not solely for pleasure. The highest rate of button pressing occurred with Patient No. B-7 when he was somewhat frustrated in his pleasurable pursuit and as he attempted to achieve an orgastic end point. In Patient No. B-10 the highest rate of button pressing also occurred with frustration, but of a different type, evolving with attempts to bring into focus a vague memory that ICSS had evoked. The subject's emotional state in this instance built into strong anger. It was interesting that the patient would button press to stimulate the region within the centromedial thalamus for a prolonged period, but at a slower rate when buttons providing more pleasurable septal and tegmental stimulation were also available. Depression of the septal button, with resultant pleasant feelings, alleviated the painful emergency state, according to the subject's report, and thereby provided him comfort to pursue his quest for the fleeting memory.

With septal stimulation in other patients, as well as the two subjects discussed here, a sexual motive state has frequently been induced in association with pleasurable response. This sexual state has not developed in association with pleasurable feelings during stimulation to other regions.

* * *

NOTE 2.

SIR JOHN ECCLES
EXPERIMENTS ON MAN IN
NEUROPHYSIOLOGY*

* * *

There is another kind of investigation that is often carried out and which I am extremely concerned about—investigations involving so-called indwelling electrodes. These are placed deep in various parts of the brain and X-ray controlled to see where they are. The electrodes are often as much as 2 or 3 millimetres in diameter and have multiple channels on them. They are inserted through a trephine hole in the skull and often stay in for weeks or months; the subjects

_____

* V. Fattorusso, ed.: *Biomedical Science and the Dilemma of Human Experimentation.* Paris: Council for International Organizations of Medical Sciences 22–23 (1967). Reprinted by permission.

who go home have a little cap on their skull and you can at any time have them back in the laboratory and lead from the hippocampus, the thalamus, or any part of the cortex where the electrodes happen to be lodged.

This, I think, causes fantastic damage to the brain. I do not believe that the subjects have been informed at all of what has been done; they are often under treatment for psychosis and various kinds of epilepsy and so on. This kind of investigation simply horrifies me. I do not believe that this damage to the brain is justifiable on any consideration whatsoever. At least, there should be a tremendous investigation on anthropoid apes using these techniques before they are used on human subjects. And, if there is going to be an investigation on human subjects, then I believe the investigators themselves should be the people who take the electrodes, at least in the first instance. I make this statement categorically.

*   *   *

NOTE 3.

MARTIN J. REIMRINGER, STERLING W. MORGAN, AND PAUL F. BRAMWELL
SUCCINYLCHOLINE AS A MODIFIER OF ACTING-OUT BEHAVIOR*

Atascadero State Hospital is a maximum security facility designed to treat mentally disordered sex offenders, the acting-out mentally ill patient, and the criminally insane. Concentrated within its buildings are those individuals whose behavior has been such as to have them considered acute dangers to society.

Within the 1500 patient population, there exists a small number of individuals who continue their aggressive, acting-out behavior during their hospitalization. These patients have frequently been engaged in fights, verbal threatening, deviant sexual behavior, and stealing. Usually, they are not cooperative and are not involved with the hospital treatment program. The procedure followed to curb this unacceptable behavior has been to transfer the patient to a ward for the acutely disturbed, medicate him and, if necessary, place him in restraint until the acute stage was past. Such a technique while having historical precedent is both time consuming and costly in terms of individual benefit. A search for another technique was begun.

The drug, succinylcholine (anectine), is a neuromuscular blocking agent used primarily as

* *Clinical Medicine* 28–29 (July 1970). Reprinted by permission.

an adjuvant to electroshock treatment and surgical anesthesia. A single intravenous dose of 20 to 35 mg. becomes maximally effective within 34–40 seconds, progressively producing fasciculations and paralysis first in the small, rapidly moving muscles of the fingers, toes and eyes through to the intercostal muscles and the diaphragm. At this point, a period of apnea is produced. During the entire period of muscular paralysis there is neither loss of memory and consciousness nor clouding of the sensorium. Due to the rapid hydrolysis of the anectine by the pseudocholinesterase of the liver and the plasma the effect of succinylcholine is very rapid and complete recovery from a single dose is usually within five minutes. The general psychological effect is to produce a decidedly unpleasant and fearful sensation.

Succinylcholine offers an easily controlled, quickening, fear-producing experience during which the sensorium is intact and the patient rendered susceptible to suggestion.

Ninety male patients were used in an exploratory study to determine the effectiveness of succinylcholine as an agent in behavior modification. The criteria of selection varied, but included persistent physical or verbal violence, deviant sexual behavior, and lack of cooperation and involvement with the individual treatment program prescribed by the patient's ward team. The subjects included overtly psychotic mentally retarded and sociopathic patients.

The number of treatments was predetermined by the ward doctors. The patient was administered an initial intravenous dose of 20 mg. of succinylcholine. Subsequent treatments sometimes required an increase in the dosage in order to meet the desired criteria of 1¼ minute period of apnea. Positive pressure breathing equipment was at the treatment site if the patient's pulse slowed during period of apnea.

After respiration stopped, the talking phase of the treatment began. Both negative and positive suggestions spoken in a confident, authoritarian manner were made by the male technician. The negative suggestions concerned the obliteration of unacceptable behaviors such as fighting and stealing. Positive suggestions focused upon the patient's becoming involved with patient government, the taking of individual responsibility and an increase in constructing socialization. These suggestions continued throughout the period of apnea and until the patient could verbally respond to the technician. After the treatment was completed, the patient was returned to his ward and no other special attention formally given to him.

The data revealed the following results: Improvement was noted in 61 of 90 patients, or 68 per cent; 16 patients, or 18 per cent, were considered temporarily improved; no change was noted in 12 men, or 13 per cent; and in one patient (one per cent) the result was increased violence.

The subjects were rated on the basis of the frequency of acting-out behavior subsequent to the treatments. At Atascadero State Hospital special incident reports are made for each episode of aggressive and/or unacceptable behavior. The subjects were rated as improved if no incident reports appeared in their record for a period exceeding three months. Temporary improvement was given when there were no incident reports for a one-to-three-month period. The "no change" category included those patients whose frequency of acting-out behavior remained approximately the same after treatments as prior to the use of anectine. Only one patient appeared to have shown an adverse reaction to the treatments. Some patients have extended their trouble-free behavior to eighteen months.

* * *

2.

Interferences with Human Evolution

a.

Bentley Glass
Human Heredity and Ethical Problems*

The discoveries of molecular biology and genetics during the past twenty years are now generally acclaimed as the most significant scientific advances of our present generation, just as the understanding of the forces of nuclear energy in the atom were those of the preceding generation. Like the application of nuclear energy to both destructive and constructive purposes, the application of the spectacular finding that deoxyribonucleic acid (DNA) is the chemical basis of heredity offers man a magnificent extension of power over nature and at the same time lays

* First Annual Address to the Society for Health and Human Values, Los Angeles, California 1–15 (Oct. 29, 1970). Unpublished manuscript printed by permission of the author who retains all rights.

on his conscience a frightening responsibility lest that power be misused.

Within these past twenty years it has been demonstrated conclusively how the DNA of the cell replicates and how errors in replication, errors producible either by high-energy radiation or by certain chemical agents, give rise to mutations, that is, produce permanent hereditary changes most of which are detrimental. Next was discovered the way in which the genetic code which is formed by the sequence of nucleotides in the DNA molecule is transcribed to ribonucleic acid (RNA) and the way in which the messenger molecules of RNA, after migrating from the nucleus of the cell to the cytoplasm, are transcribed on the ribosomes into specific sequences of amino acids in a polypeptide molecule. The problem of protein synthesis, which lies at the basis of all formation of living structures and all control over living processes, has been clarified beyond wildest expectations. The "one gene—one enzyme" hypothesis has become the well established "one gene (or cistron) —one polypeptide" theory, transformed into doctrine or dogma, so quickly has it become a basic concept of biology.

[R]apidly and step by step, the way has been opened to producing a great variety of genes which might be introduced into living cells in order to supply various hereditary deficiencies. Maybe by using a harmless virus as a carrier for such genes, in the manner known to geneticists as transduction, genes can be introduced into particular organs where they are needed and made a part of the regular replicating genome of the cell. Or perhaps, like the original classical transformation experiments of Avery, McCloud, and McCarty with Pneumococcus in the 1940's, treatment of deficient cells and organs with the isolated or synthesized active genes will be feasible. In either case, what Joshua Lederberg has called euphenics, the specifically desired modification of the phenotype of a defective organism by treatment, will have advanced a major stride.

The earlier stages of euphenics involved finding out just what gene product was missing in the body, or just what gene substrate, accumulating unused, was proving to be toxic. . . . Later developments of euphenics involved identification of the specific enzymes which are wholly or partly missing in particular hereditary conditions, in the hope that introduction of the enzymes into the body might allay the malady. This hope proved not well grounded, since most enzymes are large protein molecules, and are either digested when administered by mouth or are likely to produce allergic hypersensitivity if obtained from sources other than man himself. Or, if neither of these difficulties arises, the enzyme molecule is often unable to enter the cells where it must function. Hence only relatively small proteins, such as insulin, or enzymes which function extracellularly, such as serum cholinesterase, can be effectively administered, and even in these cases treatment is limited by the available supply.

The newest phase of euphenics, just beginning, may well surmount these difficulties by transferring to the defective person the missing gene itself. As in the case of proteins, the problem is first to get the effective gene into the cell and next to replace the incapacitated allele in the recipient's chromosomes. By means of carrier viruses this may turn out to be feasible. Recent successes in infecting mice with transducing viruses offer considerable encouragement. It may become possible to infect with the virus the specific organs or tissues which require the activity of the gene, without endeavoring to transform the entire body of the recipient genetically.

Since there is still no hint that we will ever be able to produce desired mutations to order, or indeed to eliminate the occurrence of mutations we do not want, we must in coping with genetic disease resort either to methods of euphenics or to eugenic measures that prevent the birth of the genetically handicapped. Recent advances in the detection of the normal, heterozygous carriers of genes producing recessive disorders and of the affection of a fetus at an early age greatly enhance our opportunities to reduce specific disorders. As for the former, the list of heterozygous "inborn errors of metabolism" which can be detected biochemically or by karyotype analysis is increasing so rapidly, at a rate of three or more each year, that already over sixty can be detected and the identity of the critical marriages in which two carriers are wed could theoretically be established. However, even in the case of the most prevalent of these, cystic fibrosis, which affects about one birth in each 2000, the frequency in the population of heterozygous persons (1 in 22) signifies that only one in 484 matings, random with respect to the possession of the gene, will run the high genetic risk, one in four, of producing an affected child. This frequency is not enough to require that all marrying persons be screened to determine the carriers among them, although perhaps all first cousins who marry should be tested, since the rarer the condition the greater the probability of consanguinity among the parents. But when, a few years from now, the number of heterozygous conditions which can be detected exceeds one hundred, and tests can be made both cheaper and simpler, multiple testing will become routine. The legal requirement in some states at the present time that all newborn infants be tested routinely for phenylketonuria points the way. This condition, the adverse effects of which upon mental development can be counteracted by controlled diet if detected and treated early enough in life, affects only about one child in 40,000. The heterozygous carriers, on the other hand, are at a ratio in the population of one per cent. If the test for the heterozygous condition were as simple and as cheap as that for the homozygous defect, it would be far better to test everyone for presence of the recessive gene, much as we test and identify everyone in respect to their ABO and Rh blood groups. Such tests, carried out in the maternity hospital for each baby and recorded in a computer system, would enable appropriate measures to be taken. What would these be?

Before grappling with this difficult question, let me describe another scientific advance of the past fifteen years that, like the biochemical detection of heterozygous carriers, opens the way to new eugenic and euphenic measures. Cytological methods enabling the investigator to examine the karyotype, that is, the chromosome constitution, of a person with minimal difficulty are now available. After the first development in 1955 of the techniques for examination of smears of whole cells treated to spread out the chromosomes, to stop cells just prior to metaphase during cell division, and to stain them appropriately, great advances were made in the detailed identification and characterization of the normal human chromosome complement, or karyotype. Lejeune and his colleagues pioneered in the detection of chromosome abnormalities of the karyotype by discovering in 1959 that Down's syndrome, familiarly called mongolism, is regularly characterized by the presence of an extra chromosome, one of the smallest in the set, known as Chromosome 21. . . . Usually these chromosome conditions can be identified from cultured skin cells. . . . Most recently, a technique known as amniocentesis has been developed. By means of a hypodermic needle, inserted into the amniotic fluid surrounding a fetus, amniotic fluid containing cells which may be cultured and examined can be withdrawn. Thus prenatal diagnosis may be performed, either chromosomal or biochemical. Puck has recently stated that one per cent of all human births carry a chromosome abnormality, and that the cost of caring for the Down's syndrome "mongols" in the United States is alone estimated, according to the National Foundation, to be $1.7 billion annually. Obviously, the cost of developing reliable and inexpensive methods of detecting the carriers of such conditions, when transmissible, and of coding the population genetically could be largely offset by savings from the elimination of even one such defect.

It is necessary, however, to examine the difficulties that stand in the way. In the case of Down's syndrome and other monosomic or trisomic conditions of the karyotype, most affected individuals are sterile or lack normal sexual drives. Hence most affected cases arise through errors in chromosome distribution (*i.e.* non-disjunction) occurring in the reproductive cells of the parents. In this respect they resemble fresh mutations of the genes, especially dominant mutations. Two alternative approaches may be taken. One may attempt, by treatment, to correct the condition and restore development to normality. In the case of a dominant mutant such as retinoblastoma, a condition once invariably fatal in childhood, surgical removal of the affected eye, if performed soon enough and with full removal of the cancerous condition, permits the child to retain the vision of one eye and to grow normally to adulthood. The sequel is alarming, since most of these patients then marry and pass on to half of their children, on the average, the devastating genetic disorder which will again require radical surgery. One is forced to ask whether it would not be better in some way, in these circumstances, to force the person involved to remain childless. The second alternative is more applicable to a condition such as mongolism, in which reproduction of the affected person is very unlikely but the cost of care—the burden upon family and upon society—is very great. Early diagnosis of the condition by amniocentesis would permit surgical abortion of the affected fetus.

Mongolism, and probably chromosomal abnormalities in general, increase sharply in frequency with advancing age of the parents, particularly the mother. In mothers over 35 years of age the incidence of Down's syndrome among births rises to 2 per cent, and in mothers over 40 years of age to 10 per cent or higher. It follows that even if universal fetal testing cannot

be legally prescribed, the testing of all prospective births to mothers over the age of 35 years would be unquestionably desirable. For other conditions it is the more advanced age of the father which is involved. The ethical question at once becomes clear. Inasmuch as no effective treatment for mongolism or other chromosomal abnormalities capable of surviving birth is known, and inasmuch as the social and psychological cost to both family and society is in general so high, abortion is regarded by many geneticists as the best way to handle the matter. Yet where society has banned abortion no improvement in the quality of the population by reducing the one per cent of births with chromosome abnormalities is to be expected.

The ethical problem is more acute in the case of a simple dominant gene of malignant character, such as that which produces retinoblastoma. By permitting the survival and reproduction of an affected person in this case there is inevitably a rise in the frequency of the condition in future generations, unless stern measures such as sterilization of the surviving retinoblastoma cases is made mandatory or unless by genetic counsel they are indeed persuaded not to have children. In the latter case, since contraceptive measures are not perfect and may be carelessly utilized, offspring may be produced in spite of good intentions.

. . . Most serious of all is the fact that many socially undesirable traits depend upon multiple genes. General mental inferiority, grading down into imbecility and idiocy, is of this nature. In such cases it may in time be possible to learn how to modify the environment so as to prevent any manifestation of overt disease or inferiority. Yet by surrounding ourselves with an ever more artificial environment, we unwittingly modify the rigor of natural selection in many ways. The price we must pay, in the end, for the mercies of medical care and surgical aid is a dysgenic increase in the frequencies of certain detrimental genes the effects of which we have learned to ameliorate. Thousands of diabetics who in a former day would have died early in life are now saved by insulin to live relatively normal lives, and of course to pass on to their descendants the genes responsible for their diabetes. Myopia is no longer, as it may have been in man's early hunting existence, a grave handicap in life; hearing aids alleviate certain types of deafness. No one, I think, would have it otherwise. Yet to contemplate the man of tomorrow who must begin his day by adjusting his spectacles and his hearing aid, inserting his false teeth, taking an allergy injection in one arm and an insulin injection in the other, and topping off his preparations for life by taking a tranquillizing pill, is none too pleasant. To say the least, medical science steadily increases the load it must carry.

A still more serious difficulty in the analysis of the genetic load of detrimental genes and in the choice of policies to be pursued toward that load lies in the existence of genes which are detrimental in one environment but confer a benefit in another, or of genes in which the heterozygote is more highly favored by selection than either of the homozygous types. A now classic example of both of these situations is that of sickle hemoglobin. The homozygote with two sickle hemoglobin alleles almost invariably dies of a fatal anemia, in spite of the utmost that can be done for him by means of blood transfusions. The homozygote with only standard hemoglobin falls prey, in heavily malarial regions, to that once greatest of human killers. The heterozygote, possessing half sickle hemoglobin and half standard hemoglobin, in such regions far surpasses in survival and reproductive capacity the two homozygotes.

*　　*　　*

The measures of negative eugenics prove ineffective, just as those of euphenics prove self-defeating in a long-term evolutionary sense. Segregating defectives in institutions where they cannot reproduce is temporary, and too often occurs only after the act. Sterilization would be effective only in the case of a simple, readily detected dominant condition, but is of little use in the far more numerous cases of irregularly expressed dominant conditions, recessive traits, and especially multifactorial traits. It cannot discriminate between the alleles whose heterozygote is superior to the homozygous types. Free birth control and contraceptives may be important in population control, but would have little to contribute to the genetic well-being of a population unless accompanied by a level of genetic understanding, counselling, and conscience that today seems remote. . . .

We must turn, then, from negative aspects to positive eugenics, more popularly termed "genetic engineering" today. . . .

For any program of positive selection or genetic manipulation we must clearly establish goals and standards. Difficult, yet easiest, would be to determine that a certain allele A^1 was inferior in quality to its competitor, allele A. Then we might substitute allele A for allele A^1 either euphenically, by introducing the effective gene into the tissues of the recipient whose own allele is A^1, or eugenically, by substituting A for A^1 in the same individual's reproductive cells. It has not been demonstrated at the present date that the latter transformation is feasible, but conceivably a harmless virus carrier might transduce immature sperm cells or ova as readily as cells of liver or kidney. Let us concede that, could this be done in the case of a sufferer from retinoblastoma, the action would be laudable. For the overwhelming majority of genetically conditioned traits, however, no such simple solution is possible. Clearly, for the most significant traits the values and goals are not for science alone to impose—we are concerned with social values, and which of these, we must ask, is preeminent? I once suggested that we might agree upon such goals as "freedom from gross physical or mental defects, sound health, high intelligence, general adaptability, integrity of character, and nobility of spirit." I did not imply that these characteristics were in any case fully or even partially genetic in nature. H. J. Muller selected a different list: "genuine warmth of fellow feeling and a cooperative disposition, a depth and breadth of intellectual capacity, moral courage and integrity, an appreciation of nature and art, and an aptness of expression and of communication;" on the physical side, "to better the genetic foundations of health, vigor, and longevity; to reduce the need for sleep; to bring the induction of sedation and stimulation under more voluntary control; and to develop increasing physical tolerances and aptitudes in general." I suspect that any other scientist will select a different, though overlapping, list.

Nor can we select for such qualities without having ways and means of defining them precisely and measuring them at least roughly in a quantitative way. Obviously, the psychologist and the sociologist will need to do a great deal of preliminary work before genetic analysis and understanding of these traits become possible. At present, human behavior genetics is still a young, rather undeveloped field.

*　　*　　*

It should be feasible, long before the year 2000, to bank human reproductive cells of both sexes in frozen state, as we now do with the sperms of domestic animals, especially sheep and cattle. In this way the reproductive cells of selected individuals might be utilized, even long after death, to produce in the laboratory embryos that might be implanted in the womb of a foster mother, or even, after sufficient development of techniques, to be grown in bottle cultures. The latter "brave new world" technique I do not expect to see realized by the turn of the century. On the other hand, I do expect that techniques will be developed for the cultivation in the laboratory of portions of human ovary and testis permitting successful continuous production of mature ova or sperms. Recent successes in the production of mature ova from cultured mouse ovaries lead me to expect that only persistence by a sufficient number of skilled biologists is needed to attain successful cultivation of human reproductive organs, continuous production of eggs and sperms, and formation by fertilization in the laboratory of as many human embryos as may be wished.

In 1970 piglets conceived in Canada were flown across the Atlantic Ocean in a tube and implanted in a sow of a different breed. The parents were three sows and a boar of the Canadian Yorkshire breed, and the embryos were conceived on March 16 on a Canadian Department of Agriculture farm at Hull, Quebec. The foster mother, at Weybridge, Surrey, has delivered her litter of "improved" piglets. It seems quite clear that the techniques I am describing need only to be applied to mankind, and improved in minor ways.

Geneticists are looking forward to the day when they can practice genetic surgery, that is, really reach in and transform a defective gene and make it functional again. That will not be easy. In the first place, it would have to be done either in the very young embryo, before the cells have begun to multiply, or in the reproductive cells that actually function in making new individuals. . . .

* * *

Another new technique that has extraordinary possibilities lies in the extension to man of the vegetative propagation of the individual. In frogs it has proved possible to implant the nucleus of a skin cell or an intestinal cell in a fertilized frog egg whose own nucleus has been surgically removed or inactivated by ultraviolet light. Young frogs have now been reared to adulthood from such eggs, and prove to have all the genetic characteristics of the strain that provided the implanted nucleus, not those of the original strain or species from which came the egg. It is thus plausible to think that human individuals

might be multiplied from tissues—even long-stored frozen cells—by implantation of the somatic nucleus from such cells into freshly obtained ova. A multiplied clone of Einsteins or Sophia Lorens might turn out to be disappointing on the average, although as identical genetically as any monozygous twins. The experiment would be intriguing.

I am frequently asked why anyone should wish to pursue these goals: "Aren't the age-old ways of making babies good enough?" Several reasons may be given why exploration of such new possibilities is desirable. Only by studying the development of the human embryo and fetus under continuous observation and under various conditions can life scientists really learn what factors produce particular kinds of abnormalities and how these may be corrected or avoided. Moreover, the practice of "prenatal adoption," that is, the implantation of a healthy selected embryo in a foster mother's womb, appears to have fewer religious and legal objections than the present practice of artificial insemination of a woman, without consent of her husband, or even with it. For prenatal adoption is clearly a true *adoption* of a child, *not* a usurpation of a husband's or wife's right to procreate. The development of the implanted fetus within the mother and its normal delivery at full term will surely engender the maternal and paternal feelings of the "parents" far more fully than adoption of a child already several years old. Moreover, most couples who are sterile might in this way have the full experiences of parenthood, apart from transmitting their own genes.

There are other reasons why such practices might be adopted, if not in the United States, then possibly in other countries. Banking of reproductive cells taken from individuals around 20 years of age may serve to prevent the accumulation of detrimental mutations with advancing age. . . . In the presence of the threat of nuclear war, the safest way to ensure the survival and genetic health of future generations would be to carry on these artificial reproductive practices of banking and culture selection, fertilization, and subsequent implantation in subterranean laboratories safe from direct nuclear radiation and fallout.

* * *

Now we come to the most serious aspect of what I term our present crisis of values and goals. How can one select good strains of reproductive cells? If the same material is used to produce a great many embryos which are reared into babies, they will be too much alike, like members of the same caste in *Brave New World*. This difficulty might be avoided by never using a single line of reproductive cells more than a few times. There is another difficulty. Nearly all of us carry some defective genes. The average is probably around eight. We lack visible signs of defect only because most defective genes are recessive; that is, must be inherited in a double dose, coming from both father and mother, in order to produce an evident defect. As long as we have one working gene belonging to any particular pair of genes, enough of the protein it controls is made to satisfy general needs. Close relatives, however, have a greatly heightened probability of carrying the same defective gene because of possessing a common ancestor. It would therefore be necessary to have strict rules to prevent offspring being produced by persons derived from the same lines of banked or cultured reproductive cells, and careful records on the lineage of each person would have to be kept.

In a population suffering severely from overcrowding and subject to rigorous limitations of births, eugenics might be related rather simply to the measures for population control. For example, if a couple that has used up its coupons for two babies wanted additional children they might be required to meet certain genetic tests before receiving a special permit. Some additional children, above the limitation of two per couple, would be needed in some families to maintain the population at the same level, since some women have no children or only one, for a variety of reasons. The simplest eugenic test, yet one that in the long run might be quite effective in improving the population, would be simply to examine the first two children in order to assure that neither one was physically or mentally below average. Beyond the application of so simple a test, eugenic selection runs into frightful dilemmas. Who really possesses a "good" genotype? . . .

. . . When I read in the Bill of Human Rights of the United Nations that one incorrigible right of the individual is to reproduce, and that the right of every person to have a family is a basic human right that must not be infringed, I wonder whether this "right" is indeed to remain unrestricted. Is it not equally a right of every person to be born physically and mentally sound, capable of developing fully into a mature individual? Has society, which must support at great cost the burden of genetic misfortune resulting from mutation, chromosomal accident, and prenatal harm inflicted by trauma or virus, no right at all to protect itself from the increasing misfortunate? Should not the abortion of a seriously defective fetus be obligatory? Should not the loss of a defective child be recompensed by the opportunity to have another, a sound, child by prenatal or postnatal adoption? Can we not devise laws and practices that will improve, even though slowly, the quality of our population while we retain individual choice and freedom to a great extent? Cannot the substitution of a greater freedom of choice in new respects compensate for the restriction of some time-honored privileges?

*   *   *

I wonder what will be the effect of a complete liberation of the sexual life from its relationship to reproduction upon society and upon the family in particular. Recently Robert Morison of Cornell University has pointed out the grave threat to the continuance of the family as the basic social unit. Can we safely, after a million years of human and prehuman evolution during which the family has been the basis of all protection, education, and nurture, give it up? What will be the psychological consequences of a population with no personal ties either to the older generation or to the younger generation? Can we look forward to a brotherhood of mankind when there are no more parents, brothers, or children, only unrelated people?

*   *   *

b.

Joshua Lederberg
Experimental Genetics and
Human Evolution*

*   *   *

The elaboration of euphenics is, however, not the main purpose of a discussion of human evolution, except for the one point—the added difficulties it creates for any measure of human value. If this subject were not at the heart of the eugenic controversy, it would be arrogant to insist on the discussion of it.

Reconsider how we must reevaluate the cumulative score of a human genotype regarded over a lifetime, and for its contribution to the

* 100 *American Naturalist* 519, 522–529, 531 (1966). Copyright © 1966 by the American Naturalist. Reprinted by permission.

human future. Besides present perplexities, look to future perturbations:

1) *Durability*. The mere extension of life-span alters the scores. Performance must be measured over the whole term of life, not based only on youthful precocity.

2) *The euthenic context*. Educational opportunity and practice are changing rapidly. Consider

Recognition of individual diversity. Educators have begun to learn, and exercise the knowledge, that children vary widely in the details of their information-processing machinery, e.g., the relative acuity of their sensory modalities. Many "dull" children must be reclassified as over-specialized; we might well make virtue out of necessity in enabling each child to exploit his inherent skills. . . .

* * *

Western culture and its limited population is being succeeded by a much broader world culture. Is there much point in setting eugenic standards relevant only to a small minority of the world's population even as we watch the unprecedented breakdown of intercultural barriers? The jet airplane has already had an incalculably greater effect on human population genetics than any conceivable program of calculated eugenics.

3) *The world situation*. The central problem for the species must bias any momentary evaluation. Until recently, this was perceived as agricultural efficiency. Hunger still haunts the earth, but we might just manage to marshal the technical resources to assuage it. The specter of the industrialized world is suddenly nuclear suicide, and this has already led to some concern as to the biological adaptation of the species most appropriate to an age dominated by nuclear power. Political institutions are likely to change course much more rapidly than any biological response. As has been pointed out repeatedly, adaptability is man's unique adaptation.

This begs the question how to anticipate future needs, how far adaptability can be generalized, and how well it can compete, in any well-defined microniche, with more rigorous specialization. To put it another way, how do we identify the most adaptable genotypes now living and what is the price, to the detriment in special skills, of this adaptability?

4) *Response to euphenics*. The medico-technological context of human performance is more predictable than the socio-political. We are already committed to the attempted eradication of infectious agents like malaria, tuberculosis, cholera, variola, and poliovirus. In consequence, any breakdown of public health services can be castastrophic by exposing large, imperfectly immunized populations to these parasites. If the interplay of Hemoglobin S and malaria is a useful model, genetic adaptations to a germ-free environment are taking place too; chemical pollution might replace germs as a major selective factor except that its cumulative impact on adults is less cogent than acute infanticide. The context of modern man, in fact, includes steadily increasing reliance on medicine, i.e., euphenics, from ovulation onwards. It makes as little sense to decry genetic adaptations to this as to other components of civilized life. The quality of a genotype cannot now be evaluated in terms of a hypothetical state of nature (wherein we would quickly grunt in chilly displeasure at our unfurred skins), but must match the pragmatic expectations of the milieu of the individual and his descendants. In fact selection is so slow, especially for rare genes, as to make this a theoretical issue for some time. It would be a tour-de-force to demonstrate any change in the frequency of a specific deleterious gene in a human population that could be unambiguously traced to a relaxation of natural selection against it. In comparison to the pace of medical progress, these exigencies are trivial.

As medical practice evolves so does the evaluation of health and vigor. What has happened to pancreatic diabetes is happening to phenylketonuria, and is bound to happen to many other biochemical and developmental diseases. Indeed, it would be no surprise to find compensating advantages, in certain contexts, for some of these genotypes.

* * *

Recall that the most successful exercises in plant breeding have not established pure lines of vigorous individuals. Instead, somewhat over-specialized strains are nutured and the latent resources of individually unpromising parents are merged in vigorous hybrid off-spring. (A good farmer has learned how common sense conflicts with reality when he tries to use ears of hybrid corn as seed for another generation.)

5) *Social adjustment*. We are on the shakiest ground trying to sort out the genetic basis of such social diseases as crime and delinquency. In any case we have a long way to go in elucidating how nature and nurture interact in this field; e.g., what penalty the species would suffer

by extirpating every gene that might in some environment contribute to crime and rebellious behavior. Instability of family life, the estrangement of the generations, and the shallowness of human communication are more prevalent and cumulatively more serious diseases than violent crime, and must be given equal account in any effort to define the "good man," or in any lament of human deterioration.

* * *

6) *The sexual dimorphism.* Most eugenic discussions have been overwhelmingly male-oriented, as is academic life. Western culture is more paradoxical than ever in its assignment of roles to women, and thereby in the design of their education and the advertised criteria of feminine success, stressed by conflicting demands for decoration and utility, dependence and initiative. The lack of useful occupation for many older women is a premonition of the leisure society where "work may become the prerogative of a chosen elite." Half the beneficiaries of eugenic design will be women. Will their creativity and happiness be augmented in a genotype that recombines XX and a set of male-oriented autosomes? Or shall we bypass the dimorphism and evolve a race where this does not matter? To shout "Vive la différence" and then ignore it is hypocrisy.

* * *

7) *The leisure society.* This discussion has been dominated by criteria of performance at work. The whole framework may be obsolescent on the time scale of a few generations. As machines come to do almost all of the work, and this must include managerial and inventive tasks as well as clerical and manual, what are the relevant human values? Will not boredom be the most pernicious disease, and a zest for life without the compulsion of labor the rare essential for the species? Play rather than work will be the substratum of human activity, and the transmutation of play into cultural progress will replace the underpinning by industrial and military technology of its superstructure of basic science.

Perhaps the scientist who works for his joy in it is the most nearly pre-adapted for that topsy-turvy world, obviously an impeccable criterion for eugenic choice.

This leads us finally to algeny. Man is indeed on the brink of a major evolutionary perturbation, but this is not algeny, but *vegetative propagation.* . . .

* * *

Vegetative or clonal reproduction has a certain interest as an investigative tool in human biology, and as an indispensable basis for any systematic algenics; but other arguments suggest that there will be little delay between demonstration and use. Clonality outweighs algeny at a much earlier stage of scientific sophistication, primarily because it answers the technical specifications of the eugenicists in a way that Mendelian breeding does not. If a superior individual (and presumably then genotype) is identified, why not copy it directly, rather than suffer all the risks of recombinational disruption, including those of sex. The same solace is accorded the carrier of genetic disease: why not be sure of an exact copy of yourself rather than risk a homozygous segregant; or at worst copy your spouse and allow some degree of biological parenthood. Parental disappointment in their recombinant offspring is rather more prevalent than overt disease. Less grandiose is the assurance of sex-control; nuclear transplantation is the one method now verified.

Indeed, horticultural practice verifies that a mix of sexual and clonal reproduction makes good sense for genetic design. Leave sexual reproduction for experimental purposes; when a suitable type is ascertained, take care to maintain it by clonal propagation. The Plant Patent Act already gives legal recognition to the process, and the rights of the developer are advertised "Asexual Reproduction Forbidden."

Clonality will be available to and have significant consequences from acts of individual decision—Medawar's piecemeal social engineering—given only community acquiescence or indifference to its practice. But here this simply allows the exercise of a minority attitude, possibly long before its implications for the whole community can be understood. Most of us pretend to abhor the narcissistic motives that would impel a clonist, but he (or she) will pass just that predisposing genotype intact to the clone. Wherever and for whatever motives close endogamy has prevailed before, clonism and clonishness will prevail.

Apogamy as a way of life in the plant world is well understood as an evolutionary cul-de-sac, often associated with hybrid luxuriance. It can be an unexcelled means of multiplying a rigidly well-adapted genotype to fill a stationary niche. So long as the environment remains static, the members of the clone might congratulate themselves that they had outwitted the genetic load;

and they have indeed won a short-term advantage. In the human context, it is at least debatable whether sufficient latent variability to allow for any future contingency were preserved *if* the population were distributed among some millions of clones. From a strictly biological standpoint, tempered clonality could allow the best of both worlds—we would at least enjoy being able to observe the experiment of discovering whether a second Einstein would outdo the first one. How to temper the process and the accompanying social frictions is another problem.

The internal properties of the clone open up new possibilities, e.g., the free exchange of organ transplants with no concern for graft rejection. More uniquely human is the diversity of brains. How much of the difficulty of intimate communication between one human and another, despite the function of common learned language, arises from the discrepancy in their genetically determined neurological hardware? Monozygotic twins are notoriously sympathetic, easily able to interpret one another's minimal gestures and brief words; I know, however, of no objective studies of their economy of communication. For further argument, I will assume that genetic identity confers neurological similarity, and that this eases communication. This has never been systematically exploited as between twins, though it might be singularly useful in stressed occupations—say a pair of astronauts, or a deep-sea diver and his pump-tender, or a surgical team. It would be relatively more important in the discourse between generations, where an older clonont would teach his infant copy. A systematic division of intellectual labor would allow efficient communicants to have something useful to say to one another.

The burden of this argument is that the cultural process poses contradictory requirements of uniformity (for communication) and heterogeneity (for innovation). We have no idea where we stand on this scale. At least in certain areas—say soldiery—it is almost certain that clones would have a self-contained advantage, partly independent of, partly accentuated by, the special characteristics of the genotype which is replicated. This introverted and potentially narrow-minded advantage of a clonish group may be the chief threat to a pluralistically dedicated species.

* * *

My colleagues differ widely in their reaction to the idea that anyone could conscientiously risk the crucial experiment, the first attempt to clone a man. Perhaps this will not be attempted until gestation can be monitored closely to be sure the fetus meets expectations. The mingling of individual human chromosomes with other mammals assures a gradualistic enlargement of the field and lowers the threshold of optimism or arrogance, particularly if cloning in other mammals gives incompletely predictable results.

* * *

Paradoxically, the issue of "subhuman" hybrids may arise first, just because of the touchiness of experimentation on obviously human material. Tissue and organ cultures and transplants are already in wide experimental or therapeutic use, but there would be widespread inhibitions about risky experiments leading to an object that could be labelled as a human or para-human infant. However, there is enormous scientific interest in organisms whose karyotype is augmented by fragments of the human chromosome set, especially as we know so little in detail of man's biological and genetic homology with other primates. This is being and will be pushed in steps as far as biology will allow, to larger and larger proportions of human genome in intact animals, and to organ combinations and chimeras with varying proportions of human, subhuman, and hybrid tissue (note actual efforts to transplant primate organs to man). . . .

NOTE

DAVID M. RORVIK
THE TEST-TUBE BABY IS COMING*

* * *

[W]e are poised for the performance of a medical procedure as dramatic as, and almost certainly more far-reaching than, the heart transplants of the 1960's—embryo implants and transplants. . . . Some recent announcements of successful test-tube fertilizations have been received by the press as "firsts" when, in fact, Dr. John Rock of Harvard, the birth-control pioneer, achieved this back in the 1940's.

He obtained ripe eggs from female patients and then exposed them to sperm in the test tube. No special medium was used to incubate the eggs, and success was slight. None of Dr. Rock's "test-tube babies" grew beyond the three-cell stage. . . .

---

* *Look* 83–86 (May 18, 1971). Reprinted by permission of David M. Rorvick.

Beginning in the 1950's, Dr. Landrum B. Shettles, an assistant professor of obstetrics and gynecology at Columbia University's College of Physicians and Surgeons, refined Dr. Rock's experiments to an art. He became the first to demonstrate conclusively that *in vitro* ("in glass") fertilization of the human ovum is possible. In the course of performing various operations requiring abdominal incision into the peritoneal cavity of the female, Dr. Shettles pierced the ovaries of his patients with a syringe and aspirated, or drew up into the syringe, some of the eggs from their follicles. At the same time, without harming the patient in any way, he drew off some of the follicular fluid, excised tiny pieces of the tubal fimbriae, the fingerlike projections at the end of the Fallopian tubes that "pick up" the egg when it is ejected from the ovary, and aspirated some of the mucosa that abounds within the tubes. From all of this, he formulated the culture mediums in which the egg could mature and undergo fertilization in the test tube.

When the egg, bathed in follicular fluid, was ready for fertilization, Shettles placed it in a sterile Petri dish containing another culture medium. Here the prime ingredient was ovulation mucus taken from the mid-cervical canal of the woman who provided the egg. Into this, he "unleashed" millions of sperm cells and let them fight their way to the egg—just as they would in nature. At the right moment, he added tubal mucosa and the tiny bits of tubal fimbriae in order, again, to provide the chemical components that the sperm cells normally encounter when they pass from the uterus into the tubes, still in pursuit of the egg.

Thus, he became the first man in the world to witness the drama of human fertilization. . . .

* * *

Dr. Shettles . . . grew several of his test-tube babies to the so-called blastocyst stage (64 cells and up). It is at this stage that the egg would normally attach itself to the lining of the uterus, having first made a leisurely five-day trip down the Fallopian tube. When Dr. Shettles first began experimenting, however, too little was known to attempt implanting one of his test-tube embryos in the uterus. Therefore he was forced to sacrifice what he had created.

* * *

Dr. Rock, writing in the *American Journal of Obstetrics and Gynecology* in 1958, said: . . . "The time may be rapidly approaching when the poor woman whose tubes have been excised, yet who still wants a baby, will rejoice that Dr. Shettles will be able to extract an ovum from her ovary . . . then fertilize the egg *in vitro* . . . and finally put it back in the uterus. Thus will he impregnate the woman in spite of the fact that she has no tubes."

Experiments in the 1960's, demonstrating that embryos could, with good results, be transferred from one animal to another, suggested still other possibilities. It appeared that an egg produced by one woman could be implanted in another for any of a number of reasons. Perhaps the donor of the egg, in one instance, has viable tubes but, because of a heart condition, cannot risk the rigors of pregnancy. Still, she *could* procure another woman (probably a sister or other close relative) to carry her child for her. A woman who has viable tubes and normal uterus but nonfunctioning ovaries, on the other hand, could seek out an egg donor, have the ovum fertilized in the test tube by her husband's sperm and then implanted in her uterus. This projected procedure is called "prenatal adoption" and is simply an extension of artificial-insemination techniques already in wide use. Finally, a completely healthy young woman, reluctant to remove herself from a rewarding career for even a few months, might still produce a child by *hiring* another woman to carry her embryo to term.

* * *

Understandably . . . the leaders in the field are maneuvering with great caution. Neither Dr. Shettles nor his chief competitor, a British team led by Dr. Patrick Steptoe of Oldham General Hospital, Lancashire, and Dr. R. G. Edwards of Cambridge University, are presently granting interviews. They prefer, instead, to work quietly behind the scenes while they perfect their techniques. Some of their recent results, however, have been reported in various technical journals, and it has now become possible to make some assessment of their progress.

The British, though they have only recently duplicated Dr. Shettles' decade-old success with *in vitro* fertilization, now appear to be making rapid progress, thanks to a concerted team effort and ample research funds. In 1970, they were at last able to grow several test-tube babies to the blastocyst stage. Since then, they have been examining advanced embryos for cellular defects, to be certain that test-tube fertilization does not result in anomalies that could cause birth defects. The embryos they finally implant, however, will not have the benefit of such examinations, since these would be disruptive to normal growth. "It will probably call for a brave decision," Dr. Steptoe has said, referring to the first implant attempt. . . .

Dr. Shettles, meanwhile, continues to solo, and has only recently applied for Federal funds to help his research. Nonetheless, he has just revealed . . . that he has *already* performed an embryo-transplant operation in the human, a historic step. The circumstances, however, were such that the embryo was not permitted to develop for any length of time. As Dr. Shettles reports it, a nearly mature egg was aspirated from its follicle in the ovary of a woman undergoing an operation to correct a defect in one of the Fallopian tubes. The egg was matured *in vitro*, fertilized with sperm from the woman's husband, grown in a culture for five days to the blastocyst stage and then implanted in the uterus of a second woman. The menstrual cycles of the two women had already been synchronized to insure a hospitable reception for the transplanted embryo.

Two days after the transplant, a previously scheduled hysterectomy (for cancer of the cervix) was performed on the recipient. The implanted embryo was then located, with a dissecting microscope, in the lining of the excised uterus. An examination showed that it had implanted properly. It consisted of several hundred cells at this point and, in Dr. Shettles' words, "no contraindication for continued development was discernible." The objective of the procedure was not to produce a term baby but to determine whether implantation could even occur, given the circumstances of *in vitro* fertilization, and to provide various data before proceeding to "the real thing."

*   *   *

c.

Charles L. Remington
An Experimental Study of Man's Genetic Relationship to Great Apes, by Means of Interspecific Hybridization*

Introduction

Experimental crosses between separate species are becoming a principal source of biological knowledge of evolutionary relationships. Important hybridization studies have been carried

* Unpublished manuscript (1971). Reprinted by permission of the author who retains all rights.

out among mammals, birds, reptiles, amphibians, fishes, several phyla of invertebrates, and most plant groups, but the one species that most interests us, *Homo sapiens,* is not known to have ever been tested in crosses. By contrast, *Homo sapiens* is among the few best-studied species in almost every biological discipline, including anatomy, biochemistry, cytology, ecology, embryology, endocrinology, ethology, epidemiology, genetics, histology, neurobiology, paleontology, parasitology, pathology, physiology, population genetics. Humans are interested in biology because they want and need to know themselves, their relationships to the rest of present day life, and the history of their species. The very great scientific value of well-performed hybridization experiments emphasizes the high priority that should be given to a thorough study of the interspecific genetics of *Homo* with one or more of the three types of pongids (chimpanzee, gorilla, orang) most similar to *Homo.* Because there is a strong possibility that hybrid analysis will significantly clarify and alter present views of our relationships and our past history, such an analysis will not be neglected much longer.

In humane cultures, biomedical researchers have been reluctant to experiment with man, and the philosophical taboos linked with this reluctance have surely been a major factor in postponing hybridization studies until now. However, two other causes may be even more important in the delay: (1) only relatively recently have zoologists in general begun to do sophisticated hybridization research and thereby to perfect the experimental design; (2) for the unique problems of *Homo* x pongid crosses, much of the useful technology mentioned later under "Procedure" is only now being worked out by biomedical specialists in such fields as human and bovine artificial insemination and human tissue culture.

The scientific importance of a *Homo* hybridization experiment is primarily in the great value scientists generally give to knowledge of ourselves. As with every area of biology except the study of mentality, so with hybridization, experiments involving *Homo* are not necessary for our development of generalizations about organisms. Other species of animals with hybridizable relatives would tell us as much about speciation theory, and many such groups would be easier and less expensive to hybridize.

The experiment's human interest value is too obvious to deserve much justification. In fact, an obstacle and distraction to the fullest accomplishment of the ideal *Homo* experiment would be the universal interest there would be in the progress and results of the study. The world press, if aware of the research, would perhaps try to report it as fully as moon exploration or the first heart transplants, an alarming prospect to a scholar in the ivory tower.

The human welfare value of hybridization is not easy to predict. There are dimly perceived biomedical applications that would probably be worth exploring once the initial results of hybridizing *Homo* were available. There are even vaguer speculations on the cultural uses of half-human livestock which are not the forte of the hybridizing biologist but which deserve some debate by thinkers of various backgrounds; at least one famous novel has this theme.

Basic Protocol for Hybridization Experiments

Step 1: Cross ♂ Species A with ♀ Species B. Measure hybrids' developmental rate and physiological normalcy in comparison with non-hybrid Species A and Species B. Record in hybrids the external appearance of all characters likely to alter during growth, such as hair character, color, and distribution. (If possible, actual parents should be tested for fertility by also being mated with their own species; for long-lived animals such as mammals, this would be satisfied if the ♀ parents were chosen from young individuals that have already had offspring and the ♂ parents were proven sires.) Mating even one pair of parents provides significant data, but it is important to try to have at least three replications (i.e., three different pairs of parents), to minimize the possibility that the findings from a single pair were atypical. (For example, suppose that sperm in a single human ejaculate were nonfunctional one time in five; there would thus be a twenty percent likelihood that a single *Homo* x pongid mating would appear sterile from this cause alone. Getting this result twice in a row would only have a four percent likelihood, and thrice in a row less than one percent. Consistent results in three replicates would thus reduce to a negligible level the chance of aberrancy in each of the many results of the experiment.) If hybrids fail to mature, determine the precise development stage at death. If ♂ hybrids do mature sexually, analyze chromosome homology by observing synapsis at meiosis I, from testicular samples (needle biopsies need not harm ♂ mammals).

Step 1A. Cross ♂ Species B with ♀ Species A. Same procedures as in Step 1.

Step 2. Backcross hybrids to both parental species, mating ♂ F₁ with ♀ Species A and ♀ Species B, and ♀ F₁ with ♂ Species A and ♂ Species B. (Do not waste hybrids by doing genetic F₂'s, *i.e.*, sib matings of F₁ hybrids.) Same procedures as with Step 1. This step provides the crucial measure of interspecific hybrid sterility. The backcross offspring provide essential data on heredity of discrete interspecific differences (color, form, electrophoresable enzymes, behavior, etc.).

Plan of this Experiment

1. Species to Be Used.

Because specialists in taxonomy, anatomy, and paleontology are agreed that *Homo* is more closely related to the Pongidae than to any other kind of primate, the ultimate aim of the experiment is to cross *Homo* with at least one pongid species. The gibbons (Hylobatidae) are less similar to *Homo* and are much smaller, so they are less promising than pongids. Using the dissimilarity criterion (but not size), the orangutan (*Pongo pygmaeus*) also ranks rather low. Of the three remaining species, the pigmy chimpanzee (*Pan paniscus*) is both smaller and much rarer than the chimpanzee and is not a prime candidate. That leaves the gorilla, *Gorilla gorilla* (of which there are at least two general geographic types that appear so unlike that they may ultimately prove to be separate species) and the common chimpanzee (*Pan troglodytes*). The gorilla appears to be anatomically and biochemically the most similar to *Homo* and has the best size range, but it has become rare and very expensive and is not ideally suited for breeding in captivity, even of its own kind. By elimination, therefore, *Pan troglodytes* best combines the characteristics of an optimal parental species of the *Homo* hybridization: (1) taxonomic similarity to *Homo;* (2) ease of breeding in captivity; (3) abundant availability; (4) reasonable similarity in size; (5) familiarity to psychologists, anatomists, physiologists, cytologists, and biochemists, so that characteristics of the F₁ hybrid *Homo sapiens* x *Pan troglodytes* could be compared immediately with both parents without new research on an unknown parent. In the rest of this account, the generic name *Pan* will refer only to *P. troglodytes*. Should this cross fail, however, it would still be necessary to attempt the *Homo* x *Gorilla* cross before concluding that *Homo* is not hybridizable with any other species. Although this last combination would always be of great interest, if the *Homo* x *Pan* cross succeeds, trying the *Gorilla* cross would be much less important. For a modern analysis of relatedness, all of the following should eventually be carried out, in about this priority ranking: (1) *Homo* x *Pan;* (2) *Pan* x *Gorilla;* (3) *Pan* x *Pongo;* (4) *Homo* x *Gorilla;* (5) *Homo* x *Pongo;* (6) *Gorilla* x *Pongo;* (7) *Pan* x *Hylobates.*

2. *Procedure.*

A classical hybridization experiment usually includes reciprocal crosses; e.g., ♂ *Homo* x ♀ *Pan* and ♀ *Homo* x ♂ *Pan.* However, a recent survey of interspecific hybrids throughout the animal kingdom shows that reciprocal crosses usually give the same or nearly the same results. Therefore, it is probably satisfactory for this experiment to make only the Step 1 cross: female chimpanzee inseminated with human sperm. However, when tissue-culturing techniques are developed (probably soon) allowing mammalian zygotes to be formed and reared in culture, *Homo* ova should obviously be treated with *Pan* (and *Gorilla, Pongo, Hylobates,* and even *Macaca*) sperm, in order to study at least the early stages of embryonic development in the reciprocal hybrid.

This experiment would include the involvement of specialists in several fields, in order to obtain all the important types of data and to maximize chances for success in Steps 1 and 2. In addition to the principal investigator, a speciation geneticist, the following collaborators would be arranged:

(a) primate-care specialists, probably in one of the National Regional Primate Laboratories, to care for the mothers and to be prepared to bottle-raise hybrid infants;

(b) an obstetrical surgeon, available should caesarian section of hybrids be required, and possibly to perform abortions if necessary to remove and analyze embryos that do not develop to parturition;

(c) artificial insemination specialists to treat the *Homo* sperm, inseminate the *Pan* females, and attempt to use known fertility treatments should fertilization be difficult to produce;

(d) a human cytologist to analyze the hybrids' chromosomes, especially during meiotic synapsis after obtaining bioptic testicular samples;

(e) a protein specialist, to investigate electrophoretically the enzymes and other proteins

of the hybrids (DNA and cytochrome sequencing might be needed as well);

(f) psychometrists or ethologists, to assay behavioral characteristics of the hybrids, including learning, memory, emotions, facial expressions, and manipulative ability;

(g) specialists in dermatoglyphics, hair micro-structure, hair pigmentation, and other details of the hybrid phenotype;

(h) a mammalian tissue-culture specialist already working on fertilization and early development in culture.

Ethical and Legal Aspects

In the course of many years of gathering together the world's scientific literature related to animal hybridization, I have been able to discern several patterns that recur in so many different kinds of animals that they are probably applicable to *Homo* x pongid crosses: (1) mammals this similar probably can be cross-fertilized, and there is a reasonable likelihood that the embryos will develop fully and that the infants will grow past the nursing stage; (2) there is a small chance that sexually mature hybrids will show at least some successful gametogenesis and therefore allow a measure of fertility; (3) in line with Haldane's "Rule," it is fairly likely that maturing F_1 hybrids will all be female (the homogametic sex); (4) conspicuous interspecific differences tend to exhibit simple Mendelian heredity, and the hybrids therefore will tend to be like one parent in some prominent characters, the other parent in some, and to show blending inheritance in a few, and none of these characters can have its dominance relations reliably predicted prior to experimental tests; (5) size tends to be polygenic, however, and the foetus would therefore tend to be intermediate in size between *Homo* and pongid foetuses, making it desirable to use genetically small *Homo* as the sperm source; (6) many hybrids show heterosis (hybrid vigor), including long life. These guesses suggest that *Homo* can be hybridized and hybrids reared, that they may all be females, that they will resemble *Homo* in some characters and the pongid parent in others, unpredictably, and that the hybrid will be largely but perhaps not totally sterile and may have a long life-potential.

Ethically, the scientist might be expected to have the same responsibilities for humane care of these hybrids as for any other experimental mammals. He should also have the same freedom to operate on the hybrids and to sacrifice them for study, although most of the essential data could probably be obtained without sacrificing.

Legally, it appears appropriate that the contribution of one-half of the genetical material by *Homo* should not make the hybrid subject to the legal protections and obligations of a human in the nation in which the experiment is carried out. However, if a hybrid were successfully backcrossed to *Homo*, the new offspring would of course be 0.75 *Homo*, and very interesting legal and ethical questions would then arise. Backcross hybrids, incidentally, would be likely to have substantially higher fertility than F_1 hybrids. If a hybrid were successfully backcrossed to the pongid species, on the other hand, backcross hybrids would raise even fewer questions of legal humanness than would the F_1 hybrids.

Other challenging questions in this realm might be raised if the ♀ parent of the cross were a human female volunteer, but the present experimental design is not concerned with this reciprocal combination except in the future situation in which human ova could be cultured and fertilized outside the uterus.

NOTE

Sir William Blackstone
Commentaries on the Laws of England*

*   *   *

A monster, which hath not the shape of mankind, but in any part evidently bears the resemblance of the brute creation, hath no inheritable blood, and cannot be heir to any land, albeit it be brought forth in marriage: but, although it hath deformity in any part of its body, yet if it hath human shape it may be heir. This is a very ancient rule in the law of England; and its reason is too obvious and too shocking to bear a minute discussion. . . . [Those who are born with a form not human are not considered children; as when a woman by a perversion of nature brings forth something monstrous or prodigious. Nevertheless the offspring to which nature has only added or from which withheld something, as if it should have six or only four fingers, ought to be reckoned among children, and though its limbs be useless or distorted, yet it is not a monstrous birth. (Bracton)]

*   *   *

———
* *Book the Second—of the Rights of Things* 246–247 (1756).

3.
Interferences with Mores and Laws

a.

John McLean Morris and
Gertrude van Wagenen
Compounds Interfering with Ovum
Implantation and Development—
The Role of Estrogens*

In an effort to discover an effective postcoital antifertility agent, a variety of compounds . . . have been studied. A number of these which have proved extremely effective in inhibiting ovum implantation and development in the rabbit and other species have been found to have little or no effect in the primate.

Three years ago, work was commenced on the first compound which met the fundamental requirements of being nontoxic, nonteratogenic, and 100 per cent effective: ORF-3858 (2-methyl-3-ethyl-4phenyl-Δ-cyclohexenecarboxylic acid). The "all-or-none" nature of the response in the rabbit and the absence of any fetal abnormalities in marginal doses suggested the value of trial in the primate.

The similarity of the menstrual cycle of the rhesus monkey (*Macaca mulatta*) to that of the female human being makes any data concerning mating and pregnancy in this animal of significant interest. ORF-3858 proved effective in the macaque. When administered orally in 10 mg. doses for the first six days following positive mating (three days for possible sperm survival plus three for effective period of action) there were no pregnancies.

Investigations to study the mechanism of action of this compound revealed that it had certain estrogenic properties, prompting a further evaluation of estrogens themselves.

It has been known for many years that estrogens interfere with early pregnancy in the rabbit and other species. With the control of conception assuming today such tremendous importance, it is surprising to note, as Parkes does, that "there has been, so far as I know, no determined effort to see whether the administration of estrogen during the third week of the human cycle would prevent any implantation that might otherwise take place."

———
* 96 *American Journal of Obstetrics and Gynecology* 804–808, 810–812 (1966). Reprinted by permission.

Estradiol-17β, stilbestrol, ethinyl estradiol, and mestranol (as well as ORF-3858) will not only prevent implantation, but when given to the rabbit later, in larger doses, will also result in placental separation and death of the fetus. . . .

In spite of such observations in lower species, it is obvious that human pregnancy cannot be interrupted in such fashion by the administration of estrogens. Similarly, in the macaque, the oral or intramuscular administration of stilbestrol or estradiol dipropionate after implantation (on days 18 to 167) appeared to have little effect on the development of the fetus. . . . Of 20 animals so treated, 3 aborted, an incidence of 15 per cent. This does not vary significantly from the 10 per cent expected abortion rate in this colony. There were no fetal abnormalities produced.

Efforts were undertaken, however, to see if estrogens in sufficient dosages in the primate might prevent implantation if administered immediately after mating. Observations on the timing of ovulation in macaques in our laboratory indicate that days 11 and 12 constitute the mode, and that 32 per cent of the first positive matings at this time were followed by pregnancy when the monkeys were carefully selected (on the basis of such factors as age) for probable fertility.

Experimental animals. A total of 28 monkeys were employed in this study, 26 multiparous females and 2 nulliparous. For the 26 multiparous monkeys, 42 pregnancies were recorded during the 3 years before the experiments on contraception were begun, and 18 were pregnant in the year that immediately preceded the experiments. Although identical breeding conditions have been maintained during the period of contraceptive trial, no pregnancies have occurred when ORF-3858 (10 mg.), stilbestrol (1 to 25 mg.), or estradiol (10 mg.) was given orally for 6 days following positive mating. In 3 years of normal breeding, there were 204 positive matings with 42 pregnancies; in up to 2 years of normal breeding with treatment, there were 321 positive matings without pregnancy. . . .

*　　*　　*

Preliminary clinical trials

In spite of confidence that success in the macaque should be paralleled by success in man, initial human experimentation was undertaken with some trepidation.

The first cases were rape cases. All of the subjects received 50 mg. of stilbestrol for 4 to 6 days after exposure. The chance of pregnancy following rape is uncertain for many obvious reasons. Sometimes no sperm could be found in the cervix or vagina. In a few instances, temperature charts were started; if no rise occurred, no drug was given. In most of the cases accepted for treatment, exposure occurred near midcycle and fern crystallization of cervical mucus as well as presence of sperm were demonstrated. In this small series of patients, none has become pregnant so far. . . .

A limited number of courageous volunteers furnished an opportunity for further and more adequate observation. Coitus took place at midcycle near the time of the temperature rise. . . .

*　　*　　*

In these preliminary trials there have been no pregnancies. While of interest, these clinical studies are incomplete and have as yet no statistical significance.

*　　*　　*

Just how these compounds prevent implantation is unknown. Accelerated tubal transport may be a factor, but this does not explain their effectiveness in the rabbit after implantation. . . .

*　　*　　*

Regardless of the mechanism involved, the implication of these observations is apparent: the administration of these agents in the third week of the menstrual cycle in women may inhibit implantation of the fertilized ovum. . . .

*　　*　　*

NOTE

CONNECTICUT GENERAL STATUTES (1958)

*　　*　　*

Sec. 53–29. *Attempt to procure miscarriage or abortion.* Any person who gives or administers to any woman, or advises or causes her to take or use anything, or uses any means, with intent to procure upon her a miscarriage or abortion, unless the same is necessary to preserve her life or that of her unborn child, shall be fined not more than one thousand dollars or imprisoned in the State Prison not more than five years or both.

Sec. 53–30. *Abortion or miscarriage.* Any woman who does or suffers anything to be done, with intent thereby to produce upon herself miscarriage or abortion, unless necessary to preserve her life or that of her unborn child, shall be fined not more than five hundred dollars or imprisoned not more than two years or both.

Sec. 53–31. *Encouraging the commission of abortion.* Any person who, by publication, lecture or otherwise or by advertisement or by the sale or circulation of any publication, encourages or prompts to the commission of the offenses described in section 53–29 or 53–30, or who sells or advertises medicines or instruments or other devices for the commission of any of said offenses except to a licensed physician or to a hospital approved by the state department of health, or who advertises any so-called monthly regulator for women, shall be fined not more than five hundred dollars or imprisoned not more than one year or both.

Sec. 53–32. *Use of drugs or instruments to prevent conception.* Any person who uses any drug, medicinal article or instrument for the purpose of preventing conception shall be fined not less than fifty dollars or imprisoned not less than sixty days nor more than one year or be both fined and imprisoned.

*   *   *

b.
William H. Masters and Virginia E. Johnson
Human Sexual Inadequacy*

While developing therapy concepts and procedural patterns at onset of the clinical investigative approach to sexual dysfunction in 1959, there were many severe problems to be faced. One of the most prominent concerns was the demand to develop a psychosocial rationale for therapeutic control of unmarried men and women that might be referred for treatment. During the past 11 years, 54 men and 3 women were unmarried when referred by their local authority with complaints of sexual dysfunction. In a statistical breakdown relative to intake diagnosis, 16 men were premature ejaculators, one was an incompetent ejaculator, 21 were primarily impotent, and 16 were secondarily impotent. The three women were orgasmically dysfunctional, one primarily and two situationally (coital orgasmic inadequacy).

The immediate problem to be faced was the obvious clinical demand for a female partner

—a partner to share the patient's concerns for successful treatment, to cooperate in developing physically the suggestions presented during sessions in therapy, and, most important, to exemplify for the male various levels of female responsivity. All of these factors are essential, if effective sexual functioning is to be returned to the sexually inadequate man. In brief, someone to hold on to, talk to, work with, learn from, be a part of, and above all else, *give to* and *get from* during the sexually dysfunctional male's two weeks in the acute phase of therapy.

The term *replacement partner* is used to describe the partner of his or her choice brought by a sexually inadequate unmarried man or woman to share the experiences and the education of the clinical therapy program. *Partner surrogate* has been reserved to indicate the partner provided by the cotherapists for an unmarried man referred for treatment who has no one to provide psychological and physiological support during the acute phase of the therapy. . . .

Thirteen of the 54 nonmarried men brought replacement partners of choice who were most willing to cooperate with the therapists to enable their sexually dysfunctional men to establish effective sexual performance. The three nonmarried women also brought replacement partners of their choice to participate in therapy. These replacement partners were men with whom they had established relationships of significant duration, as well as the personal warmth and security that develops from free exchange of vulnerability and affection.

Partner surrogates have been made available for 41 men during the last 11 years. This situation has involved basic administrative and procedural decisions. Should the best possible climate for full return of therapeutic effort be created for the incredibly vulnerable unmarried males referred for constitution or reconstitution of sexual functioning; or should there be professional concession to the mores of society, with full knowledge that if a decision to dodge the issue was made, a significant increase in percentage of therapeutic failure must be anticipated? Unmarried impotent men whose dysfunctional status could be reversed to allow assumption of effective roles in society would continue sexually incompetent. From a clinical point of view there really was only one alternative. Either the best possible individual return from therapeutic effort must be guaranteed the patient, or the Foundation must refuse to treat unmarried men or

---

* Boston: Little, Brown & Co. 146–155 (1970). Reprinted by permission.

women for the symptoms of sexual inadequacy. Either every effort must be made to meet the professional responsibility of accepting referrals of severely dysfunctional men and women from authority everywhere in or out of the country, or admission to clinical procedure must be denied. It would have been inexcusable to accept referral of unmarried men and women and then give them statistically less than 25 percent chance of reversal of their dysfunctional status by treating them as individuals without partners. This figure has been reached by culling the literature for material published from other centers, since it is against Foundation policy to treat the sexually dysfunctional individual as a single entity. If the concept that therapy of both partners for sexual inadequacy has great advantage over prior clinical limitations to treatment of the sexually dysfunctional individual without support of marital partner, then partners must be available. Statistically there no longer is any question about the advantage of educating and treating men and women together when attacking the clinical concerns of male or female sexual inadequacy. For these reasons the therapeutic technique of replacement partners and partner surrogates will continue as Foundation policy.

It should be emphasized that no thought was ever given to employing the prostitute population. For reasons that will become obvious as the contributions of the replacement-partner and partner-surrogate populations are described, so much more is needed and demanded from a substitute partner than effectiveness of purely physical sexual performance that to use prostitutes would have been at best clinically unsuccessful and at worst psychologically disastrous.

Women volunteered for this assignment of partner surrogate. Over the last 11 years, 13 women have been accepted from a total of 31 volunteers for assignment as partner surrogates. Their ages ranged from 24 to 43 years when they joined the research program. Although all but two of the women have been previously married, none of the volunteers were married when living their role as a partner surrogate.

The levels of formal education for the partner surrogates were high-school graduate (3), additional formal secretarial training (2), college matriculation (2), college graduates (4), and post-graduate degrees in biological and behavioral sciences (2). Nine of the 13 women had a child or children before joining the program. Ten of these women also were committed

to full-time employment outside of their role as partner surrogate; one did part-time volunteer work and the remaining two were caring for very young children.

Every effort has been made to screen from this section of the total research population women with whom the cotherapist did not feel totally secure attitudinally or socially, and approximately 60 percent of those women voluntering for roles as partner surrogate were not accepted. Of the 13 women accepted, 6 had previously served as members of the study-subject population during the physiological investigative phase of the research program, and 7 volunteered their services for this specific clinical function.

The reasons expressed for such voluntary cooperation were varied but of real significance. During the screening process, each woman was interrogated in depth while the interviewers were acquiring medical, social, and sexual histories from which to evaluate the individual's potential as a partner surrogate. The investigation was conducted by male and female interrogators both singly and in teams. If interrogation indicated potential as a substitute partner, the three involved individuals (volunteer and interrogators) discussed this concept in detail, examining both the positive and the negative aspects of such a service. No attempt ever was made to persuade any women to serve as a partner surrogate. Volunteers who showed hesitancy or evidence of personal concern were eliminated from this potential role in the research program.

Of major interest was the fact that 9 of the 13 volunteers were interested in contributing their services on the basis of personal knowledge of sexual dysfunction or sex-oriented distress within their immediate family. . . .

*   *   *

Of the remaining four volunteers, three women had more prosaic reasons for essaying the role of a partner surrogate. The expressed needs were unresolved sexual tensions, a need for opportunity of social exchange, and an honest interest in helping dysfunctional men repair their ego strengths as sexually adequate males. Finally, a physician, frankly quite curious about the partner-surrogate role, offered her services to evaluate the potentials (if any) of the role. When convinced of the desperate need for such a partner in the treatment of sexual dysfunction in the unmarried male, she continued as a partner surrogate, contributing both personal and professional experiences to develop the role to a peak of effectiveness.

*   *   *

The specific function of the partner surrogate is to approximate insofar as possible the role of a supportive, interested, cooperative wife. Her contributions are infinitely more valuable as a means of psychological support than as a measure of physiological initiation, although obviously both roles are vitally necessary if a male's inadequacies of sexual performance are to be reversed successfully. . . .

*   *   *

When assuming an active role in the clinical therapy of any sexually incompetent man, the partner surrogate is given detailed information of the individual male's psychosexual background and the cause for and specifics of his sexual dysfunction, and is kept thoroughly informed on a day-to-day basis as to the professional teams' concept of therapeutic progress. No other identifiable personal details of the involved male other than name are ever provided. Even this is masked if the name is well-known. The patient is cautioned against providing relevant personal information. In the same vein, the partner surrogate never exchanges any personal information that might lead to her identification in the future.

Shortly after the roundtable discussion . . . , the first meeting between the patient and his partner surrogate is arranged. The first meeting is always limited to a social commitment. Usually the couple go to dinner and spend a casual evening in order to develop communication and comfort in each other's company. . . .

*   *   *

Once social exchange has been established, the partner surrogate moves into a wife's role as the treatment phase is expanded. She joins the sexually inadequate male in both social and physical release of the tensions that accrue during the therapy. With the exception of attending the individual therapy sessions, every step that a wife would take as a participant with her husband in the therapeutic program is taken with the dysfunctional nonmarried male by his partner surrogate.

*   *   *

In view of the statistics there is no question that the decision to provide partner surrogates for sexually incompetent unmarried men has been one of the more effective clinical decisions made during the past eleven years devoted to the development of treatment for sexual inadequacy.

*   *   *

Thirteen women have accompanied unmarried men to the Foundation, agreeing to serve as replacement partners to support these men during treatment for sexual dysfunction. In all instances both individuals were accepted in therapy with full knowledge of the referring authority. Since the women were selected by the men involved, they were accepted as if they were wives. They were interrogated in depth and attended all therapy sessions. They lived with the unmarried males as marital partners, in contrast to the partner surrogate, who spent only specific hours during each day with the sexually dysfunctional male. Details of treatment for the various forms of male sexual dysfunction need not be repeated; clinical situations with replacement partners are managed in the same way as with wives.

*   *   *

Three unmarried women referred to the Foundation brought with them replacement partners of their choice. In each instance the current relationship was one of significant duration. The shortest span of mutual commitment was reported as six months. Two of the three women have previously been married. The replacement partners were treated as husbands of sexually inadequate wives. They attended all sessions and went through in-depth history-taking to provide information sufficient to define their roles in providing relief for their distressed women companions.

NOTES

NOTE 1.
SEX RESEARCHERS ARE SUED BY EX-PATIENT FOR $750,000*

Dr. William Masters and Mrs. Virginia Johnson, the sex researchers, have been sued for $750,000 on the ground that they used the plaintiff's wife to give sexual treatment to two men patients.

The suit was filed yesterday in United States District Court in St. Louis by George E. Calvert,

* *The New York Times* 20, col. 1 (August 26, 1970). © 1970 by the New York Times Co. Reprinted by permission.

who stated in his complaint that he lived in New Hampshire.

Dr. Masters and Mrs. Johnson issued a statement saying "Our reaction is that any such charge is ridiculous. We can prove it."

Mr. Calvert alleged that he and his wife, Barbara, had been patients of Dr. Masters and that the doctor had "breached the patient-doctor relationship in procuring the said Barbara Calvert to engage in sexual intercourse" with two co-defendants identified as "John Doe 1" of New York and "John Doe 2" of Virginia.

Mr. Calvert alleged that Dr. Masters and Mrs. Johnson had paid Mrs. Calvert $500 and $250 for her services to the two John Doe defendants. He contended that they charged John Doe 1 $3,000 for his treatment and John Doe 2 an unspecified amount.

* * *

The husband charged that Dr. Masters and Mrs. Johnson had induced Mrs. Calvert to keep her activities a secret from him.

* * *

NOTE 2.

MISSOURI REVISED STATUTES (1949)

§563.010. [A]ny person who procures a female inmate for a house of prostitution; or who shall induce, persuade, encourage, inveigle or entice a female person to become a prostitute; or who by promises, threats, violence or by any device or scheme, shall cause or influence a female person to become an inmate of a house of . . . assignation, . . . or any person who . . . by abuse of any position of confidence or authority shall cause or influence any female person to enter any place within this state in which prostitution is practiced, encouraged, or allowed, . . . or who shall receive or give, or agree to receive or give any money or thing of value for procuring or attempting to procure any female person to become a prostitute or to come into this state or leave this state for the purpose of prostitution shall be guilty of pandering, and upon conviction shall be punished by a fine of not less than one hundred dollars nor more than one thousand dollars or by imprisonment in the penitentiary for a term of not less than two years nor more than five years.

§563.130. [A]ny person or persons or corporation who shall directly or indirectly establish, keep, permit or maintain any . . . assignation house . . . in this state shall in addition to other penalties prescribed by the laws of the state of Missouri be deemed guilty of a nuisance, and all buildings, erections, rooms and places, and the ground itself in or upon which such . . . assignation house . . . is conducted, permitted, carried on, maintained or continued are also declared nuisances, and all such nuisances shall be enjoined and abated as herein provided.

NOTE 3.

HUSBAND AND WIFE—
CRIMINAL CONVERSATION*

* * *

§476. [W]henever a third person commits adultery with either spouse, he or she commits a tortious invasion of the rights of the other spouse, from which a cause of action for criminal conversation arises. At common law such a cause of action exists in favor of the husband against one who commits adultery with his wife, and this right of action is not affected by the Married Women's Property Acts. The wife also, under the Married Women's Acts, according to the weight of authority, may maintain an action for criminal conversation with her husband. . . .

The causes of action for criminal conversation and for alienation of affections are alike in that each arises from the marriage relation, and each is for a tort against the right to consortium; but they differ in that the latter is for loss of consortium or affection and does not necessarily, though it may, involve adulterous intercourse, whereas the former is for the adulterous intercourse or criminal conversation, and the alienation of affections and other consequent injuries to the consortium, such as loss of service, are only matters of aggravation and not necessary to the cause of action. . . .

* * *

§478. [I]t is no defense to an action for criminal conversation that the defendant was led into the adulterous intercourse through the acts and practices of the plaintiff's spouse instead of being himself the seducer, although that fact may be shown in mitigation of damages.

* * *

---

* 41 *American Jurisprudence* 2d §§476, 478. Rochester, N.Y.: The Lawyers Co-operative Publishing Company 402–404 (2d ed. 1968). Copyright © 1968 by Jurisprudence Publishers, Inc. Reprinted by permission.

c.
State v. Daniel Richard Martin*

SUPERIOR COURT
LITTLETOWN COUNTY
OCTOBER 4 & 5, 1955
LITTLETOWN, CONNECTICUT
STATE
v.
DANIEL RICHARD MARTIN

Before
Honorable ELMER W. RYAN, Judge
Appearances
THOMAS F. WALL, ESQ., State's Attorney
CHARLES R. EBERSOL, ESQ., Defendant's
Counsel

* * *

THE CLERK: How old are you, Mr. Martin?
THE ACCUSED: Fifty-two.
THE CLERK: You are charged in the first count of the information of the State's Attorney with the crime of indecent assault. How do you wish to plead?
MR. EBERSOL: May it please the Court, we would like permission to file a plea of *nolo contendere* to this and on the second count of the information.
MR. WALL: No objection by the State's Attorney, Your Honor.
THE COURT: Well, no objection by the State; plea of *nolo contendere* is accepted. . . .
MR. WALL: In view of the plea, I move, Your Honor, that a finding of guilty be entered on the basis of the plea.
THE COURT: Finding of guilty is entered on both counts.
MR. WALL: The defendant, Your Honor, is a physician. He was born in Bloomington, Illinois in 1902. Comes from a very good family. He has been known fairly generally as Richard Martin although his name is stated correctly in the substitute information. He has never married. He attended the elementary and high schools of his home town, graduated from college, graduated from a prominent medical school in 1927. He served as House Officer in training at his medical school at the hospital connected therewith two years; and he came to Connecticut in 1929 where he was physician for a private school

* Richard C. Donnelly, Joseph Goldstein, and Richard D. Schwartz: *Criminal Law*. New York: The Free Press 11–28 (1962). Reprinted by permission of The Macmillan Company.

in this county for five years. For five years after that, he taught pediatrics at a medical school and then he taught the same subject at another medical school from 1939 to 1946, and he returned to Littletown in 1946, and he has practiced pediatrics there until his arrest. He maintained an office in Littletown although his name did not appear at the office on the door. He was in the same office with three other physicians. These charges originated during the month of August, a complaint to my office concerning the Doctor by a mother of three children aged nine, ten and thirteen.

In the Spring of this year, one of these three children, the middle one, aged ten—I believe he was probably nine years of age when he was first treated—went to a clinic as a result of a very severe, chronic condition involving an extreme case of stuttering—stuttered to such an extent that he barked like a dog; and he went for psychiatric treatments and took them for a short period of time at this clinic; and, at that time, it was recommended that he be under the care of Dr. Martin.

Now as I have stated, Dr. Martin practiced pediatrics in his office. . . . He lived pretty generally in the woods about two or three miles away from his office at a very beautiful spot on top of a mountain in Littletown owned by a public-spirited person, well-known in the community who had confidence in the Doctor and felt that he could use her land for what you might call a "camp" or a "clinic." . . .

The Doctor had, for a number of years, taken boys and, sometimes, girls to this camp; and so far as any of the clinics or outside agencies . . . knew, the Doctor was using psychiatric treatment of his own on these boys although he made it plain that he was not a psychiatrist; and his treatment, so far as anyone knew, was to have these boys reside in a cabin which was very, very crude on the side of the lake. . . .

And the theory as stated to agencies and institutions who came in contact with Dr. Martin was that these boys would get back to nature, that they would take care of their physical needs chopping wood, cooking their own meals, and making their own beds; and that personal observation on the part of the Doctor, and supervision upon his part, and the beautiful surroundings, and taking advantage of keeping these boys busy at their occupations of maintaining themselves at the camp would have some therapeutic value; and over the years, the Doctor acquired a very good reputation for caring for these boys;

and he evidently had some results that were looked upon as—by others as having been good. As a matter of fact, the case of this ten-year-old boy was also a case which was widely talked of in psychiatric circles as attesting to the Doctor's reputation. He was told on a number of occasions that this young boy had been cured, or very nearly cured, of his habit of barking like a dog, and that the Doctor was given some credit for it.

. . . In the early Spring, probably in April, when recommendation was made that the—this nine- or ten-year-old boy be sent to Dr. Martin, he went down there to the camp; and he remained there fairly steadily from April until the summer for quite some time. The Doctor told him that—and told the family—that it was best for them not to go near him, or not to take him away from the camp; and after he had been there for a number of months, the Doctor asked the family to send down his older brother aged thirteen and the younger brother aged nine to the camp in order that he might study their case histories to give him a better understanding of the case of the ten-year-old, the middle of the three.

Shortly after the arrival of the ten-year-old boy, about a week after he went to the cabin, the doctor started to commit homosexual acts upon the ten-year-old boy: and according to the statement of the ten-year-old boy, these acts took place twice a week over a period of four months which would indicate approximately, according to my calculations from this statement, approximately thirty-two homosexual acts. Those were acts where the Doctor, himself, committed acts upon the boy and had the boy commit acts upon him; and upon one occasion, there was an act described by the boy as an act by the Doctor attempting to commit sodomy.

*   *   *

The thirteen-year-old boy stayed down there for about a week; and he made other visits which lasted, all together, about three weeks.

The nine-year-old boy went there for a week in the early part of the summer, and he was there from August first to August seventh, the week before the arrest. When the nine-year-old boy got back to his home after a visit there, through an incident of the mother warning the nine-year-old boy to stay away from a certain person in their neighborhood, having nothing to do with this case, who was considered by the mother as being queer, the young boy—nine-year-old—made a statement to his mother in answer to this caution. Quote, "Why, is he a pig like Dr. Martin?"

She then questioned the nine-year-old boy, and the nine-year-old boy related circumstances to the mother of a disgusting nature of the very same conduct as has been related, and—.

THE COURT: What you say "the very same type of conduct," are you referring to homosexual practices?

MR. WALL: They were, Your Honor. There were at least three acts during August with this nine-year-old boy and one act that was either sodomy or bordered upon sodomy; and this nine-year-old boy was also involved—which is not accountable, necessarily, to the Doctor—with an act with a fifteen-year-old boy who was also down there for treatment. In other words, it was—as far as this nine-year-old boy being there a week or two, he just got into a nest of homosexuality over which the Doctor evidently presided. He didn't see these acts, but nevertheless, having participated in them also, in an approving way, it was not to be expected that the children, themselves, would refrain from them between themselves; and this fifteen-year-old boy did molest the nine-year-old boy while he was there.

All this was told to the mother by the nine-year-old boy. Perhaps not all of it, but enough that the mother immediately notified the authorities, and she got the other children back from there without exciting suspicion; and statements were taken from the children—the three of them; and the thirteen-year-old boy told a similar story of at least six acts over a two-week period that he was there, all with Dr. Martin, all upon his solicitation.

. . . There was also this fifteen-year-old boy who had been at the camp for one year and three months; and there was another sixteen-year-old who had been there for a number of years; and there were acts related between the fifteen-year-old boy and the sixteen-year-old boy. Now, there is no act between the Doctor and the fifteen-year-old boy, but there was of the sixteen-year-old boy.

Now, this sixteen-year-old boy had acts with the ten-year-old boy, with the one who was being treated there; and he also had acts with the fifteen-year-old boy, and he also had acts with Dr. Martin once a month over a period of the two years that he was there; and the acts with the sixteen-year-old boy at some times were either sodomy or very close to sodomy. . . .

*   *   *

The information which we have concerning the ten-year-old boy concerning his—the progress of his stuttering was that while there appeared to be a slight improvement while he was there for a while, that, actually, the trouble got worse and the trouble is worse than ever at the present time.

However, this particular case has been cited as showing some of the remarkable cures that the Doctor effects. I don't say that the Doctor doesn't effect some cures in some phases of medicine. I believe he is quite a capable man in his own field. He certainly has a very good reputation in his field; and he, aside from his homosexual proclivities, is able to treat people rather well and has an understanding of human nature. . . .

* * *

MR. EBERSOL: [I]n my talks with Mr. Wall, the question of sodomy never came up; and had there been any such charge, they would have been denied.

I believe, as he stated—he was certainly speaking the truth—that the statement made by these youths might be so interpreted. As he said, they were susceptible of several interpretations.

There is a host of people who would like to be in my shoes right now—other lawyers, doctors, clergymen, teachers, heads of schools, public officials, social workers, leaders in the field of working with disturbed children, prominent people in public life, rich and intellectual, poor, humble and uneducated, mothers and fathers of radically sick children, and some of these once-derelict and lost boys, themselves, would like to be here in Court to speak; and all these and many others who would fill this courtroom many times over would attest to Dr. Martin's medical skill, to his integrity and courage, and attest to his living selfless and untiring ministrations to children and parents alike; and, in a sense, I am their agent as well as the attorney for the defendant.

Never, I am sure, in the history of Little-town County Jail, has one of its involuntary guests received so many visitors or such a flood of mail. I have here just a few of the letters the doctor has received. These letters are the sincere outpourings of people—of people of all ages and from every walk of life who knew the accused or his good works or both; and what do they say with one accord?

Simply stated it is, "We have faith in your integrity and know that you never did anything which you did not feel was in the very best interests of your boys." Would that all of them might speak for themselves, but the nature of our plea does not permit it. Therefore, I would like to give

The Court a few excerpts of representative letters.

* * *

From a mother in Wilberham: "Our prayers are with you, and we hope that they and those of so many people in Wilberham help a little." There is a postscript. "As I have said to you before, we have felt that one of the finest memories of childhood we could give our youngsters is knowing Dr. Martin. How long will the world take to realize that all the great advancements of science have been made by men working alone?"

* * *

From a master in a private school: "We think of you constantly and are desperately sorry that your wonderful work has had to be interrupted. I want to add that our belief in your personal integrity has not been changed. We realize that your medical skill and knowledge caused you to take steps not readily understood by a layman."

From a foster-mother: "We have felt deeply grateful to you these past years for the kind, considerate care you have given our young—the foster children and our own two—and have been impressed and inspired by the work you have been doing in rehabilitating disturbed and unhappy children. I wish all parents could come to talk to you a couple of times a year. It's like getting one's tires retreaded, everything goes along so much more smoothly."

And finally, a very thoughtful letter from parents in Massachusetts—one, a PTA President. . . .

"It appears to us that you are suffering the penalty that often lands on forerunners, both in science or art. The threat of popular disapproval or of law-infringement is set up to warn off the faint-hearted or the criminal. It is an effective barrier to all but the incurably courageous and the incurably vicious individuals. So, in the dog-house or the jailhouse, we find the best and the most mixed-up together, or, rather, to use a less harsh term, the most creative and the most destructive. How can human justice tell them apart? In a sense, both are threats to stable status quo society; and yet the first group are the seeds of tomorrow's best harvest.

"This is all rather trite and obvious, but it is in these terms that we see your offense. We start from the basis that if a man is to be judged by the fruits of his work, you must be rated as an exceptionally successful healer of radically sick children. The product, where human spirits are concerned, bespeaks the process; hence, we have always been quite content that you should work your magic in your own way, feeling that only the soundest sort of therapy could bring about the clarity or serenity which you seem to be able to leave in your patients and their parents.

"If other doctors, using more conservative methods, could match your score, then it might be said that radical procedures were not justified. But the size and character of your practice is evidence enough that your ways are sound and practical. No doubt, it would be easy to find points where your methods carried you across the frontiers of the legal or the moral codes and make you vulnerable to accusations like the present ones; but we do not see that such pin-point out-of-context challenges have any validity. They may be true but, lacking the whole truth, they are a kind of lie about you and your purposes.

"And, of course, we, ourselves, always come back to the hard practical fact that we have in our own family evidence of your skill, first-hand knowledge of the good you have done. No accusations made by others will ever outweigh this, for us."

This last letter clearly defines the purpose of our defense; namely, to give these acts which, out of context, the State regards as deeds of a lecherous homosexual, their true background and context in which we firmly believe they are the acts of a skillful, highly experienced professional and a serious student of difficult medical problems who has helped some very sick children and who may help other doctors to cure such sick children.

* * *

As Mr. Wall has stated, the project involved a woods cabin on a lake, part of an old farm, four miles from the village of Littletown. During nine years, twenty-two children stayed there for long periods of time—two to four years, and many more for a shorter time. This project, let me emphasize, was separate from his clinical pediatric office practice in Littletown.

Patients at the cabin project were referred by various children's agencies, both public and private, by clinics, by courts, hospitals, schools, physicians, clergymen, nurses, and by the friends or relatives of patients who had been there.

Except in the very beginning, almost all of the referrals came because the referring agency

or the person had direct knowledge of the result in the case of a patient who had been there. No publicity or promotion methods were used ever. As Mr. Wall stated, he didn't even have his name on the door of the clinic office; didn't have a registered telephone. No record was kept of the numerous applications.

The accused has estimated for me that the children accepted in this project were less than one percent of those for whom some sort of application was made. This demand reflected, not only the lack of resources for such children, but also the knowledge of the results that he was achieving.

As for the financing of the cabin project, the parents or the agencies were expected to pay the expenses of the child's care, if they were able. No child was ever refused for lack of money. Occasionally, it was necessary, not only to keep the child for nothing, but to send money home for his family in order to insure his having a family when he needed one.

* * *

Most of the cabin children were those who were—who are currently called "disturbed"....

* * *

... Other terms that might be or have been applied to them are "worried," "lost," "frightened," "defeated," "discouraged," "crazy," "neglected," "confused," "delinquent," and "bad." Disturbed children might, from the Doctor's point of view, be viewed as those who have stepped out of the pattern or path of growth far enough or for long enough time that they have become a worry to themselves, to their families, their teachers, or their neighborhoods.

The people of this Village of Littletown became accustomed to seeing derelict children such as these become respectable junior citizens of the community. At one time, three of the cabin boys were heads of young people's groups in the three churches in the community. Only on Thursday, last, did a county newspaper report that one of the boys who was at the cabin at the time of the Doctor's arrest—and who is still in Littletown in a foster home—had just been elected head of his church young people's group after the arrest of the Doctor.

There never was a routine program—the methods used to accomplish these results were experimental and unorthodox. The approach was to induce the child to go back in his life to the age when his trouble started, and then to guide him anew up to his present age along lines which would be more comforting to him and more acceptable to others—regression, and then progression or re-education.

There never was a routine program of management of a patient at the cabin. In each case, the program was improvised to fit the needs of the child, whatever they were. To induce the regression, what might be called a "permissive environment" was created. In his first few weeks, the child was usually with the Doctor continuously, night and day, and was allowed—even encouraged—to do about as he pleased. Introduced to this exceedingly free environment, not every child regressed. As soon as he was really sure that no one really cared what he did and that no one was going to try to make him behave himself, and that adult approval was not going to be meted out according to his acts, a child might show signs of real relief and immediately begin to behave in accordance with social standards which he had continually flouted before.

Usually, after an initial period of permissiveness, the Doctor closed in on a child slowly, very slowly, much as he describes he used to harness a colt when he was young—a little restraint, a small requirement, mild denials, and this while the child was more or less alone with the Doctor.

However, permissiveness was not the only technique that was used. Both public and private schools were attended by the cabin children. Inducting a cabin child into the elementary public school life by degrees was made easier because Dr. Martin was the school physician and spent many hours there in certain seasons. Being neither teacher nor parent, and not in a position of authority, he had unusual freedom and opportunity to observe the children, both normal and disturbed. In addition to the schools, the almost weekly dances at the community house were part of the laboratory where the Doctor made his studies of these cabin children.

Now it is time for me to move from the general background to the specific charges of this information; and Mr. Wall has had complete freedom, as we had agreed previously, in mentioning cases not included in this information. So will I.

In March of this year, the cabin project included eight children—four in full, actual residence in the cabin, itself, and four in foster homes in the Village. With the exception of one child who had returned to the cabin because of a school failure, all of these children were fairly advanced in their course, sufficiently stable so that they could attend school successfully and avoid overt anti-social acts.

This, then, was the situation at the cabin when the ten-year-old boy—unnamed by Mr. Wall but, for the purposes of my statement I shall call George—came at the request of his mother and the Salisbury Health Center. Being people of small income and large family expenses, the parents could not pay the child's expenses—and here we must bear in mind that the payments for the child were always for bare expenses, not one cent for professional services by the Doctor. The importunities of the family and the plight of the child were such that the Doctor agreed to take him, money or no money; and, later, after some negotiations, it was arranged that the Torrington Welfare Department should pay the cost of his care and the Diocesan Bureau would supervise his case.

Let me now describe the boy's arrival in the clinic in the accused's own words. "He stood in the center of the main waiting room, scrubbed, brushed, polished, carefully dressed, erect, healthy looking, smiling; not merely smiling, but actually radiant with enthusiastic excitement, the living picture of every parental person's dream of a child. Before I could say a word, he greeted me in as winning a way as I have ever seen. Handsome looks, good-will, charm, self-confidence, poise—perfection in a child not yet ten years old. This, the picture, then, save for one detail. Every few seconds, this perfection would be ripped by a yelp, bloodcurdling, inhuman, feral, his mouth and throat retching open as if turning inside out to rid him of something, unbelievably horrid. As abruptly as it came, this spasm passed, the perfect child, apparently unaware that anything had happened, going right on with his prattle. To the beholder, his yelp was no more shocking than his eerie ignorance of it."

This little boy, the Doctor later learned, had not only been excluded from public school in his town, never advancing beyond the first grade, but also from his church because of his affliction. He could not go to the movies, he could not be taken in the stores or even on the streets without extreme embarrassment to his companions.

From that first day, the Doctor and George, awake and asleep, spent more than three thousand hours in each other's company, through many of which the Doctor was striving to think himself into George, studying his every movement, every word, every facial expression with utter absorption. How many psychiatrists that we know would be willing to make such an intensive study while at the same time conducting a busy clinical practice in the mornings and maintaining a simple cabin life for four to eight boys? How many of us fathers in this courtroom have ever devoted so much time, energy and love to one of our own children?

*   *   *

[At] the cabin, then, in this first period, most of the other boys were three to six years older than George. His eating, his sleeping habits taught the Doctor nothing about him. He showed exaggerated modesty, never undressing before the other children even when they went swimming. A hard player, he liked rough-housing, tackling, wrestling, and was an astonishingly good baseball player. In this type of play, it never seemed to occur to him or to the other children that he was weaker or smaller or younger.

In sedentary play, or in almost any other relationship, they relegated him to his little boy status. Building something was one of his favorite forms of solitary play, and he was both persistent and good at it. In handling smaller children at the clinic, he was almost as proficient as an experienced adult. At the cabin, he would cut wood, build a fire, try to cook a meal, do all sorts of difficult things—and without being asked to do them. He was most gregarious, every new face a new friend. Active as he was, he seldom had any accident; and in the first few months, the Doctor does not remember his ever crying. He talked excessively and took over the whole conversation of the cabin. Even so, he had difficulty in expressing himself. Words just wouldn't come when he called them. He was totally unable to read and could not even recognize his own name in print.

When George was alone with the Doctor, he occasionally treated the Doctor as a contemporary playmate; occasionally, as a father, more often as a fellow-worker, perhaps, but most of the time as a physician; and he would present his own case to the Doctor almost as intently as if he were some elderly, chronic invalid in the hospital.

In the first period of ten weeks at the cabin, his chief symptom, this abrupt outcry, did not change appreciably; if anything, for the worse. The Doctor's most intent study of it showed him no connection between this terrible noise and any aspect of his life, his mood, his companions, his activity, anything. After a day or two at the

cabin, when he had grown easy with the Doctor, he began to show two more habits, as he called them. He would double his right fist and hit his pubic region hard; and he would, at the same time, raise and twist his left leg and kick his buttocks with the whole inner surface of his foot. Throughout this first period of ten weeks, these two phenomena appeared and disappeared without any apparent rhyme or reason.

At about the end of the first ten weeks which had been spent in close observation of George, the Doctor was then estimating that it would take two years for him to get much result, and maybe five years to get well, if he ever could. At that time, the Doctor might be said to have thought of George like this: if one overlooked his main symptom, he was a marvelously adjusted child—good, obedient, perfect in almost every department of behavior, unbelievably effectual in all sorts of activities except school, and in all sorts of relationships. But, to the Doctor's mind, he was a brave, long-practiced, tested and durable fake, a fabricated construction after what he thought his world expected of him, a shell of a boy; and deep inside this shell was some hidden, unrecognizable something, pressing uncontrollably and senselessly up to the surface to explode in this yelp.

Now we come to a May evening—and in this, we do not agree with the presentation of the State that these acts occurred within a few weeks after [George] had been there. . . .

*   *   *

. . . He had been playing about the clinic while the Doctor was at work there in the morning; and they worked together in the garden and cabin in the early afternoon. In the late afternoon, after school, he played with the other children while the Doctor was preparing their dinner in the cabin on the stove which The Court has a picture of. The meal over, the dishes washed, two children studying in the cabin, two children studying in the farm house kitchen. The Doctor and George have tended to the evening chores, feeding rabbits and chickens. The air is raw; and, rather than disturb the boys studying in the cabin and in the kitchen, they go into the barn—again, only fifty or seventy-five feet from the farmhouse; and the Doctor dropped down on some loose hay in the barn, George beside him.

The Doctor was lying on his back, half-asleep, his arm around George's shoulders; George beside him, his arm—his right arm across the Doctor's chest. His hand wandered inside the Doctor's shirt, stroked his belly; and, up to this time, it was accidental, drowsy, much like as though he were casually petting a friendly dog; and then George grew tense and purposeful as if some inhibition had been suddenly removed; and in the permissive pattern, the Doctor kept patting his back as if he were still absent-minded. As compulsively as if nothing could stop it, George's hand explored the Doctor's genitals, grabbed his penis firmly, and began a masturbatory movement. This act, as it grew in crescendo, was suddenly interrupted by the sound of the boys leaving the farmhouse.

And never had the Doctor been more alert to a child's looks and actions than he was to George throughout the next two days. The only change that he could detect was an increased, if anything, a small increase in his yelping, and a sort of unwillingness to meet the Doctor's eye, most unlike his usual open gaze. Two nights later, the chores over and the setting much like two evenings before, George said to the Doctor in a subdued way, quite without his usual brash confidence, "I'm tired. Can't we lie on the hay?"

This time, George quickly had the Doctor's penis in his hand and wasted no time, both manually and orally, bringing on an orgasm; the Doctor patted his back encouragingly. He then went to sleep on the hay, and the Doctor went in the farmhouse to take the night telephone calls.

When George awoke the next morning, he found the Doctor cooking his breakfast; and no matter how hard he studied the Doctor's face, George could find nothing there but loving approval. Not then did they mention this sex act nor have they ever since; but as the Doctor stood there, cooking breakfast in the early dawn, George seemed to shake himself free of something, not unlike a dog shaking himself as he comes out of a pond.

Perhaps an hour elapsed before the Doctor realized that James [sic] was no longer yelping; and as the usual day wore on, there was still no yelping. Others in the clinic and the village and, finally, James [sic] himself, toward noon, realized that he was no longer yelping. Never, after that time, did the Doctor hear the full cry again; and as if at a turn of a switch, George entered the second phase of his cabin life.

Almost a complete metamorphosis came over George. His shiny, outer shell almost visibly crumpled. He could with ease, now, go to the movies, go to his church Mass, to the school commencement. He no longer made himself work. Before imperturbable, he now sulked and fretted over any little act that didn't please him,

weeping real tears if there was some hurt to his feelings. His effectiveness with small children at the clinic ceased, and he could no longer be trusted with them. His skill in baseball was no use to him, any more, because he preferred to push little sticks around little trucks in the dust. His exaggerated modesty disappeared, and he needed to talk less. He suddenly showed the first steps toward ability to read.

And the second week of June, the Doctor let George go home for a time, explaining to his family and to George, himself, that he considered the ending of the noise to be just the end of his symptom and not the end of his disease. Apparently, they were so excited about it that they told the social worker in charge that he was cured and home for good. At this time, it was the Doctor's intention to spend the rest of the summer preparing George for school.

The third phase for George began with his return from his rather unsuccessful visit home in June. This period marked the beginning of his progression or re-education. As part of the Doctor's program, life grew harder and harder for George. Reading lessons took on a fixed schedule. Hating walking as he did, he was required to walk a mile to his tutor's house. Many little obligations were imposed, and many privileges denied. The sexual activity with the Doctor which occurred several times during the second period was not conspicuously refused by the Doctor, but he saw to it there was no time for it.

George used to tag along up to the Hague apartment where the Doctor would retreat to read a while, occasionally. Merely coming to sit on the edge of the old cot as the Doctor lay there, reading, seemed to be an intimacy sufficient to keep down the old anxiety of George. If the Doctor had said in so many words that the old genital activity was over, especially if he had shown any disgust or disapproval at this time, the Doctor thought that George would not have done so well.

With this harder program, though he showed numerous tics and other evidences of strain, he tolerated the steadily increasing pressure of the regimen, very well. He still kept his easy friendliness, with the Doctor; and in George's eye, the accused believes, he was always a doctor. Such, then, was the beginning of the rebuilding, the progression of George in this third period when it was abruptly halted on August fourteenth by the Doctor's arrest.

So far, I have said nothing about the other members of the family with whom George had lived. It is axiomatic that, in working with children, that a ten-year-old child, if he has lived with them, is as much a product of his family that he can not be considered apart from them. From years of practice and experience, the Doctor had become an astute observer of people; and his report on George's family certainly demonstrates it. Father, mother, uncle, aunt, two sisters, sixteen and eighteen years of age, three brothers, one of whom I shall refer to as "Peter," the thirteen-year old; one, nine, whom I shall call "Mark"; and one, four, whom I shall call "Philip." Peter, the thirteen-year-old; Mark, nine; and Philip, four.

Of these nine people, although they made a complex, perhaps trying, family group for George, only three seemed to the Doctor to really stir him; namely, his mother, his uncle and Mark, the nine-year-old.

It was an important part of the Doctor's work with the cabin-child to invite the relatives in and to associate them with the child in varying combinations and situations which were calculated to show the structure of the relationship. Although Peter, thirteen, did not appear to upset George, he threw some light on George's case. He first came to the cabin to visit George along with the other children, the mother and the uncle in April, one month after—approximately one month after George came there. After that, he began coming to the cabin whenever possible —and not as Mr. Wall has suggested on invitation of the Doctor; by his own request. Every time he would leave, he would ask if he could come back again; and there were dozens of times —for an hour, a day, overnight, a weekend; and in the summer, for two continuous weeks. All this time, the Doctor was carefully studying him and his relationship to George.

After the Doctor's first sexual experience with George, he was quite busy with the clinic, and Peter was not invited to the cabin for some time; and when he was, for the first time, afterwards, the Doctor saw to it that he and George did not have a moment together unless the Doctor was within earshot. He was, then, convinced that Peter could not have heard of George's experience before Peter had almost exactly a similar one with the Doctor. That is, it was not the Doctor being the aggressor, but the permissive environment, and the boy taking the initiative. After that, further acts of this nature with Peter had only—were only in continuance and furtherance of this study.

Mark, the nine-year-old, had much greater impact on George. Historically, he was conceived unintentionally while George was just a

few months old; and when George was five or seven months old, still almost an integral part of his mother, he was sent to his uncle and aunt who were childless. Thus, for George, the world fell apart when he was, in a sense, put out of his home by Mark, this now almost perfect little boy—I am speaking of Mark, age of nine, healthy, bright, successful in school, the kind of child that George was trying so desperately to be.

Helping George in his relationship with Mark, the Doctor considered to be a fundamental step in his recovery. As these boys, in George's third period, were going to be dumped together like puppies within a litter in a few weeks, and as the Doctor had discovered that both George and Peter were practiced in sex play —I think it's important to emphasize that it was the type of sex play that was not phantasy, and neither were they able to know of the acts which they did without having done it with someone older than themselves before the Doctor found this out—so it was of importance for the Doctor to learn whether or not Mark had had any of this experience because he felt that George's yelp had a sex-guilt expression—or had been a sex-guilt expression, and that this sex-guilt was pretty well now gone as far as George was concerned. So that this perfect younger brother, Mark, was just the one who would make George feel most guilty if he were in the habit of sex play with him, and then the symptoms might return.

As Mark was such a snuggling child with the Doctor and so demonstrative physically, it was easy for the Doctor to learn whether he had the same desire for genital play as his two older brothers had shown. It seemed quite clear to the Doctor that he had not. He would lie beside the Doctor with his hands on the Doctor's genitals with no apparent interest, excitement or revulsion much as he might have considered the Doctor's ear or nose. After a little of this, the Doctor was sure that Mark did not know of the sort of sex play which his brothers knew so well; and, further, the Doctor believed that he had learned this knowledge of Mark without arousing or scaring or harming him, at all, as he continued to maintain his same affectionate, trusting ways with the Doctor. Here, I do not wish to imply that all the sexual acts of the Doctor with the boys, on his part, were merely permissive; but I do assert that they were all engaged in by him with the same purpose in mind.

*   *   *

These acts are condemned and prohibited

by law as indecent, unchaste, impure, obscene. This, the Doctor knew and understood when he engaged in them; but it appears to me, the motive and intent of the actor may and does change the whole character of the act and its consequences. Killing on the battlefield is sanctioned in wartime; and, often, the killer is rewarded with medals while killing in peacetime is murder, punishable by death.

With The Court's indulgence, I would like to read from a letter I received last week from an outstanding authority in the field of child guidance and family life who, with her husband, both psychologists, have conducted a school for disturbed children for more than twenty years. These people are in Court, here, today, Your Honor.

After several talks with the Doctor and reading his report of the cabin project, she wrote me of her great concern about the possibility of the Doctor's pleading guilty to these charges. I am quoting. "It would seem to me that he had every professional and human urgency to do exactly as he did, and I would wish that he would fight for that right. Perhaps I can make myself clearer with a simple example. Two men may cut open a woman's stomach. The one, Jack, the Ripper, commits a criminal act of assault. The other, Dr. John Doe, Surgeon, performs a lifesaving miracle. Both men have performed, essentially, the same act. The intent of one is sadistic. The intent of the other is lifesaving and knowledge-seeking for the purpose of further lifesaving. The result of one is death; the result of the other is a chance for life. Are both these men to be regarded in the same light?

"Must the surgeon when attacked by ignorant, if well-meaning persons, plead guilty to assault along with Jack, the Ripper; and, if he does, does this not help to identify his act, in the public mind, with that of Jack?

"The Law necessarily follows, rather than precedes human experience. But if scientific exploration ceases until legal processes catch up, where would human progress be? History has presented us, again and again with the dilemma of brave men of insight and vision who have elected to proceed at whatever personal cost with the task of blazing new trails. The legal challenge to establish the right of such men to work must be one of the powerful inducements that attracts men like yourself to the legal profession.

"There is evidence, and lots of evidence, that Dr. Martin was on the right track. To take just one small bit—for years, there have been available to therapists, and even to educators,

flexible dolls, male and female, adult and child and baby, equipped with the appropriate genitalia for their sex and age. These have been used by psychiatrists, therapists and some nursery school teachers to permit distressed children to act out their sexual perplexities and to vent their sexual feelings. Often enough, there has been relief of anxiety symptoms; providing, of course, that the therapist has lovingly accepted all acts performed upon the dolls and between the dolls as manipulated by the child.

"Young children, and children not yet seriously disturbed, might respond reasonably well to this ventilation of anxiety, but one could hardly imagine that the seriously disturbed children brought to Dr. Martin, the so-called hopeless cases, could respond to anything or any person external to him. To use psycho-lingo, their transference was to him. It seems obvious that these youngsters had to work through their anxiety in the acquiescence and acceptance of his own person.

"Knowing what small amount I do about children, it seems to me that Dr. Martin did an enlightened act of professional and personal giving of himself that could be conjectured to have made cure possible for these children. And the indisputable fact is that the children did, thereafter, take the clearly recognizable first steps toward recovery."

*   *   *

"Scientifically, he has given us clues to understanding children and the deep roots of their disturbances that few other scientists have even dared to look at, let alone expose. I feel that my own knowledge of children and effectiveness to them in time of trouble has been vastly increased by these observations and perceptions." That's all.

May I respectfully call to The Court's attention the fact that members of the accused's family, his two brothers, one a college president, one a physician, another a sister who has come on from Illinois, his home state, are here. They, who would be his severest critics, if they believed him to be wrong, they don't have their heads lowered in shame because they have seen him before on the forefront of progress.

In addition to the members of his family, two of the physicians who were associated with him in his office practice in Littletown are in Court; and since they cannot testify here, I asked one of them for his Credo on the Doctor which he has given me permission to read to The Court since he cannot testify.

"To my knowledge, Dr. Martin has been an outstanding practitioner of medicine for many years. He has been at the head of two departments of pediatrics at major university colleges of medicine. He has maintained a large practice of pediatrics locally, doing much charity work. He has been sought after as advisor and lecturer on pediatrics and family problems. He has a tremendous number of devoted proteges, many of whom occupy positions of importance in public life. He is a man of many diverse talents and has done much of basic importance in bacteriology and serology, has published work of fundamental importance on undulant fever and streptococcal diseases.

"He has always been known as a fearless pioneer in new fields. He has never sought favor, wealth or self-aggrandizement. He is primarily interested in fundamental biologic processes.

"He has been active and effective in the field of pediatric psychiatry for many years. He has intentionally taken on only a few, but the most challenging and difficult cases for psychiatric treatment. He has had real success in rehabilitation of seriously diseased minds.

"His actions, as described by himself, represent the exploration of little known problems with equally little known techniques. The problems were unorthodox; the approach equally so. To assume that he allowed himself to indulge in self-gratification ignores a completely selfless past and loses sight of the incredible amount of time and energy devoted to maintaining, feeding and teaching the boys under his care. This was a twenty-four hour, seven-day job without interruption. This was the work of an exceptionally devoted man, for a man with very unusual singleness of purpose.

"There is no doubt in my mind, speaking as a physician, but that Dr. Martin's actions represent an extension of scientific research into the sexual problems of adolescents. I am not competent to judge as to the value of what he accomplished with them or discovered. I have no doubt as to his motive."

* * *

In answer to the charge of the state that the accused is a lecherous pervert preying on young children, his friends, his neighbors, parents and children would answer that his Spartan existence four miles from town without a car, in all seasons of the year, his selfless and untiring dedication to his desire to help children and to pierce and throw back the darkness of ignorance and the unknown, his remarkable self-discipline, his

infinite patience and understanding refute and belie that charge. In his own words, the accused's own reply is that he is a serious student of difficult medical problems, who has helped some very sick children and who may help other doctors to cure such sick children.

Already, his punishment has been extreme for, as soon as he was arrested and the accusations against him made public, the Doctor he was, was ruined; and the man he was, was broken. In losing his license,[*] sure, he has lost, not only his means of livelihood, but more important, his opportunity to go on serving children and parents as he had done so unselfishly and so successfully in the past.

In jail for only seven weeks, but dishonored for a lifetime, and already gravely punished at the age of fifty-two, he has, I sincerely believe, discharged his debt to society. Therefore, I re-

[*] The license or certificate of registration of any licensed or registered practitioner of the healing arts in this state may be revoked, suspended, or annulled, or such practitioner may be reprimanded or otherwise disciplined, after notice and hearing, on the recommendation of the examining board representing the branch of the healing arts practiced by such practitioner for any cause named below. . . . The causes for which a license or certificate of registration may be revoked, suspended or annulled or for which a practitioner may be reprimanded or otherwise disciplined are as follows: Conviction in a court of competent jurisdiction, either within or without this state, of any crime involving moral turpitude, of any infamous crime or any crime in the practice of his profession; immoral, fraudulent, dishonorable or unprofessional conduct; illegal, incompetent or habitually negligent conduct in the practice of the healing arts; habitual intemperance in the use of spirituous stimulants or addiction to the use of morphine, cocaine or other habit-forming drugs; advertising in connection with the practice of the healing arts which is found by the board representing the branch of the healing arts practiced by the practitioner to be deceptive, misleading, extravagant, improbable or untrue; aiding or abetting the unlawful practice of any branch of the healing arts; failure to record a license or certificate of registration as required by law; insanity of the practitioner; fraud or deception in obtaining a license or certificate of registration. The clerk of any court in this state in which a person practicing any branch of the healing arts has been convicted of any crime as described in this section shall, immediately after such conviction, transmit a certified copy, in duplicate, of the information and judgment, without charge, to the state department of health, containing the name and address of the practitioner, the crime of which he was convicted and the date of conviction. [Conn. Gen. Stat. §20–45 (1958)]

spectfully recommend to The Court that there be imposed a suspended sentence with probation. Thank you for your kindness.

THE COURT: May I ask one question so that I may fully understand Counsel's claims? As you related the story, these children were, in a sense, the aggressors. Do you claim that at no time was the defendant the aggressor?

MR. EBERSOL: No, Your Honor, I did not.

THE COURT: I didn't think you did. I thought you made it clear, but I wanted to be—I wanted to be certain of the position of the defense.

MR. EBERSOL: I made the statement that he was the aggressor but that the aggressions were for the same purpose and in the same medical pattern as the permissiveness, that he considered them just as necessary.

THE COURT: I am speaking of acts other than those which you have taken the trouble to describe.

MR. EBERSOL: That's right, Your Honor; and so am I.

THE COURT: Very well. Thank you.

MR. EBERSOL: Thank you.

MR. WALL: My brother has made a remarkable defense of this man. As I gather it, the crux of his defense is that, at all times, he was acting for the interests of these children and that these acts upon the children were in the nature of therapy—described as "blazing new trails," "spiritualization of the sexual act," making these young men—these boys—or "freeing these boys of their infantile needs"—I quote these things—"unlearning homosexuality". . . .

*   *   *

. . . Now, as to therapy, in the first place, it is inconceivable to me that such acts can constitute therapy. Course, I am not the greatest physician or scientist in the world, and I don't set myself up against psychiatrists of great renown; but I don't see that there is any psychiatrist of great renown who is advancing any such theory here. We have just a defendant who is accused of these most repulsive acts in connection with young children, trying to defend himself; and he says it's "therapy."

If there is any great mind, any great psychiatrist who can—who has advanced any such theory, and that appears in the literature, anywhere, why, I presume that that might have some bearing upon the Court.

Actually, we, with the limited facilities available to us, to the State, did consult a psychiatrist.

We consulted the very psychiatrist who was connected with the clinic which referred this ten-year-old boy to the defendant; and he advises us that there is nothing in the literature of psychiatry which supports any such fantastic theory.

Now, also, as to his claim of therapy, he had a ten-year-old boy that he was treating for an unfortunate condition to which he was subject. I have no doubt that he did try to rid that young boy of his condition. I have no doubt that he may have had some skill in that regard; but I have no doubt, either, Your Honor, that the—as to the effect of the homosexual acts upon the boy. I don't believe that it's possible for any—I wouldn't have believed it possible to have anyone come into a court of law and state that the—that such acts with a ten-year-old boy could constitute, by a man of fifty-two years of age, theretofore respected in his profession, that such acts could be considered as therapy; and to prove that he didn't consider it as therapy, Your Honor, and to prove, also, that to use the defendant's attorney's statement that "the State assumed he indulged for self-gratification," and to prove that he did indulge in these acts for self-gratification, Your Honor, the nine-year-old boy didn't need the therapy.

The nine-year-old boy didn't bark like a dog. The thirteen-year-old boy didn't bark like a dog. There was no necessity for any therapy between the Doctor and the nine-year-old boy and the thirteen-year-old. There was no expectation of any continuation of treatment in the future. They were only there to visit for a few days at a time, coming there for a few days at a time. All he could be considered to be doing was debauching them, getting them into the type of vice which is—up until today, Your Honor, I thought definitely was disgraceful conduct; and I thought it was generally so regarded. Certainly, it is against the law. Certainly, parents who entrust their children to physicians for treatment should not be expected to hear from that physician, at a later time, "that I committed homosexual acts on your boy for your boy's own good, and that I committed homosexual acts upon the boy to whom you entrusted me for treatment, and also his older brother, and also his younger brother because I thought it would help the boy entrusted to me for treatment." It just is inconceivable, Your Honor, that parents should have to accept any such statement.

*   *   *

. . . Your Honor. I feel that, despite the brilliance of my brother's statement to the Court in defense of the indefensible, that by having a defendant ask an attorney to make a statement such as that before the Court, that is a fraud upon the Court, Your Honor, to have the defendant ask an attorney to tell a story such as—I believe my brother is very, very well-intentioned; but to my mind, it adds insult to the injury here to have a defendant insist upon that type of a defense being made, that he was in the course of a scientific investigation, that it was therapy; and under those circumstances, Your Honor, he doesn't stand before Your Honor as someone sorry that he has disobeyed the law and telling Your Honor that he wishes no longer to continue to disobey the law. He comes before Your Honor to say, "I am a scientist. This is just a portion of my science. This is the way that I treated these children." And he takes credit for some of his undoubted skill as a physician in the past and by claiming that the homosexual activities were integrated with other treatments which he gave to his charges. I don't say that the Doctor hasn't done things for people in the past. He undoubtedly has done a great many things for people in the past; but to have prostituted children aged nine, ten, thirteen, and to claim that they—that he was completely justified in doing so is not coming before your Court—before this Court with the type of defense which would involve the extension of any mercy to him.

I think, Your Honor, that the only possible disposition of this case is a long State's Prison sentence. . . .

*   *   *

MR. EBERSOL: If it please the Court, I would like the privilege of remarking only with respect to Brother Wall's final statement—that I think, from my earlier statement, it should be apparent to the Court that, with the exception of the nine-year-old brother, that each and every one of these boys had a previous history of sexual perversion, that they were not learning new tricks from the Doctor.

THE COURT: I beg your pardon. I didn't hear the last—.

MR. EBERSOL: They were not learning new tricks from the Doctor. I have already stated the reason and purpose for the involvement of the two boys; and although there are five statements there, there are statements from only three of the cabin boys.

MR. WALL: I might say, Your Honor, that any previous sexual interest these boys may have

had is based entirely upon what the defendant, himself, states. There is nothing in our file that indicates any previous sexual experience by these children, absolutely nothing.

*   *   *

THE COURT: I went over the Doctor's notes in full, and very thoroughly, last night. I spent a great deal of time reading and studying these documents; and they are very, very revealing. There isn't any question in my mind—and I say this, not to rub salt in the wound, but as a matter of fact—that the defendant is a sex pervert. There isn't any question in the mind of the Court, either, that the defendant was the aggressor in these acts.

I think, however, that Defense Counsel stated well and accurately that this man is a man of outstanding ability, that he is a man who, unquestionably, could be a healer among these children.

I was impressed with his deep-seated knowledge of these youngsters, of the time that he spent with them and of the effort that he put into it.

I was also impressed with the fact that he has this very sad affliction which makes him a subject not fit to be associated with children. That's the sad part of it because there, probably, is where his greatest ability lies—in treating children.

With reference to punishment, these matters I consider very difficult ones to deal with. I think every judge does. The matter is serious as far as using these homosexual acts as therapy; as far as the claim that he is a pioneer in this field, the Court must reject that. That just isn't so. The facts indicate that the acts took place with two children who are in no way involved in treatment. The excuse or justification that these things took place to determine what had been the child's experience prior thereto for the purpose of therapy for the child—that, the Court can't agree with. In considering punishment, I recognize the fact that here is a man of great ability, that no matter how small the punishment or how great, he has been severely punished by the public disgrace and humiliation to which he has been subjected already. At the same time, I recognize the fact that he just can't resist these tendencies. I wish there were a physician to which I could send this defendant. I don't know of any. He's the only physician who can do anything for himself; and I hope he can because I sentence him with the utmost regret because of his outstanding ability, because of what could well be a genuine interest in children and the treatment of them; but the public is entitled to some protection.

The sentence is to the State prison for a term on the first count of not less than one nor more than three years. On the second count, three years.

That means that you have a sentence of not less than one nor more than six years. The length of time that you stay there depends upon you and depends upon the judgment of the Parole Board and the authorities in the prison. I hope that you will do the things which will get you out of there and into productive work as soon as possible; and I wish that there were a physician who could do something for you.

NOTE

CONNECTICUT GENERAL STATUTES (1949)

* * *

Sec. 8359. *Indecent assault.* Any person who shall commit an indecent assault upon another person shall be imprisoned not more than ten years. The overt act or acts of which such assault consists need not be otherwise described in a complaint under this section than as an inde-

cent assault, unless the accused shall request the court that it be particularly described in such complaint. It shall be no defense to a complaint under this section that the person assaulted shall consent to the act of violence or to the act of indecency, and this section shall not affect the penalty for sodomy.

Sec. 8369. *Injury or risk of injury to children.* Any person who shall wilfully or unlawfully cause or permit any child under the age of sixteen years to be placed in such a situation that its life or limb is endangered, or its health is likely to be injured, or its morals likely to be impaired, or shall do any act likely to impair the health or morals of any such child, shall be fined not more than five hundred dollars or imprisoned not more than ten years or both.

Sec. 8544. *Beastiality and sodomy.* Any person who shall have carnal copulation with any beast, or who shall have carnal knowledge of any man, against the order of nature, unless forced or under fifteen years of age, shall be imprisoned in the State Prison not more than thirty years.

Sec. 8553. *Fornication or lascivious carriage.* Any person who shall be guilty of fornication or lascivious carriage or behavior shall be fined not more than one hundred dollars or imprisoned not more than six months or both.

B.
In Determining the Investigator's Authority, What is the Relevance of:

1.

Choice of and Attitude toward Subjects?

a.

Vernon H. Mark and Frank R. Ervin
Violence and the Brain*

The problem that modern biological and social scientists have in trying to deal with violence is much like the problem that 19th century neurologists and psychiatrists had with "insanity"—learning enough about its causes and natural history to be able to assess individual cases and treat each patient properly. In the 19th century the insane asylums were full of people

lumped together as "crazy," but who in reality had many different diseases. Some actually had pellagra. Once doctors could recognize vitamin deficiencies, and know how to prevent and treat them, people no longer developed pellagra-related symptoms of mental illness. Others were suffering from the late stages of syphilis, and still others from undiscovered brain tumors; both conditions became accessible to diagnosis and treatment, thereby shrinking the "crazy" category still further. In short, the more psychiatrists and neurologists learned about the various causes of "insanity," the more effectively were they able to differentiate between mental conditions that appeared to be the same, but, because they had different causes, required very different methods of treatment.

We are in the same state today vis-a-vis violence: we need to find out more about the condition and learn how to sort out its different causes, so that we can decide which are the most important biological and/or social factors in each in each individual case, and then treat each patient appropriately.

* * *

If detecting a potentially violent individual is the first order of business for meaningful investigation, the second is to improve our treatment methods. This could well start with a re-evaluation of the kinds of psychotherapy given to violent patients. As certain forms of conditioning (i.e., conditional reflex therapy—à la Pavlov) have been shown to improve or alleviate special kinds of temporal lobe epilepsy, applications of improved techniques in behavior therapy might have important consequences for the psychotherapeutic treatment of impulse disorders.

The recent pharmacologic advances in anti-convulsants and tranquilizers presage not the end but the beginning of a psychopharmacological revolution. Many new and important chemical agents and drugs will be added to our armamentarium for the treatment of impulsive and violent behavior. But even with these new psychotherapeutic and medicinal tools, some people with brain disease may still require surgical treatment for the control of violence. How can we improve our surgical operations? By making smaller and more precise lesions within the brain? By using electrical stimulation . . . instead of making destructive brain lesions? Perhaps a prolonged therapeutic effect can be obtained by the introduction of chemical agents into focal areas of the brain to produce chronic chemical stimulation over a long period of time.

[A]s long as senseless killings and brutality are acceptable events in our cities, on our highways, and in our foreign relations, then identifying any violent individual as unique will continue to be very difficult indeed. How, in fact, can society even define what is "abnormal" under these circumstances? Only when our society—through its educational, religious, family, and governmental structures—clearly defines and uniformly reacts to violence as being unacceptable, will we be able to approach the situation in a truly rational way.

The definition of "unacceptable violence" is, of course, a major stumbling block. What is "unacceptable violence"? The "law and order" faction of our society might define any liberal group protest as falling into this category, while protesting groups might label any action of police against demonstrators as "police brutality"—a clear-cut case of "unacceptable violence." Some minority groups have gone even further and, having identified the deprivation of civil rights as a form of violence, have equated this term with physical violence, and justified physically violent retaliation.

* * *

b.

Herman J. Muller
Means and Aims in Human Genetic Betterment*

The main thesis I wish to uphold . . . is the following. For any group of people who have a rational attitude toward matters of reproduction, and who also have a genuine sense of their own responsibility to the next and subsequent generations, the means exist right now of achieving a much greater, speedier, and more significant genetic improvement of the population, by the use of selection, than could be effected by the most sophisticated methods of treatment of the genetic material that might be available in the twenty-first century. The obstacles to carrying out such an improvement by selection are psychological ones, based on antiquated traditions from which we can emancipate ourselves, but the obstacles to doing so by treatment of the genetic material are substantive ones, rooted in the inherent difficulties of the physicochemical situation.

* * *

[T]he earlier stages of genetic surgery, if it does come into use, will doubtless be concerned mainly with repairing germ cells having certain rare and extreme genetic defects, such as the idiocy caused by failure in handling the amino acid phenylalanine. In this negative role of the technique there will be no more question of values than there is for a surgeon of the more usual kind, for everyone would agree that such marked defects are undesirable. There is nevertheless a problem of values or ethics in deciding for which people it is justifiable to make an effort if, as seems likely, the effort were too great to be applicable to every such case. But in making these decisions we would be thrown back on the whole ethical question of who should reproduce, and to what extent. And until genetic

---

* T. M. Sonneborn, ed.: *Control of Human Heredity and Evolution.* New York: The Macmillan Co. 100, 109–115 (1965). Reprinted by permission.

surgery acquires such finesse as readily to make a sage out of a simpleton, a saint out of a scamp, and a Samson out of a shrimp, we will continue to have this problem with us.

Conceivably, we might some day achieve such seeming miracles of genetic metamorphosis as these, by manipulating certain specific genetic sites or chromosomes and thus providing genes that exerted major influences on the general abilities in question. It would at the same time be desirable, in such cases, to obtain as high concentrations as possible of the very numerous correlative or modifying genes that act, sometimes very subtly, to support the major ones, as by regulating and giving balance to their expression. However, it would be a task of transcendent magnitude, intricacy, and reconditeness to do all this by genetic surgery for any one individual. Moreover, every individual to be operated on would present his own unique complex of labyrinthine problems of this sort.

If at length, however, the techniques were mastered that did enable genetic surgeons to tackle in a really practicable way the stupendous tasks of producing to order genetically improved types of human beings, then they would find themselves face to face with the age-old problem of what human values they should strive for—a problem here couched in genetic terms. This problem, even in its genetic form, is not unique for genetic surgery, however. It applies equally to any conceivable scheme for genetic betterment, and it has been used by critics as an argument against any such attempt.

For persons who would concede the desirability of human genetic betterment, or at least the need of merely preventing genetic deterioration, the possibility of conducting it by some kind of parental selection should not be overlooked, for the technical difficulties of such an approach are incomparably less than those of genetic surgery, in view of the enormous wealth of diverse genetic combinations that are already in existence in any human population. Moreover, the potentialities of these combinations can be assessed in a rough and ready way by methods similar to those obtaining under natural selection, namely, by using the criterion of the given individual's performance. It seems truly perverse for people to wait until they can take the long way around and manufacture genetic constitutions to order, when they are, in large measure, already available. Let us then consider in what ways the genetics of existing populations might be influenced through parental selection, so as to de-

crease the frequency of genetic defects and to increase the abundance of traits that are considered desirable.

We may first dismiss as obviously biased and pernicious the claims of racists who see in their own race a markedly superior type of humanity or who, conversely, single out certain other races for special condemnation. We may likewise give short shrift to those old-style eugenists who, regarding economic, social, or educational status as a reliable enough criterion of genetic fitness, have advocated measures that would make it easier for the so-called upper classes to have children and harder for the so-called lower classes.

A recent, rather sophisticated modification of the last-mentioned notion is the proposal that certain types of occupations should be so designed as to be attractive to persons of genetically less desirable types, and that the circumstances of these jobs should be so arranged as to make it relatively inconvenient and unattractive for these workers to have children. On the other hand, conversely, certain other types of occupations should, in this view, be so contrived as to be attractive to persons of more fortunate endowments, and these occupations should be associated with ways of living made conducive to the rearing of large families. It is hard to criticize this proposal seriously unless it is spelled out much more concretely. We should, however, point out that exactly this matter of finding a suitable concrete form for it would be a source of much difficulty, especially since the system of values of genetic traits implied in the given concrete arrangement would have to be one that people could agree on. We should also point out that it is highly unlikely that any democratic society would consent to having such intentional restraints imposed on it.

In general, any type of eugenics in which, as in this proposed case, the standards and values are decided upon by governmental bodies is to be regarded with suspicion, even if the government is of some democratic form, for, as yet at least, governments, including relatively enlightened ones, represent in some respects the lowest common denominator of progressive thinking. (In fact, a distinguished scientist on reading this remark has commented that it is in his opinion an understatement.) Nevertheless, it can be heartily agreed that enlightened governments, by their support of free public education, freedom of expression, and scientific research, do indirectly fill a highly useful function in human advancement. That is, they can increase people's opportunities for finding roads to progress.

Now among the most important educational needs of modern populations are those in the area of genetics and evolution. The so-called "common man" already has sufficient native intelligence and social consciousness to be able, when suitably taught, to appreciate the importance of both a good heredity and a good environment, to realize that the betterment of both is to be sought for, and to find gratification in contributing efforts of his own for these common purposes of mankind. Moreover, he is so constituted as readily to adopt a value system in which high regard is given to such primary human psychological attributes as those of sympathy, moral courage, reasonableness, and creativity. This being the case, the most fundamental basis is at hand, through education, for preparing people to follow, voluntarily, courses of action that will on the whole be conducive to the genetic betterment of the species.

Among such courses of action the type most commonly thought of consists of the exercise of more restraint in having children on the part of the genetically less well endowed and the raising of larger families by the better endowed. To this recommendation it should be answered, first, that few people of inferior mentality are willing to appraise themselves as below the average in this respect. Second, those of lower-than-average moral fiber can hardly be expected to exercise unusual restraint in the interest of a higher moral fiber for mankind in general. On the other hand, third, persons of higher-than-average mental ability or of unusually conscientious or considerate disposition are often the very ones most likely to limit their families, in order to enable both themselves, their spouses, and the children whom they do have to live a life more rewarding in other respects. Certainly people's estimates of themselves and of those closest to them are notoriously biased and unrealistic.

At best, then, the attempt to inculcate policies of this kind could have but a small positive effect on genetic trends. Perhaps this effect would be hardly enough to counteract fully the trend toward genetic deterioration that must exist today in technically advanced countries, with their low death and birth rates. . . .

*　　　*　　　*

[F]or the present and a considerable period to come our knowledge of what genetic defects people carry in hidden form will be so fragmen-

tary as to be of little use for the purpose of substantially reducing the frequency of severe genetic defects—the main objective of negative eugenics today. Of far greater consequence for the population, however, than the avoidance of the sporadic outcroppings of such hidden defects would be the raising of the genetic level in regard to the abilities and proclivities of greatest human importance. In order to achieve major practical results along these lines it would not be necessary, nor would it for a long time be possible, to arrive at an exact knowledge of the genes and gene-differences involved. They are undoubtedly very numerous, but they give evidence of having, on the whole, a fair amount of dominance. Thus—except for the confusing influence of cultural and other environmental differences—a kind of over-all estimate of an individual's genetic level in regard to these attributes, one having considerable validity, could be obtained by considerations of his actual performance or, as the geneticist would say, his phenotypic classification (not meaning merely his looks!). This is in fact how nature operates in the process of natural selection and how man has operated in past times in the artificial selection of other animals and of plants, and the method has obviously worked. In such overall appraisals, moreover, one or more highly valuable traits often more than make up for considerable shortcomings.

A heredity clinic would hardly dare to offer advice along these lines to people in general, and, if it did, the advice would probably be discounted and resented. Many people would hold, and often quite rightly, that the fact of the advisor's being a geneticist or a physician does not necessarily make him a good judge of what constitute the higher human values, or of the degree to which they, the judged, measure up to reasonable standards in these respects. Yet, as we have noted previously, their own judgments of themselves would also tend to be biased, as they might well admit themselves during moods of unusual calm and objectivity. Does this situation force us to conclude, then, that all doors to parental selection of a salutary and significant kind are closed for the human species?

There has for some time been still another possible method of parental selection, which in large measure avoids these difficulties. This is a method I . . . have recently called germinal choice. . . .

Unlike what is true of other forms of parental selection that have been suggested for man, this method does not work by attempting to influence either the size of families that people have or their choice of marriage partners. Neither does it attempt to influence people's evaluations of themselves. Its proposed mode of procedure is to establish banks of stored germ cells (spermatozoa), eventually ample banks, derived from persons of very diverse types but including as far as possible those whose lives had given evidence of outstanding gifts of mind, merits of disposition and character, or physical fitness. From these germinal stores couples would have the privilege of selecting such material, for the engendering of children of their own families, as appeared to them to afford the greatest promise of endowing their children with the kind of hereditary constitution that came nearest to their own ideals.

As an aid in making these choices there would be provided as full documentation as possible concerning the donors of the germinal material, the lives they had led, and their relatives. The couples concerned would also have advice available from geneticists, physicians, psychologists, experts in the fields of activity of the donors being considered, and other relevant specialists, as well as generalizers. In order to allow a better perspective to be obtained on the donors themselves and on their genetic potentialities, as well as to minimize personality fads and to avoid risks of personal entanglements, it would be preferable for the material used to have been derived from donors who were no longer living, and to have been stored for at least 20 years. The technique of preparing semen in a medium containing glycerine and keeping it at the temperature of liquid nitrogen . . . provides a reliable and relatively inexpensive means of maintaining such material for an unlimited period without deterioration.

*   *   *

c.

Frank J. Ayd, Jr.
Fetology—Medical and Ethical Implications of Intervention in the Prenatal Period*

*   *   *

. . . Dr. Geoffrey Chamberlin at King's College Hospital, London, England . . . has conducted experiments with living human fetuses. . . . In his initial experiments, eight living human fetuses, weighing from 300 to 980 grams, were obtained by hysterotomy for the therapeutic

---

* 169 *Annals of the New York Academy of Sciences* 376, 379 (1970). Reprinted by permission.

abortion. In seven cases the amniotic sac was removed intact from the uterus; the other fetus was placed in normal saline solution at the operating table. To prevent any respiration, Dr. Chamberlin reported, the fetuses were kept under artificial liquor amnii in a tank. Within 12 minutes after removal from the womb, the umbilical vessels—vein and both arteries, where possible—were cannulated. In each fetus, Dr. Chamberlin said, "The cannulas were passed well beyond the abdominal wall, along the hypogastric arteries, and hopefully into at least the internal iliac vessels." Then the eight fetuses were kept alive for varying intervals on total perfusion via the artificial placenta.

Dr. Chamberlin reported that "the longest survival in this series came with the largest fetus." Delivered from a 14-year-old girl, this 980-ram male fetus . . . "was cannulated without trouble about 11 minutes after the placenta was separated. A brisk spontaneous flow was noted 22 minutes postpartum; the fetus was kept on the circuit for 5 hours and 3 minutes.

"Only when a cannula slipped out by accident and could not be reintroduced was the experiment halted.

" 'Irregular gasping movements, twice a minute, occurred in the middle of the experiment,' Dr. Chamberlin declared. 'Once the perfusion was stopped, however, the gasping respiratory efforts increased to 8 to 10 per minute.' The fetus's death was recorded 21 minutes after disconnection from the artificial placenta.

"Continuous electrocardiographic monitoring throughout the experiment, using standard I leads, revealed a regular pulse that varied from 120 to 90. When the circuit was stopped, the heart slowed, fibrillated and eventually ceased beating.

"Maintained at 39° to 42° C in a water bath, with 15-to-40-ml-per-minute extracorporeal flow rates, the fetus seemed undisturbed. He made 'occasional stretching limb movements, very like the ones in other human work,' reported by a Swedish team under Dr. Bjorn Westin."

Although none of the living human fetuses connected to the artificial placenta survived for more than five hours and three minutes, these human experiments were rated as successful. . . . The human fetuses used in these experiments are alive. What are their rights? Since they are incapable of giving consent to their use as experimental subjects, who can morally and legally give consent for them—their mothers, their fathers, both parents, or the state? . . .

*   *   *

NOTE

PAUL RAMSEY
THE ETHICS OF GENETIC CONTROL*

*   *   *

. . . In the case of cloning a man, the question is what to do with mishaps, whether discovered in the course of extracorporeal gestation in the laboratory or by monitored uterine gestation. In case a monstrosity, a subhuman or parahuman individual, results, shall the experiment simply be stopped and this artfully created human life killed? In mingling individual human chromosomes with those of the "higher" mammals (given sufficient dosage and "a few years"), what shall be done if the resulting individual lives seem remarkably human? Moreover, Lederberg not only contemplates experiments "augmenting" animal cell cultures with "fragments of the human chromosome set," the reverse is also to be done: "Clonal reproduction and *introduction of genetic material from other spheres*" are two paths already opened up in *human* evolution (italics added). Lederberg "infers" these twin genetic policies instead of taking the other and somewhat longer road to genetic engineering. But surely these are paths no less fraught with mishaps knowingly if not intentionally created. We must face the grave moral question of what to do with them.

*   *   *

2.

Benefits to Individuals?

a.

Robert L. Sinsheimer
The Prospect of Designed Genetic Change†

"It has now become a serious necessity to better the breed of the human race. The average citizen is too base for the everyday work of modern civilization. Civilized man has become possessed of vaster powers than in old times for good or ill but has made no corresponding advance in wits and goodness to enable him to direct his conduct rightly." This was written in

1894 by Sir Francis Galton. The concerns of the present are clearly not new.

It has long been apparent that you and I do not enter this world as unformed clay compliant to any mold. Rather, we have in our beginnings some bent of mind, some shade of character. The origin of this structure—of the fiber in this clay—was for centuries mysterious. In earlier times men sought its trace in the conjunction of the stars or perhaps in the momentary combination of the elements at nativity. Today, instead, we know to look within. We seek not in the stars but in our genes for the herald of our fate.

. . . For the first time in all time a living creature understands its origin and can undertake to design its future. . . . Even in the ancient myths man was constrained by his essence. He could not rise above his nature to chart his destiny. Today we can . . . envision that chance—and its dark companion of awesome choice and responsibility.

*   *   *

It is worthwhile to consider specifically wherein the potential of the new genetics exceeds that of the old. To implement the older eugenics of Galton and his successors would have required a massive social program carried out over many generations. Such a program could not have been initiated without the consent and cooperation of a major fraction of the population, and would have been continuously subject to social control. In contrast, the new eugenics could, at least in principle, be implemented on a quite individual basis, in one generation, and subject to no existing social restrictions.

The old eugenics would have required a continual selection—for breeding—of the fit, and a culling out of the unfit. The new eugenics would permit in principle the conversion of all of the unfit to the highest genetic level.

The old eugenics was limited to a numerical enhancement of the best of our existing gene pool. The horizons of the new eugenics are in principle boundless—for we should have the potential to create new genes and new qualities yet undreamed. But of course the ethical dilemma remains. What are the best qualities, and who shall choose?

It is a new horizon in the history of man. Some may smile and may feel that this is but a new version of the old dream of the perfection of man. It is that, but it is something more. The old dreams of the cultural perfection of man were always sharply constrained by his inherent, inherited imperfections and limitations. Man is

* Kenneth Vaux, ed.: *Who Shall Live? Medicine, Technology, Ethics.* Philadelphia: Fortress Press 92–93 (1970). Copyright © 1970 by Fortress Press. Reprinted by permission.

† 32 *Engineering and Science* 8, 13 (April 1969). Reprinted by permission of the California Institute of Technology.

all too clearly an imperfect and flawed creature. Considering his evolution, it is hardly likely that he could be otherwise. To foster his better traits and to curb his worse by cultural means alone has always been, while clearly not impossible, in many instances most difficult. It has been an Archimedian attempt to move the world, but with the short arm of a lever. We now glimpse another route—the chance to ease the internal strains and heal the internal flaws directly, to carry on and consciously perfect far beyond our present vision this remarkable product of two billion years of evolution.

I know there are those who find this concept and this prospect repugnant—who fear, with reason, that we may unleash forces beyond human scale and who recoil from this responsibility. I would suggest to them that they do not see our present situation whole. They are not among the losers in that chromosomal lottery that so firmly channels our human destinies. This response does not come from the 250,000 children born each year in this country with structural or functional defects, of which it is estimated 80% involve a genetic component. And this figure counts only those with gross evident defects outside those ranges we choose to call natural. It does not include the 50,000,000 "normal" Americans with an IQ of less than 90.

We who are among those who were favored in the chromosomal lottery and, in the nature of things, it will be our very conscious choice, whether as a species we will continue to accept the innumerable, individual tragedies inherent in the outcome of this mindless, age-old throw of dice, or instead will shoulder the responsibility for intelligent genetic intervention.

As we enlarge man's freedom, we diminish his constraints and that which he must accept as given. Equality of opportunity is a noble aim given the currently inescapable genetic diversity of man. But what does equality of opportunity mean to the child born with an IQ of 50?

* * *

b.

José M. R. Delgado
Physical Control of the Mind—Toward a Psychocivilized Society*

* * *

The most alarming aspect of ESB [electrical stimulation of the brain] is that psychological

* New York: Harper & Row 213–217, 220, 238–241, 244 (1969). Copyright © 1969 by José M. R. Delgado. Reprinted by permission.

reactivity can be influenced by applying a few volts to a determined area of the brain. This fact has been interpreted by many people as a disturbing threat to human integrity. In the past, the individual could face risks and pressures with preservation of his own identity. His body could be tortured, his thoughts and desires could be challenged by bribes, by emotions, and by public opinion, and his behavior could be influenced by environmental circumstances, but he always had the privilege of deciding his own fate, of dying for an ideal without changing his mind. Fidelity to our emotional and intellectual past gives each of us a feeling of transcendental stability— and perhaps of immortality—which is more precious than life itself.

New neurological technology, however, has a refined efficiency. The individual is defenseless against direct manipulation of the brain because he is deprived of his most intimate mechanisms of biological reactivity. In experiments, electrical stimulation of appropriate intensity always prevailed over free will; and, for example, flexion of the hand evoked by stimulation of the motor cortex cannot be voluntarily avoided. Destruction of the frontal lobes produced changes in affectiveness which are beyond any personal control.

The possibility of scientific annihilation of personal identity, or even worse, its purposeful control, has sometimes been considered a future threat more awful than atomic holocaust. Even physicians have expressed doubts about the propriety of physical tampering with the psyche, maintaining that personal identity should be inviolable, that any attempt to modify individual behavior is unethical, and that methods—and related research—which can influence the human brain should be banned. The prospect of any degree of physical control of the mind provokes a variety of objections: theological objections because it affects free will, moral objections because it affects individual responsibility, ethical objections because it may block self-defense mechanisms, philosophical objections because it threatens personal identity.

These objections, however, are debatable. A prohibition of scientific advance is obviously naive and unrealistic. It could not be universally imposed, and, more important, it is not knowledge itself but its improper use which should be regulated. A knife is neither good nor bad; But it may be used by either a surgeon or an assassin. Science should be neutral, but scientists should take sides. . . .

. . . It is accepted medical practice to try and

modify the antisocial or abnormal reactions of mental patients. Psychoanalysis, the use of drugs such as energizers and tranquilizers, the application of insulin or electroshock, and other varieties of psychiatric treatment are all aimed at influencing the abnormal personality of the patient in order to change his undesirable mental characteristics. The possible use, therefore, of implanted electrodes in mental patients should not pose unusual ethical complications if the accepted medical rules are followed. Perhaps the limited efficiency of standard psychiatric procedures is one reason that they have not caused alarm among scientists or laymen. Psychoanalysis requires a long time, and a person can easily withdraw his cooperation and refuse to express intimate thoughts. Electroshock is a crude method of doubtful efficacy in normal people. Although electrical stimulation of the brain is still in the initial stage of its development, it is in contrast far more selective and powerful; it may delay a heart beat, move a finger, bring a word to memory, or set a determined behavioral tone.

When medical indications are clear and the standard therapeutic procedures have failed, most patients and doctors are willing to test a new method, provided that the possibility of success outweighs the risk of worsening the situation. The crucial decision to start applying a new therapeutic method to human patients requires a combination of intelligent evaluation of data, knowledge of comparative neurophysiology, foresight, moral integrity, and courage. Excessive aggressiveness in a doctor may cause irreparable damage, but too much caution may deprive patients of needed help. The surgical procedure of lobotomy was perhaps applied to many mental patients too quickly, before its dangers and limitations were understood; but pallidectomy and thalamotomy in the treatment of Parkinson's disease encountered formidable initial opposition before attaining their present recognition and respected status.

While pharmacological and surgical treatment of sufferers of mental illness is accepted as proper, people with other behavioral deviations pose a different type of ethical problem. They may be potentially dangerous to themselves and to society when their mental functions are maintained within normal limits and only one aspect of their personal conduct is socially unacceptable. The rights of an individual to obtain appropriate treatment must be weighed with a professional evaluation of his behavioral problems—and their possible neurological basis—which necessitates a value judgment of the person's behavior in com-

parison with accepted norms. One example will illustrate these considerations.

In the early 1950s, a patient in a state mental hospital approached Dr. Hannibal Hamlin and me requesting help. She was an attractive 24-year-old woman of average intelligence and education who had a long record of arrests for disorderly conduct. She had been repeatedly involved in bar brawls in which she incited men to fight over her and had spent most of the preceding few years either in jail or in mental institutions. The patient expressed a strong desire as well as an inability to alter her conduct, and, because psychiatric treatment had failed, she and her mother urgently requested that some kind of brain surgery be performed in order to control her disreputable, impulsive behavior. They asked specifically that electrodes be implanted to orient possible electrocoagulation of a limited cerebral area; and if that wasn't possible, they wanted lobotomy.

Medical knowledge and experience at that time could not ascertain whether ESB or the application of cerebral lesions could help to solve this patient's problem, and surgical intervention was therefore rejected. When this decision was explained, both the patient and her mother reacted with similar anxious comments, asking, "What is the future? Only jail or the hospital? Is there no hope?" This case revealed the limitations of therapy and the dilemma of possible behavioral control. Supposing that long-term stimulation of a determined brain structure could influence the tendencies of a patient to drink, flirt, and induce fights; would it be ethical to change her personal characteristics? People *are* changing their character by self-medication through hallucinogenic drugs, but do they have the right to demand that doctors administer treatment that will radically alter their behavior? What are the limits of individual rights and doctors' obligations?

*   *   *

When an individual's behavior is judged unfit by members of a society, the consequences may be forceful deprivation of liberty and incarceration. If the individual is confined to a mental hospital, his undesirable conduct may cause the authorities to administer drugs, by forceful injection if necessary, in order to change or control his behavioral responses. In the early 1950s an historical precedent was established for the deliberate destruction of part of the brain as a legal treatment for criminals. A man apprehended in Pittsburgh after committing a series of robberies was given the alternative of a long jail sentence or submission to frontal lobe surgery which might curb or eliminate his future criminal behavior. Lobotomy was performed, and, although initially the patient appeared better adjusted socially, several months later he committed more thefts. When he realized that the police were closing in, he wrote a letter to the surgeon expressing appreciation for his efforts and regret that the operation had not been successful. Hoping that the study of his case might help others, he donated his brain to the surgeon and committed suicide by shooting himself through the heart. In spite of this therapeutic failure, the possibility of surgical rehabilitation of criminals has been considered by several scientists as more humane, more promising, and less damaging for the individual than his incarceration for life.

* * *

[T]he desires and mechanisms for choice are determined mainly by early childhood experiences, cultural imprinting, and learned patterns of response. Newborn babies are completely dependent on parental care for the quality and quantity of sensory inputs as well as for food and warmth. The elements offered by the environment are almost infinite, but only a limited number are used to structure each individual. Their selection depends on chance, which among many variables includes the presence and behavior of parents and teachers. We must recognize that initially an individual has no control over the sensory inputs which mold his mind, and that during the decisive years of childhood, when each of us receives emotional impacts, behavioral formulas, and ideological frameworks, we are unable to search independently for alternatives. Our initial personality is structured in a rather automatic way when our capacity for intelligent choice has not developed.

If we accept that early experience is decisive for the establishment of personal identity, then we must accept that individual mental structure is not self-determined but hetero-determined by the interaction of genes received from our ancestors and information received from the environment and culture. Where, then, is the freedom to construct personal identity? To clarify these ideas, let us remember that liberal societies are based on the principle of individual self-determination, with the assumption that each human being is *born free* and has the *right* to de-

velop his own mind, to construct his own ideology, to shape his own behavior, and to express his personality without external pressures or indoctrination. The role of education, which involves both parents and schools, is to help these processes evolve with due respect for the individual. One of the main goals in these societies is "to find ourselves," and to develop our potential while remaining independent and self-sufficient. Privacy has a high priority in its intellectual, emotional, material, and territorial aspects, and personal freedom stops with interference in the rights of others.

This kind of liberal orientation has great appeal, but unfortunately its assumptions are not supported by neurophysiological and psychological studies of intercerebral mechanisms. The brain of the newborn lacks the stored information, neuronal circuits, and functional keyboards prerequisite to the formulation of choice. The infant may have the right to be free, but he has neither the option nor the biological mechanisms for free behavior. Confrontation with a multiplicity of choices may create confusion and anxiety in a child who does not yet possess the necessary mental sophistication to choose. This frustrating situation of inadequacy may have a traumatic and deforming effect rather than a constructive and positive one. The brain of an adult usually possesses the capacity to select a response but even it is not self-sufficient; for the brain needs constant environmental inputs in order to preserve mental normality, and a flow of information is necessary to make each judgment against the background of experience.

* * *

The brain, per se, with all its genes, is not sufficient for the development of a mind in the absence of external information, and the content of this information is decisive in the establishment of mental structure. Even the withdrawal of parental care is a factor which can irrevocably shape future behavior of the young, as demonstrated by Harlow's neurotic motherless monkeys and by the emotional and mental handicap suffered by homeless children.

* * *

Whatever we do or fail to do when we are in charge of a baby will influence his future mental structure. Our attitude, therefore, should not be to close our eyes and accept chance, but to investigate the extracerebral and intracerebral elements which intervene in the formation of personality. To study what is going on inside of the brain is as important as to consider the other aspects of education and behavior.

These remarks are intended both to demonstrate that we should not base our interpersonal relations on false or unproved assumptions and to indicate the need to study these problems experimentally within the framework of intracerebral physiology. As our power to influence the mental structure of man continually increases, we face the question of the kind of people we would like to create. We must realize that parents and educators are imprinting and manipulating the minds and personalities of young people in any case, and that we are responsible for giving coherent form and ethical purpose to the psychogenetic elements transmitted to the child. The issue is whether violence and other behavioral patterns are inborn and inevitable or whether they are mainly related to a cultural learning which may be influenced by intelligent planning.

Ecological forces cannot be ignored or destroyed. Liberation from and domination of the environment became possible when we discovered the laws of nature and directed them with our intelligence. We cannot ignore the biological laws of the mind either. We should use our intelligence to direct our behavior, rather than accept its determination by unknown forces. Through education we should provide awareness of the elements, including intracerebral mechanisms, which intervene in the formation of personal identity, and we should teach the processes of decision-making and intelligent choice. Personal freedom is not a biological gift but a mental attribute which must be learned and cultivated. To be free is not to satisfy sexual drive, to fill an empty stomach, or to quarrel with our wives because of our repressed fears or mother-infant relations. Freedom requires the recognition of biological drives and their intelligent direction through processes of sublimation, substitution, postponement, or simply their satisfaction with civilized refinement and enjoyment. Individual freedom will increase when we understand the setting of our personality in early childhood and when we develop means for the intelligent evaluation and emotional interpretation of the information reaching us from the environment.

*　　*　　*

The old temple inscription "Know Thyself" is often repeated today, but perhaps it is not adequate. It should declare "Construct Thyself" as well. Shape your mind, train your thinking power, and direct your emotions more rationally; liberate your behavior from the ancestral burden of reptiles and monkeys—be a man and use your intelligence to orient the reactions of your mind.

*　　*　　*

NOTES

NOTE 1.

FRANK J. AYD, JR.
FETOLOGY—MEDICAL AND ETHICAL
IMPLICATIONS OF INTERVENTION IN THE
PRENATAL PERIOD*

*　　*　　*

. . . Edwards and his associates at Cambridge University reported that they had fertilized human egg cells *in vitro,* after overcoming the problem of sperm incapacitation. They inseminated 56 eggs, but only seven were truly fertilized, five of which were abnormal. There are several possible explanations for the abnormalities, one of which is that the experimental techniques themselves damaged otherwise healthy human oocytes. Obviously, many difficulties must be surmounted, but the hope of growing a human embryo in a test tube has been stimulated, and more efforts to achieve this growth can be expected. The objective is not to create a test-tube baby, but to gain more understanding of infertility and sterility problems, of human reproduction and growth, and ultimately to implant laboratory-grown blastocysts into women who are infertile because they lack ovaries or because their fallopian tubes are blocked. The latter may be a laudable goal, but are the means ethically unobjectionable? At present, there is no possible way of sustaining the life and development of human embryos *in vitro;* hence, their death or deliberate destruction is inevitable. This being so, should not scientists, out of respect and reverence for human life, refrain from this form of human experimentation and seek to attain their objectives in other ways? Purposely to initiate human life while knowing that it cannot survive cannot be justified by extolling the knowledge acquired and its potentially useful applications. However desirable, a good end does not authorize the use of any means. We must ask not only if *in vitro* fertilization of human

* 169 *Annals of the New York Academy of Sciences* 376–378 (1970). Reprinted by permission.

ova for these ends is immoral, but also if it is a warning of a dehumanizing trend in science.

For many valid reasons, scientists desire to know the sex of a human embryo as early as possible and to chart fetal maturation until birth. Not only are some doing cytological examinations of ova from women with somatic chromosome mosaicism, but some also are contemplating sexing the blastocyst by removing it before nidation in the uterus, excising a fragment of trophoblast and determining the sex-chromatin score of stained trophoblast cells. If the blastocyst is of the desired sex, it would be returned to the mother or to the uterus of a suitable foster parent, hopefully, to implant and grow. This has not been done in humans, but, if it becomes feasible, it would be used to control the sex of human babies, not merely to satisfy a parental whim, but to control or eradicate serious sex-linked diseases. If it should be demonstrated that a blastocyst has a sex-linked disease (for example, hemophilia), it would not be replaced in the womb. Edwards and Gardner justify this by asking: "Would not the non-replacement of a blastocyst be (socially and ethically) far more acceptable than a full-scale abortion of the implanted, thriving fetus—the only alternative today?" Implicit in this question is the conviction that there is no alternative to abortion, that the handicapped should be denied the right to life, and that physicians should have the authority to make and act on this judgment. This compels me to ask: What kind of medical scientist is he who prefers to eradicate suffering rather than face the responsibility of relieving it? What kind of a society would condone such conduct by medical scientists? . . .

*   *   *

NOTE 2.

HAROLD M. SCHMECK, JR.
VIRUS IS INJECTED INTO TWO CHILDREN IN
EFFORT TO ALTER CHEMICAL TRAIT*

Scientists here and abroad are watching with interest the progress of two little girls in West Germany who have been infected deliberately with a virus that causes harmless wart-like growths in rabbits.

The two girls, one about 2 years old and the

---

* *The New York Times* 28, col. 3 (September 21, 1970). © 1970 by The New York Times Company. Reprinted by permission.

other about 7, were given the virus in the hope that it might correct a serious hereditary defect. The project is one attempt to alter intentionally an inborn chemical trait, a feat that has never been achieved or even been considered a practical possibility.

The feat seems theoretically possible because the virus is believed to carry a genetic blueprint for making an important enzyme that the two sisters lack. If the virus infection introduces these genetic instructions into the children's cells, the girls might begin to manufacture the missing enzyme.

The two girls were born with a hereditary biochemical defect that left them unable to make the enzyme arginase. The enzyme normally breaks down the chemical arginine from ordinary food. Lacking the enzyme, the girls accumulate large excesses of arginine in their blood. This has produced mental retardation and other serious problems in the older girl, and the younger is developing in the same fashion.

*   *   *

Dr. Rogers [of Oakridge National Laboratory in Tennessee] said it was probably too late to do anything for the older girl. The main hope is that the progression of ill effects in the younger sister can be arrested.

The possibility arises because of the discovery years ago of a peculiarity of the Shope papilloma virus, the virus being given to the two girls. The discoverer of the virus, Dr. Richard Shope of the Rockefeller Institute for Medical Research, injected himself with it in the mid-1930's and suffered no ill effects then or later, but his blood levels of arginine did drop noticeably and stayed low for a long time.

During the mid-1960's Dr. Rogers and his co-workers published a report noting that about half the laboratory workers in laboratories studying the virus also had low arginine levels. It appeared that accidental infections with the virus had given the workers an excessive ability to make arginase.

*   *   *

The prospect of using a virus to make an essentially genetic change of this sort has long been discussed as a theoretical possibility for the distant future. Two children whose inborn defect matches the possible corrective action of the virus may be providing an eary test of that idea.

c.

Louis Jolyon West
Ethical Psychiatry and Biosocial Humanism*

*   *   *

A member of the APA was expelled because he publicly described and justified sexual intimacies with female patients as beneficial therapeutic procedures. But no complaint had been made by a patient in this case. What, therefore, was the written and published criterion for ethical behavior that this physician violated? Was it the Oath of Hippocrates? Other facets of that oath have recently fallen in the face of legal reforms, for example, concerning abortions. The former member in question could not really be accused of advertising, since his revelation was made in a professional journal. Even a challenge that he was administering a valueless procedure in the name of therapy could be argued, since clinicians from Hippocrates to Freud have noted the beneficial effects of sexual intercourse in certain cases.

Even if the Ethics Committee turned to the community for support in the form of laws forbidding extramarital sexual congress, it appears that such statutes may soon fall before the growing acceptance of the principle set forth in the Wolfenden Report that sexual acts between consenting adults in private are not a matter for concern under the criminal code. Nevertheless, I feel certain that the overwhelming majority of psychiatrists would agree that it is unethical to seduce patients and foolish (if not outrageous) to call it treatment.

3.

Pursuit of Knowledge

a.

Robert Reinhold
Psychologist Arouses Storm by Linking I.Q. to Heredity†

A storm is brewing over a suggestion by a leading educational psychologist that intelligence is determined largely by heredity and cannot be altered significantly by improving environment.

For this reason, argues the psychologist, Dr. Arthur R. Jensen of the University of California at Berkeley, compensatory education programs designed to raise the intelligence of disadvantaged children by enriching their cultural surroundings are misdirected.

Further, he theorizes, the measured mental differences between racial and ethnic groups are rooted in inborn genetic differences that are as much a part of group identity as skin color, hair texture and blood chemistry.

Such hereditary factors, he believes, may account for the fact that Negroes average 15 points below whites on I.Q. tests. Recent evidence, he adds, indicates that children from Negro and other disadvantaged groups do poorly in "cognitive" learning—the ability to reason abstractly—while they do well in "associative" learning, which involves rote learning and memory.

If this theory can be substantiated, says Dr. Jensen, then "the next step will be to develop the techniques by which school learning can be most effectively achieved in accordance with different patterns of ability."

This is the chief conclusion of a controversial 123-page study by Dr. Jensen in the current issues of *The Harvard Educational Review*, a student-run publication of the Harvard Graduate School of Education.

Dr. Jensen's theories are not new, but the force with which he presents them has rekindled issues that have long divided geneticists, psychologists and educators. . . .

*   *   *

Predictably, the Jensen article has prompted heated reaction from those who say it lends support to racist claims that Negroes are inferior to whites intellectually.

*   *   *

In addition, a number of geneticists and psychologists believe Dr. Jensen may have overinterpreted the limited scientific evidence available—particularly on the question of racial differences.

"From the standpoint of methodology, this is as difficult an issue as geneticists confront today," said a leading human geneticist. "It is conceivable there are signficant mental differences between blacks and whites—but we simply do not have the information to reach a valid conclusion. Negroes have been subjected to so many subtle kinds of discrimination that we cannot compare the two groups."

However, Dr. Jensen says his study was intended as an objective scientific analysis of an area that he feels has long been taboo.

* * *

In an interview, Dr. Jensen indicated that he would not recommend widespread use of his ideas without further research. "I'm trying to stimulate more research," he said. "There should not be any fear in finding biological differences between groups."

Reaction to the article has been swift. . . .

Another leading geneticist, Prof. James F. Crow of the University of Wisconsin, said he agreed "for the most part" with Dr. Jensen's analysis of the high heritability of I.Q. but disagreed on the interpretation.

"No matter how high the heritability," Dr. Crow said "there is no assurance that a sufficiently great environmental difference does not account for the differences in the two means [between Negro and white I.Q.'s], especially when one considers that the environmental factors may differ qualitatively in the two groups."

* * *

NOTES

NOTE 1.

LAWRENCE E. DAVIES
HARRASSMENT CHARGED BY AUTHOR OF
ARTICLE ABOUT NEGROES' I.Q.'s*

An educational psychologist who describes himself as a liberal and a strong civil rights advocate has been the subject in the last month of what he calls a campaign of harrassment depicting him as bent on promoting racism.

Repeated calls for the dismissal of Dr. Arthur L. Jensen from the faculty of the University of California, Berkeley, have been sounded since an article by him was published in the winter issue of the *Harvard Educational Review*.

* * *

The militant Students for a Democratic Society began in mid-April to attack the 45-year-old educator, a Berkeley faculty member for 11 years. A sound truck operating in the vicinity of the campus demanded "Fight racism, fire Jensen," and circulars described him as "Berkeley's white supremacist crusader."

* * *

In the last three weeks hardly an issue of *The Daily Californian*, the campus newspaper, has been published without one to three letters from students and faculty members assailing or defending Dr. Jensen. News articles and editorials have also kept the issue alive.

Dr. John Searle, professor of philosophy and chairman of the Berkeley academic freedom committee, said that the committee members had discussed the Jensen case.

"Any attempt to fire him would be a violation of academic freedom," Professor Searle told an inquirer, "but no such attempt has been made. . . ."

* * *

NOTE 2.
COUNCIL OF THE SOCIETY FOR THE
PSYCHOLOGICAL STUDY OF SOCIAL ISSUES
STATEMENT*

As behavioral scientists, we believe that statements specifying the hereditary components of intelligence are unwarranted by the present state of scientific knowledge. [W]e believe that such statements may be seriously misinterpreted, particularly in their applications to social policy.

The evidence of four decades of research on this problem can be readily summarized. There are marked differences in intelligence test scores when one compares a random sample of whites and Negroes. What is equally clear is that little definitive evidence exists that leads to the conclusion that such differences are innate. The evidence points overwhelmingly to the fact that when one compares Negroes and whites of comparable cultural and educational background, differences in intelligence test scores diminish markedly; the more comparable the background, the less the difference. There is no direct evidence that supports the view that there is an innate difference between members of different racial groups.

[A] more accurate understanding of the contribution of heredity to intelligence will be possible only when social conditions for all races are equal and when this situation has existed for several generations. . . . Social inequalities deprive large numbers of black people of social, economic, and educational advantages available to a great majority of the white population. The exist-

* *The New York Times* 33, col. 1 (May 19, 1969). © 1969 by The New York Times Company. Reprinted by permission.

* 39 *Harvard Educational Review* 625–627 (1969). Reprinted by permission.

ing social structures prevent black and white people even of the same social class from leading comparable lives. In light of these conditions, it is obvious that no scientific discussion of racial differences can exclude an examination of political, historic, economic, and psychological factors which are inextricably related to racial differences.

* * *

[A] number of Jensen's key assumptions and conclusions are seriously questioned by many psychologists and geneticists.

The question of the relative contributions of heredity and environment to human development and behavior has a long history of controversy within psychology. Recent research indicates that environmental factors play a role from the moment of the child's conception. The unborn child develops as a result of a complex, little understood, interaction between hereditary and environmental factors; this interaction continues throughout life. To construct questions about complex behavior in terms of heredity *versus* environment is to over-simplify the essence and nature of human development and behavior.

* * *

The Council . . . reaffirms its long-held position of support for open inquiry on all aspects of human behavior. We are concerned with establishing high standards of scientific inquiry and of scientific responsibility. Included in these standards must be careful interpretation of research findings, with rigorous attention to alternative explanations. In no area of science are these principles more important than in the study of human behavior, where a variety of social factors may have large and far-reaching effects. When research has bearing on social issues and public policy, the scientist must examine the competing explanations for his findings and must exercise the greatest care in his interpretation. Only in this way can he minimize the possibility that others will overgeneralize or misunderstand the social implications of his work.

NOTE 3.

DARTMOUTH BLACKS BAR PHYSICIST'S TALK*

Dr. William Shockley, a Nobel prize winner in physics, was prevented from delivering a

* *The New York Times* 37, col. 2 (Oct. 16, 1969). © 1969 by The New York Times Company. Reprinted by permission.

paper on genetic racial differences today when about 30 Negro students applauded continuously and would not stop.

Dr. Shockley was to have delivered the paper at the fall meeting of the National Academy of Sciences at Dartmouth College.

Dr. Shockley, a professor of engineering science at Stanford University, had provoked controversy in the last year with his views that inheritance, rather than environment, may be the major factor in intelligence.

* * *

There had been some speculation that Dr. Shockley would not be well received on the campus. A letter from the National Academy of Sciences was read before Dr. Shockley's introduction. It read in part: "As a member of the National Academy of Sciences, Dr. William Shockley has the privilege of addressing the academy on matters he believes deserving of its interest. For several years he has used this opportunity to attempt to persuade the academy to sponsor or encourage research to determine the relative importance of genetic inheritance as a factor in human intelligence, separate and apart from environmental factors."

"However," the letter continued, "the academy considers that the field is already being actively pursued. Whereas the academy encourages work in this, as in all other legitimate fields of inquiry, it regards all studies in this area with great reservation. Since Dr. Shockley has offered no new research program and no new approach . . . the N.A.S. does not endorse his recommendations."

NOTE 4.

LUTHER J. CARTER
NAS AGAIN SAYS NO TO SHOCKLEY*

For more than 4 years now, William Shockley, a Stanford physicist who shared a Nobel Prize for his part in inventing the transistor, has been carrying on a dogged campaign to have the National Academy of Sciences encourage research in "dysgenics." As he defines it, dysgenics has to do with the "retrogressive evolution" of a population through the reproduction, in disproportionately large numbers, of its genetically inferior elements. Specifically, Shockley is afraid that the U.S. population is declining

* 168 *Science* 685 (1970). Copyright 1970 by the American Association for the Advancement of Science. Reprinted by permission.

in quality through the reproduction of large numbers of Negroes of low I.Q., a view which he says can in no sense be ascribed to a "racist" motivation. Last week, the academy rebuffed Shockley's latest attempt to have it go on record as favoring dysgenics research. His proposed resolution to that effect was not seconded. He found some satisfaction, however, in the as yet unreleased report of an academy committee.

This committee was appointed by Philip Handler, president of the academy, after an academy meeting last October at which Shockley had again raised the dysgenics research issue. Kingsley Davis, a sociologist at Berkeley, was named chairman. According to Shockley, the report of the Davis committee, which the academy received but took no action on, acknowledges that study of racial and hereditary differences is "proper and socially relevant."

"The report indicates that members of the committee 'variously' regarded the impact of suppressive attitudes on research in this area," Shockley told *Science*. "The difference in viewpoints on research taboos about human quality problems are enormous in my opinion. I think the word 'variously' does not portray this."

Shockley added, however, that "my general reaction is that this report represents enormous progress over the one issued in 1967." Here Shockley was alluding to a 1967 report of the academy which concluded in part by questioning "the social urgency of a crash program to measure genetic differences in intellectual and emotional traits between racial groups." "In the first place, if the traits are at all complex [as the report had said they would surely be], the results of such research are almost certain to be inconclusive," this report said. "In the second place, it is not clear that major social decisions depend on such information; we would hope that persons would be considered as individuals and not as members of groups."

*   *   *

NOTE 5.

SCOTT THACHER
SHOCKLEY STICKS BY RACE THEORIES*

Professor William B. Shockley proposes scientific research to determine whether the genetic potential for intelligence of black people differs from whites. Because of his insistence on spreading this view, he is probably one of the most dis-

* *Stanford Daily* 4, col. 1 (Dec. 2, 1970). Reprinted by permission.

liked and controversial figures on campus, a person many prefer to ignore.

*   *   *

Joshua Lederberg, chairman of the Department of Genetics, and a Nobel Prize winner claims Shockley has already made his own conclusions about black-white differences. "He has chosen to ventilate his own inflammatory prejudgement of the results of research thinly disguised as a 'question.' "

However, the crux of Shockley's disagreement with many other scientists lies in the emphasis he places on heredity, as opposed to environment, in determining the intelligence and motivation of an individual.

On the nature-nurture argument, he says, "there is one piece (of evidence) that it's irresponsible not to accept." He states it as follows: "Heredity is more than twice as important as environment in determining intelligence as measured by IQ tests in families that adopt one of a pair of white identical twins."

He does not extrapolate this to the difference in average intelligence between races. The distribution of black IQ's is offset downwards by about 15 points from the IQ's of whites. However, Shockley's opinion is that less than half of this difference is accounted for by a different environment.

It is a nonfact that simply "blames the Negro IQ deficit on cultural disadvantages," says Shockley. "There is a whole pattern of relationships which appear to be explainable far more simply on the basis of racial genetic differences than in any other way."

He cites evidence which shows that blacks perform better on tests of verbal skills than they do on reasoning, numerical, or spatial ones, compared to the relative levels for whites. In addition, he observes that socially valuable character traits may be correlated with IQ. He says this correlation "can be four times greater for whites than for Negroes."

Shockley submits that these things may be evidence for racial genetic differences that are not greatly affected by environmental ones. He has proposed to study this further by comparing the racial compositions and average IQ's of different black populations living in uniform slum environments.

This could be done by measuring the frequency of a certain blood type that is very rare among the Africans from which the blacks came, but found in 43 per cent of all Caucasians. In a letter to *Scientific American* he writes that "my own preliminary research suggests that an increase of 1 per cent in Caucasian ancestry raises Negro IQ about one point on the average for low IQ populations."

* * *

Shockley's ideas are contested by academicians here in two main areas. First, they challenge his view that genetic factors pretty well limit intelligence to the level we observe. This idea implies that the difference in black and white IQ distributions cannot be eliminated solely by educational means.

* * *

The other area of disagreement is over the possibility of a genetic basis for racial IQ differences. A member of the Department of Genetics, suggested in *Scientific American* that this question "will be almost impossible to answer satisfactorily before the environmental differences between U.S. blacks and whites have been substantially reduced."

Dr. John L. Black, director of the Counseling and Testing Service, agrees with both views. While the study of racial differences in intelligence "might be interesting research, this has little practical significance."

In addition, he is of the opinion that the difference would be far more difficult to find than Shockley thinks. "What little talents we have might better be put more directly to the solution of educational problems."

* * *

NOTE 6.

Scott Thacher
Self-Esteem Plays Part in Shockley's Research*

Professor William Shockley is quite candid about why he pursues the topic of worsening heredity among black people. "It's what I will think of myself. . . . It's very self-oriented."

The decline of genetic potential among all races, "might well be the most important single factor in the future of the nation, maybe even the future of the world. No one else of equal eminence is tackling this one."

He feels pride is not unnatural when one undertakes a difficult project. "In the end you will be very concerned with your self-esteem

and this seems to be the nature of man or thinking man."

This is one of the conclusions that Shockley the philosopher draws from his three humanistic postulates. The first postulate is that a humane civilization depends on "man's concern for the emotions experienced by his fellow creatures." The second is that "The truth shall make you free."

He states the third, "Terminal Self-Esteem," as follows: "During the last rational five minutes of my life, I hope to consider that since 1967 I have used my capacities close to their maximum potential, in keeping with the objectives of Nobel's Will, of conferring the greatest benefit on mankind."

* * *

"His whole thrust is for rational criteria," says [Professor William] Spicer, who has known him for several years. "His whole conflict comes from people who use arguments he feels don't have a rational basis." When dealing with social questions, "He has more faith than I do that you can isolate all the variables."

A student who worked for Shockley last summer concurs: "The simplicity of his models is very nice to use." But he is unsure "whether you can really compute human intelligence with one or two variables. . . . His (Shockley's) limitation to the direct and physical sciences is his greatest danger."

Other men, such as Joshua Lederberg, feel that Shockley's advent into the fields of sociology and genetics has been something less than professional. Lederberg calls Shockley's recent pronouncements "an abuse of his privilege as a scientist."

* * *

NOTE 7.

John Walsh
National Academy of Sciences— Awkward Moments at the Meeting*

* * *

The Academy grappled again with the controversial subject of "behavioral genetics" and voted by a decisive margin not to encourage expanded federal research on the effects on intelligence of genetic differences. At the same time

* *Stanford Daily* 3, col. 3 (Dec. 3, 1970). Reprinted by permission.

* 172 *Science* 539–541 (1971). Copyright 1971 by the American Association for the Advancement of Science. Reprinted by permission.

that members turned down a committee recommendation that the Academy form an internal working group to study the feasibility of long-term research on the subject. The Academy members did, however, approve a recommendation favoring cooperation to put research in behavioral genetics in a broader scientific context.

*   *   *

Academy action on the behavioral genetics issue came in response to persistent efforts by William Shockley, co-developer of the transistor, to persuade the Academy to back research to establish the scientific basis of what he has called the "racial genetic intellectual disadvantages of the nation's black minority"....

A Shockley proposal for Academy action in 1969 led to formation of a blue-ribbon Academy study group headed by Kingsley Davis of the University of California at Berkeley. The report of the Davis committee was circulated to the Academy membership in advance of this year's meeting and last Wednesday was accepted by the members after the second and third of three recommendations had been rejected.

*   *   *

The first recommendation,† which the membership approved is, according to [Academy president Philip] Handler, addressed "to the academic world in a general way." Despite its vagueness, the recommendation appears to go somewhat further than previous Academy statements on the issue, and Shockley has been quoted as saying he feels the action indicated the Academy has "faced down the road" toward further action.

In the body of its brief report, the committee stresses that "the genetic aspects of behavioral characteristics in men are very inadequately known." And Handler in commenting on the report said "the important aspects of human behavioral genetics have to do with individual differences rather than differences between groups." Knowledgeable observers say the Academy faced the dilemma on the behavioral genet-ics issue of appearing to limit scientific inquiry on the one hand or of backing research on the other and sought to steer between the two shoals.

*   *   *

b.

President's Commission on Obscenity and Pornography Report and Model Statute*

*   *   *

Section 2. Sale and display of explicit sexual material to young persons. (a) Purpose. It is the purpose of this section to regulate the direct commercial distribution of certain explicit sexual materials to young persons in order to aid parents in supervising and controlling the access of children to such material. The legislature finds that whatever social value such material may have for young persons can adequately be served by its availability to young persons through their parents.

(b) Offenses Defined. A person is guilty of a misdemeanor if he

(i) knowingly disseminates explicit sexual material . . . to young persons. . . .

*   *   *

(e) Defenses. It shall be an affirmative defense to a prosecution under this section for the defendant to show:

(i) That the dissemination was made with the consent of a parent or guardian of the recipient. . . .

*   *   *

A primary basis for the Commission's recommendation for repeal of adult legislation is the fact that extensive empirical investigations do not indicate any causal relationship between exposure to or use of explicit sexual materials and such social or individual harms such as crime, delinquency, sexual or nonsexual deviancy, or severe emotional disturbances. The absence of empirical evidence supporting such a causal relationship also applies to the exposure of children to erotic materials. However, insufficient research is presently available on the effect of the exposure of children to sexually explicit materials to enable us to reach conclusions with the same degree of confidence as for adult exposure. Strong ethical feelings against experimentally exposing children to sexually explicit materials considerably reduced the possibility of gathering the necessary data and information regarding young persons.

---

† We recommend exploration of means for closer cooperation among those concerned with research and training in psychology, education, behavioral genetics, and neurobiology. Such cooperation will be especially valuable to the extent that it contributes to broader training and the extension of competent research that combines the insights and techniques of behavioral genetics with those of other fields. [*Ibid* at 540.]

---

* Washington, D.C.: U.S. Government Printing Office 56–57, 66–67 (1970).

In view of the limited amount of information concerning the effects of sexually explicit materials on children, other considerations have assumed primary importance in the Commission's deliberations. The Commission has been influenced, to a considerable degree, by its finding that a large majority of Americans believe that children should not be exposed to certain sexual materials. In addition, the Commission takes the view that parents should be free to make their own conclusions regarding the suitability of explicit sexual materials for their children and that it is appropriate for legislation to aid parents in controlling the access of their children to such materials during their formative years. The Commission recognizes that legislation cannot possibly isolate children from such materials entirely; it also recognizes that exposure of children to sexual materials may not only do no harm but may, in certain instances, actually facilitate much needed communication between parent and child over sexual matters. The Commission is aware, as well, of the considerable danger of creating an unnatural attraction or an enhanced interest in certain materials by making them "forbidden fruit" for young persons. The Commission believes, however, that these considerations can and should be weighed by individual parents in determining their attitudes toward the exposure of their children to sexual materials, and that legislation should aid, rather than undermine, such parental choice.

* * *

4.

Values of Investigator?

a.

Carl R. Rogers and B. F. Skinner
Some Issues Concerning the Control of Human Behavior*

I. SKINNER

* * *

[T]he control of human behavior has always been unpopular. Any undisguised effort to control usually arouses emotional reactions. We hesitate to admit, even to ourselves, that we are engaged in control, and we may refuse to

* 124 *Science* 1057–1065 (1956). Reprinted by permission.

control, even when this would be helpful, for fear of criticism. . . . Intelligent men and women, dominated by the humanistic philosophy of the past two centuries, cannot view with equanimity what Andrew Hacker has called "the specter of predictable man." Even the statistical or actuarial prediction of human events, such as the number of fatalities to be expected on a holiday weekend, strikes many people as uncanny and evil, while the prediction and control of individual behavior is regarded as little less than the work of the devil. I am not so much concerned here with the political or economic consequences for psychology, although research following certain channels may well suffer harmful effects. We ourselves, as intelligent men and women, and as exponents of Western thought, share these attitudes. They have already interfered with the free exercise of a scientific analysis, and their influence threatens to assume more serious proportions.

Three broad areas of human behavior supply good examples. The first of these—*personal control*—may be taken to include person-to-person relationships in the family, among friends, in social and work groups, and in counseling and psychotherapy. Other fields are *education* and *government*. A few examples . . . will show how nonscientific preconceptions are affecting our current thinking about human behavior.

People living together in groups come to control one another with a technique which is not inappropriately called "ethical." When an individual behaves in a fashion acceptable to the group, he receives admiration, approval, affection, and many other reinforcements which increase the likelihood that he will continue to behave in that fashion. When his behavior is not acceptable, he is criticized, censured, blamed, or otherwise punished. In the first case the group calls him "good"; in the second, "bad." This practice is so thoroughly ingrained in our culture that we often fail to see that it is a technique of control. Yet we are almost always engaged in such control, even though the reinforcements and punishments are often subtle.

* * *

[C]oncepts of choice, responsibility, justice, and so on, provide a most inadequate analysis of efficient reinforcing and punishing contingencies because they carry a heavy semantic cargo of a quite different sort, which obscures any attempt to clarify controlling practices or to improve techniques. In particular, they fail to prepare us for techniques based on other than aversive techniques of control. Most people would object to forcing prisoners to serve as subjects of dangerous medical experiments, but few object when they are induced to serve by the offer of return privileges—even when the reinforcing effect of these privileges has been created by forcible deprivation. In the traditional scheme the right to refuse guarantees the individual against coercion or an unfair bargain. But to what extent *can* a prisoner refuse under such circumstances?

We need not go so far afield to make the point. We can observe our own attitude toward personal freedom in the way we resent any interference with what we want to do. Suppose we want to buy a car of a particular sort. Then we may object, for example, if our wife urges us to buy a less expensive model and to put the difference into a new refrigerator. Or we may resent it if our neighbor questions our need for such a car or our ability to pay for it. We would certainly resent it if it were illegal to buy such a car (remember Prohibition); and if we find we cannot actually afford it, we may resent governmental control of the price through tariffs and taxes. We resent it if we discover that we cannot get the car because the manufacturer is holding the model in deliberately short supply in order to push a model we do not want. In all this we assert our democratic right to buy the car of our choice. We are well prepared to do so and to resent any restriction on our freedom.

But why do we not ask *why* it is the car of our choice and resent the forces which made it so? Perhaps our favorite toy as a child was a car, of a very different model, but nevertheless bearing the name of the car we now want. Perhaps our favorite TV program is sponsored by the manufacturer of that car. Perhaps we have seen pictures of many beautiful or prestigeful persons driving it—in pleasant or glamorous places. Perhaps the car has been designed with respect to our motivational patterns: the device on the hood is a phallic symbol; or the horsepower has been stepped up to please our competitive spirit in enabling us to pass other cars swiftly (or, as the advertisements say, "safely"). The concept of freedom that has emerged as part of the cultural practice of our group makes little or no provision for recognizing or dealing with these kinds of control. Concepts like "responsibility" and "rights" are scarcely applicable. We are prepared to deal with coercive measures, but we have no traditional recourse with respect to other measures which in the long run (and especially with the help of science) may be much more powerful and dangerous.

*   *   *

Government has always been the special field of aversive control. The state is frequently defined in terms of the power to punish, and jurisprudence leans heavily upon the associated notion of personal responsibility. Yet it is becoming increasingly difficult to reconcile current practice and theory with these earlier views. In criminology, for example, there is a strong tendency to drop the notion of responsibility in favor of some such alternative as capacity or controllability. But no matter how strongly the facts, or even practical expedience, support such a change, it is difficult to make the change in a legal system designed on a different plan. When governments resort to other techniques (for example, positive reinforcement), the concept of responsibility is no longer relevant and the theory of government is no longer applicable.

*   *   *

The uneasiness with which we view government (in the broadest possible sense) when it does not use punishment is shown by the reception of my utopian novel, *Walden Two*. This was essentially a proposal to apply a behavioral technology to the construction of a workable, effective, and productive pattern of government. It was greeted with wrathful violence. *Life* magazine called it "a travesty on the good life," and "a menace . . . a triumph of mortmain or the dead hand not envisaged since the days of Sparta . . . a slur upon a name, a corruption of an impulse." Joseph Wood Krutch devoted a substantial part of his book, *The Measure of Man,* to attacking my views and those of the protagonist, Frazier, in the same vein, and Morris Viteles has recently criticized the book in a similar manner in *Science*. Perhaps the reaction is best expressed in a quotation from *The Quest for Utopia* by Negley and Patrick:

"Halfway through this contemporary utopia, the reader may feel sure, as we did, that this is a beautifully ironic satire on what has been called 'behavioral engineering.' The longer one stays in this better world of the psychologist, however, the plainer it becomes that the inspiration is not satiric, but messianic. This is indeed the behaviorally engineered society, and while it was to be expected that sooner or later the principle of psychological conditioning would be made the basis of a serious construction of utopia —Brown anticipated it in *Limanora*—yet not even the effective satire of Huxley is adequate preparation for the shocking horror of the idea when positively presented. Of all the dictatorships espoused by utopists, this is the most profound, and incipient dictators might well find in this utopia a guidebook of political practice."

One would scarcely guess that the authors are talking about a world in which there is food, clothing, and shelter for all, where everyone chooses his own work and works on the average only 4 hours a day, where music and the arts flourish, where personal relationships develop under the most favorable circumstances, where education prepares every child for the social and intellectual life which lies before him, where—in short—people are truly happy, secure, productive, creative, and forward-looking. What is wrong with it? Only one thing: someone "planned it that way." If these critics had come upon a society in some remote corner of the world which boasted similar advantages, they would undoubtedly have hailed it as providing a pattern we all might well follow—provided that it was clearly the result of a natural process of cultural evolution. Any evidence that intelligence had been used in arriving at this version of the good life would, in their eyes, be a serious flaw. . . .

The dangers inherent in the control of human behavior are very real. The possibility of the misuse of scientific knowledge must always be faced. We cannot escape by denying the power of a science of behavior or arresting its development. It is no help to cling to familiar philosophies of human behavior simply because they are more reassuring.

*   *   *

If the advent of a powerful science of behavior causes trouble, it will not be because science itself is inimical to human welfare but because older conceptions have not yielded easily or gracefully. We expect resistance to new techniques of control from those who have heavy investments in the old, but we have no reason to help them preserve a series of principles that are not ends in themselves but rather outmoded means to an end. What is needed is a new conception of human behavior which is compatible with the implications of a scientific analysis. All men control and are controlled. The question of government in the broadest possible sense is not how freedom is to be preserved but what kinds

of control are to be used and to what ends. Control must be analyzed and considered in its proper proportions. No one, I am sure, wishes to develop new master-slave relationships or bend the will of the people to despotic rulers in new ways. These are patterns of control appropriate to a world without science. They may well be the first to go when the experimental analysis of behavior comes into its own in the design of cultural practices.

II. ROGERS

*   *   *

I am sure we agree that men—as individuals and as societies—have always endeavored to understand, predict, influence, and control human behavior—their own behavior and that of others.

I believe we agree that the behavioral sciences are making and will continue to make increasingly rapid progress in the understanding of behavior, and that as a consequence the capacity to predict and to control behavior is developing with equal rapidity.

I believe we agree that to deny these advances, or to claim that man's behavior cannot be a field of science, is unrealistic. . . .

I believe we are in agreement that the tremendous potential power of a science which permits the prediction and control of behavior may be misused, and that the possibility of such misuse constitutes a serious threat.

*   *   *

With these several points of basic and important agreement, are there then any issues that remain on which there are differences? I believe there are. They can be stated very briefly: Who will be controlled? Who will exercise control? What type of control will be exercised? Most important of all, toward what end or what purpose, or in the pursuit of what value, will control be exercised?

*   *   *

[L]et us review very briefly the various elements that are involved in the usual concept of the control of human behavior as mediated by the behavioral sciences. . . .

1) There must first be some sort of decision about goals. Usually desirable goals are assumed, but sometimes, as in George Orwell's book *1984*, the goal that is selected is an aggrandizement of individual power with which most

of us would disagree. In a recent paper Skinner suggests that one possible set of goals to be assigned to the behavioral technology is this: "Let men be happy, informed, skillful, well-behaved and productive." In the first draft of his part of this article, which he was kind enough to show me, he did not mention such definite goals as these, but desired "improved" educational practices, "wiser" use of knowledge in government, and the like. In the final version of his article he avoids even these value-laden terms, and his implicit goal is the very general one that scientific control of behavior is desirable, because it would perhaps bring "a far better world for everyone."

Thus the first step in thinking about the control of human behavior is the choice of goals, whether specific or general. It is necessary to come to terms in some way with the issue, "For what purpose?"

2) A second element is that, whether the end selected is highly specific or is a very general one such as wanting "a better world," we proceed by the methods of science to discover the means to these ends. We continue through further experimentation and investigation to discover more effective means. The method of science is self-correcting in thus arriving at increasingly effective ways of achieving the purpose we have in mind.

3) The third aspect of such control is that as the conditions or methods are discovered by which to reach the goal, some person or some group establishes these conditions and uses these methods, having in one way or another obtained the power to do so.

4) The fourth element is the exposure of individuals to the prescribed conditions, and this leads, with a high degree of probability, to behavior which is in line with the goals desired. Individuals are now happy, if that has been the goal, or well-behaved, or submissive, or whatever it has been decided to make them.

5) The fifth element is that if the process I have described is put in motion then there is a continuing social organization which will continue to produce the types of behavior that have been valued.

Are there any flaws in this way of viewing the control of human behavior? I believe there are. In fact the only element in this description with which I find myself in agreement is the second. It seems to me quite incontrovertibly true that the scientific method is an excellent way to discover the means by which to achieve our

goals. Beyond that, I feel many sharp differences, which I will try to spell out.

I believe that in Skinner's presentation here and in his previous writings, there is a serious underestimation of the problem of power. To hope that the power which is being made available by the behavioral sciences will be exercised by the scientists, or by a benevolent group, seems to me a hope little supported by either recent or distant history. It seems far more likely that behavioral scientists, holding their present attitudes, will be in the position of the German rocket scientists specializing in guided missiles. First they worked devotedly for Hitler to destroy the U.S.S.R. and the United States. Now, depending on who captured them, they work devotedly for the U.S.S.R. in the interest of destroying the United States, or devotedly for the United States in the interest of destroying the U.S.S.R. If behavioral scientists are concerned solely with advancing their science, it seems most probable that they will serve the purposes of whatever individual or group has the power.

But the major flaw I see in this review of what is involved in the scientific control of human behavior is the denial, misunderstanding, or gross underestimation of the place of ends, goals, or values in their relationship to science. . . .

In sharp contradiction to some views that have been advanced, I would like to propose a two-pronged thesis: (i) In any scientific endeavor —whether "pure" or applied science—there is a prior subjective choice of the purpose or value which that scientific work is perceived as serving. (ii) This subjective value choice which brings the scientific endeavor into being must always lie outside of that endeavor and can never become a part of the science involved in that endeavor.

Let me illustrate the first point from Skinner himself. It is clear that in his earlier writing it is recognized that a prior value choice is necessary, and it is specified as the goal that men are to become happy, well-behaved, productive, and so on. I am pleased that Skinner has retreated from the goals he then chose, because to me they seem to be stultifying values. I can only feel that he was choosing these goals for others, not for himself. I would hate to see Skinner become "well-behaved," as that term would be defined for him by behavioral scientists. His recent article in the *American Psychologist* shows that he certainly does not want to be "productive" as that value is defined by most psychologists. And the most awful fate I can imagine for him would be to have him constantly "happy." It is the fact that he is very unhappy about many things which makes me prize him.

In the first draft of his part of this article, he also included such prior value choices, saying for example, "We must decide how we are to use the knowledge which a science of human behavior is now making available." Now he has dropped all mention of such choices, and if I understand him correctly, he believes that science can proceed without them. He has suggested this view in another recent paper, stating that "We must continue to experiment in cultural design . . . testing the consequences as we go. Eventually the practices which make for the greatest biological and psychological strength of the group will presumably survive."

I would point out, however, that to choose to experiment is a value choice. Even to move in the direction of perfectly random experimentation is a value choice. To test the consequences of an experiment is possible only if we have first made a subjective choice of a criterion value. And implicit in his statement is a valuing of biological and psychological strength. So even when trying to avoid such choice, it seems inescapable that a prior subjective value choice is necessary for any scientific endeavor, or for any application of scientific knowledge.

I wish to make it clear that I am not saying that values cannot be included as a subject of science. It is not true that science deals only with certain classes of "facts" and that these classes do not include values. It is a bit more complex than that, as a simple illustration or two may make clear.

If I value knowledge of the "three R's" as a goal of education, the methods of science can give me increasingly accurate information on how this goal may be achieved. If I value problem-solving ability as a goal of education, the scientific method can give me the same kind of help.

Now, if I wish to determine whether problem-solving ability is "better" than knowledge of the three R's, then scientific method can also study those two values but only—and this is very important—in terms of some other value which I have subjectively chosen. I may value college success. Then I can determine whether problem-solving ability or knowledge of the three R's is most closely associated with that value. I may value personal integration or vocational success or responsible citizenship. I can determine

whether problem-solving ability or knowledge of the three R's is "better" for achieving any one of these values. But the value or purpose that gives meaning to a particular scientific endeavor must always lie outside of that endeavor.

* * *

My point then is that any endeavor in science, pure or applied, is carried on in the pursuit of a purpose or value that is subjectively chosen by persons. It is important that this choice be made explicit, since the particular value which is being sought can never be tested or evaluated, confirmed or denied, by the scientific endeavor to which it gives birth. The initial purpose or value always and necessarily lies outside the scope of the scientific effort which it sets in motion.

Among other things this means that if we choose some particular goal or series of goals for human beings and then set out on a large scale to control human behavior to the end of achieving those goals, we are locked in the rigidity of our initial choice, because such a scientific endeavor can never transcend itself to select new goals. Only subjective human persons can do that. Thus if we chose as our goal the state of happiness for human beings (a goal deservedly ridiculed by Aldous Huxley in *Brave New World*), and if we involved all of society in a successful scientific program by which people became happy, we would be locked in a colossal rigidity in which no one would be free to question this goal, because our scientific operations could not transcend themselves to question their guiding purposes. And without laboring this point, I would remark that colossal rigidity, whether in dinosaurs or dictatorships, has a very poor record of evolutionary survival.

If, however, a part of our scheme is to set free some "planners" who do not have to be happy, who are not controlled, and who are therefore free to choose other values, this has several meanings. It means that the purpose we have chosen as our goal is not a sufficient and a satisfying one for human beings but must be supplemented. It also means that if it is necessary to set up an elite group which is free, then this shows all too clearly that the great majority are only the slaves—no matter by what high-sounding name we call them—of those who select the goals.

Perhaps, however, the thought is that a continuing scientific endeavor will evolve its own goals; that the initial findings will alter the directions, and subsequent findings will alter them still further, and that science somehow develops its own purpose. Although he does not clearly say so, this appears to be the pattern Skinner has in mind. It is surely a reasonable description, but it overlooks one element in this continuing development, which is that subjective personal choice enters in at every point at which the direction changes. The findings of a science, the results of an experiment, do not and never can tell us what next scientific purpose to pursue. Even in the purest of science, the scientist must decide what the findings mean and must subjectively choose what next step will be most profitable in the pursuit of his purpose. And if we are speaking of the application of scientific knowledge, then it is distressingly clear that the increasing scientific knowledge of the structure of the atom carries with it no necessary choice as to the purpose to which this knowledge will be put. This is a subjective personal choice which must be made by many individuals.

Thus I return to the proposition with which I began this section of my remarks—and which I now repeat in different words. Science has its meaning as the objective pursuit of a purpose which has been subjectively chosen by a person or persons. This purpose or value can never be investigated by the particular scientific experiment or investigation to which it has given birth and meaning. Consequently, any discussion of the control of human beings by the behavioral sciences must first and most deeply concern itself with the subjectively chosen purposes which such an application of science is intended to implement.

*   *   *

III. SKINNER

I cannot quite agree that the practice of science *requires* a prior decision about goals or a prior choice of values. The metallurgist can study the properties of steel and the engineer can design a bridge without raising the question of whether a bridge is to be built. But such questions are certainly frequently raised and tentatively answered. Rogers wants to call the answers "subjective choices of values." To me, such an expression suggests that we have had to abandon more rigorous scientific practices in order to talk about our own behavior. In the experimental analysis of other organisms I would use other terms, and I shall try to do so

here. Any list of values is a list of reinforcers—conditioned or otherwise. We are so constituted that under certain circumstances food, water, sexual contact, and so on, will make any behavior which produces them more likely to occur again. Other things may acquire this power. We do not need to say that an organism chooses to eat rather than to starve. If you answer that it is a very different thing when a man chooses to starve, I am only too happy to agree. If it were not so, we should have cleared up the question of choice long ago. An organism can be reinforced by—can be made to "choose"—almost any given state of affairs.

Rogers is concerned with choices that involve multiple and usually conflicting consequences. I have dealt with some of these elsewhere in an analysis of self-control. Shall I eat these delicious strawberries today if I will then suffer an annoying rash tomorrow? The decision I am to make used to be assigned to the province of ethics. But we are now studying similar combinations of positive and negative consequences, as well as collateral conditions which affect the result, in the laboratory. Even a pigeon can be taught some measure of self-control! And this work helps us to understand the operation of certain formulas—among them value judgments—which folk-wisdom, religion, and psychotherapy have advanced in the interests of self-discipline. The observable effect of any statement of value is to alter the relative effectiveness of reinforcers. We may no longer enjoy the strawberries for thinking about the rash. If rashes are made sufficiently shameful, illegal, sinful, maladjusted, or unwise, we may glow with satisfaction as we push the strawberries aside in a grandiose avoidance response which would bring a smile to the lips of Murray Sidman.

People behave in ways which, as we say, conform to ethical, governmental, or religious patterns because they are reinforced for doing so. The resulting behavior may have far-reaching consequences for the survival of the pattern to which it conforms. And whether we like it or not, survival is the ultimate criterion. This is where, it seems to me, science can help—not in choosing a goal, but in enabling us to predict the survival value of cultural practices. Man has too long tried to get the kind of world he wants by glorifying some brand of immediate reinforcement. As science points up more and more of the remoter consequences, he may begin to work to strengthen behavior, not in a slavish devotion to a chosen value, but with respect to the ultimate survival of mankind Do not ask me why I want mankind to survive. I can tell you why only in the sense in which the physiologist can tell you why I want to breathe. Once the relation between a given step and the survival of my group has been pointed out, I will take that step. And it is the business of science to point out just such relations.

The values I have occasionally recommended (and Rogers has not led me to recant) are transitional. Other things being equal, I am betting on the group whose practices make for healthy, happy, secure, productive, and creative people. . . .

* * *

If we are worthy of our democratic heritage we shall, of course, be ready to resist any tyrannical use of science for immediate or selfish purposes. But if we value the achievements and goals of democracy we must not refuse to apply science to the design and construction of cultural patterns, even though we may then find ourselves in some sense in the position of controllers. Fear of control, generalized beyond any warrant, has led to a misinterpretation of valid practices and the blind rejection of intelligent planning for a better way of life. In terms which I trust Rogers will approve, in conquering this fear we shall become more mature and better organized and shall, thus, more fully actualize ourselves as human beings.

b.

Arthur J. Dyck
Ethical Issues in Community and Research Medicine*

. . . What tasks and what judgments accrue to physicians as physicians? What are they trained to do and what ought they be trained to do? By what primary principles and modes of ethical reasoning is and ought their practice to be governed? Let us briefly examine a specific instance in which current medical practice is involved sometimes implicitly, sometimes explicitly, in conflicting ways of answering these questions.

In a recent series of articles in the *Journal*, Milunsky et al. review the current state of prenatal genetic diagnosis and argue for the widespread use of amniocentesis. As they use the

* 284 *New England Journal of Medicine* 725–726 (1971). Reprinted by permission.

term, amniocentesis refers to the aspiration of fluid from the amniotic sac for the purpose of making cytogenetic studies. The immediate rationale for this use of amniocentesis is to advance the practice of genetic counseling by basing predictions of an increasing number of diseases upon actual diagnoses in utero instead of calculated probability risks. The advantages that they cite for this more accurate counsel is that it reassures couples regarding the normality of the fetus, it permits the decision to intervene through abortion where abnormalities are detected, and it provides a way of preventing the births of infants with irreparable genetic defects and fatal genetic diseases. Milunsky and his co-workers recognize that this last use of amniocentesis changes the traditional role of the physician so far as he can now predict diseases accurately before birth and provide the means of preventing the birth of a child with mental defects or fatal diseases. Hence, we enter a new era of social and preventive medicine.

Throughout the discussion of the diagnostic use of amniocentesis as advocated by Milunsky et al., there is no explicit recognition of the fetus as a patient. Apparently, genetic counseling does not include the task of preparing a family to accept and care for a defective child. "Therapy" at the present time is aimed at the family and not the fetus. In an earlier essay, John W. Littlefield spoke specifically to this issue:

Prenatal genetic diagnosis will constitute a major medical advance only if therapy can be given once a diagnosis is made. Eventually and occasionally, this may be prenatal therapy for the fetus. . . . But society and the professions must appreciate and accept that the proper therapy now is for the family, and at times that means abortion.

Clearly, neither reassurance for the family nor abortion provides therapy for the fetus. The hope is held out for eventual and occasional therapy for the fetus, with no explicit reference to the kinds of postnatal therapy presently available. For now, the treatment of the diseases of this "sometime patient" is, in this view, achieved by its elimination as a patient and as a living entity.

Suppose a physician argues that deciding whether to treat the fetus as a patient is a judgment that a physician as physician is not in a position to make. In effect, this is the view taken by Milunsky et al. when they suggest that physicians and society are, and should remain, impartial or neutral regarding decisions by families about whether to use amniocentesis and whether to abort the fetus where deformities are detected. This point of view is strange considering both the traditional role of physicians and current medical practice.

As the physician's role was traditionally depicted in the Hippocratic Oath and many subsequent codes, he was expected to be the physician advocate of both the pregnant woman and developing life within the womb. If, as Milunsky et al. suggest, both physician and society should be impartial regarding the use of amniocentesis to prevent diseases by eliminating the diseased, what advocate is left for defenseless life? Are physicians about to abandon also their time-honored role as advocates on behalf of the hopelessly ill, the unconscious and the experimental subject who is uninformed? And even if one wishes to leave the exact status of the fetus as a human life an open question, should it not be part of the special responsibility of the physician, as it certainly has been traditionally, to err on the side of saving and fostering human life rather than to develop or encourage programs that selectively prevent such life?

To drop the fetus as a patient at this time in history is also incongruous with the aims and increasing accomplishments of contemporary fetology. Furthermore, why should physicians claim increasing responsibility for defining and specifying the end of human life, and decreasing responsibility for defining and specifying the beginning of human life? Why, for example, should the absence of signs of brain activity spell death while signs of brain activity in the eight-week-old fetus are largely unheralded as signs of human life? If physicians nevertheless insist that specifying when human life begins is not a medical decision, by what warrant do they decide that the fetus is not a patient and that his life is dispensable? As Ramsey has indicated, the medical warrant for recommending abortion occurs only when a fetus threatens the life or the health of a pregnant woman.

To decide that a given set of diseases is to be eliminated by elimination of the diseased is one of the principles on which programs of eugenics and euthanasia rest. Decisions of this kind are surely not morally neutral. What special competence does a physician have to decide that a society ought to prefer death to giving custodial or remedial care for those who require it? Milunsky et al. cite the costs of care for the mentally retarded in Massachusetts. What a meager sum this is as compared to the amount of money being spent for destroying lives in Vietnam! If saving money is important, why not save much more money and save lives as well by thinking of other costs that could be cut? One of the problems here is that, as the physicians strive to contribute to social well-being, they find that only certain kinds of actions are predictably within their power as physicians. Hence, they look to the surest way in which they can affect social policy. Their warrant for doing so is very unclear, and, whereas we can vote out those who might suggest legislation that permits or encourages selective killing, including capital punishment and the like, our recourse in forming the conscience of physicians is less certain. Heretofore, in the area of abortion, we have generally put constraints upon physicians and others on behalf of the fetus. The assumption that the use and application of amniocentesis is a neutral sphere for physicians and society presupposes that, for physicians and society, abortion is not a moral issue, and that existing or future laws do or will assure that abortions are decided solely by families and physicians. To go that way is not morally neutral, and it is not life affirming.

*   *   *

NOTE

James K. Glassman
Harvard Genetics Researcher Quits
Science for Politics*

Last November a team of Harvard scientists announced that it had isolated a pure gene from a strain of bacterial virus for the first time in history. Now, one of the principal members of the team has decided to give up science and become a full-fledged political activist. The scientist is James Shapiro, who is 26 years old and a research fellow in bacteriology and immunology at the Harvard Medical School. . . . Nobelist Salvador E. Luria and other experts in Shapiro's field consider him one of the most promising molecular geneticists in the nation.

Shapiro discussed his three main reasons for quitting science in a recent interview. First, he believes that the work he does will be put to evil uses by the men who control science—in government and in large corporations—in the way that atomic energy, for example, was put to evil uses. Second, he refuses to contribute to a

* 167 *Science* 963 (1970). Copyright 1970 by the American Association for the Advancement of Science. Reprinted by permission.

system that does not allow "the people" to have a say in deciding what work scientists do. Third, he thinks that the most important problems the country faces, such as health care and pollution, need political solutions more urgently than scientific ones.

*   *   *

Shapiro's decision was foreshadowed by statements he made when isolation of the gene was announced. With Beckwith and Lawrence Eron, a third-year Harvard Medical School student, he warned that the work could be perverted and used for evil purposes, such as genetic manipulation in human beings. Shapiro said at the press conference, "We did this work for scientific reasons, also because it was interesting to do. But scientists generally have the tendency not to think too much about the consequences of their work while doing it. But now that we have, we are not entirely happy about it. This is a problem in all scientific research, the bad consequences we cannot control. Many of us are upset that science and technology have been used, as in Vietnam, on innocent people. I don't think we necessarily have the right to pat ourselves on the back."

*   *   *

5.

Interests of Science?

**J. Kenneth Benson and James Otis Smith
The Harvard Drug Controversy—
A Case Study of Subject Manipulation
and Social Structure***

*   *   *

In 1960 Dr. Leary and Dr. Alpert obtained a supply of psilocybin from Sandoz Pharmaceuticals, Inc., and began research on the "consciousness-expanding" properties of the drug. The research began as a thoroughly respectable inquiry in a burgeoning field of research. Alpert was an assistant professor of Clinical Psychology and of Education and Leary a lecturer on Clinical Psychology at Harvard. Both were associated with the Center for Research in Person-

---

* G. Sjoberg, ed.: *Ethics, Politics, and Social Research.* Cambridge, Mass.: Schenkman Publishing Co. 117–119, 123–126, 128–131 (1967). Reprinted by permission.

ality, a research arm of Harvard's Department of Social Relations. Both men were respected members of their profession. . . .

In initiating the research, Leary and Alpert entered a rapidly developing field of investigation. Research on the effects of peyote, mescaline, psilocybin, d-lysergic acid diethylamide (LSD-25) and other materials with similar effects has been greatly accelerated within the last twenty years. Psychiatrists and others have been interested in the psychotomimetic properties of the materials. Some have believed that the substances produced a temporary psychosis which might be studied in search of pharmacological explanation and treatment for psychosis. Although enthusiasm for this view has waned, it is still the basis for some research. In addition, the military has been interested also in the psychotomimetic properties of the substances. Some persons have argued that these materials might be used to produce a temporary state of insanity in an enemy which would permit conquest without death and destruction.

Numerous investigators have been concerned with the mystical, insightful experiences reported to them from the ingestion of psilocybin, LSD-25, and related materials. A variety of reports of mystical insight, consciousness-expansion, and increased understanding of self as a consequence of exposure to the drugs have appeared in the literature. Some psychiatrists and clinical psychologists have been interested in the therapeutic potential of such experiences. It has been suggested that mind-altering substances might be profitably employed as an adjunct to psychotherapy or even as a therapy in itself. Other reports support the idea that these materials can be helpful in the rehabilitation of criminals, alcoholics, and narcotics addicts. It has also been suggested that the pain and anxiety of dying patients can be somewhat relieved by chemically induced insight and understanding.

Leary and Alpert were interested in the study of the mystical insight and understanding produced by LSD and related drugs. However, their interest extended beyond the strictly therapeutic potential of the drugs. They argued that exposure to the substances could provide an expansion of consciousness which would enhance one's creativity, intelligence, understanding of life, and social adjustment. While some of their research involved a rehabilitation program for criminals, the bulk of their efforts were expended in studies of "normal" subjects.

As the research progressed, the activities of

Leary and Alpert reportedly became more promotional and less restrained. Concerned for the welfare of students, Harvard University officials reached an agreement with Leary and Alpert in the fall of 1961 that undergraduates would not be used as research subjects. In March, 1962, the misgivings of some colleagues in the Department of Social Relations led to a meeting of the Center for Research in Personality, at which the Leary-Alpert research was roundly criticized. Published accounts of the meeting stimulated a widespread controversy culminating in an investigation of the project by the Massachusetts Public Health Department. The decision of the investigators to permit the research to continue, with minor changes, seemed to signal a reduction in the level of public controversy, although the efforts of Harvard officials and the Department of Social Relations to establish satisfactory arrangements for the control of the drugs were unsuccessful.

The controversy bloomed anew in the fall of 1962 when Leary and Alpert returned to Harvard after a summer of drug research in Mexico. In October they formed an organization called the International Federation for Internal Freedom (IFIF) which was to sponsor and encourage research with hallucinogenic drugs.

University officials became alarmed by reports of extensive illicit use of hallucinogens by Harvard undergraduates. Although responsibility for this development could not be readily assigned to the psilocybin researchers, two university officials—Dean John U. Monro and Health Services Director Dana Farnsworth—issued public statements warning students of possible harm and decrying the sophisticated, intellectual promotion of the hallucinogens. . . .

*   *   *

. . . Some critics, especially behavioral scientists, attacked the psilocybin research for what they regarded as a departure from the proper goals and methods of science. The overlap between research and application within the project runs counter to the view that research activity should be insulated from problems of practical application.

The psilocybin investigators were impressed with the potential benefits of the consciousness-expanding drugs. In a paper presented in 1961, Leary argued as follows:

The basic aim of physical science is to reduce human helplessness in the face of the physical environment. Physical science has other goals, of course: to understand, to explain, to control, to measure, to predict. . . . Why explain? Why predict? To lessen fearful ignorance. The technologies which have grown up around the physical sciences, engineering, medicine, also take as their goal the reducing of human helplessness . . . and the social technologies—psychiatry, social work, applied psychology—is not their goal the reduction of confusion and the increase in human freedom?

When people come to us and ask us to change their behavior, why can't we do it? Why can't we teach them to see the game structure of human society?

Change in behavior can occur with dramatic spontaneity once the game structure of behavior is seen. The visionary experience is the key to behavior change.

The most efficient way to cut through the game structure of Western life is the use of drugs, consciousness-expanding drugs.

Leary and Alpert contended that consciousness-expanding drugs would eventually produce extensive changes both in individuals and in social systems. They sometimes interpreted opposition to their research as an attempt to defend the status quo. For example, in a paper entitled "The Politics of Consciousness-Expansion" they argued that because LSD can change the functioning of the nervous system it proves a threat to the established social order and therefore challenges "every branch of the Establishment." They characterized the fear consciousness-expansion caused among the Establishment as "more frightening than the Bomb!" They argued that this fear was the result of potential socio-political change rather than of physical or physiological change occurring in individual subjects. "Man" they state "is about to be changed . . ." and the ". . . present social establishments had better be prepared for the . . . floodtide, two billion years building up. The verbal dam is collapsing. Head for the hills, or prepare your intellectual craft to flow with the current."

It is, of course, not necessarily unscientific to believe that one's research is of practical value. As clinical psychologists, Leary and Alpert were members of a profession highly committed to the practical application of research findings. Researchers in other areas, e.g., the sociology of deviant behavior, have been much concerned with the utilization of research findings in prevention and rehabilitation. However, Leary and Alpert went even further, attempting to engage in research and in practical application concurrently:

The goal of the research sessions run by the Harvard-IFIF group was not to produce and study frightening disturbances of consciousness (which was the goal of most psychiatric investigations of model psychoses), but to produce the ecstatic experiences, to expand consciousness, to provide the subject with the most memorable, revelatory, life-changing experience of his life. . . .

From the beginning of our research, our attention was directed to the engineering of ecstasy, the preparation for, the setting for, the architecture of ecstasy.

Apparently, the production of ecstatic experiences was both a means to the discovery of the causes of such experiences and a desired end-product of the research. Such a combination of theoretical and practical interests is, of course, not unique to the psilocybin project. Frequently, in drug experimentation the investigator hopes that his research will cure or prevent illness among research subjects while at the same time providing valuable knowledge. In studies of delinquency control and prevention one may hope not only to discover causes and cures but also to reduce delinquency within the population studied.

The combination of research and application becomes objectionable to many when the applied concerns of the investigator interfere with his search for valid knowledge. Such interference was alleged by critics of the Harvard psilocybin project. Some contended that the scientific goals of the psilocybin investigation were eventually obscured in the attempt to produce mystic ecstasy as an end in itself. Consider, for example, the comments of Brendan A. Maher, chairman of the Center for Research in Personality at the time of the controversy:

Taking a drug, sitting in a fox-hole, falling in love, or falling out of an airplane all provide experiences. To the extent that we engage in any of these activities because the experience is an end in itself, then we are doing it—to speak colloquially—for "kicks." A university is an institution intended to provide a rather special set of experiences; experiences that lead to increased competencies, capacities for intellectual self-discipline, interest in examining all of the evidence and an understanding of the intellectual history of man. Experience *per se* is not part of a University's commissariat. . . .

Among the members of the faculty at the Center there was serious concern when it became apparent that not only were students being indoctrinated in the belief that communicable knowledge was the end-product of some kind of pointless "game," but that the drug experience was being held out to them as a kind of redemption from the rigors of rationality.

Similar concern was reportedly voiced by Dr. Herbert C. Kelman (then a lecturer in Social Psychology at Harvard) at a meeting of the faculty and students of the Center for Research in Personality. He contended that "the program has an anti-intellectual atmosphere. Its emphasis is on pure experience, not on verbalizing findings."

The methods as well as the aims of the psilocybin research were criticized. The setting in which drugs were administered and the participation of research workers in the drug sessions led to considerable opposition.

Drug sessions were often held in private homes and apartments. Research subjects were led to expect and to prepare for pleasant, insight-provoking experiences. The research setting was pleasant, relaxed, and supportive. Music, paintings, books, and drinks were sometimes provided. Research workers often took the drug with the subjects.

The careful arrangement of the research setting was based on several considerations. First, the investigators believed the expectations of research subjects and the social context of the drug sessions to be important determinants of reaction to psilocybin. They argued that many of the negative reactions reported by some other investigators were consequences of negative pre-exposure attitudes and of threatening research settings. Second, the investigators felt that the participation of research workers in the drug sessions facilitated favorable reactions by eliminating the social distance between the subject and the observer. Third, the investigators thought that reactions to psilocybin were properly understood only by persons who had themselves been exposed to the drug.

The procedures intended by Leary and Alpert to be provocative of desirable psilocybin reactions and of valid scientific data were seen by some critics as conducive to a party-like atmosphere inappropriate to scientific research. The critics charged that the participation of research workers in the drug sessions precluded rather than facilitated the collection of reliable information.

The negative reactions of behavioral scientists to the psilocybin project included criticism of goals and methods in conjunction with concern for the well-being of research subjects and the control of drugs. The matter of subject health was not dealt with separately as an ethical issue apart from other issues. Instead, behavioral scientists reacted to the combination of potentially harmful operations and questionable purposes and methods. If the research had been regarded as both worthy in its aims and rigorous in its methodology, there might have been far less furor over subject health. Similarly, if the research had not involved a potential threat to subject health, there probably would have been far less controversy over its methods and purposes.

* * *

. . . Another issue in the Harvard controversy concerns the limits of academic freedom. It is clear that the activities of Leary and Alpert were restricted to some extent by social control measures. Early in the research, the Harvard administration reached an agreement with the psilocybin investigators that undergraduates would not be used as research subjects. Later, at the insistence of the Massachusetts Public Health Department, the presence of a medical doctor at each drug administration became mandatory. At several junctures, Harvard officials issued public statements which were construed as criticism of the promotional activities of the psilocybin investigators. Still later, the psilocybin research was separated from Harvard because of the failure to devise control measures satisfactory both to the research workers and to representatives of the Laboratory of Social Relations. Finally, both Leary and Alpert were dismissed from their appointments on the Harvard faculty.

Despite the restrictions described above, it has been argued in some quarters that the principle of academic freedom was not violated. Obviously, the argument hinges upon one's concepts of academic freedom. In fact, much of the Harvard psilocybin controversy consists of a protracted, though muted, debate over the meaning of academic freedom.

The debate concerns two major issues. First, what kinds of activities are protected by the guarantees of academic freedom? Second, what types of control may be exercised over research activities without violating academic freedom?

The controversy can be partly understood as a debate concerning the scope of the term "research." Psilocybin investigators were given occasionally to very broad usage of that term. For example, in a mimeographed form letter of April, 1963, and appearing under an IFIF letterhead, Leary argued in effect that these substances are powerful agents for developing human potentialities. Because they are funda-

mentally educational rather than medical instruments, their use and availability should follow the educational model. Leary also stated that anyone who could benefit from the experience and who had some training in the area should be able to undertake *research* into the expansion of his consciousness.

By contrast, various social control agents seem to have been intent upon utilizing a narrower concept of "research." A distinction between research and nonresearch activities seems implicit in the responses of Harvard officials. To our knowledge, administrative officials never publicly criticized the formal research activities of Leary and Alpert. They did, however, on several occasions criticize the intellectual promotion of the hallucinogens. . . .

A clear attempt to delimit the concept of research was apparent in the negotiations within the Laboratory of Social Relations intended to establish acceptable conditions for the control of the drug. Robert F. Bales, Director of the Laboratory, and others, felt that the Laboratory could not continue to assist the psilocybin investigators in any way unless promotional uses of the project's psilocybin supply (e.g., to impress prospective financial supporters) were eliminated. The "non-research" uses of psilocybin led to severance of the connection between the psilocybin project and the Laboratory of Social Relations.

* * *

. . . Brendan A. Maher argued that academic freedom should not be construed to mean that incompetence is approved. As Maher put it in a general statement preceding his description of the Harvard controversy,

It is difficult to see how academic freedom is threatened by the expectation that a scholar demonstrate his competences, especially where there is the slightest possibility that harm may be caused to others by an unskilled performance. . . . Academic freedom does not include a license to be incompetent where it is possible for competence to be provided.

* * *

Thus, in many quarters there seems to have been an attempt to define the guarantees of academic freedom so as to exclude some of the activities of Leary and Alpert from their protection.

In addition, those dealing with the psilocybin research came to grips with the problem of research control. Does the principle of academic freedom mean that the investigator should be free to investigate any and all topics without interference? In the case at hand, the attempt to establish control led to severance of the connection between Harvard and the psilocybin project. Efforts were made to establish a committee within the behavioral science faculty which would oversee the psilocybin research, at least to the point of determining the conditions under which the drug was to be administered. Since an agreement satisfactory to all parties could not be reached, the proposed committee was not established. However, the effort to establish such a committee indicates an apparent preference on the part of some persons involved for controls from within the behavioral science discipline rather than from administrative officers of the university. Intra-professional controls were apparently perceived as more palatable than extra-professional ones.

*   *   *

NOTE

THE EDITORS OF NATURE
WHAT COMES AFTER FERTILIZATION*

Test tube babies may not be just round the corner, but the day when all the knowledge necessary to produce them will be available may have been brought a stage nearer by the work reported by Dr. R. G. Edwards and his colleagues. . . .

*   *   *

The advantage of having these blastocysts in culture will be that it will then be possible to make a thorough study of the early stages of human embryology, for example to find out when different enzymes become active. There will be the opportunity to investigate the nature and time of onset of various biochemical abnormalities which are now attracting considerable attention in the medical world. So little is known about the vital early stage of human embryology that any efforts that are likely to lead to an increase in knowledge are surely praiseworthy. Any research that may help to show why embryonic development sometimes goes wrong seems to be a laudable enterprise. The fact that the techniques might one day be developed to make it possible to produce a fully grown human embryo *extra utero* should not be a restraint to progress. The day of the test tube

baby is not here yet, and the advantages of this work are clear. These are not perverted men in white coats doing nasty experiments on human beings, but reasonable scientists carrying out perfectly justifiable research. One of the possible benefits of this research could be the treatment of some forms of infertility, probably in older women, who are thought to produce a high proportion of abnormal embryos which fail to develop.

But because the virtues of work like this seem self-evident to those most immediately involved, they should not fall into the trap of believing that everybody else feels the same. There is, for work like this, a real need to explain that the purposes of scientists are very different from those of Big Brother in George Orwell's *1984*. Unless this is done, there is a danger that the public may come to lose faith in science.

6.

Interests of Society?

a.

Joshua Lederberg
Curbs on Human Engineering
Can Create Thought Control*

*   *   *

A pluralistic society must make the same response to the calculated use of human biochemistry against the overcentralization of power. On the same argument that we now universally accept for leaving the responsibility for the details of child-rearing and education in the hands of the family, I would advocate the utmost permissiveness with respect to individual use of biological innovations.

Effective sanctions on the part of the state to enforce Dr. Nirenberg's cautions would generate a police and thought-control bureaucracy exactly contrary to his fundamental humanistic aims. We have already experienced the sad consequences of the confusion of law with private morals in such areas as contraception and abortion and have only begun to extricate ourselves from their attendant hypocrisy and class discrimination.

Social order must, of course, place some limits on individual discretion. We do not, for

* 221 *Nature* 613 (1969). Reprinted by permission.

* *The Washington Post* A 13 (Oct. 21, 1967). © 1967 The Washington Post. Reprinted by permission.

example, allow a parent to leave a child utterly without education, partly because of the economic stress on the community, partly because of the way this alienates the child from his culture to what we regard as the child's disadvantage.

It is doubtful, however, whether we will ever know which knowledge is for the benefit of mankind. Was the invention of printing, autos, airplanes, radio, TV, nuclear energy? If we make the most energetic, immediately beneficial use of molecular biology in medicine, as I believe we should, we must also vigilantly pursue the further research and education needed for the utmost harmony of social and technological development.

b.

Marshall W. Nirenberg
Will Society Be Prepared?*

New information is being obtained in the field of biochemical genetics at an extremely rapid rate. Thus far, this knowledge has had relatively little effect upon man. More information must be obtained before practical application will be possible, and the technical problems that must be overcome are formidable. However, when these obstacles have been removed this knowledge will greatly influence man's future, for man then will have the power to shape his own biologic destiny. Such power can be used wisely or unwisely, for the betterment or detriment of mankind.

Salvador Luria has said: "the progress of science is so rapid that it creates an imbalance between the power it places in the hands of man and the social conditions in which this power is exerted. Then neither warnings of scientists, nor breadth of public information, nor wisdom of citizens may compensate for inadequacies of the institutional framework to cope with the new situations."

*   *   *

What may be expected in the future? Short but meaningful genetic messages will be synthesized chemically. Since the instructions will be written in the language which cells understand, the messages will be used to program cells. Cells will carry out the instructions, and the program may even be inherited. I don't know

how long it will take before it will be possible to program cells with chemically synthesized messages. Certainly the experimental obstacles are formidable. However, I have little doubt that the obstacles eventually will be overcome. The only question is when. My guess is that cells will be programmed with synthetic messages within 25 years. If efforts along those lines were intensified, bacteria might be programmed within 5 years.

The point which deserves special emphasis is that man may be able to program his own cells with synthetic information long before he will be able to assess adequately the long-term consequences of such alterations, long before he will be able to formulate goals, and long before he can resolve the ethical and moral problems which will be raised. When man becomes capable of instructing his own cells, he must refrain from doing so until he has sufficient wisdom to use this knowledge for the benefit of mankind. I state this problem well in advance of the need to resolve it, because decisions concerning the application of this knowledge must ultimately be made by society, and only an informed society can make such decisions wisely.

NOTE

Joshua Lederberg
Dangers of Reprogramming Cells*

*   *   *

. . . Nirenberg's . . . underlying concern, which I share, is that biological control might be used by a malevolent government to the peril of individual freedom. . . .

Presumably we have to be even more concerned about subtler mistakes. A well-intentioned government might impose rash commitments for the sake of short-term advantages. Plainly we must be very sensitive about innovations that, once introduced, constitute irreversible evolutionary deviations.

*   *   *

. . . Our educational systems are certainly a form of psychological engineering scarcely different in fundamental principle from the biological interventions that our knowledge of nucleic acids is likely to bring about.

Our main concern must be to maximize the

---

role of individual decision. This could be defeated by overenthusiastic policing of personal initiative and experimentation as well as by premature positive measures imposed by the State.

In point of fact, we already practice biological engineering on a rather large scale by use of live viruses in mass immunization campaigns. While these are of indubitable value for preventing serious diseases, their global impact on the development of human beings of a wide range of genotypes is hard to assess at our present stage of wisdom. Crude virus preparations, such as some in common use at the present time, are also vulnerable to frightful mishaps of contamination and misidentification.

Live viruses are themselves genetic messages used for the purpose of programming human cells for the synthesis of immunogenic virus antigens. Nirenberg's cautions are just as relevant to considerations of contemporary policy as they are for the ever-widening applications of molecular biology in the near future.

c.

Andrei D. Sakharov
Thoughts on Progress, Peaceful Co-Existence, and Intellectual Freedom*

Modern technology and mass psychology constantly suggest new possibilities of managing the norms of behavior, the strivings and convictions of masses of people. This involves not only management through information based on the theory of advertising and mass psychology, but also more technical methods that are widely discussed in the press abroad. Examples are biochemical control of the birth rate, biochemical control of psychic processes and electronic control of such processes.

It seems to me that we cannot completely ignore these new methods or prohibit the progress of science and technology, but we must be clearly aware of the awesome danger to basic human values and to the meaning of life that may be concealed in the misuse of technical and biochemical methods and the methods of mass psychology.

Man must not be turned into a chicken or a rat as in the well-known experiments in which elation is induced electrically through electrodes inserted into the brain. Related to this is the question of the ever increasing use of tranquil-

* The New York Times 15 (July 22, 1968). © 1968 by The New York Times Company. Reprinted by permission.

izers and antidepressants, legal and illegal narcotics, and so forth.

We also must not forget the very real danger mentioned by Norbert Wiener in his book "Cybernetics," namely the absence in cybernetic machines of stable human norms of behavior. The tempting, unprecedented power that mankind, or, even worse, a particular group in a divided mankind, may derive from the wise counsels of its future intellectual aides, the artificial "thinking" automata, may, as Wiener warned, become a fatal trap; the counsels may turn out to be incredibly insidious and, instead of pursuing human objectives, may pursue completely abstract problems that had been transformed in an unforeseen manner in the artificial brain.

NOTE

JOSHUA LEDERBERG
GENETIC ENGINEERING, OR
THE AMELIORATION OF GENETIC DEFECT*

*   *   *

What . . . are the problems to which genetic science can be applied? Some may think of rescuing man from the prospect of nuclear annihilation by recasting the genes for aggression—or acquiescence—that are supposed to predestine a future of territorial conflict. Even if we postulate for sake of argument that we know the genetics of militarism, we have no way to apply it without solving the political problem that is the primary difficulty to begin with. If we could agree upon applying genetic (or any other effective) remedies to global problems in the first place, we probably would need no recourse to them in the actual event.

The converse argument applies to the gloomier predictions of totalitarian abuse of a genetic technology. The scenario of Brave New World is well advertised by now, and no one doubts that a modern slave state would reinforce its class stratification by genetic controls. But it could not do so without having instituted slavery in the first place, for which the control of the mass media presents much more immediate dangers than knowledge of DNA. It is indeed true that I might fear the control of my behavior through electrical impulses directed into my brain, but (possibly excepting television) I do not accept the implantation of the electrodes

* 34 The Pharos of Alpha Omega Alpha 9, 10 (1971). Reprinted by permission.

except at the point of a gun: the gun is the problem.

* * *

7.

Limits of Prediction?

a.

Francis D. Moore
Therapeutic Innovation—Ethical Boundaries in the Initial Clinical Trials of New Drugs and Surgical Procedures*

* * *

A familiar though remarkable historic example of therapeutic innovation which took place in Brookline, Massachusetts, about 250 years ago raised questions as appropriate for review in 1969 as they originally were in 1721.

An epidemic of smallpox had carried away many of the colonists in Boston and eastern New England in 1702. Accounts vary as to what brought word of smallpox inoculation to the keen ear of the Reverend Cotton Mather. But to this enterprising clergyman belongs the full credit for stimulating physicians to activity. Whether he saw accounts of the Turkish experiments or learned from talks with his own Negro slave that the practice of inoculation had been tried among primitive African populations (the latter being the more dramatic version which he himself preferred), the fact remains that he stimulated others to action with such promptness that the inoculation in Britain carried out by Lady Montagu took place only a few weeks prior to his, and the much larger New England experience became the prototype for widespread application both in this country and abroad.

The practice of inoculation against smallpox in the early eighteenth century consisted in the intentional infection of a normal person with virulent unattenuated smallpox virus obtained from a patient who himself might later die of the disease. This inoculation was done with the hope that the recipient would be afflicted with a mild case of smallpox—a "distinct case" as it was then called—and that the resultant "nonsusceptibility" would last the rest of his life. By

---

* 98 *Daedalus* 504–507 (1969). Reprinted by permission of Daedalus, Journal of the American Academy of Arts and Sciences, Boston, Massachusetts.

contrast, the practice of vaccination introduced seventy-five years later by Jenner in England and, following his lead, by Waterhouse in the United States consisted in inoculating the recipient with the virus of the cowpox. This mild and rarely lethal disease confers immunity to smallpox by virtue of an antigen shared by the two viruses.

Cotton Mather could find none of his Boston medical cronies interested in such a heterodox undertaking. So he turned to the nearby town of Brookline where he discussed the matter with Zabdiel Boylston, then thirty-seven years of age. Boylston was the son of a doctor who had studied at Oxford, yet he himself had no medical degree. He was still a young man who had not emerged as a medical figure in a society that was already teeming with strong medical characters. Among these were the men who, a few years later, were to found the Harvard Medical School and the Massachusetts Medical Society. This large conservative wing of practitioners would have no part of the Reverend Mather's suggestion. But Zabdiel Boylston saw it for what it was—a chance to reduce the mortality from smallpox epidemics.

Accordingly, Zabdiel fetched some pus from a pock and proceeded to inoculate his thirteen-year-old son by rubbing this material on a scarification on the boy's arm. This epic experiment occurred on June 26 or 27, 1721. It is generally conceded that Boylston did not select himself for this experiment because he had already suffered the disease and was immune. In any event, the deed was successfully accomplished—at least the son did not die of the disease—and Boylston inoculated 247 persons in the next few months. Of these, six died. There was a clamorous and riotous opposition to the procedure both among fellow practitioners and among the laity who were aroused by their friends the doctors. Not long thereafter, out of a group of 5,759 cases of the naturally occurring disease, 844 died, according to Boylston's own account. Other figures from contemporary literature state that Boylston inoculated 242 persons of whom six died, and that there were 5,889 cases in the epidemic of whom 844 died. Whichever figures are correct, it was evident that the mortality was lower in the inoculated form of the disease, and that those who had been successfully inoculated rarely, if ever, contracted the naturally occurring epidemic form of smallpox.

After a time of persecution, Boylston won out. He was acclaimed and honored here and in England. The practice spread to the other colonies. Benjamin Franklin, who had been a severe critic, later became a strong proponent. . . .

This was a lethal experiment. It carried a mortality of over 2 per cent. It was undertaken to protect the individual, and through him the larger group, from the ravages of an epidemic disease. It was undertaken by people who had little idea of the nature either of the disease or the infectious agent, although Mather wrote of the "animalculi" that were involved. The basis for any confidence that this experiment would be successful was in large part hearsay from the Middle and Far East. There was no animal trial or laboratory work. A cloud of fantasy and petty controversy surrounded the actual details of inoculation techniques. Little effort was made to isolate those who had been inoculated with the disease, and they could become carriers of a virulent virus. Curiously enough, opponents of the procedure based their claims on the assertion that inoculation would not protect against the epidemic disease; they were not so interested in its public hazards or mortality, although this hazard to society was quite evident at the time. (Princess Caroline, for example, following the lead of Lady Montagu, inoculated convicted criminals and pauper children before she did her own family. She evidently hesitated to inflict an experiment that she considered hazardous on people whom she considered to be of great importance.) Finally, and most remarkably, the entire mass experiment carried out in Boston and Brookline was proposed and urged by a man of the church and was opposed almost to a man by the medical profession.

Could this experiment be conducted in 1969? Certainly not. The mortality was prohibitive. There was no scientific basis or preliminary laboratory work. It is quite evident that both Cotton Mather and Zabdiel Boylston perceived a potential social benefit that was greater in their minds than the immediate sacrifice of six lives. From this experiment was born the initial awareness of active immunization as a means of protecting society against the scourge of epidemic disease. The first mass trials of the Salk polio vaccine and all the other inoculations from Pasteur to Enders went through moments when they shared precisely the same ethical problems faced by Mather and Boylston.

* * *

The first use of ether anesthesia, the first injection of insulin, the first use of liver extract, and the first application to a patient of any one of a host of new drugs are all part of the same ethical family. At the present time, we are engaged in one of the largest mass human experiments of this type ever considered: the widespread use of oral contraceptives. . . . Oral contraception has certain features that set it apart from ordinary therapeutic innovation because it is a medicinal treatment given to a healthy person to prevent a normal occurrence, rather than an inoculation given to prevent fatal epidemic disease or a drug (or operation) employed to treat human illness. Oral contraception must, therefore, be even more free of taint than innovations involved with the treatment of disease.

b.

Panel Discussion
Eugenics and Genetics*

* * *

BRONOWSKI: I find myself out of sympathy with much that has been said in Muller's and Lederberg's papers. That is because I really do not understand what problem you are trying to solve. If you are trying to upset violently the present gene frequencies in the population, then nothing that Muller proposes could do this. Just as Haldane has shown long ago that sterilization of the unfit would hardly have any influence on the proportion of recessive genes, so the multiplication of what we choose to call the fit can really have very little effect on the presence of recessives. (And no one who has known the children of accepted geniuses would suppose that the population would greatly benefit by there being several hundred of them.) If you are trying radically to change the gene frequencies, of course you can only do that in Crick's way, that is by forcibly preventing all but a few genes from reproducing. Even this supposes that you know (a) why you think a particular gene is good, and (b) what tests to apply in order to identify it.

However, I took Crick's remarks to be a *reductio ad absurdum* of the method of direct control of the gene frequencies. Indeed, we might achieve the same effect in a simpler way— by eating the children of the unfit, as Jonathan Swift suggested that the Irish poor should eat their own children. But what problem are we

---

* Gordon Wolstenholme, ed.: *Man and His Future.* Boston: Little, Brown and Co. 284–297 (1963). Reprinted by permission of J. & A. Churchill, London.

trying to solve? What genes are we trying to boost? Muller asserts in his paper that there are reasons to believe that the human population is deteriorating, and Huxley in one phrase in his paper also implied this. I know of no evidence for that. I know of no evidence that the present human population is inferior, in any respect that one could quantify, to the human population 50 years ago. On the contrary, the only important experimental test of this assertion—the experimental intelligence testing of Scottish children which has been carried out over the past 25 years—produced exactly the opposite results. The human race seems to be improving itself by those natural means which I propose to continue to enjoy so long as I can!

MacKay: I have been thinking of Shaw's mischievous remark: "What has posterity done for me that I should do anything for posterity?" Since the relation between individual responsibility and that of "society" is in fact still unclear, the notion of "our" responsibility to tinker with the genetic composition of posterity is doubly obscure. Without a much deeper analysis, the unguarded transfer to "society" of ideas proper to individual responsibility can mislead us into talking—and selling—moral nonsense.

That such nonsense has proved saleable, especially in Nazi Germany, should warn us against evaluating our plans for the race solely in terms of technical feasibility. We should, however, note one technical snag in any proposal to make the human genetic constitution self-regulating. I mean the difficulty of preventing the "goal-setting" from drifting or oscillating as time goes on, under the influence of external or even internal factors. Suppose, for example, that "we" (biologists? or politicians?) decided (and had the power) to make the next human generation of type "X." So far, perhaps, so good. But when we die, our place must presumably be taken by a new committee—which would presumably be of type "X." The question we must ponder is what kind of changes these men of type "X" would think desirable in their successors—and so on, into the future. If we cannot answer it, then to initiate such a process might show the reverse of responsibility, on any explication of the term.

In short, to navigate by a landmark tied to your own ship's head is ultimately impossible. If we are ever to make proper use of our growing eugenic powers, we shall need a wisdom greater than our own.

Here let us be quite candid. There is little agreement today that such wisdom is available, let alone as to its origin. But I believe strongly that this does not make discussion at this level pointless or impossible. For the beginning of wisdom is to ask the right questions; and it is by each faithfully drawing attention to—and listening to—questions which from a different viewpoint might not be raised, that we can most fruitfully cooperate for human welfare.

Brock: I would like to echo Bronowski's question: What is the problem that Crick and Muller are trying to solve? And are they thinking about some other problems which would arise out of the solution of what they think they are trying to solve? Are we going to bring to humanity the happiness which undoubtedly we all want? Sir Julian asked the question: What are people for? I don't believe that any of us really knows the answer, but I suppose that self-expression and self-fulfillment must be among the objectives of mankind. This brings me to the psycho-emotional aspect of the woman who is denied children. Even where childlessness is inevitable, even when she is married to an impotent husband to whom she is devoted, the psycho-emotional effect of this situation on her is devastating. Admittedly the need to have children can be met up to a point by adoption, but not when there is another alternative. In my opinion no woman is going to be emotionally satisfied by the adoption of children, when she knows that she could have had children by her own parturition. If we are to have a healthy society, we must have a society in which such psycho-emotional upsets are reduced to the minimum. When it comes to the solution that Muller proposes I doubt that, even with improved biological education, many men will be emotionally satisfied by children not their own, if they are also able to have children in the normal way. And without this emotional satisfaction and fulfillment I doubt that we would have a healthy society. There may be a small group of "advanced" or otherwise abnormal people who would be satisfied, but the average man in my opinion would not be. I agree with Pirie that perhaps for many men it is the fun rather than the children that they desire, but this is not true of all men and is certainly not true of the average woman.

Trowell: Speaking as a physician, I should like to emphasize the very profound psychological effect on both men and women who cannot have progeny by the natural method. It has played havoc with many of my patients and some of my friends.

KLEIN: I agree that the psycho-emotional reaction of a man who cannot have children is very strong. There are a number of married people who have no children because although the man is potent, he is sterile; this is a most unhappy situation and it is very difficult to explain to a couple that a man can be both potent and sterile. I think more research is needed on the problem of sterility in the male.

If we ever adopt Muller's techniques, we shall have to have biographies, not only of the great man whom we are considering as a sperm donor, but also of his antecedents. However, the present state of our knowledge of human inheritance is extremely fragile. I think we are still at the beginning of the study of human heredity, and before applying it I feel we must know it much better.

May I finish with a story by the German biologist, von Uexküll, about a man who discovered his own shadow. This man came to believe that his shadow was a living thing. At first he imagined his shadow to be his servant, because it copied all his movements; but he gradually began to doubt this and to believe that he was imitating the shadow. Thereafter he showed more and more consideration for his shadow, allowing it to have his seat or bed while he himself remained uncomfortably to one side. This man was eventually reduced to being the shadow of his shadow. Perhaps we also are too conscious of our shadows and forget what we are ourselves.

LEDERBERG: In answer to Dr. Bronowski's question about our motivation, I think that most of us here believe that the present population of the world is not intelligent enough to keep itself from being blown up, and we would like to make some provision for the future so that it will have a slightly better chance of avoiding this particular contingency. I am not saying that our measures will be effective, but I think this is our motivation; it is not the negative but the positive aspects of genetic control that we are dealing with here.

On the other hand I have serious doubts about the proposals for controlling reproduction that have been presented to us. The aspects of *social* control that seem to be necessary to make these proposals technically effective are I think extremely offensive and extremely dangerous, certainly in our present social context. But leaving the matter to individual choice, which from a social standpoint is the most ideal, is certainly not going to be technically effective. And if people are allowed to choose the fathers of their children, will they not choose just the more notorious projections of their own images, exaggerated by the publicity given to advertised donors?

COMFORT: Dr. Lederberg, what makes you think that we could make ourselves less likely to blow ourselves up by a genetic increase in intelligence?

LEDERBERG: I didn't say I thought we would succeed; I said I think this is our underlying motivation for attempting genetic control.

COMFORT: I should think that it is not so much low I.Q.'s, but personality problems and emotional disturbances which were the cause of our liability to blow ourselves up.

LEDERBERG: These are just as likely to be under genetic control.

COMFORT: They may be, but in man there is a large latitude for training. Dr. Trowell spoke about breeding a generation that displayed cruelty and efficiency. I think one could do this—or for that matter do the opposite—much more simply by *upbringing* than one can by trying to alter genetic constitution.

BRONOWSKI: I would still like an answer to my question. What is the evidence that genetically the human population is deteriorating?

HUXLEY: The evidence is mainly deductive, based on the fact that we are preserving many more genetically defective people than before, and are getting a lot of radioactive fallout. Meanwhile, the study of intelligence in Scottish children which you cited is not valid evidence. During the period between the first and the second tests, children generally were becoming larger, were developing more rapidly, and therefore were becoming more intelligent for their chronological age.

The important point, however, as Lederberg said, is not the negative one of deterioration (although it might become so if there were greatly increased fallout); the main thing is to aim at positive improvement. . . .

But the basic point was raised by MacKay, that you will have to nail your colours to some moral mast. In the present state of the world you will have to find a new moral mast to nail them to, and this will only come about by more knowledge and more education and more thinking; and this is a feedback process. At the moment the population certainly wouldn't tolerate compulsory eugenic or sterilization measures, but if you start some experiments, including some voluntary ones, and see that they work and if you make a massive attempt at educating people and making them understand what is at issue, you might be able, within a generation, to have an effect on the general population. After all, our moral values evolve like everything else and they evolve largely on the basis of the knowledge we have and share.

GLIKSON: Like Dr. Bronowski I do not see why we need the application of biological technology in changing the quantitative and qualitative composition of whole communities or of humanity. But I think emphasis should be laid on the dangers involved in the very development of such biological technology, because its application would most probably fall into the hands of political forces which would use it for quite different purpose than those anticipated here. . . .

PRICE: I would like to go further than Bronowski, and suggest that the psychosocial system might in its own bumbling homoeostatic way actually be doing the right job. We know that a great deal of the performance of man depends as much on social environment as on genetics, and this environment might act in a way completely opposite to that which would be produced by the mechanisms of genetic control which we might introduce. For example, creativity, intelligence, and the leaning towards science are apparently, on the basis of historical evidence, enormously helped by such things as being first or only children, and by losing a parent before the age of ten; these things together improve your chance of being a good and creative scientist by something like a factor of ten. Now, if the better people are having small families, they are increasing the frequency of only children, thereby giving their group an increased chance of success; and to increase the number of people carrying these genes by encouraging larger families among the more intelligent people might be to deny the possibility of the very environment which would let these factors work.

PINCUS: I am very surprised to hear some people here say that genetics has taught us nothing about nature and that if we breed in a random manner by the old-fashioned methods, we shall get good genes. This is nonsense genetically: you don't get good genes by breeding in random fashion; you get good genes by selection. If, however, you want to emphasize the phenom-

enon of heterosis or hybrid vigour, as Huxley has done, and argue that the real reason for the success of the human race is that there is so much interbreeding that you are always getting heterosis phenomena, then I accept that you have an argument there. But if we are talking about *genetic* improvement, you have to select good genes.

TROWELL: Could I put in very briefly the point of view of the Roman Catholic church (speaking as someone who is not a Roman Catholic and who does not subscribe completely to that point of view)—their great emphasis on natural law. I think they would say that we should be very careful before we distrust what has worked for about a million years in the human species and for longer than that in the animal creation, for this is one aspect of natural law. . . .

* * *

CLARK: Dr. Trowell used the phrase "natural law" in the sense of something which has been going on for a very long time. I would define it differently; it may coincide with what has been the practice of mankind or it may not. Several people have raised the question of what is the purpose of man on earth. I feel a bit hesitant at entering this field and would have preferred a professional to have tackled it—but the main purpose of man on earth is to love God and obey his commandments. I know that poses a difficulty for people who deny God's existence but I think they ought to take a look at this view, and consider how other conclusions follow from it. Cultural fulfilment and enjoyment are secondary purposes in man's existence, not his primary purpose.

* * *

CRICK: I disagree strongly with Dr. Clark's remarks and with the standpoint from which he made them. It is clear that if we take the broad ethical question of ultimate ends we shall never reach any agreement. Moreover, those of us who are humanists have a great difficulty in that we are unable to formulate our ends as clearly as is possible for those of us who are Christians. Nevertheless there are some ends that we can all share, even though we have these differences. It is surely clear that good health, high intelligence, general benevolence—the qualities Muller listed —are desirable qualities which we would all agree on. We would agree also that these qualities are not uniformly distributed. There are people who are deficient in intelligence, for example (I mention intelligence because this is something we can to some extent measure). Surely it is a very reasonable aim for us to try to increase that. Some of the arguments that "nature is doing it all right" may possibly be correct but they seem to me only to reflect conservatism and to have no real basis of fact. We are now in an environment that is changing very rapidly, and has been changing for the last few thousand years, but we evolved, as was made clear by Muller, over a much longer period of time in very different circumstances. Consequently, we should not *necessarily* go on as we are.

Are the methods for improvement which we have at our disposal effective? Now there are difficult technical questions here, but my point, which Huxley made rather strongly, is that we are likely to achieve a considerable improvement —not perhaps as fast as we could do by other methods or even as fast as may turn out to be necessary—by using a very primitive knowledge of genetics; that is, by simply taking the people with the qualities we like, and letting them have more children. Nobody is suggesting, at least it would be foolish if they did, that we should have *enormous* numbers of people all with one father; one should have a wide selection of donors and so get diversification. The difficulty I see concerns the techniques that are *socially* possible, in the present social context, and in the social context of the next twenty or thirty years—a context which will change and which to some extent our views may help to change. For example, psychological problems may arise in families with children who are not the children of the father. Whereas I reject utterly arguments about natural law, I am much concerned that evidence on the psychological problems in such families should be collected. We already have examples of families where the father is infertile and the mother has had a child by artificial insemination by a donor; I understand that the disturbance to family life is often not great in such cases. I agree entirely with Huxley that what is wanted here is some sort of limited programme to try and find the difficulties. Let us define our broad aims and then tackle the practical details.

MEDAWAR: I agree with a good deal of what Crick has just said, but I think we ought to be warned by the very diversity of opinion in this room. We all have a pretty good opinion of our own intellect and our worthiness to be sperm donors. But our opinions are extremely diverse, and my feeling at the moment is that human be-

ings are simply not to be trusted to formulate long-term eugenic objectives—least of all Roman Catholics. What frightens me about Muller and to some extent Huxley is their extreme self-confidence, their complete conviction not only that they know what ends are desirable but also that they know how to achieve them. I can perhaps imagine approving of the kind of scheme Muller has outlined if he put it this way: "we don't really know a great deal about human inheritance but with the co-operation of a number of volunteers let us put my scheme into practice and perhaps we shall learn from it."

HUXLEY: But surely Muller's point, and certainly mine, is not to think in terms of any definite eugenic ideal; the aim that I have in mind is the very general one of gradual improvement.

MEDAWAR: But you don't know how to do it! May I challenge you to explain Evelyn Hutchinson's paradox about homosexuality? The proportion of homosexuals has probably not declined over the period of recorded history; yet according to all selection theories which we are so confident about, the proportion should have declined on the reasonable grounds (a) that homosexual tendencies are to some extent genetically determined and (b) that homosexuals are on the whole less fertile (even if fractionally less fertile) than normal people. It follows that the genetic endowments that make for homosexuality or parasexuality in general should have declined. In fact they have done nothing of the kind. This means either that so deep-seated a trait as parasexuality or homosexuality is not genetically determined or that we don't really understand the mechanism of its inheritance.

HUXLEY: I didn't know about this paradox, and am afraid I can't answer that point. In any case I want to look at the problem from another angle. You say we must know more about the details of human genetics before we can think about improvement. I really don't see why. Darwin knew nothing about the details of reproduction, still less about genetics, and yet he was able to deduce a set of principles and a general theory of evolutionary transformation which have stood up to the test of time. Our new knowledge is merely permitting us to fill in the details and add a few minor modifications. What I want to stress is that if we can find the right method of exerting selective pressure, we could make for human genetic improvement. We must do it by way of experiment.

Dr. Trowell talked about breeding for efficiency. This is very important because, as psychosocial organizations get more and more complicated, we need more and more good brains at the top to run them. If you assume as a first approximation that intellectual efficiency or intelligence has a strong genetic component, and that it is distributed according to the ordinary type of symmetrical frequency curve, you can calculate that a very small increase in the mean will produce a large percentage increase in the upper values; so far as I remember, if you could raise mean I.Q. from 100 to 101.5 you would raise the percentage of people with an I.Q. of 160 and over by nearly 50 per cent. The increased social and cultural efficiency resulting from a small difference in the number of outstandingly gifted people is also very important in considering the problem of possible racial differences.

LEDERBERG: The converse of Huxley's calculation is that in order to shift the mean I.Q. by 1.5/100 you must increase the production of geniuses by 50 per cent. It is perhaps better to aim at just increasing the variance. The question is not whether we should think about doing eugenics; we certainly should, and should collect just as much information as possible. The point is whether we should embark on a concrete programme that is very costly in social and political stresses for an aim which isn't very well crystallized yet.

*   *   *

PART THREE

The Authority of the Subject as Guardian of His Own Fate

In Part Two we explored the investigator's authority in the human experimentation process. We sought to specify the nature and degree of harm to subjects, science and society as well as other identifiable elements of research design and objectives which suggest that other decisionmakers, besides the investigator, should participate in this process. We now focus on the subject in order to examine the extent and limits of his ability and authority to make decisions on his own behalf.

Belief in the idea of individual freedom is a cornerstone of the Western concept of man and society. The common law nurtures and protects individual freedom through the doctrine of self-determination, which confers on each person the right to pursue his own ends in his own way so long as he does not interfere with specified rights of other individuals or of the community. The requirement of consent is the primary means for implementing the abstract notion of self-determination. Tort law, for example, guards a man's property and person against interferences to which he has not consented. Similarly, a contract comes into being when two or more persons agree with each other that certain terms should govern their relationship.

In most commercial transactions, each party is responsible for informing himself about the terms and implications of the contract. However, when professionals intervene in the lives of others, a higher standard is imposed upon them. They may be held responsible not only for obtaining the layman's consent, but also for informing him of the consequences of their agreement.

The doctor-patient relationship has been the primary arena for the development of the rule that a professional is liable for damages if he intervenes (even if he acts with utmost care and for benevolent reasons) without his patient's "informed consent." From its origins in therapeutic settings, the requirement of informed consent has been adopted for experimental situations. In Chapter Eight we examine its history and the functions which it can serve in investigator-subject relationships, in order to analyze why and how it should be safeguarded by the participants in the human experimentation process.

The doctrine of self-determination and the requirement of consent have always had to contend with doubts about man's capacity to consent and with conflicts between man and society about society's prerogative to override consent in its own interests. These doubts and conflicts have not escaped the human experimentation process but, at present, are reflected only in a number of "exceptions" to the rule of consent rather than in an overall theory of consent which encompasses these issues. Chapters Nine and Ten examine the limits of self-determination and consent inherent in the nature of man and in the investigator-subject relationship as well as the limits imposed by the "claims" of society and the subject's own "best interests." This inquiry should begin both to define the authority and capacity of man to give consent and to identify the assumptions about man and society on which a theory of consent for human experimentation should rest.

Throughout we ask:

1. What values do law and the professions attempt to nurture and protect through the concept of self-determination and the requirement of "informed consent"?

2. How should self-determination and informed consent be defined in order to protect these values?

3. Under what circumstances is informed consent either ill-adapted or insufficient to protect these values?

4. Under what circumstances do self-determination and informed consent conflict with other values which the participants—investigator, subject, professions, and society—seek to protect and advance?

5. How should a subject's inability to consent affect his participation in the human experimentation process?

Since, under some circumstances, informed consent alone may not adequately safeguard the rights of subjects or provide the best means for resolving conflicts between the participants, the study of these materials should raise questions about additional rules and procedures for the control of human experimentation as well as about who should be given authority to formulate, administer, and review them.

CHAPTER EIGHT

What Are the Functions of Informed Consent?

The concept of informed consent is a legal hybrid. The traditional function of consent was to differentiate those medical interventions which were legally permissible from those which would subject a physician to liability for an unauthorized "offensive touching" of his patient. Recently courts have concluded that a patient's assent to a medical procedure is valid—a "voluntary" product of his "free will"—only if it is based on adequate information about the intervention including its attendant risks. The engrafting of the "information" component moved the concept beyond simple assault and battery law. A physician may now be held liable either for negligence in a malpractice suit, if he breaches his duty to inform a patient, or for battery, if his failure to inform is found to have vitiated the patient's consent.

From these beginnings, the concept of informed consent has been accepted in case and commentary as a cardinal principle for judging the propriety of research with human beings. Yet law has neither defined sufficiently well the substance and ambit of informed consent in therapeutic settings nor determined clearly its functional relevance for human experimentation. Thus, in invoking informed consent like a talisman, lawyers, investigators, and courts often seem to overlook the fact that it lacks specific construction and remains an ill-defined concept.

This chapter examines first the constructions which courts and commentators have given to informed consent. It then explores the functions which informed consent could serve for the human experimentation process; these have been grouped into four categories. Most clearly, requiring informed consent serves society's desire to respect each individual's autonomy and his right to make choices concerning his own life. Second, providing a subject with information about an experiment and encouraging him to be an active partner in the process may also increase the rationality of the experimentation process.

Third, securing informed consent protects the experimentation process by encouraging the investigator to question the value of the proposed project and the adequacy of the measures he has taken to protect subjects, by reducing civil and criminal liability for non-negligent injury to the subjects, and by diminishing adverse public reaction to an experiment. Finally, informed consent may serve the function of increasing society's awareness about human research. For instance, the need to obtain consent from large numbers of potential donors for the removal of their kidneys after death has led to an extensive program of information about renal transplantation. While the motivation for the information campaign was to recruit individual donors, it also enlightens the public at large.

The functions of informed consent, which are identified in this chapter, do not necessarily conflict with and may in some contexts reinforce one another. Nevertheless, each function suggests different substantive and procedural requisites for the definition of "consent." Thus an important task of this chapter is to arrive at a comprehensive functional definition of informed consent, in light of the competing theories and attitudes about individuals' right to and capacity for self-determination.

In studying the materials in this chapter, consider, in addition to the general questions posed in the introduction to this Part, the following specific questions:

1. What functions should informed consent serve in the human experimentation process? In seeking an answer to this question, must the "informing" and "consenting" components of this concept be considered separately?

2. What are the requisite elements of informed consent to implement these functions?

3. To what extent can the elements of informed consent, developed in therapeutic settings, be carried over by analogy to experimental contexts?

4. Under what circumstances and to what extent should the elements of informed consent be modified?

5. Should additional or alternative elements of consent be required when the experimental subject is also a patient?

A.
An Historical Perspective

1.

From Status to Contract

a.

Friedrich Kessler and Grant Gilmore
Contracts—Cases and Materials*

*   *   *

Within the framework of a free-enterprise system the essential prerequisite of contractual

---

* Boston: Little, Brown and Co. 3–6 (2nd ed., 1970). Reprinted by permission.

liability is volition, that is, consent freely given, and not coercion or status. Contract, in this view, is the "meeting place of the ideas of agreement and obligation." As a matter of historical fact, the rise of free and informal contract within western civilization reflected the erosion of a status-organized society; contract became, at an ever-increasing rate, a tool of change and of growing self-determination and self-assertion. Self-determination during the nineteenth century was regarded as the goal towards which society progressed; the movement of progressive societies, in the words of Sir Henry Maine, is a movement from status to contract. "It is through contract that man attains freedom. Although it appears to be the subordination of one man's will to another, the former gains more than he loses." Contract, in this view, is the principle of order par excellence and the only legitimate means of social integration in a free society. Translated into legal language this means that in a progressive society all law is ultimately based on contract. And since contract as a social phenomenon is the result of a "coincidence of free choices" on the part of the members of the community, merging their egoistical and altruistic tendencies, a contractual society safeguards its own stability. Contract is an instrument of peace in society. It reconciles freedom with order, particularly since with increasing rationality man becomes less rather than more egoist.

*   *   *

Small wonder that freedom of contract, as evolved in the spirit of laissez-faire, has found repeated expression in Anglo-American case law. It became the paramount postulate of public policy. "[I]f there is one thing which more than another public policy requires," Sir George Jessel, M.R., assures us, "it is that men of full age and competent understanding shall have the utmost liberty of contracting, and that their contracts entered into freely and voluntarily shall be held sacred and shall be enforced by Courts of Justice." True, fraud, misrepresentation and duress must be ruled out by the courts in the exercise of their function of making sure that the "rules of the game" will be adhered to. But these categories were narrowly defined (at least by the nineteenth century common law) due to the strong belief in the policing force of the market. Oppressive bargains, it was taken for granted, can be avoided by careful shopping around. Contracting parties are expected to look out for their own interest and their own protection. "Let the bargainer beware," as we were told, was (and to some extent still is) the ordinary rule of contract. It is not the function of courts to strike down improvident bargains. Courts have only to interpret contracts made by the parties. They do not make them. Within this framework contract justice is commutative and not distributive justice. This attitude is in keeping with liberal social and moral philosophy according to which it pertains to the dignity of man to lead his own life as a reasonable person and to accept responsibility for his own mistakes. . . .

*   *   *

NOTES

NOTE 1.

Friedrich Kessler
Contracts of Adhesion—Some Thoughts about Freedom of Contract*

With the development of a free enterprise system based on an unheard of division of labor, capitalistic society needed a highly elastic legal institution to safeguard the exchange of goods and services on the market. Common law lawyers, responding to this social need, transformed "contract" from the clumsy institution that it was in the sixteenth century into a tool of almost unlimited usefulness and pliability. Contract thus became the indispensable instrument of the enterpriser, enabling him to go about his affairs in a rational way. Rational behavior within the context of our culture is only possible if agreements will be respected. It requires that reasonable expectations created by promises receive the protection of the law or else we will suffer the fate of Montesquieu's Troglodytes, who perished because they did not fulfill their promises. This idea permeates our whole law of contracts, the doctrines dealing with their formation, performance, impossibility and damages.

Under a free enterprise system rationality of the law of contracts has still another aspect. To keep pace with the constant widening of the market the legal system has to place at the disposal of the members of the community an ever increasing number of typical business transactions and regulate their consequences. But the law cannot possibly anticipate the content of an infinite number of atypical transactions into which members of the community may need to enter. Society, therefore, has to give the parties freedom of contract; to accommodate the business community the ceremony necessary to vouch for the deliberate nature of a transaction has to be reduced to the absolute minimum. Furthermore, the rules of the common law of contract have to remain *Jus dispositivum*—to use the phrase of the Romans; that is, their application has to depend on the intention of the parties or on their neglect to rule otherwise. (If parties to a contract have failed to regulate its consequences in their own way, they will be supposed to have intended the consequences envisaged by the common law.) Beyond that the law cannot go. It has to delegate legislation to the contracting par-

* 43 *Columbia Law Review* 629–630 (1943). Reprinted by permission.

ties. As far as they are concerned, the law of contract has to be of their own making.

Thus freedom of contract does not commend itself for moral reasons only; it is also an eminently practical principle. It is the inevitable counterpart of a free enterprise system. As a result, our legal lore of contracts reflects a proud spirit of individualism and of *laissez faire*. This is particularly true for the axioms and rules dealing with the formation and interpretation of contracts, the genuineness and reality of consent. . . .

*   *   *

NOTE 2.

SCHLOENDORFF V. NEW YORK HOSPITAL
211 N.Y. 127, 129, 105 N.E. 92, 93 (1914)

CARDOZO, J.
. . . Every human being of adult years and sound mind has a right to determine what shall be done with his own body; and a surgeon who performs an operation without his patient's consent commits an assault, for which he is liable in damages. (*Pratt v. Davis*, 224 Ill. 300; *Mohr v. Williams*, 95 Minn. 261.) This is true except in cases of emergency where the patient is unconscious and where it is necessary to operate before consent can be obtained. . . .

b.

Slater v. Baker and Stapleton, C.B.
95 Eng. Rep. 860 (1767)

[PER CURIAM]

*   *   *

Special action upon the case, wherein the plaintiff declares that the defendant Baker being a surgeon, and Stapleton an apothecary, he employed them to cure his leg which had been broken and set, and the callous of the fracture formed; that in consideration of being paid for their skill and labour, &c. they undertook and promised, &c; but the defendants not regarding their promise and undertaking, and the duty of their business and employment, so ignorantly and unskilfully treated the plaintiff, that they ignorantly and unskilfully broke and disunited the callous of the plaintiff's leg after it was set, and the callous formed, whereby he is damaged. The defendants pleaded not guilty, whereupon issue was joined, which was tried before the Lord Chief Justice Wilmot, and a verdict found for the plaintiff, damages 500*l*. The substance of the evidence for the plaintiff at the trial was, first a sur-

geon was called, who swore that the plaintiff having broken both the bones of one of his legs, this witness set the same; that the plaintiff was under his hands nine weeks; that in a month's time after the leg was set, he found the leg was healing and in a good way; the callous was formed; there was a little protuberance, but not more than usual, upon cross examination he said he was instructed in surgery by his father, that the callous was the uniting the bones, and that it was very dangerous to break or disunite the callous after it was formed.

John Latham, an apothecary, swore he attended the plaintiff nine weeks, who was then well enough to go home; that the bones were well united; that he was present with the plaintiff and defendants, and at first the defendants said the plaintiff had fallen into good hands; the second time he saw them all together the defendants said the same; but when he saw them together a third time there was some alteration; he said the plaintiff was then in a passion, and was unwilling to let the defendants do any thing to his leg; he said he had known such a thing done as disuniting the callous, but that had been only when a leg was set very crooked, but not where it was straight.

*   *   *

The daughter of the plaintiff swore, that the defendant Stapleton was first sent for to take off the bandage from the plaintiff's leg; when he came he declined to do it himself, and desired the other defendant Baker might be called in to assist; when Baker came he sent for the machine that was mentioned; plaintiff offered to give Baker a guinea, but Stapleton advised him not to take it then, but said they might be paid all together when the business was done; that the third time the defendants came to the plaintiff, Baker took up the plaintiff's foot in both his hands and nodded to Stapleton, and then Stapleton took the plaintiff's leg upon his knee, and the leg gave a crack, when the plaintiff cried out to them and said, "You have broke what nature had formed"; Baker then said to the plaintiff, "You must go through the operation of extension," and Stapleton said, "We have consulted and done for the best."

*   *   *

Another surgeon was called, who swore, that when the callous is formed to any degree, it is difficult to break it, and the callous in this case must have been formed, or it would not have given a crack, and said extension was improper; and if the patient himself had asked him to do it, he would have declined it; and if the callous had not been hard, he would not have done it without the consent of the plaintiff; that compression was the proper way, and the instrument improper: he said the defendant Baker was eminent in his profession. . . .

* * *

. . . When we consider the good character of Baker, we cannot well conceive why he acted in the manner he did; but many men very skilful in their profession have frequently acted out of the common way for the sake of trying experiments. Several of the witnesses proved that the callous was formed, and that it was proper to remove plaintiff home; that he was free from pain, and able to walk with crutches. We cannot conceive what the nature of the instrument made use of is: why did Baker put it on, when he said that plaintiff had fallen into good hands, and when plaintiff only sent for him to take off the bandage? It seems as if Mr. Baker wanted to try an experiment with this new instrument.

2dly, it is objected, that this is not the proper action, and that it ought to have been trespass vi & armis. In answer to this, it appears from the evidence of the surgeons that it was improper to disunite the callous without consent; this is the usage and law of surgeons: then it was ignorance and unskilfulness in that very particular, to do contrary to the rule of the profession, what no surgeon ought to have done; and indeed it is reasonable that a patient should be told what is about to be done to him, that he may take courage and put himself in such a situation as to enable him to undergo the operation. It was objected, this verdict and recovery cannot be pleaded in bar to an action of trespass vi & armis to be brought for the same damage; but we are clear of opinion it may be pleaded in bar. That the plaintiff ought to receive a satisfaction for the injury, seems to be admitted; but then it is said, the defendants ought to have been charged as trespassers vi & armis. The Court will not look with eagle's eyes to see whether the evidence applies exactly or not to the case, when they can see the plaintiff has obtained a verdict for such damages as he deserves, they will establish such verdict if it be possible. For any thing that appears to the Court, this was the first experiment made with this new instrument; and if it was, it was a rash action, and he who acts rashly acts ignorantly: and although the defendants in

general may be as skilful in their respective professions as any two gentlemen in England, yet the Court cannot help saying, that in this particular case they have acted ignorantly and unskilfully, contrary to the known rule and usage of surgeons.

Judgment for the plaintiff per totam Curiam.

NOTES

NOTE 1.

CARPENTER v. BLAKE
60 BARB. 488 (N.Y. SUP. CT. 1871),
reversed on other grounds, 50 N.Y. 696 (1872)

By the Court, MULLIN, P. J.

* * *

Much was said on the argument, as to the right of a surgeon to exercise his own judgment as to the mode of treatment he will adopt in the case of a wound, or of a disease which he is called upon to treat; that neither the rules prescribed by writers, nor those acted upon by other physicians or surgeons, can apply to every case, and hence latitude must be allowed for the application of remedies which the attending physician or surgeon has found to be beneficial. If this is not allowed, the argument is, that all progress in the practice of surgery or physic must cease, and the afflicted lose altogether the benefits of experience and of remedies that science furnishes for the alleviation of human suffering. It must be conceded that if a surgeon is bound, at the peril of being liable for malpractice, to follow the modes of treatment which writers and practitioners have prescribed, the patient may lose the benefits of recent improvements in the treatment of diseases, or discoveries in science, by which new remedies have been brought into use; but this danger is more apparent than real. Some standard, by which to determine the propriety of treatment, must be adopted; otherwise experience will take the place of skill, and the reckless experimentalist the place of the educated, experienced practitioner. If the case is a new one, the patient must trust to the skill and experience of the surgeon he calls; so must he if the injury or the disease is attended with injury to other parts, or other diseases have developed themselves, for which there is no established mode of treatment. But when the case is one as to which a system of treatment has been followed for a long time, there should be no departure from it, unless the surgeon who does it is prepared to take the risk of establishing, by his success, the propriety and safety of his experiment.

The rule protects the community against reckless experiments, while it admits the adoption of new remedies and modes of treatment only when their benefits have been demonstrated, or when, from the necessity of the case, the surgeon or physician must be left to the exercise of his own skill and experience.

* * *

NOTE 2.

JACKSON V. BURNHAM
20 COLO. 532, 39 PAC. 577 (1895),
reversing 28 PAC. 250 (1891)

GODDARD, J.

* * *

In this connection . . . we notice instruction No. 16 . . . : "That, if writers on . . . treatment . . . , or practical surgeons prescribe a mode of treatment, it is incumbent on surgeons called on to treat such an ailment to conform to the system of treatment thus established, and, if they depart from it, they do so at their peril." The learned writer of the opinion of the court of appeals condemns this instruction, because it contravenes the rule that the criterion by which to judge of the correctness of a particular mode of treatment must be one universally adopted by the profession, and that the language used in the instruction may be construed to mean that a treatment prescribed by some writers or some surgeons may not be departed from without peril, and for the further reason that, if sustained, the rule announced will prohibit further progress in surgery. We do not think the language used should be construed, or that the jury could have understood it to mean, that a treatment laid down by some writers or practiced by some surgeons should control, but that it clearly conveys the idea that the mode of treatment meant is one which writers and the profession universally commend. With this construction the rule announced is correct. There must be some criterion by which to test the proper mode of treatment in a given case; and, when a particular mode of treatment is upheld by a consensus of opinion among the members of the profession, it should be followed by the ordinary practitioner; and, if a physician sees fit to experiment with some other mode, he should do so at his peril. In other words, he must be able, in the case of deleterious results, to satisfy the jury that he had reason for the faith that was in him, and

justify his experiment by some reasonable theory. . . .

* * *

NOTE 3.

ALLEN V. VOJE
114 WIS. 1, 12, 89 N.W. 924, 931 (1902)

DODGE, J.

* * *

The tenth assignment of error is predicated upon certain instructions to the jury. . . .

. . . The asserted vice in the first of these appears most strongly in the following quotation: "A departure from approved methods in general use, if it injures the patient, will render him [the physician] liable, however good his intentions may have been." This is criticised because it makes the physician liable in case he adopts new methods, although improved ones, and counsel suggest that no progress in medicine is possible if physicians must adhere to ancient methods; that vaccination or the use of antitoxin, however wise and generally helpful, would, under that doctrine, have been malpractice originally. The instruction, viewed in the light of the rest of the charge, of course, excludes the idea of liability for variations from customary practice merely in the way of increased precautions, recognized as such. Its only application, in the light of the evidence, must have been to the omission of precautions such as it was testified other physicians uniformly took, or in the deviation from such practice by making an operation or curettement under the circumstances presented. . . .

We have little doubt that, if the first case of vaccination had proved disastrous and injured the patient, the physician should have been held liable. Nor do we believe that a physician of standing and loyalty to his patients will subject them to mere experiment, the safety or virtue of which has not been established by experience of the profession, save possibly when the patient is in extremis, and fatal results substantially certain unless the experiment may succeed.

* * *

NOTE 4.

FORTNER V. KOCH
272 MICH. 273, 261 N.W. 762 (1935)

EDWARD M. SHARPE, JUSTICE

* * *

It is the duty of a physician or surgeon in diagnosing a case to use due diligence in ascertaining all available facts and collecting data essential to a proper diagnosis. The instant case, not being an emergency and the defendant not having used such diligence in availing himself of various methods of diagnosis for discovering the nature of the ailment as are practiced by physicians and surgeons of skill and learning in the community in which he practiced, he must be held liable for the damages due to his negligence.

We recognize the fact that, if the general practice of medicine and surgery is to progress, there must be a certain amount of experimentation carried on; but such experiments must be done with the knowledge and consent of the patient or those responsible for him, and must not vary too radically from the accepted method of procedure. One who claims to be a specialist insofar as diagnosing a case is concerned must also be held to the above rule.

*   *   *

NOTE 5.

FIORENTINO V. WENGER
26 APP. DIV.2D 693, 272 N.Y.S.2D 557 (SUP. CT. 1966), *reversed as to defendant hospital,* 19 N.Y.2D 407, 227 N.E.2D 296 (1967)

MEMORANDUM BY THE COURT.

*   *   *

It was virtually undisputed that plaintiff's decedent, her fourteen-year-old son, was caused to suffer an exsanguinating hemorrhage as the result of an operation performed upon him by the defendant physician at the defendant hospital for the purpose of correcting the decedent's scoliotic condition. The surgery performed was not the generally accepted medical treatment in the community for scoliosis, but was a procedure utilized in this country only by the defendant physician, who had first developed it five years before the operation and death in the case at bar.

It was also virtually undisputed that over the course of those five years, in at least five of the thirty-five instances in which the procedure was utilized by the defendant physician prior to the operation here involved, there had been unexpected and untoward results. Approximately one year before the operation herein, one of the defendant physician's patients had been caused to suffer an immediate paralysis when one of the screws inserted into her vertebral column to anchor the steel bar or "spinal jack" (which was in-

tended to support and hold the spine in a straight position) pierced the spinal canal and severed the spinal cord. As a result, the hospital where that operation had been performed withdrew permission for the defendant physician's use of its facilities for this type of procedure.

We are of the opinion that, under the facts and circumstances disclosed by this record, including the fact that no immediate emergency existed, the defendant physician was obligated to make a disclosure to the parents of his infant patient that the procedure he proposed was novel and unorthodox and that there were risks incident to or possible in its use. . . .

*   *   *

2.

The Genesis of "Informed Consent"

a.

Natanson v. Kline
186 Kan. 393, 350 P.2d 1093 (1960)

SCHROEDER, JUSTICE.

This is an action for malpractice against a hospital and the physician in charge of its radiology department to recover for injuries sustained as the result of radiation therapy with radioactive cobalt, alleged to have been given in an excessive amount.

The plaintiff (appellant), Irma Natanson, suffering from a cancer of the breast, had a radical left mastectomy performed on May 29, 1955. At the direction of Dr. Crumpacker, the surgeon who performed that operation, the plaintiff engaged Dr. John R. Kline, a radiologist, for radiation therapy to the site of the mastectomy and the surrounding areas.

Dr. Kline, a licensed physician and specialist in radiation therapy, was head of the radiology department at St. Francis Hospital at Wichita, Kansas. The plaintiff seeks damages for injuries claimed to have been sustained as a result of alleged acts of negligence in the administration of the cobalt radiation treatment. Dr. Kline and the hospital were named as defendants (appellees).

The case was tried to a jury which returned a verdict in favor of both defendants. The plaintiff's motion for a new trial having been denied, this appeal followed specifying various trial errors.

*   *   *

One of the alleged grounds of negligence, concerning which there was evidence before the jury, was that Dr. Kline failed to warn the appellant the course of treatment which he undertook to administer involved great risk of bodily injury or death.

The appellant requested and the trial court refused to give the following instruction:

You are instructed that the relationship between physician and patient is a fiduciary one. The relationship requires the physician to make a full disclosure to the patient of all matters within his knowledge affecting the interests of the patient. Included within the matters which the physician must advise the patient are the nature of the proposed treatment and any hazards of the proposed treatment which are known to the physician. Every adult person has the right to determine for himself or herself whether or not he will subject his body to hazards of any particular medical treatment.

You are instructed that if you find from the evidence that defendant Kline knew that the treatment he proposed to administer to plaintiff involved hazard or danger he was under a duty to advise plaintiff of that fact and if you further find that defendant Kline did not advise plaintiff of such hazards then defendant Kline was guilty of negligence.

There was evidence from which the jury could have found that the appellant fully appreciated the danger and the risk of the radiation treatment. The appellant's husband testified:

Q: Yes, how did it happen you went there for the conference with Dr. Kline? A: We, of course, made a periodic visit to Dr. Crumpacker after the operation, and he told us that as a precautionary measure Mrs. Natanson should go to the St. Francis Hospital and take the cobalt treatment. He explained to us that the cobalt was a new therapy; that it was much more powerful than the x-ray they had used previously. He suggested we see Dr. Kline.

On cross examination he testified:

Q: Just a question or two. Mr. Natanson, when you and your wife went to see Dr. Crumpacker, did you have a discussion with him about the purpose of the irradiation? A: Yes.
Q: And, was the general objective of irradiation explained to you? A: Yes.
Q: And, that was when Mrs. Natanson was with you? A: Yes.
Q: Now, did you consult any radiologist other than Dr. Kline in determining anything about this irradiation? A: No, sir.

*   *   *

Q: Now, I take it that it was Dr. Crumpacker's thought or suggestion at least to you that Dr. Kline be consulted? A: Yes.

Q: And, up to the time you engaged Dr. Kline, Dr. Crumpacker had been the doctor on the case? A: Yes.

There was also testimony from the appellant and her husband that Dr. Kline did not inform the appellant the treatment involved any danger whatever. The testimony of Dr. Kline, a radiologist with special training in cobalt irradiation, was that he knew he was "taking a chance" with the treatment he proposed to administer and that such treatment involved a "calculated risk." He testified there was always a danger of injury in the treatment of cancer. Insofar as the record discloses Dr. Kline did not testify that he informed the appellant the treatment involved any danger. His only testimony relevant thereto was the following:

Q: Now, tell us what transpired when you first met with the Natansons? A: I could not completely recall that meeting. It was such a long time ago.
Q: Just tell us what you can recall of it? A: I remember Mr. and Mrs. Natanson coming in to see me. I can't remember if I met them in my office or whether we were downstairs. I remember in a very vague way. I remember in a vague way that we discussed the treatment, about how long it took, the number of areas we would irradiate. I have a recollection of that. I remember we took her into the treatment room. She was marked out, measured. I believe the marking out and measurement was done by Mr. Darter. Her first treatment occurred the first day she came. I am not sure of that but I think so.
Q: Have you told us everything you recall? A: Yes.

No other evidence appears in the record concerning the subject.

The appellees argue that we are here concerned with a case where the patient consented to the treatment, but afterwards alleges that the nature and consequences of the risks of the treatment were not properly explained to her. They point out this is not an action for assault and battery, where a patient has given no consent to the treatment.

What appears to distinguish the case of the unauthorized surgery or treatment from traditional assault and battery cases is the fact that in almost all of the cases the physician is acting in relatively good faith for the benefit of the patient. While it is true that in some cases the results are not in fact beneficial to a patient, the courts have repeatedly stated that doctors are not insurers. The traditional assault and battery involves a defendant who is acting for the most part out of malice or in a manner generally considered as "anti-social." One who commits an assault and battery is not seeking to confer any benefit upon the one assaulted.

The fundamental distinction between assault and battery, on the one hand, and negligence such as would constitute malpractice, on the other, is that the former is intentional and the latter unintentional. . . .

We are here concerned with a case where the patient consented to the treatment, but alleges in a malpractice action that the nature and consequences of the risks of the treatment were not properly explained to her. This relates directly to the question whether the physician has obtained the informed consent of the patient to render the treatment administered.

The treatment of a cancer patient with radioactive cobalt is relatively new. Until the use of atomic energy appeared in this country, X ray was the type of radiation treatment used for such patients. Radioactive cobalt is manufactured by the Atomic Energy Commission in a neutron pile by bombarding the stable element of cobalt in its pure state. This makes the cobalt unstable and by reason thereof it is radioactive. The radioactive cobalt emits two homogeneous beams of pure energy called gamma rays, very close in character, which are far more powerful than the ordinary X rays. It produces no other rays to be filtered out. This makes it desirable for use in the treatment of cancer patients. The cobalt machine may be compared to a three-million volt X ray machine.

Radioactive cobalt is so powerful that the Atomic Energy Commission specifies the construction of the room in which the cobalt unit is to be placed. The walls of the room are made of concrete forty inches thick and the ceiling, also concrete, is twenty-four inches thick. The room is sunken down in a courtyard outside the hospital. A passageway off the control room about ten feet long leads to the treatment room. All controls are placed in the outer control room and, when the radiation treatment is administered to a patient, the operator in the outer room looks through a specially designed thick lead quartz glass which gives a telescopic view. A periodic report of radiation outside the room must be made to the Atomic Energy Commission in accordance with regulations. These facts were given by Dr. Kline in his testimony.

These facts are not commonly known and a patient cannot be expected to know the hazards or the danger of radiation from radioactive cobalt unless the patient is informed by a radiolo-

gist who knows the dangers of injury from cobalt irradiation. While Dr. Kline did not testify that the radiation he gave the appellant caused her injury, he did state cobalt irradiation could cause the injury which the appellant did sustain.

What is the extent of a physician's duty to confide in his patient where the physician suggests or recommends a particular method of treatment? What duty is there upon him to explain the nature and probable consequences of that treatment to the patient? To what extent should he disclose the existence and nature of the risks inherent in the treatment?

We have been cited to no Kansas cases, nor has our research disclosed any, dealing directly with the foregoing questions. A recent article by William A. Kelly published in the *Kansas Law Review* entitled "The Physician, The Patient, And The Consent" (8 *Kan. L. Rev.* 405) reviews many malpractice cases dealing with the consent of the patient, but the article fails to deal with the problem of disclosure involving on one hand the right of the patient to decide for himself and on the other a possible therapeutic ground for withholding information which may create tension by depressing or exciting the patient. . . .

The courts frequently state that the relation between the physician and his patient is a fiduciary one, and therefore the physician has an obligation to make a full and frank disclosure to the patient of all pertinent facts related to his illness. We are here concerned with a case where the physician is charged with treating the patient without consent on the ground the patient was not fully informed of the nature of the treatment or its consequences, and, therefore, any "consent" obtained was ineffective. An effort will be made to review the cases from foreign jurisdictions most nearly in point with the question presently at hand, although none may be said to be directly in point.

In 1958 the Supreme Court of Minnesota, in *Bang* v. *Charles T. Miller Hospital*, 251 Minn. 427, 88 N.W.2d 186, had an assault case before it, and though not alleged as a malpractice action for negligence, a new trial was granted on the ground that a fact issue was presented for the jury to determine whether the patient consented to the performance of the operation. There the patient went to a urologist because of urinary trouble and apparently consented to a cystoscopic examination and a prostate operation. He was not informed that part of the procedure of a transurethral prostatic resection would be the tying off of his sperm ducts. In the opinion the court said:

> While we have no desire to hamper the medical profession in the outstanding progress it has made and continues to make in connection with the study and solution of health and disease problems, it is our opinion that a reasonable rule is that, where a physician or surgeon can ascertain in advance of an operation alternative situations and no immediate emergency exists, a patient should be informed of the alternative possibilities and given a chance to decide before the doctor proceeds with the operation. By that we mean that, in a situation such as the case before us where no immediate emergency exists, a patient should be informed before the operation that if his spermatic cords were severed it would result in his sterilization, but on the other hand if this were not done there would be a possibility of an infection which could result in serious consequences. Under such conditions the patient would at least have the opportunity of deciding whether he wanted to take the chance of a possible infection if the operation was performed in one manner or to become sterile if performed in another. 251 Minn. at pages 434, 435, 88 N.W. 2d at page 190.

A malpractice action was before the Fifth Circuit Court in *Lester* v. *Ætna Casualty & Surety Company,* 240 F.2d 676. The patient was given electro-shock treatments prescribed by a psychiatrist and suffered a bad result. In affirming the jury's finding the court held the patient's wife gave sufficient legal consent, and said:

> The basic, the fundamental, difficulty which confronts plaintiff on this appeal is that he presents his case as though it were one of a person being deprived by another of due proces of law instead of grounding it upon the well settled principles that a physician must, except in real and serious emergencies, acquaint the patient or, when the circumstances require it, some one properly acting for him, of the diagnosis and the treatment proposed, and obtain consent, thereto express or implied, and, consent obtained must proceed in accordance with proper reasonable medical standards *and in the exercise of due care.* . . . 240 F.2d at page 679. (Emphasis added.)

The appellees rely upon the Canadian case of *Kenny* v. *Lockwood* [1932], I D.L.R. 507, where a patient alleged the defendants falsely and recklessly, without caring whether it was true or false, and without reasonable ground for believing it to be true, represented the operation to be "simple," and that her hand "would be all right in three weeks." No evidence was presented to suggest fraud or recklessness and the plaintiff's argument proceeded mainly upon the duty which

it was said the defendants owed to the plaintiff, due to the peculiar relation set up between a surgeon and his patient. The Ontario trial judge concluded that it was the duty of the defendant doctors to "enlighten the patient's mind in a plain and reasonable way as to what her ailment was, as to what were the risks of operating promptly, what were the risks of delaying the operation, and what the risks of not operating at all. Having discharged that duty, it was their further duty to secure from the patient a decision or consent as to what course is to be followed, and if that decision or consent is not had and the surgeons operate and the operation turns out badly the surgeons are liable. Such a relationship is established between a person of special skill and knowledge and a person of no skill or knowledge upon the facts required for the making of a decision that, unless the person with the special skill and knowledge discharges the duty which he owes of placing the patient in a position to make a decision, that person, when he is employed and paid because of his special skill and knowledge, has failed to perform his duty, and that breach of duty makes him liable in damages for untoward results." (*Kenny* v. *Lockwood Clinic Ltd.* [1931], 4 D.L.R. 906, 907.)

The trial court found for the plaintiff but on appeal the judgment was reversed, the appellate court saying there was some testimony that the doctors had explained all details to the plaintiff, although the extracts contained in the opinion indicate that the doctor admitted to having said that the operation was not a very serious one and that he had not clearly presented the alternatives to the plaintiff. In the court's opinion it was said:

> [T]he duty cast upon the surgeon was to deal honestly with the patient as to the necessity, character and importance of the operation and its probable consequences and whether success might reasonably be expected to ameliorate or remove the trouble, but that such duty does not extend to warning the patient of the dangers incident to, or possible in, any operation, nor to details calculated to frighten or distress the patient. (p. 525.)

The court concluded upon the evidence presented:

> That the defendant Stoddart reasonably fulfilled the duty laid upon him arising out of the relationship of surgeon and patient, not being guilty of "negligence in word" or "economy of truth" nor of misleading the plaintiff, and so is not liable for breach of the duty. . . . (p. 526.)

In the opinion it was said the duty of a surgeon is to be honest in fact and to express his honest belief, and if he does so he ought not to be judged as if he had warranted a perfect cure nor to be found derelict in his duty on any meticulous criticism of his language.

The conclusion to be drawn from the foregoing cases is that where the physician or surgeon has affirmatively misrepresented the nature of the operation or has failed to point out the probable consequences of the course of treatment, he may be subjected to a claim of unauthorized treatment. But this does not mean that a doctor is under an obligation to describe in detail all of the possible consequences of treatment. It might be argued, as indicated by the authors of the various law review articles heretofore cited, that to make a complete disclosure of all facts, diagnoses and alternatives or possibilities which may occur to the doctor could so alarm the patient that it would, in fact, constitute bad medical practice. There is probably a privilege, on therapeutic grounds, to withhold the specific diagnosis where the disclosure of cancer or some other dread disease would seriously jeopardize the recovery of an unstable, temperamental or severely depressed patient. But in the ordinary case there would appear to be no such warrant for suppressing facts and the physician should make a substantial disclosure to the patient prior to the treatment or risk liability in tort.

Anglo-American law starts with the premise of thoroughgoing self-determination. It follows that each man is considered to be master of his own body, and he may, if he be of sound mind, expressly prohibit the performance of life-saving surgery, or other medical treatment. A doctor might well believe that an operation or form of treatment is desirable or necessary but the law does not permit him to substitute his own judgment for that of the patient by any form of artifice or deception.

The mean between the two extremes of absolute silence on the part of the physician relative to the treatment of a patient and exhaustive discussion by the physician explaining in detail all possible risks and dangers was well stated by the California District Court of Appeal in *Salgo* v. *Leland Stanford, Etc. Bd. Trustees,* 1957, 154 Cal. App. 2d 560, 317 P.2d 170. There the court had before it a malpractice action wherein the defendants were charged with *negligence.* The patient, his wife and son testified that the patient was not informed anything in the nature of an aortography was to be performed. Two of the

doctors contradicted this, although admitting that the details of the procedure involving injection of a radio-opaque substance into the aorta and the possible dangers therefrom were not explained. As a result of the aortography the patient was paralyzed from the waist down. The trial court gave a rather broad instruction on the duty of the physician to disclose to the patient "all the facts which mutually affect his rights and interests and of the surgical risk, hazard and danger, if any." 154 Cal. App. 2d at page 578, 317 P.2d at page 181. On appeal, the instruction was held to be overly broad, the court stating:

> . . . A physician violates his duty to his patient and subjects himself to liability if he withholds any facts which are necessary to form the basis of an intelligent consent by the patient to the proposed treatment. Likewise the physician may not minimize the known dangers of a procedure or operation in order to induce his patient's consent. At the same time, the physician must place the welfare of his patient above all else and this very fact places him in a position in which he sometimes must choose between two alternative courses of action. One is to explain to the patient every risk attendant upon any surgical procedure or operation, no matter how remote; this may well result in alarming a patient who is already unduly apprehensive and who may as a result refuse to undertake surgery in which there is in fact minimal risk; it may also result in actually increasing the risks by reason of the physiological results of the apprehension itself. The other is to recognize that each patient presents a separate problem, that the patient's mental and emotional condition is important and in certain cases may be crucial, and that in discussing the element of risk a certain amount of discretion must be employed consistent with the full disclosure of facts necessary to an informed consent. . . .

The instruction given should be modified to inform the jury that the physician has such discretion consistent, of course, with the full disclosure of facts necessary to an informed consent. 154 Cal.App.2d at page 578, 317 P.2d at page 181.

The appellees rely upon *Hunt* v. *Bradshaw,* 1955, 242 N.C. 517, 88 S.E.2d 762, a North Carolina case. This was a malpractice action against a physician wherein the patient sought damages alleged to have resulted from the negligent failure of the defendant (1) to use reasonable care and diligence in the application of his knowledge and skill as a physician and surgeon, and (2) to exercise his best judgment in attempting to remove a small piece of steel from plaintiff's body. On these allegations of negligence the plaintiff contended, among other things, that the defendant advised the plaintiff the operation was simple, whereas it was serious and involved undisclosed risks. The plaintiff's evidence was sufficient to justify a finding the operation was of a very serious nature. The court after reviewing the evidence said:

 . . . Upon Dr. Bradshaw's advice the operation was decided upon. It is understandable the surgeon wanted to reassure the patient so that he would not go to the operating room unduly apprehensive. Failure to explain the risks involved, therefore, may be considered a mistake on the part of the surgeon, *but under the facts* cannot be deemed such want of ordinary care as to import liability.

Proof of what is in accord with approved surgical procedure and what constitutes the standard of care required of the surgeon in performing an operation, like the advisability of the operation itself, are matters not within the knowledge of lay witnesses but must be established by the testimony of qualified experts. . . .

Plaintiff's expert testimony is sufficient to justify the finding the injury and damage to plaintiff's hand and arm resulted from the operation. But, as in cases of ordinary negligence, the fact that injury results is not proof of the act which caused it was a negligent act. The doctrine *res ipsa loquitur* does not apply in cases of this character. . . .

Of course, it seems hard to the patient in apparent good health that he should be advised to undergo an operation, and upon regaining consciousness finds that he has lost the use of an arm for the remainder of his life. Infallibility in human beings is not attainable. The law recognizes, and we think properly so, that the surgeon's hand, with its skill and training, is, after all, a human hand, guided by a human brain in a procedure in which the margin between safety and danger sometimes measures little more than the thickness of a sheet of paper.

The plaintiff's case fails because of lack of expert testimony that the defendant failed, either to exercise due care in the operation, or to use his best judgment in advising it. . . . 242 N.C. at pages 523, 524, 88 S.E. 2d at page 766.

*   *   *

In our opinion the proper rule of law to determine whether a patient has given an intelligent consent to a proposed form of treatment by a physician was stated and applied in *Salgo* v. *Leland Stanford, Etc. Bd. Trustees,* supra. This rule in effect compels disclosure by the physician in order to assure that an informed consent of the patient is obtained. The duty of the physician to disclose, however, is limited to those disclosures which a reasonable medical practitioner would make under the same or similar circumstances. How the physician may best discharge his obligation to the patient in this difficult situation involves primarily a question of medical judgment. So long as the disclosure is sufficient to assure an informed consent, the physician's choice of plausible courses should not be called into question if it appears, all circumstances considered, that the physician was motivated only by the patient's best therapeutic interests and he proceeded as competent medical men would have done in a similar situation.

Turning now to the facts in the instant case, the appellant knew she had a cancerous tumor in her left breast which was removed by a radical mastectomy. Pathological examination of the tissue removed did not disclose any spread of the cancer cells into the lymphatics beyond the cancerous tumor itself. As a precautionay measure the appellant's ovaries and fallopian tubes were removed, which likewise upon pathological examination indicated no spread of the cancer to these organs. At the time the appellant went to Dr. Kline as a patient there was no immediate emergency concerning the administration of cobalt irradiation treatment such as would excuse the physician from making a reasonable disclosure to the patient. We think upon all the facts and circumstances here presented Dr. Kline was obligated to make a reasonable disclosure to the appellant of the nature and probable consequences of the suggested or recommended cobalt irradiation treatment, and he was also obligated to make a reasonable disclosure of the dangers within his knowledge which were incident to, or possible in, the treatment he proposed to administer.

Upon the record here presented Dr. Kline made no disclosures to the appellant whatever. He was silent. This is not to say that the facts compel a verdict for the appellant. Under the rule heretofore stated, where the patient fully appreciates the danger involved, the failure of a physician in his duty to make a reasonable disclosure to the patient would have no causal relation to the injury. In such event the consent of the patient to the proposed treatment is an informed consent. The burden of proof rests throughout the trial of the case upon the patient who seeks to recover in a malpractice action for her injury.

In considering the obligation of a physician to disclose and explain to the patient in language as simple as necessary the nature of the ailment, the nature of the proposed treatment, the probability of success or of alternatives, and perhaps the risks of unfortunate results and unforeseen conditions within the body, we do not think the administration of such an obligation, by imposing liability for malpractice if the treatment were administered without such explanation where explanation could reasonably be made, presents any insurmountable obstacles.

The appellant's requested instruction on the duty of a physician to make a disclosure to his patients was too broad. But this did not relieve the trial court of its obligation to instruct on such issue under the circumstances here presented, since the issue was raised by the pleadings. On retrial the instruction should be modified to inform the jury that a physician has such discretion, as heretofore indicated, consistent with the full dislcosure of facts necessary to assure an informed consent by the patient.

On retrial of this case the first issue for the jury to determine should be whether the administration of cobalt irradiation treatment was given with the informed consent of the patient, and if it was not the physician who failed in his legal obligation is guilty of malpractice no matter now skillfully the treatment may have been administered, and the jury should determine the damages arising from the cobalt irradiation treatment. If the jury should find an informed consent was given by the patient for such treatment, the jury should next determine whether proper skill was used in administering the treatment.

* * *

The judgment of the lower court is reversed with directions to grant a new trial.

b.

Natanson v. Kline
187 Kan. 186, 354 P.2d 670 (1960)

SCHROEDER, JUSTICE.

Within the time allotted after the decision of the court herein was announced the appellees filed motions for rehearing. Thereafter, pursuant to request, leave was granted the Kansas Medical Society on May 12, 1960, to file its brief amicus curiae in support of the appellees' motions for rehearing. Finding nothing, upon consideration of the motions for rehearing and the brief of amicus curiae in support thereof, which warrants a reconsideration of the case, the motions for rehearing are denied.

Recognizing, however, that this is a case of first impression in Kansas and one establishing judicial precedent of the highest importance to the medical profession, an attempt will be

made to clarify [the] portion of the opinion concerning which counsel are apprehensive.

Perhaps in preoccupation over the *legal* obligation of a physician to his patient, the court has not adequately emphasized procedural aspects of the case, or reiterated fundamental doctrine in the law of negligence sufficiently to completely avoid efforts to misconstrue the opinion.

It is charged that the court has confused a malpractice suit, where negligence is an essential element, with an assault and battery case, where negligence is not an essential element, thereby giving rise to a hybrid action which is neither one of negligence nor one of assault and battery, but may be a combination of the two.

It is argued the only way the court's opinion can be justified is to say that the duty of a physician to disclose to his patient the risks and hazards of a proposed form of treatment is an absolute one, and the matter is not to be judged by such disclosures as a reasonable medical practitioner would make under the same or similar circumstances.

In support of the argument, that the court has imposed an absolute duty upon the physician, the following paragraph is isolated from context:

On retrial of this case the first issue for the jury to determine should be whether the administration of cobalt irradiation treatment was given with the informed consent of the patient, and if it was not the physician who failed in his legal obligation is guilty of malpractice no matter how skillfully the treatment may have been administered, and the jury should determine the damages arising from the cobalt irradiation treatment. If the jury should find an informed consent was given by the patient for such treatment, the jury should next determine whether proper skill was used in administering the treatment. *Natanson* v. *Kline,* 186 Kan. 393, 411, 350 P.2d 1093, 1107.

A casual reading of this paragraph in context would indicate that reference is there being made to the *order* in which the jury is to consider the issues presented on retrial of the case, and not to an enumeration of the various elements which must be established by the evidence to prove each of the issues stated.

The gravamen of the plaintiff's complaint was malpractice or the failure of the defendants to properly perform the duties which devolved upon them—a failure which resulted in the alleged injuries to the plaintiff. Thus it was incumbent upon the plaintiff to prove and establish (1) that the defendants failed to perform their duty; and (2) that the plaintiff's injuries were the direct and proximate result of such failure.

The petition alleged that the injuries were "a direct and proximate result of the defendants' negligence and carelessness" and then set forth eight specific grounds of negligence, including:

(g) He [Dr. Kline] failed to warn plaintiff that the course of treatment which he undertook to administer involved great risk of bodily injury or death.

The answers of both defendants denied generally the allegations of asserted negligence, and in addition thereto, affirmatively pleaded that the plaintiff "assumed the risk and hazard of the treatment." Thus, at the trial the defendants were fully aware that *the informed consent of the patient to the hazards of the treatment was an issue of fact in the case.* This is true because as a defense assumption of risk is applicable only where the plaintiff is equally competent with the defendant to judge concerning the risks and hazards. See, *Taylor* v. *Hostetler,* 186 Kan. 788, 352 P.2d 1042, and cases cited therein. These affirmative allegations of the defendants presupposed an informed consent by the patient with full knowledge of the risks and hazards of the treatment.

The court held after reviewing the record presented on this appeal that a physician violates his duty to his patient and *subjects himself to liability for malpractice,* where no immediate emergency exists *and upon facts and circumstances particularly set forth in the opinion,* if he makes *no disclosure* of significant facts within his knowledge which are necessary to form the basis of an intelligent consent by the patient to the proposed form of treatment.

In other words, on the facts and circumstances presented by the record the appellant was entitled to some explanation concerning the risks and hazards inherent in the administration of cobalt irradiation treatment which Dr. Kline proposed to administer to her. For this treatment she was Dr. Kline's patient and not the patient of Dr. Crumpacker by whom she was referred to Dr. Kline.

The appellant was entitled to a reasonable disclosure by Dr. Kline so that she could intelligently decide whether to take the cobalt irradiation treatment and assume the risks inherent therein, or in the alternative to decline this form of precautionary treatment and take a chance that the cancerous condition in her left breast had not spread beyond the lesion itself which had been removed by surgery. There was no emergency calling for immediate attention. The appellant had recovered from the surgery. In addition to the evidence related in the opinion her husband testified:

Q: Now directing your attention to approximately the 5th or 6th day of June, 1955, I would like to have you describe for us the general apparent condition of the health of Mrs. Natanson. A: Mrs. Natanson at that particular time was very, very well. She had gone through the two operations and had made a very, very fine recovery. She was able to use her arm because of the therapy; she had almost the complete use of the left arm again. The breast had healed fully. There were actually no scars—just the one large scar but there was a thickness there. We were living a very normal life after the big scare we had.

Q: Now, directing your attention to the first week of June, 1955, I will ask you whether or not Mrs. Natanson ever recovered to the point where she was able to do her own housework? A: Yes, she had.

But contrary to the legal obligation imposed upon a physician to make a reasonable disclosure to his patient of the inherent risks and hazards of a proposed form of treatment, Dr. Kline gave the appellant no explanation whatever. He made no disclosures. He was silent. On this state of the record Dr. Kline failed in his legal duty to make a reasonable disclosure to the appellant who was his patient *as a matter of law.*

Conceivably, in a given case as indicated in the opinion, no disclosures to a patient may be justified where such practice, under given facts and circumstances, is established by expert testimony to be in accordance with that of a reasonable medical practitioner under the same or similar circumstances. But on the state of the record here presented the appellant was not required to produce expert medical testimony to show that the failure of Dr. Kline to give any explanation or make any disclosures was contrary to accepted medical practice. To hold otherwise would be a failure of the court to perform its solemn duty.

Whether or not a physician has advised his patient of the inherent risks and hazards in a proposed form of treatment is a *question of fact* concerning which lay witnesses are competent to testify, and the establishment of such fact is not dependent upon expert medical testimony. It is only when the facts concerning the actual disclosures made to the patient are ascertained, or ascertainable by the trier of the facts, that the expert testimony of medical witnesses is required to establish whether such disclosures are in accordance with those which a reasonable medical practitioner would make under the same or similar circumstances.

The question then remains whether such failure on the part of Dr. Kline to make a reasonable disclosure to the appellant was a proximate cause of her injury. As indicated in the opinion the mere fact that Dr. Kline was silent does not compel a verdict for the appellant. It was said:

. . . Under the rule heretofore stated, where the patient fully appreciates the danger involved, the failure of a physician in his duty to make a reasonable disclosure to the patient would have no causal relation to the injury. In such event the consent of the patient to the proposed treatment is an informed consent. The burden of proof rests throughout the trial of the case upon the patient who seeks to recover in a malpractice action for her injury. *Natanson* v. *Kline,* supra, 186 Kan. at page 410, 350 P.2d at page 1106.

Negligence is an essential element of malpractice, and the foregoing statement recognizes that a causal relation must be established by the patient, between the negligent act of the physician and the injury of the patient, to sustain the burden of proof where damages are sought in a malpractice action for injury. Prior to a discussion of the manner in which the court instructed the jury it was said in the opinion:

. . . At best it may be said, upon all the facts and circumstances presented by the record, there was evidence from which a jury could find that the proximate cause of the appellant's injury was the negligence of the defendants. On the other hand a jury, *properly instructed,* would be justified in finding for the appellees. *Natanson* v. *Kline,* supra, 186 Kan. at page 398, 350 P.2d at page 1098.

After making the foregoing statement in the opinion, discussion was directed to the instructions of the court without further specific attention to the issue of proximate cause. If, of course, the appellant would have taken the cobalt irradiation treatments even though Dr. Kline had warned her that the treatments he undertook to administer involved great risk of bodily injury or death, it could not be said that the failure of Dr. Kline to so inform the appellant was the proximate cause of her injury. While the appellant did not directly testify that she would have refused to take the proposed cobalt irradiation treatments had she been properly informed, we think the evidence presented by the record *taken as a whole* is sufficient and would authorize a jury to infer that, had she been properly informed, the appellant would not have taken the cobalt irradiation treatments.

Two days after the decision of this court was announced, the Supreme Court of Missouri handed down its opinion in *Mitchell* v. *Robinson,* 334 S.W.2d 11, 12, on April 11, 1960, wherein the Missouri court reached the same conclusion as this court on the duty of a physician to inform his patient of the hazards of treatment. There the patient had a rather severe emotional illness but was not mentally incompetent. The treatment prescribed was "combined electro-shock and insulin subcoma therapy." A sharp conflict developed in the testimony as to whether the patient was informed of the risks of the treatment. Serious hazards incident to shock treatment were admitted, to wit: fractured bones, serious paralysis of limbs, irreversible coma and even death, and further that there were no completely reliable or successful precautions. The patient as a result of treatment went into convulsions which caused the fracture of several vertebrae and sued the physicians in a malpractice action on the ground that he was not informed of the risks inherent in the treatment. The "essentially meritorious problem" before the court was whether upon the record there was any evidence to support the jury's finding of negligence. In the opinion the court said:

In the particular circumstances of this record, considering the nature of Mitchell's illness and this rather new and radical procedure with its rather high incidence of serious and permanent injuries not connected with the illness, the doctors owed their patient in possession of his faculties the duty to inform him generally of the possible serious collateral hazards; and in the detailed circumstances there was a submissible fact issue of whether the doctors were negligent in failing to inform him of the dangers of shock therapy. [At page 19.]

As always, an effort is made by the court to present an opinion in logical sequence, so that consideration of subsequent issues is dependent upon the disposition of issues previously determined, and if opinions are analyzed in this manner misinterpretations will be minimized.

NOTES

NOTE 1.

WILLIAMS V. MENEHAN
191 KAN. 6, 8, 379 P.2D 292, 294 (1963)

WERTZ, JUSTICE.

*   *   *

. . . We said in the Natanson case [that] it is the duty of a doctor to make a reasonable disclosure to his patient. . . . But this does not mean that a doctor is under an obligation to describe in detail all of the possible consequences of treatment. To make a complete disclosure of all facts, diagnoses and alternatives or possibilities which might occur to the doctor could so alarm the patient that it would, in fact, constitute bad medical practice.

. . . So long as the disclosure is sufficient to assure an informed consent, the physician's choice of plausible courses should not be called into question if it appears, all circumstances considered, that the physician was motivated only by the patient's best therapeutic interests and he proceeded as competent medical men would have done in a similar situation.

* * *

NOTE 2.

AIKEN V. CLARY
396 S.W. 2D 668 (Mo. 1965)

FINCH, JUDGE.

* * *

We . . . have concluded that the question of what disclosure of risks incident to proposed treatment should be made in a particular situation involves medical judgment and that expert testimony thereon should be required in malpractice cases involving that issue.

* * *

The question is not what, regarding the risks involved, the juror would relate to the patient under the same or similar circumstances, or even what a reasonable *man* would relate, but what a reasonable *medical practitioner* would do. Such practitioner would consider the state of the patient's health, the condition of his heart and nervous system, his mental state, and would take into account, among other things, whether the risks involved were mere remote possibilities or something which occurred with some sort of frequency or regularity. This determination involves medical judgment as to whether disclosure of possible risks may have such an adverse effect on the patient as to jeopardize success of the proposed therapy, no matter how expertly performed.

NOTE 3.

HUNTER V. BROWN
4 WASH. APP. 899, 484 P.2D 1162 (1971)

* * *

JAMES, JUDGE:

Plaintiff, Mrs. Chung Hunter, claims damages suffered as a result of an allegedly unsuc-

cessful dermabrasion procedure performed by defendant, Walter S. Brown. Dr. Brown is a medical doctor whose specialty is plastic and reconstructive surgery. At the close of Mrs. Hunter's case, the trial judge sustained Dr. Brown's challenge to the sufficiency of the evidence. Mrs. Hunter appeals from the judgment of dismissal which followed. . . .

* * *

[W]e find that there was substantial evidence which, if believed, would tend to establish that during pregnancy Mrs. Hunter became concerned about dark spots of increased pigmentation which appeared upon her face. She consulted Dr. Brown who diagnosed her condition as chloasma. . . .

Dr. Brown recommended and thereafter performed a surgical procedure known as "dermabrasion." Dermabrasion is a mechanical procedure whereby the epidermis is removed by sandpapering. Although performed under local anesthetic, the recovery period was for Mrs. Hunter a painful, prolonged and embarrassing experience. Rather than improving Mrs. Hunter's appearance, the dermabrasion resulted in increased pigmentation in her face.

* * *

The evidence upon which Mrs. Hunter relies would permit findings that: Dr. Brown is a recognized expert in the treatment of chloasma by the dermabrasion process; that he knew (1) that the probability of a good result was only 50 per cent; (2) that there was a possibility of resulting hyperpigmentation—a worsening of the chloasma condition; (3) that the risk of hyperpigmentation is greater when the patient is of Oriental origin; and (4) that he considered Mrs. Hunter to be a "borderline case." Mrs. Hunter is of Korean extraction.

The evidence would further support a finding that Dr. Brown did not inform Mrs. Hunter that there was any possibility that the operation would not be successful, and that Mrs. Hunter was justified in assuming that there was no question but what the dark spots on her face would disappear.

Dr. Brown was called as an adverse witness. He testified that it was not good standard medical practice within the specialty of plastic and reconstructive surgery to inform a patient of the risk involved in a dermabrasion operation. He said:

Now, if we go into the risks involved, I would be talking the rest of the day about the risks. . . .

* * *

[R]isks are minimal, and they are never mentioned to a patient. . . .

*   *   *

. . . A patient would walk out of everybody's office if you would say there is a danger of anything. This is never done.

*   *   *

It is not good practice to frighten a patient by telling them a dozen different things that might happen as a result of dermabrasion.

Mrs. Hunter produced no evidence to contradict Dr. Brown's testimony.

Dr. Brown was not interrogated as to whether there was a recognized medical standard as to disclosure to a patient of the percentage probability of success. Mrs. Hunter presented no other testimony concerning medical standards.

*   *   *

The trial judge felt that he was compelled to dismiss Mrs. Hunter's case because she produced no evidence of a medical standard of disclosure.

*   *   *

The physician-patient relationship is of a fiduciary character. The inherent necessity for trust and confidence requires scrupulous good faith on the part of the physician. *Lockett* v. *Goodill,* 71 Wash.2d 654, 430 P.2d 589 (1967). His duty of disclosure extends beyond the realm of *risks.* He must disclose to his patient all material *facts* which reasonably should be known if his patient is to make an informed and intelligent decision. The availability of alternatives to surgery is an example of the kind of information required.

Whether the failure to disclose was willful or attributable to negligence is immaterial. The causal wrong is the violation of the fiduciary duty to disclose.

We cannot agree that the matter of informed consent must be determined on the basis of medical testimony any more than that expert testimony of the standard practice is determinative in any other case involving a fiduciary relationship. We agree with appellant that a physician's duty to disclose is not governed by the standard practice of the physicans' community, but is a duty imposed by law which governs his conduct in the same manner as others in a similar fiduciary relationship. To hold otherwise would permit the medical profession to determine its own responsibilities. . . .

Berkey v. *Anderson,* 1 Cal.App.3d 790, 805, 82 Cal.Rptr. 67, 78 (1969).

Reasons why the physician withheld facts are a matter of defense. Evidence that the patient was not uninformed or that the facts undisclosed were immaterial or that disclosure might be harmful would properly be matters of defense. It is at this juncture that evidence of medical standards of disclosure might become relevant and material.

*   *   *

Dr. Brown testified that the "risks" in a dermabrasion procedure were minimal. And, as he also observed, the contemplated surgery was "an elective thing." There was no emergency. His patient's health was not at stake. Arguably, one of the *facts* which Mrs. Hunter needed for an informed and intelligent decision was the percentage probability that the contemplated surgery would improve her appearance. Whether or not Dr. Brown violated his fiduciary duty in withholding the information is a question of fact to be judged by reasonable man standards.

*   *   *

We hold that if a patient-plaintiff presents substantial evidence that (1) his physician failed to disclose material *facts* reasonably necessary to form the basis of an intelligent consent, and (2) he has been injured as a result of submitting to a surgical procedure, he has made out a prima facie case.

Accordingly, we reverse and remand for a new trial.

NOTE 4.

DOW V. KAISER FOUNDATION
12 CAL. APP.3D 488, 503–508, 90 CAL. RPTR.
747, 756–759 (1970)

COMPTON, ASSOCIATE JUSTICE.

Plaintiff Dorothy Dow sued defendants Dr. Paul Harmon, Permanente Medical Group, a partnership, Southern California Permanente Medical Group, a partnership, and Kaiser Foundation Hospital, a non-profit corporation, seeking damages for injuries allegedly resulting from medical malpractice and the lack of an informed consent to lower back surgery performed by Dr. Harmon.

*   *   *

Plaintiff presented to the jury through her pleadings and evidence [a] theory of liability designed to demonstrate that the operation was performed without her "informed" consent and that therefore she should recover for her injuries.

* * *

It is well established that a doctor has a duty to inform his patient concerning contemplated medical procedure and the inherent risks therein. . . .

* * *

In California, contrary to the conclusion reached in *Kline,* the cause of action which arises from medical treatment based on an uninformed consent sounds in battery and not negligence.

The jury here was instructed that "Failure to obtain consent when and as required renders the physician and surgeon liable in damages for any injury *proximately resulting* from the operation or treatment. . . . The failure to disclose in all instances does not necessarily suggest a *neglect* of duty." (Emphasis added.)

Furthermore, the court instructed the jury that the doctor's duty was to make those "Disclosures *which a competent medical practitioner would make under the same* or similar circumstances. . . ." (Emphasis added.)

* * *

A surgeon's negligence in performing an operation may be the cause of the resultant injuries but it does violence to logic, however, to say that the failure to inform a patient about certain risks is the proximate cause of those subsequent injuries. If the lack of sufficient information vitiates a consent the cause of action is the same as if no consent had ever been given. Thus a doctor who breaches his duty to inform, as we shall define it below, is liable for *all* injuries sustained by the patient whether the result of negligence in the performance of the operation or not.

* * *

Inasmuch as the patient is already well protected where the treatment itself is negligently performed and recovery on the basis of uninformed consent will generally occur where such negligence cannot be proved; we hold that in order for a patient to vitiate his voluntary consent to treatment on the basis that the doctor breached his duty of disclosure, it must be proved that the doctor *wilfully,* and *without good medical reason,* withheld *material* information.

Battery being an intentional tort requires in this situation proof of a higher degree of culpability than ordinary negligence in failing to inform a patient of some aspect of proposed medical treatment.

Further, the plaintiff must establish as part of his burden of proof that the information which was withheld was of such significance that, had it been disclosed, consent would not have been given.

It is our opinion that these standards comport squarely with the fiduciary nature of the doctor-patient relationship.

* * *

In the final analysis the court's instructions did not accurately inform the jury on the law of uninformed consent. This error was prejudicial. Moreover, the evidence was insufficient to support the verdict in light of the requirements enunciated above.

* * *

The judgment is reversed.

B.
To Promote Individual Autonomy

1.

Safeguarding the Concept of Freedom

a.

John S. Mill
On Liberty*

* * *

The object of this Essay is to assert one very simple principle, as entitled to govern absolutely the dealings of society with the individual in the way of compulsion and control, whether the means used be physical force in the form of legal penalties, or the moral coercion of public opinion. That principle is, that the sole end for which mankind are warranted, individually or collectively, in interfering with the liberty of action of any of their number, is self-protection. That the only purpose for which power can be rightfully exercised over any member of a civilised community, against his will, is to prevent harm to others. His own good, either physical or moral, is not a sufficient warrant. He can-

* London: John W. Parker & Son 21–23 (1859).

not rightfully be compelled to do or forbear because it will be better for him to do so, because it will make him happier, because, in the opinions of others, to do so would be wise, or even right. These are good reasons for remonstrating with him, or reasoning with him, or persuading him, or entreating him, but not for compelling him, or visiting him with any evil in case he do otherwise. To justify that, the conduct from which it is desired to deter him must be calculated to produce evil to someone else. The only part of the conduct of anyone, for which he is amenable to society, is that which concerns others. In the part which merely concerns himself, his independence is, of right, absolute. Over himself, over his own body and mind, the individual is sovereign.

It is, perhaps, hardly necessary to say that this doctrine is meant to apply only to human beings in the maturity of their faculties. We are not speaking of children, or of young persons below the age which the law may fix as that of manhood or womanhood. Those, who are still in a state to require being taken care of by others, must be protected against their own actions as well as against external injury. . . .

*   *   *

b.

Patrick Devlin
The Enforcement of Morals*

*   *   *

The core of [Mill's] principle is that a man must be allowed to pursue his own good in his own way. Its opposite has come to be identified as paternalism. But an identifying mark is not a line. To secure the citadel of freedom Mill flung a line beyond which the law must not trespass. The law was not to interfere with a man unless what he did caused harm to others. What Mill included in "harm to others" was chiefly physical harm to other individuals.

Now if a man lives in society it is not simply his own concern whether or not he keeps himself physically, mentally, and morally fit. He owes in these respects a duty to others as well as to himself. Mill accepted the duty as owing to "assignable individuals," such as a man's family or his creditors. He did not see it as a debt due to society at large. The only right he allowed to society as a collective entity, i.e., to the State, and

* London: Oxford University Press 103–105, 121–123, 132–136 (1965). Reprinted by permission.

which it might enforce by law, was the right to exact contributions to common defence and protection. "But with regard to the merely contingent, or, as it may be called, constructive injury which a person causes to society, by conduct which neither violates any specific duty to the public, nor occasions perceptible hurt to any assignable individual except himself, the inconvenience is one which society can afford to bear, for the sake of the greater good of human freedom."

Yet if apart from his assignable duties a man does not observe some standard of health and morality, society as a whole is impoverished for such a man puts less than his share into the common well-being. The enforcement of an obligation of this sort can be distinguished from paternalism. The motive of paternalism is to do good to the individual; the motive of the other is to prevent the harm that would be done to society by the weakness or vice or too many of its members. Mill did not overlook the distinction; he overrode it in the interests of individual freedom. If a man knew his own true interest and pursued it as he ought to, he would make himself as virtuous as he could and by so doing make his contribution to society's well-being. The right to exact such a contribution must be sacrificed on the altar of freedom. . . .

As Mill noted, this conception of liberty was not accepted in his own time which we now look back upon as an age of individualism triumphant. In the hundred years that have passed since then it has over and over again been decisively rejected in economic matters. Its weakness in practice is that it enables one man in a hundred to hold up indefinitely projects which would benefit the other ninety-nine. So we have laws that allow the compulsory acquisition of property. We have also social schemes that an individual is not allowed to contract out of because he cannot be excluded from the benefits of the scheme without wrecking it. Contracting out may be an expression of individuality and proceed from the pure desire for liberty, but we have come to think that it proceeds from selfishness or laziness, indifference to the common good, or a desire to get something for nothing. So we have health laws, thinking it wrong that a man should receive the benefit of modern sanitation in the town in which he lives and keep his own home as a pigsty.

In short, the great majority of our fellow citizens may be as highminded as Mill expected them to be but we have not yet got rid of the troublesome minority who will yield only to compulsion. Perhaps in the course of several centuries, teaching and example will lift the minority to the common level and in the end it might have been better for us all if we had waited for that to happen. But social reformers are not as patient as philosophers and we have not waited.

This does not mean that necessarily we have witnessed the triumph of paternalism. We would still, I think, most of us deeply resent a law that was passed avowedly for our own good and treated us as if we were in need of care and protection. What it means is that the citadel has not been secured from attack in the way in which Mill proposed. His outer line enclosed territory which has had to be yielded, and authority has not decisively, as he hoped, been kept at bay.

*　　*　　*

. . . What Mill demands is that we must tolerate what we know to be evil and what no one asserts to be good. He does not ask that in particular cases we should extend tolerance out of pity: he demands that we should cede it for ever as a right. Because it is evil we may protect youth from corruption by it, but save for that we must allow it to spread unhindered by the law and infect the minds of all those who are not strong enough to resist it. Why do ninety of us have to grant this licence to the other ten or, it would be truer to say, ninety-nine to the other one? Because, the answer is, we are fallible. We are all quite convinced that what we call vice is evil but we may be mistaken. Although no one asserts that it is not evil, yet we may be mistaken. True it is that if the waters of toleration are poured upon the muck, bad men will wallow in the bog: but it may be—how can we tell otherwise?— that it is only under such conditions that seed may flourish which some day some good man may bring to fruit and that otherwise the world would lose and be the poorer for it.

This is the kernel of Mill's freedom. This is why we must not suppress vice. It is not because it is not evil; Mill thought that it was. It is not because legal suppression would be futile; this argument, favoured by some of Mill's followers, is not one that he advanced. Nor because Mill thought, that in the battle between virtue and vice, virtue would be bound to triumph without the aid of the law. In some cogent passages he refuted the argument that in spite of persecution truth would always prevail against error; and if truth can be suppressed, so can error and so can vice. When all this is stripped away, the kernal

of Mill is just this—that he beseeches us to think it possible that we may be mistaken. Because of this possibility, Mill demanded almost absolute freedom for the individual to go his own way, the only function of society being to provide for him an ordered framework within which he might experiment in thought and in action secure from physical harm.

There is here, I humbly believe, a flaw in Mills' thinking which, even assuming that we accept his ideal, renders it unacceptable to the lawmaker as a basis for action. It lies in the failure to distinguish sufficiently between freedom of thought and freedom of action. It may be a good thing for a man to keep an open mind about all his beliefs so that he will never claim for them absolute certainty and never dismiss entirely from his mind the thought that he may be wrong. But where there is a call for action, he must act on what he believes to be true. . . .

*　　*　　*

. . . For better or worse the law-maker must act according to his lights and he cannot therefore accept Mill's doctrine as practicable even if as an ideal he thought it to be desirable.

But I must say for my part that I do not accept it as an ideal. I accept it as an inspiration. What Mill taught about the value of freedom of inquiry and the dangers of intolerance has placed all free men for ever in his debt. His admonitions were addressed to a society that was secure and strong and hidebound. Their repetition today is to a society much less solid. As a tract for the times, what Mill wrote was superb, but as dogma it has lost much of its appeal. For Mill's doctrine is just as dogmatic as any of those he repudiates. It is dogmatic to say that if only we were all allowed to behave just as we liked so long as we did not injure each other, the world would become a better place for all of us. There is no more evidence for this sort of Utopia than there is for the existence of Heaven and there is nothing to show that the one is any more easily attained than the other. We must not be bemused by words. If we are not entitled to call our society "free" unless we pursue freedom to an extremity that would make society intolerable for most of us, then let us stop short of the extreme and be content with some other name. The result may not be freedom unalloyed, but there are alloys which strengthen without corrupting.

*　　*　　*

The second fundamental principle has to do

with the function of consent in the criminal law. Mill's doctrine should make it always a good defence because the law should be concerned only with harming another against his will. But in general, consent is no defence, though there are crimes, such as rape and larceny, in which the absence of consent is an ingredient of the offence and has to be proved by the prosecution accordingly. One example of the ordinary crimes to which consent is no defence is murder in cases of euthanasia, duelling, and suicide pacts. Another is assault; some form of masochism would perhaps today be the most likely case of a willing submission to an assault.

The conclusion which I drew from this . . . was that a breach of the criminal law was regarded as an offence not merely against the person injured but against society as a whole; and that an act done by consent, such as euthanasia, could be prohibited only as the breach of a moral principle which society required to be observed. Professor Hart says roundly that this "is simply not true." The emphasis suggests that I have overlooked the obvious. What, alas, I did not foresee was that some of the crew who sail under Mill's flag of liberty would mutiny and run paternalism up the mast. Professor Hart considers that it is paternalism and not moral principle that is the justification of the law in these matters and he is thereby enabled to accept the second principle. "The rules excluding the victim's consent as a defence to charges of murder or assault may perfectly well be explained as a piece of paternalism, designed to protect individuals against themselves."

"Mill no doubt might have protested," Professor Hart goes on in a meiosis which deserves to be commemorated. This tears the heart out of his doctrine. "His own good either physical or moral is not a sufficient warrant. He cannot rightfully be compelled to do or forbear because it will be better for him to do so, because it will make him happier, because in the opinions of others, to do so would be wise or even right."

Professor Hart suggests that Mill might have objected not quite as much to paternalism as to the enforcement of moral principle. He bases this on Mill's particularization of the three grounds on which compulsion would be wrongful. These, he says, are separate, the first two as I understand it, referring to paternalism, and the third to enforcement of morality. This seems to me a forced reading. Mill states his reasons cumulatively and not alternatively. If a man does what is wise and right, surely in Mill's view it would make him better and happier; he would not have distinguished between them. . . .

*   *   *

. . . When dealing with the exclusion of consent as a defence to murder or assault, Professor Hart uses a phrase which suggests that he might be drawing a distinction between physical and moral paternalism. He refers to "using the law to protect even a consenting victim from *bodily* harm." But I do not think that—at least in this connexion—he can mean the word "bodily" to be distinctive. It would be quite unrealistic to treat the crimes with which Professor Hart is dealing as offences against the body of the consenting party and not against morals. The most common case of a man willingly submitting to assault would, as I have suggested, be a case of masochism. To say that the law should intervene there not because of the vice but to protect the man in his own best interests from getting bodily hurt hardly seems sense. So in euthanasia. It cannot seriously be suggested that, if there were no moral principle involved, the law in a free country would tell a man when he was and when he was not to die, obtaining its mandate from its paternal interest in his body and not in his soul. Or that in euthanasia the crime lies not in the moral decision to seek death but purely in the physical and no doubt painless act that causes it.

If however there is an element of physical paternalism in the law that forbids masochism and euthanasia these crimes seem to me as good examples as any that could be selected to illustrate the difficulty in practice of distinguishing between physical and moral paternalism. Neither in principle nor in practice can a line be drawn between legislation controlling the individual's physical welfare and legislation controlling his moral welfare. . . .

The terms in which Professor Hart justifies the sort of paternalism he advocates lead to the same conclusion. There is, he says, "a general decline in the belief that individuals know their own interests best." There can be no reason to believe that if unable to perceive their own physical good unaided, they can judge of their own moral good. He continues: "Choices may be made or consent given without adequate reflection or appreciation of the consequences; or in pursuit of merely transitory desires; or in various predicaments when the judgment is likely to be clouded; or under inner psychological compulsion; or under pressure by others of a kind too subtle to be susceptible of proof in a law court."

... It is moral weakness rather than physical that leads to predicaments when the judgement is likely to be clouded and is the cause of inner psychological compulsion.

These considerations drive one to the conclusion that a distinction between moral and physical paternalism is not what Professor Hart has in mind. But the alternative hypothesis seems even more unacceptable. If it is difficult to draw a line between moral and physical paternalism, it is impossible to draw one of any significance between moral paternalism and the enforcement of the moral law. A moral law, that is, a public morality, is a necessity for paternalism, otherwise it would be impossible to arrive at a common judgement about what would be for a man's moral good. If then society compels a man to act for his own moral good, society is enforcing the moral law; and it is a distinction without a difference to say that society is acting for a man's own good and not for the enforcement of the law. . . .

*   *   *

c.

Isaiah Berlin
Two Concepts of Liberty (1958)*

To coerce a man is to deprive him of freedom—freedom from what? Almost every moralist in human history has praised freedom. Like happiness and goodness, like nature and reality, the meaning of this term is so porous that there is little interpretation that it seems able to resist. . . . I propose to examine no more than two of these senses—but those central ones, with a great deal of human history behind them and, I dare say, still to come. The first of these political senses of freedom or liberty (I shall use both words to mean the same), which I shall call the "negative" sense, is involved in the answer to the question "What is the area within which the subject—a person or group of persons—is or should be left to do or be what he wants to do or be, without interference by other persons?" The second, which I shall call the positive sense, is involved in the answer to the question "What, or who, is the source of control or interference, that can determine someone to do, or be, one thing rather than another?" The two questions are clearly different, even though the answers to them may overlap.

---

* *Four Essays on Liberty*. Oxford: Clarendon Press 118–138 (1969). Reprinted by permission of the Clarendon Press, Oxford.

The notion of "negative" freedom

. . . If I am prevented by other persons from doing what I want I am to that degree unfree; and if the area within which I can do what I want is contracted by other men beyond a certain minimum, I can be described as being coerced, or, it may be, enslaved. Coercion is not, however, a term that covers every form of inability. If I say that I am unable to jump more than 10 feet in the air, or cannot read because I am blind, or cannot understand the darker pages of Hegel, it would be eccentric to say that I am to that degree enslaved or coerced. Coercion implies the deliberate interference of other human beings within the area in which I wish to act. You lack political liberty or freedom only if you are prevented from attaining your goal by human beings.

*   *   *

. . . If my poverty were a kind of disease, which prevented me from buying bread or paying for the journey round the world, or getting my case heard, as lameness prevents me from running, this inability would not naturally be described as a lack of freedom at all, least of all political freedom. It is only because I believe that my inability to get what I want is due to the fact that other human beings have made arrangements whereby I am, whereas others are not, prevented from having enough money with which to pay for it, that I think myself a victim of coercion or slavery. In other words, this use of the term depends on a particular social and economic theory about the causes of my poverty or weakness. If my lack of means is due to my lack of mental or physical capacity, then I begin to speak of being deprived of freedom (and not simply of poverty) only if I accept the theory. If, in addition, I believe that I am being kept in want by a definite arrangement which I consider unjust or unfair, I speak of economic slavery or oppression. . . .

*   *   *

[T]here ought to exist a certain minimum area of personal freedom which must on no account be violated, for, if it is overstepped, the individual will find himself in an area too narrow for even that minimum development of his natural faculties which alone makes it possible to pursue, and even to conceive, the various ends which men hold good or right or sacred. It follows that a frontier must be drawn between the area of private life and that of public authority.

Where it is to be drawn is a matter of argument, indeed of haggling. Men are largely interdependent, and no man's activity is so completely private as never to obstruct the lives of others in any way. "Freedom for the pike is death for the minnows"; the liberty of some must depend on the restraint of others. Still, a practical compromise has to be found.

*   *   *

. . . The answer to the question "Who governs me?" is logically distinct from the question "How far does government interfere with me?" It is in this difference that the great contrast between the two concepts of negative and positive liberty, in the end, consists.[1] For the "positive" sense of liberty comes to light if we try to answer the question, not "What am I free to do or be?" but "By whom am I ruled?" or "Who is to say what I am, and what I am not, to be or do?" The connexion between democracy and individual liberty is a good deal more tenuous than it seemed to many advocates of both. The desire to be governed by myself, or at any rate to participate in the process by which my life is to be controlled, may be as deep a wish as that of a free area for action, and perhaps historically older.

---

[1] "Negative liberty" is something the extent of which, in a given case, it is difficult to estimate. It might, *prima facie,* seem to depend simply on the power to choose between at any rate two alternatives. Nevertheless, not all choices are equally free, or free at all. If in a totalitarian state I betray my friend under threat of torture, perhaps even if I act from fear of losing my job, I can reasonably say that I did not act freely. Nevertheless, I did, of course, make a choice, and could, at any rate in theory, have chosen to be killed or tortured or imprisoned. The mere existence of alternatives is not, therefore, enough to make my action free (although it may be voluntary) in the normal sense of the word. The extent of my freedom seems to depend on (*a*) how many possibilities are open to me (although the method of counting these can never be more than impressionistic. Possibilities of action are not discrete entities like apples, which can be exhaustively enumerated); (*b*) how easy or difficult each of these possibilities is to actualize; (*c*) how important in my plan of life, given my character and circumstances, these possibilities are when compared with each other; (*d*) how far they are closed and opened by deliberate human acts; (*e*) what value not merely the agent, but the general sentiment of the society in which he lives, puts on the various possibilities. All these magnitudes must be "integrated," and a conclusion, necessarily never precise, or indisputable, drawn from this process. . . .

But it is not a desire for the same thing. So different is it, indeed, as to have led in the end to the great clash of ideologies that dominates our world. For it is this—the "positive" conception of liberty: not freedom from, but freedom to—which the adherents of the "negative" notion represent as being, at times, no better than a specious disguise for brutal tyranny.

The notion of "positive" freedom

The "positive" sense of the word "liberty" derives from the wish on the part of the individual to be his own master. I wish my life and decisions to depend on myself, not on external forces of whatever kind. I wish to be the instrument of my own, not of other men's, acts of will. I wish to be a subject, not an object; to be moved by reasons, by conscious purposes which are my own, not by causes which affect me, as it were, from. outside. I wish to be somebody, not nobody; a doer—deciding, not being decided for, self-directed and not acted upon by external nature or by other men as if I were a thing, or an animal, or a slave incapable of playing a human role, that is, of conceiving goals and policies of my own and realizing them. This is at least part of what I mean when I say that I am rational, and that it is my reason that distinguishes me as a human being from the rest of the world. I wish, above all, to be conscious of myself as a thinking, willing, active being, bearing responsibility for his choices and able to explain them by reference to his own ideas and purposes. I feel free to the degree that I believe this to be true, and enslaved to the degree that I am made to realize that it is not.

The freedom which consists in being one's own master, and the freedom which consists in not being prevented from choosing as I do by other men, may, on the face of it, seem concepts at no great logical distance from each other—no more than negative and positive ways of saying the same thing. Yet the "positive" and "negative" notions of freedom developed in divergent directions until, in the end, they came into direct conflict with each other.

One way of making this clear is in terms of the independent momentum which the metaphor of self-mastery acquired. "I am my own master"; "I am slave to no man"; but may I not . . . be a slave to nature? Or to my own "unbridled" passions? Are these not so many species of the identical genus "slave"—some political or legal, others more or spiritual? Have not men had the experience of liberating themselves from spiritual slavery, or slavery to nature, and do they not in the course of it become aware, on the one hand, of a self which dominates, and, on the other, of something in them which is brought to heel? This dominant self is then variously identified with reason, with my "higher nature," with the self which calculates and aims at what will satisfy it in the long run, with my "real," or "ideal," or "autonomous" self, or with my self "at its best"; which is then contrasted with irrational impulse, uncontrolled desires, my "lower" nature, the pursuit of immediate pleasures, my "empirical" or "heteronomous" self, swept by every gust of desire and passion, needing to be rigidly disciplined if it is ever to rise to the full height of its "real" nature. Presently the two selves may be represented as divided by an even larger gap: the real self may be conceived as something wider than the individual (as the term is normally understood), as a social "whole" of which the individual is an element or aspect: a tribe, a race, a church, a state, the great society of the living and the dead and the yet unborn. This entity is then identified as being the "true" self which, by imposing its collective, or "organic," single will upon its recalcitrant "members," achieves its own, and, therefore, their, "higher" freedom. The perils of using organic metaphors to justify the coercion of some men by others in order to raise them to a "higher" level of freedom have often been pointed out. But what gives such plausibility as it has to this kind of language is that we recognize that it is possible, and at times justifiable, to coerce men in the name of some goal (let us say, justice or public health) which they would, if they were more enlightened, themselves pursue, but do not, because they are blind or ignorant or corrupt. This renders it easy for me to conceive of myself as coercing others for their own sake, in their, not my, interest. I am then claiming that I know what they truly need better than they know it themselves. What, at most, this entails is that they would not resist me if they were rational, and as wise as I, and understood their interests as I do. But I may go on to claim a good deal more than this. I may declare that they are actually aiming at what in their benighted state they consciously resist, because there exists within them an occult entity—their latent rational will, or their "true" purpose—and that this entity, although it is belied by all that they overtly feel and do and say, is their "real" self, of which the poor empirical self in space and time may know nothing or little; and that this inner spirit is the only self that deserves

to have its wishes taken into account. Once I take this view, I am in a position to ignore the actual wishes of men or societies, to bully, oppress, torture them in the name, and on behalf, of their "real" selves, in the secure knowledge that whatever is the true goal of man (happiness, fulfilment of duty, wisdom, a just society, self-fulfilment) must be identical with his freedom—the free choice of his "true," albeit submerged and inarticulate, self.

This paradox has been often exposed. It is one thing to say that I know what is good for X, while he himself does not; and even to ignore his wishes for its—and his—sake; and a very different one to say that he has *eo ipso* chosen it, not indeed consciously, not as he seems in everyday life, but in his role as a rational self which his empirical self may not know—the "real" self which discerns the good, and cannot help choosing it once it is revealed. This monstrous impersonation, which consists in equating what X would choose if he were something he is not, or at least not yet, with what X actually seeks and chooses, is at the heart of all political theories of self-realization. It is one thing to say that I may be coerced for my own good which I am too blind to see; and another that if it is for my good, I am not being coerced, for I have willed it, whether I know this or not, and am free even while my poor earthly body and foolish mind bitterly reject it, and struggle against those who seek to impose it, with the greatest desperation.

This magical transformation, or sleight of hand . . . can no doubt be perpetrated just as easily with the "negative" concept of freedom, where the self that should not be interfered with is no longer the individual with his actual wishes and needs as they are normally conceived, but the "real" man within, identified with the pursuit of some ideal purpose not dreamed of by his empirical self. And, as in the case of the "positively" free self, this entity may be inflated into some super-personal entity—a state, a class, a nation, or the march of history itself, regarded as a more "real" subject of attributes than the empirical self. But the "positive" conception of freedom as self-mastery, with its suggestion of a man divided against himself, lends itself more easily to this splitting of personality into two: the transcendent, dominant controller, and the empirical bundle of desires and passions to be disciplined and brought to heel. This demonstrates (if demonstration of so obvious a truth is needed) that the conception of freedom directly derives from the view that is taken of what constitutes a self, a person, a man. Enough manipulation with the definitions of man, and freedom can be made to mean whatever the manipulator wishes. Recent history has made it only too clear that the issue is not merely academic.

* * *

For if the essence of men is that they are autonomous beings—authors of values, of ends in themselves, the ultimate authority of which consists precisely in the fact that they are willed freely—then nothing is worse than to treat them as if they were not autonomous, but natural objects, played on by causal influences, creatures at the mercy of external stimuli, whose choices can be manipulated by their rulers, whether by threats of force or offers of rewards. To treat men in this way is to treat them as if they were not self-determined. "Nobody may compel me to be happy in his own way," said Kant. "Paternalism is the greatest despotism imaginable." This is so because it is to treat men as if they were not free, but human material for me, the benevolent reformer, to mould in accordance with my own, not their, freely adopted purpose. This is, of course, precisely the policy that the early utilitarians recommended. Helvetius (and Bentham) believed not in resisting, but in using, men's tendency to be slaves to their passions; they wished to dangle rewards and punishments before men —the acutest possible form of heteronomy—if by this means the "slaves" might be made happier. But to manipulate men, to propel them towards goals which you—the social reformer— see, but they may not, is to deny their human essence, to treat them as objects without wills of their own, and therefore to degrade them. That is why to lie to men, or to deceive them, that is, to use them as means for my, not their own, independently conceived ends, even if it is for their own benefit, is, in effect, to treat them as sub-human, to behave as if their ends are less ultimate and sacred than my own. In the name of what can I ever be justified in forcing men to do what they have not willed or consented to? Only in the name of some value higher than themselves. But if, as Kant held, all values are the creation of men, and called values only so far as they are so, there is no value higher than the individual. Therefore to do this is to coerce men in the name of something less ultimate than themselves—to bend them to my will, or to someone else's particular craving for happiness or expediency or security or convenience. I am aiming at something desired by me or my group, to which I am

using other men as means. But this is a contradiction of what I know men to be, namely ends in themselves. All forms of tampering with human beings, getting at them, shaping them against their will to your own pattern, all thought control and conditioning, is, therefore, a denial of that in men which makes them men and their values ultimate.

NOTES

NOTE 1.

GINSBERG v. NEW YORK
390 U.S. 629 (1968)

Mr. JUSTICE BRENNAN delivered the opinion of the Court.

This case presents the question of the constitutionality on its face of a New York criminal obscenity statute which prohibits the sale to minors under 17 years of age of material defined to be obscene on the basis of its appeal to them whether or not it would be obscene to adults.

Appellant and his wife operate "Sam's Stationery and Luncheonette" in Bellmore, Long Island. They have a lunch counter, and, among other things, also sell magazines including some so-called "girlie" magazines. Appellant was prosecuted under two informations, each in two counts, which charged that he personally sold a 16-year-old boy two "girlie" magazines on each of two dates in October 1965, in violation of § 484-h of the New York Penal Law. He was tried before a judge without a jury in Nassau County District Court and was found guilty on both counts. . . .

* * *

The "girlie" picture magazines involved in the sales here are not obscene for adults, *Redrup* v. *New York*, 386 U.S. 767. But § 484-h does not bar the appellant from stocking the magazines and selling them to persons 17 years of age or older, and therefore the conviction is not invalid under our decision in *Butler* v. *Michigan*, 352 U.S. 380.

Obscenity is not within the area of protected speech or press. *Roth* v. *United States*, 354 U.S. 476, 485. . . .

The New York Court of Appeals "upheld the Legislature's power to employ variable concepts of obscenity". . . . In sustaining state power to enact the law, the Court of Appeals said,

[M]aterial which is protected for distribution to adults is not necesssarily constitutionally protected from restriction upon its dissemination to children. In other words, the concept of obscenity or of unprotected matter may vary according to the group to whom the questionable material is directed or from whom it is quarantined. Because of the State's exigent interest in preventing distribution to children of objectionable material, it can exercise its power to protect the health, safety, welfare and morals of its community by barring the distribution to children of books recognized to be suitable for adults.

Appellant's attack is not that New York was without power to draw the line at age 17. Rather, his contention is the broad proposition that the scope of the constitutional freedom of expression secured to a citizen to read or see material concerned with sex cannot be made to depend upon whether the citizen is an adult or a minor. He accordingly insists that the denial to minors under 17 of access to material condemned by § 484-h, insofar as that material is not obscene for persons 17 years of age or older, constitutes an unconsitutional deprivation of protected liberty.

*   *   *

. . . We do not regard New York's regulation in defining obscenity on the basis of its appeal to minors under 17 as involving an invasion of such minors' constitutionally protected freedoms. Rather § 484-h simply adjusts the definition of obscenity "to social realities by permitting the appeal of this type of material to be assessed in terms of the sexual interests . . ." of such minors. *Mishkin* v. *New York,* 383 U.S. 502, 509; *Bookcase, Inc.* v. *Broderick, supra,* at 75, 218 N.E.2d, at 671. That the state has power to make that adjustment seems clear, for we have recognized that even where there is an invasion of protected freedoms "the power of the state to control the conduct of children reaches beyond the scope of its authority over adults. . . ." *Prince* v. *Massachusetts,* 321 U.S. 158, 170. . . . To sustain state power to exclude material defined as obscenity by § 484-h requires only that we be able to say that it was not irrational for the legislature to find that exposure to material condemned by the statute is harmful to minors. . . . To be sure, there is no lack of "studies" which purport to demonstrate that obscenity is or is not "a basic factor in impairing the ethical and moral development of . . . youth and a clear and present danger to the people of the state." But the growing consensus of commentators is that "while these studies all agree

that a causal link has not been demonstrated, they are equally agreed that a causal link has not been disproved either." We do not demand of legislatures "scientifically certain criteria of legislation." *Noble State Bank* v. *Haskell,* 219 U.S. 104, 110. We therefore cannot say that § 484-h, in defining the obscenity of material on the basis of its appeal to minors under 17, has no rational relation to the objective of safeguarding such minors from harm.

*   *   *

MR. JUSTICE STEWART, concurring in the result.

*   *   *

The First Amendment guarantees liberty of human expression in order to preserve in our nation what Mr. Justice Holmes called a "free trade in ideas." To that end, the Constitution protects more than just a man's freedom to say or write or publish what he wants. It secures as well the liberty of each man to decide for himself what he will read and to what he will listen. The Constitution guarantees, in short, a society of free choice. Such a society presupposes the capacity of its members to choose.

When expression occurs in a setting where the capacity to make a choice is absent, government regulation of that expression may co-exist with and even implement First Amendment guarantees. . . .

I think a state may permissibly determine that, at least in some precisely delineated areas, a child—like someone in a captive audience—is not possessed of that full capacity for individual choice which is the presupposition of First Amendment guarantees. It is only upon such a premise, I should suppose, that a state may deprive children of other rights—the right to marry, for example, or the right to vote—deprivations that would be constitutionally intolerable for adults.

*   *   *

Mr. JUSTICE DOUGLAS, with whom Mr. JUSTICE BLACK concurs, dissenting.

*   *   *

. . . Today the Court determines the constitutionality of New York's law regulating the sale of literature to children on the basis of the reasonableness of the law in light of the welfare of the child. If the problem of state and federal regulation of "obscenity" is in the field of substantive due process, I see no reason to limit the legislatures to protecting children alone. The "juvenile delinquents" I have known are mostly over 50 years of age. If rationality is the measure of the validity of this law, then I can see how modern Anthony Comstocks could make out a case for "protecting" many groups in our society, not merely children.

While I find the literature and movies which come to us for clearance exceedingly dull and boring, I understand how some can and do become very excited and alarmed and think that something should be done to stop the flow. It is one thing for parents and the religious organizations to be active and involved. It is quite a different matter for the state to become implicated as a censor. As I read the First Amendment, it was designed to keep the state and the hands of all state officials off the printing presses of America and off the distribution systems for all printed literature. . . .

NOTE 2.

UNITED STATES CODE
TITLE 25—INDIANS (1964)

§174. The President is authorized to exercise general superintendence and care over any tribe or nation which was removed upon an exchange of territory . . . and to cause such tribe or nation to be protected, at their new residence, against all interruption or disturbance from any other tribe or nation of Indians, or from any other person or persons whatever.

§202. It shall be unlawful for any person to induce any Indian to execute any contract, deed, mortgage, or other instrument purporting to convey any land or any interest therein held by the United States in trust for such Indian, or to offer any such contract, deed, mortgage, or other instrument for record in the office of any recorder of deeds. . . .

§263. The President is authorized, whenever in his opinion the public interest may require the same, to prohibit the introduction of goods, or of any particular article, into the country belonging to any Indian tribe, and to direct all licenses to trade with such tribe to be revoked, and all applications therefore to be rejected. No trader to any other tribe shall, so long as such prohibition may continue, trade with any Indians of or for the tribe against which such prohibition is issued.

d.

His Holiness, Pope Pius XII
The Moral Limits of Medical Research and Treatment*

. . . You do not expect Us to discuss the medical questions which concern you. Those are your domain. . . . We wish to make Ourself the interpreter of the moral conscience of the research worker, the specialist and the practitioner and of the man and Christian who follows the same path.

. . . A serious, competent doctor will often see with a sort of spontaneous intuition the moral legality of what he proposes to do and will act according to his conscience. But there are other instances where he does not have this security, where he may see or think he sees the contrary with certainty or where he doubts and wavers between Yes and No. In the most serious and profound matters, the man in the physician is not content with examining from a medical point of view what he can attempt and succeed in. He also wants to see his way clearly in regard to moral possibilities and obligations.

We would like to set forth briefly the *essential principles* which permit an answer to be given to this question. . . .

*   *   *

[T]he basic considerations may be set out in the following form: "The medical treatment of the patient demands taking a certain step. This in itself proves its moral legality." Or else: "A certain new method hitherto neglected or little used will give possible, probable or sure results. All ethical considerations as to the licitness of this method are obsolete and should be treated as pointless."

How can anyone fail to see that in these statements truth and falsehood are intermingled? In a very large number of cases the "interests of the patient" do provide the moral justification of the doctor's conduct. Here again, the question concerns the *absolute* value of this principle. Does it prove by itself, does it make it evident that what the doctor wants to do conforms to the moral law?

In the first place it must be assumed that, as

_____
* 44 *Acta Apostolicae Sedis* 779–784 (1952); Rome: 3 *Proceedings of the First International Congress of Neuropathology* 713–725 (1952). (Translated from the French by the N.C.W.C. News Service). Reprinted by permission.

a private person, the doctor can take no measure or try no course of action without the consent of the patient. The doctor has no other rights or power over the patient than those which the latter gives him, explicitly or implicitly and tacitly. On his side, the patient cannot confer rights he does not possess. In this discussion the decisive point is the moral licitness of the right a patient has to dispose of himself. Here is the moral limit to the doctor's action taken with the consent of the patient.

As for the patient, he is not absolute master of himself, of his body or of his soul. He cannot, therefore, freely dispose of himself as he pleases. Even the reason for which he acts is of itself neither sufficient nor determining. The patient is bound to the immanent teleology laid down by nature. He has the right of use, limited by natural finality, of the faculties and powers of his human nature. Because he is a user and not a proprietor, he does not have unlimited power to destroy or mutilate his body and its functions. Nevertheless, by virtue of the principle of totality, by virtue of his right to use the services of his organism as a whole, the patient can allow individual parts to be destroyed or mutilated when and to the extent necessary for the good of his being as a whole. He may do so to ensure his being's existence and to avoid or, naturally, to repair serious and lasting damage which cannot otherwise be avoided or repaired.

The patient, then, has no right to involve his physical or psychic integrity in medical experiments or research when they entail serious destruction, mutilation, wounds or perils.

Moreover, in exercising his right to dispose of himself, his faculties and his organs, the individual must observe the hierarchy of the orders of values—or within a single order of values, the hierarchy of particular rights—insofar as the rules of morality demand. Thus, for example, a man cannot perform on himself or allow doctors to perform acts of a physical or somatic nature which doubtless relieve heavy physical or psychic burdens or infirmities, but which bring about at the same time permanent abolition or considerable and durable diminution of his freedom, that is, of his human personality in its typical and characteristic function. Such an act degrades a man to the level of a being reacting only to acquired reflexes or to a living automaton. The moral law does not allow such a reversal of values. Here it sets up its limits to the "medical interests of the patient."

Here is another example. In order to rid himself of repressions, inhibitions or psychic complexes man is not free to arouse in himself for therapeutic purposes each and every appetite of a sexual order which is being excited or has been excited in his being, appetites whose impure waves flood his unconscious or subconscious mind. He cannot make them the object of his thoughts and fully conscious desires with all the shocks and repercussions such a process entails. For a man and a Christian there is a law of integrity and personal purity, of self-respect, forbidding him to plunge so deeply into the world of sexual suggestions and tendencies. Here the "medical and psychotherapeutic interests of the patient" find a moral limit. It is not proved—it is, in fact, incorrect—that the pansexual method of a certain school of psychoanalysis is an indispensable integrating part of all psychotherapy which is serious and worthy of the name. It is not proved that past neglect of this method has caused grave psychic damage, errors in doctrine and application in education, in psychotherapy and still less in pastoral practice. It is not proved that it is urgent to fill this gap and to initiate all those interested in psychic questions in its key ideas and even, if necessary, in the practical application of this technique of sexuality.

We speak this way because today these assertions are too often made with apodictic assurance. Where instincts are concerned it would be better to pay more attention to indirect treatment and to the action of the conscious psyche on the whole of imaginative and affective activity. This technique avoids the deviations We have mentioned. It tends to enlighten, cure and guide; it also influences the dynamic of sexuality, on which people insist so much and which they say is to be found, or really exists, in the unconscious or subconscious.

Up to now We have spoken directly of the patient, not of the doctor. We have explained at what point the personal right of the patient to dispose of himself, his mind, his body, his faculties, organs and functions, meets a moral limit. But at the same time We have answered the question: Where does the doctor find a moral limit in research into and use of new methods and procedures in the "interests of the patient?" The limit is the same as that for the patient. It is that which is fixed by the judgment of sound reason, which is set by the demands of the natural moral law, which is deduced from the natural teleology inscribed in beings and from the scale of values expressed by the nature of things. The limit is the same for the doctor as for the patient because, as We have already said, the doctor as a private individual disposes only of the rights given him by the patient and because the patient can give only what he himself possesses.

What We say here must be extended to the *legal representatives* of the person incapable of caring for himself and his affairs: children below the age of reason, the feeble-minded and the insane. These legal representatives, authorized by private decision or by public authority have no other rights over the body and life of those they represent than those people would have themselves if they were capable. And they have those rights to the same extent. They cannot, therefore, give the doctor permission to dispose of them outside those limits.

* * *

NOTE

APPLICATION OF PRESIDENT AND DIRECTORS OF GEORGETOWN COLLEGE 331 F.2D 1000 (D.C.CIR.), *certiorari denied*, 377 U.S. 978 (1964)

J. SKELLY WRIGHT, CIRCUIT JUDGE.

* * *

Mrs. Jones was brought to the hospital by her husband for emergency care, having lost two thirds of her body's blood supply from a ruptured ulcer. She had no personal physician, and relied solely on the hospital staff. She was a total hospital responsibility. It appeared that the patient, age 25, mother of a seven-month-old child, and her husband were both Jehovah's Witnesses, the teachings of which sect, according to their interpretation, prohibited the injection of blood into the body. When death without blood became imminent, the hospital sought the advice of counsel, who applied to the District Court in the name of the hospital for permission to administer blood. Judge Tamm of the District Court denied the application, and counsel immediately applied to me, as a member of the Court of Appeals, for an appropriate writ.

I called the hospital by telephone and spoke with Dr. Westura, Chief Medical Resident, who confirmed the representations made by counsel. I thereupon proceeded with counsel to the hospital, where I spoke to Mr. Jones, the husband of the patient. He advised me that, on religious grounds, he would not approve a blood transfusion for his wife. He said, however, that if the court ordered the transfusion, the responsibility was not his. I advised Mr. Jones to obtain counsel immediately. He thereupon went to the telephone and returned in 10 or 15 minutes to advise that he had taken the matter up with his church and that he had decided that he did not want counsel.

I asked permission of Mr. Jones to see his wife. This he readily granted. Prior to going into the patient's room, I again conferred with Dr. Westura and several other doctors assigned to the case. All confirmed that the patient would die without blood and that there was a better than 50 per cent chance of saving her life with it. Unanimously they strongly recommended it. I then went inside the patient's room. Her appearance confirmed the urgency which had been represented to me. I tried to communicate with her, advising her again as to what the doctors had said. The only audible reply I could hear was "Against my will." It was obvious that the woman was not in a mental condition to make a decision. I was reluctant to press her because of the seriousness of her condition and because I felt that to suggest repeatedly the imminence of death without blood might place a strain on her religious convictions. I asked her whether she would oppose the blood transfusion if the court allowed it. She indicated, as best I could make out, that it would not then be her responsibility.

* * *

[I] signed the order allowing the hospital to administer such transfusions as the doctors should determine were necessary to save her life.

* * *

Before proceeding with this inquiry, it may be useful to state what this case does not involve. This case does not involve a person who, for religious or other reasons, has refused to seek medical attention. It does not involve a disputed medical judgment or a dangerous or crippling operation. Nor does it involve the delicate question of saving the newborn in preference to the mother. Mrs. Jones sought medical attention and placed on the hospital the legal responsibility for her proper care. In its dilemma, not of its own making, the hospital sought judicial direction.

* * *

If self-homicide is a crime, there is no exception to the law's command for those who believe the crime to be divinely ordained. The

Mormon cases in the Supreme Court establish that there is no religious exception to criminal laws, and state *obiter* the very example that a religiously inspired suicide attempt would be within the law's authority to prevent. . . . But whether attempted suicide is a crime is in doubt in some jurisdictions, including the District of Columbia.

The Gordian knot of this suicide question may be cut by the simple fact that Mrs. Jones did not want to die. Her voluntary presence in the hospital as a patient seeking medical help testified to this. Death, to Mrs. Jones, was not a religiously commanded goal, but an unwanted side effect of a religious scruple. . . . Nor are we faced with the question of whether the state should intervene to reweigh the relative values of life and death, after the individual has weighed them for himself and found life wanting. Mrs. Jones wanted to live.

A third set of considerations involved the position of the doctors and the hospital. Mrs. Jones was their responsibility to treat. The hospital doctors had the choice of administering the proper treatment or letting Mrs. Jones die in the hospital bed, thus exposing themselves, and the hospital, to the risk of civil and criminal liability in either case. It is not certain that Mrs. Jones had any authority to put the hospital and its doctors to this impossible choice. The normal principle that an adult patient directs her doctors is based on notions of commercial contract which may have less relevance to life-or-death emergencies. It is not clear just where a patient would derive her authority to command her doctor to treat her under limitations which would produce death. The patient's counsel suggests that this authority is part of constitutionally protected liberty. But neither the principle that life and liberty are inalienable rights, nor the principle of liberty of religion, provides an easy answer to the question whether the state can prevent martyrdom. Moreover, Mrs. Jones had no wish to be a martyr. And her religion merely prevented her consent to a transfusion. If the law undertook the responsibility of authorizing the transfusion without her consent, no problem would be raised with respect to her religious practice. Thus, the effect of the order was to preserve for Mrs. Jones the life she wanted without sacrifice of her religious beliefs.

The final, and compelling, reason for granting the emergency writ was that a life hung in the balance. There was no time for research and reflection. Death could have mooted the cause in a matter of minutes, if action were not taken to preserve the *status quo*. To refuse to act, only to find later that the law required action, was a risk I was unwilling to accept. I determined to act on the side of life.

e.

Fyodor Dostoyevsky
The Brothers Karamazov (1880)*

*   *   *

. . . Amid the profound darkness, the iron door of the prison is suddenly opened and the old Grand Inquisitor himself slowly enters the prison with a light in his hand. He is alone and the door at once closes behind him. He stops in the doorway and gazes for a long time, for more than a minute, into his face. At last he approaches him slowly, puts the lamp on the table and says to him:

*   *   *

. . . And look what you have done . . . in the name of freedom! I tell you man has no more agonizing anxiety than to find someone to whom he can hand over with all speed the gift of freedom with which the unhappy creature is born. But only he can gain possession of men's freedom who is able to set their conscience at ease. With the bread you were given an incontestable banner: give him bread and man will worship you, for there is nothing more incontestable than bread; but if at the same time someone besides yourself should gain possession of his conscience—oh, then he will even throw away your bread and follow him who has ensnared his conscience. You were right about that. For the mystery of human life is not only in living, but in knowing why one lives. Without a clear idea of what to live for man will not consent to live and will rather destroy himself than remain on the earth, though he were surrounded by loaves of bread. That is so, but what became of it? Instead of gaining possession of men's freedom, you gave them greater freedom than ever! Or did you forget that a tranquil mind and even death is dearer to man than the free choice in the knowledge of good and evil? There is nothing more alluring to man than this freedom of conscience, but there is nothing more tormenting, either. And instead of firm foundations for

* Translated by David Magarshack. Baltimore: Penguin Books 293, 298–301 (1958). Translation copyright © David Magarshack, 1958. Reprinted by permission.

appeasing man's conscience once and for all, you chose everything that was exceptional, enigmatic, and vague, you chose everything that was beyond the strength of men, acting, consequently, as though you did not love them at all—you who came to give your life for them! Instead of taking possession of men's freedom you multiplied it and burdened the spiritual kingdom of man with its sufferings for ever. You wanted man's free love so that he should follow you freely, fascinated and captivated by you. Instead of the strict ancient law, man had in future to decide for himself with a free heart what is good and what is evil, having only your image before him for guidance. But did it never occur to you that he would at last reject and call in question even your image and your truth, if he were weighed down by so fearful a burden as freedom of choice? They will at last cry aloud that the truth is not in you, for it was impossible to leave them in greater confusion and suffering than you have done by leaving them with so many cares and insoluble problems. It was you yourself, therefore, who laid the foundation for the destruction of your kingdom and you ought not to blame anyone else for it. And yet, is that all that was offered to you? There are three forces, the only three forces that are able to conquer and hold captive for ever the conscience of these weak rebels for their own happiness—these forces are: miracle, mystery, and authority. You rejected all three and yourself set the example for doing so. . . . But . . . are there many like you? And could you really assume for a moment that men, too, could be equal to such a temptation? Is the nature of man such that he can reject a miracle and at the most fearful moments of life, the moments of his most fearful, fundamental, and agonizing spiritual problems, stick to the free decision of the heart? Oh, you knew that your great deed would be preserved in books, that it would go down to the end of time and the extreme ends of the earth, and you hoped that, following you, man would remain with God and ask for no miracle. But you did not know that as soon as man rejected miracle he would at once reject God as well, for what man seeks is not so much God as miracles. And since man is unable to carry on without a miracle, he will create new miracles for himself, miracles of his own, and will worship the miracle of the witch-doctor and the sorcery of the wise woman, rebel, heretic and infidel though he is a hundred times over. You did not come down from the cross when they shouted to you, mock-

ing and deriding you: "If thou be the Son of God, come down from the cross." You did not come down because, again, you did not want to enslave man by a miracle and because you hungered for a faith based on free will and not on miracles. You hungered for freely given love and not for the servile raptures of the slave before the might that has terrified him once and for all. But here, too, your judgement of men was too high, for they are slaves, though rebels by nature. Look round and judge: fifteen centuries have passed, go and have a look at them: whom have you raised up to yourself? I swear, man has been created a weaker and baser creature than you thought him to be! Can he, can he do what you did? In respecting him so greatly, you acted as though you ceased to feel any compassion for him, for you asked too much of him—you who have loved him more than yourself! Had you respected him less, you would have asked less of him, and that would have been more like love, for his burden would have been lighter. He is weak and base. What does it matter if he does rebel against our authority everywhere now and is proud of his rebellion? It is the pride of a child and of a schoolboy. They are little children rioting in class and driving out their teacher. But an end will come to the transports of the children, too. They will pay dearly for it. They will tear down the temples and drench the earth with blood. But they will realize at last, the foolish children, that although they are rebels, they are impotent rebels who are unable to keep up with their rebellion. Dissolving into foolish tears, they will admit at last that he who created them rebels must undoubtedly have meant to laugh at them. They will say so in despair, and their utterance will be a blasphemy which will make them still more unhappy, for man's nature cannot endure blasphemy and in the end will always avenge it on itself. And so, unrest, confusion, and unhappiness—this is the present lot of men after all you suffered for their freedom! Your great prophet tells in a vision and in an allegory that he saw all those who took part in the first resurrection and that there were twelve thousand of them from each tribe. But if there were so many then, they, too, were not like men, but gods. They had borne your cross, they had endured scores of years of the hungry and barren wilderness, feeding on locusts and roots—and you can indeed point with pride to those children of freedom, freely given love, and free and magnificent sacrifice in your name. But remember that there were only a few thousand of them, and they, too, gods. But what of the rest? And why are the rest, the weak ones, to blame if they were not able to endure all that the mighty ones endured? Why is the weak soul to blame for being unable to receive gifts so terrible? Surely, you did not come only to the chosen and for the chosen? But if so, there is a mystery here and we cannot understand it. And if it is a mystery, then we, too, were entitled to preach a mystery and to teach them that it is neither the free verdict of their hearts nor love that matters, but the mystery which they must obey blindly, even against their conscience. So we have done. We have corrected your great work and have based it on *miracle, mystery, and authority*. And men rejoiced that they were once more led like sheep and that the terrible gift which had brought them so much suffering had at last been lifted from their hearts. Were we right in doing and teaching this? Tell me. Did we not love mankind when we admitted so humbly its impotence and lovingly lightened its burden and allowed men's weak nature even to sin, so long as it was with our permission? . . .

* * *

2.

Protecting the Status of the Subject as a Human Being

a.

Pratt v. Davis
118 Ill. App. 161, 166 (1905),
affirmed, 224 Ill. 30, 79 N.E. 562 (1906)

MR. JUSTICE BROWN delivered the opinion of the Court.

* * *

[U]nder a free government at least, the free citizen's first and greatest right, which underlies all others—the right to the inviolability of his person, in other words, his right to himself—is the subject of universal acquiescence, and this right necessarily forbids a physician or surgeon, however skillful or eminent, who has been asked to examine, diagnose, advise, and prescribe (which are at least necessary first steps in treatment and care), to violate without permission the bodily integrity of his patient by a major or capital operation, placing him under an anaesthetic for that purpose, and operating on him without his consent or knowledge. . . .

* * *

b.

Alfred Gellhorn
Experimental Treatment of Cancer Patients*

* * *

. . . I have little confidence in the usual interpretation of written consent as informed consent, because I believe this to be a fiction. The patient cannot be expected to understand adequately the implications of the proposed research and his consent is therefore unlikely to be informed. The written consent is important, however, because it accords to the patient the status of a person, not an experimental animal, and provides a degree of assurance that he is being considered as an end, not merely a means.

* * *

c.

Margaret Mead
Research with Human Beings—A Model Derived from Anthropological Field Practice†

* * *

. . . To fail to acquaint a subject of observation or experiment with what is happening—as fully as is possible within the limits of the communication system—is to that extent to denigrate him as a full human being and reduce him to the category of dependency in which he is not permitted to judge for himself. The various ethical ruses that are used—such as telling the subject he has been tricked, deluded, spied upon, or lied to immediately after the experiment is over—fail to take into account that when such a subject is debriefed, he can accept such debriefing only by some other ruse, such as in the identification with the lying experimenter or in the decision that social science is a bunch of confidence tricks and now he also knows a few. Alternately, if he cannot make use of satisfying self-protective devices, his dignity will have been abused and affronted. If he decides that being lied to or tricked is the price he must pay for some other benefit—health, education, political preferment, employment, or a graduate

___

* V. Fattorusso, ed., *Biomedical Science and the Dilemma of Human Experimentation.* Paris: Council for International Organizations of Medical Sciences 41 (1967). Reprinted by permission.
† 98 *Daedalus* 361, 375 (1969). Reprinted by permission of Daedalus, Journal of the American Academy of Arts and Sciences, Boston, Massachusetts.

education in a social science—he will nevertheless invest these very benefits and those who confer them upon him with some negative effect.

NOTES

NOTE 1.

GRISWOLD v. CONNECTICUT
381 U.S. 479 (1965)

Mr. JUSTICE DOUGLAS delivered the opinion of the Court.

*   *   *

The . . . cases suggest that specific guarantees in the Bill of Rights have penumbras, formed by emanations from those guarantees that help give them life and substance. . . . Various guarantees create zones of privacy. The right of association contained in the penumbra of the First Amendment is one, as we have seen. The Third Amendment is its prohibition against the quartering of soldiers "in any house" in time of peace without the consent of the owner is another facet of that privacy. The Fourth Amendment explicitly affirms the "right of the people to be secure in their persons, houses, papers, and effects, against unreasonable searches and seizures." The Fifth Amendment in its Self-Incrimination Clause enables the citizen to create a zone of privacy which government may not force him to surrender to his detriment. The Ninth Amendment provides: "The enumeration in the Constitution, of certain rights, shall not be construed to deny or disparage others retained by the people."

The Fourth and Fifth Amendments were described in *Boyd* v. *United States,* 116 U.S. 616, 630, . . . as protection against all governmental invasions "of the sanctity of a man's home and the privacies of life."

*   *   *

The present case, then, concerns a relationship lying within the zone of privacy created by several fundamental constitutional guarantees. And it concerns a law which, in forbidding the *use* of contraceptives rather than regulating their manufacture or sale, seeks to achieve its goals by means having a maximum destructive impact upon that relationship. . . .

We deal with a right of privacy older than the Bill of Rights—older than our political parties, older than our school system. Marriage is a coming together for better or for worse, hopefully enduring, and intimate to the degree of being sacred. It is an association that promotes a way of life, not causes; a harmony in living, not political faiths; a bilateral loyalty, not commercial or social projects. Yet it is an association for as noble a purpose as any involved in our prior decisions.

Reversed.

Mr. JUSTICE GOLDBERG, whom THE CHIEF JUSTICE and Mr. JUSTICE BRENNAN join, concurring.

*   *   *

[T]he right of privacy is a fundamental personal right, emanating "from the totality of the constitutional scheme under which we live." . . . Mr. Justice Brandeis, dissenting in *Olmstead* v. *United States,* 277 U.S. 438, 478, comprehensively summarized the principles underlying the Constitution's guarantees of privacy.

The protection guaranteed by the [Fourth and Fifth] amendments is much broader in scope. The makers of our Constitution undertook to secure conditions favorable to the pursuit of happiness. They recognized the significance of man's spiritual nature, of his feelings and of his intellect. They knew that only a part of the pain, pleasure and satisfaction of life are to be found in material things. They sought to protect Americans in their beliefs, their thoughts, their emotions and their sensations. They conferred, as against the government, the right to be let alone—the most comprehensive of rights and the right most valued by civilized men.

The Connecticut statutes here involved deal with a particularly important and sensitive area of privacy—that of the marital relation and the marital home. This Court recognized in *Meyer* v. *Nebraska,* supra, that the right "to marry, establish a home and bring up children" was an essential part of the liberty guaranteed by the Fourteenth Amendment. 262 U.S., at 399. . . . In *Pierce* v. *Society of Sisters,* 268 U.S. 510 . . . the Court held unconstitutional an Oregon Act which forbade parents from sending their children to private schools because such an act "unreasonably interferes with the liberty of parents and guardians to direct the upbringing and education of children under their control." 268 U.S., at 534–535. . . . As this Court said in *Prince* v. *Massachusetts,* 321 U.S. 158, at 166 . . . the Meyer and Pierce decisions "have respected the private realm of family life which the state cannot enter."

*   *   *

My Brother STEWART, while characteriz-

ing the Connecticut birth control law as "an uncommonly silly law," post, at 1705, would nevertheless let it stand on the ground that it is not
for the courts to " 'substitute their social and
economic beliefs for the judgment of legislative
bodies, who are elected to pass laws.' " Post, at
1705. Elsewhere, I have stated that "[w]hile I
quite agree with Mr. Justice Brandeis that . . .
'a . . . State may . . . serve as a laboratory; and
try novel social and economic experiments,' *New
State Ice Co.* v. *Liebmann,* 285 U.S. 262 . . .
(dissenting opinion), I do not believe that this
includes the power to experiment with the fundamental liberties of citizens. . . ." The vice of
the dissenters' views is that it would permit such
experimentation by the States in the area of the
fundamental personal rights of its citizens. I cannot agree that the Constitution grants such power
either to the States or to the Federal Government.

The logic of the dissents would sanction
federal or state legislation that seems to me even
more plainly unconstitutional than the statute
before us. Surely the Government, absent a
showing of a compelling subordinating state interest, could not decree that all husbands and
wives must be sterilized after two children have
been born to them. Yet by their reasoning such
an invasion of marital privacy would not be
subject to constitutional challenge because,
while it might be "silly," no provision of the
Constitution specifically prevents the Government from curtailing the marital right to bear
children and raise a family. While it may shock
some of my Brethren that the Court today holds
that the Constitution protects the right of marital privacy, in my view it is far more shocking
to believe that the personal liberty guaranteed by
the Constitution does not include protection
against such totalitarian limitation of family size,
which is at complete variance with our constitutional concepts. Yet, if upon a showing of a slen-
der basis of rationality, a law outlawing voluntary birth control by married persons is valid,
then, by the same reasoning, a law requiring
compulsory birth control also would seem to be
valid. In my view, however, both types of law
would unjustifiably intrude upon rights of marital privacy which are constitutionally protected.

In a long series of cases this Court has held
that where fundamental personal liberties are
involved, they may not be abridged by the
States simply on a showing that a regulatory
statute has some rational relationship to the ef-
fectuation of a proper state purpose. "Where
there is a significant encroachment upon per-

sonal liberty, the State may prevail only upon
showing a subordinating interest which is compelling," *Bates* v. *City of Little Rock,* 361 U.S.
516, 524. . . .

*   *   *

NOTE 2.

MULLER V. OREGON
208 U.S. 412 (1908)

Mr. JUSTICE BREWER delivered the opinion of
the court.

On February 19, 1903, the legislature of the
State of Oregon passed an act . . . the first section of which is in these words:

"SEC. 1. That no female (shall) be employed in any mechanical establishment, or factory, or laundry in this State more than ten hours
during any one day. The hours of work may be
so arranged as to permit the employment of
females at any time so that they shall not work
more than ten hours during the twenty-four
hours of any one day."

*   *   *

The single question is the constitutionality
of the statute under which the defendant was
convicted so far as it affects the work of a female
in a laundry. . . .

*   *   *

It is the law of Oregon that women, whether
married or single, have equal contractual and
personal rights with men. . . .

*   *   *

It thus appears that, putting to one side the
elective franchise, in the matter of personal and
contractual rights they stand on the same plane
as the other sex. Their rights in these respects
can no more be infringed than the equal rights
of their brothers. We held in *Lochner* v. *New
York,* 198 U.S. 45, that a law providing that no
laborer shall be required or permitted to work
in a bakery more than sixty hours in a week or
ten hours in a day was not as to men a legitimate
exercise of the police power of the State, but an
unreasonable, unnecessary and arbitrary interference with the right and liberty of the individual to contract in relation to his labor, and as
such was in conflict with, and void under, the
Federal Constitution. . . .

*   *   *

It is undoubtedly true, as more than once
declared by this court, that the general right to
contract in relation to one's business is part of

the liberty of the individual, protected by the Fourteenth Amendment to the Federal Constitution; yet it is equally well settled that this liberty is not absolute and extending to all contracts, and that a State may, without conflicting with the provisions of the Fourteenth Amendment, restrict in many respects the individual's power of contract. . . .

That woman's physical structure and the performance of maternal functions place her at a disadvantage in the struggle for subsistence is obvious. This is especially true when the burdens of motherhood are upon her. Even when they are not, by abundant testimony of the medical fraternity continuance for a long time on her feet at work, repeating this from day to day, tends to injurious effects upon the body, and as healthy mothers are essential to vigorous offspring, the physical well-being of woman becomes an object of public interest and care in order to preserve the strength and vigor of the race.

Still again, history discloses the fact that woman has always been dependent upon man. He established his control at the outset by superior physical strength, and this control in various forms, with diminishing intensity, has continued to the present. . . . Differentiated by these matters from the other sex, she is properly placed in a class by herself, and legislation designed for her protection may be sustained, even when like legislation is not necessary for men and could not be sustained. It is impossible to close one's eyes to the fact that she still looks to her brother and depends upon him. Even though all restrictions on political, personal and contractual rights were taken away, and she stood, so far as statutes are concerned, upon an absolutely equal plane with him, it would still be true that she is so constituted that she will rest upon and look to him for protection; that her physical structure and a proper discharge of her maternal functions—having in view not merely her own health, but the well-being of the race—justify legislation to protect her from the greed as well as the passion of man. . . .

* * *

NOTE 3.

IN RE GAULT
387 U.S. 1 (1967)

MR. JUSTICE FORTAS delivered the opinion of the Court.

This is an appeal . . . from a judgment of the Supreme Court of Arizona affirming the dismissal of a petition for a writ of habeas corpus.

. . . The petition sought the release of Gerald Francis Gault, appellants' 15-year-old son, who had been committed as a juvenile delinquent to the State Industrial School by the Juvenile Court of Gila County, Arizona. The Supreme Court of Arizona affirmed dismissal of the writ against various arguments which included an attack upon the constitutionality of the Arizona Juvenile Code because of its alleged denial of procedural due process rights to juveniles charged with being "delinquents."

* * *

. . . In their jurisdictional statement and brief in this Court, appellants do not urge upon us all of the points passed upon by the Supreme Court of Arizona. They urge that we hold the Juvenile Code of Arizona invalid on its face or as applied in this case because, contrary to the Due Process Clause of the Fourteenth Amendment, the juvenile is taken from the custody of his parents and committed to a state institution pursuant to proceedings in which the Juvenile Court has virtually unlimited discretion, and in which the following basic rights are denied:

1. Notice of the charges;
2. Right to counsel;
3. Right to confrontation and cross-examination;
4. Privilege against self-incrimination;
5. Right to a transcript of the proceedings; and
6. Right to appellate review.

* * *

From the inception of the juvenile court system, wide differences have been tolerated—indeed insisted upon—between the procedural rights accorded to adults and those of juveniles. In practically all jurisdictions, there are rights granted to adults which are withheld from juveniles. In addition to the specific problems involved in the present case, for example, it has been held that the juvenile is not entitled to bail, to indictment by grand jury, to a public trial or to trial by jury. It is frequent practice that rules governing the arrest and interrogation of adults by the police are not observed in the case of juveniles.

* * *

The early reformers were appalled by adult procedures and penalties, and by the fact that children could be given long prison sentences and mixed in jails with hardened criminals. They were profoundly convinced that society's duty to the child could not be confined by the concept of justice alone. They believed that society's role was not to ascertain whether the child was "guilty" or "innocent," but "What is he, how has he become what he is, and what had best be done in his interest and in the interest of the state to save him from a downward career." The child—essentially good, as they saw it—was to be made "to feel that he is the object of [the state's] care and solicitude," not that he was under arrest or on trial. The rules of criminal procedure were therefore altogether inapplicable. The apparent rigidities, technicalities, and harshness which they observed in both substantive and procedural criminal law were therefore to be discarded. The idea of crime and punishment was to be abandoned. The child was to be "treated" and "rehabilitated" and the procedures, from apprehension through institutionalization, were to be "clinical" rather than punitive.

* * *

The right of the state, as *parens patriae,* to deny to the child procedural rights available to his elders was elaborated by the assertion that a child, unlike an adult, has a right "not to liberty but to custody." He can be made to attorn to his parents, to go to school, etc. If his parents default in effectively performing their custodial functions—that is, if the child is "delinquent"—the state may intervene. In doing so, it does not deprive the child of any rights, because he has none. It merely provides the "custody" to which the child is entitled. On this basis, proceedings involving juveniles were described as "civil" not "criminal" and therefore not subject to the requirements which restrict the state when it seeks to deprive a person of his liberty.

Accordingly, the highest motives and most enlightened impulses led to a peculiar system for juveniles, unknown to our law in any comparable context. The constitutional and theoretical basis for this peculiar system is—to say the least—debatable. And in practice, as we remarked in the *Kent* case, *supra,* the results have not been entirely satisfactory. Juvenile Court history has again demonstrated that unbridled discretion, however benevolently motivated, is frequently a poor substitute for principle and procedure. In 1937, Dean Pound wrote: "The powers of the Star Chamber were a trifle in comparison with those of our juvenile courts. . . ." The absence of substantive standards has not necessarily meant that children receive careful, compassionate, individualized treatment. The absence of procedural rules based upon constitutional principle has not always produced fair, efficient, and effective procedures. Departures from established principles of due process have frequently resulted not in enlightened procedure, but in arbitrariness. The Chairman of the Pennsylvania Council of Juvenile Court Judges has recently observed: "Unfortunately, loose procedures, high-handed methods and crowded court calendars, either singly or in combination, all too often, have resulted in depriving some juveniles of fundamental rights that have resulted in a denial of due process."

Failure to observe the fundamental requirements of due process has resulted in instances, which might have been avoided, of unfairness to individuals and inadequate or inaccurate findings of fact and unfortunate prescriptions of remedy. Due process of law is the primary and indispensable foundation of individual freedom. It is the basic and essential term in the social compact which defines the rights of the individual and delimits the powers which the state may exercise. . . .

It is claimed that juveniles obtain benefits from the special procedures applicable to them which more than offset the disadvantages of denial of the substance of normal due process. As we shall discuss, the observance of due process standards, intelligently and not ruthlessly administered, will not compel the States to abandon or displace any of the substantive benefits of the juvenile process.

* * *

Ultimately . . . we confront the reality of that portion of the Juvenile Court process with which we deal in this case. A boy is charged with misconduct. The boy is committed to an institution where he may be restrained of liberty for years. It is of no constitutional consequence—and of limited practical meaning—that the institution to which he is committed is called an Industrial School. The fact of the matter is that, however euphemistic the title, a "receiving home" or an "industrial school" for juveniles is an institution of confinement in which the child is incarcerated for a greater or lesser time. His world becomes "a building with whitewashed walls, regimented routine and institutional hours. . . ." Instead of mother and father and sisters and brothers and friends and classmates, his world is peopled by guards, custodians, state employees, and "delinquents" confined with him for anything from waywardness to rape and homicide.

In view of this, it would be extraordinary if our Constitution did not require the procedural regularity and the exercise of care implied in the phrase "due process." Under our Constitution, the condition of being a boy does not justify a kangaroo court. . . .

NOTE 4.

ARTHUR ALLEN LEFF
UNCONSCIONABILITY AND THE CODE—
THE EMPEROR'S NEW CLAUSE*

* * *

When faced with the difficulties inherent in deciding the bargaining fairness of any given transaction, the equity courts . . . leaned heavily on relatively gross classifications. In effect, they seem continually to have taken a kind of *sub rosa* judicial notice of the amount of power of certain classes of people to take care of themselves, often without too much inquiry into the actual individual bargaining situation. And it is arguable that sometimes they were wrong; not all old ladies or farmers are without defenses. Put briefly, the typical has a tendency to become stereotypical, with what may be unpleasant results even for the beneficiaries of the judicial benevolence. One can see it enshrined in the old English equity courts' jolly treatment of English seamen as members of a happy, fun-loving race (with, one supposes, a fine sense of rhythm), but certainly not to be trusted to take care of themselves. What effect, if any, this had upon the sailors is hidden behind the judicial chuckles as they protected their loyal sailor boys, but one cannot help wondering how many sailors managed to get credit at any reasonable price. In other words, the benevolent have a tendency to colonize, whether geographically or legally.

* * *

d.

Geoffrey Edsall
A Positive Approach to the Problem
of Human Experimentation†

* * *

[In 1957 there] arose the landmark case concerning the consent of a minor to donate a

---

* 115 *University of Pennsylvania Law Review* 485, 556–557 (1967). © 1967. Reprinted by permission.

† 98 *Daedalus* 464–467 (1969). Reprinted by permission of Daedalus, Journal of the American Academy of Arts and Sciences, Boston, Massachusetts.

kidney for his identical twin brother, who suffered from chronic renal disease that would soon prove fatal. The question at issue was whether or not the operation to remove a kidney from the healthy brother could proceed—even with the consent of the parents and of both twins—without incurring civil or criminal liability. The judge pointed out that testimony by a psychiatrist had indicated that if the sick twin should die without the transplant, the resulting emotional disturbance could well affect the health and physical well-being of the donor twin for the rest of his life. Thus the judge found the operation was necessary "for the continued good health and future well-being of Leonard" (the healthy twin). Here we have clear reaffirmation of the principle implied in the skin graft case: If the action to be taken is at variance with traditionally or legally established procedure, it may be condoned *if it is of self-interest to the person upon whom the operation is to be performed*. On the other hand, the argument that the proposed action has a generous, humanistic, or idealistic basis is apparently inadmissible in court. Thus, in the eyes of the law, the individual is physically inviolable, *his* interests are paramount, and consent for any action that may violate the integrity of his physical being must be based upon the assumption that such action will be for his benefit.

e.

In re Brooks Estate
32 Ill. 2d 361, 205 N.E. 2d 435 (1965)

UNDERWOOD, JUSTICE.

* * *

On and sometime before May 7, 1964, Bernice Brooks was in the McNeal General Hospital, Chicago, suffering from a peptic ulcer. She was being attended by Dr. Gilbert Demange, and had informed him repeatedly during a two-year period prior thereto that her religious and medical convictions precluded her from receiving blood transfusions. Mrs. Brooks, her husband and two adult children are all members of the religious sect commonly known as Jehovah's Witnesses. Among the religious beliefs adhered to by members of this group is the principle that blood transfusions are a violation of the law of God, and that transgressors will be punished by God. . . .

Mrs. Brooks and her husband had signed a document releasing Dr. Demange and the hospital from all civil liability that might result from the failure to administer blood transfusions to Mrs. Brooks. The patient was assured that there would thereafter be no further effort to persuade her to accept blood.

Notwithstanding these assurances, however, Dr. Demange, together with several assistant State's attorneys, and the attorney for the public guardian of Cook County, Illinois, appeared before the probate division of the circuit court with a petition by the public guardian requesting appointment of that officer as conservator of the person of Bernice Brooks and further requesting an order authorizing such conservator to consent to the administration of whole blood to the patient. . . . Thereafter, the conservator of the person was appointed, consented to the administration of a blood transfusion, it was accomplished and apparently successfully so, although appellants now argue that much distress resulted from transfusions due to a "circulatory overload."

* * *

Appellees argue that society has an overriding interest in protecting the lives of its citizens which justifies the action here taken. . . .

* * *

We believe Jefferson's fundamental concept that civil officers may intervene only when religious "principles break out into overt acts against peace and good order" has consistently prevailed. . . .

* * *

. . . It seems to be clearly established that the First Amendment of the United States Constitution, as extended to the individual States by the Fourteenth Amendment to that constitution, protects the absolute right of every individual to freedom in his religious belief and the exercise thereof, subject only to the qualification that the exercise thereof may properly be limited by governmental action where such exercise endangers, clearly and presently, the public health, welfare or morals. Those cases which have sustained governmental action as against the challenge that it violated the religious guarantees of the First Amendment have found the proscribed practice to be immediately deleterious to some phase of public welfare, health or morality. The decisions which have held the conduct complained of immune from proscription involve no such public injury and no danger thereof.

Applying the constitutional guarantees and the interpretations thereof heretofore enunci-

ated to the facts before us we find a competent adult who has steadfastly maintained her belief that acceptance of a blood transfusion is a violation of the law of God. Knowing full well the hazards involved, she has firmly opposed acceptance of such transfusions, notifying the doctor and hospital of her convictions and desires, and executing documents releasing both the doctor and the hospital from any civil liability which might be thought to result from a failure on the part of either to administer such transfusions. No minor children are involved. No overt or affirmative act of appellants offers any clear and present danger to society—we have only a governmental agency compelling conduct offensive to appellant's religious principles. Even though we may consider appellant's beliefs unwise, foolish or ridiculous, in the absence of an overriding danger to society we may not permit interference therewith in the form of a conservatorship established in the waning hours of her life for the sole purpose of compelling her to accept medical treatment forbidden by her religious principles and previously refused by her with full knowledge of the probable consequences. In the final analysis, what has happened here involves a judicial attempt to decide what course of action is best for a particular individual, notwithstanding that individual's contrary views based upon religious convictions. Such action cannot be constitutionally countenanced.

* * *

While the action of the circuit court herein was unquestionably well-meaning, and justified in the absence of decisions to the contrary, we have no recourse but to hold that it has interfered with basic constitutional rights.

Accordingly, the orders of the probate division of the circuit court of Cook County are reversed.

3.

Avoiding Fraud and Duress

a.

Stammer v. Bd. of Regents, University of N.Y. 262 App. Div. 372, 29 N.Y.S. 2d 38 (1941), affirmed, 287 N.Y. 359, 39 N.E. 2d 913 (1942)

PER CURIAM.

Petitioner was licensed to practice medicine in New York State on September 19, 1919.

He is now charged with violations of paragraphs (a) and (d) of subd. 2, § 1264, of the Education Law, which provide among other things that a physician's license to practice may be suspended if he is guilty of fraud and deceit in the practice of medicine or that he undertook to cure or treat a disease by a secret formula.

One Gladys Brower was suffering from a very bad cancer on the side of her face. The photographs show that it had advanced to immense size and nearly covered one side of her face. She had received both radium and surgical treatments without avail and her family had been told that there was no hope for her, and that she would live but a short time.

Petitioner had a patient named Blakeney who had told him that he had a formula that was used in the treatment of cancer. A friend of Mrs. Brower heard about Blakeney and this treatment and went to see him. Blakeney had given this formula to petitioner who was familiar with its ingredients and knew that some of them were used in treatment of cancers of this type. Petitioner also applied the treatment to portions of his own body to make certain that there would be no ill effects from it when applied to healthy tissue. Petitioner was consulted and he examined Mrs. Brower. The patient was informed that the treatment might do some good and that it could not do any harm and consented to its use. The treatment was thus applied under petitioner's directions and in due time a complete cure was effected. Blakeney was present at some of the treatments but took no part therein. The cancerous growth disappeared entirely, the sore was completely healed and there has been no reappearance. Petitioner never submitted a bill and has never received any pay whatsoever for his services, although he made something over a hundred calls. He testified that if the formula proved satisfactory he intended to write the case up for the medical profession, that the treatment was an experiment on his part and that both he and the patient knew that. He gave the contents of the formula and made no effort to conceal the same.

At least one member of the sub-committee which conducted the hearing evidenced a wholly unfair and partial attitude. This sub-committee had the duty to conduct the hearing and weigh the testimony in a manner that should have been at least quasi-judicial. Such attitude was entirely lacking in at least the one member. This doctor effected a cure when the so-called orthodox methods of treatment had failed and now he

has been punished for it. It is not fraud or deceit for one already skilled in the medical art, with the consent of the patient, to attempt new methods when all other known methods of treatment had proved futile and least of all when the patient's very life has been despaired of. Initiative and originality should not be thus effectively stifled, especially when undertaken with the patient's full knowledge and consent, and as a last resort. Under these circumstances we fail to find fraud or deceit on the part of the petitioner or that he undertook to treat or cure disease by a secret treatment and the determination is against the weight of the evidence.

The determination should be annulled and the matter remitted.

*   *   *

b.

John P. Dawson
Economic Duress—An Essay in Perspective*

The boundaries of common law duress have been gradually expanding for more than a century. The processes of expansion are themselves of interest, as illustrating methods of growth in a system of case law. More important is the goal toward which this movement aims. For it is through duress and related ideas that private law has dealt most directly with problems raised by inequality in bargaining power. . . .

*   *   *

The concept of duress which first appeared in common law sources was merely a by-product of legal controls over crime and tort. In Bracton's treatise the specific content given duress was physical assault, exerted or threatened, by means of which transfers (in particular, transfers of land) were extorted. . . . The cancellation of transfers induced by such means was a natural supplement to the sanctions then being evolved for the control of private violence.

*   *   *

Even harder to eliminate was another restrictive formula, the requirement that the pressure or threat must be sufficient to overcome a "constant" man. The standard of "ordinary firmness" was borrowed by Bracton from the glossators, through whom it was likewise transmitted to the legal systems of continental Eu-

* 45 *Michigan Law Review* 253–255, 261–267, 272–274, 279–280, 288–290 (1947). Reprinted by permission.

rope. . . . In American cases of the nineteenth century this formula was frequently reproduced; even in the twentieth century it has occasionally put in an appearance. . . . Its chief effect was to preserve emphasis on the misconduct of the coercing party, thus distracting attention from the specific consequences to the party coerced.

* * *

Equity doctrines of undue influence had been concerned from the outset with a different type of inequality of bargaining power. They were never conceived, like common law doctrines of duress, as a corollary of the law of crime and tort. They were aimed instead at protection for the mentally or physically inadequate, whose inadequacy fell short of a total lack of legal capacity. Protection for such persons did not need to be justified through some violation, accomplished or threatened, of the law of tort or crime; indeed it was seldom that the pressure used would include any element of "wrong" as defined by damage action or criminal prosecution. It was enough that the extraction of economic gain from persons mentally or physically handicapped was condemned by prevailing standards of ethics, defined and applied by equity courts through their own independent tests.
. . . Throughout the formative period doctrines of undue influence were frequently reinforced by other protective doctrines of equity, particularly those evolved for "confidential" and "fiduciary" relationships. Close family relationships frequently provided opportunity for the exercise of "influence"; or if the parties were not related by blood or marriage, a condition of dependence by the weaker party might provide the elements of a "confidential" relationship which supplemented undue influence as ground for overhauling the transaction. . . .
It was not until the nineteenth century that serious efforts were made to explain the undue influence cases in terms of a larger objective. The objective chiefly employed soon acquired a remarkable appeal, since it coincided with main movements in nineteenth century thought. The "wrong" involved in undue influence, it was said, was the interference with another's will, which should ideally be free. The test for the existence of undue influence became the presence or absence of "free agency," whether or not the individual will have been "overpowered." From this it was easy to move to the broader thesis that, whatever the means of pressure used, "the inequity of the act consists in compelling a per-

son to do what he does not want to do." The objective defined for cases of mental or physical weakness began to seem equally appropriate for situations included in common law duress, such as threats of criminal prosecution and even duress of goods. Inspired by this new conception, the nineteenth century cases seemed to have set off in pursuit of an ideal as attractive as it was unattainable.
Even in the undue influence cases themselves, the ideal of complete freedom for the individual will was incompletely realized. In the first place, it was clear that no legal agencies would entirely eliminate the pressures that operate on the physically, mentally, or emotionally handicapped, or insulate them from all the multiplied stimuli of a complex social environment. The problem, here as elsewhere, is to select the means of pressure that are permissible and to regulate the manner in which they may be exercised. . . .
. . . It was the undue influence cases that helped most to exorcise the ghostly figure of the "constant man," who had stalked the fields of common law duress since the time of Bracton; for in the undue influence cases it was abundantly clear that the weak, the timid, the anxious and submissive were precisely the ones who should and did receive the greatest legal protection. By posing the problem of individual freedom and condemning some of the subtler forms of compulsion, the undue influence cases suggested to many courts a new approach to those other types of pressure, particularly economic pressure, which were being brought within the scope of common law duress.
Toward the end of the nineteenth century the effects of the undue influence cases were increased by the breakdown of procedural distinctions between law and equity. So long as doctrines of undue influence could be confined to "equity" cases, there remained at least a procedural distinction which preserved the purity of common law doctrine. But in the late nineteenth century and increasingly in the twentieth, undue influence was made available in law actions, both by way of defense and by way of affirmative action for restitution.
Accompanying the breakdown of divisions between law and equity there came an expansion of the content of undue influence to include various cases of psychological pressure without extreme disparities in mental or physical condition of the parties. Precise definition of the elements of undue influence had never been undertaken, indeed, had been carefully avoided. But it was

clear that the doctrine was being extended to numerous peripheral situations, just as common law duress was being pushed out beyond the typical cases on which attention had been mainly focussed. This widening range of application obscured still further the boundaries between undue influence and other types of coercion.

More rapid growth was prevented, however, by a basic contradiction in the concepts of "freedom" which were now at work. On the one hand, doctrines of undue influence were attempting to "free" the individual by regulating the pressures that restricted individual choice; on the other hand, theories of economic individualism aimed at an entirely different kind of freedom, a freedom of the "market" from external regulation. . . . From this point of view, where urgent need or special disadvantage compelled agreement to the terms proposed, these circumstances must be disregarded since they differed only in degree from the basic conditions which governed the exchange of goods and services throughout society.

To resolve this major dilemma more perspective was needed than was supplied by the materials of individual cases or the techniques of refined distinction in a system of case law. Indeed it appears that the insight gained through a close analysis of the undue influence cases helped to postpone the needed perspective, through directing attention toward a false issue. Lacking a general theory to explain the results desired, the courts approached the undue influence problem through analysis of the "will" which undue influence destroyed. It is true that in some of the more extreme cases the condition of the person "unduly" influenced might almost be described as one of complete subjection, with a "substitution" of the will of another. But even in the more extreme cases, it was usually inaccurate to say that the transfer or agreement did not result from an exercise of volition, however narrow the range within which volition could operate. In the cases of less extreme disparity, the search for evidence that the "will" had been destroyed confused the reasoning of the undue influence cases. More important than this, it left a legacy in the broader field of duress and helped to confirm the impression that relief for any type of pressure depends on a showing of complete absence of consent. This impression had filtered down from the cases of threats of physical violence, the original source of duress doctrines. Even in this type of case, courts had been slow to realize that the instances of more extreme pressure were precisely those in which the consent expressed was *more* real; the more unpleasant the alternative,

the more real the consent to a course which would avoid it.

*　　*　　*

In the meantime another body of doctrine had taken shape out of the haze which surrounds the earlier activities of the English Chancery. This doctrine, giving relief to expectant heirs, promised at first no major contribution. It aimed at a narrow objective, the protection of a landed aristocracy against its own improvidence. . . .

[The] very vagueness of Chancery doctrines . . . helped greatly in their extension to related situations. The process of extension was easiest in those cases where bargain transactions were made with persons who were physically and mentally weak. Such elements of personal disability occasionally appeared in the reversioner cases themselves, and in such cases the relations between doctrines as to sales of reversions and "undue influence" were particularly close. The contribution of the reversioner cases is more directly traceable in other situations where disparity in worldly experience was coupled with extreme poverty or pressing economic need. The English cases, in considerable variety, which awarded cancellation, could spell out no reason more precise than "fraud," "surprise," or the "unconscionable" character of the bargain. Taken together they constituted an important departure from the class bias which first inspired the reversioner cases. They also established a source, from which American courts were to draw, for a broad doctrine that inadequacy of consideration would justify cancellation when coupled with extreme disparity in knowledge, experience, or economic and social position.

*　　*　　*

[O]ne should not neglect the special rules developed in equity for the so-called "confidential" and fiduciary" relationships. Throughout this large and important group it is clear that ordinary processes of bargaining are considered inappropriate, because of unusual reliance on personal honesty and good faith that exists in fact or that is thought necessary for performance of "fiduciary" functions. In enforcing such expectations of honesty and good faith, the technique commonly used is the one already encountered in the English reversioner cases, a shift in the burden of proof. The person securing an advantage from a confidential or fiduciary relationship is required to prove not only his own full disclosure of all the relevant facts, but the fairness of the transaction as a whole. The attempt to frame substantive doctrines in terms of purely procedural handicap, together with the murky language employed in the equity cases, has disguised the main policies that are at work. Though discussion is largely in terms of false motivation ("fraud" and associated ideas), the effect is a standard of equivalence, that applies in a wide variety of personal relationships and to many types of legal transactions.

In addition there survived some broader and still vaguer doctrines of equity which admitted mere inadequacy of consideration as ground for cancellation. The language used was characteristic. After denying that equity possesses its own independent tests of adequacy of price, it was usual to add that the result was otherwise where the inadequacy was so great as to "shock the conscience." In such cases the inadequacy was said to raise a presumption of "fraud" (often expressed as a conclusive presumption), so that relief could be rested on an ancient and respectable ground of equity jurisdiction, rather than on the doubtful ground of inadequacy as such. . . .

The preceding survey was intended to suggest that the modern American law of duress reflects the convergence of several lines of growth, originally moving from sources quite distinct. The symptom of this convergence has been an increasing interplay and transfer of ideas. Its result has certainly not been a coherent body of doctrine, unified around some central proposition; on the contrary, the conflict and confusion in results of decided cases seem greater than ever before. This conflict and confusion must be attributed in part to the fact that the processes of growth are still continuing and the effects of earlier history are not yet dissipated. In part, however, they are due to the complex issues of ethics and economic policy that constantly intrude themselves and on which courts, like other agencies of organized society, must take a positive stand.

*   *   *

c.

Friedrich Kessler
Contracts of Adhesion—Some Thoughts about Freedom of Contract*

The development of large scale enterprise with its mass production and mass distribution

* 43 *Columbia Law Review* 629, 631–633, 640–642 (1943). Reprinted by permission.

made a new type of contract inevitable—the standardized mass contract. A standardized contract, once its contents have been formulated by a business firm, is used in every bargain dealing with the same product or service. The individuality of the parties which so frequently gave color to the old type contract has disappeared. The stereotyped contract of today reflects the impersonality of the market. It has reached its greatest perfection in the different types of contracts used on the various exchanges. Once the usefulness of these contracts was discovered and perfected in the transportation, insurance, and banking business, their use spread into all other fields of large scale enterprise, into international as well as national trade, and into labor relations. It is to be noted that uniformity of terms of contracts typically recurring in a business enterprise is an important factor in the exact calculation of risks. Risks which are difficult to calculate can be excluded altogether. Unforseeable contingencies affecting performance, such as strikes, fire, and transportation difficulties can be taken care of. The standard clauses in insurance policies are the most striking illustrations of successful attempts on the part of business enterprises to select and control risks assumed under a contract. The insurance business probably deserves credit also for having first realized the full importance of the so-called "juridical risk," the danger that a court or jury may be swayed by "irrational factors" to decide against a powerful defendant. Ingenious clauses have been the result. Once their practical utility was proven, they were made use of in other lines of business. It is highly probable that the desire to avoid juridical risks has been a motivating factor in the widespread use of warranty clauses in the machine industry limiting the common law remedies of the buyer to breach of an implied warranty of quality and particularly excluding his right to claim damages. . . .

The use of standard contracts has, however, another aspect which has become increasingly important. Standard contracts are typically used by enterprises with strong bargaining power. The weaker party, in need of the goods or services, is frequently not in a position to shop around for better terms, either because the author of the standard contract has a monopoly (natural or artificial) or because all competitors use the same clauses. His contractual intention is but a subjection more or less voluntary to terms dictated by the stronger party, terms whose consequences are often understood only in a vague way, if at all. Thus, standardized contracts are frequently contracts of adhesion; they are *à prendre ou à laisser....*

And yet the tremendous economic importance of contracts of adhesion is hardly reflecting the great texts on contracts or in the Restatement. As a matter of fact, the term "contract of adhesion" or a similar symbol has not even found general recognition in our legal vocabulary. This will not do any harm if we remain fully aware that the use of the word "contract" does not commit us to an indiscriminate extension of the ordinary contract rules to all contracts. But apparently the realization of the deepgoing antinomies in the structure of our system of contracts is too painful an experience to be permitted to rise to the full level of our consciousness. Consequently, courts have made great efforts to protect the weaker contracting party and still keep "the elementary rules" of the law of contracts intact. As a result, our common law of standardized contracts is highly contradictory and confusing, and the potentialities inherent in the common law system for coping with contracts of adhesion have not been fully developed. The law of insurance contracts furnishes excellent illustrations. Handicapped by the axiom that courts can only interpret but cannot make contracts for the parties, courts had to rely heavily on their prerogative of interpretation to protect a policy holder. To be sure many courts have shown a remarkable skill in reaching "just" decisions by construing ambiguous clauses against their author even in cases where there was no ambiguity. Still, this roundabout method has its disadvantages....

*   *   *

The individualism of our rules of contract law, of which freedom of contract is the most powerful symbol, is closely tied up with the ethics of free enterprise capitalism and the ideals of justice of a mobile society of small enterprisers, individual merchants and independent craftsmen. This society believed that individual and cooperative action left unrestrained in family, church and market would not lessen the freedom and dignity of man but would secure the highest possible social justice. It was firmly convinced of a natural law according to which the individual serving his own interest was also serving the interest of the community. Profits can be earned only by supplying consumable commodities. Freedom of competition will prevent profits from rising unduly. The play of the market if left to itself must therefore maximize net satisfactions.

Justice within this framework has a very definite meaning. It means freedom of property and of contract, of profit making and of trade. Freedom of contract thus receives its moral justification. The "prestabilized harmony" of a social system based on freedom of enterprise and perfect competition sees to it that the "private autonomy" of contracting parties will be kept within bounds and will work out to the benefit of the whole.

With the decline of the free enterprise system due to the innate trend of competitive capitalism towards monopoly, the meaning of contract has changed radically. Society, when granting freedom of contract, does not guarantee that all members of the community will be able to make use of it to the same extent. On the contrary, the law, by protecting the unequal distribution of property, does nothing to prevent freedom of contract from becoming a one-sided privilege. Society, by proclaiming freedom of contract, guarantees that it will not interfere with the exercise of power by contract. Freedom of contract enables enterprisers to legislate by contract and, what is even more important, to legislate in a substantially authoritarian manner without using the appearance of authoritarian forms. Standard contracts in particular could thus become effective instruments in the hands of powerful industrial and commercial overlords enabling them to impose a new feudal order of their own making upon a vast host of vassals. This spectacle is all the more fascinating since not more than a hundred years ago contract ideology had been successfully used to break down the last vestiges of a patriarchal and benevolent feudal order in the field of master and servant. Thus the return back from contract to status which we experience today was greatly facilitated by the fact that the belief in freedom of contract has remained one of the firmest axioms in the whole fabric of the social philosophy of our culture.

*   *   *

In the happy days of free enterprise capitalism the belief that contracting is law making had largely emotional importance. Law making by contract was no threat to the harmony of the democratic system. On the contrary it reaffirmed it. The courts, therefore, representing the community as a whole, could remain neutral in the name of freedom of contract. The deterioration of the social order into the pluralistic society of our days with its powerful pressure groups was needed to make the wisdom of the contract

theory of the natural law philosophers meaningful to us. The prevailing dogma, on the other
hand, insisting that contract is *only* a set of
operative facts, helps to preserve the illusion that
the "law" will protect the public against any
abuse of freedom of contract. This will not be
the case so long as we fail to realize that freedom
of contract must mean different things for different types of contracts. Its meaning must
change with the social importance of the type of
contract and with the degree of monopoly enjoyed by the author of the standardized contract.

NOTES

NOTE 1.
NEW YORK GENERAL OBLIGATIONS LAW (1964)
AGREEMENTS EXEMPTING LESSORS
FROM LIABILITY FOR NEGLIGENCE VOID
AND UNENFORCEABLE

§ 5–321. Every covenant, agreement or
understanding in or in connection with or collateral to any lease of real property exempting the
lessor from liability for damages for injuries to
person or property caused by or resulting from
the negligence of the lessor, his agents, servants
or employees, in the operation or maintenance
of the demised premises or the real property containing the demised premises shall be deemed to
be void as against public policy and wholly unenforceable.

NOTE 2.
FEDERAL COMMUNICATIONS COMMISSION
ADVERTISEMENT OF CIGARETTES*

*   *   *

The Commission's previous action [with regard to the advertisement of cigarettes] was designed to carry out the Congressional policy embodied in the 1965 [Cigarette Labeling and
Advertising] Act of not, in effect, barring cigarette advertisements and at the same time promoting intensive smoker-education during the
life of the Act.
    . . . It required that a broadcast licensee
presenting cigarette commercials—which convey
". . . any number of reasons why it appears desirable to smoke . . ."—must ". . . devote a significant amount of time to informing the listeners of the other side of the matter—that
however enjoyable smoking may be, it repre-

* Notice of Proposed Rule Making, 34 *Federal
Register* 1959 (1969).

sents a habit which may cause or contribute to
the earlier death of the user."

*   *   *

. . . As stated in the 1967 Report to Congress on
the Health Consequences of Smoking by the Department of Health, Education, and Welfare:

In the 3½ years since the publication of [the 1964]
report, an unprecedented amount of pertinent research has been completed, continued, or initiated in
this country and abroad under the sponsorship of
governments, universities, industry groups, and other
entities. This research has been reviewed and no
evidence has been revealed which brings into question
the conclusions of the 1964 report. On the contrary,
the research studies published since 1964 have
strengthened those conclusions and have extended
in some important respects our knowledge of the
health consequences of smoking.

The present state of knowledge of these health consequences can, in the judgment of the Public Health
Service, be summarized as follows:
    1. Cigarette smokers have substantially higher
rates of death and disability than their non-smoking
counterparts in the population. This means that
cigarette smokers tend to die at earlier ages and
experience more days of disability than comparable
non-smokers.
    2. A substantial portion of earlier deaths and
excess disability would not have occurred if those
affected had never smoked.
    3. If it were not for cigarette smoking, prac-
tically none of the earlier deaths from lung cancer
would have occurred; nor a substantial portion of the
earlier deaths from chronic bronchopulmonary diseases (commonly diagnosed as chronic bronchitis or
pulmonary emphysema or both); nor a portion of
the earlier deaths of cardiovascular origin. Excess
disability from chronic pulmonary and cardiovascular
diseases would also be less.
    4. Cessation or appreciable reduction of ciga-
rette smoking could delay or avert a substantial portion of deaths which occur from lung cancer, a substantial portion of the earlier deaths and excess disability from chronic bronchopulmonary diseases, and
a portion of the earlier deaths and excess disability of
cardiovascular origin.

*   *   *

[P]resentation of commercials promoting
the use of cigarettes is inconsistent with the obligation imposed upon broadcasters to operate in
the public interest. One of the foremost facets of
the public interest standard is public health, as
the Court pointed out in *Banzhaf* v. *F.C.C.* . . .
We are here faced with a most serious, unique
danger to public health "authenticated by official
and Congressional action. . . ." It would thus ap-

pear wholly at odds with the public interest for broadcasters to present advertising promoting the consumption of the product posing this unique danger—a danger measured in terms of an epidemic of deaths and disabilities.

The commercials do promote the use of cigarettes. As we developed in our 1967 document, that is understandably their purpose. We also note that in its 1968 report to Congress, the Federal Trade Commission concluded:

In 1964 and again in 1967, the Commission found that three principal themes dominate cigarette advertising. These are that (1) smoking and particularly the taste derived from it are satisfying; (2) smoking is associated with that which is desirable or even good; and (3) it is an activity relatively free of hazard.

A review of specimen 1967 and early 1968 advertising, obtained through the Commission's continuous monitoring program and also directly from cigarette advertisers, reveals that these three themes, the "satisfaction" theme, the "associative" theme, and the "assuaging of anxiety" (relative to the danger of cigarette smoking) theme, continue to dominate.

There is no question but that cigarette commercials have significant impact. Here we note initially that the broadcast industry is the recipient of more than 75 percent of the advertising dollar of cigarette manufacturers, in the amount of $244.4 million in 1967. This expenditure, when measured in terms of "exposures" on television to members of the broadcast audience (i.e., the number of cigarette commercials times the estimated program audience), resulted in 13.3 billion exposures in January, 1968 alone. Finally, we note that the commercials reach children to a very significant extent. . . .

*   *   *

This brings up a most important consideration—that of voluntary industry action to eliminate cigarette commercials. We specifically listed this possibility in our 1967 decision. We again stress it, and indeed regard it as a threshold matter—ahead of any final consideration of the issue by either the Commission or Congress. The broadcast industry does not accept the advertising of hard liquor. . . . Why, then, should this same industry accept cigarette commercials in the face of the public health findings. . . .

*   *   *

The proposed rule would simply provide that after a certain date, broadcast licensees shall not present cigarette advertising. . . .

The proposed rule does not affect the presentation of broadcast material concerning cigarette smoking in any other form, such as in newscasts, documentaries, roundtable discussions, etc. Licensees might adjudge that there is a controversial issue to be discussed or explored, and here we refer to all facets of the matter (including the issue of this notice, a ban on radio and TV advertising). They, of course, might well conclude that the anti-smoking messages, which contribute to an informed public in this critical area, should continue unabated, with the cigarette manufacturer afforded the opportunity to present his side in newscasts, documentaries, roundtable discussions, and other formats. . . .

*   *   *

NOTE 3.
WILLIAMS v. WALKER-THOMAS FURNITURE CO.
350 F.2d 445 (D.C.Cir. 1965)

J. SKELLY WRIGHT, CIRCUIT JUDGE:

*   *   *

[W]e hold that where the element of unconscionability is present at the time a contract is made, the contract should not be enforced.

Unconscionability has generally been recognized to include an absence of meaningful choice on the part of one of the parties together with contract terms which are unreasonably favorable to the other party. Whether a meaningful choice is present in a particular case can only be determined by consideration of all the circumstances surrounding the transaction. In many cases the meaningfulness of the choice is negated by a gross inequality of bargaining power. The manner in which the contract was entered is also relevant to this consideration. Did each party to the contract, considering his obvious education or lack of it, have a reasonable opportunity to understand the terms of the contract, or were the important terms hidden in a maze of fine print and minimized by deceptive sales practices? Ordinarily, one who signs an agreement with full knowledge of its terms might be held to assume the risk that he has entered a one-sided bargain. But when a party of little bargaining power, and hence little real choice, signs a commercially unreasonable contract with little or no knowledge of its terms, it is hardly likely that his consent, or even an objective manifestation of his consent, was ever given to all the terms. In such a case the usual rule that the terms of the agreement are not to be questioned should be abandoned and the court should consider whether the terms of the contract are so unfair that enforcement should be withheld.

*   *   *

d.

Miranda v. Arizona
384 U.S. 436 (1966)

Mr. Chief Justice Warren delivered the opinion of the Court.

The cases before us raise questions which go to the roots of our concepts of American criminal jurisprudence: the restraints society must observe consistent with the Federal Constitution in prosecuting individuals for crime. More specifically, we deal with the admissibility of statements obtained from an individual who is subjected to custodial police interrogation and the necessity for procedures which assure that the individual is accorded his privilege under the Fifth Amendment to the Constitution not to be compelled to incriminate himself.

*   *   *

Today . . . there can be no doubt that the Fifth Amendment privilege is available outside of criminal court proceedings and serves to protect persons in all settings in which their freedom of action is curtailed in any significant way from being compelled to incriminate themselves. We have concluded that without proper safeguards the process of in-custody interrogation of persons suspected or accused of crime contains inherently compelling pressures which work to undermine the individual's will to resist and to compel him to speak where he would not otherwise do so freely. In order to combat these pressures and to permit a full opportunity to exercise the privilege against self-incrimination, the accused must be adequately and effectively apprised of his rights and the exercise of those rights must be fully honored.

*   *   *

At the outset, if a person in custody is to be subjected to interrogation, he must first be informed in clear and unequivocal terms that he has the right to remain silent. For those unaware of the privilege, the warning is needed simply to make them aware of it—the threshold requirement for an intelligent decision as to its exercise. More important, such a warning is an absolute prerequisite in overcoming the inherent pressures of the interrogation atmosphere. It is not just the subnormal or woefully ignorant who succumb to an interrogator's imprecations, whether implied or expressly stated, that the interrogation will continue until a confession is obtained or that silence in the face of accusation is itself damning and will bode ill when presented to a jury. Further, the warning will show the individual that his interrogators are prepared to recognize his privilege should he choose to exercise it.

The Fifth Amendment privilege is so fundamental to our system of constitutional rule and the expedient of giving an adequate warning as to the availability of the privilege so simple, we will not pause to inquire in individual cases whether the defendant was aware of his rights without a warning being given. Assessments of the knowledge the defendant possessed, based on information as to his age, education, intelligence, or prior contact with authorities, can never be more than speculation; a warning is a clearcut fact. More important, whatever the background of the person interrogated, a warning at the time of the interrogation is indispensable to overcome its pressures and to insure that the individual knows he is free to exercise the privilege at that point in time.

The warning of the right to remain silent must be accompanied by the explanation that anything said can and will be used against the individual in court. This warning is needed in order to make him aware not only of the privilege, but also of the consequences of foregoing it. It is only through an awareness of these consequences that there can be any assurance of real understanding and intelligent exercise of the privilege. Moreover, this warning may serve to make the individual more acutely aware that he is faced with a phase of the adversary system—that he is not in the presence of persons acting solely in his interest.

The circumstances surrounding in-custody interrogation can operate very quickly to overbear the will of one merely made aware of his privilege by his interrogators. Therefore, the right to have counsel present at the interrogation is indispensable to the protection of the Fifth Amendment privilege under the system we delineate today. Our aim is to assure that the individual's right to choose between silence and speech remains unfettered throughout the interrogation process. A once-stated warning, delivered by those who will conduct the interrogation, cannot itself suffice to that end among those who most require knowledge of their rights. . . . [T]he need for counsel to protect the Fifth Amendment privilege comprehends not merely a right to consult with counsel prior to questioning, but also to have counsel present during any questioning if the defendant so desires.

*   *   *

An individual need not make a pre-interrogation request for a lawyer. While such request affirmatively secures his right to have one, his failure to ask for a lawyer does not constitute a waiver. . . .

*   *   *

In order fully to apprise a person interrogated of the extent of his rights under this system then, it is necessary to warn him not only that he

has the right to consult with an attorney, but also that if he is indigent a lawyer will be appointed to represent him. Without this additional warning, the admonition of the right to consult with counsel would often be understood as meaning only that he can consult with a lawyer if he has one or has the funds to obtain one. . . .

*   *   *

If the interrogation continues without the presence of an attorney and a statement is taken, a heavy burden rests on the government to demonstrate that the defendant knowingly and intelligently waived his privilege against self-incrimination and his right to retained or appointed counsel. . . .

*   *   *

C.
To Encourage Rational Decisionmaking

1.
Allowing the Subject to Know

a.
Halushka v. University of Saskatchewan
52 W.W.R. 608 (Sask. 1965)

HALL, J. A.—The appellants, Wyant and Merriman, were medical practitioners employed by the appellant, University of Saskatchewan. The appellant, Wyant, was professor of anaesthesia and chief of the department of anaesthetics at the University Hospital. The appellant, Merriman, was director of the cardio-pulmonary laboratory. As part of their duties in the employ of the appellant, University of Saskatchewan, the appellants, Wyant and Merriman, conducted and carried out medical research projects, some of which involved the comparative study of anaesthetics. When anaesthetics were administered, the subjects were obtained from the employment office.

The respondent, a student at the University of Saskatchewan, had attended summer school in 1961. On August 21, 1961, he went to the employment office to find a job. At the employment office he was advised that there were no jobs available but that he could earn $50 by being the subject of a test at the University Hospital. The

respondent said that he was told that the test would last a couple of hours and that it was a "safe test and there was nothing to worry about."

The respondent reported to the anaesthesia department at the University Hospital and there saw the appellant, Wyant. The conversation which ensued concerning the proposed test was related by the respondent as follows:

Dr. Wyant explained to me that a new drug was to be tried out on the Wednesday following. He told me that electrodes would be put in my both arms, legs and head and that he assured me that it was a perfectly safe test, it had been conducted many times before. He told me that I was not to eat anything on Wednesday morning and I was to report at approximately nine o'clock, then he said it would take about an hour to hook me up and the test itself would last approximately two hours, after the time I would be given fifty dollars, pardon me, I would be allowed to sleep first, fed and then given fifty dollars and driven home on the same day.

The appellant, Wyant, also told the respondent that an incision would be made in his left arm and that a catheter or tube would be inserted into his vein.

The respondent agreed to undergo the test and was asked by the appellant, Wyant, to sign a form of consent. This form, entered as Ex.D.1, reads as follows:

Intensive Care
460–57–2

Halushka, Walter
72756 Jan 2 '40 MR.
Dr. Nanson

Consent for Tests on Volunteers

I, Walter Halushka, age 21 of 236–3rd Street, Saskatoon hereby state that I have volunteered for tests upon my person for the purpose of study of
Heart & Blood Circulation Response under General Anaesthesia
The tests to be undertaken in connection with this study have been explained to me and I understand fully what is proposed to be done. I agree of my own free will to submit to these tests, and in consideration of the remuneration hereafter set forth, I do release the chief investigators,
Drs. G. M. Wyant and J. E. Merriman, their associates, technicians, and each thereof, other personnel involved in these studies, the University Hospital Board, and the University of Saskatchewan from all responsibility and claims whatsoever, for any untoward effects or accidents due to or arising out of said tests, either directly or indirectly.
I understand that I shall receive a remuneration of $50.00 for *one* test
Witness my hand and seal.
[Sgd.] WALTER HALUSHKA
[Sgd.] IRIS ZAECHTOWSKI (Witness)
Date: Aug. 22/61

The respondent described the circumstances surrounding the signing of D.1, saying:

He then gave me a consent form, I skimmed through it and picked out the word "accident" on the consent form and asked Doctor Wyant what accidents were referred to, and he gave me an example of me falling down the stairs at home after the test and then trying to sue the University Hospital as a result. Being assured that any accident that would happen to me would be at home and not in the hospital I signed the form.

The test contemplated was known as "The Heart and Blood Circulation Response under General Anaesthesia," and was to be conducted jointly by the appellants, Wyant and Merriman, using a new anaesthetic agent known commercially as "Fluoromar." This agent had not been previously used or tested by the appellants in any way.

The respondent returned to the University Hospital on August 23, 1961, to undergo the test. The procedure followed was that which had been described to the respondent and expected by him, with the exception that the catheter, after being inserted in the vein in the respondent's arm, was advanced towards his heart. When the catheter reached the vicinity of the heart, the respondent felt some discomfort. The anaesthetic agent was then administered to him. The time was then 11:32 A.M. Eventually the catheter tip was advanced through the various heart chambers out into the pulmonary artery where it was positioned.

The appellants, Wyant and Merriman, intended to have the respondent reach medium depth of surgical anaesthesia. However, an endotracheal tube which had been inserted to assist the respondent in breathing caused some coughing. In the opinion of the appellant, Wyant, the coughing indicated that the respondent was in the upper half of light anaesthesia—on the verge of waking up. At 12:16 P.M., therefore, the concentration of the mixture of the anaesthetic was increased. The respondent then descended into deeper surgical anaesthesia.

At about 12:20 P.M. there were changes in the respondent's cardiac rhythm which suggested to the appellants, Wyant and Merriman, that the level of the anaesthetic was too deep. The amount of anaesthetic was then decreased, or lightened.

At 12:25 P.M. the respondent suffered a complete cardiac arrest.

The appellants, Wyant and Merriman, and their assistants took immediate steps to resuscitate the respondent's heart by manual massage. To reach the heart, an incision was made from the breastbone to the line of the armpit and two of the ribs were pulled apart. A vasopressor was administered as well as urea, a drug used to combat swelling of the brain. After one minute and 30 seconds the respondent's heart began to function again.

The respondent was unconscious for a period of four days. He remained in the University Hospital as a patient until discharged 10 days later. On the day before he was discharged, the respondent was given $50 by the appellant, Wyant. At that time the respondent asked the appellant, Wyant, if that was all he was going to get for all he went through. The appellant said that $50 was all that they had bargained for but that he could give a larger sum in return for a complete release executed by the respondent's mother or elder sister.

As a result of the experiment, the appellants concluded that as an anaesthetic agent "Fluoromar" had too narrow a margin of safety and it was withdrawn from clinical use in the University Hospital.

The respondent brought action against the appellants, basing his claim for damages on two grounds, namely, trespass to the person and negligence. The action came on for trial before Balfour, J., sitting with a jury. The respondent called Dr. Mark Baltzan, whose testimony regarding medical practice and whose expert opinion were supplemented by, and in some areas confirmed by, questions and answers from the examinations-for-discovery of the appellants, Wyant and Merriman.

The medical evidence established that the use of any anaesthetic agent involves a certain amount of risk and should be accompanied by care and caution. In general medical practice the risk involved in the use of an anaesthetic agent is balanced against the threat to life presented by the ailment to be treated. It is standard procedure to obtain a medical history of the patient and in some cases to conduct a complete physical examination before administering a general anaesthetic. The medical history is for the most part obtained by interrogating the patient himself. The taking of a medical history usually involves investigation of the functioning of certain of the organic systems. Included are questions primarily related to the heart, to ascertain whether the patient has had any specific heart disease, such as high blood pressure or rheumatic fever, in the past.

In the instant case the appellants, Wyant and Merriman, admit that the cardiac arrest would not have occurred if the respondent had not undergone the test, the arrest being caused by the anaesthetic agent used. Dr. Baltzan was of the opinion that the test itself had been well conducted. He also gave his opinion that the insertion of a catheter into the heart is not a dangerous procedure.

If a patient does not die immediately from cardiac arrest, the damage which might ensue can vary in degree from none at all to eventual death with all intermediate degrees possible. Brain damage is the usual cause of death and most of the intermediate damage occurring will be to the brain. The brain cells can be damaged either permanently or temporarily. The portion of the brain most susceptible to damage under these circumstances is that which controls the highest functions, that is, the thinking functions as contrasted to the lowest or automatic functions. Major damage is objective as the patient is totally oblivious to his surroundings. Minor degrees of damage are more subjective as they are confined to emotional and intellectual attributes and are difficult to detect clinically. Dr. Baltzan had examined the respondent prior to the trial and could find no abnormality but he stated that he knew of no equipment available today which would necessarily and unequivocally determine whether there had been minor brain damage.

In Dr. Baltzan's opinion a certain amount of pain would be associated with the incision necessary for the open massage of the heart and expected general discomfort at the site of the incision for a month or two. The respondent himself testified that he experienced a considerable amount of pain in the chest area and that a portion of his left arm was numb for approximately six weeks.

*   *   *

The respondent returned to the university in the fall of 1961. He testified that he became very tired every day and that he had to rest for about three hours before doing his homework. Although this condition did gradually improve, the respondent said that he was never able to complete his homework because of it. The respondent failed in six or seven subjects that year. He said he could not think or concentrate on problems as he had before. He therefore did not try to continue with his university course.

At the time of the trial the respondent was employed as an electrician at Thompson, Man., earning $376 per month. He stated that it was difficult for him to think or concentrate and that he could not understand instructions given to him in the course of the employment unless they were given very slowly.

The appellants, at the close of the respondent's case, moved a non-suit. The motion was denied by the trial judge. The questions then put to the jury and the answers to them were as follows:

1. Q: Did the plaintiff consent to the performance of the test made by the defendant doctors? A: No.

2. Q: If the answer to Question 1 is no, did the defendant doctors commit a trespass in the performance of the test? A: Yes.

3. Q: Were the defendant doctors or either of

them negligent in the performance of the test? A: Yes.

4. Q: If the answer to Question 3 is yes, in what respect was there negligence? A: (1) Lack of full explanation to the plaintiff of the test at the time of the so-called consent. (2) Failure to acquire medical history of the plaintiff and to perform a physical examination of the plaintiff. (3) Lack of liaison between the two defendant doctors throughout this test.

5. Q: If the answer to Question 2 or Question 3 is yes, then at what amount do you assess the plaintiff's damage? A: $22,500.00.

From these findings and the judgment thereon the appellants appeal on the grounds:

1. That the learned trial judge erred in refusing to withdraw the plaintiff's claim from the jury on the ground that there was no evidence upon which the jury could find liability against the defendants or either of them.

2. That the learned trial judge misdirected the jury in respect of the consent which had been signed by the plaintiff and further erred in instructing them that this was a case of a doctor and patient relationship whereas he should have charged the jury that it was a contractual relationship.

3. That the findings of the jury on all the questions submitted to them were perverse.

*　　*　　*

The main issue before the jury concerning the respondent's claim of trespass to the person was that of consent. The attachment of the electrodes, the administration of anaesthetic and the insertion of the catheter were each an intentional application of force to the person of the respondent. When taken as a whole they certainly constitute a trespass which would be actionable unless done with consent: See *Parmley* v. *Parmley and Yule* [1945] SCR 635, reversing (*sub nom. Yule* v. *Parmley*) [1945] 1 WWR 405, 61 BCR 116. The appellants rely upon Ex.D.1 and the conduct of the respondent as evidence of consent.

In ordinary medical practice the consent given by a patient to a physician or surgeon, to be effective, must be an "informed" consent freely given. It is the duty of the physician to give a fair and reasonable explanation of the proposed treatment including the probable effect and any special or unusual risks. . . .

*　　*　　*

It was on the basis of the ordinary physician-patient relationship that the learned trial judge charged the jury on the matter of consent. In dealing with this part of the case he said:

In the circumstances of this case I will say that before signing such a document the plaintiff was entitled to a reasonably clear explanation of the proposed test and of the natural and expected results from it.

In my opinion, the duty imposed upon those engaged in medical research, as were the appellants, Wyant and Merriman, to those who offer themselves as subjects for experimentation, as the respondent did here, is at least as great as, if not greater than, the duty owed by the ordinary physician or surgeon to his patient. There can be no exceptions to the ordinary requirements of disclosure in the case of research as there may well be in ordinary medical practice. The researcher does not have to balance the probable effect of lack of treatment against the risk involved in the treatment itself. The example of risks being properly hidden from a patient when it is important that he should not worry can have no application in the field of research. The subject of medical experimentation is entitled to a full and frank disclosure of all the facts, probabilities and opinions which a reasonable man might be expected to consider before giving his consent. The respondent necessarily had to rely upon the special skill, knowledge and experience of the appellants, who were, in my opinion, placed in the fiduciary position described by Lord Shaw in *Nocton* v. *Ashburton* (*Lord*) [1914] AC 932, 83 LJ Ch 784, when he said at p. 969:

Once . . . the relation of parties has been so placed, it becomes manifest that the liability of an adviser upon whom rests the duty of doing things or making statements by which the other is guided or upon which that other justly relies can and does arise irrespective of whether the information and advice given have been tendered innocently or with a fraudulent intent.

And at p. 972:

. . . [O]nce the relations of parties have been ascertained to be those in which a duty is laid upon one person of giving information or advice to another upon which that other is entitled to rely as the basis of a transaction, responsibility for error amounting to misrepresentation in any statement made will attach to the adviser or informer, although the information and advice have been given not fraudulently but in good faith.

Although the appellant, Wyant, informed the respondent that a "new drug" was to be tried out, he did not inform him that the new drug was, in fact, an anaesthetic of which he had no previous knowledge, nor that there was risk involved with the use of an anaesthetic. Inasmuch as no test had been previously conducted using the anaesthetic agent "Fluoromar" to the knowledge of the appellants, the statement made to the respondent that it was a safe test which had been conducted many times before, when considered in the light of the medical evidence describing the characteristics of anaesthetic agents generally, was incorrect and was in reality a non-disclosure.

The respondent was not informed that the catheter would be advanced to and through his heart but was admittedly given to understand that it would be merely inserted in the vein in his arm. While it may be correct to say that the advancement of the catheter to the heart was not in itself dangerous and did not cause or contribute to the cause of the cardiac arrest, it was a circumstance which, if known, might very well have prompted the respondent to withhold his consent. The undisclosed or misrepresented facts need not concern matters which directly cause the ultimate damage if they are of a nature which might influence the judgment upon which the consent is based.

The explanation of Ex.D.1 given by the appellant, Wyant, to the respondent could be misleading and could well serve to distract the respondent from a proper appraisal of his position.

In view of the foregoing, there was no misdirection on the question of consent of which the appellants can complain and there was evidence upon which the jury could find that the respondent gave no effectual consent or release to the appellants. The appellants cannot, therefore, succeed on their first three grounds of appeal in so far as they relate to the respondent's claim of trespass.

* * *

NOTES

NOTE 1.

Food and Drug Administration Consent for Use of Investigational New Drugs (IND) on Humans—Statement of Policy*

(a) Section 505 (*i*) of the act provides that regulations on use of investigational new drugs on humans shall impose the condition that investigators "obtain the consent of such human beings or their representatives, except where they deem it not feasible or, in their professional judgment, contrary to the best interest of such human beings."

(b) this means that the consent of such humans (or the consent of their representatives) to whom investigational drugs are administered primarily for the accumulation of scientific knowledge, for such purposes as studying drug behavior, body processes, or the course of a disease, must be obtained in all cases and, in all but exceptional cases, the consent of patients under treatment with investigational drugs or the consent of their representatives must be obtained.

(c) "Under treatment" applies when the administration of the investigational drug for diagnostic, therapeutic, or other purpose involves medical judgment, taking into account the individual circumstances pertaining to the patient to whom the investigational drug is to be administered.

(d) "Exceptional cases" as used in paragraph (b) of this section are those relatively rare cases in which it is not feasible to obtain the patient's consent or the consent of his representative, or in which, as a matter of professional judgment exercised in the best interest of a particular patient under the investigator's care, it would be contrary to that patient's welfare to obtain his consent.

(e) "Patient" means the person under treatment.

(f) "Not feasible" is limited to cases wherein the investigator is not capable of obtaining consent because of inability to communicate with the patient or his representative; for example, the patient is in a coma or is otherwise incapable of giving consent, his representative cannot be reached, and it is imperative to administer the drug without delay.

(g) "Contrary to the best interests of such human beings" applies when the communication of information to obtain consent would seriously affect the patient's well-being and the physician has exercised a professional judgment that under the particular circumstances of this patient's case, the patient's best interests would suffer if consent were sought.

(h) "Consent" means that the person involved has legal capacity to give consent, is so situated as to be able to exercise free power of choice, and is provided with a fair explanation of pertinent information concerning the investigational drug, and/or his possible use as a control, as to enable him to make a decision on his willingness to receive said investigational drug. This latter element means that before the acceptance of an affirmative decision by such person the investigator should carefully consider and make known to him (taking into consideration

---

* 32 *Federal Register* 8753 (1967); *see* 21 *Code of Federal Regulations* §130.37 (1971).

such person's well-being and his ability to understand) the nature, expected duration, and purpose of the administration of said investigational drug; the method and means by which it is to be administered; the hazards involved; the existence of alternative forms of therapy, if any; and the beneficial effects upon his health or person that may possibly come from the administration of the investigational drug.

When consent is necessary under the rules set forth in this section, the consent of persons receiving an investigational new drug in Phase 1 and Phase 2 investigations (or their representatives) shall be in writing. When consent is necessary under such rules in Phase 3 investigations, it is the responsibility of investigators, taking into consideration the physical and mental state of the patient, to decide when it is necessary or preferable to obtain consent in other than written form. When such written consent is not obtained, the investigator must obtain oral consent and record that fact in the medical record of the person receiving the drug.

NOTES

NOTE 1.

WATSON V. CLUTTS
262 N.C. 153, 159, 136 S.E. 2d 617, 621 (1964)

HIGGINS, JUSTICE.

*   *   *

Difficulty arises in attempting to state any hard and fast rule as to the extent of the disclosure required. The doctor's primary duty is to do what is best for the patient. Any conflict between this duty and that of a frightening disclosure ordinarily should be resolved in favor of the primary duty. And yet, the consent of the patient or of someone duly authorized to consent for him, except in emergencies, is required before the operation is undertaken. The surgeon should disclose danger of which he has knowledge and the patient does not—but should have—in order to determine whether to consent to the risk.

*   *   *

NOTE 2.

PUTENSEN V. CLAY ADAMS, INC.
12 CAL. APP.3d 1062, 1084, 91 CAL. RPTR. 319, 333 (1970)

MOLINARI, ASSOCIATE JUSTICE.

*   *   *

Plaintiff requested that the jury be instructed that a doctor-patient relationship is one fiduciary in nature and a doctor accordingly must reveal all pertinent information to his patient. Such request was refused. Plaintiff urges such refusal was error since there was evidence that Dr. Paley failed to apprise plaintiff of the risks involved in the heart catheterization.

It is the duty of a doctor to properly explain a contemplated procedure or operation to his patient in a manner which the patient can reasonably comprehend in order for the patient to give his informed or knowledgeable consent to the procedure or operation. Here, the evidence does not show that Dr. Paley withheld any information from plaintiff. Although plaintiff testified that Dr. Paley failed to explain the operation and its risks, she also testified that she had specifically requested not to be told about the intricacies of heart catheterization. Moreover, plaintiff, prior to the operation, looked into heart catheterization and stated she was aware of what it involved. . . . Under the circumstances of this case it may not be said that plaintiff's consent to the procedure was not an informed one. Rather, the evidence was such that Dr. Paley's attempts at explanation were prevented by plaintiff's insistence on remaining ignorant of the risks involved and that Dr. Paley acceded to this request in the exercise of his discretion on the basis that an explanation of any risk involved might result in actually increasing the risks by reason of the psychological results of the apprehension itself. Accordingly, we perceive no error in refusing the requested instruction.

*   *   *

b.

Alexander M. Capron
The Law of Genetic Therapy*

*   *   *

[A] distinction is sometimes drawn between the kind of consent needed from a patient in treatment as against that required of a subject in research. Some have argued, however, that there is no basis for a distinction between therapy and experimentation. A. C. Ivy has written that

Even after the therapy of a disease is discovered, its application to the patient remains, in part, experimental. Because of the physiological variations in the response of different patients to the same therapy, the therapy of disease is, and will always be, an ex-

---

* M. Hamilton, ed.: *The New Genetics and the Future of Man*. Grand Rapids, Michigan: Eerdmans Publishing Co. (1972). © 1971. Reprinted by permission.

perimental aspect of medicine. [T]he patient is always to some extent an experimental subject of the physician. . . .

On the theory that the medical profession agrees with Ivy that the distinction is bogus, Jay Katz has carried this argument one step further. He finds in physicians' collective "reluctance to examine" the ethics of medical experimentation a "conscious or unconscious realization that any resolution of the problems posed by human experimentation cannot be limited to research settings, but instead has far-reaching consequences for medical practice."

While there is certainly at least a grain of truth in the position that all treatment is experimentation, I do not agree that there is no distinction between the conditions for consent in the two settings. However, I take a rather heretical view of which situation sets a higher standard. As suggested by the quotation from Katz, it is usually assumed that "more" consent is needed from experimental subjects than from patients; thus, physicians fear that the standards developed for subjects will be extended to their patients, for whom physicians have traditionally been allowed to make many decisions on "best interests" grounds.

Yet if we look at these contexts carefully and focus on the psychological stance of the patient or subject, it seems to me that the standard approach has it backwards. Higher requirements for informed consent should be imposed in therapy than in investigation, particularly when an element of honest experimentation is joined with the therapy. The "normal volunteer" solicited for an experiment is in a good position to consider the physical, psychological and monetary risks and benefits to him in consenting to participate. How much harder that is for the patient to whom an experimental technique is offered during a course of treatment. The man proposing the experiment is one to whom the patient may be deeply indebted (emotionally us well as financially) for past care and on whom he is probably dependent for his future well-being; the procedure may be offered, despite its unknown qualities, because more conventional modalities have proved ineffective. Even when a successful, but slow, recovery is being made, patients offered new therapy often have eyes only for its novelty and not for its risks. To paraphrase an observation of Dr. Francis D. Moore:

People in this country have been weaned on newspaper accounts of exciting new cures. Particularly in

the field of [genetics], patients are pressing their doctors to be the subjects of innovation.

How many of those of us who heard Dr. Anderson describe the process of virus-instigated changes in genes would volunteer to have that procedure performed on ourselves tomorrow? Yet what would our responses be if we suffered from a rare genetic anomaly? The answer was given by Dr. Anderson's example of the German girls who are being treated for argininemia: "Many parents . . . would not only allow [previously untried genetic therapy], they would urge its use." Certainly, part of the difference in response of subjects and patient-subjects is based on the obvious difference in the potential benefits which may be derived from participation. But that would not entirely explain the far greater favorable response in the second situation. And while, as I argued previously, we may not wish *in any particular instance* to override the consent given by a patient whose strong desire for treatment causes him to overrate the benefits and underestimate the risks of a research technique, I believe we should nevertheless decide *as a general rule* to set higher requirements for consent and to impose additional safeguards on experimentation-with-therapy lest investigators (even unwittingly) expose "consenting" patient-subjects to unreasonable risks.

The disinterested weighing of risks and benefits suggested here is not intended to imply that patients usually ought to be excluded as subjects; in some research it may be necessary to have persons manifesting a disease or defect in order to study that condition. Yet this is not always the case. For example, the ova for research on *in vitro* human development *need not* be obtained from infertile women; these women merely provide a more compliant subject population for the necessary laproscopies (surgery on the egg follicles) than normal women would.

* * *

c.

Daedalus—NIH Working Party Ethical Aspects of Experimentation on Human Subjects*

MOORE: It does not help the surgeon one whit to have talked to the patient because the

* Sponsored by *Daedalus* and the Department of Health, Education, and Welfare, Public Health Service, National Institutes of Health. Proceedings of Working Party #3 (December 5, 1966). Reprinted by permission of Daedalus, Journal of the American Academy of Arts and Sciences, Boston, Massachusetts.

patient has no concept of the hazard involved in taking out a small piece of liver. Let me ask you, what is the hazard to the patient in taking out a small piece of liver?

KATZ: I would turn to you for the answer.

MOORE: In other words, if you cannot even answer this question, what real good is consent doing—this is an informed consent. The hazard of taking out a small piece of liver is very peculiar; it is that of a bile leak. How could the patient possibly know that? In fact, the surgeon probably doesn't know that himself.

KATZ: Could you translate what we ought to communicate to the patient about this into ordinary language?

MOORE: Well, I like your question because my answer is a categorical, "It's ridiculous." By telling that to a patient and somehow assuaging yourself, all you are doing is making yourself feel better. There has been no ethical transaction. It is a vacuum because the patient does not know anything about the hazard of taking out a bit of his liver. All you have done is to make yourself feel better because you have talked to him and he has signed something.

KATZ: What are the hazards?

MOORE: I have just told you.

KATZ: What does it mean?

MOORE: In effect, . . . [it] is a tiny hazard, but it is the hazard and it is there. All I am saying is that you have made a brushstroke, but there is nothing in the brush, nothing. You have stroked yourself, and you have stroked the patient, by having this little talk with him, but there is no advantage. Ethically the problem has been unchanged by saying to the patient, "Mr. Jones, we are planning to take your gall bladder out in the morning, do you mind terribly if we take a bit of liver out for my old friend Gus?"

KATZ: But let me carry this a step further. You have to tell him about the hazards. . . .

MOORE: Well you say, what's the hazard? and I say there have not been a great many done so I cannot give you a significant figure. I suppose if this were done in a thousand patients, one or two might have quite a sore belly for a few days. That is about all you could say. All I am trying to say is that here the patient's assumed confidence in his doctor is being taken advantage of. So where are you? You have not moved. You are still on home base.

*   *   *

RUTSTEIN: I feel that on this matter of informed consent, the majority of patients, re-gardless of educational level, probably will not understand what you are talking about. That is true. I think you have a responsibility. This does not mean that you should try to do something to a patient without explaining to him what you are going to do. You should explain to him not only what you are going to do, but what the hazards are. I think the hazards for a liver biopsy are a little more specific than Dr. Moore would imply at the moment. In any event, you ought to tell the patient the story insofar as he is able to understand it. On the other hand, I do not set much store by informed consent as an important part of this problem, because I think that any doctor who is a good doctor and who has the confidence of his patient can get his patient to do practically anything he wants. So I do not think this really has much meaning. I think the problem is to make sure that the person who is talking to the patient is honest and objective. . . .

*   *   *

Informed consent, however you look at it, has so many liabilities. I still think the doctor ought to tell a patient, as part of the job of being the patient's doctor, what the risks are. But I do not set very much store by this as a protection for the patient. Not if the doctor is also an investigator. Even though you do all of this mumble-jumble—and I still think it is fine to do it, I am in favor of doing it—but I do not think it means anything. I agree with Dr. Moore. I do not think it means anything in terms of making medical research more ethical in the long run.

*   *   *

. . . I think the patient needs other controls. I do not think [this explanation is] a control. It is a good thing to do, but I do not think it is a control.

*   *   *

BLUMGART: What you say is true but it is only an element. The patient when asked about this might come back to the doctor and say, "Is this necessary to take a piece of my liver out?" And the doctor says, "No." "Well then, I do not want to have it taken out if it is not necessary." That might also be an answer.

*   *   *

RUTSTEIN: If I may try to answer your [comment] indirectly. I think you [must distinguish between] the question of being informed [and] that of consent because you get shocking situations. [I]n New York, they actually injected living cancer cells into human beings without telling them anything about it. [T]he need for informing the patient [in such a situation] is evident. People feel very strongly that these individuals should have been told that they were being given living cancer cells. . . .

FREUND: The investigator may [perhaps] be ashamed to explain and therefore he refrains. I do not think he could bring himself to say, "My friend Gus wants a piece of liver."

KATZ: Dr. Rutstein just made a very important distinction. The concept of informed consent may have to be studied from two aspects: what needs to be disclosed and what importance to place on consent. [W]hatever [the] reasons which eventually will make the patient agree, the physician has a duty and obligation to inform [the patient] that he wants to take out a piece of liver. I think it is good for the patient, and it is good for the physician.

MOORE: I agree with that. [Moreover, from] a legal point of view, it is . . . essential for the physician to protect himself.

d.

Oliver Cope
Breast Cancer—Has the Time Come for a Less Mutilating Treatment?*

In May, 1958, a physician called and asked me to come immediately to his office to see a patient with a lump in her breast. He had arranged for her to enter the hospital the following day under the care of a well-known cancer surgeon, but at lunchtime she had dismissed him and was now asking for me. Would I please take care of her?

*   *   *

There was, indeed, a lump in one of her breasts which felt as if it were malignant. Not knowing why she had dismissed the other surgeon, I was wary in what I said. I began by reminding her that I was not sure about the nature of the lump, and that as the first step she should have a biopsy to establish its identity. I told her that we did not need to go beyond a biopsy until we had a chance to consult with each other. She agreed.

When I saw her alone at the hospital the next day, she said, "I expect you are surprised that I have asked you to care for me. I first noticed the lump in my breast several months ago. It has been slowly increasing in size. I had decided that I would do nothing about it and accept the consequences. But, recently my arthritis flared up and I had to see my physician. I did not tell him about the lump, but he, of course, found it. As I expected, he insisted that I be operated upon, and the surgeon he first chose for me unequivocally advised that I have my breast removed.

"It may seem strange to you, but I have a horror of losing my breast. I am 62, my husband is dead, and I have no thought of marrying again. However, I am still horrified by the thought of losing my breast, and I asked for you because I thought you might help me find a way to keep it."

I examined her again. The mass was large. Above the breast, under the fold of her pectoral muscles, was a smaller lump consistent with spread of cancer into the nearby lymph nodes of the axilla. Together, these two masses meant that the growth was already advanced, and, according to the criteria of the day, even radical surgery would probably only delay, not cure, the disease.

At this point, I recalled that two years before another woman in her sixties had consulted me about a lump in her breast. The lump had been a small one with a good outlook if treated by the traditional surgical operation. She had refused, however, to have her breast removed. In view of her refusal, I had asked Dr. Laurence Robbins, chief of the radiology department at Massachusetts General Hospital, to treat her by radiation. She was well and free of evidence of any residual cancer now at the time of this current patient.

I told my [patient] that I would ask Dr. Robbins to treat her with radiation if the lump proved to be malignant, as indeed it did. I also followed my promise to her to remove only the lump and not the breast. Her physician was very upset when I did not do the traditional mastectomy, and her son-in-law, also a physician, was outraged at my neglect.

After radiation of the breast and adjacent areas, the secondary lump melted away, and my patient was remarkably well for the next six years. Then suddenly she felt poorly, lost strength and weight, and died within a month at the age of 68. An autopsy revealed that no cancer cells were within the breast or the lymph nodes in the axilla, showing that the radiation had been successful in these irradiated areas. Cancer cells, however, were widely distributed

* 54 *Radcliffe Quarterly* 6–11 (No. 4, 1970). Reprinted by permission of Maryel Finney Hartung Locke, editor.

throughout her body, having escaped from the area of the breast either before or during the treatment.

*   *   *

With the knowledge which we now possess in 1970, how should cancer of the breast be treated? . . . I favor a considerable change in attitude toward treatment. Unfortunately, there are still large gaps in our knowledge which must be filled in before we will have solid, accountable treatments. For example, until the forces giving rise to cancerous tumors are identified, we will not have a vaccination or inoculation such as we now possess for poliomyelitis or a drug with the specificity that penicillin has against the streptococcus. There is room for much optimism on these points, however, since a number of investigators are pursuing leads which may prove successful in the foreseeable future. But we cannot wait for this more complete knowledge. How should we treat tumors at present?

Until physicians know more about the origin of cancer, there is room for disagreement as to what constitutes the best treatment. With this incomplete knowledge in mind, I suggest the following:

Women should know that there are alternatives. There is room now for them to have a say. They don't need to be railroaded into having their breast removed.

The physician needs to know the full diagnosis, including every bit of knowledge that can be obtained. Diagnostic procedures such as roentgenographic mammograms are helpful in directing the physician's attention.

A biopsy is essential. Under special circumstances, a needle biopsy may suffice, but since the needle offers the pathologist so little tissue to study, an open biopsy is much to be preferred. The surgeon and pathologist should examine not only the type of cell involved and the rate of proliferation, but also the cell distribution. Can cells be seen entering the blood vessels of the tumor itself? Are they confined to the tumor, or are they spreading widely through the lymph spaces? These important details cannot be identified on frozen sections. The tissue has to be properly prepared for study, which takes at least 24 hours, and then time is needed for study and consultation. The patient has the right to ask of her surgeon that he delay decision regarding definitive therapy until these questions have been answered and their meaning discussed with her. It is true that biopsy theoretically carries a risk of disseminating cancer cells

and that on this basis the breast should be removed immediately after the biopsy. But it has been shown that this danger of biopsy is slight and shrinks to unimportance when compared with the knowledge gained by waiting for the pathologist's more seasoned study.

Regarding the definitive therapy, it is to be remembered that surgery still has its good points. For those tumors of sluggish growth, it is probably the best treatment, since slowly growing types of cells are not so sensitive to radiation as are the rapidly proliferating cells.

Another argument in favor of operation is that some patients prefer psychologically to be done with the problem. The removal of the breast with the tumor in it seems to some to have eliminated the problem—out-of-sight, out-of-mind. This is, of course, a short view. In this sophisticated world, women know well that a cancer can catch up with them later. Also, some women are not aware, psychologically, of what the loss of the breast may mean to them later on, either as a mutilation or as a daily reminder that they once had cancer.

The advantages of non-surgical treatment, making use of modern radiation, are obvious. First, the two-to-three-day pause between biopsy and definitive decision enables the doctors to be sure the tumor is really malignant. From time to time, haste to get rid of the tumor has led pathologist and surgeon to believe it malignant, whereas in retrospect it was benign. A frozen section isn't good enough in the borderline cases, and unnecessary mastectomies are sometimes carried out by the overly anxious surgeon, fearful of neglecting his patient.

Second, if there is blood vessel invasion, any therapy may well be too late. Therapy should not be withheld, however, since the cells in the blood stream may not have taken root in distant organs. Nothing will have been sacrificed. If cells have taken root, palliative treatment is still indicated, and radiation is a more reasonable, less destructive palliation than surgery.

The third point is that modern radiation theoretically offers a better chance of eradicating all of the cancer than surgery. The radical mastectomy removes only the primary tumor and the nodes in the axilla. Radiation can also destroy primary tumor and axillary nodes, and in addition it may be able to eradicate cells in the internal chest nodes.

It is essential to realize that radiation, like surgery, is not without hazard. Radiation is a powerful tool and can burn healthy organs if not properly directed. The radiotherapist has to be watchful that his beam does not injure the lung or the spinal cord. The patient also must realize that during the course of the radiation there may be discomfort in swallowing as the rays hit the esophagus. Cough may also develop from the radiation's hitting the borders of the lungs. It is usually slight and transient. Some fibrosis of the breast is also to be expected. Usually minimal, it goes unnoticed by most patients; occasionally considerable, it can be alarming until its nature is understood.

A disadvantage of the radiation program is that it takes time, at least six weeks and sometimes a good deal longer. The radiation has to cover the middle of the chest on both sides, and if the esophagus feels a little hot and painful, the therapy has to be slowed up or delayed. The length of the time required, however, is not theoretically disadvantageous, since more of the cells are given the chance to come into the phase of mitosis when they are theoretically more sensitive to the radiation.

Finally, there is the psychological advantage to the woman of keeping her breast. The breast is part of woman's beauty; the art of our civilization tells us this. Woman's breasts are also a part of her sexuality. It is she who builds the infant and nourishes it after it is born. The breast is inherently part of the survival of the race. What is so strange is that the surgeon has been so slow to realize how woman feels about her breasts. The only adequate explanation for his lack of feeling is that the problem of mutilation is too much for him to manage. Only when mutilation is put to him in terms of an analogy—the loss of his masculinity—does he react to it.

Woman has been willing to put up with a mastectomy when she was told there was no other way to rid her of the tumor. Now that there is a feasible alternative, the efforts of medicine should be directed toward improving the non-mutilating therapy. She has a right to demand this of the profession.

NOTE

Jon R. Waltz and Thomas W. Scheuneman
Informed Consent to Therapy*

*   *   *

The informed consent concept, clearly enough, separates into two elements: informa-

* 64 *Northwestern University Law Review,* 628, 637–640, 643–645 (1969). Reprinted by special permission of the Northwestern University Law Review. Copyright © 1970.

tion and consent. A two-fold duty is imposed: the physician must disclose certain information about collateral risks, and he must not proceed without consent to the risks which were, or should have been, disclosed. The cases have been concerned primarily with the duty of information disclosure but the scope and content of both duties must be analyzed since each poses separate and difficult legal puzzles. Ideally, a patient will be informed of all possible collateral risks of contemplated therapy and his consent to confronting them will then insulate his physician from liability if any described risk materializes. The broad problems for analysis are the necessary and the acceptable limitations on the realization of this ideal.

The "information" element of informed consent concerns the scope of the physician's duty to disclose collateral risks. This duty becomes relevant when the patient neither knows nor could be expected to know of particular collateral risks. There is no need to disclose risks that either ought to be known by everyone or that are in fact known to the patient because of prior experience with the therapy in question.

*   *   *

A physician probably need not disclose every risk which *could* be disclosed, if only because of the time required to disclose every remote risk. Less than "total" disclosure will satisfy the law's demands, but how much less?

*   *   *

The question of what risks of therapy should be disclosed to the patient must take two interests into account. The first interest is the patient's desire and right, at least under other than life-preserving conditions, to make his own decision whether to undergo a particular therapy. The law, to serve this interest, must assess the significance of a risk in terms of the potential effect of knowledge of it on the patient's decision. The law must, as a matter of policy, set the level of effect which will be deemed significant. The traditional legal litmus for measuring the significance of information in decision-making is "materiality." Since the patient's interest in making an informed decision is paramount, the first principle is that all material risks should be disclosed to him. The content of the standard of materiality of risks will therefore determine the scope of the duty to disclose. Materiality of risk is thus the first issue in the duty to disclose.

The second interest, sometimes at odds with the first, is the physician's desire to withhold information about risks the disclosure of which may have a harmful effect on the well-being of the patient. . . .

Materiality is the keystone of the physician's duty to disclose. The first task, then, is to determine what risks are material and, therefore, to be disclosed in the absence of a privilege to withhold. While the cases have not clearly articulated standards of materiality, two have been proposed by commentators. It has been suggested, at one extreme, that only risks which would cause the patient to forego the therapy need be disclosed. At the other extreme, it has been argued that any risk which might have any influence, however slight, on the patient's decision to accept a therapy should be disclosed.

The first standard is myopic. It does not take into account the fact that although a single risk of a given magnitude may not cause a patient to forego a therapy, two or more such risks in combination might have that result. A standard of materiality limited to risks which, in isolation, would cause a patient to refuse a therapy deprives the patient of the opportunity to contemplate possible combinations of risks. Conversely, a rule inflexibly dictating disclosure of all risks, however unlikely they are to affect a patient's judgment, is unrealistic. We must reach middle ground.

The materiality of a risk must be determined in the first instance by the physician. Since he must first know how much impact a risk must have on the patient's judgment before its disclosure is dictated, the issue should be approached from the physician's point of view. The ideal rule would require that a risk be disclosed when the patient would attach importance to it, alone or in combination with others, in making his decision whether or not to consent to the therapy in question. But a physician obviously cannot be required to know the inner workings of his patient's mind. He can, however, employ his general experience with people. He can be required to exercise a sense of how the average, reasonable man would probably react. Additionally, he will know, or can reasonably be required to know, his particular patient's background, present circumstances and prognosis. In resolving the materiality issue, the physician—and the courts—can apply the standard of the reasonable man who finds himself in the position of the patient.

A risk is thus material when a reasonable person, in what the physician knows or should know to be the patient's position, would be likely to attach significance to the risk or cluster of risks in deciding whether or not to undergo the proposed therapy.

*　*　*

Consent . . . connotes the dual elements of awareness and assent. To establish consent to a risk, it must be shown both that the patient was aware of the risk and that he assented to encounter it. The hard question involves the kind of evidence that will be admitted to establish these elements.

Preliminarily, it is obvious that a risk must have been understandably communicated before the element of awareness can be established. Communication involves the manner in which the physician must disclose risks—the vocabulary he must adopt and the degree of elaboration in which he must engage. While the cases rightly indicate that technical language will not ordinarily suffice to disclose a risk to an untutored layman, they are unclear as to what more is required. To require the physician, absolutely, to use language which his patient will in fact understand calls, once again, for clairvoyance. Furthermore, any such requirement would be logically untenable within the concepts of semantics. One can only communicate in terms which, based on experience and perceptions of the recipient's capacity, one believes he will understand. Translated to the legal framework, the physician should be required to disclose risks in such terms as a reasonable man would believe the patient would understand. The disclosure should elaborate, in the same sort of terms, the nature and severity of the risk and the likelihood of its occurrence.

Some courts apparently take the approach that only the subjective state of mind of the patient should be considered in establishing the elements of awareness and assent. Under this approach, a physician could proceed only where the patient subjectively understood a risk and subjectively intended to manifest his assent to it. One difficulty with this view is that the patient's testimony, undeniably admissible at trial, in fact controls the issue of consent. And the trial lawyer's healthy cynicism tells him that a claimant's testimony is sometimes susceptible to modification based upon hindsight. Another difficulty is that it leaves no room for reasonable communication or interpretation mistakes by the physician; he assumes the risk of incorrectly concluding that the patient in fact understood and assented to the risks communicated. As the entire history of contract law attests, legal relationships based on communication cannot practically be made to depend on the vagaries of the parties' subjective intent.

*   *   *

2.

Helping the Subject to Decide

a.

Russell v. Harwick
166 So. 2d 904 (Fla. 1964)

CARROLL, JUDGE.

The appellee Charlotte Harwick fell and broke her hip. Following an operation and treatment by the appellant Dr. Lyle Russell, an orthopedic surgeon, Mrs. Harwick sued Dr. Russell and others charging negligence and trespass to the person. . . . A jury trial resulted in a verdict against Dr. Russell. . . . Dr. Russell has appealed.

The complaint alleged that Dr. Russell was negligent in failing to inform the plaintiffs as to the alternate methods of surgical treatment he contemplated, and in proceeding without the informed consent of the plaintiffs; that had they been informed of such alternative procedures they would not have consented to the procedure utilized. . . .

*   *   *

Mrs. Harwick was treated by Dr. Harris, an internist, and Dr. Russell, the orthopedic surgeon. Dr. Harris was a friend of the plaintiffs and had rendered professional service to them in the past. They engaged him to take charge of the case. His training fitted him to supervise the medication, but not the surgical processes. There was an issue and conflicting evidence on whether the plaintiffs were informed as to the nature of the operative processes contemplated and recommended by the surgeon, and their risks, dangers, and outcome probabilities. A jury question was presented as to whether the consent given for surgery by Mrs. Harwick was an informed consent.

The doctor attempted as a first process to reduce the fracture by manipulation to be secured with the use of a nail. Unable to obtain the proper positional result in that process, Dr. Russell proceeded with an alternative process

in which he performed an operation of severing the head of the femur and substituting therefor a metal (Austin Moore) prosthesis. This operation amounted to major surgery, and one which was calculated to result in some change in the length of the leg. The plaintiffs stated that had they known this was the intended or contemplated procedure they would have insisted on an orthopedic consultation, and would not have been in favor of the process.

. . . There was also an issue and conflicting evidence from which the jury could have found for or against the defendant doctor as to the need or propriety of the process undertaken in view of the lack of emergency and the circumstances of the injury as then present.

*   *   *

Basically, this appeal amounts to a contention of want of evidence or of sufficient evidence on the material issues. We find no such deficiency in the record, and our examination of the record leads to the conclusion that the verdict was justified and had adequate evidentiary support.

*   *   *

Affirmed.

DUVAL, ASSOCIATE JUDGE (dissenting).

I can not agree with the conclusions reached in the majority opinion.

*   *   *

Dr. Russell was personally retained by Mrs. Harwick on the evening of her accident for the purpose of caring for her condition. After examining the x-rays he informed her it would be necessary for him to operate in order to repair her hip, to which she consented.

Mrs. Harwick had sustained a complicated fracture of the neck of the femur with damage to the head. All the medical testimony agreed there were two generally accepted procedures to repair such a break. One was to try and manually reduce the fracture and fasten it with a nail or pin. The other was to remove the head of the femur and substitute a metallic prosthesis. All medical witnesses testifying agreed that if a correct alignment could not be accomplished that nailing could not be used.

In this case Dr. Russell first attempted to manually reduce the fracture and failed. If he had succeeded he would have opened the hip, drilled a hole up through the femur into the head of the femur, inserted a pin, closed the incision completing the operation. After being unable to obtain a manual reduction of the fracture he proceeded with the alternative method of removing the head of the femur and replacing it with a metallic prosthesis.

There was a difference of opinion between the doctors testifying as to what action they would have taken after manual reduction failed, a failure quite common in this type of fracture. Several testified they would have cut open the hip capsule and attempted to reduce the fracture manually and, if successful, drill and place a pin through the top of the head of the femur down into the femur. Others testified that they would have opened the capsule, but instead of attempting to drill and pin through the top of the head of the femur would remove the head and replace it with a metallic prosthesis, using the same procedure followed by Dr. Russell.

All the medical testimony recognized both alternative procedures of repair, after manual reduction failure, to be recognized and approved methods of treatment and would leave the procedure selected to the judgment of the individual doctor performing the operation. Each of the procedures described entailed complicated and major surgery.

The fact that certain physicians would have proceeded in a different manner than the defendant is not a basis for malpractice. The Supreme Court of Florida has held that the courts cannot hold a defendant in a malpractice suit to the theory of one physician to the exclusion of the contrary opinion by another physician, if the treatment used is approved by a respectable minority of the medical practice. The treatment afforded by Dr. Russell was approved by the majority of physicians testifying in this case and was not disapproved by any.

*   *   *

Mrs. Harwick's third count alleged that the defendants were liable on a theory of trespass to the person for the reason that in adopting the surgical procedure utilized they failed to inform the plaintiff of the alternative procedures available and the potential consequences involved in the repair of the hip operation.

Liability for failure to fully inform a patient as to all the alternative procedures available and the potential consequences in an operation is relatively new in Florida. . . .

*   *   *

The question is whether or not Dr. Russell was legally required, under the circumstances of this case, to detail to Mrs. Harwick all of the procedures involved and did such a failure cause him to be liable under the theory of operating without the informed consent of the patient.

*   *   *

This is not a case where the doctor misrepresented any material facts or used false misrepresentation in an attempt to gain the consent of his patient to operate.

In reviewing this record it is found that in addition to the alternative methods of repair discussed, there were other recognized and acceptable methods as well as a great number of individual techniques used in the performance of these operative procedures. In addition, the record discloses that there are many different types of nails or pins used and a number of different metallic prosthesis available (at least thirty) for use. Would it, in order to have the informed consent of the patient, have been necessary to detail each of the many methods, techniques and appliances which could be used? Would such information assist a patient in making an intelligent choice? I think not.

*   *   *

In this case Mrs. Harwick personally retained Dr. Russell's services for the purpose of repairing her hip. Dr. Russell advised her of the necessity to operate in order to accomplish her wishes. She was advised of the necessity of the operation thirty-six (36) hours prior to the surgery. During the elapsed time she spoke with Dr. Harris; she had her husband by her side for most of the day; she was alert and knew what the situation was. She testified that she relied on Dr. Russell to do whatever was necessary to relieve her condition. She did not request him or anyone to advise her of what specific method of repair was going to be attempted. Mrs. Harwick was not limited in any way in making inquiry concerning the details of the surgery. It was her prerogative to rely on the professional judgment of the Defendant without making further inquiry, which she did.

*   *   *

There are no cases, that I have been able to find, which require a physician having consent, not gained by misrepresentation, to describe to his patient each technique or procedure available before proceeding with a required and necessary operation. If a patient must have an operation, it is not required that a physician describe all of the gory details and further disturb the patient. The patient in most cases has no desire to have the physician describe all of the details. However, if the patient wishes to have such a description, it would be his duty to inquire and the physician's duty to give reasonable and prudent answers.

The issue of informed consent should not have been submitted to the jury.

* * *

NOTES

NOTE 1.

MICHAEL JUSTIN MYERS
INFORMED CONSENT IN MEDICAL MALPRACTICE*

* * *

It is submitted that the law's strong predisposition toward personal control over bodily invasions has been violated by the current judicial treatment of informed consent. That predisposition could be more effectively served if the following standard were adopted:

A physician is under an obligation (1) to make a full disclosure of all known material risks in a proposed operation or course of treatment except for those risks of which the patient is likely to know or (2) to prove the reasonableness of any lesser disclosure or the immateriality of the undisclosed risk.

* * *

Where there is no problem of consent, and where harm results from an operation, the doctor need only compensate the patient for negligence. Since the patient bears the entire risk of nonnegligent injury and is concerned with his own interests as no other person can be, it is only fair to allow him to choose between accepting or rejecting the hazards of a proposed treatment even if his choice is irrational.

If a squeamish individual would rather not know about the potential hazards of treatment, he may delegate control to his physician through a conscious, knowing waiver. The physician presumably desires the best for his patient. But the doctor who proceeds under the doctor-knows-best theory without securing a deliberate waiver from his patient and without disclosing collateral hazards substitutes his judgment about the de-

* 55 *California Law Review* 1396, 1407–1410 (1967). Copyright, © 1967, California Law Review, Inc. Reprinted by permission.

sirability of undergoing a risk for that of his patient. Such substitution is inconsistent with the law's respect for the patient's control over his own body. . . .

It is objectionably paternalistic for a physician to justify nondisclosure of risks on the ground that otherwise "both the patient and [physician] would back out." To tolerate such argument is to subordinate the patient's control of his body to his physician's absolute discretion.

* * *

NOTE 2.

HENRY K. BEECHER
CONSENT IN CLINICAL EXPERIMENTATION—
MYTH AND REALITY*

* * *

There is the disturbing and widespread myth that "codes" (all of which emphasize, above all else, consent) will provide some kind of security. While there is value, doubtless, to be gained from their examination as guides to the thinking of others on the subject, the reality is that any rigid adherence to codes can provide a dangerous trap: no two situations are alike; it is impossible to spell out all contingencies in codes. When an accident occurs, in the course of experimentation, it will be easy for the prosecution to show failure to comply fully, and an endless vista of legal actions opens up. It is a curious thing that lawyers for even the greatest institutions are much more likely, in my experience, to cripple themselves and their institutions with inevitably imperfect codes than are the investigators involved, who usually understand the pitfalls represented by the codes. Security rests with the *responsible* investigator who will refer difficult decisions to his peers.

Most codes dealing with human experimentation start out with the bland assumption that consent is ours for the asking. This is a myth. The reality is that informed consent is often exceedingly difficult or impossible to obtain in any complete sense. The difficulties inherent in this complex situation are no excuse for giving up the effort: informed consent is a goal toward which we strive. . . . Imperfect as our attempts to get informed consent may be, an important reality nevertheless invariably emerges from such effort: The patient involved then knows he is to be the subject of an experiment—too often not

* 195 *Journal of the American Medical Association* 34–35 (1966). Reprinted by permission.

otherwise the case—and, knowing, can reject the opportunity if he chooses to do so.

* * *

A different kind of myth is that propounded by some critics; namely, that if the investigator *says* he got consent all is well. . . . Far more dependable evidence of right or wrong is to be found in examination of the given investigation itself. It is clear that many published studies never should have been undertaken in the first place.

* * *

A particularly pernicious myth is the one that depends on the view that ends justify means. A study is ethical or not at its inception. It does not become ethical merely because it turned up valuable data. Sometimes such a view is rationalized by the investigator as having produced the most good for the most people. This is blatant statism. Whoever gave the investigator the god-like right of choosing martyrs?

Is the patient, then, without hope for honest, responsible care? Not at all. His great safeguard in experimentation as in therapy is the presence of the skillful, informed, intelligent, honest, responsible, compassionate physician. And one hopes and believes these are in the majority.

b.

Ralph J. Alfidi
Informed Consent—
A Study of Patient Reaction*

I have questioned a number of physicians concerning their reactions to obtaining an informed consent from the patient who is about to undergo a diagnostic or therapeutic procedure. Their reactions vary from (1) "I always inform my patients of what is coming, and the possible complications," to (2) "I never do it; it's a waste of time," to most frequently, (3) "If I give my patients a comprehensive explanation of what is to be done and what possible complications might ensue, the result would be the wholesale refusal of patients to undergo the procedure." For many years, I advocated the latter.

* * *

. . . When this statistical study of informed consent was begun, it was expected to prove that

* 216 *Journal of the American Medical Association* 1325–1329 (1971). Reprinted by permission.

patients would indeed refuse angiography after they were informed of its possible complications. Much to my surprise it proved the opposite.

Two forms were used in this study. The second form was prepared because of the objections of my colleagues to the content and construction of the first form. . . . The first form was presented to 132 patients before angiography.

FORM I
DEPARTMENT OF HOSPITAL RADIOLOGY—
SPECIAL PROCEDURE SECTION
INFORMED CONSENT FOR ARTERIOGRAPHY
AND PHLEBOGRAPHY

Dear Patient,
Your doctor has referred you to us for an angiogram (a study of your blood vessels). We would like to inform you of what we are going to do and of possible complications that might result from this procedure.

A small tube (catheter) will be introduced into one or several of your blood vessels. Later we will inject a dye which is opaque to x-rays. This will enable us to see blood vessels in your body which may be diseased. The catheter will be introduced into an artery either in your groin or at times in your arm, just above the elbow. This is done either by puncturing the artery with a needle, or through the means of minor surgery. The study is done under local anesthesia.

Although the possibility of clotting the vessel used is small, it does happen occasionally. In addition, it is possible that an artery or arteries feeding an organ could also be clotted. In either of these circumstances, it may be necessary to perform surgery to remove the clot or to treat you with certain medications which may dissolve the clot. I am sure you realize that although the risk is very small, clotting the blood supply to an organ can result in the loss of that organ and, remotely, in the loss of life. The latter is true of other complications but is just as rare.

During the procedure, it is possible that dye (contrast medium) might result in an adverse reaction causing hives, shortness of breath, extremely low blood pressure, and, rarely, temporary or permanent paralysis.

Upon removing the catheter, it is occasionally difficult to stop bleeding; a small lump (hematoma) may form at the point where the catheter was introduced into the blood vessel. These generally subside in several days; however, large hematomas may have to be treated with surgical evacuation and the hole in the artery sewed shut. More rarely, but another possibility, a small tear may develop in the blood vessel resulting in what we call pseudoaneurysm, which acts like a bulge in a weakened rubber tire. This may also require corrective surgery.

There are still more unusual complications which we could mention, but because they are so rare it would be impractical to list them. If you desire, these will be discussed with you.

Our overall "serious" complications rate is approximately 1 in 500 cases. Your chances of being injured in an auto accident in the United States during 1969 were 1 in 100.

Unfortunately, this information may have alarmed you, but I believe it to be in your best interests to know what is involved.

Sincerely,

This form was presented to patients by the residents or nursing staff of our department. In general, no explanation was given until the form was read and completed. Anxious patients and patients who refused on the basis of the information given were approached by members of the professional staff to allay apprehension and to dissuade those who had refused the procedure. Form 1 most frequently was given to the patients about an hour before the angiogram and before any premedication had been administered.

Initial objections to this form by colleagues were: (1) too strongly worded; (2) too weakly worded; (3) did not provide actual mortality statistics and therefore no reference point of ultimate risks; (4) did not state that the referring physician had weighed the risks vs the advantages, and that the latter were much greater than the former; (5) objections to inclusion of the questionnaire within the form. Some felt that the questions should be appended on the last page. Because of the objections and questions concerning the above, a revised form was substituted and presented to the next 100 patients on whom angiograms were performed.

FORM II
CONSENT FOR ANGIOGRAPHY

Dear Patient,

Your doctor has referred you for an angiogram, which is a study of your blood vessels. This is one of the most accurate studies we can make concerning the condition of your blood vessels. As with all medical procedures, it carries some risks, about which we think you should be informed. Your doctor is aware of these risks and has determined that the benefit in diagnostic information which may be obtained from the arteriogram outweighs the potential risk of the procedure.

In this procedure, a small tube (catheter) is introduced into one or several of your blood vessels. Through this tube, a solution will be injected which will enable us to see your blood vessels on x-rays. This tube is introduced into a blood vessel, either in your arm or your groin, by means of minor surgery under local anesthesia.

Patients, understandably, wonder what complications can occur from this procedure. It does involve some minor surgery and it does involve entering the body and the blood stream. The usual complications which we would consider relatively minor, but nevertheless can be distressing to patients, are accumulations of blood in the tissues where the catheter has been introduced (hematoma) or a small outpouching of the artery at the site where it was entered by the catheter. There are less frequent complications which we consider more serious, which might lead to serious damage or to loss of an organ. Surgery may be required to correct the complication.

Very rarely, complications from the procedure have resulted in death. This has occurred four times in the 6,500 angiograms we have performed.

Our overall serious complications rate is approximately one in 500 angiograms.

It would be impractical, and probably misleading to the average person, to describe here in detail all of the complications which might possibly result from this procedure. If you would like more detailed information, we will be glad to discuss it with you.

Sincerely yours,

An attempt was made to give this form to each patient as early as possible either on the night or day before the angiogram. This was partially successful but a number of patients received the forms shortly before the angiograms because they had not been prescheduled, and angiography had been requested only a few hours before. In one emergency situation no attempt was made to obtain an informed consent.

*   *   *

TABLE 1

Responses of 132 Patients to Questionnaire for Informed Consent Form 1*

Questions	Yes	No	Not Checked	Incompletely Checked
1. Did you appreciate receiving this information?	107	12	6	7
2. Has this information disturbed you?	46	69	6	11
3. Do you desire further information regarding very rare complications?	8	109	6	9
4. Has this information caused you to change your mind as to whether to go through with this procedure?	5	113	6	8
5. Would you have preferred that we withheld information concerning possible complications?	21	103	6	2

* One hundred thirty patients consented; 5 patients refused consent, but after personal discussion with physician, 3 consented, leaving 2 patients who ultimately refused. Six patients checked none of questions but gave consent. Remaining disparity is due to incomplete checking.

The straightforward and perhaps even harsh statements of the possible complications of angiography were accepted and desired by the majority of patients. Eighty percent of patients responding to form 1 and 89 percent of patients responding to form 2 answered question 1 affirmatively (the context of both questions is essentially the same).

In responding to form 1, question 2, approximately 35 percent of the patients were disturbed by the information; nevertheless all but two consented. This question was modified and included in section 4C of form 2, where 27 percent of patients stated that they were made less comfortable by this information. In both forms only a few patients asked for more information concerning the complications. The incidence of these questions in form 2 is twice that in form 1 and may be related to the fact that the content of form 2 was generally felt less likely to cause apprehension.

Questions 1 and 5 in form 1 are similar but expressed differently. At first glance there seems to be considerable disparity, but comparing the incompletely checked portion of Table 1, this disparity is greatly lessened. I have interpreted this to mean that seven patients who did not complete question 1 did not wish to express their distaste for this information, but when it came to question 5, they felt it easier to say what they wanted.

In all, 228 of 232 patients consented to an-giography after a straightforward disclosure of possible complications. Four refused the procedure; their reasons for refusal will be commented upon.

*   *   *

Approximately 2 percent of the patients in this study refused angiography on the basis of the consent form itself. It must be remembered that this is a diagnostic procedure and it is possible that no additional diagnostic information might be gained from it. This is in contrast to the necessity for a therapeutic procedure such as cholecystectomy or appendectomy when the patient's plight would probably produce a higher percentage of consent; probably few would refuse.

The four patients who refused this procedure cannot be placed in any specific category. One patient expressed hostility. There is the hypothetical question of whether this patient would have brought suit if a complication had occurred during angiography without informed consent. Another patient who refused seemed to be a reasonable individual; yet when he weighed the risks vs the advantages and benefits of the angiogram, he elected not to have the angiogram. Still another patient refused on the basis of fear of complications. . . . The form had been presented to the patient at a time when we knew that only a pulmonary angiogram was requested. Upon examining the patient and his chart, as

TABLE 2
Responses of 100 Patients to Questionnaire for Informed Consent Form 2*

Questions	Yes	No	None Checked	Incompletely Checked
1. Do you regard the above information as useful?	89	3	4	11
2. Do you think all patients should receive the above information?	74	12	4	8
3. Do you desire further information regarding specifics of possible medical complications of this procedure?	15	73	4	6
4. Has this information caused you to change your mind as to whether to go through with this procedure? (a) Makes me more comfortable going ahead with it, 34. (b) Did not affect me one way or the other, 30. (c) Makes me less comfortable going ahead with the procedure, 27. (d) Has caused me to decide not to go ahead with the procedure, 2.			4	3

* Ninety-eight patients consented, two refused. One patient refused after further discussion with physician. No attempt was made to discuss second patient's refusal, as there was only questionable indication for procedure. Four patients checked none of questions but gave consent.

we do normally before an angiogram, we found questionable indications for a pulmonary angiogram and made no effort to change this patient's mind.

The following paragraph was included in both of the informed consent forms.

It would be impractical and probably misleading to the average person to describe here in detail all the complications which might possibly result from this procedure. If you would like more detailed information we would be glad to discuss it with you.

We felt it necessary to add this paragraph for three reasons. First, we felt that to list all of the known complications which we have thus far encountered would simply increase apprehension. Secondly, [we felt] that, although rare, new complications are reported now and then, and that the form itself would be invalid should one of these very rare complications occur. Third, it would be impossible to list all possible complications. . . .

* * *

. . . We believe that we have proven that the majority of patients not only have a right to know but want to know what possible complications may be expected from any given procedure. The concern that informing a patient of possible complications will result in his refusal of the procedure is now outmoded.

NOTE

ELEANOR S. GLASS
RESTRUCTURING INFORMED CONSENT—
LEGAL THERAPY FOR THE DOCTOR-PATIENT
RELATIONSHIP*

* * *

In assessing whether the doctor acted reasonably, courts should adopt a patient's, or layman's, standard of care. The jury would decide whether the doctor disclosed enough information for the reasonable patient to make an intelligent decision. The jury should not undertake a subjective inquiry into what the individual patient actually understood or whether he acted intelligently. Presumably the plaintiff will present evidence regarding material facts that were not disclosed. The jury's task is to determine whether the information actually withheld would have been relevant for the jury members themselves, for their judgment is by definition that of the reasonable patient. They make this deter-

* 79 *Yale Law Journal* 1533, 1559–1562 (1970). Reprinted by permission of the Yale Law Journal Company and Fred B. Rothman & Company.

mination in the light of the knowledge about a given procedure which is available to the medical profession. Thus whether a piece of undisclosed information would have been relevant for their own decision is the only question which the jury need resolve, unless the doctor claims that the patient was for some reason "unreasonable." If the jurors find the information irrelevant, the doctor acted reasonably in withholding it. If they find it relevant, the doctor acted unreasonably and will be held liable for failure to obtain informed consent.

* * *

In addition to a different standard of care, the restructured law of informed consent also should have at its center formal rules of disclosure stipulating the minimum amount of information that a reasonable patient must be told before his consent is requested. The doctor ought to initiate discussion with his patient on the following substantive topics: the diagnosis; the physician's choice of treatment; the physician's experience with this treatment; the methods to be used; the risks involved, major and collateral; expected pain and discomfort; the benefits of this treatment; alternatives to this treatment; prognosis. Any omission from this list would constitute a prima facie violation of the physician's duty to disclose and liability would ensue. The physician must at least mention basic facts within each category.

Determinations about the relevance of collateral methods, risks, pains or alternatives are within the province of the jury. Expert testimony should be received only to inform the jury about specific treatments. No inquiry should be permitted into the "practice" of professionals in disclosing these procedures. Under a restructured law of informed consent, the job of the medical professional will be the job of the traditional expert witness—to inform the jury about facts, not to establish the rule which governs the interpretation of facts.

These substantive requirements should not deter doctors from expressing their uncertainties about the course of treatment. Doctors should convey their uncertainties as clearly as possible, so that the patient will not rely on vague probabilities as facts. . . .

In administering the substantive requirements, the court should be prepared to look beyond *pro forma* compliance. At the request of the plaintiffs, it should allow evidence that the patient was told information that apparently satisfied the requirements but was informed in a manner which did not allow him to understand —and to question—the analysis imparted by the doctor. The court could allow an inquiry into whether the doctor asked for questions from the patient about what he had disclosed, and whether he indicated a willingness to continue the discussion at the patient's request.

The patient should also be allowed the right to waive the doctor's compliance with the substantive requirements. But the law must provide safeguards against the doctor's abuse of this waiver—an abuse which would subvert the restructured law of informed consent. The problem, of course, is how to determine whether the patient's waiver is based on a genuine understanding that he is giving up his right to be informed. Two safeguards should be required, at least. The doctor should give an explicit statement indicating what the waiver entails and that he is willing to continue the discussion, before he accepts the waiver. A third party, preferably friend or relation, should also be present to corroborate, in so far as possible, that the waiver was given voluntarily and knowingly.

* * *

D.
To Protect the Experimental Process

1.

Increasing Investigator-Subject Communication

Paul Ramsey
The Patient as Person—
Explorations in Medical Ethics*

* * *

[A]ny human being is more than a patient or experimental subject; he is a *personal* subject—every bit as much a man as the physician-investigator. Fidelity is between man and man in these procedures. Consent expresses or establishes this relationship, and the requirement of consent sustains it. Fidelity is the bond between consenting man and consenting man in these procedures. The principle of an informed consent is the cardinal *canon of loyalty* joining men together in medical practice and investigation. In this requirement, faithfulness among men—the faithfulness that is normative for all the covenants or moral bonds of life with life—gains specification for the primary relations peculiar to medical practice.

Consent as a canon of loyalty can best be exhibited by a paraphrase of Reinhold Niebuhr's celebrated defense of democracy on both positive and negative grounds: "Man's capacity for justice makes democracy possible; man's propensity to injustice makes democracy necessary." Man's capacity to become joint adventurers in a common cause makes the consensual relation possible; man's propensity to overreach his joint adventurer even in a good cause makes consent necessary. In medical experimentation the common cause of the consensual relation is the advancement of medicine and benefit to others. In therapy and in diagnostic or therapeutic investigations, the common cause is some benefit to the patient himself; but this is still a joint venture in which patient and physician can say and ideally should both say, "I cure."

Therefore, I suggest that men's capacity to become joint adventurers in a common cause makes possible a consent to enter the relation of patient to physician or of subject to investigator. This means that *partnership* is a better

term than *contract* in conceptualizing the relation between patient and physician or between subject and investigator. The fact that these pairs of people are joint adventurers is evident from the fact that consent is a continuing and a repeatable requirement. We can legitimately appeal to permissions presumably granted by or implied in the original contract only to the extent that these are not incompatible with the demands of an ongoing partnership sustained by an actual or implied *present* consent and terminable by any present or future dissent from it. For this to be at all a human enterprise—a covenantal relation between the man who performs these procedures and the man who is patient in them—the latter must make a reasonably free and an adequately informed consent. Ideally, he must be constantly engaged in doing so. This is basic to the cooperative enterprise in which he is one partner.

At the same time, just as Lincoln said concerning political covenants among men that "no man is good enough to govern another without his consent," so there is also this same negative warrant for the requirement of consent in the relation between those who perform and those who are the patients in medical procedures. No man is good enough to experiment upon another without his consent. . . .

* * *

[E]xperimentation involving human subjects should be undertaken only when an informed consent has been secured. There are enormous problems, of course, in knowing how to subsume cases under this moral regulation expressive of respect for the man who is the subject in medical investigations no less than in applying this same moral regulation expressive of the meaning of medical care. What is and what is not a mature and informed consent is a preciously subtle thing to determine. Then there are questions about how to apply this rule arising from those sorts of medical research in which the patient's knowing enough to give an informed consent may alter the findings sought; and there is debate about whether the use of prisoners or medical students in medical experimentation, or paying the participants, would not put them under too much duress for them to be said to consent freely even if fully

* New Haven: Yale University Press 5–11 (1970). Copyright © 1970 by Yale University. Reprinted by permission.

informed. Despite these ambiguities, however, to obtain an understanding consent is a minimum obligation of a common enterprise and in a practice in which men are committed to men in definable respects. The *faithfulness*-claims which every man, simply by being a man, places upon the researcher are the morally relevant considerations. This is the ground of the consent-rule in medical practice, though obviously medical practice has also its consequence-features.

Indeed, precisely because there are unknown future benefits and precisely because the results of the experimentation may be believed to be so important as to be overriding, this rule governing medical experimentation upon human beings is needed to ensure that for the sake of those consequences no man shall be degraded and treated as a thing or as an animal in order that good may come of it. In this age of research medicine it is not only that medical benefits are attained by research but also that a man rises to the top in medicine by the success and significance of his research. The likelihood that a researcher would make a mistake in departing from a generally valuable rule of medical practice because he is biased toward the research benefits of permitting an "exception" is exceedingly great. In such a seriously important moral matter, this should be enough to rebut a policy of being open to future possible exceptions to this canon of medical ethics. On grounds of the faithfulness-claims alone, we must surely say that future experience will provide no morally significant exception to the requirement of an informed consent—although doubtless we may learn a great deal more about the meaning of this particular canon of loyalty, and how to apply it in new situations with greater sensitivity and refinement—or we may learn more and more how to practice violations of it.

Doubtless medical men will always be learning more and more about the specific meaning which the requirement of an informed consent has in practice. Or they could learn more and more how to violate or avoid this requirement. But they are not likely to learn that it more and more does not govern the ethical practice of medicine. It is, of course, impossible to demonstrate that there could be *no* exceptions to this requirement. But with regard to unforeseeable future possibilities or apparently unique situations that medicine may face, there is this rule-assuring, principle-strengthening, and practice-upholding rule to be added to the requirement of an informed consent. *In the grave moral matters of life and death, of maiming or curing, of the violation of persons or their bodily integrity, a physician or experimenter is more liable to make an error in moral judgment if he adopts a policy of holding himself open to the possibility that there may be significant, future permissions to ignore the principle of consent than he is if he holds this requirement of an informed consent always relevant and applicable.* If so, he ought as a practical matter to regard the consent-principle as closed to further morally significant alteration or exception. In this way he braces himself to respect the personal subject while he treats him as patient or tries procedures on him as an experimental subject for the good of mankind.

The researcher knows that his judgment will generally be biased by the fact that he strongly desires one of the consequences (the rapid completion of his research for the good of mankind) which he could hope to attain by breaking or avoiding the requirement of an informed consent. This, too, should strengthen adherence in practice to the principle of consent. If every doer loves his deed more than it ought to be loved, so every researcher his research—and, of course, its promise of future benefits for mankind. The investigator should strive, as Aristotle suggested, to hit the mean of moral virtue or excellence by "leaning against" the excess or the defect to which he knows himself, individually or professionally, and mankind generally in a scientific age, to be especially inclined. To assume otherwise would be to assume an equally serene rationality on the part of men in all moral matters. It would be to assume that a man is as able to sustain good moral judgment and to make a proper choice with a strong interest in results obtainable by violating the requirement of an informed consent as he would be if he had no such interest.

Thus the principle of consent is a canon of loyalty expressive of the faithfulness-claims of persons in medical care and investigation. Let us grant that we cannot theoretically rule out the possibility that there can be exceptions to this requirement in the future. This, at least, is conceivable in extreme examples. It is not logically impossible. Still this is a rule of the highest human loyalty that ought not in practice to be held open to significant future revision. To say this concerning the there and then of some future moral judgment would mean here and now to weaken the protection of coadventurers from violation and self-violation in the common cause of medical care and the advancement of medical science. The material and spiritual pressures upon investigators in this age of research medicine, the collective bias in the direction of successful research, the propensities of the scientific mind toward the consequences alone are all good reasons—even if they are not all good moral reasons—for strengthening the requirement of an informed consent. This helps to protect coadventurers in the cause of medicine from harm and from harmfulness. This is the edification to be found in the thought that man's propensity to overreach a joint adventurer even in a good cause makes consent necessary.

This negative aspect of the ethics of medical research is essential even if only because the constraints of the consent-requirement serve constantly to drive our minds back to the positive meaning or warrant for this principle in the man who is the patient and the man who performs these procedures. An informed consent alone exhibits and establishes medical practice and investigation as a voluntary association of free men in a common cause. The negative constraint of the consent-requirement serves its positive meaning. It directs our attention always upon the man who is the patient in all medical procedures and a partner in all investigations, and away from that celebrated "nonpatient," the future of medical science. Thus consent lies at the heart of medical care as a joint adventure between patient and doctor. It lies at the heart of man's continuing search for cures to all man's diseases as a great human adventure that is carried forward jointly by the investigator and his subjects. Stripped of the requirement of a reasonably free and an adequately informed consent, experimentation and medicine itself would speedily become inhumane.

* * *

2.

Diminishing Unfavorable Public Reaction

Oscar M. Ruebhausen and Orville G. Brim, Jr. Privacy and Behavioral Research*

* * *

There is no doubt as to the community reaction to the administration, even in the name

* 65 *Columbia Law Review* 1184, 1192–94 (1965). Reprinted by permission.

of research, of live cancer cells to unwitting patients. Nor should we expect that the community will be any more tolerant of behavioral research that subjects non-consenting persons to the risk of injurious, though non-fatal, after-effects. Indeed, community sensitivity as to what is reasonable, or tolerable, is not limited to situations where physical or psychic injury may be involved.

While neither the most representative nor serious intrusion, a well-known example of privacy invasion in the field of behavioral research is the so-called "jury bugging" experiment conducted by the University of Chicago. Financed by the Ford Foundation, this was a scientific inquiry conceived and carried out with the best of professional motivation and skill. Although the consent, in advance, of the court and of opposing counsel was obtained, the surreptitious probing of the individual and institutional privacy of the members of the jury shocked the community when the experiment became public knowledge in October, 1955. . . .

* * *

Another example where neither physical injury nor emotional trauma is necessarily involved is found in personality testing. It requires no Cassandra to predict lawsuits by parents, and a spate of restrictive legislation, if those who administer these tests in schools—even for the most legitimate of scientific purposes—do not show a sensitive appreciation for both individual and group claims to a private personality.

The lesson is plain. Unless the advances of science are used with discrimination by scientists engaged in behavioral research—as well as by other professions, by industry and by government—the constructive and productive uses of these advances may be drastically and unnecessarily restricted by a fearful community.

* * *

NOTES

NOTE 1.

GWYNN NETTLER
TEST BURNING IN TEXAS*

By a 5–1 vote the governing board of the Houston Independent School District, one of the largest in the nation, in June 1959 ordered burned the answer sheets to six sociopsycho-

* 14 *American Psychologist* 682–83 (1959). Reprinted by permission.

metrics administered to some 5,000 ninth graders. Four of these instruments were taken from a pilot study of the National Talent Project to be administered by the University of Pittsburgh and the American Institute for Research in 1960; the remaining instruments were added by local psychologists interested in forecasting the realization of talent and in the assessment of psychological health.

* * *

The Houston test burning came as a result of few telephone calls (no one knows how many) from parents complaining, at the outset, to two of the seven trustees concerning the content and purport of the tests. The metropolitan press was alerted and published stories in advance of the school board meeting promising a ruckus. . . .

According to newspaper accounts parents were objecting to having their children respond to such items as:

I enjoy soaking in the bathtub.

A girl who gets into trouble on a date has no one to blame but herself.

If you don't drink in our gang, they make you feel like a sissy.

Sometimes I tell dirty jokes when I would rather not.

Dad always seems too busy to pal around with me.

* * *

It seems advisable that future large-scale testing programs be preceded by a public "warm up" explaining to as broad a segment of the public as possible the purposes and methods of such research. For example, effort spent in the education of PTAs and boards of education in advance of such surveys may prevent such loss as Houston has suffered.

Psychologists are behaving "ethnocentrically" in assuming that their ethic is shared by the people they study. The statement of "Ethical Standards of Psychologists" carried in the June issue of the *American Psychologist* holds:

As a scientist, the psychologist believes that society will be best served when he investigates where his judgment indicates investigation is needed. . . .

The psychologist in the practice of his profession shows sensible regard for the social codes and moral expectations of the community in which he works. . . .

When the student of behavior works in a xenophobic and individualistic community, he cannot assume that his scientifically honorable intentions will be considered morally justifiable by those whom he seeks to help. Even though the scientist says, in effect, "I am studying you, and asking you these questions, for your own good," his subject may respond, "It is part of my 'good' that you desist from your intrusion of my privacy."

* * *

NOTE 2.
LEONARD D. ERON AND LEOPOLD O. WALDER
TEST BURNING II*

This is a report on public reaction to a community-wide psychological research program. . . .

* * *

The research has been conducted by staff members in the research department of the Rip Van Winkle Foundation, an organization which sponsors a group practice of medicine providing comprehensive medical care on both a prepaid and fee-for-service basis. . . . This organization . . . was founded in an attempt to provide the population of a relatively poor rural community with high quality medical care at a cost that at least 90 percent of the people could afford. Since 1954 there has been a continuous mental health unit including psychologists, psychiatrists, and psychiatric social workers integrated into the comprehensive medical program. Demand for mental health services which are provided to both children and adults has steadily increased since inception of the service. . . .

The research program sponsored by the foundation started in 1955 and has been concerned with mental health in rural areas. The content selected for one study was the development of aggression in children. For purposes of this research it was decided to study all third grade children in their classrooms and to interview the parents of each child. . . .

* * *

. . . At this time plans were completed for our final data collection year in which we were to see all third grade children and parents in the county. A meeting was held with the county school administrators and our plans completely

---

* 16 *American Psychologist* 237 (1961). Reprinted by permission.

outlined to them. Because of the good response we had been getting up until then, the school personnel suggested that it was not necessary to send home notices with the children. They considered our testing program like any other routine school procedure.

*   *   *

. . . The testing of the children was completed without incident. Simultaneously and subsequently parents were contacted for interviews. A day after letters were sent out to the Chatham area, the supervising principal of that district phoned the director of the research and said she received a number of calls from irate parents concerning the letter from the Mental Health Research Center about their child in school. The parents reported that they had engaged a lawyer to see what action could be taken to prevent this study from going any further. The principal felt that the words "Mental Health" in our letterhead had scared them and that we had made a tactical error in not sending the initial contact letters out on school letterheads over the signature of the individual principals. Thus to the parents in the succeeding four school districts, letters went out on school letterheads over the supervising principal's signature. The letter remained the same with some minor changes in pronouns. After that there were only two direct complaints made to a supervising principal.

In the meantime, however, the situation in the Chatham district had blown up. The parents demanded a public meeting with the school authorities and the research team. At the meeting, held on a snowy evening, only 18 parents showed up. Questions were asked primarily by two mothers, one of whom was secretary to the aforementioned lawyer. . . . The questions had to do primarily with what authority the school could allow an outside agency to come in and test their children, who was behind the study, who financed it, who was making money out of it. There were vague references to personal questions being asked of the children and parents but the wording of these purported questions could not be ascertained at the meeting by either the school authorities or the researchers. We were frank and candid in our replies and offered to show the procedures which we had with us to the parents who were present. After describing each of the children's tests and giving sample items, one of the speakers then started to read the parents' questionnaire, item by item;

after three pages, the audience lost interest. No one asked to look at the materials afterwards. Many of the parents did come up to us and say that the fuss was all much ado about nothing.

*   *   *

However, a week later during a routine meeting of the Chatham Board of Education, without warning the opposition appeared in force. . . . The board was unprepared for the uninterrupted barrage of questions. The report of the meeting which made the front pages the next day made the school board look foolish and the researchers sinister. We were accused of asking the third graders such questions as "How often do you have sexual relations?" "Do you get suicidal thoughts?" "Do you prefer your mother to your father?" "Is your father a tyrant?" etc. Needless to say, none of these questions had ever been asked in our survey procedures, either with the children or the parents. The matter of confidentiality, invasion of privacy, lack of parental permission, etc. were all brought up. The penny candy which we gave the children as prizes after each session was alleged to be a bribe. One mother said: "I give my children strict training never to take candy from strange men." The president of the board asked for and received a motion to suspend any further testing until a subcommittee of the board could investigate the whole matter and make a recommendation.

*   *   *

From that point on, publicity became more favorable. The subcommittee of the Chatham Board of Education drew up a recommendation to continue wholehearted support of the research effort with the proviso that, in the future, permission from the parents should be obtained before testing the children in school. This recommendation was then presented at a well-advertised board meeting at which no one of the objectors appeared and it was unanimously approved by the board after no opposition from the floor. A petition against continuation of the research purportedly signed by many parents was not presented. A very fine statement was made at this meeting by the executive director of the foundation, supporting the research and its place in a community-oriented organization. . . .

*   *   *

What has been the effect of this entire controversy on the data gathering? Actually, the ruckus did not blow up until the period of data collection from the children was in its last week. Data from only three children were destroyed in compliance with the wishes of their parents. The effect on interview acceptance by the parents is really unassessable. The controversy exploded midway in our 6-month field period and extended until the end. However, there did not seem to be a lessening of cooperation on the part of parents; in fact, the publicity may have helped. For the total sample of 875 third graders, we successfully interviewed at least one parent in 83 percent of the cases and both parents in 75 percent. Thus we feel confident we had the support of the majority of parents.

* * *

. . . Despite our careful preparation and groundwork and our indefatigible efforts in public relations and our striving to be candid at all times, there was a lot of misunderstanding about just what we were doing. This is perhaps inevitable when psychological concepts which have restricted meanings to psychologists have to be communicated to the lay public in an open meeting. The words are in English and carry the extra freight of both conventional and personal meaning to each individual. . . . How many . . . times such terms were used blithely by us and misinterpreted by our audiences is uncertain. This is illustrated by the following quotation from a newspaper account of one board meeting:

Some parents want another meeting with the research director. Others charge that this would do no good. "All he would do," one said, "would be to stand up there and turn on the charm and give us a bunch of vague and meaningless terms about norms and statistics and such, and none of us would find out anything."

* * *

NOTE 3.

ALEXANDER M. KIDD
LIMITS OF THE RIGHT OF A PERSON TO
CONSENT TO EXPERIMENTATION ON HIMSELF*

* * *

[I]t may be that, on the maxim *"De minimis non curat lex"*—"The law does not regard trifles"—an extra drop of blood to build up a control group for a research study, or the use of

---

* 117 *Science* 211, 212 (1953). Reprinted by permission.

tissue that has been properly severed would not be condemned by the court. But the medical profession should consider carefully whether, as a matter of good public relations, nothing should be done to a patient except for his benefit, and whether he should not be used either directly or indirectly as a guinea pig without his consent. A doctor who has the reputation of experimenting with his patients is avoided by those who know that reputation.

* * *

3.

Removing Civil and Criminal Liability

a.

Barnett v. Bachrach
34 A. 2d 626 (D.C. Mun. Ct. App. 1943)

* * *

CAYTON, ASSOCIATE JUDGE.

Defendant engaged Dr. Joseph Harris to treat his wife during her period of pregnancy. There was evidence that in the course of such treatment she complained of certain pains in her lower right abdomen, and of nausea. Dr. Harris made a diagnosis of tubal pregnancy. He called in the plaintiff, a surgeon, for consultation. Plaintiff took the history and made a pelvic examination, in the presence of Dr. Harris. He found a mass the size of a small orange in the right ovarian region; from that and other symptoms he made a diagnosis of a tubal or extra-uterine pregnancy, confirming the diagnosis of Dr. Harris. Plaintiff recommended an immediate operation.

Plaintiff's testimony was taken by deposition and is not too clear as to precisely what authority he received. On direct examination he said, "[A] diagnosis of extra-uterine pregnancy was made. . . . I discussed the importance of immediate operation with the patient in the presence of Dr. Harris. *Permission for operation was granted* and the patient was operated on by me." In answer to one question on cross examination he said: "I was engaged to perform an abdominal operation *and do whatever was necessary to cure the patient.* I was not engaged to do an appendectomy per se." But to the next question his answer was: "Mrs. Lillian Barnett engaged me *to perform an operation on her to remove a possible tubal pregnancy,* however an acute appendix was found instead and removed." These answers can fairly be taken to mean that the only express authority he received was to remove the tubal pregnancy. If plaintiff had more specific authority the evidence does not show it.

The operation was performed under anaesthesia, and upon opening the abdomen, plaintiff found that his and Dr. Harris' original diagnosis of tubal pregnancy was mistaken and that a normal pregnancy was present in the uterus. Also he found a very unusual condition in that the patient, instead of having one uterus, had a double uterus. Also he found a very acute appendix. Deciding that this had caused patient's abdominal pains, he removed the appendix. He testified that she made an uneventful recovery and that he and Dr. Harris were satisfied that the source of her trouble had been removed.

Defendant's wife contended that as a result of the operation she had difficulty in getting about the house and going up and down stairs and was confined to bed for a "considerable" length of time. There is no denial that she gave birth in the usual course to a normal child in a normal way.

Defendant resisted the surgeon's claim for his fee on the sole ground that the appendix had been removed without the consent of himself or wife. He has disavowed any charge of malpractice, any claim of negligence, either in the original diagnosis or in the operation itself. He rests his defense entirely upon the claim that the operation, having gone further than was authorized, constituted a trespass or assault upon his wife.

* * *

The question for our decision is whether an emergency existed so as to justify the removal of the appendix without the express consent of the patient. To answer the question we must look at the picture through the eyes of the surgeon. The patient lay before him on the operating table, her abdomen laid open, and unconscious from the anaesthetic. Her pregnancy was a normal one in the uterus and not tubal as he and Dr. Harris had thought it was. She did reveal a very unusual structural condition in the form of a double uterus. More immediately important, he beheld a very acute appendix with all its potentially dangerous consequences.

What was the surgeon to do? Should he have left her on the operating table, her abdomen exposed, and gone in search of her husband to obtain express authority to remove the appendix? Should he have closed the incision on the inflamed appendix and subjected the patient, pregnant as she was, to the danger of a general

spread of the poison in her system, or to the alternative danger and shock of a second, independent operation to remove the appendix? Or should he have done what his professional judgment dictated and proceed to remove the offending organ, regarded as it is as a mere appendage serving no useful physiological function and causing only trouble, suffering, and ofttimes death?

Defendant does not say that the plaintiff used bad judgment, or that the operation was not dictated by sound surgical procedure, or that it was a failure. He says only that it was unauthorized, and makes no real showing of resulting injury or damage. . . .

This case is not one where a patient was rendered barren; on the contrary, her foetus was not disturbed and she achieved motherhood in a normal manner. Nor was she crippled or otherwise mutilated; on the contrary the operation was a success, and she is forever relieved from the fear and danger of appendicitis.

And yet we are asked to deny the plaintiff's fee because he comes into court unable to show express authority for the excision he made. It seems to us that to adopt that view would be granting poor reward indeed for faithful professional service. Moreover this would require us to shut our minds and eyes, as judges, to "truths that all others can see and understand."

To accept this view, we would have to deny that it was an emergency and declare a rule which would tend to make every surgeon litigation-conscious instead of duty-conscious as he stands, scalpel in hand, over his unconscious patient. This we decline to do. We hold the law to be that in case of emergency a surgeon may lawfully perform, and it is his duty to perform, such operation as good surgery demands even when it means extending the operation further than was originally contemplated; and that for so doing he is neither to be held in damages, or denied recovery of his fee.

The law should encourage self-reliant surgeons to whom patients may safely entrust their bodies, and not men who may be tempted to shirk from duty for fear of a law suit. The law does not insist that a surgeon shall perform every operation according to plans and specifications approved in advance by the patient, and carefully tucked away in his office-safe for courtroom purposes.

We do not attempt to mark off the line which will define the type of emergency which will create implied consent in every case; that is a question for the jury, or, as here, for the judge who sat as trier of the facts. Here we hold only that on the showing made, authority was born of the emergency, and conferred upon the surgeon the legal right to proceed as he did.

Affirmed

NOTE

MILTON OPPENHEIM
INFORMED CONSENT TO MEDICAL TREATMENT*

* * *

It is submitted that the public interest requires that the physician be permitted to exercise his discretion in good faith, knowing that the

_____
* 11 *Cleveland-Marshall Law Review* 249, 251, 261–263 (1962). Reprinted by permission.

physician-patient relation is one of fiduciary requirements of trust and confidence. This is important, for if one is to explain to the patient every risk attendant upon surgical or therapeutic procedures, no matter how remote, it may well result in unduly alarming the patient, who is already apprehensive, fearful, and dejected.

* * *

The absurdity of the trend towards a "more informed patient" is evident in the attempts of physicians to comply, even where compliance is not in conformance with good medical practice. This required "informed" consent may create delay, apprehension, and restrictions on the use of new techniques that will impair the progress of medicine. It is questionable whether the "average prudent man" will understand and comprehend the following examples of informed consent forms used by a prominent neuro-surgeon in his practice:

CONSENT AND OPERATIVE PERMIT FOR CAESAREAN GANGLION OPERATION

1. The side of the face (operation) may be numb.
2. There may be a loss of sensation on the cornea of the eye on the side operated, with the possibility of ulceration leading to possible loss of the eye.
3. There may be impaired hearing on the operated side.
4. There may be residual weakness in chewing movements on the operated side.
5. There may be weakness of the muscle of facial expression on the operated side.
6. There may be residual pain on the operated side.
7. There may be weakness of the body—hemiplegia—on the operated side of the body.

The above has been read and explained to me, and I accept responsibility for these or any other complications which may arise or result during or following this surgical procedure, which is performed at my request.

WITNESS: _____   _____

(Patient's Signature)

* * *

CONSENT AND OPERATIVE PERMIT

PATIENT _____ AGE _____ PLACE _____

DATE _____ TIME _____ A.M. P.M.

1. I hereby authorize Dr. _____ and whomever he may designate as

his assistants to perform upon _____
(State name of person or "myself")

the following operation: "THYROIDECTOMY" that is,
(State procedures(s) to be performed)

"SURGICAL REMOVAL OF THYROID GLAND—SUBTOTAL" and if any unforeseen condition arises in the course of
(State full explanation of procedure)
this operation calling in his judgment for procedures in addition to or different from these now contemplated,
I further request and authorize him to do whatever he deems advisable and necessary in the circumstances.

2. The clinical outcome in my case is directly in proportion to the nature of the pathology, that is, the condition revealed, disclosed, or discovered by the procedure or procedures. The nature, purpose, and risk of the operation and procedures and possible alternative methods of treatment, possibility of complications have been fully explained to me. I acknowledge that no guarantee or assurance has been made as to the results that may be obtained. Further, I consent to the disposal of any tissue which may be removed.

3. My condition therefore, may:
   (a) Be improved;
   (b) Remain stationary; or
   (c) Become aggravated with respect to *"Weakness or Hoarseness of Voice: Prominence of Eyes may persist: Calcium Metabolism may be disturbed, with resulting muscle weakness."*

4. I consent, authorize and request the administration of such anesthetic or anesthetics as is deemed suitable by the physician-anesthetist who shall be chosen by the surgeon. It is the understanding of the undersigned that the physician-anesthetist will have full charge of the administration and maintenance of the anesthesia, and that this is an independent function from the surgery.

The above has been read and explained to me and I accept responsibility for these or any other complications which may arise or result during or following the above procedure, which is to be performed at my request.

       Signature of Patient _____

       Signature of Patient's
         husband or wife _____
       When patient is a minor or incompetent to give consent:
       Signature of Person Authorized to consent for the patient. _____

WITNESS: _____

RELATIONSHIP TO PATIENT _____

* * *

b.

Bang v. Charles T. Miller Hospital
251 Minn. 427, 88 N.W.2d 186 (1958)

FRANK T. GALLAGHER, JUSTICE.

* * *

This was an action for damages for alleged assault or unauthorized operation by the defendant on his patient, Helmer Bang, referred to herein as plaintiff. The latter contends that the question as to whether he expressly or impliedly consented to the operating procedures involved was one of fact for the jury. At the close of plaintiffs' case, the defendant moved for a direct verdict upon the grounds that plaintiffs had failed to prove any actionable negligence or any cause of action against him. This motion was treated by the trial court as a motion for dismissal on the merits, which motion was granted. . . .

* * *

[P]laintiff began having urinary trouble in 1951 to 1952. He consulted a doctor in his home town of Austin, Minnesota, who sent him to the hospital for a cystoscopic examination which was made by two local doctors in Austin. Plaintiff testified that they informed him of an enlargement of the prostate gland and bladder soreness and recommended either Rochester or defendant in St. Paul as places he could go to have some tissue removed from the gland to overcome the trouble.

* * *

The important question for determination of the matter presently before us is whether the evidence presented a fact question for the jury as to whether plaintiff consented to the severence of his spermatic cords when he submitted to the operation. Defendant testified on cross-examination under the rules that he did not tell plaintiff at the time of the office visit, April 6, that any examination defendant had made or was going to make had anything to do with the spermatic cord, nor did he recall explaining to his patient what a prostate gland operation involved. He also said that plaintiff's life was in no immediate danger because of his condition on that day.

*   *   *

On the following day the operation was performed. When defendant was asked as to the procedure used, he replied:

A: [T]he cysto-urethroscopic examination was made; following that I went over to the head of the table and talked to Mr. Bang, told him what the findings were, and that in my opinion the transure-thral prostatic resection should be done and I had his consent that we proceed with that operation.

Q: Did you at that time as I understand it now ask him for his consent?   A: Yes.

*   *   *

Q: Did you inform Helmer Bang that in his specific case of a prostate gland resection that you intended to sever the spermatic cords of him as a part of the operation or that it was necessary to do so in his specific case?   A: I did not inform Helmer Bang that as a part of the prostate gland resection it would be necessary to sever the spermatic cords of his.

*   *   *

Q: Did you also answer, severance of the spermatic cords—bilateral was section [vas section] and ligation—is a routine part of this procedure in all cases of patients the age of Mr. Bang?   A: Yes.

*   *   *

The patient recalled the start of the operation and, when questioned on direct examination, stated:

Q: Did he at any time before the operation began tell you that he was going to cut your spermatic cords?   A: No.

Q: Did he at any time before the operation began tell you that it was necessary to cut your cords?   A: No.

When questioned as to whether he had any conversation with the defendant at the operating table or during the entire period when he was in the operating room, plaintiff replied that with the exception of a morning greeting "and stuff like that" nothing was said to him with reference to the operation.

When being questioned on cross-examination with reference to consent, the plaintiff was asked:

Q: And you certainly did consent, didn't you, Mr. Bang, to Dr. Foley doing anything to correct your trouble which in his medical knowledge he felt should be corrected?   A: Not anything he wanted to, no.

Q: Did you put any limitation on his job as a surgeon?   A: No.

Q: When he said, if I find anything that needs correction I will do it at the same time and you said that was all right, that was all of the conversation there was, wasn't it?   A: That was all of the conversation there was.

It is plaintiff's claim that he thought he was discussing his bladder because he understood from his Austin physicians something about burning out the ulcers if there were any ulcers in there. He admitted, however, that defendant said nothing to him about ulcers. Plaintiff also admitted that he did not expect to tell the doctor what to do; that he had faith in him; and that he did not expect to tell him how to perform the operation. He said that he expected the doctor would operate to do what was necessary to right and cure his condition. He testified that he did not ask the doctor what he intended to do and left it up to him to do the right thing.

It is our opinion that under the record here the question as to whether plaintiff consented to the severance of his spermatic cords was a fact question for the jury and that it was error for the trial court to dismiss the action.

*   *   *

While we have no desire to hamper the medical profession in the outstanding progress it has made and continues to make in connection with the study and solution of health and disease problems, it is our opinion that a reasonable rule is that, where a physician or surgeon can ascertain in advance of an operation alternative situations and no immediate emergency exists, a patient should be informed of the alternative possibilities and given a chance to decide before the doctor proceeds with the operation. By that we mean that, in a situation such as the case before us where no immediate emergency exists, a patient should be informed before the operation that if his spermatic cords were severed it would result in his sterilization, but on the other hand if this were not done there would be a possibility of an infection which could result in serious consequences. Under such conditions the patient would at least have the opportunity of deciding whether he wanted to take the chance of a possible infection if the operation was performed in one manner or to become sterile if performed in another.

Reversed and a new trial granted.

c.

Marcus L. Plant
An Analysis of "Informed Consent"*

* * *

The legal wrong conventionally called "battery" or "assault and battery" consists of an unpermitted touching of the person of another; by definition a touching is not tortious if there has been consent to it by the one touched. Consent can be rendered nugatory under some circumstances. One of these circumstances is inducement of the consent by a certain kind of misrepresentation. Not every misrepresentation will have this vitiating effect. In order to negate consent the misrepresentation must relate to the nature and character of the touching. If it does, the touching is tortious (a battery) because it is no longer with the consent of the one touched. Misrepresentation that does not relate to the nature and character of the touching but merely concerns some collateral matter does not have the fatal effect. . . .

* * *

. . . In *Bang*, plaintiff thought he was going to be touched in a certain way (operation on his prostate gland, possibly surgery on the bladder) but was subjected to a touching of a substantially different character (severance of spermatic cords). In *Mitchell*, plaintiff thought he was going to be touched in a certain way (insulin injection). He *was* touched in *exactly* that way, but there was a harmful result arising from a collateral risk he had not been warned about. The fundamental point is not what name we give to the two categories of cases as long as what we call them depicts two basically different wrongs which call for quite different treatment by the courts and quite different self-protective steps to be taken by the physician. It is fatal to clear understanding to intermingle the two under some broad heading such as "malpractice" or to state that both involve "informed consent." For pur-

* 36 *Fordham Law Review* 639, 648–655 (1968). © 1968 by Fordham University Press, Lincoln Center, New York, N.Y. Reprinted by permission of copyright holder.

poses of this discussion I will refer to the first type of case (*Bang*) as a "battery" and to the second type of case (*Mitchell*) as "medical negligence."

* * *

It is clear in the battery cases that a patient has virtually an absolute right to be free from touchings of a substantially different nature and character from those to which he has consented. It is the patient's prerogative to accept medical treatment or to take his chances of living without it. . . .

* * *

Wall v. *Brim* presents a variation of the general theme involving a failure to disclose. Plaintiff underwent a procedure involving an incision in the neck just under the back of the ear for removal of a cyst. When it was finished she had suffered a serious injury which caused considerable facial disfigurement with disability of her mouth, tongue and eyes. Plaintiff had been told by the surgeon before surgery that it was a "very simple operation" which would not take more than five or ten minutes and the cyst could be pulled out "like hulling a pea out of a pod." After the incision was made, the surgeon discovered that the cyst was deeply embedded and in close proximity to the facial nerve. He continued with the operation without any disclosure of these facts to plaintiff who was fully conscious, the operation being performed under a local anesthetic. Plaintiff sued on a negligence theory. The jury verdict was for plaintiff and from judgment thereon defendant appealed. The Fifth Circuit Court of Appeals held that there was insufficient evidence to establish negligence because under the applicable law (Georgia) expert evidence was required and had not been adduced. However, the evidence suggested what appeared to be an operation without the consent of plaintiff, and the case was remanded for trial and development on that theory. The court's reasoning was that the surgeon, having previously described the operation as a simple one and then having discovered that it was a complicated and different one, had a duty so to advise plaintiff, particularly as she was conscious at the time. While his failure to do so would not support a negligence action, it could support an action for unpermitted operation.

* * *

When the case involves no substantial misunderstanding of the nature and character of the touching, but plaintiff claims he was not fully or correctly informed as to collateral hazards attendant upon the procedure, the judicial approach is quite different from that found in battery cases. Here defendant-physician's obligation and plaintiff-patient's corresponding right is less certain in nature, more flexible in character and subject to considerable variation. While it is often stated as a general proposition that the patient has the right to be advised of collateral hazards and the physician has the duty so to advise him, most cases have recognized, starting with *Salgo*, that this obligation is not rigid and cannot be prescribed with specificity. It is only a part of the broad obligation of the physician to use reasonable care, but as any sophisticated person knows, the elasticity in that concept is more than negligible.

*   *   *

One consideration often mentioned is whether the case is an emergency requiring immediate treatment. This aspect usually appears in a negative fashion; i.e., in buttressing the conclusion that defendant owed a duty to disclose collateral hazards, the court emphasizes that no emergency made it impractical to perform the duty. For example, in *Bowers* v. *Talmage,* the claim was that parents had not been warned of a hazard to their nine-year-old child from an arteriogram, an exploratory surgical process. The procedure was considered dangerous since three percent of the cases had injurious results. It caused partial paralysis of the boy. In holding that it was error to direct a verdict for defendant, the court emphasized that there was no emergency.

*   *   *

A second factor, and perhaps the one most frequently referred to by courts in delineating the physician's duty, is the danger of alarming the patient or causing other adverse psychological effects on him. . . .

*   *   *

A third factor that influences the decision as to whether there is a duty to disclose collateral dangers is the likelihood that the danger will materialize. The greater the frequency of injury from it, the greater the obligation of the physician to mention it and vice-versa. . . .

*   *   *

d.

Gramm v. Boener
56 Ind. 497 (1877)

WORDEN, J.—This was an action by the appellee, against the appellant, to recover damages for alleged negligence and unskilfulness on the part of the defendant, in the performance of his undertaking, as a surgeon, to set a broken arm and a broken leg of the plaintiff, whereby the plaintiff lost the use of his arm, and his leg became crooked, deformed and permanently lame.

Trial by jury; verdict and judgment for the plaintiff . . .

*   *   *

It seems to us to be the duty of a surgeon, when called upon to perform some surgical operation, to advise against it, if, in his opinion, it is unnecessary, unreasonable, or will result injuriously to the patient. The patient is entitled to the benefit of his judgment, whether asked for or not. If the surgeon, when called upon, should proceed to the performance of the operation, without expressing any opinion as to its necessity or propriety, the patient would have a right to presume, that, in the opinion of the surgeon, the operation was proper.

But if a surgeon, when thus called upon, advises the patient, who is of mature years and of sound mind, that the operation is unnecessary and improper, in short advises against the performance, and the patient still insists upon the performance of the operation, in compliance with which the surgeon performs it, we do not see upon what principle the surgeon can be held responsible to the patient for damages, on the ground that the operation was improper and injurious. In such case, the patient relies upon his own judgment, and not upon that of the surgeon, as to the propriety of the operation; and he can not complain of an operation performed at his own instance and upon his own judgment, and not upon that of the surgeon. The maxim, *volenti non fit injuria,* we think, well applies to such a case. The principle is quite analogous to that which prevents a recovery for injuries consequent upon unskillful or negligent treatment by a physician, if the plaintiff's own negligence directly contributed to them.

There is evidence in the record tending to show that the plaintiff, who was a married man and may be supposed to have been of mature years, repeatedly desired to have his arm re-broken, when the defendant visited him. He said positively that he wanted it re-broken. The defendant advised against it. He told them it would be of no use; that it had better be left alone, and that they ought not to think of it. In short, there is enough in the evidence, if the jury believed it, to justify them in finding that the arm was re-broken at the sole instance of the plaintiff, and against the advice of the defendant.

* * *

The judgment below is reversed . . . and the cause remanded, for a new trial.

NOTES

NOTE 1.

CHAMPS v. STONE
58 N.E. 2d 803 (1944)

ROSS, PRESIDING JUDGE.

This is an appeal on questions of law from a judgment of the Court of Common Pleas of Hamilton county, in favor of the defendant, entered upon a verdict which such court instructed after the opening statement of counsel for plaintiff and his stipulation as to what his evidence would show.

MR. SCHEAR: If the court please and ladies and gentlemen of the jury, the action here is one for personal injuries. . . .

* * *

I believe the evidence will show to you ladies and gentlemen of the jury that . . . the doctor was so grossly intoxicated and under the influence of alcohol that he could (not) comprehend to carry through a proper treatment. In other words, he was physically unfit to administer any aid to a patient.

* * *

THE COURT: . . . It is agreed in this case as follows: That the plaintiff went to the defendant for the purpose of having a blood test made by the defendant physician; that the defendant at said time was grossly intoxicated; that the plaintiff saw that the defendant was grossly intoxicated and refused to be treated by him; that the defendant insisted upon treating the plaintiff and the plaintiff submitted to being treated by him, and that the plaintiff claims that as a result of the treatment, which was improper and not according to what an ordinary physician— that by reason of not exercising the skill a physician should exercise he was damaged.

* * *

On the opening statement, the defendant moves for a directed verdict and I grant that motion on the ground that if I myself take the chance of being treated by someone whom I ought not to take the chance of being treated by, [in] other words, if I go to a doctor who is drunk and I know he is drunk and let him treat me because he insists on treatment (treating) me I take the consequences thereof and that is my own fault, in plain language, and I am guilty of negligence in law which contributes to a proximate cause of an injury. That is the reason why I direct you all to sign the verdict. . . .

The questions presented here are: Whether such conduct on the part of the plaintiff constituted contributory negligence as a matter of law, or an assumption of the risk presented by the physician's condition.

Contributory negligence is such an act or omission on the part of the plaintiff, constituting a failure to exercise the care which ordinarily prudent persons are accustomed to employ for their own safety, which, concurring or cooperating with the negligent act of the defendant is a proximate cause or occasion of the injury of which the plaintiff complains. . . .

* * *

It is claimed the intoxicated condition of defendant was the proximate cause of plaintiff's injuries. Such condition was apparent to plaintiff before he permitted the defendant to inject the needle in his arm. Had the plaintiff the right to rely upon the skill of defendant when grossly intoxicated? Plaintiff must have concluded that, although defendant was in such condition, he could still administer treatment without harmful results to him. Could reasonable minds differ on the conclusion that reasonably prudent persons would not permit a physician to act under such circumstances?

It would seem that any reasonable person would naturally ask: Why did you let the physician proceed? Why did you not at once leave his office? You certainly saw he was in no condition to use a needle upon you.

It must have been apparent to any reasonable person that the physician in such a condition might even select the wrong drug or inject an overdose. . . .

The only possible argument against the conclusion that plaintiff was either guilty of contributory negligence or assumed the risk of the physician's evident incapacity to properly perform his duties is that, under any such circumstances, a patient has the right to rely upon the professional representation of ability contained in the fact that the physician holds himself out as such and insists upon his ability to properly practice his profession.

Such implied ability and even definitely professed ability certainly may not be accepted by a patient in the presence of "gross intoxication" of which plaintiff is fully aware. Ordinary care for one's safety would impel the ordinary careful and prudent person to seriously doubt the physician's ability and cause the patient to refuse treatment.

The judgment of the trial court is affirmed.

*   *   *

MATTHEWS, JUDGE (dissenting).

Manifestly, the plaintiff concluded that the defendant was not so drunk as to preclude him from safely performing the injection by means of a hypodermic needle. The defendant, by holding himself out as a physician, represented that he had the required training and skill, and, at the time of this treatment, represented that he was in such physical and mental condition as to enable him to apply his training and skill. He occupied the dominant position in relation of trust and confidence. I do not think we are justified in holding that the patient was negligent as a matter of law in relying on the physician's assurance that he was in condition to safely use a hypodermic needle.

It is my opinion that the opening statement of counsel was a sufficient statement of a cause for submission to the jury, and that the court erred in instructing a verdict for the defendant upon such statement.

NOTE 2.
FOWLER V. HARPER AND FLEMING JAMES, JR.
THE LAW OF TORTS*

The term assumption of risk has led to no little confusion because it is used to refer to at least two different concepts, which largely overlap, have a common cultural background, and often produce the same legal result. But these concepts are nevertheless quite distinct rules involving slightly different policies and different conditions for their application. (1) In its primary sense the plaintiff's assumption of a risk is only the counterpart of the defendant's lack of duty to protect the plaintiff from that risk. In such a case plaintiff may not recover for his injury even though he was quite reasonable in encountering the risk that caused it. *Volenti non fit injuria*. (2) A plaintiff may also be said to as-

_____
* Boston: Little, Brown and Co. 1162, 1168–1170, 1173–1174 (1956). Reprinted by permission.

sume a risk created by defendant's breach of duty towards him, when he deliberately chooses to encounter that risk. In such a case, except possibly in master and servant cases, plaintiff will be barred from recovery only if he was unreasonable in encountering the risk under the circumstances. This is a form of contributory negligence. Hereafter we shall call this "assumption of risk in a secondary sense."

*   *   *

It is sometimes said that knowledge or comprehension of the risk by plaintiff is the watchword of assumption of risk. In many types of situations this is true; in others it is not. Unless the limitations which should be put on such a statement are fully appreciated, it may be very misleading. There may be assumption of a specific risk of which the plaintiff is completely ignorant. On the other hand the plaintiff does not assume, in the primary sense, many risks which he knows and fully appreciates. Thus the borrower of a chattel or the licensee on land takes the risk of dangers that he does not and cannot know about. And the rescuer or traveler on the highway, for instance, does not assume the most open and obvious risks (though he may be negligent in encountering them under the circumstances of any given case). The key to the problem lies in the relationship between the parties, and the duty owed by defendant to plaintiff under all the circumstances. It is only where (1) defendant knows of the danger, or (2) is under a duty to plaintiff to use care to discover the danger, *but* (in either event) *will fully discharge his duty to plaintiff by complete disclosure of the danger,* that plaintiff's knowledge and comprehension of the risk will spell assumption of risk in the primary sense. The commonest examples of this are cases of invitor and invitee on real property and (formerly, at least) master and servant. In these situations plaintiff is viewed as having no right to enter into or remain within the relationship, but only to be apprised of its risks so he can choose intelligently whether to encounter them. And if the risks are such that he who runs may read them, defendant owes no further duty with respect to them. Here, indeed, comprehension of the risk is the watchword of the doctrine.

In such a situation at least *actual* comprehension of a risk by a plaintiff means that if he voluntarily encounters it, he assumes it. But actual comprehension implies more than knowledge of the defect that constitutes the danger. It also includes an appreciation and an understanding of the dangers that lurk in the defect and result in the injury, and it is usually a jury question whether there was such appreciation in fact.

A different and more difficult question concerns a defendant's duty with respect to defects which are obvious and visible or to conditions pregnant with risks which most men would appreciate, but which this plaintiff does not see or does not comprehend. . . . There an attempt was made to examine the extent to which his own shortcomings would be considered in evaluating the plaintiff's conduct as negligent or not. Now our problem is the different one of deciding the extent to which certain defendants may assume a minimum of knowledge and perceptiveness on the part of others and act on that assumption. For example, the owner of a baseball park owes no duty to warn the experienced spectator of the dangers of foul balls in the unscreened part of the bleachers; and an analogous situation is presented by hockey. But does the proprietor of either sporting event owe such a duty to the uninitiated? Except for a few situations the rule does not seem clear and opinions are too often clouded with talk about presumptions. It seems fairly safe to say, however, that there are at least some situations whose dangers are so obvious, so customary, and so commonly known that a defendant need give no warning of them. Here again a plaintiff may assume a risk that he does not in fact comprehend. Yet by no means all the dangers which would be obvious to the attentive or appreciated by the experienced are thus assumed. Whether they are depends upon the kind of relationship, the character of the place, the likelihood that attention will be distracted, the customary behavior of people who frequent the place, the likelihood that inexperienced, young, or handicapped people will be there, and the like. These are of course the same factors which are to be considered on the issue of defendant's duty, for, as we have seen, the issue is the same.

*   *   *

We have said that the voluntary character of the association between plaintiff and defendant is the gist of the defense. This needs further elucidation. Plaintiff may voluntarily encounter a risk in one sense, yet not assume it. An example is the case of the traveler who chooses the more dangerous but shorter route on the highway. On the other hand plaintiff may assume a risk which in a very real sense he does not voluntarily encounter, as where a fireman in the line of duty enters a factory which is dark and full of dangerous machinery, or where a tenant leases premises in a dangerous state of disrepair because no other quarters are available. The key is to be found in the character of the relationship between the parties and their respective duties in the light of it. The plaintiff takes a risk *voluntarily* (within the meaning of the present rule) where the defendant has a right to face him with the dilemma of "take it or leave it"—in other words, where defendant is under no duty to make the conditions of their association any safer than they appear to be. In such a case it does not matter that plaintiff is coerced to assume the risk by some force not emanating from defendant, such as poverty, dearth of living quarters, or a sense of moral responsibility. If, on the other hand, defendant is not privileged to put plaintiff to the choice of taking or leaving a danger, the mere posing of the dilemma takes away the voluntary character of any assumption there may be of the risk.

*   *   *

4.

Encouraging Self-Scrutiny by the Investigator

a.

Paul Freund
Legal Frameworks for
Human Experimentation*

*   *   *

Throughout this discussion of legal frameworks the criterion of consent has emerged in one guise or another. It may sound for investigators a jarring note, as if a *prima facie* assault were proposed, which was made lawful by the victim's consent. The concept of participation may have greater semantic appeal, suggesting as it does a common enterprise in which the various parties share. Nevertheless the concept of agreement in one form or another seems inescapable, as an earnest of the law's concern for voluntarism in private hazardous undertakings that, in fact, serve public purposes.

The concept of consent has been much derided as unrealistic and artificial, and of course it

* 98 *Daedalus* 322–324 (1969). Reprinted by permission of Daedalus, Journal of the American Academy of Arts and Sciences, Boston, Massachusetts.

embraces a range of responses that differ in their degree of autonomy and understanding. The psychological constraints or compulsions that operate on a seriously ill patient are different from those that affect a person attracted to an experiment through an advertisement. Nevertheless a requirement of "voluntary, informed consent" does have values beyond the symbolic one of respect for individual autonomy and personality. It is far from the be-all and end-all of legal and ethical safeguards, but it is a valuable ultimate check, reminding one of Keynes' rationale for the gold standard: that it is a safeguard in case the managers of the currency should all go mad at once.

Not the least of the functions of consent is its reflexive effect on the management of the experiment itself. To analyze an experiment in terms of risks and benefits to particular groups by way of presentation for consent is a salutary procedure for self-scrutiny by the investigator—like the preparation of a registration statement by a corporation issuing securities.

An example in the field of medical experimentation can be taken from the tests of magnesium as a remedy for a serious form of nutritional deficiency in infants, which is fatal in perhaps 20 per cent of the cases and for which no effective treatment had been found. Magnesium appeared to give good results, but had not been subjected to a controlled experiment on human infants. Assume that such an experiment is, in fact, considered. What is the role of consent? Four possibilities suggest themselves. First, no consent might be required, in the view that a physician could conscientiously employ or decline to employ the drug in the interest of sound patient care. Secondly, consent might be thought irrelevant for an opposite reason, that good practice would call for use of the drug even without a controlled trial, in view of the seriousness of the illness, the drug's promise, the lack of an alternative, and no indication of deleterious side effects. The drug might thus be accepted, like aspirin or digitalis, on a basis lacking in scientific rigor. Assuming the experiment is to be tried, two further alternatives are open. The patients' parents, after an explanation, might be asked to consent to the use of the drug or to its non-use. It seems likely that it would be more difficult to secure the latter consent than the former. Finally, the parents might be asked to consent to the inclusion of their children in a randomly designed experiment.

One additional element of consent might enter into the calculus—namely, termination of consent. How should a physician measure his responsibility to continue the experiment for the sake of scientific rigor against preliminary indications during the experiment that the drug is effective and safe? There is an inescapable element of choice, judgment, or will in every inductive experiment; there is no "logical" stopping point so long as the hypothesis tested has not (yet) been disproved. Consequently scientific rigor is at best an imprecise canon, to be weighed along with economy of time, effort, and other pragmatic judgments concerning appropriate termination. The making of this kind of analysis does not, to be sure, depend on a requirement of consent, but that requirement will make more vivid to the investigator the options that he must weigh in order to be candid with himself and his patient.

NOTE

HEDIN v. MINNEAPOLIS
MEDICAL AND SURGICAL INSTITUTE
62 MINN. 146, 64 N.W. 158 (1895)

*   *   *

. . . The plaintiff, an illiterate man, badly injured in an accident, and physically a wreck, consulted with the physician and surgeon in charge of a medical and surgical institute or hospital as to his condition and the probability of a recovery. After an examination by the surgeons, he was positively assured, if he told the truth as to what was said (and the jury found that he did), that he could be cured, and by treatment at the institute could and would be made sound and well. Considering the circumstances, and the relations of the parties, there was something more in defendants' statements than the mere expression of his opinion upon a matter of conjecture and uncertainty. It amounted to a representation that plaintiff's physical condition was such as to insure a complete recovery. The doctor, especially trained in the art of healing, having superior learning and knowledge, assured plaintiff that he could be restored to health. That the plaintiff believed him is easily imagined; for a much stronger and more learned man would have readily believed the same thing. The doctor, with his skill and ability, should be able to approximate to the truth when giving his opinion as to what can be done with injuries of one year's standing, and he should always be able to speak with certainty before he undertakes to assert positively that a cure can be effected. If he cannot speak with certainty, let him express a doubt.

If he speaks without any knowledge of the truth or falsity of a statement that he can cure, and does not believe the statement true, or if he has no knowledge of the truth or falsity of such a statement, but represents it as true, of his own knowledge, it is to be inferred that he intended to deceive. The deception being designed in either case, and injury having followed from reliance upon the statements, an action for deceit will lie.

*   *   *

b.
Jon R. Waltz and Thomas W. Scheuneman
Informed Consent to Therapy*

*   *   *

In the case of risks unknown to the patient, a distinction must be drawn between risks that a physician *could* disclose and those that he *should* disclose. The cases and commentators have focused on the second facet, without emphasizing that the class of risks which *should* be disclosed is limited to those which *could* be disclosed. Blurred analysis of the disclosure duty has resulted.

A simple proposition provides a starting point for analysis of risks a physician could disclose: it is impossible to disclose something of which one is unaware. This point is not made in the cases because most informed consent cases have involved collateral risks attaching to widely-used therapies; thus the courts have probably been correct in assuming that the physician-defendants actually knew of them. If a risk is not actually known to the physician, however, it is inappropriate to speak solely of a duty to disclose. Instead, a second dimension of the class of risks that a physician could disclose appears: the physician's duty to have known of a risk so that he could have disclosed it.

The duty to know of a risk has two branches: the duty to learn of risks known to others in the profession, and the duty to investigate to discover whether there are risks unknown to others in the profession. When a risk is known to some part of the profession but not to the treating physician, the question is whether he should be legally held to a standard of equal knowledge. Here, familiar notions of a physician's duty provide a relatively easy solution. A physician is duty-bound to have the knowledge

of a reasonably well-trained and knowledgeable physician practicing under like circumstances. If his knowledge of collateral risks does not meet this standard, liability will be based on that shortcoming, not on failure to disclose. Although the distinction as to source of liability is usually unimportant, it becomes crucial if the physician was not required to know of a risk, and was therefore not required to make disclosure.

The logical first step to liability for failure to disclose a collateral risk is the demonstration that the defendant doctor either knew or, because of the state of knowledge in the medical profession, should have known of the particular risk. It is fair to impute this breadth of knowledge to the modern-day physician—medical knowledge is highly accessible. It is, therefore, reasonable to say that the class of collateral risks that could be disclosed should extend this far. Beyond this point, however, the situation does not present an orthodox problem of informed consent since the duty to disclose particular risks must presuppose either actual or imputed knowledge. Risks that were unknown to the medical profession pose different problems which will arise most frequently in cases of innovative therapy. By "innovative" we mean a therapeutic procedure which is not one customarily used by the profession in treating a particular condition. The distinction drawn is between "customary" and "innovative" therapy. We use the term "innovative" rather than "experimental" because the distinction is basically one of frequency of use and because the term "experimental" is freighted with irrelevant overtones.

The duty to know what a reasonable physician under like circumstances would know can only extend to risks of which some segment of the profession is aware. Beyond that point the problem becomes one of initial discovery. Although no reported informed consent case has involved an undiscovered risk, the problem must be analyzed because of its obvious significance for therapeutic innovation.

The problem of risk-discovery poses the two-pronged question whether existing medical knowledge was sufficient or whether further investigation should have been made to explore the possibility of unknown additional risks. The standard of reasonable medical practice will provide the answer.

In the case of a customary therapy, the reasonableness of the level of knowledge of collateral risks will already have been determined. In the case of innovative therapy, however, a major issue is whether enough has been discovered

* 64 *Northwestern University Law Review* 628, 630–635 (1969). Reprinted by special permission of the Northwestern University Law Review. Copyright © 1970.

about collateral risks to justify the conclusion that the innovation accords with reasonable medical practice. In the area that lies beyond the physician's knowledge about an innovative therapy, then, the duty to discover risks for the purpose of disclosure involves the same problem as does the question whether enough is known about the procedure's collateral risks to justify its use. The answer to both puzzles depends on whether a practitioner in the position of the innovator could reasonably conclude that enough was known about the collateral risks of the proposed therapy to warrant its use, or that, on the other hand, he should have postponed its use in order to investigate the possibility of previously unknown risks.

If a known risk of an innovative therapy is disclosed and subsequently materializes, the effect of a patient's consent will depend on the propriety of using the procedure. If use of the innovative therapy constituted reasonable medical practice under the circumstances, consent to disclosed collateral risks should relieve the innovator of liability. The result, however, should be different if use of the therapy was itself unreasonable. We accept the principle that a patient's consent to a therapy and its collateral risks will not relieve the physician of liability for negligence in performing the therapy. The same principle should apply in a case where use of an innovative therapy is negligent in light of knowledge of its collateral risks. In both cases the physician has breached his duty of care to the patient in the manner of treatment, and consent to a disclosed collateral risk becomes irrelevant.

Inevitably, innovative therapy will also raise the problem of consent to unknown risks. Two principal problems are posed. Should there be disclosure of the possibility of unknown risks? What will be the effect of the patient's consent to the possibility of unknown risks if one in fact materializes?

As to the first inquiry, it seems axiomatic that in all cases of optional innovative therapy the possibility of unknown risks should be disclosed, since this will bear heavily on the patient's decision whether to consent to use of the therapy. However, the effect of consent to unknown risks which later materialize is somewhat more troublesome. It could be maintained that a blanket agreement to confront the possibility of unknown risks will constitute consent to any unknown danger that may later materialize. The difficulty with this proposition, however, is that it does not accord with orthodox concepts of consent. The consent concept has traditionally

involved two elements: awareness and assent. Just as one cannot disclose something he does not know, so one cannot assent to something of which he is unaware. It may therefore seem both anomalous and unfair to suggest that agreement to accept the unknown constitutes knowing, binding consent.

The threshold question must again be whether the decision to employ an innovative therapy was reasonable in light of the physician's level of knowledge concerning it. Where use of an innovative technique is unreasonable because it prompts too many unanswered questions, introduction of a concept of consent to unknown risks assumes that advance consent relieves an innovator of liability for negligence in going forward with a therapy. No such concept obtains in cases of customary therapy, and none should apply in cases of innovative treatment. Consent is simply irrelevant. If a physician acted improperly by going ahead with an innovative technique as to which there were too many unplumbed questions involving its potential risks, liability will flow from the physician's unreasonable conduct. If, on the other hand, he acted reasonably in going forward on the basis of existing knowledge, the patient's consent even to the possibility of unanticipated risks is again irrelevant since the physician had no legal duty to disclose risks about which he neither knew nor should have known, and for that reason alone he is immune from liability. Maintaining the traditional meaning of consent in this context permits the question of liability for use of an innovative procedure to be resolved on a proper basis.[22]

---

[22] It could be argued that the concept of consent should be expanded to provide for "consent to unknown risks," thus holding a patient who consents in the face of disclosure of the possibility of unknown risks to have consented to any unknown risk that may later materialize. The difficulty with this redefinition of the consent concept is that it would do away with the distinction between innovative procedures the use of which constitutes due care in light of available knowledge and those whose use does not constitute due care. In either case, the patient would be held to have consented to the particular unknown risk, whether or not it was consistent with reasonable medical practice to employ the therapeutic procedure. If this course were adopted, the only limits to the effectiveness of consent would be set by criminal sanctions, where use of an innovative therapy would constitute a crime. It is usually held that consent to a criminal act is ineffective. . . . The traditional consent concept permits the law to stop short of this relatively crude position and assess effectiveness of consent to unknown risks on a more particularized basis.

NOTE

FRANCIS D. MOORE—
THERAPEUTIC INNOVATION—
ETHICAL BOUNDARIES IN THE INITIAL
CLINICAL TRIALS OF NEW DRUGS AND
SURGICAL PROCEDURES*

* * *

[An] aspect of "informed consent" that is so limiting in its application to therapeutic innovation (as indeed it is also in experimental investigation of any sort) is the obvious fact that there is no means of becoming informed other than by the experiment itself, even if there is a desire to give consent. The very fact that the procedure has not previously been carried out in man indicates that the scientist himself lacks the critical information required for informed consent. If the doctor knew the most likely outcome of the procedure, such information could only have come from previous experience, and in that event the patient would hardly be at risk.

* * *

E.
To Increase Society's Awareness

**William J. Curran
Professional Controls—
Internal and External†**

* * *

We now have four transplant programs in [Boston] with a large number of patients awaiting transplants in each one of the hospitals, and we do not yet have a developed public program of donation. We need a public program. We need public acceptance. We need an administrative mechanism for getting the donation programs off the ground. Legislation is only the start. Legislation is only the opportunity to move; it is not movement in itself. To date, not a single cadaver organ transplant has been made in this country as a result of a personal donation before death. All have been next-of-kin donations. Individual personal donation still isn't off the ground. If it doesn't proceed, if individual voluntary donation prior to death does not begin to occur, then the Dukeminier type of proposal [that organs and tissues be considered authorized for use, unless specifically denied or disallowed by the decedent prior to death, or by his next-of-kin thereafter] will receive a great deal more support. I think there will also be more support for authorizing a medical examiner to donate organs, at least those that he perhaps would have to destroy anyway, or at least sever, in his procedures.

As a result of this very fine piece of legislation, the Uniform Anatomical Gift Act, we can have a national effort in the field of donations, via a voluntary program. Both the Federal Government's reluctance to impose rules or regulations on conduct, as expressed by Dr. Confrey, and the general attitude that those of us working in the medical-legal field have tried to adopt, suggest that voluntariness is the preferred approach. We have encouraged it with regard to matters of consent as part of our professional feelings, and we want to extend it to other programs.

* * *

NOTES

NOTE 1.

WILLIAM W. FRYE
COMMUNITY INFORMATION PROGRAM
FOR TISSUE AND ORGAN DONATION*

* * *

Kidney transplantation now leads the field of successes in total organ transplants. The first successful kidney transplantation ever performed in the world was accomplished in Boston in 1954. Since that time, research in all aspects of organ and tissue transplantation has made possible the transfer of a number of organs. The kidney, cornea of the eye, and skin are now being transplanted routinely to restore health of the patient, due to the generous support of normal organs and tissues by healthy donors. . . . Today, heart, liver, lung, and pancreas transplantation procedures are now in the early stage of development, and we face a similar situation that is even

* 98 *Daedalus* 502, 510 (1969). Reprinted by permission of Daedalus, Journal of the American Academy of Arts and Sciences, Boston, Massachusetts.

† 169 *Annals of the New York Academy of Sciences* 555 (1970). Reprinted by permission.

* 169 *Annals of the New York Academy of Sciences* 560–563 (1970). Reprinted by permission.

more critical. Two major problems exist: one that must be solved by the scientist and the physician; and the other, by procurement of organs that must come from an enlightened public willing to donate their organs and tissues. There are also legal, ethical, and moral problems that must be solved. We are now at the stage where the public is becoming increasingly aware of today's scientific and medical accomplishments, the potential benefits, and the extraordinary contributions that can and need to be made by individuals willing to donate their tissues and organs to help restore others to health.

The need, at the present time, for organs for transplantation is unlimited. Approximately three-forths of the deaths in the United States result from kidney, liver, and heart disease. Thousands of patients have benefited from the use of transplants of cornea of the eye to restore vision; the use of transplanted skin in the treatment of deep burns caused by fire or scalding water; and the more recent successes with kidney transplantation. The availability of kidneys from living donors or the availability of livers, hearts, and kidneys immediately after death is severely limited because the pressing need for such organs is not generally known. . . . The public must be kept informed, and the public attitudes must be revised to keep pace with medical advances in transplantation. Individuals must be convinced of the great benefits obtained from organs if they can be removed promptly after death. . . .

For more than a year, the United Health Foundations Inc. has had a special committee investigating what function a private voluntary organization might have in the tissue and organ transplant program. . . . [T]he UHF Board of Directors, at its annual meeting in December 1968, authorized the staff to develop a National Transplant Information Center. The main function of the center will be to develop a national voluntary program relating to organ transplantation and tissue utilization. The program will combine the development of national and local services, public and professional education, community-related research and demonstrations, and legislative information.

*   *   *

[A] function of the National Transplant Information Center will be to develop, for the general public, information about who can be a donor, what the cost of a transplant is, what kinds of tissues are needed, where information can be obtained in any given community, and many other questions. These will be made available through community agencies, medical organizations, and other concerned groups.

*   *   *

NOTE 2.

JOHN M. PRUTTING
NEW YORK'S NEW UNIFORM ANATOMICAL
GIFT ACT—WHAT IT MEANS*

Many physicians have been reluctant in the past to ask the next-of-kin's permission for organ transplantation. In some measure this may have been caused by uncertainty over the legal implications as well as by fear of hostility and criticism from their patients' families. Valid excuses should be extremely rare now that the Uniform Anatomical Gift Act has clarified matters and established legally acceptable procedures. Hospitals and physicians in New York State no longer have cause to hesitate about undertaking this privileged responsibility. The transplantation of many organs is increasingly successful, and the physician or hospital not making a sincere effort to obtain these is remiss in the performance of basic medical responsibilities.

In short, the time is here for all of us to acquaint our patients with the need for donating organs and tissues by inviting them to fill out the new donor cards. Once the benefits have been clearly explained, an informed public will more readily grant permission for these procedures that can bring life to others after the donor's death. The importance of contributing toward the conquest of disease should be stressed. And families should be made to understand the dignity and care with which organs are removed, just as in a surgical operation, with respect for the body and its preservation. With implementation of the Uniform Anatomical Gift Act, there is no longer any excuse for letting inertia, apathy or unawareness deprive the needy of organs and tissues which can now be readily and legally available. By the same token, it becomes our collective obligation to overcome with logic the objections of the emotional or superstitious who would deny these great inherent benefits to their fellow human beings.

---

* 1 *New York State Journal of Medicine* 2359, 2361 (1970). Copyright by the Medical Society of the State of New York. Reprinted by permission.

CHAPTER NINE

What Limitations Are Inherent in Informed Consent?

To give effective protection to the subject's rights and the integrity of the human experimentation process, the concept of informed consent must take into account the limitations on the subject's ability to make "intelligent" and "insightful" decisions. In this chapter we examine the impediments to self-determination and informed consent inherent in the intellectual capacities, psychological forces, and social pressures operating in and on man. More specifically, we ask whether an awareness of these problems on the part of investigators and subjects can overcome the failures of communication, understanding, and intelligent decisionmaking which now plague the research process.

The limitations of informed consent discussed in this and the following chapters raise questions which go far beyond the human experimentation process. Like the larger issues underlying experimentation, which were presented in Chapter Three, the definitions of these limits reflect contradictory assumptions about the nature and rights of man. These assumptions are only touched upon here, but they should be kept in mind in order not to isolate human experimentation from other societal practices nor, in turn, to neglect questioning those practices in light of our explorations.

In studying these materials, re-evaluate the answers already given to the questions posed in Chapter Eight. In addition, consider the following questions:

1. How and to what extent should the dynamics of the inner and outer world, inherent in the nature of man as an individual and social being, be taken into account in defining his capacity for self-determination and informed consent?

2. How and to what extent are these dynamics affected by the nature and extent of the communications given to subjects?

3. To what extent can and should the investigator ascertain from the subject that informed consent has been obtained?

4. How should the authority of the subject to make decisions be affected by any limitations inherent in informed consent?

5. What implications do the answers to the previous questions have for the formulation, administration, and review of the human experimentation process?

A.
Barriers to Achieving Autonomy

1.

The Impact of the Inner World

a.

Sigmund Freud
Introductory Lectures on Psycho-analysis
(1916)*

[M]ental processes are in themselves unconscious and . . . of all mental life it is only certain individual acts and portions that are conscious. [P]sychoanalysis . . . cannot accept the identity of the conscious and the mental. It defines what is mental as processes, such as, feeling, thinking, and willing, and it is obliged to maintain that there is unconscious thinking and unapprehended willing. . . . The question whether we are to make the psychical coincide with the conscious or make it extend further sounds like an empty dispute about words; yet I can assure you that the hypothesis of there being unconscious mental processes paves the way to a decisive new orientation in the world and in science.

*   *   *

We will not start with postulates but with an investigation. Let us choose as its subject certain phenomena which are very common and very familiar but which have been very little examined, and which, since they can be observed in any healthy person, have nothing to do with illnesses. They are what are known as "parapraxes," to

———————
* James Strachey, ed.: 15 *The Standard Edition of the Complete Psychological Works of Sigmund Freud.* London: The Hogarth Press and the Institute of Psychoanalysis 21–22, 25–26, 33–35, 44–45, 52–53, 57–58, 60, 64–66, 72–74 (1963). Reprinted by permission of George Allen & Unwin Ltd., London, and Liveright Publishing Corp., N.Y.

which everyone is liable. It may happen, for instance, that a person who intends to say something may use another word instead (a *slip of the tongue*) . . . or he may do the same thing in writing, and may or may not notice what he has done. Or a person may read something, whether in print or manuscript, different from what is actually before his eyes (a *misreading*) . . . or he may hear wrongly something that has been said to him (a *mishearing*). . . . Another group of these phenomena has as its basis *forgetting* . . . not, however, a permanent forgetting but only a temporary one. Thus a person may be unable to get hold of a *name* which he nevertheless knows and which he recognizes at once, or he may forget to carry out an *intention*, though he remembers it later and has thus only forgotten it at that particular moment. In a third group the temporary character is absent—for instance, in the case of *mislaying* . . . when a person has put something somewhere and cannot find it again, or in the precisely analogous case of *losing*. . . . Here we have a forgetting which we treat differently from other kinds of forgetting, one at which we are surprised or annoyed instead of finding it understandable. . . .

*   *   *

The most usual, and at the same time the most striking kind of slips of the tongue . . . are those in which one says the precise opposite of what one intended to say. Here, of course, we are very remote from relations between sounds and the effects of similarity; and instead we can appeal to the fact that contraries have a strong conceptual kinship with each other and stand in a particularly close psychological association with each other. There are historical examples of such occurrences. A president of the Lower House of our Parliament once opened the sitting with the words: "Gentlemen, I take notice that a full quorum of members is present and herewith declare the sitting *closed.*"

* * *

[W]hat results from the slip of the tongue has a sense of its own. What do we mean by "has a sense"? That the product of the slip of the tongue may perhaps itself have a right to be regarded as a completely valid psychical act, pursuing an aim of its own, as a statement with a content and significance. So far we have always spoken of "parapraxes [faulty acts]," but it seems now as though sometimes the faulty act was itself quite a *normal* act, which merely took the place of the other act which was the one expected or intended.

The fact of the parapraxis having a sense of its own seems in certain cases evident and unmistakable. When the president of the Lower House with his first words *closed* the sitting instead of opening it, we feel inclined, in view of our knowledge of the circumstances in which the slip of the tongue occurred, to recognize that the parapraxis had a sense. The president expected nothing good of the sitting and would have been glad if he could have brought it to an immediate end. We have no difficulty in pointing to the sense of this slip of the tongue. [Or] we are told that a lady who was well known for her energy remarked on one occasion: "My husband asked his doctor what diet he ought to follow; but the doctor told him he had no need to diet: he could eat and drink what I want." Here again the slip of the tongue has an unmistakable other side to it: It was giving expression to a consistently planned program.

* * *

[P]arapraxes . . . are not chance events but serious mental acts; they have a sense; they arise from the concurrent action—or perhaps rather, the mutually opposing action—of two different intentions. . . .

* * *

[I]s this the explanation of *all* cases of slips of the tongue? I am very much inclined to think so, and my reason is that every time one investigates an instance of a slip of the tongue an explanation of this kind is forthcoming. But it is also true that there is no way of proving that a slip of the tongue cannot occur without this mechanism. It may be so; but theoretically it is

a matter of indifference to us, since the conclusions we want to draw for our introduction to psychoanalysis remain, even though—which is certainly not the case—our view holds good of only a minority of cases of slips of the tongue. The next question—whether we may extend our view to other sorts of parapraxis—I will answer in advance with a "yes". . . .

* * *

[A] lady inquired from her doctor for news of a common acquaintance, but called her by her maiden name. She had forgotten her friend's married name. She admitted afterwards she had been very unhappy about the marriage and disliked her friend's husband.

* * *

The forgetting of intentions can in general be traced to an opposing current of thought, which is unwilling to carry out the intention. But this view is not only held by us psychoanalysts; it is the general opinion, accepted by everyone in their daily lives and only denied when it comes to theory. A patron who gives his protégé the excuse of having forgotten his request fails to justify himself. The protégé immediately thinks: "It means nothing to him; it's true he promised, but he doesn't really want to do it." For that reason forgetting is banned in certain circumstances of ordinary life; the distinction between the popular and the psychoanalytic view of the parapraxes seems to have disappeared. Imagine the lady of the house receiving her guest with the words: "What? Have you come today? I'd quite forgotten I invited you for today." Or imagine a young man confessing to his fiancée that he had forgotten to keep their last rendezvous. He will certainly not confess it; he will prefer to invent on the spur of the moment the most improbable obstacles which prevented his appearing at the time and afterwards made it impossible for him to let her know. We all know, too, that in military affairs the excuse of having forgotten something is of no help and is no protection against punishment, and we must all feel that that is justified. Here all at once everyone is united in thinking that a particular parapraxis has a sense and in knowing what that sense is. . . .

* * *

. . . The governing condition of these cases, it will be realized, is that the present psychical situation is unknown to us or inaccessible to our inquiries. Our interpretation is consequently no more than a suspicion to which we ourselves do not attach too much importance. Later, however, something happens which shows us how well-justified our interpretation had been. I was once the guest of a young married couple and heard the young woman laughingly describe her latest experience. The day after her return from the honeymoon she had called for her unmarried sister to go shopping with her as she used to do, while her husband went to his business. Suddenly she noticed a gentleman on the other side of the street, and nudging her sister had cried: "Look, there goes Herr L." She had forgotten that this gentleman had been her husband for some weeks. I shuddered as I heard the story, but I did not dare to draw the inference. The little incident only occurred to my mind some years later when the marriage had come to a most unhappy end.

*   *   *

. . . We may take it as the outcome of our efforts so far and the basis of our further investigations that parapraxes have a sense. Let me insist once again that I am not asserting—and for our purposes there is no need to do so—that every single parapraxis that occurs has a sense, even though I regard that as probably the case. It is enough for us if we can point to such a sense relatively often in the different forms of parapraxis. Moreover, in this respect these different forms behave differently. Cases of slips of the tongue and of the pen, etc., may occur on a purely physiological basis. I cannot believe that this is so in the types depending on *forgetting* (forgetting names or intentions, mislaying, etc.). It is very probable that there are cases of *losing* which can be regarded as unintended. It is in general true that only a certain proportion of the *errors* that occur in ordinary life can be looked at from our point of view. . . .

*   *   *

We can now turn . . . . to the main question, which we have long postponed, of what sort of intentions these are, which find expression in this unusual fashion as disturbers of other intentions. Well, they are obviously of very different sorts, among which we must look for the common factor. If we examine a number of examples with this in view, they will soon fall into three groups. The first group contains those cases in which the disturbing purpose is known to the speaker and, moreover, had been noticed by him before he made the slip of the tongue. . . . A second group is made up of other cases in which the disturbing purpose is equally recognized as his

by the speaker, but in which he was unaware that it was active in him just before he made the slip. Thus, he accepts our interpretation of his slip, but nevertheless remains to some extent surprised at it. . . . In a third group the interpretation of the disturbing intention is vigorously rejected by the speaker; he not only denies that it was active in him before he made the slip, but seeks to maintain that it is entirely foreign to him. . . .

*   *   *

[W]hat distinguishes these three groups from one another is the differing extent to which the intention is forced back. In the first group the intention is there and makes itself noticed before the speaker's remark; only then is it rejected; and it takes its revenge in the slip of the tongue. In the second group the rejection goes further; the intention has already ceased to be noticeable before the remark is made. Strangely enough, this does not in the least prevent it from playing its part in causing the slip. But this behavior makes it easier for us to explain what happens in the third group. I shall venture to assume that a purpose can also find expression in a parapraxis when it has been forced back and not noticed for a considerable time, for a very long time perhaps, and can for that reason be denied straight out by the speaker. But even if you leave the problem of the third group on one side, you are bound to conclude from the observations we have made in the other cases that *the suppression of the speaker's intention to say something is the indispensable condition for the occurrence of a slip of the tongue.*

[P]arapraxes are the outcome of a compromise: They constitute a half-success and a half-failure for each of the two intentions; the intention which is being challenged is neither completely suppressed nor, apart from special cases, carried through quite unscathed. . . .

*   *   *

The instances of forgetting an intention are in general so uniform and so perspicuous that for that very reason they are of no interest for our investigation. Nevertheless there are two points at which we can learn something new from a study of these parapraxes. Forgetting—that is, failure to carry out—an intention points, as we have said, to a counter-will that is hostile to it. this is no doubt true; but our inquiries show that the counter-will can be of two kinds—direct or indirect. What I mean by the latter will best appear from one or two examples. . . . [S]upposing someone forgets an appointment which he has promised someone else to keep, the most frequent reason for it will be, no doubt, a direct disinclination to meeting this person. But in such a case analysis might show that the disturbing purpose did not relate to him but was directed against the place at which the meeting was planned to happen and was avoided on account of a distressing memory attaching to it. Or, again, if someone forgets to post a letter, the counter-purpose may be based on the contents of the letter; but it is by no means out of the question that the letter may be harmless in itself and may only be subject to the counter-purpose because something about it recalls another letter which had been written on some earlier occasion and which offered the counter-will a direct point of attack. It can be said, therefore, that here the counter-will was transferred from the earlier letter, which justified it, to the present one, which it had in fact no grounds for concern about. . . .

Phenomena such as these last may seem to you most unusual, and you will perhaps be inclined to suppose that an "indirect" counter-will already indicates that the process is a pathological one. But I can assure you that it occurs as well within the limits of what is normal and healthy. . . .

The second point I have in mind is this. If in a large majority of instances we find confirmation of the fact that the forgetting of an intention goes back to a counter-will, we grow bold enough to extend the solution to another set of instances in which the person under analysis does not confirm but denies the counter-will we have inferred. Take as examples of this such extremely common events as forgetting to return books one has been lent or to pay bills or debts. We shall venture to insist to the person concerned that an intention exists in him to keep the books and not to pay the debts, while he will deny this intention but will not be able to produce any other explanation of his behavior. Thereupon we shall go on to say that he has this intention but knows nothing about it, but that it is enough for us that it reveals its presence by producing the forgetting in him. He may repeat to us that he has in fact forgotten. You will now recognize the situation as one in which we found ourselves once before. If we want to pursue our interpretations of parapraxes, which have so frequently proved justified, to a consistent conclusion, we are forced to the inescapable hypothesis that there are purposes in people which can become operative without their knowing about them. . . .

*   *   *

NOTES

NOTE 1.

ERNEST JONES
THE REPRESSION THEORY IN ITS
RELATION TO MEMORY*

. . . In working with psychoanalysis one finds that the unconscious material in the mind is very much more extensive than might have been surmised, that the assimilative capacity of the complexes, due to the radiation of affect, is very much greater, and that, therefore, the number of associations that are established in the unconscious is simply enormous. That being so, it is extremely difficult, and at present impossible, to set any limits to the extent to which operations characteristically applying to unconscious material, such as repression does, are in action. One is practically never in a position, for instance, to assert that such and such an idea cannot have been associated with any "unpleasant" buried complex, for to be so would necessitate a most searching investigation of all its associations, both conscious and unconscious. It is rather like the question of the alleged destruction or fading of forgotten memories, a negative proposition that it is impossible to prove. One can only say, with considerable emphasis, that the more extensive the investigation the greater is the number of forgotten ideas that prove to be affectively connected with repressed complexes, so that the possibility is at least open that they all are.

NOTE 2.

SIGMUND FREUD
A DIFFICULTY IN THE PATH OF
PSYCHO-ANALYSIS (1917)†

*   *   *

[T]he universal narcissism of men, their self-love, has up to the present suffered three severe blows from the researches of science.

(a) In the early stages of his researches, man believed at first that his dwelling-place, the earth, was the stationary centre of the universe,

* *Papers on Psychoanalysis.* London: Bailliére, Tindall & Cox 117 (1920). Reprinted by permission of Bailliére, Tindall & Cassell, Ltd.

† James Strachey, ed.: 17 *The Standard Edition of the Complete Psychological Works of Sigmund Freud.* London: The Hogarth Press and the Institute of Psychoanalysis 139–143 (1955). Reprinted by permission of Sigmund Freud Copyrights, Ltd., the Institute of Psychoanalysis and the Hogarth Press, Ltd., London, and of Basic Books, Inc., N.Y.

with the sun, moon and planets circling round it. In this he was naively following the dictates of his sense-perceptions, for he felt no movement of the earth, and wherever he had an unimpeded view he found himself in the centre of a circle that enclosed the external world. The central position of the earth, moreover, was a token to him of the dominating part played by it in the universe and appeared to fit in very well with his inclination to regard himself as lord of the world.

The destruction of this narcissistic illusion is associated in our minds with the name and work of Copernicus in the sixteenth century. . . .

(b) In the course of the development of civilization man acquired a dominating position over his fellow-creatures in the animal kingdom. Not content with this supremacy, however, he began to place a gulf between his nature and theirs. He denied the possession of reason to them, and to himself he attributed an immortal soul, and made claims to a divine descent which permitted him to break the bond of community between him and the animal kingdom. . . .

We all know that little more than half a century ago the researches of Charles Darwin and his collaborators and forerunners put an end to this presumption on the part of man. . . .

(c) The third blow, which is psychological in nature, is probably the most wounding.

Although thus humbled in his external relations, man feels himself to be supreme within his own mind. Somewhere in the core of his ego he has developed an organ of observation to keep a watch on his impulses and actions and see whether they harmonize with its demands. If they do not, they are ruthlessly inhibited and withdrawn. His internal perception, consciousness, gives the ego news of all the important occurrences in the mind's working, and the will, directed by these reports, carries out what the ego orders and modifies anything that seeks to accomplish itself spontaneously. For this mind is not a simple thing; on the contrary, it is a hierarchy of superordinated and subordinated agencies, a labyrinth of impulses striving independently of one another towards action, corresponding with the multiplicity of instincts and of the relations with the external world, many of which are antagonistic to one another and incompatible. For proper functioning it is necessary that the highest of these agencies should have knowledge of all that is going forward and that its will should penetrate everywhere, so as to exert its influence. And in fact the ego feels secure both as to the completeness and trustworthi-

ness of the reports it receives and as to the openness of the channels through which it enforces its commands.

In certain diseases—including the very neuroses of which we have made special study—things are different. The ego feels uneasy; it comes up against limits to its power in its own house, the mind. Thoughts emerge suddenly without one's knowing where they come from, nor can one do anything to drive them away. These alien guests even seem to be more powerful than those which are at the ego's command. They resist all the well-proved measures of enforcement used by the will, remain unmoved by logical refutation, and are unaffected by the contradictory assertions of reality. Or else impulses appear which seem like those of a stranger, so that the ego disowns them; yet it has to fear them and take precautions against them. The ego says to itself: "This is an illness, a foreign invasion." It increases its vigilance, but cannot understand why it feels so strangely paralysed.

Psychiatry, it is true, denies that such things mean the intrusion into the mind of evil spirits from without; beyond this, however, it can only say with a shrug: "Degeneracy, hereditary disposition, constitutional inferiority!" Psycho-analysis sets out to explain these uncanny disorders; it engages in careful and laborious investigations, devises hypotheses and scientific constructions, until at length it can speak thus to the ego:—

"Nothing has entered into you from without; a part of the activity of your own mind has been withdrawn from your knowledge and from the command of your will. That, too, is why you are so weak in your defence; you are using one part of your force to fight the other part and you cannot concentrate the whole of your force as you would against an external enemy. And it is not even the worst or least important part of your mental forces that has thus become antagonistic to you and independent of you. The blame, I am bound to say, lies with yourself. You over-estimated your strength when you thought you could treat your sexual instincts as you liked and could utterly ignore their intentions. The result is that they have rebelled and have taken their own obscure paths to escape this suppression; they have established their rights in a manner you cannot approve. How they have achieved this, and the paths which they have taken, have not come to your knowledge. All you have learned is the *outcome* of their work—the symptom which you experience as suffering. Thus you do not recognize it as a derivative of your own rejected instincts and do not know that it is a substitutive satisfaction of them.

"The whole process, however, only becomes possible through the single circumstance that you are mistaken in another important point as well. You feel sure that you are informed of all that goes on in your mind if it is of any importance at all, because in that case, you believe, your consciousness gives you news of it. And if you have had no information of something in your mind you confidently assume that it does not exist there. Indeed, you go so far as to regard what is 'mental' as identical with what is 'conscious'— that is, with what is known to you—in spite of the most obvious evidence that a great deal more must constantly be going on in your mind than can be known to your consciousness. Come, let yourself be taught something on this one point! What is in your mind does not coincide with what you are conscious of; whether something is going on in your mind and whether you hear of it, are two different things. In the ordinary way, I will admit, the intelligence which reaches your consciousness is enough for your needs; and you may cherish the illusion that you learn of all the more important things. But in some cases, as in that of an instinctual conflict such as I have described, your intelligence service breaks down and your will then extends no further than your knowledge. In every case, however, the news that reaches your consciousness is incomplete and often not to be relied on. Often enough, too, it happens that you get news of events only when they are over and when you can no longer do anything to change them. Even if you are not ill, who can tell all that is stirring in your mind of which you know nothing or are falsely informed? You behave like an absolute ruler who is content with the information supplied him by his highest officials and never goes among the people to hear their voice. Turn your eyes inward, look into your own depths, learn first to know yourself! Then you will understand why you were bound to fall ill; and, perhaps you will avoid falling ill in future."

It is thus that psycho-analysis has sought to educate the ego. But these two discoveries—that the life of our sexual instincts cannot be wholly tamed, and that mental processes are in themselves unconscious and only reach the ego and come under its control through incomplete and untrustworthy perceptions—these two discoveries amount to a statement that *the ego is not master in its own house.* Together they represent the third blow to man's self-love, what I may call

the *psychological* one. No wonder, then, that the ego does not look favourably upon psycho-analysis and obstinately refuses to believe in it.

* * *

NOTE 3.

ROBERT P. KNIGHT
DETERMINISM, "FREEDOM," AND
PSYCHOTHERAPY*

* * *

The first step in extricating ourselves from the confusion inherent in the determinism versus free will debate lies in clarifying the terms. Determinism in the physical world is no longer seriously questioned by scientists or philosophers. Its alternative, indeterminism—pure chance, accident, unpredictability—represents chaos. "Indeterminacy" in modern (post-Newtonian) physics, simply refers to the fact that human limits of perception and their intrusion into the field of the experimental measuring instruments make absolute precision impossible. Rigorous physical determinism is not contested by Heisenberg's principle of indeterminacy. In the psychological and philosophical realm there is also no real alternative to psychic determinism. To defend "free will" as an alternative is to be guilty of semantic confusion. Determinism refers to the complex of causal factors, hereditary and environmental, internal and external, past and present, conscious and unconscious, which combine to produce a certain resultant in a given individual. Determinism is thus a theoretical construct which fits the observed data, as demonstrated by predictions which were fulfilled, and which is essential to any psychology which claims to be scientific. The antithesis to this construct is the construct, indeterminism—pure chance, chaos. "Free will," on the other hand, is not on the same conceptual level as are these constructs. It refers to a subjective psychological experience, and to compare it to determinism is like comparing the enjoyment of flying to the law of gravity.

. . . A scrutiny of this matter of "choice" may lead us to further understanding. When such choices involve only trivial matters, the mentally healthy person has the subjective sense of complete freedom of choice, and hence feels

———
* 9 *Psychiatry* 251–259 (1946). Copyright 1946 by the William Alanson White Psychiatric Foundation. Reprinted by special permission of the William Alanson White Psychiatric Foundation, Inc.

that he has acted of his own free will. Indeed, were a person not to feel free to choose in trivial matters, but instead feel powerfully compelled toward a single course, and experience anxiety if prevented from completing his choice, we would suspect him of suffering from a compulsion neurosis. Or if he were unable to choose quickly and lightheartedly—that is, with a sense of freedom of choice—in unimportant matters we would suspect the presence of obsessional doubt. In weightier matters, however, the healthy person has a combined feeling of freedom and of inner compulsion. He feels that his course is determined by standards, beliefs, knowledge, aspirations that are an integral part of himself and he can do no other; yet at the same time he feels free. A decision or course of action that is in harmony with his character seems to carry with it the reward of a pleasurable sense of freedom. It is not easy to analyze the sense of freedom as it is used in this context but it can be described more fully. In a negative sense it means absence of anxiety, of irrational doubt, and of those inhibitions and restrictions which paralyze both choice and action. In a positive sense it connotes feelings of well-being, of self-esteem, of confidence, of inner satisfaction based on successful use of one's energies for achievement that promotes the best interests of one's fellow men as well as one's own.

It is a part of the thesis of this essay that this kind of "freedom" is experienced only by emotionally mature, well-integrated persons; it is the goal sought for one's patients in psychotherapy; and this freedom has nothing whatever to do with free will as a principle governing human behavior, but is a subjective experience which is itself causally determined. This subjective experience, however, is subjective in a special sense, not in the one which equates "subjective" with "spurious." The behavior of a well-integrated, civilized person can be objectively assessed as "free." Observers see that such a person makes ego syntonic choices, that his motives are "good," and that he is able to carry out what he wills to do.

There are, however, experiences of freedom which are illusions to the persons experiencing them. They are subjective in the sense of spuriousness. Critical examination of the nature of such varieties of the subjective experience of freedom, and objective assessment of their relationship to the actualities of life, distinguish them readily from the freedom defined above. There is, for example, the sense of freedom in children or immature adults which occurs with the removal of external pressure or with solitary flights of fantasy of being omnipotent. The release from inner checks and restraints that occurs in mania likewise conveys a sense of complete freedom. There is a spurious sense of freedom in those persons, who, unconsciously driven by intense defiance, carry out criminal acts, acts of libertinism, and acts of spurious independence and self-assertion. One of the first tasks in the psychotherapy of such persons is to show them that they are not free, as they have thought, but are enslaved and driven by their compulsion to defy others. There is also the spurious sense of freedom that accompanies the hypocritically righteous decision in a person who perceives that a nefarious purpose may be executed under the cloak of righteousness. In such persons closer scrutiny will reveal a complicated scheme of balances between well-rationalized, sadistically motivated acts of aggression and compulsive acts and rituals of penance. Many other examples could be cited to illustrate varieties of subjective freedom which are illusions to the subject, and are vulnerable to objective assessment.

The genuine freedom which is a mark of mental health and emotional maturity is best expressed by the following quotation, whose authorship I do not know: "That man is free who is conscious of being the author of the law that he obeys." This definition includes both the sense of freedom and the sense of inner compulsion which we have designated as inseparable subjective feelings in matters of real importance in life. It also includes the concept of integration of the personality, that is, the individual's energies and impulses are subject to conscious control but are capable of satisfying discharge according to standards which the ego accepts. If it is correct to assume that this linkage of subjective freedom with inner acceptable compulsion is a criterion of mental health and of emotional and intellectual maturity in human beings, and that other experiences of subjective freedom which do not meet the test of linkage with acceptable inner compulsion and of objective assessment are psychiatrically suspect, then we have narrowed down the problem of freedom by eliminating from further consideration the spurious varieties of subjective freedom. It is sufficient to say, then, that all of the subjective experiences of freedom are, like every other psychological datum, understandable as causally determined products of many factors—hereditary, experiential, biological, cultural, and so on. "Free will" is thus reduced from its presumptuous position as a real threat or alternative to determinism, and is demoted to the position of a variety of subjective experience—one which is itself causally determined.

[D]ynamic psychology has been able to develop constructs which fit the observable clinical data, which provide a scientific theory based on the axiom of psychological determinism. . . .

The first construct is that there is an unconscious part of the self, the id, containing the instinctual forces which are rooted in biology, and molded by infantile emotional experience. These forces are aggressive, selfish, lustful, and seek immediate gratification. But their full satisfaction in each individual, were there no external or internal controls, would result in collision with the external laws and limitations of the physical world on the one hand, and with the attempts of other individuals to fulfill their instinctual strivings on the other hand. The result would be chaos. We are saved from such chaos in organized society by the inevitable operation of natural laws and by man-made restrictive rules (laws) under which unlimited freedom for each individual is sharply curtailed so that the interests of each person are protected. The aim of man-made laws is—or, at least, should be—to guarantee the maximum degree of gratification of individual needs which is consistent with the protection of the rights of others. Civilization thus sacrifices individual freedom of action to promote collective security.

The second construct of dynamic psychology is that out of the original infantile unorganized mass of instinctual wishes there develops an organized portion of the self, the ego, which is largely conscious. It co-ordinates the faculties of perception, intelligence, judgment, memory, discrimination, learning, and so on. The ego has the task of achieving what satisfactions it can of the instinctual drives of the id, while taking cognizance of the nature of the environment and its natural and man-made restrictions. The ego is the feeling, experiencing, aware portion of the personality.

The third construct is that there also develops, in early childhood, as an internalization of the restricting, frustrating, disciplining parents and their surrogates, a third portion of the psyche called the superego, or conscience, which is largely unconscious. It is an internal master to which the ego is subject, so that the ego's adjustive task becomes one of managing the instinctual drives from within against the limitations and frustrations of the outer world, while being compelled to obey also the forbidding directives of the superego.

The development and operation of each of these portions of the self, and thus of the total personality, is causally determined in accordance with the psychological laws governing the inherited endowment, biological drives, physiological and emotional experiences, and external, natural, cultural, and interpersonal pressures affecting each individual in the milieu in which he is reared. In the healthy person there is a harmonious interrelationship between the various parts of the self and with the environment, and one of the important by-products of such harmonious integration is a subjective sense of freedom. Viewed in this way, the feeling of freedom is also determined, and is possible to be experienced only to the extent that there exists within the individual a harmonious integration of his instinctual drives, his superego standards and restrictions, his ego perceptions and discriminative faculties, and the possibilities provided by the environment. Such a theoretically healthy, integrated person will then feel free, and, to some extent, will be "free." That is, his flexibility of adaptation will be greater than that of the neurotic person, and what behavior he "chooses" will conform to the laws and standards, internal and external, which he accepts, but his choices will *feel* free.

NOTE 4.

ERNST LEWY
RESPONSIBILITY, FREE WILL,
AND EGO PSYCHOLOGY*

*   *   *

[David] Rapaport in a personal communication [states]:

"Man has developed an anticipatory apparatus which is far more effective than any other animal's. This apparatus is very effective for outside events and fairly effective (anxiety and other affect signals) for internal events. These events play a causal role in behavior. But man himself (and every organism to some degree) is a source of causes. Man's anticipatory apparatus is a particularly effective mobilizer of man's own causal role. Man isn't freed from internal and external causes by means of his anticipatory apparatus, that is, by dint of his being

* 42 *International Journal of Psychoanalysis* 260, 267–268 (1961). Reprinted by permission.

also a source of causes. But he certainly can within limits avoid, evade, cushion, and counteract causes which would determine his behavior. Some of these causes he is less adept at avoiding or cushioning (instinctual drives)—but to the extent that he has a relatively autonomous ego, he can do even some of that. Instinctual drives are causes and motives; other causes of the same sort (neutralized to various degrees) he can cushion better. Non-motivational causes he can yet easier evade or cushion, somatic ones less so than environmental ones.—So to the degree to which he is within these limits, he is a free agent. To this degree (and to the degree he fails to use this ability) he is responsible in the broadest sense."

In addition to the above . . . there is the question of how the acceptance of one's responsibility is achieved and transmitted. I submit that if responsibility of the individual for himself is considered traditionally and conventionally an established reality factor, this very fact acts as a sufficiently strong adaptive force to determine the individual's choice. Assuming the capacity of the ego to adapt its operations and reactions to the environment and its realities, we can expect that the ego can be purposefully influenced by reality factors. Thus, specifically the reality fact that traditionally, conventionally, and tacitly every individual is considered to be responsible for his acts by the society in which he lives, and that this is inculcated in the child through the educational and rearing process, constitutes a powerful reality factor to which the ego has to adapt itself and is capable of adapting itself. The established standard provides the environmental setting to which the adaptable ego responds. I am referring to what Erikson calls our "institutionalized attitude". . . .

*   *   *

An important part of the dynamics of adaptation is played, of course, in particular in the course of growing up, by the process of the formation of the superego through identification with the authority figures, their introjection and the subsequent internalization of accepted standards. . . .

*   *   *

. . . We not only can, we also must hold man responsible, in order to establish the necessary and correct environment. To put it bluntly, I should like to re-state Voltaire's famous saying

about God with the appropriate alteration: "If free will and responsibility did not exist, they would have to be invented". . . .

*   *   *

b.

Benjamin N. Cardozo
The Nature of the Judicial Process*

I have spoken of the forces of which judges avowedly avail to shape the form and content of their judgments. Even these forces are seldom fully in consciousness. They lie so near the surface, however, that their existence and influence are not likely to be disclaimed. But the subject is not exhausted with the recognition of their power. Deep below consciousness are other forces, the likes and the dislikes, the predilections and the prejudices, the complex of instincts and emotions and habits and convictions, which make the man, whether he be litigant or judge. . . . There has been a certain lack of candor in much of the discussion of the theme, or rather perhaps in the refusal to discuss it, as if judges must lose respect and confidence by the reminder that they are subject to human limitations. I do not doubt the grandeur of the conception which lifts them into the realm of pure reason, above and beyond the sweep of perturbing and deflecting forces. Nonetheless . . . they do not stand aloof on these chill and distant heights; and we shall not help the cause of truth by acting and speaking as if they do. The great tides and currents, which engulf the rest of men, do not turn aside in their course and pass the judges by. We like to figure to ourselves the processes of justice as coldly objective and impersonal. The law, conceived of as a real existence, dwelling apart and alone, speaks, through the voices of priests and ministers, the words which they have no choice except to utter. That is an ideal of objective truth toward which every system of jurisprudence tends. It is an ideal of which great publicists and judges have spoken as of something possible to attain. "The judges of the nation," says Montesquieu, "are only the mouths that pronounce the words of the law, inanimate beings, who can moderate neither its force nor its rigor." So Marshall, in *Osborne* v. *Bank of the United States*, 9 Wheat. 738, 866: The judicial department "has no will in any case. . . . Judicial power is never exercised

* New Haven: Yale University Press 167–170 (1921). Reprinted by permission.

for the purpose of giving effect to the will of the judge; always for the purpose of giving effect to the will of the legislature; or, in other words, to the will of the law." It has a lofty sound; it is well and finely said; but it can never be more than partly true. Marshall's own career is a conspicuous illustration of the fact that the ideal is beyond the reach of human faculties to attain. He gave to the constitution of the United States the impress of his own mind; and the form of our constitutional law is what it is, because he moulded it while it was still plastic and malleable in the fire of his own intense convictions. At the opposite extreme are the words of the French jurist, Saleilles, in his treatise "De la Personnalité Juridique": "One wills at the beginning the result; one finds the principle afterwards; such is the genesis of all juridical construction. Once accepted, the construction presents itself, doubtless, in the ensemble of legal doctrine, under the opposite aspect. The factors are inverted. The principle appears as an initial cause, from which one has drawn the result which is found deduced from it." I would not put the case thus broadly. So sweeping a statement exaggerates the element of free volition. It ignores the factors of determinism which cabin and confine within narrow bounds the range of unfettered choice. Nonetheless, by its very excess of emphasis, it supplies the needed corrective of an ideal of impossible objectivity. . . .

*   *   *

c.

Carl H. Fellner and John R. Marshall
Kidney Donors—
The Myth of Informed Consent*

*   *   *

[W]e undertook to study all available previous [kidney] donors to find out how they had become involved [and] how they had made their decision. . . .

*   *   *

Of the 20 donors interviewed, 14 were seen at five weeks to 24 months after surgery, with a mean of 11 months, and six were seen before as well as after surgery. In addition, a number of

* 126 *American Journal of Psychiatry* 1245–1250 (1970). Copyright 1970, the American Psychiatric Association. Reprinted by permission.

potential donors were interviewed who were subsequently rejected as medically unsuitable. Another ten potential donors who were interviewed are currently awaiting surgery. . . .

The process of making a decision to give up a kidney for a close relative begins when the first communication about the seriousness of the recipient's illness is received. It continues when the first demand for participation in the medical selection process is made and must be sustained through the long-drawn-out medical investigation and usually through a waiting period even after the decision-making process of the renal transplantation team has been concluded, the potential donor is considered a candidate for transplantation, and has been permitted to give his consent. In addition, there appears to be a third or family system, which also tends to influence the selection of a donor but which is very difficult to demonstrate.

1. The medical selection system. When a transplant situation arises, all possible donor relatives of the patient are asked to come to the clinic for blood tests (ABO typing). Great care is taken at this point by the medical staff to inform the volunteer subjects that this is an exceedingly preliminary procedure and that no commitment whatsoever is involved by their appearing at this clinic, or elsewhere, to have their blood samples drawn. Those potential donors who are not ruled out on the basis of blood grouping are then asked to come to the renal clinic for a brief history-taking and complete physical examination, including routine laboratory studies.

Somewhat later, those of the possible donors who still remain are asked to return to the clinic for histocompatability tests. The results of the mixed leucocyte culture tests (MLCT) are not known until several weeks later and may have to be repeated before they can be read conclusively. Only after this stage does it become possible for the renal transplant team to select from among the available possible donors that most suitable one. He is then asked to come to the special studies unit at the hospital for a complete work-up, careful evaluation of renal status, and so on. During this brief hospitalization he is evaluated independently by at least three of the team physicians. Only at the end of this evaluation and after intensive, repeated briefing on the risks involved and the chances for success is the potential donor asked to make a decision, and permitted, if he desires, to give his informed consent. A final chance to refuse any time in a dignified and comfortable manner is offered in the team's expressed willingness to supply a plausible medical excuse to the recipient and family.

2. Donor decision. The medical selection system as described assumes that the future donor will make his decision only at the conclusion of the medical work-up and after intensive and repeated briefing. It is assumed that the decision will occur only at the end of adequate information-gathering and weighing of the pros and cons. Actually, members of the renal transplant team were aware that most of the potential donors were ready to make a commitment earlier than that and had to be held off until the team had made its selection. It was thought that this point of commitment was reached perhaps halfway through the evaluation process.

Our findings were surprising. Not one of the donors weighed alternatives and rationally decided. Fourteen of the 20 donors and nine of the ten donors waiting for surgery stated that they had made their decision immediately when the subject of the kidney transplant was first mentioned over the telephone, "in a split-second," "instantaneously," and "right away." Five said they just went along with the tests hoping it would be someone else. They could not recall ever really having made a clear decision, yet they never considered refusing to go along either. As it became clear to each of them toward the end of the selection process that he was going to be the person most suited to be the donor, each had finally committed himself to the act. However, this decision too occurred before the sessions with the team doctors in which all the relevant information and statistics were put before these individuals and they were finally asked to decide.

Of all the subjects who made their initial decision on the telephone upon first hearing of the possibility of the kidney transplant, none had consulted his or her spouse. When questioned about this particular circumstance each explained that the spouse later on had either been neutral or reinforced the decision. To the hypothetical question of "What would you have done if your spouse had said no?" each answered, "I would have gone ahead and done it anyway." One 48-year-old woman had a good deal of trouble in making her decision. The recipient was her son and the first communication that a renal transplantation would be necessary came from the doctor who had treated her son

for some time. The immediate family consisted of the donor, her husband, and four children, two of whom were under 18. The older daughter, who might have been a potential donor, immediately refused to participate in any way. The husband was a diabetic and was therefore disqualified. The woman's own doctor advised her not to do it. However, she went along with the preliminary tests, feeling very ambivalent about them. All her tests were fine and she was finally asked to make a decision before the renal arteriograms would be taken. At that point she felt she wanted to go home for another family conference to ask her husband what she should do. This was a very frightened woman, organized along strict obsessive-compulsive lines, who said, "I get worked up over every little thing, and I have never had surgery before." In the end she did decide to donate her kidney after her family consultation, saying, "I guess I had some encouragement from my husband now."

Of all the people asked to come for the preliminary blood tests, there were about eight who did not show up. Of all those who participated in the initial screening tests, only one subject later refused to participate in further tests. None of the final potential donors availed themselves of the "last-out" opportunity, although there were one or two subjects who seemed glad when they were rejected for medical reasons after the last test (arteriogram). This leads us to believe that for all participants, and by the same token for all those who refused to participate from the beginning, decision making is an early event preceding all information-gathering and clarification offered by the renal team.

Supportive evidence for the instantaneous character of the decision making came from a rather unexpected quarter. We spoke to a resident physician whose blood had been used as a control in the MLC test. By the merest chance he had proved to be compatible with the potential kidney recipient patient. When he was informed of this finding he immediately refused without even having been asked to be a donor. He was subsequently able to tell us that this had been an immediate decision and that he had later spent much time marshalling evidence in support of this decision.

The immediacy of the decision making with regard to donorship often contrasts markedly with the usual way in which the person makes other important decisions. When questioned more closely about this contrast, all our subjects clearly expressed their opinion that this was a rather special situation that could not be compared to ordinary decision making.

3. The family system of donor selection. The role the family plays in the selection of donors was very difficult to demonstrate. In retrospect, this difficulty arose perhaps from the general feeling, which we shared, that the family would tend to select a likely donor in the sense of a sacrifice or scapegoat under threat of family ostracism. We could not demonstrate such dynamics in our sample, except possibly in one case.

What we did see, once we had become aware of its possibility, was that a family would *exclude* certain members from participation. This was done most commonly at the level of the initial contact. In only one case was the donor given the first communication about the possibility of renal transplant by a member of the transplant team, and in two cases by the family physician. All the others heard about it first from a family member. Usually the communication was by telephone call, the informant telling the future donor about the seriousness of the future recipient's illness and explaining that the doctors were considering a kidney transplantation and that all close relatives would be invited in the near future to come to the clinic or the hospital for some blood samples to be taken for initial tests. Usually, the informant followed this up with a brief discussion of who among the other family members should be asked to participate, who should not, and for what reasons. The same route was subsequently used to transmit the results of tests and make further appointments and could also serve to discourage further participation.

* * *

The fact remains that all the donors and potential donors interviewed by us reported a decision-making process that was immediate and "irrational" and could not meet the requirements adopted by the American Medical Association to be accepted as an "informed consent." Actually, the medical renal transplant team did not permit these donors to volunteer until a prolonged process of repeated information (or indoctrination?) had been completed. The effectiveness of this procedure must, however, be questioned by the investigators, if for no other reason than that it did not dissuade one single volunteer.

* * *

NOTE

JEAN HAMBURGER
PROTECTION OF DONOR RIGHTS IN
RENAL TRANSPLANTATION*

What is a real volunteer? I consider this very important, for it is related to the question of "informed consent" discussed this morning. I think that four conditions should exist for a real volunteer. First, he should be fully aware of the exact dangers he is running. Second, he should have a reasonable motive for wishing to donate his kidney; that is why, at Paris and at many other centres, we have adopted the habit of considering a volunteer acceptable if he is a relative of the patient to be saved and inacceptable if he is not. There are immunological reasons also. Third, the offer should be at the free will of the volunteer; it is for the doctor and for the organization dealing with the problem to verify whether there has been pressure from the family or elsewhere, such as the promise of payment. Finally, it seems to me that mental balance must be required and that, therefore, there should be a psychological, if not a psychiatric, examination to verify that the volunteer is in a full possession of his mental faculties. This psychological examination seems to us to be mandatory, both to verify that the decision is free and to say to the volunteer that if he wishes to withdraw his offer of his kidney nobody will ever know that he himself is responsible for that decision and the doctors will assume full responsibility towards the family. The examination will also ensure whether the mental balance of the donor is fully satisfactory.

These seem to me to be reasonable requirements at present: a balance of the risks and a real volunteer. Is the wish of the donor as thus expressed always completely satisfactory? This is to me a most important point, for it seems to me capable of transcending this particular case of the kidney donor. I think that in addition the doctor should put himself in the place of the donor and carry out what might be called a "motivation check."

Since it is certain that neither a patient nor a donor will ever be completely informed, I think that it is our duty to understudy the donor by a kind of check placing of ourselves in his

* V. Fattorusso, ed.: *Biomedical Science and the Dilemma of Human Experimentation.* Paris: Council for International Organizations of Medical Sciences 44 (1967). Reprinted by permission.

situation. Now that I know the donor and his behaviour, I should morally put myself in his position and see if it is reasonable for him to take that decision, since I, the doctor, am more objectively placed for assessing the safety of the donor than if I were in his necessarily subjective circumstances.

* * *

d.

Harold Esecover, Sidney Malitz, and Bernard Wilkens
Clinical Profiles of Paid Normal Subjects Volunteering for Hallucinogen Drug Studies*

* * *

Our study dealt with clinical psychiatric evaluations of 56 subjects volunteering for hallucinogen studies at the New York State Psychiatric Institute from 1956 to 1959. Our focus in this work was on motivations for volunteering, incidence and types of psychopathology, relationship between psychopathology and motivations, and personality patterns.

The sample was composed of 46 males and 10 females ranging in age from 21 to 38 with a median age of 23.4, with varying occupations but a high preponderance of students. All subjects had some college and 46 had varying degrees of post-graduate training. Volunteers were recruited by posting an announcement on the bulletin boards of a university medical school and a university undergraduate school. . . .

WANTED

Volunteers. Between 21 and 30 in good physical health for special medication studies involving temporary alterations in perceptions. Subjects should be prepared to sleep in the hospital overnight. Fee $25.

For further information and screening interview call Dr. Malitz, N.Y. State Psychiatric Institute, LO8-4000, Ext. 96.

All volunteers received an initial 1-hour psychiatric screening interview. The interview was a semi-structured one, with sufficient latitude given so that spontaneous material could emerge. . . .

* * *

A. *Motivations:* Motivations for volunteering were frequently quite complex and could be seen as operating simultaneously on 2 levels.

---

* 117 *American Journal of Psychiatry* 910–914 (1961). Copyright 1961, the American Psychiatric Association. Reprinted by permission.

Consciously stated motivations on one level; preconscious and unconscious ones on another. In only certain instances did we feel that we could determine the pre-conscious and unconscious roots. We felt that the subjects' conscious motivations could generally be broken down into the following broad categories: 1. Financial need; 2. Scientific interest and curiosity; 3. Seeking new experiences (adventure); 4. Indirect seeking of psychiatric help; 5. Symptomatic relief from tension, depression or anhedonia; 6. Searching for insights into personal problems; 7. Desires for status or prestige; 8. Employing the study as a vehicle for the expression of socially unacceptable impulses; and 9. Hope of stimulating creativity through drug-induced perceptions. The following brief examples will serve to illustrate some of these categories:

Seeking relief from anhedonia: A 21-year-old single male undergraduate volunteer majoring in physics described obsessive fears of dying and of pointed instruments piercing his eyes. He was undergoing a classical analysis 5 times a week at the time of volunteering. He openly expressed his feelings of boredom and anhedonia as follows: "I'm bored by nearly everything in life. I'm looking for new forms of excitement. The only reason I don't take heroin is that it's addicting. One of the happiest days of my life was the day I took mescaline." This subject was not accepted for drug studies. He revealed in a follow-up interview that he had begun to take mescaline regularly. It seems clear that he consciously sought relief from anhedonia through means of the anticipated "pharmacogenic pleasure effect" of the drug.

* * *

Indirect seeking of psychiatric help: A 22-year-old married female with highly competitive strivings toward masculine figures volunteered for the study with the consciously stated motivation of "being interested only in the money." She had a good deal of suppressed and repressed rage toward female authority figures stemming dynamically from an unresolved conflict with a controlling, domineering mother. She developed a post-drug reaction of mild depression, anxiety, and irritability, with obsessive angry ruminations about her mother-in-law. She was seen by one of us for 5 psychotherapeutic sessions, and during the third session spontaneously stated that she was able to recognize that in volunteering she had been looking for some psychiatric help to aid her in solving her marital problems. As a result of the drug experience she felt that she "got not only what I was looking for, but much more than I bargained for." The subject was referred for private treatment and is now receiving psychotherapy.

Seeking new experiences (adventure): A 38-year-old schizoid bachelor poignantly expressed his feelings of disappointment in his search to alleviate the isolation of his daily living as follows: "I somehow feel that I missed out on many things in my life. I was never in the service because of my deafness and I've tried to make up for this by traveling. But I've felt a further need for such experiences and the drug seemed to be able to supply this to me."

Desires for status and prestige: A 27-year-old oriental student married to a white woman had sought for identification with whites throughout his life. He attempted to deny his own racial origins and tended to think of himself as white. He felt that he had gained prestige through participating in the study because "very few people have gone through this and I am in good company—people like Aldous Huxley." Huxley was much admired by this subject.

*   *   *

B. *Psychopathology:* Diagnoses were made on 26 subjects. Twenty-three of these 26 subjects were evaluated as "needing psychiatric treatment." The degree of concordance between the evaluating psychiatrists in their estimations of psychopathology was quite high. One indication of the degree of psychopathology in the group was the relatively large number of volunteers exposed to psychiatric treatment. Twelve subjects either had a history of previous treatment, were in treatment, or entered treatment after volunteering. . . .

C. *Relationship between Motivation and Psychopathology:* The group of subjects with better life adaptations were motivated mainly by financial need, scientific interest and curiosity, or combinations of these. Subjects with significant psychopathology tended frequently to volunteer for reasons related to maladaptive patterns. They often perceived drug effect and the milieu of the study as having a problem-solving function. Some saw the study as a means of making contact with psychiatrists; others as fulfilling frustrated needs for excitement and adventure. Those with symptoms of anxiety, depression, or anhedonia sought magical relief from these painful feelings. Some subjects hoped to undergo transcendental experiences. Inhibited, repressed subjects fantasied being able to act out forbidden impulses. Subjects with high addic-

tive potentials looked forward to the "pharmacogenic pleasure effect" of the drug. Several of these subjects reported using mescaline regularly and deriving from it incomparable feelings of excitement and enjoyment.

*   *   *

Although diagnostic categories are admittedly rough estimations of psychopathology they can be exceedingly useful. On the basis of our clinical impressions the prevalence of psychopathology in the volunteer group seemed quite high. Psychiatric diagnoses were made on almost 50 percent of the group. More than one-third of the group were rated as "needing psychiatric treatment," and one-fifth of the group were or had been in psychiatric treatment. These results are similar to the incidence of psychopathology reported in Lasagna's study (48 percent) and in Pollin and Perlin's work (52 percent). . . .

*   *   *

NOTES

NOTE 1.

Louis Lasagna and John M. von Felsinger
The Volunteer Subject in Research*

*   *   *

In the course of certain pharmacological studies on healthy young male volunteers, routine Rorschach tests and psychological interviews were obtained on 56 subjects. These young men were from 21 to 28 years of age and (with a few exceptions) were college students. All of them received one or more drugs as a part of experiments for which they received a fixed hourly stipend.

An examination of the Rorschach data and interview material revealed what seemed to be an unusually high incidence of severe psychological maladjustment (Table 1). The nosological classification is an arbitrary one, chosen to simplify the presentation of data. The "pigeonholing" of individuals into neat psychiatric categories is admittedly an oversimplification that is intended here only to indicate, in a rough way, the magnitude or nature of the psychological disturbance. There is little question that most of the subjects listed in Table 1 would qualify as deviant, regardless of the diagnostic label affixed to them by examining psychiatrists or clinical psychologists. Of the three psychotics described,

---

* 120 *Science* 359 (1954). Reprinted by permission.

TABLE 1

Incidence of Psychological Maladjustment
in 56 Volunteers

Psychosis	3
Psychoneurosis:	
Under treatment	1
Seeking treatment	6
Others	5
Psychopathic personality	3
Alcoholism	1
Overt homosexuality	6†
Peptic ulcer, severe	1
Stutter, severe	1

† Two of these are also represented in psychotic group above.

for example, two were hospitalized for psychiatric treatment either before or after the studies in our laboratory. One of the subjects listed as neurotic suffered from increasingly severe anxiety, for which he ultimately sought treatment in a psychiatric out-patient department. There the majority of staff members considered him to be schizophrenic. The incidence of homosexuality refers only to those volunteers freely describing overt and continuing homosexual activities and excludes any volunteers for whom evidence of homosexuality was only presumptive (for example, Rorschach responses or behavior under drugs). In all cases, *both* the Rorschach data *and* the interview material had to show significant deviation of personality structure and defense mechanisms from a broadly defined norm to warrant inclusion of a volunteer in the seriously maladjusted group.

The findings described thus raised the question of whether our "normal" sample was representative even of the special population subgroup from which it was drawn—that is, college students. [O]ur subjects differed from other students by reason of the very fact of volunteering for participation in experiments. . . .

*   *   *

An examination of the reasons for volunteering in our group is also of interest. A number of volunteers undertook to participate in experiments primarily for the monetary rewards. Many others, however, volunteered for other reasons. Some hoped to find professional advice and help or a drug that might prove "the golden key" to their personality problems. Some volunteered in a search for new experiences,

much as a potential drug addict experiments with a variety of agents in a search for "thrills" or "kicks." Finally, there were certain volunteers whose primary reason for volunteering was a search for escape or release from personal problems and drives. This latter category included (among others) those who desired temporary relief fron the boredom or pressure of everyday life, those who sought sexual gratification in a relatively guilt-free environment, and those who sought to satisfy self-destructive urges.

*   *   *

NOTE 2.

EDMOND CAHN
DRUG EXPERIMENTS AND THE PUBLIC CONSCIENCE*

*   *   *

The investigator who desires a tranquil conscience must ultimately satisfy himself that the purported consents on which he acts are understanding and real. His scientific zeal should not blind him to the fact that certain individuals seek to become subjects for neurotic or masochistic motives. When motives like these come to his attention, he need not reject the consent; he need only make certain that it is based on a reasonably stable understanding rather than a violent and momentary impulse. If we were bound to reject every act and transaction in our society that might have a neurotic incentive, not much would remain for use.

*   *   *

2.

The Impact of the Outer World

a.

David Rapaport
The Theory of Ego Autonomy—
A Generalization†

*   *   *

. . . I will contrast the Berkeleian view of man with the Cartesian (Descartes). In the Berkeleian view, the outside world is the crea-

---

*Paul Talalay, ed.: *Drugs in Our Society*. Baltimore: The Johns Hopkins Press 255, 263–264 (1964). Reprinted by permission.

† 22 *Bulletin of the Menninger Clinic* 13–32 (1958). Copyright 1958 by the Menninger Foundation. Reprinted by permission.

tion of man's imagination. In this solipsistic view, man is totally *independent* of the environment, and totally *dependent* on the forces and images residing within him: he cannot envisage an external world independent of these inner forces. In turn, he need not come to terms with the outside world: since that world is created by forces inherent in man, he is a priori in harmony with it. In the Cartesian world, on the other hand, man is born as a clean slate upon which experience writes. No forces or images exist in man except for those which arise from the impingements of the outside world. In this world, man is totally *dependent* on and in harmony with the outside world. In turn, he is totally *independent* from, *i.e.,* autonomous from, internal forces, which in this conception do not exist.*

Observation confirms neither of these views. It shows that while man's behavior *is* determined by drive forces which originate in him, it is not totally at their mercy since it has a certain independence from them. We refer to this independence as *the autonomy of the ego from the id.* The most common observation which necessitated this conception was the responsiveness and relevance of behavior to external reality. But this dependence of behavior on the external world and on experience is not complete either. Man can interpose delay and thought not only between instinctual promptings and action, modifying and even indefinitely postponing drive discharge, he can likewise modify and postpone his reaction to external stimulation. This independence of behavior from external stimulation we will refer to as *the autonomy of the ego from external reality.* Since the ego is never completely independent from the id nor from external reality, we always speak about *relative* autonomy.

*   *   *

. . . I have [a] story to illuminate the autonomy of the ego from external reality. "A king returned to his capital followed by his victorious army. The band played and his horse, the army, the people, all moved in step with the rhythm. The king, amazed, contemplated the power of music. Suddenly he noticed a man who walked out of step and slowly fell behind. The king, deeply impressed, sent for the man, and told him: 'I never saw a man as strong as you are. The mu-

_____

* This sketch of Berkeley's and Descartes' views is oversimplified. Neither actually held such an extreme view. . . .

sic enthralled everybody except you. Where do you get the strength to resist it?' The man answered, 'I was pondering, and that gave me the strength'."

In other words, it is possible for man to maintain relative autonomy, *i.e.,* a degree of independence, from his environment. This relative autonomy of man from his environment is the subject of the following discussion.

*   *   *

There is actually nothing radically new in what follows. To the medical man, it is a commonplace that nonliving matter cannot escape the impact of its environment and its reactions are strictly (or statistically) predictable, but that organisms can escape such impacts, can avoid responding to them, and, when they respond, they can do so in a variety of alternative (vicarious) ways. Man's simultaneous relative dependence on and independence from his environment is an issue well within the biological tradition. While psychoanalytic theory, in general, has had a biological cast from the beginning, this did not extend to its consideration of the environment's role in determining behavior.

Our task is to seek the answers to two questions: What are the guarantees of the ego's autonomy from the environment? How is the autonomy of the ego from the environment related to the autonomy of the ego from the id?

*   *   *

To approach the relationship between the two autonomies, let us examine the conditions which interfere with either or both.

Three examples will illustrate the conditions in which the ego's autonomy from the id is impaired. *First,* there are periods of development in which the drives are intensified and threaten this autonomy of the ego. In puberty, the intensified drives interfere with ego autonomy so extensively that the ego combats them with—among other defenses—intellectualization, which is perhaps the most powerful means of enlisting environmental reality and the apparatuses of memory and thought against the encroachments of the id. The adolescent's subjectivity, his rebellion against his environment and his seclusiveness, as well as the converse of these—for instance his striving for intellectual understanding and objectivity and the quest for all-embracing companionship—indicate the pubertal intensification of id forces and the consequent decrease of the ego's autonomy. The climacteric (both male and female) often involves a similar loss of ego autonomy.

Some recent experiments will serve as the *second* example. Hebb and his students put subjects into a sound-proof, blacked-out room, in which restraints minimized tactile and kinesthetic sensations. They made two important observations: (a) the subjects experienced autistic fantasies and a decrease of their ability to pursue ordered sequences of thought; (b) repetitive verbal information given to the subjects—against the background of the stimulus-void—attained such an impact on their minds that some of them came to experience it as "truth," that is, this experience approached delusional intensity and persevered for several weeks. . . . Thus stimulus deprivation too is a condition which may interfere with this autonomy.

Our *third* example is the hypnotic state. A common technique of inducing hypnosis is to make the subject concentrate on something and thus in effect to reduce the intake of other external stimulation. The hypnotist further interferes with attention to external stimulation by pouring forth a steady patter. These measures pre-empt the attention cathexes available, and interfere not only with stimulus intake but also with organized, logical, reality-oriented thinking. Thus both the outside and inside sources of signals—which subserve reality orientation and support the ego's autonomy—are blocked. The result—in hypnotizable people—is a regressive state in which the countercathectic barriers differentiating ego and id processes become fluid; images, ideas, and fantasies representing id contents rise to consciousness, and the sense of voluntariness disappears. In the lack of other stimulation which could serve as a comparison, pivot, or means of reality-testing, the utterances of the hypnotist attain a great impact, just like the repetitive information droned at the subject in Hebb's room. The reduction of reality relationships to a single interpersonal relationship, in hypnosis, impairs the ego's autonomy from the id.

Disregarding for the moment the subject's increased susceptibility to the information given in Hebb's room and by the hypnotist, we will consider only the interferences with the ego's autonomy from the id in these . . . examples.

The generally held assumption that ego structures (controls, defenses, as well as the means used in reality-testing and action) are stable, and altered only by major disorders, is amply justified by the continuity of character and behavior, as well as by the great "resistance" these structures offer to therapeutic intervention. The very concept "structure" implies a slow rate of change in comparison to processes of drive-tension accumulation and discharge. Yet Hebb's . . . experiments suggest that these structures depend upon stimulation for their stability, or, to use Piaget's terms, they require stimulation as nutriment for their maintenance. When such stimulus-nutriment is not available, the effectiveness of these structures in controlling id impulses may be impaired, and some of the ego's autonomy from the id may be surrendered. The example of hypnotic induction seems to corroborate this inference, and the interference of intensified drives with ego autonomy may be considered as due to drive respresentations commanding attention and thus pre-empting the attention cathexes necessary for effective intake of stimulus-nutriment. The interference of passionate love and deep mourning with the ego's autonomy and reality-testing are familiar phenomena. . . . Without assuming that ego structures (other than those of primary autonomy) need stimulus-nutriment for their autonomous effectiveness and even for their maintenance, the very process of therapy would be inconceivable.

We have long known this dependence on nutriment of certain structures, *e.g.*, those underlying the conscious superego. When a man pulls up stakes and moves far away where his past is not known, he is subject to temptations: in the course of his sea voyage, the mutt he left behind may grow into a Saint Bernard, or the painting by a local amateur which he owned may turn into a Rembrandt. The super ego is a persistent structure, but its conscious parts seem to require stimulus-nutriment. In the lack of nutriment it becomes prone to compromise and corruption, and the greater their extent, the more mercilessly does the unconscious superego exact its pound of flesh: the unconscious sense of guilt. The maintenance of conscience seems to require the continuous input of the nourishment readily provided by a stable, traditional environment in which the individual is born, grows up, and ends his life; that is, the stimulus of the presence, opinions, and memories of the "others" who have always known him and always will. We seem to choose the social bonds of marriage, friendship, *etc.*, to secure that familiar (paternal, maternal) pattern of stimulation which we need as nutriment for our various superego and ego structures) for example, those which underlie our values and ideologies).

Now, some examples of interference with the ego's autonomy from the environment:

* * *

[T]ake the procedures lumped together under the term "brainwashing." Instead of reviewing the literature, I will discuss Orwell's *Nineteen-Eighty-Four,* in which the writer's intuition epitomizes the means used by most "brainwashing" procedures to bring the individual to the point where the ego's autonomy from the environment is surrendered. The aim of these procedures is not just to force a false *confession* of guilt, but rather to bring about a *profession* of, or a *conversion* to, a particular view and a *belief* in the "facts" pertaining to it.

In the world of *Nineteen-Eighty-Four,* the individual is robbed of his privacy, the environment invades it: whenever the individual is alone he is watched through "telescreens"; whenever he is not driven by his work, he is driven by the "telescreen," which constantly bombards him with information and with instructions which he *must* obey. The language is so simplified that it can convey only factual information and orders; · it carries no implications, connotations, allusions, or individual expression. Memory is undermined: when the political alliances of the state change, the books and newspaper files are destroyed and replaced by a revised version which fits the new circumstances. Finally, the fear of unknown but horrible punishment is kept constant. The lack of unobserved privacy coupled with the steady shower of information and orders, the lack of personal expression, the changing records which attack even the continuity vouchsafed by memory, and the mortal fear of punishment, are the means by which the world of *Nineteen-Eighty-Four* robs the individual ego of its autonomy and turns the person into an automaton at the command of the environment. *Nineteen-Eighty-Four* is an overdrawn caricature of our own world and a good montage of "brainwashing" procedures. The individual rebellion which Orwell describes has its roots in a yearning for tenderness, love, and sex, which—as I suggested above—are *ultimate* guarantees of the ego's autonomy from the environment. *Nineteen-Eighty-Four* is fiction, but its implications are corroborated by the evidence available concerning "brainwashing," which indicates that the measures summarized above are potent means for impairing the ego's autonomy from the environment.

[Another] example, Bettelheim's paper "In-dividual and Mass Behavior in Extreme Situations," will stand here for all the literature on concentration camps and on Nazi methods of mass psychology. Its study shows that in concentration camps two overlapping sets of conditions interfere with autonomy from the environment, both of which—though not discussed above—obtain to varying degrees in "brainwashing" situations also.

The first set of conditions includes extreme needfulness (hunger, cold, *etc.*) and danger, as well as an attack on the inmates' "identity." In extreme needfulness and danger, the drives—which are otherwise the *ultimate guarantees* of this autonomy—endow drive-satisfying objects with a power the effect of which amounts to slavery and surrender of autonomy. The attack on identity (operating through identification with the aggressor, dependence on arbitrary authority akin to the dependence of childhood, and absence of all encomia of status and other supports of identity) impairs the *proximal guarantees* of autonomy.

The second set of conditions includes curtailment of information and stimulation (though less stringent than in Hebb's room), and against the background of this stimulus-void, a steady stream of humiliating, degrading and guilt-arousing information (akin in its role to the repetitive information of the Hebb room and to the hypnotist's patter). The deprivation contributes to the surrender of autonomy both by enhancing needfulness and by providing the background for the steady and overwhelming impact of the environment.

Thus the outstanding conditions which impair the ego's autonomy from the environment are: (1) massive intrapsychic blocking of the instinctual drives which are the *ultimate guarantees* of this autonomy; (2) maximized needfulness, danger, and fear which enlist the drives (usually the guarantees of this autonomy) to prompt surrender of autonomy; (3) lack of privacy, deprivation of stimulus-nutriment, memorial and verbal supports, all of which seem to be necessary for the maintenance of the structures (thought-structures, values, ideologies, identity) which are the *proximal guarantees* of this autonomy; (4) a steady stream of instructions and information which, in the lack of other stimulus-nutriment, attain such power that they have the ego completely at their mercy.

Just as with the guarantees of autonomy from the id, neither the *ultimate* nor the *proximal* guarantees of autonomy from the environment are absolute. Both autonomies require external and/or drive stimulation of a specific intensity and quality for maintenance and effectiveness.

* * *

[T]hese extreme instances provide good models for the relationships of the autonomies. They show that the ego's autonomy from the id may be impaired either when its necessary dependence on the environment is excessively increased, or when environmental support is excessively decreased. Likewise, the ego's autonomy from the environment may be impaired when either its necessary independence from or its necessary dependence on the id becomes excessive. Since these autonomies are always relative, their extremes are never reached. Hence, a further implication of the relativity of the autonomies is: only a relative autonomy of the ego from the id—that is, only autonomy within the optimal range—is compatible with a relative—that is, optimal—autonomy of the ego from the environment, and vice versa. This conclusion is consistent with the one reached in our discussion of the autonomy guarantees. Since reality relations guarantee autonomy from the id, excessive autonomy from the environment must impair the autonomy from the id; and since drives are the ultimate guarantees of the autonomy from the environment, and excessive autonomy from the id must impair the autonomy from the environment.

* * *

The concept of nutriment is derived from Piaget. According to him, "structures of intelligence" arise by differentiation from constitutionally given sensorimotor coordinations, but require stimulus-nutriment to do so. So far no evidence exists to clarify the relationship between Piaget's structures and those structures which psychoanalytic theory has conceptualized. But since our considerations suggest that psychoanalytic "structures" require stimulus-nutriment for their *maintenance* and *effectiveness*, the question arises: does the *development* as well as the maintenance and effectiveness of psychoanalytic "structures" require stimulus-nutriment?

[T]he concentration camp and brainwashing procedures [do not] bank primarily on the withdrawal of this elementary stimulus-nutriment, though they have used that too as an auxiliary technique. The concentration camp removes first of all the nutriment of the structures

underlying dignity, self-respect, and identity. The aim of brainwashing is to remove the nutriment for the structures which underlie beliefs, political convictions, ideology, social and personal allegiances, and ultimately identity. These differences point to what psychoanalysis has already discovered about defenses, controls, etc., namely that psychological structures form a complex hierarchy within the psychic apparatus. Moreover, these differences suggest that the structures on each hierarchical level may require a different nutriment, ranging from simple, minimally organized sensory stimulations, to those complex experiences which a society provides to maintain, in its individuals, ideological beliefs and identities compatible with that society.

* * *

[W]e must at least touch on the crucial observation that structures can persist and remain effective even when deprived of external stimulus-nutriment. What are the facts and how are they to be explained?

. . . Persistence in spite of deprivation is a hallmark of autonomy. Since autonomy is relative, long-range persistence despite deprivation needs further explanation. It is known that people have spent years in solitary confinement without suffering striking impairments of either of the ego-autonomies, and that people have maintained their ego-autonomy in spite of "brainwashing," though of these only a few have survived to tell the tale. There is the familiar figure of the Englishman who, totally isolated from the setting which would provide the natural nutriment for his proprieties, traditions, outlook and values, maintains these essentially unchanged in the solitude of the jungle or the desert. Last but not least, clinical and therapeutic observation shows that defenses (in the form of both character traits and symptoms) may survive without tangible environmental nourishment, or where the person has to "provoke" nourishment from the environment.

This survival of defense structures without external stimulus-nutriment is understood by psychoanalysis: these structures are maintained, ultimately, by internal (drive) stimulus-nutriment. Clinical evidence shows that values, ideologies, and even more complex structures (like identity) too may be maintained by drive-nutriment, to the degree to which they are part of a defensive system. The explanation of the maintenance of such higher order ego structures in instances of solitary confinement seems at first glance equally obvious: the method of survival seems to be a deliberate application of physical and mental exercise to prevent weakening of ego autonomy and drifting into fearful or wishful daydreaming, or into mindless, empty surrender. . . .

*   *   *

b.

Renée C. Fox
Some Social and Cultural Factors in American Society Conducive to Medical Research on Human Subjects*

*   *   *

Clinical investigators also give special recognition to some of the persons who act as their subjects. "We celebrate our patients" was how one such investigator once described the way he and his colleagues treated their volunteer research subjects in rounds, conferences, technical medical publications, and even in releases to the lay press. Thus, in rounds and conferences in which medical investigators present their patients and their research to other physicians they often express their indebtedness and admiration for the part the patients have voluntarily played in the research:

This is Leo Angelico. . . . Leo has been assaying ACTH for us for three years now. And we've gotten some wonderful baseline studies with his help. He's been written up in many of our papers. . . .

Or, again, medical investigators speak out in letters to their patient-volunteers:

. . . You will be interested in knowing that the results from the big experiment in which you were involved are of greatest interest not only to us, but also to many scientists who work on the new steroids in Switzerland and elsewhere. . . . You are now quite a famous person. . . . The article you appeared in was a teaching paper and has proved to be of considerable value to a large number of practicing physicians.

Finally, in the prepared stories about their research activities which medical investigators sometimes release to the daily newspapers and weekly newsmagazines, and in the interviews they grant to science reporters, prestige is awarded to individual patient-volunteers:

Survives After Rare Operation: Wayne Williams is congratulated by Dr. Herbert Norton on his ability to walk after having been bedridden five years. . . . Dr. Norton said that Wayne's case was the first time in medical history that a faulty heart valve had been restored through surgery. . . .

Before the days of miracle drugs a man could not have lived more than a few weeks after surgical removal of his adrenals. . . . Last week the amphitheatre at _____ Hospital was crowded with standees as Dr. John Thomas described cases in which patients have lived as long as nine months . . . and are still going strong. . . . [One patient] Walter Cousins, 32, had been given six months to live. . . . He had the operation done months ago, responded so well that he got a job as a night orderly at the Hospital. . . .

In addition, clinical investigators often give their subjects what one physician has termed "red carpet treatment." They extend special privileges and considerations to subjects which are not accorded the "usual" hospital patient, such as free room and board in the hospital, free medical services, free supplies of new, scarce drugs, especially attractive hospital accommodations, and so on.

The manifest functions of the special personal and privileged ways in which clinical investigators treat the persons who act as their subjects, and of the ways in which they deal with them as if they were professional collaborators, are obvious.

By fully informing their subjects about the experiments in which they participate, of course, physicians are meeting the ethical and legal requirement that they obtain "the voluntary consent of the human subject," and that before they accept his "affirmative decision" they make "known to him the nature, duration and purpose of the experiment; the method and means by which it is conducted; all inconveniences and hazards reasonably to be expected; and the effects upon his health or person which may possibly come from his participation in the experiments." Reinforcing the moral reasons for which physicians give subjects a detailed explanation of the experiments in which they participate is a more pragmatic one. It is their impression that this increases their motivation to act as research subjects and makes them more cooperative about the demands and restrictions the studies impose on them. Thus, to some extent, clinical investigators provide research subjects with information about experiments in order to secure their optimal compliance.

The same thing might be said about some

* Symposium on the Study of Drugs in Man, Part IV. 1 *Clinical Pharmacology and Therapeutics* 423, 432–441 (1960). Reprinted by permission.

of the ways in which clinical investigators treat their subjects as valued colleagues and privileged friends.

In addition, there are certain more latent functions that these informal relations between medical investigators and their research subjects seem to serve. "Thank you for suffering so stoically," a research physician wrote to one of his patient-subjects after he had been discharged from the hospital. This seems to be one of the primary things the clinical investigators we observed tried to convey to the patients who acted as their subjects through the behavior described. The intimate and extra things they shared with their subjects enabled them to show their personal and professional concern over the "suffering" to which research as well as illness subjected patients. It also seemed to have given these physicians some feeling that they were compensating patients for their suffering, or at least, that they were doing something to help counterbalance it. Thus, one of the implicit functions the special ways they treated patient-subjects seems to have served for this group of clinical investigators is that it helped to relieve them of some of the anxiety and guilt they felt about subjecting their patients to the strictures and hazards of experimentation.

* * *

[W]e know that many patients serve as subjects, and that by volunteering to do so they may attain a variety of instrumental benefits. In some cases there is the possibility that new knowledge, techniques, or medicaments relevant to their maladies may result from the experiments in which they participate. Besides medical aid in this form, as we have already pointed out, patients who act as research subjects may be given free hospitalization and care, or access to otherwise rare or prohibitively expensive modes of treatment. For some patients, hospitalization as a research subject may provide a solution to a lonely or difficult home situation. The following three cases illustrate these instrumental functions:

. . . Margaret S., a widow of 54 . . . had begun to feel weak and run-down ten or twelve years before entry [into Ward 4, the research ward of the Massachusetts General Hospital]. . . . She came to Dr. Forbes at the MGH, who recognized that she had the symptom picture of classic Addison's disease. . . . Dr. Forbes at once appreciated that Margaret S. would give Dr. M. M. Pechet . . . an admirable chance to pursue his study of the relation between molecular configurations of steroid hormones and their physiologic actions on people. . . . Actually, the studies caused only temporary and slight inconvenience, and life in the ward itself she enjoyed, finding it preferable to her previously lonely existence in a lodging by herself.

Since 1950, this patient has been admitted every year to the Metabolic Ward [of a New England Hospital] as a volunteer . . . a well-developed, well-nourished, healthy-appearing, young-looking, middle-aged male who shows no abnormalities other than paraplegia of the lower extremities and flaccid paralysis of the left arm. . . . On the ward, he stays in a wheel chair during the day, and requires the help of an orderly to be put to bed at night and in his wheel chair in the morning. He is pleasant and seems to be well-adjusted. He has found a fairly satisfactory solution to his problem by serving as a permanent volunteer for metabolic studies. . . .

Mr. D. suffered from ill-health from 1922 on, which was finally diagnosed as Addison's disease in 1931, when he had a series of crises. He was treated with subcutaneous adrenaline, 6 injections a day, for a few years. From 1935 on he took Eschatin [adreno-cortical extract] twice daily at a cost of $60 a week. Mr. D. reports, "This took every cent I could lay my hands on." In 1948 he was invited to volunteer for experiments with cortisone, which was to be supplied to him free. In addition, he was to be paid all transportation costs and $10 a day while in the hospital. After one such stay he wrote to the medical investigator: "I want to thank you and Dr. T. for having me . . . for the recent tests. It was a good experience for me and the financial arrangement was most helpful, this being the first real hard cash I've been able to lay my hands on in some time. Do hope you will find an opportunity to use me again. . . ."

* * *

Another important instrumental function that acting as a research subject can have is an economic one. Under certain circumstances, persons who volunteer to serve in this capacity are financially rewarded for doing so. For some ill persons and prisoners, this may be one of the few possible ways of earning some money open to them. As for the well persons and those with good standing in the eyes of society who volunteer for this role, the money payments sometimes offered to them may be a desirable or necessary supplement either to the financial resources provided by another full-time job or some temporarily unremunerative role. . . .

For those persons in our society who are conscientious objectors, acting as a research subject may have still another kind of instrumental function. Under the United States Selective Service Act it is possible for a selectee to fulfill his military obligation for two years' service by contributing to "the maintenance of the national health, safety, or interest" as a volunteer research subject. According to one estimate, "4000 Quakers, Mennonites, members of the Assemblies of God and Church of the Brethren, or other pacifist sects . . . choose this course each year." The Clinical Center at Bethesda, for example, has established a permanent corps of normal volunteers for medical experiments by developing contractual agreements with these "peace churches." "Young people enrolled in the church public service movements are permitted to select health research as a type of citizen duty equivalent to military service for some of the candidates."

* * *

It is primarily because of some of its value-symbolic functions that the role of volunteer research subject and those who play it are so highly regarded by medical investigators and the lay public. For in a number of ways this role seems to epitomize some of the cardinal values of American society. Ours is a society with a high regard for active, rationally based mastery of life and for any sort of achievement that blends individualism and a humanitarian sense of social responsibility. We are inclined to glorify our frontier, pioneering tradition and spirit. We have a special appreciation for the pragmatic and ethical value of science in general, and also for its particular contribution to the realization of another one of our important values, good health. In the role of volunteer research subject, these values are brought together and played out in a way that is regarded with a great deal of social approval. For, of their own volition, partly with humanitarian goals in view, research subjects endure the discomforts, uncertainties, and hazards of pioneering experiments and thus make a contribution to our rational mastery of the problems of health and social welfare.

* * *

Many patient-volunteers in this situation seem to enjoy what the psychiatrist would term "secondary gains" from this role; some establish "transference" relations with medical investigators from which they derive important emotional satisfactions. Or, as Leopold indicated, the comfort, privileges, and trust that he and his fellow-prisoners were granted as volunteers made them feel that they were "on the same side of the fence . . . partners in a common endeavor" with the Army doctors for the benefit of society,

which, in turn, gave them "more solid, lasting satisfaction from what they were doing than many of them had known in some time."

* * *

NOTES

NOTE 1.

OSCAR M. RUEBHAUSEN AND
ORVILLE G. BRIM, JR.
PRIVACY AND BEHAVIORAL RESEARCH*

* * *

[A] complicating factor in the concept of consent is the determination of whether consent has been freely given or coerced. Torture is an old and well-tried technique for extracting private information—and torture need not be physical. Mental anguish can be just as searing and difficult to endure. The prospect of release from suffering, therefore, is a powerful lever for access to the private area. Its uses for the manipulation of behavior or the probing for knowledge are not unknown to sheriffs and prosecutors, to personnel directors, school teachers, and parents —indeed, to virtually anyone who has experienced authority. Conversely, its uses are very well known by the jobless, the hungry, the homeless, the ambitious and the young. The obvious cases of physical, mental, economic, or social duress are readily identifiable; but when does a subtle inducement such as the regard of your boss or even or your peers, or some inducement, not quite so subtle, such as an extra point added to your college grade in return for participation in psychological experiments—when do these become tantamount to duress? What about the vast prestige of scientific research itself as a means of persuasion upon the unsophisticated? And when does the relative disproportion between the knowledge, sophistication and talents of the investigator and his subject make the consent of the respondent questionable, however freely and explicitly given? It is all too apparent that the distinction between consent and concealed coercion may often be difficult to establish. This is, however, the type of distinction with which our social institutions, in particular our law and our courts, have a demonstrated competence to deal.

* * *

* 65 *Columbia Law Review* 1184, 1199–1200 (1965). Reprinted by permission.

NOTE 2.

Milton E. Rosenbaum
The Effect of Stimulus and Background Factors on the Volunteering Response[*]

*   *   *

. . . The general plan of the study called for creating test situations within which invitations to participate in a psychological experiment that varied in strength were tendered to Ss after they had seen the reaction of another person to the same request, with the observed reaction also being subjected to systematic variation. Three stimulus requests were used, designed to vary along an intensity continuum in terms of their capacity to produce a volunteering response. Positive and negative backgrounds and a control condition or neutral background were introduced to determine the rate of volunteering in conjunction with each of the stimulus requests.

Hypotheses. The variations of stimulus request strength and the character of social background mentioned above lead to the following hypotheses: (a) willingness to volunteer is positively related to stimulus-request intensity, and (b) willingness to volunteer is directly related to the behavior of others who are observed responding to the same invitation.

. . . The study was conducted during the regular Fall semester of 1953–54 at The University of Texas. The settings were the reading rooms of two large university libraries. The Ss, numbering 135 males, were occupants of the library going about their everyday school affairs. . . .

. . . Fifteen assistants participated and each served on six different testing occasions, once under each of the six experimental conditions requiring an assistant, to which they were randomly assigned. The assistants were all males recruited from undergraduate and graduate psychology courses. On each testing occasion the assistant was instructed concerning the response he was to give. . . .

*   *   *

Each of the requests dealt with a need for participants in a psychological experiment, but they differed in terms of length of time implied to complete the task and the compellingness of the phrasing. The high intensity request was phrased as a plea for subjects to help complete

dissertation research. The medium intensity request was a matter of fact statement of a need for Ss for departmental research. The low intensity request was stated in a form presenting a relatively weak desire to have S participate in an experiment but discouraging him from doing so.

. . . Background was created by the reaction of a person invited to participate in the presence of the naive test S. By bending over between the assistant and the test S, E first approached the assistant who had been instructed as to the response he should give. Then the test S was approached and requested to participate in the experiment. The general procedure used to create each of the background conditions was as follows:

Positive background. To the invitation to participate in the experiment, the assistant responded by saying "Okay". . . .

*   *   *

Negative background. The assistant responded to the invitation by saying, "No, I'd rather not," and he turned back to his books. The E then presented the invitation to the test S. . . .

Neutral background. The S was approached directly and tendered the invitation. He was not given the opportunity to observe the reaction of another person under this condition. . . .

*   *   *

. . . Greatest acceptance occurred under the positive background and least under the negative background. The data necessary to evaluate the similar aspects of the present experiment are presented in Table 1.

TABLE 1

Frequencies of Acceptance and Rejection under the Medium Intensity Stimulus-Request

Background Condition	Acceptance	Rejection
Positive	12	3
Neutral	7	8
Negative	0	15

*   *   *

. . . Both the stimulus and background variables are seen to be significant in their effect on the response elicited in the predicted direc-

* 53 *Journal of Abnormal and Social Psychology* 118–120 (1956). Reprinted by permission.

tion: the higher the intensity of the stimulus-request, the greater the willingness of the test S to volunteer. On the other hand, the more conducive the background conditions toward the act of volunteering in terms of the observed behavior of another person, the greater the willingness of the test S to volunteer. No significant interaction is indicated between the two variables. Both hypotheses therefore are supported by the results.

*   *   *

NOTE 3.

STUDIES WITH CHILDREN BACKED ON MEDICAL, ETHICAL GROUNDS*

*   *   *

[T]he obtaining of consent at Willowbrook [an institution for mentally retarded children] has not been without controversy. Dr. Jack Hammond, administrator of the institution, said the "biggest fuss" arose more than a year ago over a "complete misinterpretation . . . of an unfortunate coincidence."

The circumstances were set up by the closing of Willowbrook in late 1964 to all new admissions because of overcrowding. Parents who applied for their children to get in were sent a form letter over Dr. Hammond's signature saying that there was no space for new admissions and that their name was being put on a waiting list.

But the hepatitis program, occupying its own space in the institution, continued to admit new patients as each new study group began. "Where do you find new admissions except by canvassing the people who have applied for admission?" Dr. Hammond asked.

So a new batch of form letters went out, saying that there were a few vacancies in the hepatitis research unit if the parents cared to consider volunteering their child for that.

In some instances the second form letter apparently was received as closely as a week after the first letter arrived. "All of a sudden," Dr. Hammond recalled, "we had parents' meetings, calls from local politicians, calls from family physicians. . . . all sorts of kicks."

Canvassing the parents by letter "obviously was open to misinterpretation, so we stopped it more than a year ago," Dr. Hammond said.

*   *   *

NOTE 4.

SAUL KRUGMAN AND JOAN P. GILES VIRAL HEPATITIS—NEW LIGHT ON AN OLD DISEASE*

*   *   *

The study groups [at Willowbrook] have included only children whose parents gave written consent. Our method of obtaining informed consent has changed progressively. . . . At that time [1956] the information was conveyed to individual parents by letter or personal interview. More recently, we have used the group technique of obtaining consent. The following procedure has been employed: First, a psychiatric social worker discusses the project with parents during a preliminary interview. Those who are interested are invited to attend a group session at the institution to discuss the project in greater detail. These sessions are conducted by the staff responsible for the program, including the physician, supervising nurse, staff attendants, and psychiatric social workers. . . . Parents in groups of six to eight are given a tour of the facilities. The purposes, potential benefits, and potential hazards of the program are discussed with them, and they are encouraged to ask questions. Thus, all parents can hear the response to questions posed by the more articulate members of the group. After leaving this briefing session parents have an opportunity to talk with their private physicians who may call the unit for more information. Approximately two weeks after the visit, the psychiatric social worker contacts the parents for their decision. If the decision is in the affirmative, the consent is signed but parents are informed that signed consent may be withdrawn any time before the beginning of the program. . . .

NOTE 5.

EWART E. SMITH OBTAINING SUBJECTS FOR RESEARCH†

The United States Employment Service offices throughout the United States have a large continuous number of individuals entering their offices. Although we had anticipated difficulty with these subjects in filling out questionnaires developed for use with students, we have been surprised at their general literacy, and have had

---

no more difficulty using such instruments as the semantic differential than we have experienced with students. The employment service has been willing to select subjects for us on any variables we specify, such as age, sex, type of occupation, etc. An interviewer obtains subjects and delivers them to a room assigned to us. Subjects are always ready and waiting when we finish with a group, and we have completed a large study without the loss of a single hour or subject in two days.

The cooperation of the United States Employment Service was obtained by explaining the objectives of the research being performed, and stressing its potential value in terms of its application to national goals. It was pointed out that our military sponsor would be grateful for any cooperation received and would be informed of the help received from the United States Employment Service.

It was agreed that the subjects be paid $1.25 an hour. This allowed the employment service to offer the unemployed something to keep them busy, and let them earn some pocket money while waiting for job leads. It might have been possible to obtain some subjects without payment, but payment insured a constant supply of subjects standing by. The employment service did not charge us for the use of their space or the interviewer. The subjects are paid in cash immediately upon completion of a session.

One of the advantages of this subject pool has been the motivation of the subjects, who are more amenable to experimental procedures than are students. They do not anticipate or attempt to deduce the "real" independent variable as overexposed student subjects frequently do. An-

other advantage is their availability for extended periods of time. It was possible to maintain experimental control at university laboratory levels.

NOTE 6.

EDMOND CAHN
THE LAWYER AS SCIENTIST AND SCOUNDREL— REFLECTIONS ON FRANCIS BACON'S QUADRICENTENNIAL*

* * *

One of the major malpractices of our era consists in the "engineering of consent." Sometimes this is effected simply by exploiting the condition of necessitous men, as in certain Indian states where thousands of consents to sexual sterilization have been purchased by offering a trivial bounty to the members of a destitute caste. Then again, consent may be "engineered" by the kind of psychologist who takes it for granted that his assistants and students will submit to experiments and implies a threat to advancement if they raise objections. Or the total community may "engineer" a consent, as when the president, the generals, and the newspapers call with loud fanfare for a heroic crew of astronautical volunteers to attempt some ultrahazardous exploit.

It is worth considering that the destitute Indians who accept payment for sterilization can at least know what they are consenting to; the psychological and astronautical subjects cannot. Moreover, though the astronauts are fairly certain of winning some species of glory, the lady who submits to hypnosis in the interest of science is certain of scarcely anything. . . .

---

* 36 *New York University Law Review* 1, 11–12 (1961). Reprinted by permission.

B.
Barriers to Rational Decisionmaking

1.

Transferences

a.

Anna Freud
The Doctor-Patient Relationship*

*   *   *

. . . Even if the doctor contributes a good deal to [the doctor-patient relationship] I think it is only fair to say that the patient contributes more. . . . Your patients will be ill and therefore they need a doctor. They will have bodily pains; they expect you to cure them. . . . One would expect that this is a straight-forward relationship, that the doctor . . . enters the patient's life as a new person with new qualities, that the patient reacts to him as such, that the patient values his knowledge, appreciates his attitude, and chooses him like one chooses other professional people in life. . . . But curiously enough the relationship between . . . patient and doctor does not remain the same. Elements enter it which cannot be explained by the present reality at all. We are surprised by it, we have to search for the origin. For example . . . many patients over-evaluate their doctors. . . . Their doctor is the best in the world. Their dentist is the best. Enormous expectations are raised—he will help, he will cure, he will fulfill all expectations. This gives you a warm glow of satisfaction. It's nice to be thought such a remarkable person until, a week later, the scene changes. You are no good at all—such an ignorant person has never existed. You don't fulfill the expectations. You have promised something and you can't carry it out. The patient is deeply disappointed in you, and you become dejected. Am I really as bad as that? . . . Until, when this same sequence has repeated itself a number of times, you become alerted to it and you realize this is not you at all. You are neither as good, nor as bad, neither as efficient nor as inefficient as the patient sees you. He evidently has turned you into somebody else. And this belief is strengthened by further discoveries, namely that the patient doesn't only expect you to fulfill the

contract to be cured by you, but that he expects you to like him or, if it is in analysis, even to love him, to be interested in him, to prefer him to other patients. He comes to you with details of his life, which have really nothing to do with the doctor-patient relationship on a reality basis, and you realize that now you have ceased to be what you set out to be—the person to cure this particular individual; you have become an important person in his life, somebody who is loved, hated, on whom demands are made, from whom the patient wants interest, intimacy, preference, and suddenly you feel this must be somebody quite definite from the patient's past. He treats you as if you were his parent. He obeys you as if you had authority over him, or he fights against you as if he were a rebellious child. And suddenly you find that instead of having a sensible patient before you, you have become what we call an object of his transference, namely the whole load of feeling left over from earlier years —unfulfilled, disappointed—has been unloaded onto you. You are in the center of his interest, and he expects you to play the role that you are given.

[W]hat can you do with this most disturbing doctor-patient relationship? . . .

I think that all doctors use the transferred positive relationships from the patients for their own advantage. The patient is in a state of submission, admiration, obedient to the doctor. All the better. So long as this whole trend is positive, you can use it for your own ends; you will find that your prescriptions work better, your commands are obeyed, and at least the psychological side of the patient's illness—and we know there is mostly a psychological side—will be influenced favorably. Doctors have done that always. They have done it without knowing it. It's only when this attitude becomes negative that you are in trouble. . . .

[T]o understand what is going on can be of enormous help in your profession. It will save you a lot of annoyance. It will make you very careful how to act or how to make use of the patient's personal relationship. It will do something to your self-esteem when you know that this changing picture of yourself is not your fault. It will help you to stand firm and, as in so many other walks of life, understanding the difficulties of the situation will ease them. It will ease it es-

---

* Unpublished manuscript, based on a lecture to students at Western Reserve Medical School (October 29, 1964). Printed by permission of the author who retains all rights.

pecially with regard to one particular point. The patient uses the doctor . . . not only to replace people of a lost past, he also uses him to represent in the outside world parts of his own person. For instance, a patient may be quite aware of the fact that either his eating habits or his drinking habits, or any other habits are injurious to his health, but he doesn't feel that he has the strength inside to combat the injurious habits. Then he will give you the role, to represent that part of himself which should control the eating and drinking. Many women who want to lose weight look for a doctor who gives them a diet, where they could diet themselves by eating less. But that is very difficult. It is easier to have the figure of the forbidding agency outside, and then either to obey or to revolt. The same is true about drinking. The same is true about people with heart trouble who cannot bring themselves to be really careful of their bodies. It's easier to have the forbidding agency outside, which in itself does not yet guarantee obedience. . . .

But even that isn't the whole story yet. I have another point to make for you. [You will discover] how badly adult and sensible people take care of their own bodies. After all, our body, our health is one of our most valuable possessions, if not the most valuable one altogether. Wouldn't you expect all your patients to take the greatest care of their bodies, never to do anything that is injurious to their health, carefully to avoid infections, damage, dangers and, if they are ill, to take the right measures immediately. Wouldn't that be eminently sensible behavior? But there are very few adults, reasonable as they may be otherwise, who show such sensible behavior. This lack of good sense in health matters will make your future work extremely difficult. It will make it all the more difficult because you will feel, "I just can't understand it. After all it's his body. Why doesn't he take better care of it? Why does he expect me to do it instead of doing it himself?" You wouldn't be at all astonished about that point, if you had the opportunity to watch the human being's relationship to his body from the very beginning. . . .

If you have the chance to observe children in their second year of life, you will make the surprising discovery that they treat their bodies as if they were not their own. Their bodies belong to their mothers which is only natural since it is not so very long ago—in the intrauterine stage—that the infant's body was actually part of the mother's. Neither in his first nor in his second year can the infant do anything for the care of his body. There is, in the beginning, even no barrier to self-injury and the baby would draw blood from his face if the mother did not see to the cutting of his nails. What we call the pain barrier is established gradually during the first year and the child's aggression deflected with it from his own body to the world outside.

We even think that the infant begins to love and resect his own body to the degree it is loved and respected by the mother, i.e., for the mother's sake. As regards the toddler, we certainly feel that he needs more than our guardian angel to keep alive in spite of the attractions of heights, stairs, water, fire, scissors, knives, and whatever other dangerous objects he may meet. He has, at this time of life, no appreciation of danger and he will inevitably injure himself unless he is protected. Pediatricians, child analysts and other workers in the field have learned to judge the quality of mothering available to a young child by the numbers of accidents in which he has been involved.

The child's intelligence has to mature before he learns to appreciate that fire burns and water drowns, that not everything is edible, etc. What he learns last of all is submission to the rules of hygiene and obedience in medical matters. At school age even, and right up to adolescence, many children act as if it were their privilege to do the most harmful and dangerous things to their bodies, while it is the parents' duty and privilege to protect them. [You] know how difficult it is to keep a child in bed with a fever, with an infection, that the dietary rules are felt by the child as a deep offense, a deprivation, a sign of not being liked. Even the ill child would eat what is bad for him, or the child would, for its own reasons, not eat even if he were starving himself. . . .

But what about you and the doctor-patient relationship? I only tell you these stories so that you can understand where all the irrational attitudes of your adult patients towards their health and towards their bodies come from. It is true you deal with adults, but every adult who is ill, who has fever, who is in in pain, or who expects an operation, returns to childhood in some way. He feels small and helpless, and due to the ease with which he transfers feelings of the past onto you, you become the parent, you own his body. It is now your duty to look after him, and it is his privilege to be naughty about it; he feels well protected by you because he feels that somehow you will see to it that he doesn't do the wrong thing. You may get angry about it, but you will not be angry, if you remember that this adult before you is in reality a child, once more the child who has entrusted his body for safe-keeping to an adult.

This brings us to the end point and perhaps to one of the most difficult tasks of the doctor in the doctor-patient relationship. The patient, as you see from the various points I made, will do his best to push you into the place of parental authority, and he will make use of you as parental authority to the utmost. You must understand that. On the other hand, you must not be tempted to treat him as a child. You must be tolerant towards him as you would be towards a child and as respectful as you would be towards a fellow adult, because he has only gone back to childhood so far as he's ill. He also has another part of his personality which has remained intact, and that part of him will resent it deeply, if you make too much use of your authority. . . .

* * *

NOTES

NOTE 1.

PAUL SCHILDER
PSYCHOTHERAPY*

* * *

[T]he following relations between the physician and the patient are possible. We speak here primarily about the psychotherapist, but since patients go to the physician because they suffer, it is obvious that the psychotherapeutic relation is inherent in every relation between physician and patient.

(a) Physician and patient are fellow human beings. There is no fundamental difference between them. The physician merely has more knowledge in a field of experience in which the patient happens not to be so well versed. In compensation for the advice, the patient gives money to the physician as he would give it to anyone else who serves him. Relations between physician and patient are mostly not of this type.

(b) The patient wants to go to an outstanding physician. The mere fact that the patient chooses the physician gives to the latter the superiority in their relation. The patient, especially

* New York: W. W. Norton & Co. 7–9 (1938). Reprinted by permission of W. W. Norton & Company, Inc. Copyright 1938, 1951 by W. W. Norton & Company, Inc. Copyright renewed 1965 by Lauretta Bender, M.D.

when he comes with psychic problems, wants to find a leader in the physician. Human beings need a leader whom they admire and who takes a part of their responsibilities. In one type of leadership the leader is merely expected to have superior insight. If the patient expects such leadership, the relation between the two will be a relation of superiority and inferiority, and in their discussion common sense and reason will prevail.

(c) Since the discussion between patient and physician circles around the moral problems of life, it will sooner or later become apparent that purely from the point of view of reason, the physician is not greatly superior to the patient after all. Sooner or later the patient will have to add faith to his relation to the physician if he wants to get a sufficient amount of consolation out of this relation. The physician himself will eventually be compelled to demand faith from his patient, unless he discharges the patient in disgust as some practitioners do when they see that the patient cannot avail himself of the physician's advice. We may suppose that this elementary faith (not based upon reason) very often enters the psychotherapeutic relation without the knowledge of either patient or physician. . . . When faith enters the relation, the superior-inferior relation between physician and patient is obviously still more emphasized, but seemingly a new element has been added. The relation becomes similar to that between the adult and the child, or, better and more specifically, the relation is more like the one between parent and child. . . .

(d) From this relation to the complete surrender of the patient to the physician is only a short step. The physician does not only become a father, but he also becomes a father endowed with magic powers. . . . Since the physician is so far superior in this relation, reasoning obviously becomes unnecessary, and the physician has to direct the faith of his patient. He may become a mystical leader, or he may use the more definite technique of suggestion and hypnosis. When the faith of the patient in such a relation is blind, the physician himself is no less blind. He is called to take over a leadership by reason or faith: and according to the whole situation, he cannot know where he should lead the patient. The physician ultimately will become discontented with his role as a fellow adviser who does not know what to advise, and as a rational or mystical leader who does not know where to lead.

* * *

NOTE 2.

HANS JONAS
PHILOSOPHICAL REFLECTIONS ON
EXPERIMENTING WITH HUMAN SUBJECTS*

*   *   *

. . . To the question "Who is conscriptable [for experimentation]?" the spontaneous answer is: Least and last of all the sick—the most available source as they are under treatment and observation anyway. That the afflicted should not be called upon to bear additional burden and risk, that they are society's special trust and the physician's particular trust—these are elementary responses of our moral sense. Yet the very destination of medical research, the conquest of disease, requires at the crucial stage trial and verification on precisely the sufferers from the disease, and their total exemption would defeat the purpose itself. . . .

*   *   *

On the whole, the same principles would seem to hold here as are found to hold with "normal subjects": motivation, identification, understanding on the part of the subject. But it is clear that these conditions are peculiarly difficult to satisfy with regard to a patient. His physical state, psychic preoccupation, dependent relation to the doctor, the submissive attitude induced by treatment—everything connected with his condition and situation makes the sick person inherently less of a sovereign person than the healthy one. Spontaneity of self-offering has almost to be ruled out; consent is marred by lower resistance or captive circumstance, and so on. In fact, all the factors that make the patient, as a category, particularly accessible and welcome for experimentation at the same time compromise the quality of the responding affirmation that must morally redeem the making use of them. . . .

*   *   *

NOTE 3.

HENRY K. BEECHER
CONSENT IN CLINICAL EXPERIMENTATION—
MYTH AND REALITY†

*   *   *

Patients will, if they trust their doctor, accede to almost any request he cares to make.

"My doctor would not ask anything of me not for my good." In too many cases this, too, is a myth. The experienced clinician knows that if he has a good rapport with his patients they will often knowingly submit, for the sake of "science," to inconvenience and even to discomfort, if it doesn't last very long; but, excepting the extremely rare individual, the reality is, patients will not knowingly seriously risk their health or their lives for a scientific experiment. It is ridiculous to assume otherwise. They will not do it.

*   *   *

NOTE 4.

AUGUST B. HOLLINGSHEAD AND
FREDERICK C. REDLICH
SOCIAL CLASS AND MENTAL ILLNESS*

*   *   *

A deep-seated distrust of authority figures pervades class V persons [†] from childhood to old age. Suspicion is directed toward police, clergymen, teachers, doctors, public officials, public health nurses, and social workers. A class V respondent had finished a tirade on police efficiency when he switched to doctors. He told of a neighbor's wife who had developed a side reaction from a sulfa drug prescribed by a clinic doctor:

> That's a doctor for you. I wouldn't take my dog to one. To prescribe 100 pills like that for a working man's wife and not even find out if she had ever had sulfa. I can't see doctors. Maybe this one was in league with the druggist. Maybe he sells sulfa pills on the side for all I know.

Politicians are believed to operate a machine designed to exploit poor people. Non-Italians think this machine is run by Italians, "just like a gang." This statement by a person of Irish descent is typical. "The Italians stick together. The Irish don't stick together, so they can't run the machine like they used to. The machine is mostly one nationality, that is Italian." Protestants make the allegation that New Haven was run by the

* 98 *Daedalus* 219, 237–239 (1969). Reprinted by permission of Daedalus, Journal of the American Academy of Arts and Sciences, Boston, Massachusetts.
† 195 *Journal of the American Medical Association* 124 (1966). Reprinted by permission.

* New York: John Wiley & Sons, Inc. 130–135 (1958). Copyright 1958. Reprinted by permission of John Wiley and Sons, Inc.
[†] "Occupationally, class V adults are overwhelmingly semiskilled factory hands and unskilled laborers. Educationally, most adults have not completed the elementary grades. Individuals and families are concentrated in the 'tenement' and 'cold-water flat' areas of New Haven and in semirural 'slums' in two of the suburban towns. . ." [p. 134].

Catholics: "The Italians and the Irish got together with the Poles and ran the town for their advantage." Others claimed the machine politicians had "sold out" to the Catholic church and "the rich people."

Institutions for care of the disabled and the ill are believed to be run for money and one has to have "pull" to get into them. A family with a feeble-minded four-year-old child claimed that its efforts to have the child admitted to the state home had failed because of their lack of influence.

Hostility against official representatives of society is linked to convictions that they are being exploited. Some believe they have to live in the slums because the state is taking advantage of them. One veteran living in a three-room flat in a dilapidated tenement stated:

Like in other states, where a project is for a veteran who can buy his own home without such a hard down-payment. They have nice homes and we have to live like this. There's nothing in Connecticut—that somewhere, somehow—they can do things so that you don't have to live like this.

Another believed the city officials were taking advantage of the veterans living in an "emergency" housing project. He told how a child from the project had been drowned a few days before because a hole had been torn in the fence surrounding the area. The police had not made the responsible construction company repair the fence. He also explained how dredging in the harbor had led to sand being blown into the houses day after day. . . .

* * *

. . . Manifestations of a feeling of exploitation were encountered among families in other housing projects scattered through the area. In a low-cost state housing development, we were told that the people were not getting much for their money, but that nothing could be done about it.

What are they giving us in this project? And the people, they won't say anything because if they do what happens? They get thrown out. They (the state officials in the housing office) make life miserable for you so you have to move. You will probably have to move into something worse. What I mean is, well, people today, they won't work together for anything.

* * *

The struggle for existence is a meaningful reality to these people. Their level of skill is low, their jobs are poorly paid, and they have no savings to carry them over a crisis. Adults are resentful of the way they have been treated by employers, clergymen, teachers, doctors, police, and other representatives of organized society. They express their resentments freely in the home and in other primary groups.

NOTE 5.

RALPH K. SCHWITZGEBEL
ETHICAL PROBLEMS IN EXPERIMENTATION
WITH OFFENDERS*

* * *

[T]he difficulty in adequately describing the effects of certain experiments makes it difficult for the experimenter clearly to convey relevant information to prospective subjects and therefore obtain valid consent. For example, how is it possible for a delinquent unfamiliar with Freudian theory to comprehend the concept of transference? Perhaps ultimately only the experience of transference itself may be an adequate basis for valid consent.

To avoid the situation in which subjects consent only once without an adequate understanding of the experiences produced by experimental procedures, arrangements may be made for repeatedly requesting the consent of the subjects throughout the duration of an experiment. In the case of one experiment which employs delinquents as experimental subjects over a period generally of several months, the receipts signed by the subjects upon payment are also release forms reminding them in simple language of their right to quit. In this way the subject is clearly given the opportunity to terminate his participation as he becomes increasingly familiar with the experiment. At the same time, the experimenters may be quite sure that in the absence of duress they are receiving valid, voluntary consent repeatedly affirmed.

* * *

NOTE 6.

ROBERT J. SAVARD
SERVING INVESTIGATOR, PATIENT, AND
COMMUNITY IN RESEARCH STUDIES†

* * *

As many authorities have pointed out, consent is not a one-time process. The patient retains the right to reconsider his original consent

* 38 *American Journal of Orthopsychiatry* 738, 744 (1968). Copyright 1968, the American Orthopsychiatric Association, Inc. Reprinted by permission.
† 169 *Annals of the New York Academy of Sciences* 428, 433 (1970). Reprinted by permission.

at any time. But reconsideration and thoughts of withdrawal are painful experiences for most people. In the research situation, many subjects become, in effect, members of the team. Withdrawal may represent the cutting off of very meaningful allegiances. In some cases, when chronic illness is involved, patients may feel so guilty about their inadequate and parasitic-like existence, that to expiate a sense of guilt they may allow the continuation of procedures past what could be considered a reasonable point.

* * *

b.

Renée C. Fox
A Sociological Perspective on
Organ Transplantation and Hemodialysis*

* * *

. . . Clinical investigations typically are responsible for the care of many gravely ill patients, moving rapidly toward what seems likely to be their imminent deaths because their conditions are those that elude the knowledge and skills of medicine at a given historical juncture. Frequently, such a patient and the members of his family are desperately and uncritically enthusiastic about a new experimental treatment that they know the research physician might make available, and they prevail upon him to do so. As Dr. Norman Shumway, a cardiac surgeon prominent in the field of heart transplantation, explains: "When you get a very sick patient . . . to the doctor, it may be a clinical trial, but to that patient, it is very definitely therapy. When you get such a case, it is very difficult to withhold something that can be attempted." The believing hope of such a patient that an experimental measure will prove to be life-saving therapy is not only a consequence of his otherwise hopeless medical situation. In American society, it is also frequently an expression of his positive commitment to medical science and faith in the day-to-day progress it is making to stem back and "conquer" disease. This is a set of attitudes shared by many other members of the population, both sick and well. With this as a background, a strong transference relationship to the research physician may lead such a patient to see him as the charismatic personification of the dramatic, supercompetent, but thoroughly human capacities of medical science and technology

to save, if not cure, him. The research physician not only has these patient-induced emotional pressures upon him to try experimental means, but also his own professional motivation to do what he can to help a dying patient. . . .

* * *

[T]o our knowledge all kidney transplant centers intensively interview donor-candidates as part of an evaluative medical work-up. It has become a generalized norm among transplantation teams that if they discover a potential donor to be what they consider "psychologically unsuited or incorrectly motivated . . . a medical reason will be found to exclude him, the usual one being that he has not proved to be compatible with the proposed recipient." Too much ambivalence, fear, anxiety, resentment, or reluctance on the part of the donor regarding the gift he has offered are among the attitudes that might psychologically disqualify him. The rationale given for this procedure of stating that a donor is physically rather than psychologically incompatible is that it will protect him against self-condemnation and "blame" by the recipient and relatives. In medical practice as a whole, it is not uncommon for physicians deliberately to withhold information from patients or their families on the grounds that it would cause them excessive psychological pain or harm. But physicians rarely tell patients and family members calculated nontruths. The fact that such a convention has grown up in connection with kidney transplantation is an important indicator of how grave physicians feel the individual, interpersonal, and familial consequences would be if they revealed that the prospective donor was not acceptably motivated to give his kidney.

* * *

NOTE

PHILIP BLAIBERG
LOOKING AT MY HEART

* * *

. . . December 3 . . . was the day the world learned that 45-year-old Professor Christiaan N. Barnard, head of a specially trained and selected team, had transplanted a new heart, taken from a car accident victim, Denise Darvall, into Louis Washkansky, a sufferer like myself.

---

* 169 *Annals of the New York Academy of Sciences* 406, 413–415 (1970). Reprinted by permission.

---

* New York: Stein and Day 56–57, 65–66, 69, 70 (1968). Copyright © 1968 by Dr. Philip Blaiberg. Reprinted by permission.

I was feeling particularly ill and despondent at the time, but when I heard the momentous news over the radio at the lunch hour I called [my wife] Eileen. She hurried to the bedroom to find me wildly excited.

"Did you hear the news?" I asked her.

"No, what news?" she said.

"A man," I said, "has been given a new heart. Right here in Cape Town, in the Groote Schuur Hospital. His name is Louis Washkansky. Isn't that terrific?" At first, I thought, the implications of the operation did not seem to register with her.

Let her take up the story of the events of that day:

"I thought Phil's remark interesting, but somehow I could not comprehend exactly what had happened. Though I knew he was desperately ill, I had no thought that he could also be given a new heart and he certainly didn't mention it. But he remained excited and said he hoped Louis Washkansky would pull through. He just could not stop talking about it.

"By four o'clock, however, he was so ill that I was more anxious than usual. I had never telephoned Professor Schrire directly before, but I believed a call was warranted now. He walked in while I was talking to his wife. He took the receiver from her and inquired what was the matter. I replied that Phil was very ill indeed. He asked whether I had not received his message—that he had told our family doctor Phil was being considered for a second heart transplant. It appeared later that our doctor had telephoned several times but he had missed me.

"Anyhow, Professor Schrire repeated that Phil was next on the list. I was astounded. . . ."

*   *   *

The day after my admission to Ward D 1, I was lying in bed with eyes closed, feeling drowsy and thoroughly miserable when I sensed someone at the head of my bed. I opened my eyes and saw a man. He was tall, young, good-looking with features that reminded me a lot of General Jan Christian Smuts in his later years. His hands were beautiful; the hands of the born surgeon.

"Don't you know me?" he asked.

"No," I said with little interest, "I don't."

"I'm Professor Chris Barnard," he said.

"I'm sorry, Professor," I replied, "but I didn't recognize you. I have never seen you in person, and you look so different from your photographs in the Press."

He spoke earnestly. "Dr. Blaiberg, how do you feel about the prospect of a heart transplant operation? You probably know, don't you, that I am prepared to do you next?"

"The sooner the better," I said fervently, "and I promise you my full cooperation at all times."

Though our conversation was brief and he stayed only a few minutes, I was immediately impressed with the stature of the man and his air of buoyant optimism. He inspired me with the greatest confidence, an invaluable asset in the relations between a surgeon and his patient.

I felt somewhat better. Here was a man to whom I would willingly entrust my life. I came to know him well in the weeks and months that followed. He is a vital, determined, somewhat mercurial, personality, utterly dedicated to his profession.

*   *   *

On the morning of December 21, 1967, I was surprised to see my wife walk into my ward at about 9:30. Her visits had always been in the afternoons because of her morning job.

"Aren't you working today?" I asked.

"No," she said. "I just felt I wanted to see you."

"The nurses have told me that Professor Barnard is also coming to see me this morning," I said.

It seemed strange and unusual, but I did not give the matter further thought. I accepted Eileen's explanation and believed Professor Barnard's visit would be mere routine. Soon afterward he walked in. Eileen rose to excuse herself.

"No, don't go," Professor Barnard said to her. "I want to speak to you together." I looked more closely at him. He was haggard and drawn as though he had not slept all night. He no longer resembled the handsome Smuts, to whom I had compared him, but more a martyred Christ. I felt a twinge of pity for him when I noticed the pain in his face and eyes. Something, I was sure, had happened to dampen the gaiety and boundless optimism I had seen before.

*   *   *

Professor Barnard spoke in low tones. "I feel like a pilot who has just crashed," he said. "Now I want you, Dr. Blaiberg, to help me by taking up another plane as soon as possible to get back my confidence."

Still I did not know what he was driving at. "Professor," I said, puzzled, "why are you telling me this? You know I am prepared to undergo a heart transplant operation at any time you wish."

"But don't you know that Louis Washkansky is dead?" he asked. "He died this morning, of pneumonia."

It dawned on me why Eileen and Professor Barnard had paid me this unexpected visit. Now I knew the reason for his distress and agitation.

"Professor Barnard," I said at once, "I want to go through with it now more than ever—not only for my sake but for you and your team who put so much into your effort to save Louis Washkansky."

*   *   *

"Don't worry," he said a little more cheerfully now, "everything is going to be fine."

*   *   *

2.

Countertransferences

a.
O. Spurgeon English and Gerald H. J. Pearson
Common Neuroses of Children and Adults*

*   *   *

[I]t must not be overlooked that the transference process is one that works both ways. It is impossible for the physician not to have some attitude toward the patient, and this is called *countertransference*. The good psychotherapist, however, is able and willing to conceal any feelings he may have beyond desire to help the patient. Overt pity, sympathy, criticism, intolerance, affection, etc., are best kept out of the attitude of the psychotherapist. His role is to skillfully and tactfully mirror the patient's emotions and conflicts in such a way that the patient will see their origin and the futility of their endless repetition. The good psychotherapist must necessarily keep out of the therapeutic relationship any personal prejudices he may have upon arbitrary social questions such as divorce, contraception, religious belief. His attitude may be inquiring but impartial. He may discuss current opinions upon these topics but refrain from injecting his own, even though the patient asks

for it. He must be understanding of human weaknesses and fears, but firm in demanding as much adult behavior as the patient can give to his daily living.

*   *   *

b.
Anna Freud
The Doctor-Patient Relationship*

*   *   *

According to our experience, there are three different ways which urge a young person to choose the medical career. One, and a very good one, is curiosity. The wish to know, as you are probably familiar with, arises very early in the human individual. Already at the age of two, three and four, certainly later also in the school ages, you can distinguish the curious children from those who have no special interest in the mysteries, in the riddles of their surroundings. But the curious ones want to know everything. Parents and teachers are plagued by the continual "why" of the young child—a "why" that they are not always to counter with the proper answer. And very often when parents and teachers do their best to answer the child as fully as they can, the "why" continues, because it springs from rather deep sources. The child wants to know everything about his own body, about his own sex, about the workings of the different parts of himself, of other people's bodies, of the difference between the sexes, of how one becomes a father and a mother, how children are born, what intercourse is about, and from this field curiosity widens to the world as a whole, to the whole world of adults. If curiosity is blocked by the attitude of the adult world, the child may become stunted, apparently incurious and uninterested, and a bad learner. Sometimes not answering the child's questions has the opposite effect. "They don't tell me but I will find out," which means the child becomes more curious. There is somewhere in the child an insatiable wish to know, which stands him in very good stead in later life. One of the ways in which this wish reveals itself rather early, at nursery school age already, is "doctor play." Doctor play goes on between little girls and boys, by preference in secret, because it doesn't always respect the

---

* New York: W. W. Norton & Co. 302–303 (1937). Reprinted by permission.

* Unpublished manuscript based on a lecture to students at Western Reserve Medical School (October 29, 1964). Printed by permission of the author who retains all rights.

bounds set by the adult world, but it combines curiosity about the other child's body with the wish to interfere with that body. Both wishes can be only fully satisfied in later life—if they stay alive somewhere—and lead the child into medicine. So much for curiosity.

But also at these early ages you can find something else. In every nursery school, the nursery school teacher is prepared that in some corner of the room, or of the garden if there is one, a hospital will be established, and this hospital will be usually for insects, frogs or lizards or any other small animals that can be found. And these small animals will be tended carefully in boxes, fed and looked after and, as the child says, cured. Sometimes, especially when it is an insect, legs will be pulled off beforehand so that a patient is produced, and the patient is cured afterwards. Which means that the child's wish to help and to cure is still very close to the wish to hurt and to maim. The younger the child, the stronger his wish to hurt. The older and more socially adapted he becomes, the more this aggressive wish can be submerged under a strong urge to help. Both wishes can lead the growing individual straight into medicine. Naturally, no need for the doctor anymore to provide his own patients by harming them. Fate does that for him. He only needs to cure them. But the wish to deal with those who are hurt, in pain, maimed has to be there, and probably always underlies, even though hidden in the unconscious, the wish to cure and to help.

There's a third source—a very respectable one, too—for the wish to become a doctor. I remember very vividly when I was a child, myself, of being impressed by those fairy tales usually placed somewhere in the middle ages, where an unusually trained or gifted medical man took up straightforwardly the battle with death, and proved that he could conquer death at any time and save his patients. Death was his enemy. He was the savior and the hero. And this image of the medical profession being heroes strong enough and wise enough to conquer death or at least to put off and postpone death is certainly an idea which is attractive to many people. I know if I had become a doctor, it would have been very attractive to me. In your medical training I know that this interest in death as an enemy has been deflected in part to the interest in birth—birth which provides you with your patients.

I think we have every right to expect that these three sources of interest in medicine pro-duce three very different types of doctors. The one who is led to medicine by curiosity quite evidently becomes the researcher—the one who wants to know more and more, who is never satisfied with the knowledge that is handed on to him, who wants to add to it and hand on more. The second one quite evidently is the helper, much appreciated by his patients. The third, I suppose, is the autocrat because his is the wish for power. The patients, I believe, react very differently to the three types. By rights they should welcome the researcher, because he is the one who will bring new knowledge into the field, will be able to cure illnesses which have not been cured before, and will offer them the best of medicine. But instead of welcoming that attitude in the doctor, you will hear the patients complain. If you are one of the researchers later on, the patients will probably say you are inhuman—you are not interested in them, you are interested in their illness. They can't make real contact with you, because you overlook them and look at the body and the illness instead. And I suppose you will rightly feel that it is really very ungrateful of the patients. But if you become one of the helpers, the patients will appreciate you. They will appreciate it even if your knowledge of medicine should be minimal compared to the researcher, which is a danger. The one who wants to fight death brings a rather dangerous attitude to the doctor-patient relationship. Patients know it very well, that he's only interested in them if they respond well to treatment. These doctors love the patients who get well, and who thereby give obvious signs of their power and knowledge, and they resent deeply those patients who don't respond to their treatment. And this is an attitude to guard against on your side. It is not the patient's fault, if you cannot cure him.

*   *   *

c. **Carl H. Fellner and Shalom H. Schwartz
Altruism in Disrepute***

*   *   *

[W]e have become increasingly aware of another variable that seems to affect donor selection, mostly in a negative sense: the distrust and suspicion with which the medical profession regards the volunteer donor and his motiva-

* 284 *New England Journal of Medicine* 282–285 (1971). Reprinted by permission.

tion. This distrust and suspicion reaches major proportions in the genetically unrelated donor, often unacquainted with the recipient, who wants to volunteer.

Sadler et al. recently reported that of 54 world transplant centers that responded to their questionnaire, half disapproved of using the living unrelated kidney donor, and 20 per cent have used such donors themselves. [T]he replies contained "much evidence of distrust and suspicion toward the motivation of such donors and a definite repugnance concerning their use". . . .

Not only is the altruism of potential donors held suspect owing to estimates of their current psychological status, but it is feared that actual donation will produce further disturbance. Thus, Hamburger asserts that "very few types of medical interventions are as capable of disturbing the innermost core of the personality of the protagonists". . . . Finally, by the choice of vocabulary in his guidelines for the transplant physician, Hamburger implies that the would-be altruistic donation may be akin to a criminal rather than an ethical act: "The major problem is the question as to how far the physician has the right to become *the accomplice* of a person who wishes to take a risk with his or her own life. . . ."

Despite the widespread medical bias against the unrelated living transplant donor, 85 people answered a plea for a kidney to be used in a transplant in Cleveland in 1963. Does this response indicate that the medical profession is out of step with public opinion in considering unrelated transplant donation to be unreasonable? Does such willingness to be a donor reflect psychopathology, or could it reflect healthy altruism derived from genuine moral concern? . . .

Written questionnaires were completed by 116 adults in a Midwestern city of 175,000 population while they waited in bus, train and airplane terminals and in laundromats. A cover sheet provided information about the purpose, results, donors used and costs involved in heart, kidney, liver and bone-marrow transplants. . . .

*   *   *

How willing are people actually to donate a kidney to a stranger? If a substantial proportion of the public would seriously consider becoming a kidney donor, doctors would have less reason to suspect the potential volunteers they encounter. Belief in the normality of volunteering is supported by the fact that only 46 per cent of our respondents thought there was less than an

even chance that they would donate one of their kidneys to a stranger in need, with only 24 per cent definitely ruling this out. . . .

*   *   *

Is the public . . . as greatly concerned as the medical profession with the possibility that transplants are unethical and psychologically disturbing? Responses . . . suggest that this is not so. Fewer than one in five respondents thought that each of [the] ethical or psychologic objections, which were presented as "reasons that doctors and other serious critics have given for considering reductions in transplant activity," had a great deal of merit. In the light of the assumption that sensitivity to psychologic and perhaps to ethical analyses of behavior increases with education, the negative correlations between schooling and acceptance of these items as meritorious objections is especially revealing. It is the well educated in particular who dismiss the objections that members of the medical profession have raised.

*   *   *

It might be objected that answers to questions in this research . . . are hypothetical, and do not reflect accurately how members of the public would feel and what they would do when faced with a real request to donate. The one reported study in which such a request has been made suggests that the survey results may not overestimate the public's favorable attitude toward involvement in transplant activities. Schwartz has found, in an experimental study, that 83 per cent of a sample of 144 blood donors actually agreed to have their blood tested for compatibility with a stranger, with the understanding that there was at least a 50–50 chance that they would be willing to donate bone marrow if they were found compatible.

What additional reasons can be offered for the distrust and suspicion with which the medical profession regards the volunteer donor? Certainly, the reluctance to inflict irreversible damage on a healthy person can account for much of it. Every member of a surgical team that has participated in the removal of a healthy donor organ will testify to that. The point has even been made that the operation on the donor is not a medical procedure at all since it is not making a sick person well but a well person sick.

But there appear to be other, more irrational reasons on which available research bears. First of all, the spontaneous, often immediate character of the related donor's decision is interpreted as "emotional" or "impulsive," and therefore symptomatic of psychopathology. . . .

Secondly, the role of other family members in donor selection is a priori suspect by physicians; "undue pressure" and "scapegoating" are readily assumed. . . . .

A final argument against the use of live donors, the assumption that the donor cannot possibly derive any benefit from giving up an organ, completely ignores the very real increase in self-esteem and feelings of worth that result from donorship. Time and again, donors have asserted that they have no regret, that they would do it all over again, and that each derived a sense of worthwhile accomplishment from helping to save a life. And it has been shown that these positive changes in self-feeling persist irrespective of the vagaries of the donated organ and the fate of the recipient.

Regardless of the merits of the many arguments that we have discussed, the fact remains that almost uniformly the genetically unrelated, live kidney donor, and quite often also the related live donor, are excluded from donation. The almost mandatory psychiatric examination of donors in transplant centers that still use live kidney donors is most often but another expression of the same medical bias. There have been several medical conferences on the ethical and legal aspects of organ transplantation, but they have failed to pay attention to this medical bias. We believe the time has come for the medical profession to reconsider where it stands in this issue.

*   *   *

d.

H. Harrison Sadler, Leslie Davison, Charles Carroll, and Samuel L. Kountz The Living, Genetically Unrelated, Kidney Donor*

*   *   *

This survey began in late 1967 with the purpose of helping to form a local policy regarding the use of living, unrelated donors for kidney transplantation. We were aware of five general objections to using the living, unrelated donor as an organ source: (1) The prevailing statistical conclusion: "The results are no better than the cadaver series." (2) The psychological verdict:

---

* Pietro Castelnuovo–Tedesco, ed.: *Psychiatric Aspects of Organ Transplantation.* 3 *Seminars in Psychiatry* 86–88, 92–93, 98–99 (1971). Reprinted by permission of Grune & Stratton, Inc.

"He's crazy." (3) The ethics of medicine: "*Primum non nocere* (in regard to the donor)." (4) The legal implication: "Someday he will harass the recipient or the hospital." (5) The attitude of physicians: "He offends the human conscience."

*   *   *

We carried out a detailed, prospective, psychiatric study of the donors (8 in number) who were operated on after December 1967, and a retrospective study of those (10 in number) who had been operated on prior to this date. . . . All the donor candidates were interviewed for at least 10 hours and one for over 50 hours. To date we remain in touch with all of these patients and, with their permission, monitor them through friends, relatives and various agencies.

*   *   *

In the data from the donors who had experienced the transplant operation, certain universal findings appeared in every protocol: (1) No matter how they heard of the need for a kidney, their declaration to give in response to this plea was almost immediate. For example, 15 donors reported their readiness to give a kidney in less than 12 hours. (2) All were supported in their donation by their families and later by friends, although initially these supporters reported that such an act seemed "crazy." (3) None of the donors reported feeling coerced by physicians. (4) The operation itself, the hospital stay and subsequent outpatient visits were uneventful. (5) After the operation each donor reported a deep feeling of increased self-esteem (i.e., that he had done something wholesome and natural) with no indication of regret. (6) The donors reported no depression which needed special attention, nor have there been any subsequent complications, either psychological or physiological, related to the transplantation. Our data indicate that each donor lives a well-balanced life at his own level.

*   *   *

Typical . . . is the 46-year-old wife of a successful civil engineer. She lives an active personal and social life in an upper-middle class suburban community. Her four children range in age from 14 to 7; the two middle children, a brother and a sister, were adopted following a newspaper appeal by an adoption agency. Prior to her marriage at age 35, she had been a successful executive secretary in a large insurance company.

*   *   *

She had no interest in kidney disease or transplantation until by chance she read in the paper that in a nearby community a 46-year-old man with two adopted children, the ages of her own, could "have his life saved if donors with O negative blood would come forth and offer their organs." She excitingly "knew" she would volunteer: "His children are the same ages as mine. What if mine needed a father? . . . How often are you given the chance on a silver platter to save a man's life?" She immediately shared her thoughts with her whole family, discussed all of the pros and cons, extracted their cooperation, and made the experience "ours." Six hours later she called the recipient. (She chose not to meet him actually until after the operation.)

In the three-month intervening period prior to the operation, she and her entire family remained firm and energetically devoted to the work-up and study. Her children shared each phase with their school friends. She took an impish delight in "letting the secret out" and enjoyed the feedback of awe, praise, and adoration.

The operation, the hospital stay, and the postoperative course were without any serious complications. She visited the recipient on the fourth postoperative day, and they fell spontaneously into each other's arms. They have remained distant friends ever since. She continues to work for the local Kidney Foundation and as a community volunteer. Her reflections immediately after recovery were: "I feel so full of love and now know that such a feeling is humanly possible. I really have gotten so much more than I have given. I know now that it is possible that such love is a potential of the human being and that it has no other need for reward than the giving itself."

Although not all of our donors have shown this dramatic growth, we can find no examples of anyone having been injured by the experience. An example of a less integrated individual, who by our current psychological standards would not now be chosen, is a 28-year-old, former nurse who presented herself in 1966. She had read about the need for a kidney in the newspaper and was strangely moved to offer her own organ with the reason that, "It might make my own life better." She described "deeper feelings" that the recipient, as depicted in the paper, seemed a most worthy person, and there was evidence of a strange feeling of identification. She was not moved, however, to make an actual declaration until a second newspaper appeal impressed her even more: "Why don't

people want to help others?" She thought about this declaration for 2 more weeks and then called the recipient's local physician, who introduced her to the recipient's family. She then decided to go ahead.

Prior to her appearance as a donor, she had a four-year history of addiction to amphetamines and methadrine, had experienced a broken marriage and was a member of Alcoholics Anonymous. She had attempted burglary and had received a suspension of her nurse's certification because of antisocial behavior, which included being in jail. She was isolated from her family and was living an almost nomadic life.

Following the transplant there was a striking display of increased self-esteem and an increase in her actual ability to relate to people in the hospital, in the community, at AA meetings, and with her family: "The transplant has broadened my whole interest in working with people. It makes me forget the bad things of my past." In those years the publicity was great, and she had received over 50 letters of praise as well as visits from unknown people. With the many offers that came to her, she reported feeling "a new start." Two months following the transplant, the organ failed and the recipient died. The donor rapidly reverted to her former antisocial pattern and later was hospitalized at a state mental institution. Her reflections were "Why should someone like me live and someone as fine as that die?"

In the interim (4 years) she has not taken alcohol or drugs and, since her discharge from the hospital, has been living a controlled life. She is now a welfare recipient and occasionally babysits or cooks for those who need her. There is no evidence that the transplant episode injured her. She now tells us she feels it was a crisis experience from which she benefited, and the fact that she made this donation has been one wholesome experience in her life. She is gradually attempting a rehabilitation program.

*   *   *

In spite of these findings and the data supporting them, most physicians who discussed this paper at a scientific meeting, and many transplant surgeons, in responding to the prepublication article, have continued to maintain that "no matter what you show, these people must be abnormal—to do such a thing." They indicate that psychological tests and interviews may fail to reveal the presence of psychopathology. They offer as evidence for this agreement the donor's "social role." For example, for those donors with young children (10 out of 18) to jeopardize their own health by giving a kidney was an indication of "a defective sense of parental responsibility." Furthermore they declare that "if these people derived emotional gain from the experience, they must have been acting out of highly subjective neurotic motives."

Our prospective analysis of the eight donors has included free associative interviews, dream analsis, exploratory long-term psychological investigations (some continuing for 2½ years), Rorschach and Thematic Apperception projective test analyses, and a continual monitoring of their lives. These studies have revealed ample evidence for the presence of primitive masochistic trends, reaction formation against early sadism, homosexual conflict, pregnancy symbolism, penis envy in women, etc.—all the primitive and elemental forces present in mankind. However, the human mind is not a fixed and static organization, but is by its very nature capable of palpable self-awareness and possesses the capacity for synthesis and growth. Therefore, the question to be asked is not "Are these primitive factors present?", but rather, "To what degree are they present?" "Do they preempt behavior and thereby the decision to donate?" "Will the surgical procedures weaken the mind's ability to grow?"

* * *

To the question, "Have any donors been harmed, especially if they had obvious psychological problems?" the answer is "No, none of the 18 donors have been harmed." In our retrospective study, we found three candidates who would not be accepted by today's standards. Two have been diagnosed as chronic alcoholics and one has an antisocial character disorder. All three had given their "informed consent." The two alcoholics are 6-years postoperative and the one antisocial character 4-years. We found that they were not injured psychologically, socially, or physiologically. Whereas their underlying psychiatric condition has not improved, neither has there been evidence of decompensation. . . .

Perhaps the greatest discrepancy found in this study revolves around two poles: a voluntary, altruistic, and personally rewarding act of donating a kidney to an unrelated person is viewed by most physicians as impulsive, suspect, and repugnant—although the public does not share their view. It seems that these physicians base their clinical judgments on their own "view of human nature." Guided by the tone of

the letters from the various transplant centers, we interpret this viewpoint as follows: if one experiments with human beings for therapeutic reasons, one needs convincing evidence that the experiment will be successful. In as much as the evidence is not at hand, this is scientific reason not to use them as donors. There is also the unacknowledged problem that an added responsibility exists because the donor becomes another patient as a result of the surgery. The surgeon must then assume care for donor as well as recipient. The physician's own anxiety as a result of these problems gives rise to defensive statements and the tendency to legitimize.

* * *

NOTES

NOTE 1.

WILLIAM B. BEAN
A TESTAMENT OF DUTY—
SOME STRICTURES ON MORAL RESPONSIBILITIES IN CLINICAL RESEARCH*

* * *

Clinical investigators rarely meditate upon the wide cleavage which separates clinician from investigator in their split personality. As physicians, their prime concern is intimate, personal responsibility in caring for sick people. As investigators they are goaded by divine discontent and impelled by curiosity as well as ambition for renown. Such stimulus sometimes suppresses the physician altogether. The different views are seen well in the subtle but great change which occurs when a house officer becomes a research fellow. Unless wisdom and compassion are neatly blended, the friction between the excited investigator bent on research and the resident with his mind set on care for the patient may produce fire as well as acrid smoke.

* * *

Of more danger and concern is the custom now current that clinical investigators come to positions of academic responsibility by apprenticeship in laboratory science rather than by the thornier path as practitioners of the art who become wise clinicians. And the danger is not in the matter of teaching, which may be done well or poorly without exact correlation with training, but that the most praiseworthy zeal for knowledge may lead the man whose technical background overshadows his caring for the pa-

---

* 39 *Journal of Laboratory and Clinical Medicine* 3, 4–5 (1952). Reprinted by permission.

tient into a disregard for the subject of his researches. Thus, potentially dangerous experiments may be done without the subjects' knowledge or express permission. Whether it be thoughtlessness or heartlessness, such practice is a measure of the moral obliquity which exists in some high places of research today. Fortunately, it is not widely current, but it does exist. At a time when ethical standards are high, or religion elevates moral tone, this situation would have other correctives. They are not effective today. Moral necrosis is sinister in its pervasive insinuations, and all who are concerned with clinical research, that is, experiments on themselves and their fellow man, must face the implications. The recent degradation of physicians in Nazi Germany exemplifies the decline and fall of a group whose moral obligations went by default in a single generation. The house would not have fallen had not many timbers been rotten. Descent into the gas chamber by doctors of infamy had its beginning in disregard for the patient. Never forget that the difference between an experiment on human beings without clear understanding and freely granted permission, and the determination of the M.L.D. [minimum lethal dose] in man is one of degree, not of kind. . . .

*   *   *

NOTE 2.

DEPARTMENT OF PSYCHIATRY— UNIVERSITY OF PENNSYLVANIA STATEMENT OF PRINCIPLES COVERING THE USE OF VOLUNTEER SUBJECTS IN PSYCHIATRIC RESEARCH*

*   *   *

. . . The investigator, using normal human subjects, must be aware of his dual responsibility to the subject participant as well as to the scientific community. Thus, whenever possible, the purposes of the research, the procedures to be followed, and the possible risks involved must be explained to the subject; the investigator is to make certain that the subject understands the explanation. When such an explanation might bias the results, as in much psychological research, such an account may be postponed. In so doing, the investigator assumes an even greater responsibility. The subject's participation is predicated on his faith in the investigator and the institution that no harm shall befall. The investigator must be careful to pre-

---

* Memorandum to Faculty (1965). Reprinted by permission.

serve this faith. Unless it would be deleterious to the research effort, every effort should be made to indicate to the subject, at least after the experiment, something of the purpose and aims of the research. . . .

*   *   *

NOTE 3.

FROM A CORRESPONDENT PSYCHIATRY*

*   *   *

. . . Desire to alleviate suffering was, in Dr. Szent-Gyorgyi's view, of small value in research —such a person should be advised to work for a charity. "Research wants egotists, damn egotists, who seek their own pleasure and satisfaction, but find it in solving the puzzles of nature." Material success, however, also played a very small part, and most significant researchers and artists died poor. Mere knowledge did not interest him, it was *new* knowledge he sought, and he often felt ashamed of his general ignorance compared with his colleagues; but really such learning as this would only serve to weigh him down and he preferred to see things without much sophistication.

*   *   *

NOTE 4.

LORD PLATT MEDICAL SCIENCE—MASTER OR SERVANT?†

*   *   *

Patients, often hideously called the "clinical material" of teaching and research, have been drawn so far as possible from the lower social classes (everyone well brought up knows that the lower social classes have no emotional needs or feelings), and were, and still are, interrogated either in an almost open outpatient department in the presence of numerous students or recumbent in a hospital bed in an open ward; conditions chosen with unerring insight to ensure that the psychological factors in disease, even if present, cannot obtrude and disturb the proper pursuit of scientific medicine. But to make assurance doubly sure, the ward round is conducted as a ritual, the chief followed by his numerous attendants.

The advent of the professional medical departments, which should have brought with

---

* 1 *The Lancet* 1394 (1961). Reprinted by permission.
† 4 *British Medical Journal* 439, 442 (1967). Reprinted by permission.

it new attitudes towards patients consistent with the new understanding of interpersonal relations, has in some instances merely reinforced the defences by a more refined and narrow choice of the "clinical material" . . . by the development of grand rounds to replace the ritual visits of former years. I have seen a patient wheeled in and demonstrated to a large meeting and wheeled out again without a single word being said to her—not even a word of thanks. . . .

*   *   *

NOTE 5.

MOORE V. WEBB
345 S.W.2D 239, 242 (MO. 1961)

*   *   *

Dr. Webb testified he had no recollection of talking to plaintiff about what teeth were to be extracted or discussing the X-rays, with her. . . . Further testimony of Dr. Webb is quoted as follows:

Q: Isn't that pretty much up to the patients what they would do with reference to a partial plate, if they wanted a partial plate?   A: No sir.
Q: Couldn't they have that if they wanted that? A: That all depends. I don't think so. I think you should strive to do for the patient what is the best thing over a long period of time for the patient. We tried to abide by that.
Q: Isn't that up to the patient?   A: No, I don't think it should be. If they go to a doctor they should discuss it. He should decide. The patient should agree that that is what is to be done and should be done.
Q: Isn't this up to the patient? If I want to pay $800.00 for a partial, I hope the dear Lord lets me keep my teeth. If I want to keep these teeth, can't I do it?   A: You don't know whether they are causing you trouble.
Q: That is up to me, isn't it?   A: Not if you come to see me it wouldn't be."

*   *   *

NOTE 6.

FRANCIS D. MOORE
THERAPEUTIC INNOVATION—
ETHICAL BOUNDARIES IN THE INITIAL CLINICAL TRIALS OF NEW DRUGS AND SURGICAL PROCEDURES*

*   *   *

[T]he principle of informed consent has two special limitations. The first unique feature

of informed consent in therapeutic innovation is that the patient actively seeks the untried therapy with an earnest plea to become the willing subject. To those who have never dealt with such desperate patients, it may come as a surprise to witness the enthusiasm with which the patient with late cancer or the family of children with severe heart disease approach an entirely new and untried procedure. This willingness is especially notable if the family knows or suspects, with or without suggestions by the doctor, that the new procedure is the only source of hope for survival. The cancer patient himself seeks out the new drug or the new treatment; people of education and considerable scientific sophistication become blinded and will transgress the boundaries of the simplest common sense not only in accepting new drugs, but in seeking quackery in the hope of a cure. The posture of "informed consent" in therapeutic innovation is, therefore, not a matter of trying safely and sanely to explain to a volunteer what is going to be done, but rather the much more difficult task of explaining alternatives to a worried patient who wishes, above all else, to have the experiment carried out on him.

*   *   *

An intrinsic feature of consent lies in the presentation of sound alternatives to the patient. If I were to identify any one feature of the doctor-patient relationship that is most frequently colored by unconscious subjective factors on the part of the doctor, it is this question of clinical alternatives. One or two examples will illustrate. A colostomy or ileostomy is a form of diversion of the gastrointestinal tract made so that the fecal contents are emptied onto the abdominal skin. Here the discharge is received in some sort of a bag or receptacle that the patient empties from time to time. While unpleasant and unhygienic, most intelligent persons accept this as the price that they pay for the treatment of severe disease—usually malignancy. The more intelligent the patient and the more fastidious his care of his own physical person, the less difficulty he has with colostomy or ileostomy, since he takes special time each day to care for himself in a way that is acceptable to his own high standards. On many occasions I have borne witness to conversations between physicians and patients in which the picture painted of this colostomy or ileostomy was entirely the product of a physician's imagination, based on the fear that he himself might one day have to have such a procedure. A patient suffering from ulcerative co-

* 98 *Daedalus* 502, 509–511 (1969). Reprinted by permission of Daedalus, Journal of the American Academy of Arts and Sciences, Boston, Massachusetts.

litis or cancer of the rectum who is given an offensive or frightening verbal description of colostomy or ileostomy would be so biased in his approach to the operation that he may actually refuse a procedure that offers him the greatest likelihood of survival. By contrast, the over-enthusiastic description of the state of well-being which may result from the surgical treatment of ruptured intervertebral disc, bursitis of the elbow, or hypertrophy of the prostate (considering only three of many examples) will sometimes result in a patient entering into an operation for benign disease, not life-threatening, with an optimism born of the surgeon's tone of voice rather than a realistic estimate of his own response to the projected treatment.

*   *   *

NOTE 7.

MULLOY v. HOP SANG
[1935] 1 W.W.R. 714 (ALTA. APP. DIV.)

JACKSON, D.C.J.—The plaintiff's claim is for professional fees for an operation involving the amputation of the defendant's hand which was badly injured in a motor-car accident. The accident took place near the town of Cardston and the defendant was taken to the hospital there. The plaintiff, a physician and surgeon duly qualified to practice, was called to the hospital and the defendant, being a stranger and unacquainted with the plaintiff, asked him to fix up his hand but not to cut it off as he wanted to have it looked after in Lethbridge, his home city. Later on in the operating room the defendant repeated his request that he did not want his hand cut off. The doctor, being more concerned in relieving the suffering of the patient, replied that he would be governed by the conditions found when the anaesthetic had been administered. The defendant said nothing. As the hand was covered by an old piece of cloth and it was necessary to administer an anaesthetic before doing anything, the doctor was not in a position to advise what should be done. On examination he decided an operation was necessary and the hand was amputated. Dr. Mulloy said the wounds indicated an operation as the condition of the hand was such that delay would mean blood poisoning with no possibility of saving it. In this he was supported by the two other attending physicians. I am, however, not satisfied that the defendant could not have been rushed to Lethbridge where he evidently wished to consult with a physician whom he knew and relied

on. Dr. Mulloy took it for granted when the defendant, a Chinaman without much education in English and probably not of any more than average mentality, did not reply or make any objection to his statement that he would be governed by conditions as he found them, that he had full power to go ahead and perform an operation if found necessary. On the other hand, the defendant did not, in my opinion, understand what the doctor meant, and he would most likely have refused to allow the operation if he did. Further, he did not consider it necessary to reply as he had already given explicit instructions.

Under these circumstances I think the plaintiff should have made full explanation and should have endeavoured to get the defendant to consent to an operation, if necessary. . . .

3.

Regression

Edmund C. Payne, Jr.
Teaching Medical Psychotherapy in Special Clinical Settings*

*   *   *

The concept of regression is useful in explaining many of the otherwise puzzling attitudes that a patient shows in response to illness. By regression we mean the replacement of more complexly organized and more recently acquired aspects of the functioning of personality by more primitive and chronologically earlier modes of functioning. Human personality develops by changing and integrating simple forms of behavior into more highly organized patterns that possess a broader capacity for adaptation. . . . . Many of the earlier patterns, however, persist in modified form in a hierarchically ordered relation to the more highly developed and usually controlling systems. In the face of stress, whether caused by internal conflict or by external danger or frustration, a person may give up the more mature aims and ways of functioning and again seek gratification and attempt to cope with his problems in ways more in accordance with these earlier patterns. A simple example of regression is seen in the toddler who

---

* Norman E. Zinberg, ed.: *Psychiatry and Medical Practice in a General Hospital.* New York: International Universities Press, Inc. 135, 143–144 (1964). Copyright 1964, International Universities Press. Reprinted by permission.

is gaining increasing independence and self-reliance, but who periodically turns back to his mother's lap for comfort and security when the world is temporarily too much for him. When a person falls ill, some degree of regression invariably occurs, induced by a number of factors. Illness interferes with bodily functions that are necessary for the maintenance of important aspects of the personality. The patient who comes to the hospital loses freedom of movement, is deprived of his clothes, and must literally put himself into the hands of other people and depend on them to care for many of the needs that he normally attends to himself. His passive dependent needs are increased, his usual patterns of adjustment are disrupted, and he often suffers intense conflict. Illness is a threat to the integrity of his body and to his life, and consequently generates feelings of anxiety. Since he may be unable to cope with these dangers himself, his anxiety is usually accompanied by a feeling of helplessness. Thus he is forced to rely on the physician for security in ways that resemble his dependence on his parents when he was a child. All of these factors encourage regression. When regression occurs, conflicts that

were important in childhood but that may have subsequently become latent tend to regain their intensity, and the old defenses that were associated with those conflicts may be mobilized again. In many cases these unconsciously determined defensive reactions are not appropriate to reality, to the requirements of dealing with the present illness and of adapting to the necessary medical procedures; in some cases they may be diametrically opposed. The regressive process not only adds a burden of irrational anxiety to the difficulties created by the illness, but may also distort the patient's relationship with his physician. Under the pressure of regression, the patient frequently attributes to the physician characteristics that really belonged to people who were important in an earlier period of his life. In some patients this attribution will increase their confidence and trust in the doctor and thus augment the doctor's effectiveness in providing support and allaying anxiety. In other patients it may produce a negative reaction that can prove both baffling and frustrating to the physician.

*   *   *

C.
Barriers to Comprehension

1.

Failures of Communication

a.

Corn v. French
71 Nev. 280, 289 P.2d 173 (1955)

BADT, JUSTICE.

Plaintiff sued defendant for the unauthorized and unnecessary amputation of her right breast, alleging that the operation was contrary to her desire and consent and without making an appropriate diagnosis to ascertain presence of malignancy therein, it appearing from a post-operation pathological analysis that there was no malignancy. After the plaintiff had completed the presentation of her evidence, the court granted a motion for involuntary dismissal on the ground that upon the facts and the law the plaintiff had failed to prove a sufficient case for the jury. . . .

Plaintiff testified that on August 12, 1950

she had an appointment with defendant at the latter's office at Boulder City, Clark County, Nevada: ". . . We talked about the condition of my breast; that there were danger signals; and he examined me and it was my understanding that he would make a test of a lump under my breast to see if it was cancerous. . . . He didn't make X-rays or blood tests or anything like that, whatever tests you make. He did examine me with his hands, looked at my breast and examined me with his hands. . . . I asked him if he could make a test to see whether or not it was cancerous and he said he could and that he would. . . . [He] called the hospital later when I was dressed, and he said he was going to make sure that they would have a room reserved for us, myself and another patient he had in mind. . . . At that time that he was talking on the telephone, to the hospital, he was talking about preparing a tray. And he said 'for the removal of a right breast.' And I said 'If that's my breast you are talking about, you are not going to remove it.' He said 'I have no intentions of removing your breast. I wouldn't think of doing so without first making a test.' He said 'It takes the same instruments to make a test as it does to remove one.' I subsequently entered the hospital. . . . At that time I signed a consent." She then identified a document as the one which she had signed and which reads as follows: "I hereby give my consent to James B. French, M.D., to perform an operation for mastectomy and hemorrhoidectomy upon myself, and to do whatever may be deemed necessary in his judgment." It was witnessed by her husband and a hospital nurse. She testified further: "Up to that time that I signed that document I had never heard the word mastectomy that I know of. I did not know the term. . . . On the evening of the 14th I saw Dr. French at the hospital. One of the sisters in the hospital and Junelle Sherwood were also present. . . . I asked [the doctor] again to make sure that he understood he was just to make a test of the breast, and the hemorrhoidectomy. His answer was that he had no intentions of doing anything different; he was to make a test of the breast only. I remember that I just kept repeating it, and talking about it, and I did say to him that if he did go ahead and remove the breast that it could not be put back on, but if he didn't take it off, then we could make the test and it need not be taken off."

After the removal of her breast she testified to a subsequent conversation with Dr. French at the hospital and she understood him to say that she had had cancer but that he had removed it; that he had got it early and got every bit of it. "I said 'Are you sure you got it all' and he said 'yes,' and I said 'How long would it have been before it started to spread?' He said 'That I can't say, maybe two days, maybe a week.' He said it hadn't started to spread." She testified to a later conversation with the doctor at his office in Boulder City concerning some lumps on her ribs. "And I went to see if the cancer was spreading and he said that it could not be, because I didn't have cancer in the first place. That was the first time I was aware of the fact that the breast did not have cancer."

*   *   *

Plaintiff's theory of this issue is, first, that when she signed the written consent to the operation she had never heard and did not know the meaning of the word mastectomy, and, secondly, that in any event she clearly and unmistakably made known to the defendant that he was just to make a test of the breast and that his answers

showed that he completely understood such instructions; that the witness Junelle Sherwood substantially corroborated her testimony; that the jury had the right to believe this testimony and to determine that the operation was unauthorized. The trial court's reaction to this contention, when made in opposition to the motion to dismiss was as follows: "Now, if any person after signing that sort of consent, which is general in its terms as well as specific, could repudiate it after an operation, there wouldn't be any doctor in the country that would be safe from suits of this sort. She, whether or not she understood the meaning of it, by her action in giving a general consent, is estopped from denying that she gave her consent to the very operation that was performed." Plaintiff's contention however is not that she had a right to *repudiate* her consent but that, even assuming that she signed the written consent with full knowledge of its meaning, she was not precluded from canceling or withdrawing it before the operation. Such right is not seriously denied by defendant. . . .

*   *   *

[W]e are not called upon to determine whether or not defendant, in removing plaintiff's breast as the result of his original provisional diagnosis and without any pathological examination, failed to use ordinary care and diligence, but rather whether the evidence presented was sufficient to have justified a finding, or a necessary inference from the facts, to such effect, by a jury.

For over two generations pathologists and other medical men have been writing treatises on the pathological analysis of tissues for the diagnosis of cancer, and general practitioners have been sending their patients with symptoms of the disease to specialists. "What everybody knows the court must know." And this knowledge might well permit a jury to peer beneath the cloak of protection thrown about the defendant by the testimony that his diagnosis and treatment were in accordance with the standards of the profession in his community. . . .

. . . Dr. Hemmington, called by the plaintiff, but characterized by the trial court as a hostile witness, did come forward with an "explanation" that the ordinary diagnostic procedure of biopsy was not followed because there was no local pathologist in the county. This might well serve to explain why no biopsy was secured during the operation proper, preliminary to the mastectomy. It would not explain absence of a preliminary or independent pathological examination. There was no evidence that an emergency existed and no explanation as to why a specimen could not have been sent to an outside pathologist or the patient referred to another city for treatment where these services were available, or why she was not at least advised that defendant intended to make a diagnosis without the assistance of a biopsy or pathological examination, or why she was not advised of Clark County's lack of such facilities and the availability to her of these facilities in some other city that could be readily reached by air transportation within the course of a couple of hours. At this stage in the proceedings (before the defendant had made a presentation of his defense) the absence of such explanation is readily understandable. We may not, however, anticipate that it would eventually have been given or that if given it would unquestionably have served to satisfy the jury.

[W]e are convinced . . . that . . . the use of (or the failure to make use of) the pathological analysis of the tissue, in a proper case, for the purpose of diagnosis [can be taken into consideration by a jury] in its own common knowledge and experience and without the assistance of expert testimony—the knowledge, concisely expressed, that "[m]icroscopic diagnosis is the *sine qua non* of neoplastic disease. It is the only means of absolutely establishing the true nature of the disease."

For the reasons given, we conclude that the order granting the motion for involuntary dismissal was error, and that the judgment must be reversed and the case remanded for a new trial.

b.

Wilson v. Scott
412 S.W. 2d 299 (Tex. 1967)

POPE, JUSTICE.

*   *   *

Plaintiff, Frank E. Scott, sued Dr. Anthony Wilson for failure to make reasonable disclosure of risks incident to a stapedectomy operation. He alleged that his right to refuse the operation upon his left ear was violated because the preoperative warning was not sufficiently full for him to exercise an informed consent, and the operation was unsuccessful. The trial court rendered judgment for Dr. Wilson. . . .

*   *   *

In 1962 Scott consulted Dr. Wilson who correctly diagnosed the cause of the hearing defect as a bony growth on the stapes bone which inhibited its vibration and dulled Scott's hearing. He recommended a stapedectomy with a vein graft. The operation is relatively new and is regarded as a delicate and complex one. . . . Dr. Wilson is highly trained and has received special instruction in the performance of stapedectomy surgery. He had performed similar ear operations, but Scott's operation was his first stapedectomy with vein graft. . . .

*   *   *

Scott testified that Dr. Wilson, in discussing the probable results, told him about statistical experiences in terms of "we," from which he inferred that Dr. Wilson had performed this specific operation previously. Although he had performed related operations, Dr. Wilson's former experience with this specific procedure had been confined to experimental operations upon cadavers under the instruction of the originators of the procedure and the best available instructors.

*   *   *

. . . Neither Dr. Wilson nor any other witness testified about a medical standard for disclosure to a patient about the surgeon's experience with a specific operation. . . .

*   *   *

SMITH, JUSTICE [dissenting].

Scott alleged that the doctor was guilty of fraud in representing that he was thoroughly experienced in performing a stapedectomy and that a "stapedectomy with vein graft and polyethylene prosthesis was a safe and proven operation when in fact it was an experimental operation condemned by some of the most prominent experts and authorities. Had Scott been informed of this fact, he would not have submitted to the operation." Scott's third theory of recovery was that "[a]lthough Scott had specifically inquired of Dr. Wilson prior to the operation whether there was danger of disability, Dr. Wilson stated that there was none other than the normal risk of taking anesthetics and possibly some slight loss of taste. In truth and in fact the risk of nerve deafness, tinnitus, vertigo, dizziness and other nervous disorders were well-known to Dr. Wilson, and the operation was still in the experimental stage. Dr. Wilson's failure or refusal to advise and inform Scott of such facts made it impossible for Scott to know and understand the nature of the operation or to give a knowledgeable consent to such operation. Had Scott been informed of such facts, he would not have consented to said operation. *Such operation* constituted an assault and battery." [Emphasis added.]

* * *

. . . This is a case of first impression in Texas, but I find no case decided in other jurisdictions that holds a doctor is under a duty to state in precise words that there probably would be 1 percent who would sustain a complete loss of hearing as a result of the stapedectomy. Nor do I find any cases which sustain Scott's apparent theory that to be an informed consent the doctor is required to relate all of the dangers associated with the operation, such as 1 percent of patients sustain a complete loss of hearing, or that tinnitus, vertigo, dizziness and other nervous disorders probably would follow the operation.

Whether or not a physician or surgeon is under a duty to warn a patient of the possibility of a *specific* adverse result of a proposed treatment or operation depends upon *the circumstances of the particular case, and of the general practice with respect to such cases followed by the medical profession in the locality.* The custom of the medical profession to warn must be established by expert medical testimony.

It is not the duty of a physician in this type of case to relate specific adverse results that might obtain after surgery. The physician's duty to disclose is limited to those disclosures which a reasonable medical practitioner would make under the same or similar circumstances.

c.

Steele v. Woods
327 S.W.2d 187 (Mo. 1959)

JUSTIN RUARK, SPECIAL JUDGE.

This is a malpractice case. Plaintiff sought and obtained damages because of gangrene and resulting crippling by the loss of her toes and part of her feet following a varicose vein operation. . . .

. . . Defendant contended that plaintiff's gangrene and subsequent disability resulted from her refusal to submit to certain postoperative treatment which is referred to as a paravertebral block. At the close of the evidence the defendant was permitted to amend his answer by charging contributory negligence on the part of the plaintiff (among other things) in failing or refusing to have such paravertebral block when it became apparently necessary following the operation. Plaintiff abandoned her theory of negligence in failure to give preoperative tests and submitted her case to the jury upon the theory that, following the operation, plaintiff suffered an impairment of circulation, that a paravertebral nerve block was necessary, that defendant negligently failed to advise the plaintiff of the need for such paravertebral block and that it was not performed. The defendant caused the jury to be instructed on the theory that plaintiff refused to have the nerve block suggested by the defendant and thereby contributed to her own disability. Thus the sole issue which went to the jury was (a) whether the defendant advised a paravertebral nerve block and (b) whether the plaintiff refused to permit it. The plaintiff received a jury verdict for $40,000. Thereafter the court sustained the defendant's motion for judgment after verdict and also sustained defendant's motion for new trial. . . . Plaintiff has appealed.

* * *

Practically all the medical opinion, including that of the defendant himself, is to the effect that plaintiff's gangrenous condition was the result of a failure or incompetence of the inner circulation; that this was caused by spasms of the blood vessels, and that this in turn was caused by the action of automatic sympathetic nerves which constrict the vessels. Such spasms are not a usual occurrence and are not necessarily to be anticipated. They sometimes result from the trauma or shock of the operation. These spasms can be allayed by the performance of a sympathectomy (cutting of the nerves which control the constricting muscles or sheaths) or a paravertebral block, which consists of injecting the nerves with novocain or other anesthetic agent. The latter is the more conservative treatment, since its result is only a temporary anesthetization and consequent relaxation of the nerves involved. . . . Defendant's witness Graham . . . further testified that the doctor has a duty to tell the patient what treatment is necessary, and that, if necessary treatment was refused, he as a skillful and prudent physician would inform the patient that he was going to make it plain to his colleagues and to the patient's family that the proffered treatment had been refused.

In reference to the paravertebral block the plaintiff testified:

Q: Did you ever have any conversation with Dr. Woods about giving you one of those?   A: Not to my knowledge.

*   *   *

Q: Well, you were conscious at all of those times the doctor asked to have a paravertebral block, were you not?   A: I don't remember him ever asking me about a block, sir.

*   *   *

Q: Didn't Dr. Woods explain to you that a paravertebral block would release the spasm around your arteries in your legs and increase your blood circulation?   A: No, sir, he didn't.

*   *   *

The defendant testified that for the first two or three days the patient seemingly progressed all right except that she was complaining of more pain than the usual vein patient complains of, "and it wasn't until a little later on that these areas of discoloration showed up . . . and subsequently broke down;" that as this complication arose he felt that there had been a spasm and that a paravertebral block was necessary; that he desired to do this and "I discussed it, tried to explain it to her, on two or three occasions. . . . We were in rather desperate straits, and she didn't want it done". . . .

*   *   *

[T]he refusal of treatment, after reasonable explanation as to its necessity, by an adult patient who is in possession of her faculties and capable of exercising free judgment in agreeing or refusing, is a complete defense of the doctor who is accused of negligence in not giving the treatment. But whether the treatment was so offered and so refused is a question of fact for the jury.

And this brings us to the hub of the question: was there probative evidence that the paravertebral block was offered and refused? Appellant says that the testimony of plaintiff is an assertion that it was not. Respondent contends that her testimony only indicates a lack of memory as to whether or not the block was offered.

*   *   *

. . . We are of the opinion that . . . the doctor never discussed a paravertebral block with her at any time or interval when she was so sufficiently in possession of her mental faculties that it reached into her consciousness and understanding, when she knew and understood what he was talking about. [A]dvice to a patient unable to comprehend it is no advice at all. The patient who is charged with contributory negligence is to be charged in the light of what she should have known, and it is the duty of her physician to see that she is fully advised and informed as to the treatment which is necessary. And if the patient is incompetent or incapable of understanding but urgently requires the necessary treatment proffered and the doctor knows or should know of this condition, the duty of the physician to advise the treatment does not necessarily end. Depending upon the circumstances of the case, the seriousness of the need, and the urgency of the situation, perhaps the time or interval of the patient's mental incapacity, the circumstances may require and make it his duty to communicate with and advise the husband or other members of the family who are available and competent to advise with or speak for the patient or take other steps to bring understanding of the need home to the plaintiff. In this case the defendant said that he did not talk with the husband about plaintiff's condition and the need for a paravertebral block, although the husband testified that he was at the hospital almost every day.

*   *   *

So here we have the proposition from the standpoint of plaintiff's evidence. The treatment was needed; a jury could find that a reasonably careful physician should have advised it. The physician did not advise it at a time when the patient was capable of understanding, remembering, and heeding that advice. This we think is sufficient negative to make a jury issue on the affirmative defense of contributory negligence. But the question is, is it sufficient to make the plaintiff's case in chief? Under this testimony there is an "open end," an *alternative* possibility that the doctor may have (as the plaintiff's hospital records say he did) advised the operation to the patient, who was then incompetent. The doctor would not necessarily and automatically become liable upon the bare fact he had an incompetent patient who refused his treatment, but his duty to advise and treat might extend and require him to make further effort to communicate with the patient at a more propitious time or to communicate with the husband or someone in position of authority, as the circumstances demanded and the opportunity permitted. Is this, the duty which may have arisen under this alternative possibility, sufficiently within the pleadings or issues which were tried as to support the submissibility? This alternative proposition, which really arose with the development of the evidence, is ignored by both the parties here, because they both contend for and tug at the nether ends, i.e., the block was advised and refused—the block was not advised and refused. However, it is such proposition which causes us the most concern. If it is the injection of an entirely new and different violation of duty which was not pleaded or tried by consent, then it was beyond the issues which could have been submitted to the jury. But if the question of duty to take further effort at communication with the patient or to communicate necessity of treatment to some competent person (if available) in position of authority to speak for or advise the incompetent is really a part of the basic duty to communicate the necessity of the treatment, as a matter of fact a part of the treatment itself, then it is not beyond the scope of the issues which the parties tried. We think it was so in this case. Quite obviously the plaintiff was attempting to inquire during the trial of this case concerning such extended or continuing duty in this respect, so it was not foreign to her theory, and we think it is but a natural extension of the issue, which defendant himself contended for and willingly tried, i.e., that the needed treatment was by him advised. We conclude that plaintiff made a submissible case.

* * *

The judgment is reversed in respect to the sustention of the motion for judgment and affirmed in respect to the granting of a new trial, and the cause is remanded for further proceedings.

d.

Haggerty v. McCarthy
344 Mass. 136, 181 N.E.2d 562 (1962)

CUTTER, JUSTICE.

Count 1 of the declaration in an action of tort alleged that the defendant, a surgeon, failed to remove the plaintiff's appendix completely during an operation, on May 1, 1949, was doubtful whether he had done so, and negligently failed to inform the plaintiff of his doubts, with the consequence that the plaintiff later "provided an inaccurate . . . medical history to . . . [a] physician whom he subsequently consulted regarding . . . abdominal pains, and accordingly was unnecessarily subjected to a series of . . . . operations commencing . . . about January 23, 1957 . . . to his damage." Count 2 recited essentially the same averments with the

addition of allegations that the surgeon "represented . . . that the operation had been a complete success, the appendix completely removed and the danger of further appendicitis attacks removed; [and] that the plaintiff relied on . . . [the surgeon's] failure to . . . inform him as to his doubt," to the plaintiff's damage.

* * *

The operation on May 1, 1949, lasted about two hours. The surgeon in notes described the operation as follows: "Right Rectus incision. No free fluid in abdomen. Small intestine distended. Cecum tied down. *Appendix finally found* Retrocecal and at the bottom of a mushy area. *The appendix was covered with adhesions, was very small* and was tied down. . . . [T]he tissues were very friable and the clamps tore off and there was brisk bleeding for a few minutes. Vessels reclamped and tied. *Appendix removed to what appeared to be the base, but there were such dense adhesions that it was impossible to be certain and the raw oozing area at the bottom of the space was considerable.* A piece of oxycel gauze was placed at the bottom of wound over the ooze. It was dry on closing. Abdomen closed in layers with great difficulty because of [s]pasm and [t]ightness which was finally overcome with [e]ther and curare. Patient left O[perating] R[oom] in good condition" (emphasis as it appears in record). Following the operation, the surgeon informed the plaintiff that the operation had been long because "it had taken a long time to find the appendix." The surgeon "made no further report to [the plaintiff] then or later about the operation or the appendix."

The plaintiff was discharged from the hospital approximately ten days after the operation. He "had no abdominal operations or . . . pain . . . until on or about January 14, 1957," nearly eight years later. As a result of symptoms then developing, he consulted Dr. Meyer, a general practitioner in Schenectady, where the plaintiff then resided. Dr. Meyer testified that the plaintiff's symptoms "were consistent with several abdominal disorders, but were particularly suggestive of appendicitis." He, however, noted the "rectus scar, and [the plaintiff] reported . . . that his appendix had been removed . . . in 1949." As a consequence Dr. Meyer omitted certain "standard medical tests in cases of suspected appendicitis, and diagnosed [the] illness as gastroenteritis or 'intestinal grippe.' "

The pain continued during the following week increasing to acute on January 23. Dr.

Breault, a surgeon, was consulted. He "operated on [the plaintiff] locating a large abscess . . . of infectious pus, together with considerable local peritonitis, caused by a ruptured appendix. . . . He also stated "that the abscess would not have formed, and the operation to drain it would not have been necessary, if the appendicitis condition had been discovered and the diseased appendix removed before it had ruptured."

* * *

. . . There was evidence, in addition to what has already been summarized, that, following the operation, the plaintiff asked the surgeon why the operation had taken so long and that the surgeon (who "made no further report to [the plaintiff] then or later about the operation or the appendix") replied "that it had taken a long time to find the appendix." There is no evidence of any affirmative misrepresentation . . . or any statement of fact, without disclosure of other known facts which might affect that statement. . . . Any contention that there was deceit must rest upon the surgeon's failure to comply with some duty to disclose his doubts. . . . We think that whether there was a duty to disclose depends upon whether there was, in the circumstances, conduct which would have been noncompliance with the special duty . . . created by the doctor-patient relationship. . . .

. . . A verdict for the surgeon was properly directed on each count. . . .

SPIEGEL JUSTICE, with whom SPALDING and WHITTMORE, JJ., concur (dissenting).

* * *

[I]t should be borne in mind that it is the patient who is taking the risk, not the surgeon, nor a group of surgeons in the particular locality where the operation takes place. If an appendix requires removal it would seem to be a corollary that the failure to remove the complete organ might result in subsequent difficulties.

This is not a case of a dread illness. There is not the slightest suggestion that the psychological condition of the patient was such that the surgeon was justified in withholding the fact that he was uncertain as to whether he had removed the complete appendix. The failure to disclose this fact was not in the interest of the plaintiff. As to information revealed in diagnosis it has been said that "no medical privilege should be recognized to withhold the diagnosis in ordinary cases where the usual patient would feel entitled to have the information as a basis for charting his course and there being no apparent grounds for

supposing that a disclosure of the truth would engender in the patient reactions dangerous to his health or life." Smith, Therapeutic Privilege to Withhold Specific Diagnosis from Patient Sick with Serious or Fatal Illness, 19 Tenn.L.Rev. 349, 350–351. It is readily understandable why a surgeon may withhold information from a patient afflicted with cancer. However, we are not confronted with that type of situation in an operation for the removal of an appendix. Even if the possibility of the need for further medical treatment is quite remote, I can think of no sound reason for not disclosing the information to the patient. . . .

* * *

Under the circumstances of this case, I do not believe that evidence of the prevailing medical practice in the neighborhood was necessary to show that the defendant had a duty to disclose to the plaintiff his doubts as to the complete removal of the appendix. Even if there had been evidence that the practice was to maintain silence under these circumstances, this court should not be foreclosed from imposing a duty to disclose. "Courts must in the end say what is required; there are precautions so imperative that even their universal disregard will not excuse their omission." L. Hand, J., in The T. J. Hooper, 2 Cir., 60 F. 2d 737, 740.

* * *

e.

Kraus v. Spielberg
37 Misc. 2d 519, 236 N.Y.S.2d 143
(Sup.Ct. 1962)

BENJAMIN BRENNER, JUSTICE.

The defendant is a treating doctor accused of erroneously informing the plaintiff that her arrested pulmonary tubercular condition had become active and that tuberculosis germs were in her stomach. In effect, plaintiff says that this misinformation and resultant therapy have caused her to suffer from a tuberculosis phobia. . . .

There is little reason to doubt the plaintiff's testimony that, while she is a highly nervous individual and was always apprehensive about her long-standing disease, she has become exceedingly conscious of the possibility of the spread of the tuberculosis germ to her intestines and that her doctor's statements and treatment have caused her real distress. A verdict was nevertheless directed for the defendant in the light of the overwhelming evidence that the diagnosis of active tuberculosis disclosed by him to the plaintiff and his administration of effective chemotherapy were medically warranted and constituted no deviation from standard medical practice. . . .

The doctor's statement to the plaintiff that the "germs may have reached her intestines," though not then medically verified, also presented no fact question for the jury. This, too, being a statement of the well-known fact that the germ could affect the entire body, did not constitute a departure from standard medical practice or present a jury question to determine lack of care or an error of judgment, for, regardless of whether the disease was active or inactive, or whether it had invaded intestinal tissue or not, the administration of the drugs was plainly curative. On all the evidence, the statement clearly was a requisite medical technique to induce plaintiff, then suffering from stomach pains, to undergo the treatment and indeed, though she may have been badly frightened, plaintiff may be alive today because of the very chemotherapy thus administered to her.

. . . No case has been brought to my attention which holds a doctor liable for causing fright and a psychic injury brought on by a statement in the course of his diagnosis or treatment.

The reappearance of positive tubercular sputa, based on recognized tests, convinced the defendant doctor that the inactive tubercular condition had become active once more. As plaintiff was suffering from unexplained gastric pains and was again actively tubercular, he informed her, in the light of those findings and the history of her illness, of the possibility that the tuberculosis germs may have invaded the intestines and that this was an added reason why she must embark upon chemotherapy at once. He may have been mistaken and possibly he should have awaited added clinical signs and medical proof but certain it is that if he was in error, it was an understandable error, if not an error of judgment. In any case, he did not report the information to his patient capriciously or without medical foundation nor was his prescription of chemotherapy palpably an improper prescription for her condition or harmful to her, even if the tuberculosis germ had not invaded the intestines.

Doctors are sometimes held legally responsible for their failure to alert patients to the existence of disease. . . . Had this defendant failed to fully alert plaintiff he could conceivably have been subjected to censure and suit and thus, on plaintiff's reasoning, there is jeopardy both for making the disclosure and for withholding it.

Were doctors to be made conscious of the possibility of suit for honestly explaining their diagnoses to patients for purpose of swift cure they would, with so hazardous a cloud hanging over them, tend to avoid doing so. What sort of medicine would we then achieve? The practice of medicine would then become a secretive practice with doctors uncommunicative to patients, delaying therapy and witholding information for fear that frightened patients might turn upon them. Indeed, professionals in other fields would also find advice to clients most hazardous if fright were caused thereby. Think of the plight of a lawyer sued by a frightened cardiac client when informed of the poor prospects of a lawsuit or of the size of a proposed fee which could be exceeded by the client's recovery against the lawyer for fright.

[R]eason and common sense demand that in the interest of public health and safety a doctor who stands in a special relationship to his patient, even if his diagnosis be not fully verified, shall be free to inform his patient of the presence of disease if he needs to alert her to it or to induce her to embark upon safe and healing therapy. It therefore seems to me that a psychic injury suit, based upon fright from medical advice by a diagnosing doctor, should be confined to gross negligence and is not warranted if the information is well founded, not capricious and does not induce harmful therapy.

The claims of the plaintiff that the doctor erroneously interpreted the x-rays as evidence of cavity rather than of bronchiectasis and that he made a change of his diagnosis to "minimal inactivity," even if true, have no bearing on the issues and in any event are not proximately related to the psychic or other injury resulting from the chemotherapy. Upon the law and the facts the defendant is entitled to the direction of a verdict in his favor.

NOTES

NOTE 1.

PRESTON J. BURNHAM
MEDICAL EXPERIMENTATION ON HUMANS*

Having read the News and Comment headed "Human experimentation: New York verdict affirms patient's rights," I believe I under-

* 152 *Science* 448–450 (1966). Copyright 1966 by the American Association for the Advancement of Science. Reprinted by permission.

stand the situation well enough to attempt to help lay committees develop a series of forms for obtaining patients' informed consent. I am working now on forms . . . for our standard operations. . . .

*   *   *

Consent Form for Hernia Patients:

I, _____, being about to be subjected to a surgical operation said to be for repair of what my doctor thinks is a hernia (rupture or loss of belly stuff—intestines—out of the belly through a hole in the muscles), do hereby give said doctor permission to cut into me and do duly swear that I am giving my informed consent, based upon the following information:

Operative procedure is as follows: The doctor first cuts through the skin by a four-inch gash in the lower abdomen. He then slashes through the other things—fascia (a tough layer over the muscles) and layers of muscle—until he sees the cord (tube that brings the sperm from testicle to outside) with all its arteries and veins. The doctor then tears the hernia (thin sac of bowels and things) from the cord and ties off the sac with a string. He then pushes the testicle back into the scrotum and sews everything together, trying not to sew up the big arteries and veins that nourish the leg.

Possible complications are as follows:

1) Large artery may be cut and I may bleed to death.

2) Large vein may be cut and I may bleed to death.

3) Tube from testicle may be cut. I will then be sterile on that side.

4) Artery or veins to testicles may be cut —same result.

5) Opening around cord in muscles may be made too tight.

6) Clot may develop in these veins which will loosen when I get out of bed and hit my lungs, killing me.

7) Clot may develop in one or both legs which may cripple me, lead to loss of one or both legs, go to my lungs, or make my veins no good for life.

8) I may develop a horrible infection that may kill me.

9) The hernia may come back again after it has been operated on.

10) I may die from general anesthesia.

11) I may be paralyzed if spinal anesthesia is used.

12) If ether is used, it could explode inside me.

13) I may slip in hospital bathroom.

14) I may be run over going to the hospital.

15) The hospital may burn down.

I understand: the anatomy of the body, the pathology of the development of hernia, the surgical technique that will be used to repair the hernia, the physiology of wound healing, the dietetic chemistry of the foods that I must eat to cause healing, the chemistry of body repair, and the course which my physician will take in treating any of the complications that can occur as a sequela of repairing an otherwise simple hernia.

_____
Patient

_____
Lawyer for Patient

_____
Lawyer for Doctor

_____
Lawyer for Hospital

_____
Lawyer for Anesthesiologist

_____
Mother-in-Law

_____
Notary Public

NOTE 2.

FRANCIS D. MOORE
BIOLOGIC AND MEDICAL STUDIES IN HUMAN VOLUNTEER SUBJECTS—ETHICS AND SAFEGUARDS*

In approaching the study of normal man, medicolegal precautions must be taken. In our experience these have [included]:

*   *   *

A signed and witnessed *permission slip* that is completely realistic in all its details. It is not enough for the volunteer to say that he is willing to undergo study. He must specifically say that he is willing to undergo a period of seven days of semi-starvation, with four injections, sixteen blood samples . . . or whatever the details must be. We have also taken special pains to tell our subjects, often in rather discouraging terms,

_____
* Symposium on the Study of Drugs in Man, Part II. 1 *Clinical Pharmacology and Therapeutics* 149, 153 (1960). Reprinted by permission.

the actual details of our studies so that the reality would be a pleasant rather than an unpleasant surprise.

*   *   *

f.

Bradford H. Gray
Some Vagaries of Consent*

Although the informed consent of human research subjects has been a key concept and an important topic in clinical investigation, little empirical research bearing on the discussion has been reported. This is a preliminary report of some findings which emerged from interviews with actual research subjects. It is limited to a discussion of some ways informed consent can fail to occur even where currently accepted procedures are followed. The material discussed here is based on interviews with 51 subjects who participated in a single investigation conducted by a medical school faculty member (assisted by a postdoctoral fellow). The subjects were patients hospitalized in a large, research-oriented, teaching hospital. During a 6-month period in 1970–71, all English-speaking subjects were interviewed, although the project was started before and continued beyond the interviewing period.

The subjects were women having their labor induced in a double-blind drug study. One drug was the standard one used for this purpose; the other was an experimental drug in which the investigators were interested. There were no known risks with either drug, although the experimental drug was still of Phase 1 FDA status, and one of the purposes of the study was to evaluate its risks as well as its effectiveness. Fetal monitoring, customarily employed only when problems with birth are anticipated, was used on the subjects in the project; this resulted in some discomfort but had the advantage of quick detection of certain kinds of fetal problems. The research also called for the drawing of several blood samples. In a related study, the subjects were also asked to consent to having their babies observed by a pediatrician interested in the effects of the procedure on the newborn. Another important aspect of the research situation was the presence of two nurses who were part of the study team and whose duties were confined to the study. Subjects received a high degree of

pre-delivery care from very competent and experienced nurses who always cared for only that one subject.

The usual procedure (with a few exceptions) was for the woman's doctor to arrange for participation in the study a few days ahead of time. Almost one-third of the subjects had private physicians; the remainder were patients of the house staff. Patients were instructed by their doctors to come to the hospital at 7:00 A.M. on a given day for the induction to take place. There was great variation in how much subjects knew about the project before admission; only 19 to 50 reporting knew before admission that they were going to take part in research. However, after admission a standard procedure was followed in obtaining consent. When she reached the labor room, the subject would sign the consent form given to her by one of the research nurses, and, after other preparations by the nurses, one of the investigators would start the intravenous infusion of one of the drugs. Shortly thereafter, with the permission of the principal investigator, I conducted a short interview with the subject; a more extensive interview was done later, usually in the next two days. The interviews, which were recorded and transcribed, covered a series of topics centering around the decision to become involved in the study.

A widespread lack of informed consent was found among the subjects. The lack of informed consent was of three types, the first two perhaps differing only in degree. First, 20 subjects (of 51) were not aware that they were experimental subjects until their participation in the study was well underway. Most of these subjects learned of the existence of the study during the interviews done for my research. Second, many more subjects (the exact number awaits further analysis), while aware of the research, had significant gaps in their understanding of the project and consented on a more or less uniformed basis. These included women who had no knowledge of whether there were alternatives to participation, women who did not know that two drugs were involved, women who did not know of the double-blind nature of the study (it was not part of the research design to withhold this information), and women who were not aware of the fetal monitoring procedures and extra blood samples required by the research. Others were not aware beforehand that their consent to have the baby observed would be sought by a separate researcher.

---

* This is a preliminary report (1971) on data collected for the author's doctoral thesis. Printed by permission of the author who retains all rights.

The third way in which informed consent failed to occur had to do with pressure to participate. Several subjects reported that they would have preferred not to participate but felt they had no choice. Of these, two stated that pressure from their physician had been the overriding factor. In these instances, the physician involved was a private physician, and the two complied, even though they did not want to, because they felt that refusal would jeopardize their relationship with him. Both of these subjects felt later (after delivery) that it had been best for them, but both still felt that they should have been given more information about the study and their doctor's reasons for wanting them to take part, and that they should have been given more of a choice. Some other subjects felt constrained by circumstances which will be described below.

A number of different factors can be identified as contributing to the widespread lack of awareness of the research and the lack of knowledge found even where awareness was present. Since this is written at a preliminary stage in the analysis, this discussion will be limited to factors that became apparent during the interviews with the subjects. Other factors will no doubt emerge during data analysis when variables such as level of education of subjects and the presence of a private physician are systematically examined.

Lack of Explanation

Although a few subjects were well informed about the study, many subjects received the consent form with little or no prior or accompanying explanation. In some cases where an explanation was given, its purpose was not made clear, and it was not sufficiently precise; thus, for example, many subjects who knew that a "new drug" was involved in their induction did not understand that they were taking part in research. These subjects had obviously received some information but not an explanation that communicated the necessary information. A number of interrelated factors were behind the lack of an adequate explanation received by many subjects.

First, no *one* person was assigned responsibility for communicating the necessary information to the subject. Since subjects came from several sources, and responsibility for patients was shared by the researchers and each subject's physician (house staff or private), gaps in disclosure occurred which were not necessarily intended by anybody.

The principal investigator reported that he had held a meeting with residents at the beginning of the research and had asked them to inform prospective subjects before sending them in to be induced in the study; yet about two-thirds of subjects from the clinic indicated that they knew nothing about the research *qua* research until they were handed the consent form in the labor room (if they even realized then). With regard to private physicians, the principal investigator said that he felt it was not his place to suggest to them how to inform their patients. These physicians did not always choose to do so at all, although in some cases they gave detailed explanations to their patients. As to the two investigators themselves, at the time of their usual first contact with a subject, she was already in the labor room, with preliminary preparations completed, a signed consent form nearby, awaiting the start of the drug infusion to bring her baby. A natural assumption for the investigator encountering such a scene would be that the patient had already been informed. Even if such an assumption were not made, it would hardly have seemed appropriate to begin an explanation of the research at this point.

All of this meant that often the subject received no information about the research from a physician. Or if she was given information, it was not recognized for what it was.

The two research nurses seemed to have taken the responsibility for getting consent forms signed almost by default, partially because they had the first actual research contact with the subjects after their admission. The principal investigator reported that convenience was the main reason why the nurses performed this task, and that he had not given them any special instructions because they had long experience (both over 10 years) as research nurses. It was not clear how much responsibility the nurses felt they had for *informing* the subject although they clearly took responsibility for getting a signature on the consent form; it is also not clear whether the nurses were aware that many subjects knew little or nothing about the project prior to admission.

In any event, an explanation did not necessarily accompany the consent form in the labor room. This was indicated by several subjects who reported that they were given the form with instructions to "read this and sign it" or "sign this and we can get started," and was reflected in the large number of subjects who were not aware of what they had signed. The nurses were not at all reluctant to discuss the research with subjects during the long day they would spend together;

in fact, many subjects later commented enthusiastically on how much they had learned from the nurses and how much they felt a part of the whole procedure. However, several things worked against detailed explanations by the nurses (unless questioned by the subjects) at the time the consent form was presented.

First, they had no clear responsibility to give such an explanation. Second, getting the subject's signature on the consent form was only one of many tasks and procedures that had to be carried out prior to the starting of the drug infusion by one of the investigators. The more drawn out these tasks, the longer would be their day since the nurses stayed until after delivery (up to 14 hours among the subjects interviewed) or until the end of labor (the drug infusion stopped after 10 hours, but labor could continue for some time, even for those who failed to deliver). So, strong incentives to be brisk were present. Third, the nurses' job was to assist the investigators in innumerable ways, and causing difficulty with subjects would have been inconsistent with this role. Certainly they did not want to be responsible for causing a subject to refuse to participate after being admitted to the hospital. An occasional subject became upset in the labor room upon learning of the study itself or about particular details of the study, and this could be awkward and difficult to handle, so there was ample incentive to keep everything under control.

A primary method of maintaining this control was to treat everything as being routine in nature. Thus, certain words, particularly "research" and "experiment" were avoided. One of the nurses warned me against using these terms with the subjects for fear of arousing their anxieties and raising questions in their mind. The experimental drug when referred to was called a "new drug" by professionals, subjects, and this researcher. One had the feeling that the situation was very delicate and one had to be very circumspect in making references to the research. The delicacy was handled by avoiding possibly emotionally charged words in favor of terms which neither aroused the subject nor, in many cases, informed her.

Also contributing to the success of the "routinization" efforts were the fact that the research consent form was the second of two consent forms signed by the subject (the first one being truly routine), and the outward similarity of the research to a normal induction, particularly at the beginning. The procedure that subjects were undergoing did not differ markedly from what they had expected.

This suggests that the danger of leaving subjects uninformed is heightened when an investigator gives his responsibility to a subordinate. Because of the nature of superordinate-subordinate relationships, the tendency is for the subordinate to perform the visible task (getting a signed form) at the expense of the less tangible task of giving the subject a complete explanation. This is particularly true where the subordinate fears that full disclosure might jeopardize the chances of "getting the consent" by alarming the subject.

Deficiencies in the Consent Form

The consent form itself was another reason why *informed* consent did not take place in many cases. It was incomplete in that the blood samples were not mentioned. Also it made no reference to alternatives; thus, it was not clear even to most aware subjects what their alternative was, i.e., whether labor could have been induced in another way. The consent form also did not mention the planned 6-hour observation (with blood test and X-ray) of the baby; this was usually presented to the woman for her consent during her labor. Although a separate investigator was involved in that study, this was a serious omission since many of the women going into labor expressed more concern about the health of their baby than anything else.

The word "research" does not appear on the consent form although the term "study" is used. The form itself—standard at the institution—is headed "Patient Consent Form for Participation in a Clinical Investigation Project." The term "clinical investigation" may not carry the negative connotations that are perhaps associated with the terms "experiment," and "research," but it also may not communicate much to many patients, particularly since patients of relatively low educational levels are often used in such investigations. The experimental drug is initially referred to on the form as a "new drug," but the form goes on to designate it as "experimental" at one point. This was the form's strongest indication that it was not a routine form, but the clue was not picked up by 20 subjects.

Circumstantial Factors

The circumstances under which the form was presented to subjects are another set of factors which worked against *informed* consent. Preliminary figures indicate that at least 31 subjects did not know they were to be in research at the time of their admission. Of these, 20 never did find out until they were actively participating by receiving the drug, although all signed the consent form in the labor room, A number of circumstantial factors working together are involved in explaining this.

Patients came in at 7:00 A.M. prepared to be induced and prepared to sign whatever forms were necessary for this. Most had other children for whom arrangements had been made. Under these circumstances, they were in a poor position to give careful attention to anything other than the job ahead of them. Several said that they "hadn't felt like" reading the forms they were given. The inadequacies of the consent form, and the facts that it was one of two forms to be signed and was presented as routine have already been discussed.

A further consequence of the form's being presented under these circumstances was that this often took the husband out of the decision-making process, because hospital procedure had the husband at the admissions desk completing forms while preparations were being done in the labor room. Usually, by the time a husband was able to join his wife in the labor room, the form had been signed and she was receiving the drug. One woman who did refuse to sign until her husband arrived in the labor room said that she had felt very uncomfortable doing so, because everything around her had ground to a halt and she sensed impatience.

Role Relationships and Status Differences

The final main category of factors interfering with *informed* consent is perhaps less specific to this particular study than the others previously discussed. Some subjects among those who *were* aware that they were taking part in research stated that they agreed to do so because this is how the doctors wanted it done and the doctors knew what was best for them. This suggests that, to put it in sociological terms, they were not aware that they had been asked to assume a role other than the patient role.

Although there are important differences in the requirements of the role of patient and the role of subject, there is widespread lack of knowledge about the unique requirements of the subject's role—particularly that a decision-making responsibility is involved. Thus, some women did not understand that a decision was being asked of them—that consent rather than compliance was being asked—when the consent form

was handed to them; many were not aware of what information was relevant to such a decision; and most seemed unaware that the researchers had strong interests in the *research*—interests that had little to do with subjects' welfare although, in this instance, seemingly not in conflict with subjects' welfare. That is, some subjects' assumption that they were asked to participate because the doctor thought it was best for them was not necessarily the case. For example, there were elective inductions among the subjects.

Even though research is involved, prospective subjects coming into the hospital often move into the familiar role of patient when they come into contact with doctors and nurses. The tendency to react to the researcher as therapist, and only as therapist, is to the detriment of the consent process, for as patients many people are accustomed to leaving all decisions in the therapist's hands.

Related to this are the barriers raised by the wide status differential that exists between the researchers and low-status patients, particularly from the clinic. Such status differences may help account for the tendency toward acquiescence and a reluctance to raise questions found in many subjects, even if they were aware of their own lack of understanding. In the absence of any cues that consent was being asked and questions were appropriate, low-status subjects may have felt that they lacked the standing to raise questions, particularly on the professionals' home ground.

2.
Failures of Understanding

a.

Francis D. Moore
Letter to Jay Katz—September 2, 1964*

*   *   *

You ask if there ever is a situation in which "explanation of potential hazards or discomforts" is not enough. Let me give you an example.

Some years ago an individual from this country went to Nigeria to try out a new measles vaccine on a lot of small children.

Now exactly how are you going to explain to a black African jungle mother the fact that measles vaccine occasionally produces encephalitis but that more important than that it might

---

* Printed by permission.

sensitize the child for the rest of his life to some other protein in the vaccine? We now know that any sort of an immune response excites crossed-reactions. For example if a person develops a heightened immune reaction to some specific antigen such as typhoid he will be found to have other higher titers against non-specific antigens at the same time. In fact there is a suspicion that some of the so-called auto-immune diseases are aroused by exposure of the reticuloendothelial system to completely different antigens.

The possibility therefore arises that measles vaccines applied to thousands and thousands of children might excite in some of them such diseases as thyroiditis and ulcerative colitis.

Can you imagine trying to explain that to a jungle mother? I doubt as a matter of fact that you can make much sense out of the foregoing because it is a bit out of your field as a learned man.

We therefore have a problem of ethics and morality which has nothing whatsoever to do with "seeking permission."

One of the greatest assets of a good doctor is the ability to look the patient in the eye and have that patient go along with him on a hazardous course of treatment. This is something that a surgeon experiences everyday as he asks a patient to put his life in the surgeon's trusted hands for some operation or other.

This same quality is exhibited by a medical experimenter when he looks at a patient and says that he thinks everything is all right.

However there is a difference and that is that in the case of the medical experimenter he would not be doing the experiment at all if he was actually sure that he knew all the answers. So there we are.

NOTES

NOTE 1.

DAVID L. RIMOIN, THOMAS J. MERIMEE,
DAVID RABINOWITZ, L. L. CAVALLI-SFORZA,
AND VICTOR A. MCKUSICK
PERIPHERAL SUBRESPONSIVENESS TO HUMAN
GROWTH HORMONE IN THE AFRICAN PYGMIES*

The cause of the African pygmies' short stature has long been a subject of speculation. Because of their resemblance to persons with isolated growth-hormone deficiency (sexual ateliotic dwarfs), an expedition was made to the Central African Republic to assess the pygmies' abil-

ity to secrete human growth hormone (HGH). This study clearly demonstrated that the pygmies attain normal plasma concentrations of immunoreactive HGH after insulin-induced hypoglycemia and arginine infusion. Nevertheless, a number of clinical and metabolic similarities were observed between the pygmies and patients with isolated HGH deficiency. Two possible mechanisms were postulated to explain these paradoxical findings: the pygmies might secrete an altered HGH molecule that was functionally inert but antigenically intact; or they might secrete normal HGH to which their peripheral tissues were unresponsive.

In an attempt to distinguish between these two possible mechanisms, another expedition to Central Africa was made to assess the pygmies' ability to respond to exogenous HGH. . . .

*   *   *

Two expeditions were made to the M'Baiki Region of the Central African Republic, where a group of Babinga pygmies, living in typical pygmy camps, was studied. On the first trip, HGH secretion was assessed in 22 pygmies (15 males and seven females) who were subjected to insulin-induced hypoglycemia . . . or arginine infusion . . . or both. . . .

On the second expedition, 19 Babinga pygmies (13 males and six females) were studied before and after the administration of HGH. Eight pygmies received an acute intravenous infusion of HGH (4 mg over 20 minutes), as did five white control subjects of normal stature and eight ateliotics. Oral glucose tolerance tests (50 gm of glucose) were performed on 11 pygmies before and after the intra-muscular administration of 5 mg of HGH for five days. Arginine infusions (0.25 gm per pound of body weight) were given to six of these pygmies before and after this intramuscular HGH regimen. Similar studies were performed on four controls of normal stature and five ateliotic dwarfs before and after five days of intramuscular HGH administration (5 mg per day). All subjects studied were post-adolescent.

*   *   *

The mean fasting plasma HGH concentration of the pygmies . . . did not differ greatly from that of the controls. . . . After the infusion of 0.1 unit of insulin per kilogram of body weight, plasma HGH levels rose to a mean peak concentration of 29.6 ± 0.35 ng per milliliter in the pygmies, a value not markedly different from that attained by the controls (25.6 ± 3.9 ng per

* 281 *New England Journal of Medicine* 1383–1384 (1969). Reprinted by permission.

milliliter). Unlike the controls, however, in whom the plasma glucose concentrations returned to baseline values by 90 minutes, the pygmies had an exaggerated hypoglycemic response. Both the pygmies and the ateliotic dwarfs had severe hypoglycemic symptoms after insulin and maintained low blood glucose concentrations for over 90 minutes.

* * *

NOTE 2.

DANIEL P. ASNES
CONSENT FOR STUDIES ON PYGMIES*

. . . I wonder what sort of explanation of the research the subjects were given. Were they aware of the feelings they might experience after receiving insulin? The problem of maintaining high ethical standards in the recruiting of experimental subjects is difficult enough in our own culture. It seems to be even more difficult in a culture that might not have a conception of "medical research" and the tacit acceptance of its value.

* * *

NOTE 3.

DAVID L. RIMOIN
CONSENT FOR STUDIES ON PYGMIES†

I can assure Dr. Asnes that with the use of Bantu interpreters, we obtained full consent from the pygmies after a detailed explanation of the procedures. Indeed, when pygmy subjects were required to return for second and third procedures, not one refused after his first experience.

NOTE 4.

T. A. LAMBO
ASPECTS OF CLINICAL RESEARCH IN DEVELOPING COUNTRIES‡

. . . We have found in some areas of Africa that we have not only to consider or to weigh the balance between therapy and the risks to human life, but also to consider the philosophy of the dignity and rights of human beings. Not long ago, a comatose patient was picked up in the

street; while he was still unconscious, he was given a blood transfusion. A few weeks later I was called to see him on one of the wards where he was having a very severe psychotic breakdown, because he had been rejected by his own tribe for having received blood from another tribe. The patient said to me that it would be better for him to die than to remain alive; this raised another set of problems, another dilemma. Again, not long ago, we had another problem, a tribe in Nigeria taking a case to court because one of the physicians had taken postmortem material from an old man who died and they felt that this should have been explained to them. To a person of Western culture this may seem absurd, but it involves the question of ancestor worship, which is a culture-bound phenomenon in many of the African tribes: it has been prescribed by tradition that the old man should arrive upstairs with all his organs in the right place, and this was not the case. So that you see that there are many problems which in fact do not involve directly the question of risk to human life, but which may imply cultural differences, ethical differences which are of very deep emotional significance to individuals in a particular society. . . .

NOTE 5.

J. HIERNAUX
ETHICAL PROBLEMS IN ANTHROPOBIOLOGICAL RESEARCH*

* * *

Whatever the individual risk in this research, the consent of the subject is required. In a large number of populations where the hygiene and nutrition are very deficient and where the most urgent need for research exists—those on which the efforts of the International Biological Programme will be concentrated—the great majority of the people are illiterate and the cultural set-up requires the prior informed consent of the leaders of the community, whether the administrative—including the medical—leaders, the political leaders, or the customary leaders, but especially the customary religious leaders. The consent of the individuals often depends on these people, who in any case are the best placed to understand the value of the research for the community and to tell the people so in terms that they can follow (for often the investigator does not speak the language of the subjects he

* 282 *New England Journal of Medicine* 634 (1970). Reprinted by permission.
† 282 *New England Journal of Medicine* 634 (1970). Reprinted by permission.
‡ V. Fattorusso, ed.: *Biomedical Science and the Dilemma of Human Experimentation.* Paris: Council for International Organizations of Medical Sciences 63, 66–67 (1967). Reprinted by permission.

* V. Fattorusso, ed.: *Biomedical Science and the Dilemma of Human Experimentation.* Paris: Council for International Organizations of Medical Sciences 70 (1967). Reprinted by permission.

is going to examine). The prior agreement of these leaders will meet both the ethical requirements and the efficiency requirements of the research and integrate it in the cultural values of the community. . . .

* * *

NOTE 6.

MARGARET MEAD
RESEARCH WITH HUMAN BEINGS—A
MODEL DERIVED FROM ANTHROPOLOGICAL
FIELD PRACTICE*

* * *

The problem of communicating to a primitive people what will be done with the information that they have helped develop is of a different order. They may have no conception of printing or of what the publication of details about their social forms and individual behavior may mean. Consent in such cases would be even more ridiculous than it has been shown to be in the case of complicated experiments in our own society. Furthermore, it is not only their own current reputations that are at a risk they cannot estimate, but today, as primitive peoples are rapidly entering the modern world, it is the dignity and sensitivity of their descendants that must be considered. The situation is somewhat comparable to consent given by parents for the use of films made of their children in a modern country, without any real ability to predict how the children will feel about such continuing exposure to the public eye. Here, in the case of primitive peoples, of children, or of any individuals who are not in a position to evaluate the effects of publication, a heavy responsibility falls upon the research worker. . . .

* * *

b.

Mitchell v. Robinson
334 S.W.2d 11 (Mo. 1960)

BARRETT, COMMISSIONER.

William Mitchell has been awarded $15,000 damages against the Doctors Robinson and their associates, particularly Dr. Jack DeMott, for malpractice, and the essentially meritorious problem is whether upon the record there is any evidence to support the jury's finding of negligence.
. . . Mitchell had "a rather severe emotional

———————
* 98 *Daedalus* 361, 364 (1969). Reprinted by permission of Daedalus, Journal of the American Academy of Arts and Sciences, Boston, Massachusetts.

illness," process schizophrenia, but he was not mentally incompetent; his illness was characterized by serious depression and rather severe anxiety, complicated by alcoholism. It is not necessary at this point to detail his case history and symptoms; it was the opinion of the doctors that he should have "combined electroshock and insulin subcoma therapy." The general purpose of electroshock treatment is to build up the patient's "defense and controls and self-confidence" while insulin relieves "basic anxiety" and "disturbance of the mood." The desired physical reaction and intended purpose of electroshock is to induce convulsive seizures of forty to fifty seconds duration. The desired physical reaction of insulin shock is the induction of unconsciousness, a "subcoma" state, but it is neither intended nor desired, as it is with electroshock, that the patient suffer a convulsion. One of the unpredictable results of insulin shock, however, is an unpreventable convulsion and one of the hazards of convulsions, whether from insulin or electroshock, is fractured vertebrae, fractured legs and various other injuries.

[W]ith his seventh insulin treatment of 40 units, he had "a hard generalized convulsion," a grand mal seizure, which resulted in a compression fracture of the fifth, sixth and seventh dorsal vertebrae, It is to recover damages for these specific injuries that Mitchell instituted this action.

* * *

This . . . brings us to the really meritorious question of whether in the circumstances of this case, the illness and treatment involved, the doctors were under a duty to inform the plaintiff that one of the hazards of insulin treatment is the fracture of bones not involved in either the illness or the treatment. That the hazard exists is beyond question; Dr. G. Wilse Robinson, Jr., said that fractured bones, serious paralysis of limbs, irreversible coma and even death were hazards incident to shock therapy and further that there are no completely reliable or successful precautions. In their amended answer the defendants "state that the fracture of bones is a danger and risk that is inherent in insulin shock therapy, and that compression fractures of the spine, and fractures of the limbs can and frequently do occur when said insulin shock therapy is properly administered." The plaintiff's principal claim here is that "There was evidence of a negligent failure to disclose to plaintiff the hazards of insulin treatment," and, of course, evidence that plaintiff would not have consented to the treatment had he known of the dangers. . . .

[T]he serious hazards being admitted, the problem is whether in the circumstances of this record the doctors were under a duty to inform their patient of the hazards of the treatment, leaving to the patient the option of living with his illness or of taking the treatment and accepting its hazards.

*   *   *

. . . Dr. DeMott and Dr. Robinson insist that they did warn Mitchell of the dangers and risks of the treatment in great detail, including the possibilities of fractures from either intended or unintended convulsive seizures. Upon this precise point the burden of the doctors' argument is that "Mitchell's contrary testimony is not substantial and competent to sustain his verdict in view of Dr. DeMott's testimony that in the mental and emotional state that Mitchell was in at the time of the conferences, he could not possibly have an accurate memory of the conferences after the passage of a number of years." And while on this subject it is just as well to note that Mitchell testified that he did indeed remember the conferences and he said that Drs. Robinson and DeMott recommended the electroshock and insulin therapies, that he personally had no knowledge of the possibilities of fractures from insulin, that they explained the "process" to him "but there was nothing in his conversation to me that indicated any risk or disability as a result of the insulin treatment or any risk of disability at all." He categorically denied that either of the doctors advised him of the possibility of bone injuries or death from the treatments. He said that he asked Dr. DeMott if there was any danger and "His answer was that the treatments had only a temporary effect, a confusion that would last only a matter of an hour or so. He didn't say there would be any lasting effect at all"—in fact the doctor replied, "no danger."

*   *   *

In the particular circumstances of this record, considering the nature of Mitchell's illness and this rather new and radical procedure with its rather high incidence of serious and permanent injuries not connected with the illness, the doctors owed their patient in possession of his faculties the duty to inform him generally of the possible serious collateral hazards; and in the detailed circumstances there was a submissible fact issue of whether the doctors were negligent in failing to inform him of the dangers of shock therapy.

. . . Even though there was a submissible case, solely upon the indicated hypothesis, it is not possible to affirm the judgment plaintiff has obtained. The principal instruction is indeed a very sketchy submission of his basic theory and right of recovery and that theory is submitted conjunctively with extraneous matter and another hypothesis upon which he was not entitled to recover . . . one that required expert medical testimony. . . . For these indicated reasons the judgment is reversed and the cause remanded.

NOTE

Grannum v. Berard
70 Wash.2d 304, 307, 422 P.2d 812, 814 (1967)

Hunter, Judge:

*   *   *

The mental capacity necessary to consent to a surgical operation is a question of fact to be determined from the circumstances of each individual case. In *Peterson* v. *Eritsland*, 69 Wash. 2d 588, 419 P.2d 332 (1966), we stated:

The mental competency or capacity of an individual to execute an agreement, when challenged, presents a factual issue to be determined by the trier of the fact, with the test being whether the person in question, at the time of executing the contract, possessed sufficient mind or reason to enable him to understand the nature, the terms and the effect of the transaction. . . .

It is well settled that the law will presume sanity rather than insanity, competency rather than incompetency; it will presume that every man is sane and fully competent until satisfactory proof to the contrary is presented. . . . In Washington we have held that the standard of proof required to overcome this presumption, in civil cases, is that of clear, cogent and convincing evidence. . . .

c.

Hans Jonas
Philosophical Reflections on Experimenting with Human Subjects*

*   *   *

To whom should the appeal [to participate in the research project] be addressed? The natural issuer of the call is also the first natural ad-

---

* 98 *Daedalus* 219, 234–237 (1969). Reprinted by permission of Daedalus, Journal of the American Academy of Arts and Sciences, Boston, Massachusetts.

dressee: the physician-researcher himself and the scientific confraternity at large. With such a coincidence—indeed, the noble tradition with which the whole business of human experimentation started—almost all of the associated legal, ethical, and metaphysical problems vanish. If it is full, autonomous identification of the subject with the purpose that is required for the dignifying of his serving as a subject—here it is; if strongest motivation—here it is; if fullest understanding—here it is; if freest decision—here it is; if greatest integration with the person's total, chosen pursuit—here it is. . . .

*   *   *

If the properties we adduced as the particular qualifications of the members of the scientific fraternity itself are taken as general criteria of selection, then one should look for additional subjects where a maximum of identification, understanding, and spontaneity can be expected—that is, among the most highly motivated, the most highly educated, and the least "captive" members of the community. From this naturally scarce resource, a descending order of permissibility leads to greater abundance and ease of supply, whose use should become proportionately more hesitant as the exculpating criteria are relaxed. An inversion of normal "market" behavior is demanded here—namely, to accept the lowest quotation last (and excused only by the greatest pressure of need), to pay the highest price first.

As such a rule of selection is bound to be rather hard on the number-hungry research industry, it will be asked: Why all the fuss? . . . What is wrong with making a person an experimental subject is not so much that we make him thereby a means (which happens in social contexts of all kinds), as that we make him a thing—a passive thing merely to be acted on, and passive not even for real action, but for token action whose token object he is. His being is reduced to that of a mere token or "sample." This is different from even the most exploitative situations of social life; there the business is real, not fictitious. . . . The soldier's case . . . is instructive: Subject to most unilateral discipline, forced to risk mutilation and death, conscripted without, perhaps against, his will—he is still conscripted with his capacities to act, to hold his own or fail in situations, to meet real challenges for real stakes. Though a mere "number" to the High Command, he is not a token and not a thing. (Imagine what he would say if it turned out that the war was a game staged to sample observations on his endurance, courage, or cowardice.)

These compensations of personhood are denied to the subject of experimentation, who is acted upon for an extraneous end without being engaged in a real relation where he would be the counterpoint to the other or to circumstance. Mere "consent" (mostly amounting to no more than permission) does not right this reification. The "wrong" of it can only be made "right" by such authentic identification with the cause that it is the subject's as well as the researcher's cause—whereby his role in its service is not just permitted by him, but *willed*. That sovereign will of his which embraces the end as his own restores his personhood to the otherwise depersonalizing context. To be valid it must be autonomous and informed. The latter condition can, outside the research community, only be fulfilled by degrees; but the higher the degree of the understanding regarding the purpose and the technique, the more valid becomes the endorsement of the will. A margin of mere trust inevitably remains. Ultimately, the appeal for volunteers should seek this free and generous endorsement, the appropriation of the research purpose into the person's own scheme of ends. Thus, the appeal is in truth addressed to the one, mysterious, and sacred source of any such generosity of the will—"devotion," whose forms and objects of commitment are various and may invest different motivations in different individuals. The following, for instance, may be responsive to the "call" we are discussing: compassion with human suffering, zeal for humanity, reverence for the Golden Rule, enthusiasm for progress, homage to the cause of knowledge, even longing for sacrificial justification (do not call that "masochism," please). On all these, I say, it is defensible and right to draw when the research objective is worthy enough. . . .

We have laid down what must seem to be a forbidding rule. Having faith in the transcendent potential of man, I do not fear that the "source" will ever fail a society that does not destroy it—and only such a one is worthy of the blessings of progress. But "elitistic" the rule is (as is the enterprise of progress itself), and elites are by nature small. The combined attribute of motivation and information, plus the absence of external pressures, tends to be socially so circumscribed that strict adherence to the rule might numerically starve the research process. This is why I spoke of a descending order of permissibility, which is itself permissive, but where the realization that it is a *descending* order is not without pragmatic import. Departing from the august norm, the appeal must needs shift from idealism to docility, from high-mindedness to compliance, from judgment to trust. Consent spreads over the whole spectrum. I will not go into the casuistics of this penumbral area. I merely indicate the principle of the order of preference: The poorer in knowledge, motivation, and freedom of decision (and that, alas, means the more readily available in terms of numbers and possible manipulation), the more sparingly and indeed reluctantly should the reservoir be used, and the more compelling must therefore become the countervailing justification.

Let us note that this is the opposite of a social utility standard, the reverse of the order by "availability and expendability": The most valuable and scarcest, the least expendable elements of the social organism, are to be the first candidates for risk and sacrifice. It is the standard of *noblesse oblige;* and with all its counterutility and seeming "wastefulness," we feel a rightness about it and perhaps even a higher "utility," for the soul of the community lives by this spirit. It is also the opposite of what the day-to-day interests of research clamor for, and for the scientific community to honor it will mean that it will have to fight a strong temptation to go by routine to the readiest sources of supply—the suggestible, ignorant, the dependent, the "captive" in various senses. I do not believe that heightened resistance here must cripple research, which cannot be permitted; but it may slow it down by the smaller numbers fed into experimentation in consequence. This price—a possibly slower rate of progress—may have to be paid for the preservation of the most precious capital of higher communal life.

d.

John Griffiths and Richard E. Ayres
A Postscript to the Miranda Project—
Interrogation of Draft Protestors*

* * *

During the week beginning Monday, October 23, agents of the Federal Bureau of Investigation questioned about 21 undergraduate and graduate students, faculty, and staff of Yale who had earlier turned in their draft cards. . . .

* * *

On Monday morning, October 23, shortly after 9 o'clock, Dean Johnson of the Divinity

* 77 *Yale Law Journal* 300–319 (1967). Reprinted by permission of the Yale Law Journal Company and Fred B. Rothman & Company.

School learned that FBI agents intended to question Divinity School students who had turned in their cards. The interrogations began immediately thereafter. That day five Divinity School students and the Assistant to the University Chaplain were interrogated. Word spread quickly, and several persons telephoned the Law School for legal advice immediately before or after being questioned. A number of us at the Law School concluded almost at once that something should be done to inform those about to be interviewed of their rights and to help them obtain a lawyer if they felt the need. . . . Notices giving warning of the FBI's presence and emphasizing the right to silence were posted all over the campus. A meeting was organized for that evening. . . .

Of the 21 people . . . seven were members of the Yale faculty or staff, 11 were graduate or professional students, and only three were undergraduates. The oldest was 36 and the youngest 19; their average age was 25. A substantial minority of them were old enough, or enough encumbered with family obligations, to be virtually draft exempt. One had actually received an honorable discharge from the Army, along with a letter of commendation from his commanding officer. Ten held advanced degrees, and several held more than one.

* * *

The interrogations followed a standard format. Two agents arrived at the suspect's home, office or dormitory room. In eight cases their visit was unheralded; in six cases, they had telephoned beforehand; and in seven cases their impending visit was presaged by an earlier unsuccessful attempt. They confirmed the suspect's name, identified themselves, and asked to speak to the suspect alone. Two suspects insisted on having their wives or friends present; the agents successfully discouraged two others who expressed such an interest.

Unless cut off at the outset, the agents came quickly to the point. One asked the questions, while the other recorded the answers with pen and paper. When a statement was taken, the agent asked the student to sign it and to initial any changes he made in the wording. . . .

* * *

The *Journal*'s study of the impact of *Miranda* in New Haven concluded that warnings, even when given clearly and distinctly and without any attempt to discourage the suspect from exercising them, are an inadequate means to assure that he can make an informed decision whether to answer questions. The observations which led to that conclusion may have derived in part from the trauma of arrest, the "inherently coercive" stationhouse atmosphere, and the apparent inability of many ordinary criminal suspects to understand, or even to read, a printed warning. The suspects in this study—all of them well-educated and highly intelligent, and questioned in their homes or offices without an arrest—enabled us to test the *Miranda Project*'s conclusion in a situation where those other factors were not present. Under these favorable circumstances, it appears that the waiver forms effectively conveyed the limited message that one could remain silent or could ask to see an attorney. Of the five suspects interrogated on Monday, before the meeting at which rights were explained, all but one said they had learned of at least some part of their *Miranda* rights from the form the agents gave them. Most of the suspects interrogated, before and after the Monday meeting, told us that reading the form reassured them in their assertion of their rights.

However, despite the effectiveness of the forms in conveying the literal meaning of the *Miranda* advice, most of the suspects interrogated on Monday signed the waiver form, and all gave written statements to the agents. All of these told us that in the light of the explanation of rights afforded after their interrogation by the Monday night meeting, they regretted having answered the agents' questions. It should be emphasized that this regret was entirely based upon a greater understanding of the role of interrogation in the criminal process, the possible uses of admissions in a trial, and the extra-judicial uses of admissions; none of them regretted making the statement simply because, having had some legal advice, they later concluded they might be able to "beat the rap" except for their admissions under interrogation. In other words we have here a fairly pure case of admissions made simply because of a lack of *understanding* of the nature and function of the constitutional rights at stake, and of later regret based wholly upon increased understanding, not of a change of heart.

*   *   *

The Monday meeting afforded those who were interrogated thereafter a substantial degree of understanding of the nature and significance of their rights. It corrected a number of misconceptions they had about the interrogation process. The effect of the meeting was dramatic. While all those interrogated before the meeting made more or less full incriminating statements to the agents, no suspect interrogated after the meeting did so. . . .

*   *   *

The question why suspects talk to interrogators is one which has evoked many different answers in the controversy over the *Miranda* decision. . . .

*   *   *

With the suspects interrogated by the FBI, we had a chance, very shortly after they had been questioned, to ask a group of articulate people their reasons for talking to the agents. It would be unrealistic to generalize widely from such a small and atypical group, of course. Still, the reasons they gave for their decisions to answer some or all of the agents' questions may suggest factors important in other contexts as well.

One of the prime reasons why the suspects questioned Monday answered the questions of the agents was that they did not appreciate the reasons for remaining silent. Because, as we have observed above, they lacked knowledge of the legal context of the decisions they faced, they could not make an informed choice whether to exercise their rights, even though they were more or less aware of the literal meaning of the statements on the waiver form. One suspect, presented with the form by the agents, said to them, "I really don't know what I should do in a situation like this because I've never been in a situation such as this—I really don't know". . . .

*   *   *

One of the major factors preventing intelligent exercise of rights in the typical interrogation is the fact, as the *Miranda Project* expressed it, that the suspect "is in a crisis-laden situation." . . .

*   *   *

Nervousness alone, however, probably did not prevent any of those questioned after Monday from carrying through whatever resolve they had taken. What nervousness did do, we think, was to interfere with the capacity of suspects, including those interrogated after the Monday meeting, to exercise their powers of judgment in conducting themselves deliberately during their interrogations. . . . This problem was more serious for the pre-Monday-meeting group, where nervousness combined with ignorance and surprise to produce waivers of rights that were not "intelligently" made.

Most of the little that suspects said to the FBI after Monday probably flowed from their desire to appear courteous and not to offend. The most striking lesson we learned from interviewing the suspects after their interrogation is the point, obvious once noticed, that interrogation is a social situation, and suspects respond according to the normal rules of social interaction in such a situation. For middle-class suspects like ours, it seems that one of the fundamental rules is that one not be unnecessarily rude. . . .

*   *   *

The failure of the agents to overcome the determination of the few post-Monday suspects who did not answer *any* questions was determined by these suspects' ability to seize and maintain the offensive. In most of the interrogations, the agents assumed the offensive from the outset and imposed their format upon the encounter. They would begin asking questions, and, in the social situation we have described above, a question demands an answer (*Miranda* states legal, not social, rules). The suspect is thus in a position of having to *decide* whether to answer each question. In making each such decision, he is subject to all of the stresses and incapacities we have dealt with above, and above all to the disability of ignorance and the pressure of politeness. . . .

*   *   *

Our interviews reinforce the conclusions of the *Miranda Project* that the psychological interaction between the interrogator and the suspect in an interrogation is extremely subtle, and the interrogator has most of the advantages. Even when we explained their rights to silence and counsel to a group of very bright and extremely willful people, they felt pressed to answer at least some of the questions put to them by the agents. Absent such a preparatory infusion, the experience of the suspects questioned on Monday confirms the *Project*'s finding that the *Miranda* warnings are almost wholly ineffective, and this obtains even when the suspect is intelligent, and the interrogation is polite, non-custodial, and at the suspect's home.

We conclude, therefore, that if the high purposes of *Miranda* are to be effected, the warnings alone are insufficient even in the extremely favorable situation we have discussed. For full achievement of *Miranda*'s values, a suspect needs

even more than a sympathetic explanation before his interrogation—he needs a sympathetic advocate during the interrogation. Only in this way will most suspects be able to assert a measure of control over the situation, overcome inevitable nervousness, and avoid the impact of perceived (but irrelevant) social rules operating in a situation structured and manipulated by a professional interrogator.

NOTES

NOTE 1.

HENRY K. BEECHER
EXPERIMENTATION IN MAN*

*   *   *

. . . At one time Pfeiffer held the view that one should ". . . never use anyone except a volunteer who is at least at the level of a graduate student and who has investigated for himself the nature and possible dangers of the drug or procedure involved." Many would not agree with this last view. For some types of investigation, especially when subjective factors are involved, it is essential to have subjects who know nothing about the expected results and have no vested interest in the outcome. . . . Pfeiffer states his present view: "My quotation from 1951 must certainly be modified as of this date since we are using prisoners at the Atlanta Penitentiary who are not graduate students! We do screen our prisoners for psychiatric difficulties by having them complete a Rorschach examination, IQ assay and MMPI tests. We also go over their psychiatric history very carefully. My statement of 1951 represents the ideal situation rather than the practical situation."

*   *   *

NOTE 2.

SIR AUSTIN B. HILL
MEDICAL ETHICS AND CONTROLLED TRIALS†

*   *   *

. . . Surely it is often quite impossible to tell ill-educated and sick persons the pros and cons of a new and unknown treatment versus the orthodox and known? And, in fact, of course one does not know the pros and cons. The situation

---

* Springfield, Ill.: Charles C. Thomas 16–17 (1959). Reprinted by courtesy of Charles C. Thomas, Publisher, Springfield, Ill.

† 1 *British Medical Journal* 1043, 1046 (1963). Reprinted by permission.

implicit in the controlled trial is that one has two (or more) possible treatments and that one is wholly, or to a very large extent, ignorant of their relative values (and dangers). Can you describe that situation to a patient so that he does not lose confidence in you—the essence of the doctor/patient relationship—and in such a way that he fully understands and can therefore give an *understanding* consent to his inclusion in a trial? In my opinion nothing less is of value. Just to ask the patient does he mind if you try some new tablets on him does nothing, I suggest, to meet the problem. That is merely paying lip-service to it. If the patient cannot really grasp the whole situation, or without upsetting his faith in your judgment cannot be made to grasp it, then in my opinion the ethical decision still lies with the doctor, whether or not it is proper to exhibit, or withhold, a treatment. He cannot divest himself of it simply by means of an illusory or uncomprehending consent.

*   *   *

NOTE 3.

G. LONG, R. D. DRIPPS, AND H. L. PRICE
MEASUREMENT OF ANTI-ARRHYTHMIC
POTENCY OF DRUGS IN MAN—
EFFECTS OF DEHYDROBENZPERIDOL*

Among the various pharmacologic agents used in the operating room, perhaps none is more difficult to evaluate than an anti-arrhythmic drug. Species differences render animal data suspect. . . .

The belief arose—largely from the results of giving . . . large doses of epinephrine to animals —that any attempt to provoke arrhythmias during anesthesia in man would be hazardous. Yet the alternative—that of trying to study "spontaneous arrhythmias"—is probably doomed to failure because of their evanescent nature.

It occurred to us that there was no a priori reason to fear the effect of an intravenous infusion of epinephrine which was just adequate to provoke an arrhythmia. Using a calibrated constant-rate infusion pump and continuous observation of the ECG, we developed a method which we believed to be objective, accurate and safe for determining the "arrhythmic threshold" in any subject under specified conditions. . . .

*   *   *

Nine normal female patients scheduled for

elective operation were studied; they ranged in age from 29 to 51 years. . . . [The problem of obtaining valid consent always exists in an experiment performed on human beings. Despite the fact that all of our subjects were interviewed before the study and the procedure explained, we believe that an informed consent cannot be obtained for a study of this type, because of the impossibility of transmitting to a patient both the relevant information and the background needed to analyze and evaluate such information. Instead, we have accepted the role of guarantor of the patient's rights and safety. . . .]

*   *   *

The method of determining the threshold for production of ventricular arrhythmias was as follows. An initial injection at a rate of 4 g./ minute was first tried. If this did not produce an arrhythmia within 5 minutes, the infusion was terminated and restarted at a higher rate following a pause of 5 to 10 minutes. In general, rates were increased in increments of 50 per cent until an arrhythmia was observed. In every case determination of the arrhythmic threshold was repeated at least once in order to ascertain that the value was reproducible.

NOTE 4.

LORD PLATT
MEDICAL SCIENCE—MASTER OR SERVANT?*

*   *   *

To use the new aids which science has now put at his command the doctor does not have to know the scientific principles from which they have developed; and as science advances and becomes more complex it becomes increasingly impossible for him to do so. This should be accepted by medical educators without guilt or shame. The modern physician does not have to learn the engineering and physical principles on which an x-ray machine is constructed or the chemical nature of the emulsions used on the film in order to interpret an x-ray picture. (Even the interpretation is usually done for him.) He does not have to be a physicist to read an electrocardiogram. Almost none of the physicians who daily prescribe the tetracycline group of drugs knows anything about their chemical structure; or cares. . . .

*   *   *

---

* 28 *Anesthesiology* 318–319 (1967). Reprinted by permission.

* 4 *British Medical Journal* 439, 443 (1967). Reprinted by permission.

NOTE 5.

ERICH FROMM
ESCAPE FROM FREEDOM*

*   *   *

. . . With regard to all basic questions of individual and social life, with regard to psychological, economic, political, and moral problems, a great sector of our culture has just one function —to befog the issues. One kind of smokescreen is the assertion that the problems are too complicated for the average individual to grasp. On the

* New York: Holt, Rinehart and Winston, Inc. 249–250 (1941). Reprinted by permission.

contrary it would seem that many of the basic issues of individual and social life are very simple, so simple, in fact, that everyone should be expected to understand them. To let them appear to be so enormously complicated that only a "specialist" can understand them, and he only in his own limited field, actually—and often intentionally—tends to discourage people from trusting their own capacity to think about those problems that really matter. The individual feels helplessly caught in a chaotic mass of data and with pathetic patience waits until the specialists have found out what to do and where to go.

*   *   *

CHAPTER TEN

What Limitations Should Be Imposed on Informed Consent?

In this chapter we focus on the restraints which the professions and society place on informed consent to "protect" the subject's and society's "best interests." Such constraints are invoked by investigators in order to shield the subject, usually also a patient, from "unpleasant" knowledge and "unwise" choices or by lawmakers in order to shield society from troublesome choices, like euthanasia, considered offensive to the "moral sense" of the community.

Though encroachments on self-determination are traditionally viewed with disquiet, law has, without careful scrutiny, recognized, or at least acquiesced in, broadly defined limitations on informed consent. We seek to search out the conscious and unconscious assumptions about man which underlie these limitations and to compare them with observations about patient-subjects' actual behavior and desires. Materials are presented which illustrate the dilemma that arises from the conflict between the requirement of informed consent and the value of hope and blind faith in safeguarding patient-subjects' health or life. The chapter closes with a discussion of the grounds on which society either overrides a subject's choice to participate in a risky procedure or alternatively requires him to take part without his consent.

In studying these materials, reevaluate the answers already given to the questions posed in Chapters Eight and Nine. In addition, also consider:

1. To what extent should the status of being sick and dying extend or limit the right to self-determination or the capacity to give informed consent?

675

2. Who should have the authority to give consent for subjects whose "best interests" preclude their having knowledge about a research project?

3. To what extent should what kind of harm or benefit to subjects or society affect the decision to experiment without consent?

A.
In the Subject's Interests

1.
Safeguarding "Health"

a.
How Much Should the Patient-Subject Know?

[i]
L. J. Henderson
*Physician and Patient as a Social System**

*   *   *

[I]t is meaningless to speak of telling the truth, the whole truth, and nothing but the truth, to a patient. It is meaningless because it is impossible;—a sheer impossibility. Since this assertion is likely to be subjected to both objective and subjective criticism, it will be well that I should try to explain it. I know of no other way to explain it than by means of an example. Let us scrutinize this example, so far as we may be able, objectively, putting aside all our habits of moralistic thought that we acquired in early years and that arise from the theological and metaphysical traditions of our civilization.

Consider the statement, "This is a carcinoma." Let us assume in the first place that the statement has been made by a skilful and experienced pathologist, that he has found a typical carcinoma—in short, that the diagnosis is as certain as it ever can be. Let us also put aside the consideration that no two carcinomas are alike, that no two patients are alike, and that, at one extreme, death may be rapid and painful or, at another extreme, there may be but a small prospect of death from cancer. In short, let us assume, putting aside all such considerations, that the statement has nearly the same validity as the assertions contained in the nautical almanac. If we now look at things, not from the standpoint of philosophers, moralists, or lawyers, but from the standpoint of biologists, we may regard the statement as a stimulus applied to the patient.

This stimulus will produce a response and the response, together with the mechanism that is involved in its production, is an extremely complex one, at least in those cases where a not too vague cognition of the meaning of the four words is involved in the process. For instance, there are likely to be circulatory and respiratory changes accompanying many complex changes in the central and peripheral nervous system. With the cognition there is a correlated fear. There will probably be concern for the economic interests of others, for example, of wife and children. All these intricate processes constitute the response to the stimulus made up of the four words, "This is a carcinoma," in case the statement is addressed by the physician to the patient, and it is obviously impossible to produce in the patient cognition without the accompanying affective phenomena and without concern for the economic interests. I suggest, in view of these obvious facts, that, if you recognize the duty of telling the truth to the patient, you range yourself outside the class of biologists, with lawyers, and philosophers. The idea that the truth, the whole truth and nothing but the truth can be conveyed to the patient is an example of false abstraction, of that fallacy called by Whitehead, "the fallacy of misplaced concreteness." It results from neglecting factors that cannot be excluded from the concrete situation and that have an effect that cannot be neglected. Another fallacy also is involved, the belief that it is not too difficult to know the truth; but of this I shall not speak further.

I beg that you will not suppose that I am recommending, for this reason, that you should always lie to your patients. Such a conclusion from what I have said would correspond roughly to a class of fallacies that I have already referred to above. Since telling the truth is impossible, there can be no sharp distinction between what is true and what is false. But surely that does not relieve the physician of his moral responsibility. On the contrary, the difficulties that arise from

* 212 *New England Journal of Medicine* 819, 822, 823 (1935). Reprinted by permission.

the immense complexity of the phenomena do not diminish, but rather increase, the moral responsibility of the physician, and one of my objects has been to describe the facts through which the nature of that moral responsibility is determined.

Far older than the precept, "the truth, the whole truth, and nothing but the truth," is another that originates within our profession, that has always been the guide of the best physicians, and, if I may venture a prophecy, will always remain so: So far as possible, do no harm. You can do harm by the process that is quaintly called telling the truth. You can do harm by lying. In your relations with your patients you will inevitably do much harm, and this will be by no means confined to your strictly medical blunders. It will arise also from what you say and what you fail to say. But try to do as little harm as possible, not only in treatment with drugs, or with the knife, but also in treatment with words, with the expression of your sentiments and emotions. Try at all times to act upon the patient so as to modify his sentiments to his own advantage, and remember that, to this end, nothing is more effective than arousing in him the belief that you are concerned whole-heartedly and exclusively for *his* welfare.

*   *   *

NOTES

NOTE 1.

HUBERT WINSTON SMITH
THERAPEUTIC PRIVILEGE TO WITHHOLD
SPECIFIC DIAGNOSIS FROM PATIENT SICK
WITH SERIOUS OR FATAL ILLNESS*

*   *   *

Anglo-American law starts with the premise of thoroughgoing self-determination; it follows that each man is considered to be master of his own body, and he may, if he be of sound mind, expressly prohibit the performance of life-saving surgery. A doctor might well believe that an operation is medically desirable or necessary but the law does not permit him to substitute his own judgment for that of the patient by any form of artifice or deception. . . .

[I]n general, no medical privilege should be recognized to withhold the diagnosis in ordinary cases where the usual patient would feel entitled

---

* 19 *Tennessee Law Review* 349, 350–352 (1946). Reprinted by permission.

to have the information as a basis for charting his course and there being no apparent grounds for supposing that a disclosure of the truth would engender in the patient reactions dangerous to his health or life. If a broad, absolute privilege were granted to the physician to withhold medical information on allegedly therapeutic grounds, this would afford a perfect shield to cover the negligence of many who were unable to reach a timely or accurate diagnosis of the true illness. The physician could always say that he knew the diagnosis but withheld it for fear of worsening the patient's condition. Secondly, it would be dangerous in the extreme to say that a physician is entitled, either by misrepresentation or concealment, to gain the patient's consent to particular forms of treatment on the theory that "the doctor knows best" and it would only make the patient a sicker man to hear the risks.

[T]he physician should be recognized to have a therapeutic privilege to withhold part or all of the facts regarding a dread illness, when he has reason to believe that communicating them freely to the patient will involve risks of causing his death or serious impairment of his health without any countervailing gain. It is suggested that this should be in the nature of an imperfect privilege, to be passed upon by the presiding judge in the light of evidence adduced in the particular case. . . .

[T]he question was raised, to some degree, however, in the early Massachusetts case of *Twombly and wife* v. *Leach,* an action on the case against a physician for alleged malpractice in treating a felon of the thumb and consequent lymphangitis which plaintiff's wife developed after accidentally inflicting a penetrating wound upon herself with a paring knife. It appeared that defendant treated her for a considerable time without disclosing the diagnosis. On the trial of the case, the court refused to permit defendant to ask several expert witnesses: "whether or not it is good medical treatment in some cases to withhold from the patient the extent of the disease and her actual condition?" The jury returned a verdict in plaintiff's favor in the trial court, but on appeal defendant's exceptions were sustained and a new trial was granted on the ground, among others, that "upon the question whether it be good medical practice to withhold from a patient in a particular emergency, or under given or supposed circumstances, a knowledge of the extent and danger of his disease, the testimony of educated and experienced medical practitioners is material and peculiarly appropriate."

The one sovereign question by which one may fairly test the obligation of the physician is this: considering the nature of the particular physician-patient relationship, or of the employment, would the withholding of the specific diagnosis defeat the patient's just expectations or would this, under all the circumstances, really contribute to a successful performance of the physician's mission in the case?

* * *

NOTE 2.

HUNT v. BRADSHAW
242 N.C. 517, 88 S.E.2D 762 (1955)

* * *

On July 18, 1950, the plaintiff, an able-bodied man, was working in his auto repair shop near Kingsport, Tenn., when a small piece of steel, about 3/8" × 2/8" × 2/8", with sharp edges, broke off from the end of an automobile axle under a sledge hammer blow and penetrated plaintiff's body, entering the left front side of his neck just above his collar bone. He was examined by Dr. Howkins and later by Dr. Reed. There was bleeding from the entrance wound for about 15 or 20 minutes, but afterwards very little pain, no fever, and no apparent adverse effect from the accident. However, Dr. Reed had x-ray photographs made. He recommended that plaintiff consult the defendant, Dr. Bradshaw, and follow his advice as to an operation for removal of the missile.

On July 31, 1950, plaintiff consulted Dr. Bradshaw, who had five x-ray pictures made of plaintiff's upper chest. The pictures were taken from the front, back and side. On one or two the foreign body showed indistinctly. When asked for his advice after the examination, Dr. Bradshaw stated that he thought the metal was going down, that it might get into his heart, and he strongly recommended it be removed. "I asked him about the operation, if it was a very serious one, and he said it wasn't nothing to it, it was very simple."

The defendant performed the operation on the morning of August 2, 1950. Plaintiff testified: "When I woke up, I was trying to work my hand, and I couldn't use my fingers at all; I had never experienced that feeling before. At the present time (1955) I can't use my left hand at all. I can't use those fingers no way at all". . . .

At the conclusion of the plaintiff's evidence, the defendant's motion for judgment as of non-

suit was allowed, judgment entered accordingly, and the plaintiff excepted and appealed.

HIGGINS, JUSTICE.

* * *

The plaintiff's evidence is sufficient to support a finding the operation was of a very serious nature. Dr. Bradshaw, after examination, advised the plaintiff the missile might move and get to the heart, and recommended the operation. That a sharp-edged piece of steel does migrate is borne out by plaintiff's expert evidence, especially by Dr. Jeffreys. Upon Dr. Bradshaw's advice the operation was decided upon. It is understandable the surgeon wanted to reassure the patient so that he would not go to the operating room unduly apprehensive. Failure to explain the risk involved, therefore, may be considered a mistake on the part of the surgeon, but under the facts cannot be deemed such want of ordinary care as to import liability.

* * *

Of course, it seems hard to the patient in apparent good health that he should be advised to undergo an operation, and upon regaining consciousness finds that he has lost the use of an arm for the remainder of his life. Infallibility in human beings is not attainable. The law recognizes, and we think properly so, that the surgeon's hand, with its skill and training, is, after all, a human hand, guided by a human brain in a procedure in which the margin between safety and danger sometimes measures little more than the thickness of a sheet of paper.

The plaintiff's case fails because of lack of expert testimony that the defendant failed, either to exercise due care in the operation, or to use his best judgment in advising it. . . .

The judgment of nonsuit entered in the Superior Court is Affirmed.

[ii]
Ferrara v. Galluchio
5 N.Y.2d 16, 152 N.E.2d 249 (1958)

CONWAY, CHIEF JUDGE.

Plaintiff wife, who was suffering from bursitis in the right shoulder, received a series of X-ray treatments from defendants, doctors specializing in X-ray therapy. . . . At the conclusion of the sixth treatment she still had a pain in her right shoulder and one of the defendants suggested that if the pain continued she should come back for a seventh treatment. The pain persisted and three days later she returned and the seventh treatment was administered. Subsequent thereto, the shoulder began to itch, turned pink, then red, and blisters formed. These blisters ruptured and the skin peeled, leaving the raw flesh of the shoulder exposed. Scabs formed and lasted several months, a few as long as five or six months and one lasted several years. . . . This condition was diagnosed as chronic radiodermatitis which was caused by the X-ray therapy. While the blisters were still present the plaintiff went back to the defendants and showed them the condition of her shoulder. They gave her a prescription for some salve which she procured and used.

On December 3, 1951, approximately two years after the treatments, the plaintiff was referred by her attorney to a dermatologist for examination. After taking a history and making an examination the dermatologist prescribed a substance used in the treatment of radiodermatitis, and advised the plaintiff to have her shoulder checked every six months inasmuch as the area of the burn might become cancerous.

The instant action for malpractice was predicated upon (the theory) that the total number of Roentgens (1,400) applied to the plaintiff was excessive. . . . Plaintiff also introduced, on the issue of mental anguish, the testimony of a neuro-psychiatrist to the effect that she was suffering from a severe cancerophobia, that is, the phobic apprehension that she would ultimately develop cancer in the site of the radiation burn. The witness further testified that she might have permanent symptoms of anxiety.

*   *   *

The dermatologist apparently thought it essential as part of his treatment and as a protective measure for plaintiff to advise her to have her shoulder checked every six months because of the possibility of cancer. Under our law the risk of such advice and its effects on the plaintiff must be borne by the wrongdoers who started the chain of circumstances without which the cancerophobia would not have developed.

This case is somewhat novel, of course, in that it appears to be the first case in which a recovery has been allowed against the original wrongdoer for purely mental suffering arising from information the plaintiff received from a doctor to whom she went for treatment of the original injury. We have concluded, however,

that under the circumstances of the case such recovery was justified.

*   *   *

FROESSEL, JUDGE (dissenting).

*   *   *

Whatever argument may be made to the contrary, we do not feel, on balance and as a matter of public policy, that damages based upon mental anguish, engendered by a physician's statement as to a *possible* development of another ailment, are warranted under such a rule. Physicians commonly inform patients of conceivable complications which may arise from an injury, and we do not believe that so ready a road to the multiplication of damages ensuing from physical injury should be opened to plaintiffs. The unfortunate result of the rule announced by this decision, albeit disclaimed, is that a doctor's mere statement as to a possibility is a steppingstone to an increased recovery should the patient simply claim to be concerned enough to suffer worry by reason thereof. In other words, recovery would depend upon the subjective mind of the litigating plaintiff and speculation by the physician, without even the safeguard of an opinion by the latter based on reasonable certainty.

*   *   *

[iii]
Bolam v. Friern Hospital Committee
[1957] 2 All E. R. 118

MCNAIR, J. [to the jury]:

*   *   *

Let us examine those three points. Bear in mind that your task is to say whether, in failing to take the action which it is said Dr. Allfrey should have taken, he has fallen below a standard of practice recognised as proper by a competent reasonable body of opinion. First let me deal with the question of warning. There are two questions that you have to consider. First—does good medical practice require that a warning should be given to a patient before he is submitted to electro-convulsive therapy? Secondly —if a warning had been given, what difference would it have made? Are you satisfied that the plaintiff would have said: "You tell me what the risks are. I won't take those risks. I prefer not to have the treatment."

The plaintiff relies, on this aspect of the

case, on the evidence of Dr. Randall who, you may think, was a most distinguished psychiatrist, well-qualified to express an opinion. He said regarding his practice as to giving a warning:

Having assessed the patient, it is then put to him that he might benefit from electro-convulsive therapy—some people call it electro-shock therapy, but from the point of view of the patient that is not material because the patient is never aware either that he has a shock or a convulsion. Our practice at St. Thomas's Hospital, and my practice at Charing Cross Hospital is to provide the patient with a consent form.

Dr. Randall was asked whether he would warn the patient of the risks involved. He answered:

Yes, I would indeed; in fact, we do. I make a practice always of saying to the patient that, using the technique of relaxation, he would be given an injection which would put him to sleep; that he would then be given another injection which would have the effect of paralysing all his muscles so that he could not move. I explain to the patient that if he were not given a relaxant drug his body would make some strong movements.

Dr. Randall was asked about the warning:

Q: If you feel very sincerely as a doctor that it is the only hope of relieving this illness, would you think it wise to discourage the patient by describing to him the possible risk of serious fractures?   A: I suppose that one has to form some opinion whether the patient is likely to be influenced by it. Depressed patients are often deluded about their bodily health, and nothing will alter their attitude. Taking that distortion of judgment into account, it is probable that to tell a patient that a risk of fracture exists will not materially alter his attitude to treatment, or his attitude to his illness.

If it is right that to tell a patient of the risk of fracture will not materially alter his attitude to treatment or his attitude to his illness, you may ask yourselves: Is there really any great value in giving this warning? In dealing with consent forms, Dr. Randall says that these forms are provided so that the patient may be aware of the nature of the treatment, and also because it is the practice of the boards of governors of hospitals to provide them in case litigation ensues. Then Dr. Randall's evidence continued:

Q: Does it help the patient in any way to be told all the risks which are involved in electro-convulsive therapy? A: In the outcome I think that it does, because the patient takes the decision whether or not to have a treatment which might affect his whole future, and at that point he has the chance of deciding whether he will do it or whether he will not do it.   Q: Would you quarrel with a point of view as being wholly unsound if it was held that it was not beneficial to the patient to hear about that sort of thing?   A: I can believe that there would be circumstances in which it could be considered that it would not be beneficial to tell a patient of possible dangers and mishaps, subject to what I have already said.

Then I put questions to him:

Q: Do you think that other competent people might take a contrary view to the one which you have expressed?   A: I think so, my Lord; yes, they might.   Q: Other competent people might think that it is better not to give any warning at all? A: I think that that is going a little further than I could go generally, but I think that other people might consider it better not to give any warning at all.

Counsel for the plaintiff quite rightly relies on answers which Dr. Randall gave on reexamination:

Q: Do you think it ever right to give no warning of the risk to a person who can understand the warning?   A: I think that it is not right to give no warning of the risks to a patient who can understand the import of the warning.

That is the high-water mark of the case for the plaintiff in favour of the view that it was negligent, in the sense which I have used, not to give a warning.

Against that, you have to consider the evidence given by the defendants, first, by Dr. de Bastarrechea, who says:

I don't warn as to technique. I don't think it desirable to do so. If the patient asks me about the risks, I say that there is a very slight risk to life, less than in any surgical operation. Risk of fracture 1 in 10,000. If they don't ask me anything, I don't say anything about the risk.

Dr. de Bastarrechea also said that in his view there was some danger in emphasising to a patient who ex hypothesi is mentally ill any dangers which in the doctor's view were minimal, because, if he does so, the patient may deprive himself by refusal of a remedy which is the only available hopeful remedy open to him. In cross-examination Dr. de Bastarrechea agreed that when an operation is decided on, the patient should be carefully examined, but not that he should be warned of all the risks involved. He agreed that a man should be given the opportunity of deciding whether to take the risk, but it should be left to him to put questions; he should be told that there were some slight risks, but not told of the risks of catastrophe.

*   *   *

That is, in very summary form, the evidence on this point that you have to consider; and, having considered it, you have to make up your minds whether it has been proved to your satisfaction that when the defendants adopted the practice that they did (namely, the practice of saying very little and waiting for questions from the patient), they were falling below a proper standard of competent professional opinion on this question of whether or not it is right to warn. Members of the jury, though it is a matter entirely for you, you may well think that when a doctor is dealing with a mentally sick man and has a strong belief that his only hope of cure is submission to electro-convulsive therapy, the doctor cannot be criticised if he does not stress the dangers, which he believes to be minimal, which are involved in that treatment.

The second point on the question of giving a warning is this: Suppose you come to the conclusion that proper practice requires some warning to be given. If a warning had been given, would it have made any difference? Only the plaintiff can answer that question, and he was never asked it. . . .

*   *   *

. . . The question what the plaintiff would have done if he had been told that there was a one in ten thousand risk was never put. Surely, members of the jury, it is mere speculation on your part to decide what the answer would have been, and you might well take the view that unless the plaintiff has satisfied you that he would not have taken the treatment if he had been warned, there is really nothing in this point.

*   *   *

NOTE

PHYSICIAN'S DUTY TO WARN*

*   *   *

. . . The duty to warn should be based not on the doctors' practice but on the patients'

needs; that is, the inquiry should be whether a reasonable man in the doctor's position and with his knowledge of the patient would have been justified in concluding with substantial certainty that the patient, if informed of this risk, would not have withdrawn his consent. [T]he patient of average sophistication is already aware of certain dangers inherent in any surgical treatment; he may be presumed to have considered these in giving his consent, even though he has not been specifically reminded of them. The duty narrows then, in the average case, to disclosure of dangers peculiar to the treatment proposed and of which it is likely that the patient is unaware. The doctor should have little difficulty in choosing from these the risks that are sufficiently serious and likely to occur as to be essential to an intelligent decision by his patient.

Circumstances will occasionally arise, however, in which the disclosure of risks should be limited or withheld for therapeutic reasons—that is, where the patient's emotional condition is such that full disclosure would seriously complicate or hinder treatment. In other cases, the patient might justifiably be considered incapable of coping with knowledge of potential dangers and likely to distort them in such a way that rational decision would be impossible. In either of these cases, a privilege to withhold or to limit disclosure would seem justified, though it would seem desirable to require the physician to make full disclosure to a relative when possible. Disclosure, it may be noted, cannot be withheld or limited merely because the patient might, on learning of the risks, rationally decline treatment. The right to decline is the very right being protected. . . .

[Jury found defendants not negligent.]

*   *   *

[iv]
Irving L. Janis
*Psychological Stress—Psychoanalytic and Behavioral Studies of Surgical Patients**

*   *   *

To obtain observational data . . . the author has conducted systematic studies of hospitalized patients who were required to have surgical operations. . . .

A major goal of the research was to arrive at propositions that are likely to be broadly ap-

* 75 *Harvard Law Review* 1445, 1447–1448 (1962). Copyright 1962 by the Harvard Law Review Association. Reprinted by permission.

* New York: John Wiley & Sons, Inc. 8, 352–353, 367–371 (1958). Copyright 1958, Irving L. Janis. Reprinted by permission.

plicable to most people in contemporary society and that will pertain to behavior in a wide variety of danger situations. Accordingly, the main variables investigated in the surgery studies were selected on the basis of *uniformities* noted in the extensive observational reports currently available on how people in many different national and cultural subgroups tend to react to severe physical dangers—tornadoes, floods, industrial accidents, air raids, criminal assaults, concentration camp tortures, epidemics, acute illness, etc. . . .

* * *

The theoretical concepts and hypotheses which have evolved . . . have a number of important implications for the role of warnings, information about impending events, and other types of communications which can influence the adequacy of a person's psychological preparation for stressful life experiences. The case study evidence . . . suggests that the arousal of some degree of anticipatory fear may be one of the necessary conditions for developing inner defenses of the type that can function effectively when the external dangers materialize. In many of the individual case studies we have examined, the patient had received very little information about the suffering that he would undergo and, in some cases, this lack of information seems to have been a major factor in determining the relative absence of anticipatory fear. One surmises that most people ignore problematical dangers of the future unless they receive specific warnings or predictions from respected authorities. The unpleasant task of mental rehearsal, which appears to be essential for developing effective danger-contingent reassurances, is apt to be shirked, even when a person knows that he is going to be exposed to some form of suffering or deprivation.

If a person is given appropriate preparatory communications before being exposed to potentially traumatizing stimuli, his chances of behaving in a disorganized way and of suffering from prolonged sensitization effects may be greatly decreased. . . .

* * *

[A]n essential difference between the moderate and low anticipatory fear groups lies in the sphere of stress tolerance. Perhaps one reason for the difference is that the patients with moderate anticipatory fear, having greater motivation to seek information and to mentally rehearse the coming events, are in a better position to ignore a host of potentially distressing perceptions which they are able to explain away as being in the "normal course of events". . . .

The pathogenic consequences of warding off anticipatory fear by means of blanket immunity defenses . . . are not limited merely to the direct effects of being unprepared to cope with clear-cut danger stimuli but also include the indirect effects of lower tolerance for ambiguous threat stimuli. This theoretical notion carries some specific implications for psychological preparation for stress. In order to be maximally effective, preparatory communications should presumably have the goal of giving as complete a cognitive framework as possible for appraising the potentially frightening and disturbing perceptions that the person might actually experience, so as to prevent the type of surprise and ambiguity that generates unproductive, energy-consuming reactions of hypervigilance. Provided that the material is not presented in a lurid or threatening manner, and is accompanied by impressive reassuring comments, specific forecasts about future stressful experiences can probably influence most persons to engage in an imaginative mental rehearsal of the type that promotes the development of effective danger-contingent reassurances.

* * *

Probably the most effective preparatory communications would be those which give a detailed factual account of the *outstanding perceptual experiences that are most likely to occur*, concentrating especially on the vague and ambiguous events that are most likely to be misinterpreted. Communications of this type are currently being given, presumably with some success, to prepare pregnant women for the stresses of childbirth. For surgical patients, however, it is much more difficult to predict in advance the outstanding crises that may arise (e.g., unusual organic complications may drastically interfere with the normal course of recovery). Nevertheless, the patient could be told in advance about all those pains, discomforts, and unpleasant treatments which invariably do occur. And then, if unpredictable events were to take place, the patient might be given additional information early enough so that the processes of inner preparation could reduce the shock of surprise. For example, when a surgical incision turns out to be much more extensive or creates more of a cosmetic defect than the surgical staff had originally anticipated, it may be possible to give the patient appropriate information about it during the early phase of the postoperative period, before he makes the shocking discovery himself. Even for relatively minor complications, such as Mrs. R.'s discolored bruise, the patient can probably be spared some unnecessary emotional tension if information about the unexpected injury is presented and discussed as soon as the patient is capable of engaging in conversation.

The foregoing discussion has emphasized the probable advantages of giving detailed preparatory information to surgical patients so that they can anticipate correctly and become emotionally prepared for distressing stimuli which they will subsequently perceive. But this emphasis should not be construed as indicating that there is any special advantage to telling surgical patients about the medical aspects of the operation—details about the surgical procedures that will be carried out while the patient is unconscious, the potential risks from the anesthesia, the unusual complications that occasionally arise, and the factors that make for a poor prognosis. In general, there is probably little or no gain from giving any technical information which is not essential for conveying a realistic picture of what the patient will actually perceive. A small amount of background information about the medical aspects may sometimes have a beneficial effect, but only if it serves to correct a patient's misconceptions or if it subsequently contributes to the patient's understanding that nothing untoward is happening to him.

The available evidence suggests that when a physical crisis occurs, prior familarity with the fear-arousing stimuli tends to lower the chances of emotional shock. But there are some indications in the case study material that detailed medical knowledge does not necessarily help a patient's postoperative adjustment. On the contrary, he may find it much more difficult to feel reassured if he knows a great deal about the dire complications and potential risks which the surgeon is taking into account.

Too much information about the medical aspects of one's own case can create an attitude of sustained hypervigilance that serves no constructive purpose and that may increase one's sensitivity to adverse events. These negative consequences are suggested by the case study material from a number of well-informed and well-educated surgical patients. . . .

NOTE

Irving L. Janis
Emotional Inoculation—
Theory and Research on Effects
of Preparatory Communications*

* * *

In order to specify functional properties of the work of worrying, it is necessary to delineate what occurs in its absence. What happens when, because of lack of opportunity or inadequate motivation, a person remains unworried about an impending danger experience and fails to undergo any inner preparation before it materializes? At the moment when inescapable signs of danger or actual suffering are encountered, efforts at intellectual denial (by minimizing or discounting the likelihood of being personally affected by the danger) will no longer succeed. The person then suddenly finds himself unable to ward off intense fear or fright (which sometimes is experienced as anger or other affects), especially because he has not developed any means for actively protecting himself from the danger. Moreover, the crisis seems to be augmented by the fact that when more danger or suffering is encountered than had been expected beforehand, feelings of helplessness are likely to occur which drastically interfere with the ego's normal reassurance mechanisms. One of the most important sources of reassurance, markedly impaired under these conditions, is the anticipation of being protected from the full impact of the danger by the danger-control authorities or other benevolent parent surrogates.

* * *

From what has just been said about the dynamics of stress behavior, one can predict that a number of interrelated adverse effects will ensue if, for any reason, a person fails to do the work of worrying prior to being exposed to actual danger or loss:

1. The spontaneous tendency to ward off anticipatory fear remains unchecked and the person therefore remains relatively unmotivated to engage in the realistic fantasying or the mental rehearsing essential for developing two types of effective defense against fright: (a) reality-based cognitions and expectations about opportunities

* 5 *Psychoanalysis and the Social Sciences* 139–143 (1958). Reprinted by permission of the International Universities Press, Inc., New York.

for surviving the impending danger, the subsequent contemplation of which can function as a source of hope and reassurance; and (b) reality-based plans for taking protective actions in case various contingencies arise, the subsequent execution of which can contribute to reducing feelings of passive helplessness.

2. The person's overoptimistic expectations and fantasies remain uncorrected and hence the chances are increased that there will be a marked disparity between the amount of victimization expected beforehand and the amount that is actually experienced, increasing the probability of regressive aggrievement reactions (childlike rage and/or depression).

3. When the person subsequently comes to realize that the danger-control authorities failed to predict or give warnings about the suffering that was in store for him, childhood experiences of resentment against the parents (for unfair or unprotective treatment) are especially apt to be reactivated, thus increasing the likelihood that the danger-control authorities will lose their capacity to give reassurances and will be irrationally blamed for objective dangers and deprivations.

All three reactions to objective danger situations would be expected to occur whenever a person fails to engage in adequate work of worrying beforehand, whether the failure is attributable primarily to the predanger environmental conditions or to exceptionally strong personality needs which predisposed the person to deny clear-cut signs of impending danger. Sometimes absence of the work of worrying is caused by the sudden onset of an unpredictable event (e.g., an emergency operation following an automobile accident). Thus the essential factor may be that the anticipatory period is too short to allow the person time to prepare himself for the emergency. Often, however, people fail to carry out adequate inner preparation even though there is ample time between an initial warning stimulus and the onset of the crisis. In such instances, a major causal factor responsible for the incompleteness of the work of worrying is likely to be *lack of unambiguous warnings and information about the magnitude of the impending danger.* Rosen points out, for example, that surgeons sometimes will "join the patient in his denial of the unpleasant consequences of surgery with an 'everything is going to be all right just leave the worrying to me' attitude." And, of course, at the opposite extreme there are some physicians who severely frighten their patients long in advance of an operation, giving alarming information be-

fore it can properly be evaluated and assimilated, thereby stimulating defensive reactions of extreme denial which preclude the normal work of worrying. Thus, it may often happen that the adequacy of a person's emotional preparation for danger will depend upon the *adequacy and timing of the preparatory communications* to which he has been exposed.

b.

To Choose on Faith or Knowledge?

[i]
W. R. Houston
The Doctor Himself as a Therapeutic Agent*

*   *   *

The great lesson . . . of medical history is that the placebo has always been the norm of medical practice, that it was only occasionally and at great intervals that anything really serviceable, such as the cure of scurvy by fresh fruits, was introduced into medical practice. By and large, the doctors were, as reported by that sane and shrewd observer, Montaigne, a danger to their patients. The medical historian is apt to mislead us when he speaks of the learned and skilful doctors of the past. While undoubtedly exceptional instances might be unearthed to show that these physicians accomplished something for the somatic good of their patients, in the large view we are forced to realize that their learning was a learning in how to deal with men. Their skill was a skill in dealing with the emotions of men. They themselves were the therapeutic agents by which cures were effected. Their therapeutic procedures, whether they were inert or whether they were dangerous, were placebos, symbols by which their patients' faith and their own was sustained.

The history of medicine is a history of the dynamic power of the relationship between doctor and patient. Through centuries when doctors were doing more harm than good this dynamic force has sustained the medical profession in the esteem of their clientele, it has inspired their fellow citizens with such faith in its values that they were willing to give economic support to the doctor. However little the doctor had to offer, it was to him that men turned in the distress of illness. When we observe the honor and emolument bestowed on the physician throughout the ages we

---

* 11 *Annals of Internal Medicine* 1415, 1416, 1420 (1938). Reprinted by permission.

are forced to exclaim, "Oh rare cogency of the relation between doctor and patient!"

*   *   *

When thoughtfully considered, this situation is not one to be regarded with comfort. Medical men are not without misgivings about the spurious psychotherapy that they are under constant temptation to practice. Yet the path to development of a better psychotherapy is full of obstacles. The doctor's training in the laboratory and the ward has offered few opportunities for the development of any aptitude in dealing with the problems of personality. Doctors consider that their vocation is to deal with things that can be weighed and measured and that the reactions of the cerebral cortex and the autonomic nervous system are too intangible for them to deal with. As a distinguished member of this body, and contributor to this program, recently wrote me:

"I suppose that I am particularly bitter about the people whom we may as well call neurotics, who, as you say, take up so much of an internist's time. They are the people who drove me out of practice. I never could see any sense in paying any attention to them because, as your word picture of them so graphically shows, they have neither sense, nor gratitude, nor any idea of cooperation, nor any qualities that might endear them to man, woman or child.

"I cannot understand why those of us who have trained ourselves to take care of people who have organic disease can't be allowed to take care of organic disease. Why won't these people take our word for it that there is nothing the matter with them and let it go at that? I suppose I have as many somatic sensations as anybody on earth but I explain them to myself in a physiological way. Why can't an intelligent neurotic take the same sort of advice that I give myself? There seems to be no way of handling them except that sort of semi-quackery that some highly respectable members of our fraternity are able to get away with so successfully."

[*ii*]
Stewart Wolf
*The Pharmacology of Placebos**

*   *   *

Placebos have been used for centuries by physicians under pressure to "do something," but

_____
* 11 *Pharmacological Reviews* 689, 690, 692, 694, 696 (1959). © 1959, The Williams and Wilkins Co., Baltimore, Md. Reprinted by permission.

wishing to do no harm. Traditionally, the function of the placebo was to pacify without actually benefiting the patient. The benefit, however, has proved to be unexpectedly lavish. Not only has the hopeful reassurance of placebos engendered in patients a feeling of increased well-being, but recent experimental evidence has shown that placebo administration may be followed by substantial and measurable changes in bodily mechanism. Therefore, since placebos do a great deal more than placate or pacify, a new definition may be offered as follows: *Placebo effect = any effect attributable to a pill, potion, or procedure, but not to its pharmacodynamic or specific properties.* Placebo effects derive from the significance to the patient of the whole situation surrounding the therapeutic effort. . . .

*   *   *

Modell writes that the placebo effect ". . . is the only single action which all drugs have in common and in some instances it is the only useful action which the medication can exert". . . .

Dubois listed three classes of placebos. The first included simple substances, inert and unpretentious, such as lactose and starch. The second class included pseudomedicaments, extracts of herbs, poisonous metals, superfluous vitamins, and so forth. Such are the ingredients of most proprietary medicines sold over the counter. The third is the placebo effect that goes along with the pharmacodynamic action of a specific therapeutic agent.

*   *   *

Except in the case of a patient's special need, a physician's special hope, or an experimenter's deliberate manipulation of the situation by suggestion, or otherwise, there appears to be nothing predictable about placebo effects. Placebos may induce in an organ a change in one direction or in another, or no change at all. A vivid example of the way a placebo may produce changes in opposite directions in a single organ is available in the studies of gastric acid secretion in man. Two separate investigators measured gastric secretion in healthy human subjects in response to an oral placebo without verbal suggestion. In one group of 22 subjects a 12 percent increase of gastric acidity was observed and in the other group of 15 subjects an 18 percent decrease following the administration of a placebo. The difference between the two groups was significant at the 0.001 level of confidence.

Several authors have observed toxic reactions in response to the administration of placebos. Sheldon, in a study of reserpine administered to by hypertensive patients, found that the patients who were receiving placebos complained of nasal stuffiness as often as did those who were getting reserpine. Shapiro and Grollman, studying effects of antihypertensive agents given by mouth to ambulatory patients, found that one of their most troublesome and persistent . . . headaches occurred in an individual who was getting placebo at the time. . . .

*　　*　　*

It is important to realize that placebo effects are not imaginary. Neither are they necessarily suggestive in the usual sense of the word. For example, certain workers have induced changes in circulating eosinophiles, either during the discussion of meaningful topics or following the administration of placebos. . . .

*　　*　　*

There is not universal agreement as to the place of the placebo in therapeutic research. Some investigators have asserted that the placebo control is unnecessary or even misleading, but most agree that it is an indispensable step toward the establishment of the therapeutic efficacy of any new agent. The placebo by no means provides a perfect control procedure, however. Telltale side effects of a potent agent may vitiate the attempt to keep the physician or the subject unaware of what is being given. While placebos may induce almost any side effect, they do not produce them as predictably as an active agent. Furthermore, the use of a placebo control may be awkward and cumbersome when establishing a dose range or when looking for serious toxic effects of an agent. In a clinical trial, however, and before the presumed therapeutic action of the agent can be accepted, the placebo must be given and given without the knowledge of either the one who gives it or the one who gets it because, as already pointed out, drug therapy backed by unconscious enthusiasm and solicitude of the physician may result in powerful and measurable bodily changes which are not attributable to the pharmacodynamic effects of the agent in question. A case in point was that of a patient who had had chronic asthma for twenty-seven years. Having suffered almost continuous asthma for the past seventeen, he had become a favorite subject on which to test new drugs. He had become refractory even to epinephrine. Finally, the product of one pharmaceutical company seemed

effective in his case. When he was given the agent, he was free of asthma; when it was stopped, the asthma returned. Accordingly, his physician substituted a placebo without the patient's knowledge. Asthma was not relieved. Shifts from agent to placebo and back again were carried out several times with consistent results in favor of the agent. When the company was approached for an additional supply of the material, their representative acknowledged that, because they had had so much trouble with positive enthusiastic reports, they had, in this instance, sent along the placebo first. It would be hard to find a more vivid illustration of the need for placebo control to be blindly undertaken so that the doctor as well as the patient is in ignorance of what is being administered. Investigators have often been naive in failing to recognize that patients, like dogs and children, are likely to know what is in the atmosphere without our telling them and even when we try desperately to conceal our attitudes.

*　　*　　*

NOTES

NOTE 1.

HENRY K. BEECHER
SURGERY AS PLACEBO*

*　　*　　*

Various surgical procedures have been recommended and carried out for the relief of angina pectoris. One of these, ligation of the internal mammary arteries, offers material pertinent to the subject of this paper. . . .

At first when this procedure was tried in man, it was believed to be beneficial. Unfortunately, the early studies were uncontrolled; results were not for the reasons thought, and they were fleeting—lasting for a number of weeks. The procedure's relevance to this study is that the benefit was not due to changes in blood flow produced by the ligations: We are now sure of that. Benefit was due to what happened in the minds of the patients and the surgeons involved. It will be shown that both of these can produce significant change, and that the changes are both subjective and objective. . . .

Harken reported on 35 patients with angina who had had internal mammary artery ligation

---

* 176 *Journal of the American Medical Association* 1102, 1103–1104, 1106 (1961). Reprinted by permission.

with the result that "more than a third have enjoyed complete relief and there has been worthwhile palliation in almost three-fourths of the group." Significantly, how long the relief lasted is not stated. He concludes that "the present experience is indeed exciting," and that "this seems a simple but valuable therapeutic adjunct." Even if one considers only the "more than a third" who found complete relief, here are results achieved by an enthusiastic surgeon far beyond those achieved by the sceptic.

*   *   *

Adams's paper is important for its early timing since, in the midst of enthusiasm for ligation, it threw doubt on the cause of the improvement. He found that incision of the skin and placement of an untied ligature around the internal mammary arteries of 2 patients produced great subjective improvement which was not increased on subsequent tightening to obstruction of the previously placed ligatures.

Fish, Crymes, and Lovell carried out internal mammary artery ligation in 24 patients with angina pectoris. . . . they approached the procedure with scepticism. Fish and associates say: "It was explained to each patient that the operation was experimental, that there was no generally accepted physiologic basis for apparent good results and that those attending the patient had no idea whether or not the angina would be improved". . . .

In the Fish study: "In 20 of the 24 cases there was an initial period of marked improvement, which usually began in the postoperative period and lasted approximately ten to sixty days. This was reflected by increased exercise tolerance and a reduction of the quantity of nitroglycerin required and in electrocardiographic stability. . . . In the light of subsequent findings, this striking early improvement is difficult to explain." It is no more difficult to explain than all placebo effects, one might add. At the time the Fish paper was written, only 4 of the 24 patients, in their own opinion, had moderate improvement; 2 believed they were slightly improved, while "in the remaining 18, the angina syndrome has resumed its preoperative course."

The quantitative approach has been embodied in several studies, 2 of which are particularly outstanding. Cobb and co-workers set up a well-planned study to test whether any relief of symptoms was produced by the procedure and, if so, whether this was greater than a placebo effect. Seventeen patients seriously limited by angina

agreed to cooperate. They recorded the number of anginal attacks occurring, and the number of nitroglycerin tablets required before, and at specified intervals after, the operation. In addition, a standardized exercise-tolerance test was given before and after operation; so were determinations of respiratory efficiency, blood pressure, and electrocardiograms made during rest and during exercise. The procedure was done under local anesthesia, and only at the time of operation was the surgeon given a card to tell him whether to ligate the arteries or only to make skin incisions. The patients were asked to estimate their improvement, if any, at intervals during the postoperative period. They had been told merely that they were participating in an evaluation of the operation, and were not aware of the double-blind nature of it. The observers did not know, when evaluating the data, whether ligation had been carried out or whether only a skin incision was made. It was quite evident that ligation produced no greater benefit than the sham operation.

It would be a mistake to give weight to a case or 2, but in conjunction with similar material it is interesting to observe that in one patient of this series (not ligated) the skin incisions permitted 10 minutes of exercise without pain and without electrocardiographic abnormality 6 weeks after operation, whereas 4 minutes of exercise before surgery led to pain and striking inversion of T waves. Greatly increased work tolerance and remarkably decreased consumption of nitroglycerin—both easily expressed in objective terms—are the usual findings of nearly all investigators. It is of such "convincing" objective stuff that new operations are made.

*   *   *

One could argue that, since placebos have considerable therapeutic power, the benefit obtained from them is sufficiently great to justify the risk involved. This point of view hardly holds up when the price may be life itself.

Our aim in medicine is to relieve often, and to cure when we can. Placebo effects are not to be despised; they play a part—sometimes a very important part—in surgical success; but we would be deceived by our own maneuvers if we fail to find out when placebo effects may be the sole agents functioning in a given case. Having understood this, we have gone a long way to control the destructive force of bias.

*   *   *

NOTE 2.

JULIAN M. RUFFIN, JAMES E. GRIZZLE,
NICHOLAS C. HIGHTOWER, GORDON MCHARDY,
HARRISON SHULL, AND JOSEPH B. KIRSNER
A CO-OPERATIVE DOUBLE-BLIND
EVALUATION OF GASTRIC "FREEZING" IN
THE TREATMENT OF DUODENAL ULCER*

*   *   *

Gastric "freezing" for the treatment of duodenal ulcer was introduced by Wangensteen and his associates in 1962, and its usefulness was promptly supported by further investigation. Subsequently, this method of treatment was used in many small clinical groups throughout the country. However, the enthusiasm of early publications was soon followed by a wave of skepticism. . . .

In recognition of this need, a double-blind study was initiated in 1963 and conducted simultaneously in five institutions. . . . The same criteria were used by all five institutions in selection of patients, and identical methods employed in the "freezing" procedure, collection of data and evaluation of results. . . .

The specific [objective of the study was]: to evaluate the effects of gastric "freezing" on the natural history of duodenal ulcer. . . .

*   *   *

The procedure adopted for this study was that proposed by Wangensteen et al. A Swenko hypothermia machine was used in all institutions. The volume of coolant (95 per cent ethyl alcohol) in the gastric balloon ranged from 550 to 700 ml in all the patients. . . . The temperature of the coolant returning to the hypothermia machine from the gastric balloon was maintained at −10°C, and the flow rate of the coolant was maintained between 1200 and 1400 ml per minute. The duration of the procedure (time of circulation of coolant within the balloon) was 50 minutes in all patients.

*   *   *

An attempt was made to have every aspect of the sham gastric "freeze" identical to the true "freeze" with the one exception of the temperature of the coolant circulating in the balloon. Thus, the exact procedure as described for gastric "freezing"—preparation of patient, volume

of coolant in gastric balloon, duration of procedure and monitoring—was followed.

*   *   *

The follow-up study was conducted by a physician who was unaware of which procedure had been employed. Provision was made to break the code for the protection of the patient's welfare if the need arose.

*   *   *

The results of this study demonstrate conclusively that the "freezing" procedure was no better than the sham in the treatment of duodenal ulcer, confirming the work of others. There was no significant difference in relief of pain, secretory suppression, number and severity of recurrences or development of end points in the two groups. It is reasonable to assume that the relief of pain and subjective improvement reported by early investigators was probably due to the psychologic effect of the procedure.

The importance of random assignment of patients to treatment and the double-blind method in clinical trials has been emphasized repeatedly, but these features are still too frequently ignored. Only by strict adherence to such principles and resisting the urge to publish until data have been gathered by these rigorous methods will false leads be kept to a minimum and erroneous conclusions avoided.

NOTE 3.

ABRAM HOFFER
A THEORETICAL EXAMINATION OF
DOUBLE-BLIND DESIGN*

There are at least three major variables in any therapeutic program. The first is that feeling of trust or faith the patient has in his doctor and, therefore, in his therapy. The second factor is the faith or confidence the physician has in himself and in the line of therapy he proposes to use. The third factor is the therapy. The best results are obtained when all three variables are set at their optimum level. . . .

*   *   *

The double-blind technique makes it difficult to sustain these two variables at their optimum level. It is hardly likely that a doctor will have as much faith in a new drug as he does in drugs with which he is familiar, and when he

---

* 281 New England Journal of Medicine 16–19 (1969). Reprinted by permission.

* 97 Canadian Medical Association Journal 123, 124 (1967). Reprinted by permission.

is forced to work in a double-blind way his faith and enthusiasm are reduced to a very low level. It has been our tradition for centuries to abhor the use of placebo or trickery. For centuries doctors have condemned quacks. In the Middle Ages the only difference between quacks and doctors was that while the doctors were more honest, the quacks were more intelligent. Quacks knew their remedies were no good and so sold atmosphere, displays, catharsis and other trappings of non-medical faith. Doctors used similar remedies which were no more therapeutic, but they did have faith in their efficacy. In the end the doctors won because therapies in which we can justly have great faith developed.

*   *   *

NOTE 4.

David W. Meyers
The Human Body and the Law*

*   *   *

One ethical difficulty posed by much of medical experimentation is its inevitable reliance on a 'control group': those who take sugar pills, for example, instead of a penicillin derivative and are used as a measure to determine the effects of the experimental substance or treatment. These people must consent to undergo the full rigours of the experimental therapy and cannot be told they will serve only as decoys. This, of course, involves a subtle but patent series of misrepresentations and may be ethically unpalatable to some. However, it is submitted, such a practice is generally recognized as inherent in many experiments involving more than one individual, and people, in offering themselves to act as subjects for (non-therapeutic) experimentation, must be presumed to have understood and accepted this fact.

*   *   *

NOTE 5.

Chauncey D. Leake
Ethical Theories and Human Experimentation†

*   *   *

In designing an experimental study with human subjects, clinical pharmacologists usually devise some sort of a double- or triple-blind tech-

* Chicago: Aldine Publishing Co. 92 (1970). © 1970 David W. Meyers. Reprinted by permission.
† 169 *Annals of the New York Academy of Sciences* 393–394 (1970). Reprinted by permission.

nique, where neither subject, experimenter, nor observer knows whether the test drug or a placebo is being used. It is often claimed that the subject should not even know what the purpose of the experiment may be, in order not to jeopardize the objectivity of the findings. In my opinion, this is not wise. Let the subject know just as much about the design of the study as the experimenter, even to the point of explaining that drugs may be interchanged, with erroneous hints as to how they may act. Such a method could control the possible subjective notions of the experimenter as well as of the subject.

*   *   *

NOTE 6.

Louis Lasagna
Drug Evaluation Problems in Academic and Other Contexts*

*   *   *

When one is trying to diminish prejudice for or against a remedy, however, it is probably preferable, at least scientifically, for subjects and observers to be kept in the dark. To begin with, patients told that they may receive a placebo may refuse to participate in the trial. If such refusals are few, they need not inconvenience the experimenter or the experiment. But if they are frequent, not only will the trial be prolonged, but the generalizations possible at the end may be seriously limited, in view of the possibly atypical nature of the sample.

It may be argued that such problems are unfortunate but unavoidable if one is to respect an individual's freedom to say "No." Indeed so. But since society hedges on individual liberties in all sorts of other situations, is it not desirable at least to consider the possibility that individual freedom—provided serious harm is not involved—may have to yield at times to the general welfare?

Placebo trials pose no serious ethical problems for me in most situations: If the true merit and hazard of a new remedy are not established, it is unethical not to perform a proper controlled trial (which may, to be sure, use a standard drug for comparison, rather than a placebo, if such a standard is available). Too often the placebo-treated patients turn out to be the lucky ones in such a trial, "deprived" only of an ineffective and toxic chemical.

I do object, however, to such deceit as the

* 169 *Annals of the New York Academy of Sciences* 506 (1970). Reprinted by permission.

use of homeopathic doses of drug as placebo so that patients may be told that they will receive only "varying doses of active drug." It also strikes me as unacceptable to disguise the placebo treatment as " a standard and time-honored remedy that is safe and has been proven to help many people" (true though the statement is!).

On the other hand, I submit that telling patients they will or may receive a placebo changes the rules of the game, with unpredictable Heisenbergian impact. It is a bit like bugging a jury room to observe the jury process at work. It may be reprehensible to do so without asking consent of the jurors, but who would pretend that the behavior of the jurors will be unaffected by the knowledge that they are under surveillance?

* * *

NOTE 7.

THOMAS C. CHALMERS AND LOUIS LASAGNA
EXPERIENCE IN DESIGN, CONDUCT, AND
EVALUATION OF RESEARCH*

DR. CHALMERS: . . . One may explain in great detail the hazards of both procedures, stating that, because one does not know which hazard is greater for the patient, we're going to flip a coin or randomize. Objection can be raised to that technique as bad medical care, because any sensible patient could draw two conclusions from such an elaborate explanation of the technique regarding a decision for surgery; namely, that if the physician can't make up his mind about the operation, the patient will find a doctor who can, or if the difference between surgery and medicine is so small that an elaborate study is required, the patient will choose medical therapy.

In either case, the patient ends up being deprived of the operation. If it should turn out that the operation is better, then we have practiced improper medicine, because we have deprived half of the patients of the opportunity of having the operation. This probability would be an ethical argument in favor of not explaining in great detail the randomization procedure.

On the other side, there is the experience of a number of physicians who explain randomization as a method of deciding on an elective operation to a patient who is not very sick. They claim that full explanation pays off, and the explanation to the patient is proper. Obviously, it is proper, but this depends on what we call full ex-

planation in terms of the details one presents to the patient concerning the operative procedure.

So we must conclude that it depends on what the physician investigator thinks best for his patient. It may be very bad for a sick patient selected for trial of emergency surgery or portacaval surgery to be given all the gory details. In such a case, it may be better medical care or therapy not to explain fully—despite the basic obligations to disclose. However, the family must be kept fully informed.

DR. LASAGNA: The ethical problem here comes in making it clear to potential patients or volunteers what the situation is; namely, that you have two surgical techniques or a surgical technique and a nonsurgical technique of which the relative merits are not known. I assume that you don't do the experiment unless that situation pertains. Now, if that point is made clear, and the willingness of the subject to have one or the other form of therapy is clear, then I submit that it's pointless and cruel to say, "By the way, now we're going to decide by pulling cards out of the file." It seems to be that you can say, "Are you willing to take whichever one is decided for you to undergo?" If the patient then asks how that decision is to be made, you shouldn't lie about it. But why should you go out of your way to detail how the decision is made? I really don't see that. I know some people do, but I think that would be heinous.

DR. CHALMERS: This is the way I feel also.

* * *

[iii]
Lee C. Park, L. Covi, and E. H. Uhlenhuth
Effects of Informed Consent on Research
Patients and Study Results*

Recent rulings by the National Institutes of Health about research grant applications require a detailed description of the manner in which informed consent of research subjects is obtained. Many researchers have been alarmed by the possibility that informing patients of the research nature of their treatment will severely limit the validity of results. Negative effects of informed consent in patients would include: resentment about being used as research subjects or about being given supposedly inactive treatments (for instance, placebo); anxiety resulting from knowledge that treatments are assigned arbitrarily; poor response to treatments which might be

* 169 *Annals of the New York Academy of Sciences* 513–514 (1970). Reprinted by permission.

* 145 *Journal of Nervous and Mental Disease* 349–354 (1967). © 1967, The Williams and Wilkins Co., Baltimore, Md. Reprinted by permission.

effective in a positively oriented nonresearch atmosphere. Another issue would be the researcher's anxiety and guilt about "using" patients, which might be alleviated by the patient's ignorance of research goals.

With regard to the patient's resentment of inactive treatments, Liberman stated, "If subjects were forewarned of placebo administration, many would not cooperate with the experimenter—such candid statements of placebo use early in the experiment would engender suspicion and perhaps hostility in subjects, making them undesirable if not unwilling candidates for placebo research." However, he did note that when the use of placebo was revealed to patients at the end of his experiment, "Almost all the subjects reacted to the disclosure in a relaxed fashion. Some expressed surprise but most were unruffled and left the room without any sign of resentment or dismay." Bukanz stated, "Indeed, I have been told by some highly qualified investigators that their patients are increasingly reluctant to sign the required consent form, particularly if the use of placebo is involved. It is very difficult to explain to a patient why he should be the one to voluntarily agree to receive no medication if the luck of the draw runs that way. His concern, quite justifiably, is with his own health, not with the advancement of medical knowledge." Similarly, Lasagna stated, "This business of consent has already deterred some investigators from doing research." He reported that a recently proposed study was dropped because less than 20 per cent of the informed patients agree to sign the consent form and he questioned whether valid results could be obtained from such a selective population.

With regard to the possibility that premature disclosures might bring about faulty study findings, Liberman wrote, "To bring greater understanding into the dynamics of placebo reactivity, placebo research must be carried out under conditions as nearly similar to those occurring in *real* drug experiments as possible." Fisher, Cole, Rickels and Uhlenhuth stated: "Patients more often see themselves as being 'treated' rather than 'researched,' and this may provide a highly favorable setting for drug action. In many controlled experiments, the patients become definitely aware that they are participating in a research project (implying 'Let's see if the drugs will help you'), and such a perception could tend to inhibit drug action."

With such an atmosphere of negative expectations, there have been few attempts to evaluate objectively the pros and cons of these issues.

Over the last few years, we have participated in a number of clinical psycho-pharmacological studies in which careful concern was given to patients' attitudes and concerns about research procedures, although at the time it was still considered necessary for valid findings that patients be kept unaware of key facts indicating the research nature of their treatment. In this paper, we present material from some of our studies in which patients have been given information and instructions not usually given in such research and have nevertheless consented to participate. In addition, we discuss the findings of a survey in which patients were asked about their perceptions of the research procedures and goals in a drug study just completed.

In an 8-week double-blind, cross-over study of the effectiveness of imipramine and placebo on neurotic depressed outpatients, carried out in 1959–1960, Uhlenhuth and Park formulated the following statement for the patients: "The kind of trouble you have been telling me about often responds quite well to medicine. We now have two different medicines available that we know help many people with difficulties like yours. However, some people do better with one and other people do better with the other medicine. The best way to find out which of the two medicines is best for you personally is to try them both. So we have set up a treatment program which will give you the opportunity to do just that. You will be able to take each medicine for 4 weeks. At the end of 8 weeks, if necessary, you may continue to take whichever medicine works best for you." This was presented to the patients as treatment rather than as research, although such a presentation of alternative treatments is not made in the usual treatment setting. Rather, patients are usually given one medicine and advised it will help them; then, if the medicine doesn't work, the doctor subsequently may switch to another medicine.

Nevertheless, neither the 42 patients who completed the treatment nor the 8 patients who dropped out indicated any particular interest or concern about this manner of presentation. On follow-up, it was determined that 2 patients were dropped because they were hospitalized, 2 obtained jobs which interfered with appointments, 1 complained that the medicine wasn't helping, 1 complained of side effects, and 1 was ill with a medical condition. There is inadequate information on the other patient. There is some evidence of possible factors influencing drop-outs. For instance, 4 of the 8 drop-outs were patients of one of the seven treating doctors. Thus, informing patients of an experimental manipulation of medicine—in their own interests—did not appear to result in drop-outs, and, in fact, the study doctors reported that patients appeared to accept the rehearsed speech without reservation. . . .

*   *   *

To explore . . . the possibility of breaking with the traditional taboo of informing patients of the research nature of treatment, Park and Covi in 1963 carried out a brief (1-week) non-blind treatment of 15 anxious patients with placebo. Each patient was told, "Mr. Doe, at the intake conference we discussed your problems and your condition, and it was decided to consider further the possibility and the need of treatment for you before we make a final recommendation next week. Meanwhile, we have a week between now and your next appointment, and we would like to do something to give you some relief from your symptoms. Many different kinds of tranquilizers and similar pills have been used for conditions such as yours, and many of them have helped. Many people with your kind of condition have also been helped by what are sometimes called 'Sugar Pills' and we feel that a so-called sugar pill may help you, too. Do you know what a sugar pill is? A sugar pill is a pill with no medicine in it at all. I think this pill will help you as it has helped so many others. Are you willing to try this pill?"

Surprisingly, 14 patients completed the treatment and showed symptomatic improvement as a group, on a 65-item symptom checklist, to a greater degree than patients in our double-blind studies of drugs and placebos. In this study, in which patients were asked to participate for only 1 week, no patients showed the expected resentment, although some were skeptical, and some showed friendly amusement, accompanied in at least 1 patient by a report of symptomatic improvement even before the "treatment" began. Furthermore, the social worker who interviewed some of the patients after the study reported that they were very different from patients seen after other drug studies: they appeared much more verbal, comfortable, inquisitive and free with comments.

In spite of the fact that each patient was told the pills were placebos, only three patients were certain of this after the week of treatment. Five additional patients thought the pills probably were placebos. On the other hand, two patients thought the pills definitely contained drugs and four thought they probably contained drugs. Thus, there appeared to be limits in the capability of the experimenter to influence established concepts in the patients.

*   *   *

We learned that clinic outpatients come into our studies with deep feelings of trust and expectations of marked improvement, and they often do not believe they are subjected to research or are given inert medication, even when research paraphernalia are obvious or they are informed of the nature of the treatment. They will obediently perform "unusual" tasks in "unusual" settings without question. In some of our research, patients were given information usually withheld because such knowledge might have a detrimental effect on patients and study results. We found no evidence that this information had negative effects on either patients or findings.[3]

*   *   *

A basic purpose of this paper is to suggest that the present anxiety about informed consent may be based partly on preconceived bias and that the process of informing patients is worthy of research in itself. Orne pointed out, "If one were to employ any form of deception, it is crucial to find out whether it is the subject or experimenter who is deceived." We make assumptions that some information may have negative effects and even that some may have positive effects, but there has been little objective experimentation to test these assumptions with distressed patients as opposed to volunteer subjects.

2.

Safeguarding "Life"

a.

How Much Should the Dying Patient Know?

[i]
Donald Oken
What to Tell Cancer Patients—A
Study of Medical Attitudes*

No problem is more vexing than the decision about what to tell the cancer patient. . . . The manner in which such questions are handled is

---

[3] Our findings, of course, may have been biased by patients' high expectations about Johns Hopkins Hospital as a prominent medical center. Perhaps patients would be less willing to participate as informed research subjects in a small or less-known clinic.

* 175 *Journal of the American Medical Association* 1120–1126 (1961). Reprinted by permission.

crucial for the patient and may determine his emotional status and capacity for function from that time on. It is easy enough to decide to follow a course which will "do least harm," but it is far from simple to determine just what course that is. . . .

*   *   *

The research on which this report is based represents a further attempt to study physicians' approaches to the problem of what to tell cancer patients. The aim here has been not merely to learn what is done but, more importantly, to understand the attitudes which are underlying determinants of these strategies. . . .

*   *   *

The initial undertaking in this research was the determination of whether or not physicians tell their patients they have cancer. [T]here is a strong and general tendency to *withhold* this information. Almost 90 percent of the group is within this half of the scale. Indeed, a majority tell only very rarely, if ever. No one reported a policy of informing every patient. . . . No difference between specialities was uncovered. . . . These findings also cut across the hospital staff rank and age. Younger and less experienced men did not have any greater inclination to tell than their seniors.

Use of a questionnaire, of course, forces answers into an artificially rigid mold. But, information derived from the interviews strengthens the finding. Answers indicating that patients are told often turned out to mean telling the patient that he had a "tumor," with strict avoidance of the terms cancer, malignancy, and the like. These more specific words were almost never used unless the patient's explicit and insistent questioning pushed the doctor's back to the wall.

Euphemisms are the general rule. These may extend from the vaguest of words ("lesion," "mass"), to terms giving a general indication that the process is neoplastic ("growth," "tumor," "hyperplastic tissue")—often tempered by a false explicit statement that the process is benign; to a somewhat more suggestive expression (a "suspicious" or "degenerated" tumor). Where major surgical or radiation therapy is involved, especially if the patient is hesitant about proceeding, recourse may be had to such terms as "pre-cancerous," or a tumor "in the early curable stage." Some physicians avoid even the slightest suggestion of neoplasia and quite specifically substitute another diagnosis. Almost every one reported resorting to such falsification on at least a few occa-sions, most notably when the patient was in a far-advanced stage of illness at the time he was seen.

It is impossible to convey all the flavor of the diverse individual approaches. No two men use exactly the same technique. Each has his preferred plan, his select euphemisms, his favored tactics, and his own views about the optimal time for discussion and the degree of directness to be used. Some have a set pattern, while others vary their approach. But the general trend is consistent.

The modal policy is to tell as little as possible in the most general terms consistent with maintaining cooperation in treatment. Exceptions are made most commonly when the patient is in a position of financial responsibility which carries the necessity for planning. Questioning by the patient almost invariably is disregarded and considered a plea for reassurance unless persistent and intuitively perceived as "a real wish to know." Even then it may be ignored. The vast majority of these doctors feel that almost all patients really do not want to know regardless of what people say. They approach the issue with the view that disclosure should be avoided unless there are positive indications, rather than the reverse. Intelligence and emotional stability are considered prerequisites for greater disclosure only if other "realistic" factors provide a basis for doing so. For the fewer physicians who tell with some frequency, these two factors assume more primary importance.

A few additional consistent themes emerge. Agreement was essentially unanimous that some family member must be informed if the patient is not made aware of the diagnosis. Legal and ethical considerations are by no means the only points of relevance here. Repeated instances were reported of patients who, dissatisfied with the progression of their disease in the face of treatment and desperate for help, were dissuaded from fruitless and unwise shifts to a new physician (or quack) only by the cooperation of an informed relative. Beyond this is the need to have someone to share the awful burden of knowledge. As one man put it, "I just can't carry the load alone." Few responsibilities are as heavy as knowing that someone is going to die; dividing it makes it easier to bear.

Variations in approach also converge to a single major goal: maintenance of hope. No inference was necessary to elicit this finding. Every single physician interviewed spontaneously emphasized this point and indicated his resolute and determined purpose is to sustain and bolster the patient's hope. Each in his own way communicates the possibility, even the likelihood, of recovery. Differences revolve about the range of belief about just how much information is compatible with the maintenance of hope. While some doctors believe "cancer means certain death and no normal person wants to die," others hold that "knowledge is power": power which can conquer fear. The crux of the divergence centers on two issues: whether cancer connotes certain death, and whether the expectation of death insurmountably deprives the patient of hope. The data indicate that an impressively large number of physicians would answer affirmatively to both.

The approach used by a physician may derive from many sources. Perhaps he acquired it as a result of teaching in medical school or while a house officer; maybe it grows out of his own clinical experience or is a result of personal experiences with afflicted friends and family; it may arise as a result of reading; or perhaps it is a personal conviction which stems from the deeper influences of his personality and individual philosophy. . . .

*   *   *

Clinical experience would seem to be of overwhelming importance. Only 6 percent (12 of 203) failed to list this as a factor. Other sources are reported with far less frequency, and if reported at all, usually in addition to clinical experience, which is the factor accorded primary importance by more than three-quarters of the group. Medical school teaching apparently plays a minimal role. Internship and residency training is somewhat more often listed. . . . Few people could remember hearing about the subject during their training. When someone did, usually there was no recall of anything specific said, other than the emphasis of the need of the physician to deal with the problem. This silence, like the lack of research, is striking. . . .

Personal factors are reported by only a moderate number of the group. The experience of seeing a close relative (most commonly a parent) die of cancer, was a decisive occurrence for some. This experience, however, did not lead to any difference in policy between these physicians and the group as a whole; they were neither more nor less likely to tell. Less concretely derived personal feelings were reported by a small group. These responses, comprising all but two of those listed as "other," were described in such terms as "my philosophy of life," "my personal

conviction," or "projecting myself into the patient's situation." Interestingly, if such a feeling was reported at all, there was a strong likelihood that it was considered the determining factor.

*   *   *

[E]xperience can be acquired only over a span of time. A young group, whose graduation from medical school has taken place not many years earlier, might be expected to report that their policy stems largely from other sources. At least they should cite experience less often than their seniors. This is not the case. The group under 45 years of age, or those in the lower staff ranks, are just as likely to list experience as a factor as their older colleagues. Indeed, they are no less likely to cite it as the major determinant. The mean age and the staff level of those who reportedly base their policy on experience does not differ from those who do not. Nor do the policies of the two groups differ.

Experience, moreover, implies a state of knowledge based upon a range of earlier observation, with the opportunity to become familiar with the outcomes of various alternatives. Occasions for some such experience, of course, have been available to all these physicians. Yet only 27 (14 percent) have had the opportunity for first-hand knowledge based on their own trial of any policy different from their current one. More detailed exploration in the interviews cast a great deal of further doubt about the role of experience. It was the exception when a physician could report known examples of the unfavorable consequences of an approach which differed from his own. It was more common to get reports of instances in which different approaches had turned out satisfactorily. Most of the instances in which unhappy results were reported to follow a differing policy turned out to be vague accounts from which no reliable inference could be drawn.

Instead of logic and rational decision based on critical observation, what is found is opinion, belief, and conviction, heavily weighted with emotional justification. As one internist said: "I can't give a good reason except that I've always done it." Explanations are begun characteristically with such phrases as "I feel . . ." or "It is my opinion. . . ." Personal convictions were stated flatly and dogmatically as if they were facts. Thus, "Most people do not want to know," "It is my firm belief that they always know anyway," or "No one can be told without giving up and losing all hope." Highly charged emotional terms and vivid expressions were the rule, indicating the intensity and nature of feelings present. Knowledge of cancer is "a death sentence," "a Buchenwald," and "torture." Telling is "the cruelest thing in the world," "awful," and "hitting the patient with a baseball bat." It is not necessary even to read the words on the questionnaires. Heavy underlinings and a peppering of exclamation points tell the story. These are hardly cool scientific judgments. It would appear that personal conviction is the decisive factor.

There is direct confirmation of this point. *Subsequent* to the general inquiry: "How did you acquire your policy?" it was specifically asked if personal issues were determinants. Nearly three-fourths (98 of 138) reported that personal elements were involved, in contrast to the much smaller number who listed this originally. These 98 were about equally divided as to whether these factors were the most important.

*   *   *

Another relevant finding is the doctor's wish to be told if he were the patient. As expected, those who tend to tell their patients wished to be told, themselves, more often than those who do not tell. But the total number of those who said they wished to be told (73 of 122) is far greater than those who tend to tell their patients. The explanation usually given was that, "I am one of those who can take it" or "I have responsibilities." That they did not feel this to be true for all physicians, however, is attested to by their treatment of other doctor-patients. Most of the group said they were neither more nor less likely to tell physicians than other patients. Of the group who did modify their policy, it was just as likely to find that they were *less* prone to tell doctors. It is impossible to draw any precise conclusion from this type of hypothetical question about one's self. But the inconsistency is characteristic of emotionally determined attitudes.

The pros and cons of telling have been discussed so often that there is little point in doing so again. Whatever the reasons for telling, the argument against doing so centers on the anticipation of profoundly disturbing psychological effects. There is no doubt that this disclosure has a profound and potentially dangerous impact. Questions do arise about the capacity of human beings to make a satisfactory adaptation to the expectation of death. Can anyone successfully handle such news without paying a price which mitigates whatever value this knowledge brings? If so, how widespread is the ability to call forth the necessary psychological defenses? What about time: does this readjustment take place within some reasonable span? Can the emotional cost of such a shattering experience, or of the effort required for mastering it, be weighed and predicted? The truth is that we know very little about these matters.

It has been repeatedly asserted that disclosure is followed by fear and despondency which may progress into overt depressive illness or culminate in suicide. This was the opinion of the physicians in the present study. Quite representative was the surgeon who stated, "I would be afraid to tell and have the patient in a room with a window." When it comes to actually documenting the prevalence of such untoward reactions, it becomes difficult to find reliable evidence. Instances of depression and profound upsets came quickly to mind when the subject was raised, but no one could report more than a case or two, or a handful at most. This may merely follow from the rarity with which patients are told. Such an explanation must be reconciled with the fact that these same doctors could remember many instances in which the patient was told and seemed to do well. It may also reflect the selection of those told. Or perhaps the knowledge produces covert psychological changes which are no less malignant for their subtlety. But actually, the incidence and severity of depression and other psychological reactions in cancer patients, and their relation to being told, are not known.

The same situation holds with regard to suicide. Only 6 doctors could report definite known cases of suicide (2 of these reported two cases and 1 "several"), although about one-third of the group had "heard of" suicides after being told. Further investigation indicated that at least 2 of these patients had never been told. (And it is not altogether inconceivable that they would have felt better, not worse, had this been done.) Actually, the circumstances surrounding all but one or two of these cases are quite vague; it is impossible to feel any certainty about what lay behind the suicide.

*   *   *

Among the motivations for entering medicine, the wish to conquer suffering and death stands high on the list. Practicing physicians are not the kind of persons who can sit quietly by while nature pursues its course. One of the hardest things for a fledgling medical student to learn is watchful waiting. Few situations are as frustrating as sitting by impotently and "helplessly" in the face of illness. Fatal illness is felt as a major defeat. . . .

NOTE

HERMAN FEIFEL
THE FUNCTION OF ATTITUDES
TOWARD DEATH*

*   *   *

An interesting contrast emerges in comparing studies of physicians and patients as to whether the physician should tell or should not tell the patient he is dying. Sixty-nine to 90 per cent of physicians, depending on the specific study, are in favor of not telling the patient. In opposing vein, 77 to 89 per cent of the patients want to know. Our outlook as physicians may be too conditioned by the "healthy" rather than by the seriously ill and the dying.

*   *   *

[ii]
A Physician
Should Doctors Tell the Truth
to a Cancer Patient?†

*   *   *

Not so long ago I had to decide whether to tell a patient of mine—a man in his sixties who had just retired from an active, successful career—that he had cancer. I thought a lot about it. In the end I decided not to tell him. I told his children—they were all grown—and they agreed that their father should not be told. Nor should their mother. "Not yet. They've made so many plans for his retirement. If he has a little time, we would like it to be happy time."

The man did have time, he lived quite comfortably for three years. He and his wife traveled and saw a lot of the world. Together they were happy doing all the things he had been too busy to do when he was working. At the end he went pretty rapidly, without prolonged suffering. Two days before his death the children told their mother the truth. She was very angry with me because I had not told her in the beginning.

"If you had known," I asked, "could you and Bob have enjoyed these last three years?"

She looked at me for a moment. Her eyes were wet, but she went on with the honesty and insight that often come to help people through their hardest hours. "No. No, we couldn't have. Worse, I couldn't have kept the truth from Bob. I've never been able to keep a secret from him."

I think I was right in not telling that patient the truth.

When I was a young doctor I once told a patient flatly that he had inoperable cancer. He was a man in his middle years, respected and successful. He had asked for the truth and he seemed to me to be the sort of man who could take it. But when I told him, he went into shock right there in my office. He never had a happy or relaxed moment until his death some months later. It was a terrible ordeal for him and for his family. And much of it was unnecessary. If I had withheld the truth, or given him only a part of it, some of his remaining months might have been good.

I never forgot that man. I thought of him every time I had to decide whether or not to tell the truth to another patient suffering from incurable cancer. In many cases it began to seem wiser and kinder not to tell. Until one day I found myself looking a patient straight in the eye and saying in reply to a direct question, "No, of course you don't have cancer!" She was a tense, nervous person who had overcome deep apprehension, fear and dread to ask me this question. She was in no state to hear the truth and probably could not accept it without severe emotional damage. She probably had a year or more of reasonably comfortable life ahead. There was a chance of keeping it a happy time for her. Her family had been told the truth about her illness. They wanted it kept from her. And so I lied.

The patient had almost two good years. I think that somewhere in her mind she knew the truth—it is my belief that most people do—but she never asked me the direct question "Do I have cancer?" again. I think most people know without being told. They don't want it put into words. Perhaps in the beginning they do, or think they do, but later on, when they are not feeling so strong, I think they are glad those words are not there.

Now in medicine you always tell the truth—98 per cent of the time. You couldn't practice good medicine if you didn't. And if you find that a patient has cancer, his family must be told even

---

* *Death and Dying—Attitudes of Patient and Doctor* (Symposium No. 11). New York: Group for the Advancement of Psychiatry 632, 635 (1965). Reprinted by permission.

† *Ladies Home Journal* 65, 108 (May 1961). © 1961, Downe Publishing, Inc. Reprinted by special permission of the Ladies Home Journal.

if the patient himself is not. For a doctor to take on his own shoulders the responsibility of withholding such knowledge is unfair to everyone, including the doctor. . . .

*   *   *

The patient's own temperament has a lot to do with whether or not you tell him. To some highly intelligent people—like John Foster Dulles or Robert A. Taft—you can tell the simple truth and know that it is not going to destroy them as human beings. Their minds and their emotions are capable of absorbing the knowledge and adjusting to it rationally. A person with less understanding and self-control might not be able to do this. Being told the truth could prove an overpowering shock. He might become so emotionally unstable that he would have to be treated as a mental patient as well as a cancer patient. This makes it tragically harder, not only for him but for his family.

Sometimes you must tell the truth to a man who has a highly responsible job involving the welfare of other people. Or a man who owns his own business and has no relatives or partners to take over. Such men would want—and I think should have—the truth, because they must find someone to carry on for the sake of the many other people who may depend on them.

*   *   *

Recently a patient of mine, a famous athlete, had to be operated on for an intestinal ailment. We knew right away that we were too late. There was nothing to do but close the incision. His wife and I decided not to tell Jack the truth. He thought that his weakness and loss of weight were simply the aftereffects of surgery and he stayed quite cheerful. He never said a word about cancer.

One day when I stopped in to see him, he grinned and showed me a letter written to him by a friend who had had diverticulitis and made a good recovery from it. "The symptoms were just like yours, Jack," the letter said. Jack lived on that letter. He must have quoted it and showed it to me a dozen times.

Two weeks later Jack died. I had visited him on the morning of that day. "Hello, Jack," I said, "you're looking better today." I meant simply that he was looking better than he had yesterday, but Jack smiled in a pleased way. Later, when I talked to his wife, she said quietly, "Doctor, do you know what Jack told me after you

visited him this morning? He said, "Mary, the doctor says I'm getting well!" "

Mary loved him. He was my friend as well as my patient. We were both happy that Jack could die thinking he was getting well.

NOTES

NOTE 1.

ARTHUR H. BECKER
THE PATIENT WITH A FATAL ILLNESS—
TO TELL OR NOT TO TELL*

*   *   *

As a hospital chaplain, I have found, however, that the patient hesitates to ask the physician for a variety of reasons: a fear of displaying lack of trust in the doctor, the feeling that the doctor himself is threatened by the possibility of death, or the feeling that the doctor either does not have time, or is not willing to sit down and "work through" the implications of the information with the patient. . . .

*   *   *

NOTE 2.

THOMAS P. HACKETT AND AVERY D. WEISMAN
WHEN TO TELL DYING PATIENTS THE TRUTH†

*   *   *

[A] woman with a terminal breast cancer [after weeks of apparent serenity] asked her doctor whether the headache she'd been having might be due to nerves. The doctor said it might —and then asked her why she was nervous. Her reply: "I've lost sixty pounds in a year. The priest comes to see me twice a week when he hardly came at all before. And my mother-in-law's nicer to me than ever, though I'm meaner than ever to her. Wouldn't you be nervous, too?"

There was a pause. Then the doctor said, "You mean you think you're dying?" She said, "I do." He said, "You are."

The smile she gave him actually expressed relief. "Thank God," she said. "Someone's finally told me the truth!"

*   *   *

---

* 201 *Journal of the American Medical Association* 646 (1967). Reprinted by permission.

† *Medical Economics* 81, 84–85 (December 4, 1961). Copyright © 1961, by Medical Economics, Inc., A Subsidiary of Litton Publications, Inc., Division of Litton Industries, Inc., Oradell, N.J. Reprinted by permission.

NOTE 3.

J. M. HINTON
THE PHYSICAL AND MENTAL DISTRESS OF THE DYING*

* * *

As at least three-quarters of the patients here studied became aware that they were probably dying, the question "Should the doctor tell?" loses much of its force. The problem becomes rather more ordinary and more capable of solution. It resolves itself into discovering what the patient knows, and how much more he really wants to know, information that can be gathered with no distress in a quiet, unhurried conversation. Many writers, including Cappon, have felt that it is not justifiable to tell a patient a fact about his approaching death which he does not consciously want to know. This opinion against supplying such gratuitous information was supported in the present study by evidence that awareness was associated with depression and anxiety. This association was found at the initial interview; and the 34 patients who became more aware of dying became at the same time more anxious or depressed. But if a patient sincerely wanted to know his possible fate, and was met by prevarication or empty reassurance, he felt lonely and mistrustful. Then, commonly, while a young nurse was caring for the patient, the vital question was put to her, to the potential embarrassment and distress of both. In my opinion, if the awareness of the patient is so great that he has formulated the question, an honest answer which does not seek to destroy all hope will not add to his distress. Gavey has said that there is more room for frankness in intelligent patients; but in the present study the length of education and the social class, in so far as they indicated intelligence, made no significant difference to mood or to the awareness of dying. It is very probable that a doctor feels better able to tell an intelligent patient, but this does not necessarily mean that the less intelligent may not cope with this knowledge just as well. There are occasions when a patient experiences anguish, ineffectively trying to thrust out the fear that he may die, but yet vaguely aware that he may need to accept the possibility. Leading the patient into talking of this, and not denying the situation, enables an adjustment to take place with less distress. The few patients in the present series who were told that they had a tumour, or some other potentially lethal condition, were usually sad for one or two days, and then appeared to come to terms with this knowledge. If given some positive information about the plan of treatment they usually kept this in the forefront of their minds, and gained great comfort thereby. The courageous acceptance of the situation by the majority of these patients, and their appreciation of the frank discussion with their doctor, were in accord with the findings of Aitken-Swan and Easson; two-thirds of their patients were glad that they had been told that they had cancer, and only 7 per cent resented such frankness. . . .

[iii]
Paul Rhoads
Management of the Patient with Terminal Illness*

* * *

[H]e must tell the patient the facts of his physical condition as truthfully and as fully as the patient wishes to know them—always with a liberal admixture of understanding and hope. Just how and how soon this is to be done will vary with each individual, but it is my firm conviction that, with few exceptions, it must be done. Many patients will make it clear that they do not want to be told the whole truth, whether they say it in so many words or not. And, of course, their wishes must be respected. Most will, in the end, have to be told by someone.

* * *

I was astonished to learn of a survey of the views of a liberal sampling of physicians on this point, in which more than 70 percent stated that they usually did not inform patients that they were facing a terminal illness. Some even attempted to justify giving false information about the diagnosis if they felt patients were unprepared to accept the truth. . . . My own conviction is that never, under any circumstances, should patients be told untruths. This is the surest way to destroy the mutual trust and respect which, in the end, may prove to be the most important therapeutic asset the physician possesses.

William Bean in his essay "On Death" has stated well the attitude I share:

I cannot conceive of the practice of medicine in which there is any breach of absolute trust and confidence between patient and doctor. A good physician cannot lie to his patient. If the truth be bitter he must help the patient face it. On the other hand, I could

* 32 *Quarterly Journal of Medicine* 1, 19 (1963). Reprinted by permission of the Clarendon Press, Oxford.

* 192 *Journal of the American Medical Association* 661–662 (1965). Reprinted by permission.

not bear the practice of medicine if I felt obliged to tell the patient everything I know or think I know. . . .

* * *

NOTE

PAUL TALALAY
A SUMMARY OF COMMENTS*

* * *

In many instances, a serious medical condition may admit of several therapeutic decisions. Suppose that a young woman consults her physician with a sarcoma of the arm. The doctor is confronted with the possibility of giving no therapy, in which case she will certainly die, or of amputating the arm, or of administering various chemotherapeutic agents, or of giving radiation therapy. In practice, the physician selects what appears to him to be the wisest of these alternatives. He sensitively and delicately communicates this decision to the patient. In fact, he is experimenting. The code requires that the nature, the reason, and the risks of the experiment should be fully explained to the patient, who should in turn have complete freedom to decide whether or not to take part in this experiment. But no respected physician who is considerate of his patient would think of telling her all the implications of the disease. The essence of the good doctor is that he must assume responsibility for the management of the patient's illness, and an essential part of this responsibility is not to burden the patient with unnecessary anxieties which would inevitably result from a full exposition of the disease, its implications, and the therapeutic experiment. The good physician must continually interpret the ethical codes and the legal requirements in terms of the best interests of the patient.

* * *

[iv]
Avery D. Weisman
The Patient with a Fatal Illness—
To Tell or Not To Tell†

* * *

The central question is not whether or not to tell a patient about his dim outlook, but *who*

* P. Talalay, ed.: *Drugs in Our Society*. Baltimore: The Johns Hopkins Press 269–278 (1964). Reprinted by permission.

† 201 *Journal of the American Medical Association* 646, 647–648 (1967). Reprinted by permission.

shall tell, *how much* to tell, *what* to tell, *how* to tell, *when* to tell, and *how often* to tell.

Who Shall Tell?—Telling a patient is only the beginning, certainly not the end. It is not a painful task to be gotten out of the way, or to be relinquished gladly to someone else, such as to a minister or another family member. For everyone concerned, it is a genuine opportunity to reaffirm the reality of a human relationship. For the physician, it is an obligation and probably a necessary step, if the patient is to have a reasonably tranquil terminal period. Physicians who are most reluctant to talk about death with their patients are sometimes those who are also most reluctant to order sufficient analgesics and tranquilizers in the terminal stage. This suggests that, on both counts, these doctors avoid direct confrontation with death, perhaps to spare anguish for themselves, not for their patients.

How Much to Tell?—Telling a patient about his terminal illness is certainly not like giving him neutral information. A patient should be told only as much as he can use and absorb at the moment. A doctor should give information gradually, often over a series of visits, watching for individual responses and inquiries, allowing for idiosyncratic reactions, and being prepared to modulate the conversation to correct for unexpected complications. Rules and standard policies only approximate the facts; individual variations are the only rules.

What to Tell?—Most patients already have a fairly accurate intimation about the trend of illness by the time the physician and family get around to telling them. When a patient denies concern, he usually does so in order to preserve a relationship with someone on whom he is dependent, and cannot afford to alienate—and this includes the physician taking care of him. It is by no means rare for terminal patients to conceal the extent of their awareness, lest the doctor or family become upset!

Initially, most patients should be advised of the doctor's findings *and the treatment planned.* Frankness does not mean hopelessness, nor does unrealistic denial do more than foster temporary reassurance. At the beginning, the patient need not be told more than the facts of the illness. His doctor's directness should convey a more important, nonverbal message that he will not be abandoned. Gratuitous reassurances, overly precise predictions, and philosophical precepts are to be avoided.

How to Tell?—Plenty of time is needed for a significant human interchange. Information that involves a strong emotion can be given openly, but in the direction of the patient's strengths. Avoid technical terms, because the doctor's concern about the histological type of tumor, for example, may not be the patient's concern. The predominant concerns of dying patients are usually not with the fact of dying, but with fears of isolation, abandonment, intractable pain, or of being sent off to a nursing home to languish and die. The physician, then, should be prepared for responses that seem to be accepting but are not, for delayed responses, and for anxieties not literally expressed that actually refer to something else. As a rule, the doctor cannot recognize the difference between true acceptance and outright denial without knowing the patient for a long time. Simple sincerity is a better guide to *how to tell* than are clichés or standard formulas which tend to protect the doctor without helping the patient.

When to Tell?—Although families may at first protest about giving the patient any information, lest he give up, become insane, or commit suicide, let them know that these reactions are decidedly uncommon. If the patient does not already know or suspect, families must be assured that soon it will be impossible and even undesirable to keep the "secret." Let them know also that dissimulation risks alienation and abandonment long before the patient is, in fact, ready to die. Families who have been the least accessible to the patient during health are often those who show the most opposition to telling the patient the truth about his illness.

How Often to Tell?—After the initial step of candor and confidence has been taken, subsequent discussions become easier. Because communication is uncluttered with rationalizations and unnecessary apologies, patients can be told about new symptoms and why older symptoms have not responded to treatment. Openness means that patients are told that they will have enough medication to reduce pain and that they will be consulted when procedures which merely prolong survival are being considered. By damaging a patient's sense of being a person, unnecessary procedures may inflict more suffering and exact a greater price than the biological extension of life in terms of days or weeks can justify.

Few patients persist in talking about dying. They accommodate to awareness of death, especially in the advanced stages of illness, and still more when they can face death with their doctor's help. Availability of the doctor leads to acceptance by the patient, even though acceptance may come gradually. Conversely, efforts by the

doctor to encourage denial in the patient may lead to the doctor's denial of the patient as a person. After all, the physician's prime consideration, once death can no longer be postponed, should be to help the patient live as effectively as possible until he dies.

NOTES

NOTE 1.

SAMUEL B. WOODWARD
MEDICAL ETHICS*

* * *

Is it ethical to lie outright to a patient? Has one a right to deceive a patient as to his condition? Must one make public a prognosis if it be unfavorable or bolster up vain hopes of a recovery when the physician well knows that this is impossible? Every tub, medical or otherwise, must stand on its own bottom and these questions can be answered in individual cases according to individual circumstances. Personally I can, I think, truthfully say that in a practice of forty years I never, so far as I can remember, found it necessary to tell an outright lie to a patient about his condition. Tactful and skillful explanations with their ifs and ands, side issues and suggestion of possibilities always sufficiently befogged the issue, satisfied the patient and left my conscience unseared. Few are the patients that really wish to be told that their cases are hopeless. . . .

* * *

NOTE 2.

RICHARD A. KALISH
DEATH AND RESPONSIBILITY—
A SOCIAL-PSYCHOLOGICAL VIEW†

I would suggest that [the patient] not only has the right to know, but he has the right *not* to learn everything all at once. More to the point, he has the right to learn a little bit at a time, to eliminate alternatives as he becomes psychologically able to eliminate them. [The patient] most certainly has the right to get honest answers to direct questions, but he may ask these questions one at a time over a period of weeks. Then he has the right to withdraw and deal with the new bit of evidence. The physician has the obligation to

---

* 202 *New England Journal of Medicine* 843, 852 (1930). Reprinted by permission.

† 3 *Psychiatric Opinion* 14, 16–17 (June 1966). Reprinted by permission.

answer these questions honestly, but his task will also be less painful because [the patient] is likely to ask only those questions to which he can anticipate the answers.

Thus, I feel, the physician should inform [the patient] that his illness is serious, perhaps very serious, and that he may never fully recover. After that, he can take his cue from [the patient]. If asked to give a date of death, he can be honest in saying he does not know, that medical science is just not that accurate; if pressed, he can speak in terms of "sooner rather than later," or "perhaps before Christmas." If asked about pain and suffering, the physician can answer generally, then more specifically as more specific questions are put to him, always explaining—of course—that individual cases vary. As these questions occur, the physician might open the discussion to what [the patient] would like done for his pain; he might explain something of the effects of various sedatives and let [the patient] consider the pros and cons of being heavily sedated. However, these discussions should not be formal lectures of planned duration, but brief comments and responses to questions. The main point is that [the patient] be made to feel that the channel of communication to his physician remains open.

NOTE 3.
BARNEY G. GLASER AND ANSELM L. STRAUSS
AWARENESS OF DYING*

* * *

Many conditions reduce a doctor's inclination to make a separate decision for each case. Few doctors get to know each terminal patient well enough to judge his desire for disclosure or his capacity to withstand the shock of it. . . . Even when a doctor has had many contacts with a particular patient, class or educational differences, or personality clashes, may prevent effective communication. Some doctors simply feel unable to handle themselves well enough during disclosure to make a complicated illness understandable. If a doctor makes a mistake, he may be liable for malpractice. Some doctors will announce an impending death only when a clear-cut pathologist's report is available. Others do not tell because they fear the patient might become despondent or mentally ill or commit suicide, because they do not want him to "lean" on

them for emotional support, or because they simply wish to preserve peace on the ward by preventing a scene.

At the same time, a number of other conditions encourage disclosure regardless of the individual patient's capacity to withstand it. Some doctors disclose to avoid losing the patient's confidence if he should find out through cues or accidentally. Telling also justifies radical treatment or a clinical research offer; it also reduces the doctor's need to keep up a cheerful but false front. Some tell so that the patient can put his affairs in order and plan for his family's future, or reduce his pace of living; others, because family members request it. Of course, if the chances for recovery or successful treatment are relatively good, a doctor is naturally more likely to disclose an illness that is possibly terminal; disclosing a skin cancer is easier than disclosing bone cancer.

The combined effect of these conditions—some of which may induce conflicting approaches to the same patient—is to make it much easier for doctors to apply to all patients a flat "no, he should not be told." For when people are in doubt about an action, especially when the doubt arises from inability to calculate the possible effects of many factors about which there is little information, it is almost always easier and safer not to act.

* * *

Many of the standard arguments given by doctors both for and against disclosure anticipate a single, permanent impact on the patient. He is expected to "be brave," "go to pieces," "commit suicide," "lose all hope," or to "plan for the future" and such. But the impact is not so simple. Disclosing the truth sets off a generalized response process through which the patient passes. To base the decision about disclosure on a single probable impact is to focus on only one stage in the response process; not only does it neglect the other stages, but also it omits how each stage may be controlled by the staff through appropriate forms of interaction. For example, to predict that the patient will become too despondent is to neglect the possibility that he might overcome this despondency and, with the aid of a chaplain or social worker, prepare adequately for his death and for his family's future. But to expect a patient simply to settle his affairs is to fail to evaluate his capacity for overcoming an initial depression, as well as the capacity of the staff to help him at this stage.

The generalized response process is stim-

* Chicago: Aldine Publishing Co. 119–122 (1965). Reprinted by permission.

ulated by a doctor's *disclosure* to the patient. The patient's initial response is almost invariably *depression,* but after a period of depression he either *accepts* or *denies* the disclosure; and his ensuing behavior may be regarded as an affirmation of his stand on whether he will, in fact, die. Acceptance of the doctor's disclosure may lead to active preparation, to passive preparation, or to fighting the illness. A particular patient's response may stop at any stage, take any direction, or change directions. The outcome depends first on the manner in which he is told, and then on his own inclinations combined with staff management.

A doctor deciding whether to tell the patient, therefore, cannot consider a single impact, but how, in what direction, and with what consequences the patient's response is likely to go; as well as what types of staff are available and how they will handle the patient at each stage. A doctor who says "no" to disclosure because the patient will "lose hope" need not be in conflict with one who says "yes" to give the patient a chance to plan for his family. Each is merely referring to a different stage of the same process. For both, the concern should be with judging whether the patient can achieve the acceptance-active preparation stage.

*   *   *

b.

Death—At Whose Choosing?

[i]
Glanville Williams
The Sanctity of Life and the Criminal Law*

*   *   *

The object of the bill [sponsored by the English Euthanasia Society] was to legalize voluntary euthanasia. The patient desiring euthanasia must be over twenty-one years of age and suffering from an incurable and fatal disease accompanied by severe pain. The bill excluded any question of compulsory euthanasia, even for hopelessly defective infants. . . .

. . . The promoters of the bill hoped that they might be able to mollify the opposition by providing stringent safeguards. Now, they were right in thinking that if they had put in no safeguards—if they had merely said that a doctor could kill his patient whenever he thought it right —they would have been passionately opposed on this ground. So they put in the safeguards. Un-

der the proposals of the bill, the patient must sign a statutory form, in the presence of two witnesses, requesting euthanasia. The form, accompanied by two medical certificates, goes up to an official euthanasia referee appointed by the Minister of Health; he interviews the patient to make sure that he really wants it. Then euthanasia is administered in the presence of an official witness, who must be a justice of the peace, barrister, solicitor, doctor, minister of religion, or registered nurse.

Did the opposition like these elaborate safeguards? On the contrary, they made them a matter of complaint. The safeguards would, it was said, bring too much formality into the sickroom, and destroy the relationship between doctor and patient. So the safeguards were wrong, but no one of the opposition speakers said that he would have voted for the bill without the safeguards.

Much the most important of these opposition speeches were delivered by two of the acknowledged leaders of the medical profession, the late Lord Dawson of Penn and the late Lord Horder. . . .

Lord Dawson for the greater part of his speech seemed to be in sympathy with the views of the bill. He scouted the opposition notion that the only duty of the doctor is to save life. That, he said, was the nineteenth-century view, but medical opinion has changed; we now think that it is also the doctor's duty to relieve pain. Hence anaesthesia in childbirth and dentistry, and all the new drugs to assuage pain and bring sleep and forgetfulness to the troubled mind. Lord Dawson proceeded: "I would say that this is a courageous age, but it has a different sense of values from the ages which have gone before. It looks upon life more from the point of view of quality than of quantity. It places less value on life when its usefulness has come to an end." So "there has gradually crept into medical opinion, as it has crept into lay opinion, the feeling that one should make the act of dying more gentle and more peaceful even if it does involve curtailment of the length of life."

Then Lord Dawson went on: "If once you admit that you are going to curtail life by a single day, you are granting the principle that you must look at life from the point of view of its quality rather than from its quantity under these special circumstances. . . . I would give as my deliberate opinion that there is a quiet and cautious but irresistible move to look at life and suffering from the more humane attitude, and in face of a disease which is undoubtedly incurable, and

* New York: Alfred A. Knopf 333–340 (1957). Reprinted by permission.

when the patient is carrying a great load of suffering, our first thoughts should be the assuagement of pain even if it does involve the shortening of life." This means that the physician will, at the end, drug the patient even though he knows that this will shorten the patient's life. But what if death is still far off? Lord Dawson said: "When the gap between life burdened by incurable disease and death becomes wider, then greater difficulty presents itself, and greater variety in practice holds among individual doctors and patients. None the less there is in the aggregate an unexpressed growth of feeling that the shortening of the gap should not be denied when the real need is there. This is due, not to a diminution of courage, but rather to a truer conception of what life means and what the end of its usefulness deserves."

This remarkable speech seemed not merely to concede the case for euthanasia but to admit that it was actually practised, consciously or subconsciously, by the medical profession. Moreover, the concluding reference to "shortening the gap" seems to be a cautious admission of the principle that euthanasia is permissible, and is practised, not only where this is the only way of avoiding pain, but also where it is the only way of avoiding the prolongation of a life burdened by an incurable disease and robbed of all the quality that makes life worth while. This is a concession of the first importance to the cause of euthanasia.

Although he went thus far with the promoters of the measure, Lord Dawson opposed the bill on the ground that he preferred the present position under which everything was left to the discretion of the doctor. The Archbishop of Canterbury seized upon this idea with approval and relief; at the end of his speech he guardedly admitted that "cases arise in which some means of shortening life may be justified"; but he thought that Parliament should fold its hands because these cases were best left to the medical profession. Apparently the Primate thought that the consent of the patient would not be necessary, for one of his points was that a man racked with pain and full of drugs may be incapable of making a moral judgment. Thus these opponents of the bill, in allowing the doctor to end life without seeking the patient's consent, were in an important way prepared to go further than the proponents of the measure.

Lord Horder's argument was broadly similar to Lord Dawson's, though he did not elaborate it in the same way. He declared that it is outside a doctor's reference to put an end to life; but

"the good doctor is aware of the difference between prolonging life and prolonging the act of dying." The former comes within his terms of reference, the latter does not. On this it may be commented that there must obviously be room for a good deal of difference of opinion on what is meant by "not prolonging the act of dying." It is not, really, a very satisfactory formula, because it appears, misleadingly, to point to simple inactivity. A doctor who is engaged in giving large doses of a narcotic is not merely "not prolonging the act of dying"; he is doing something positive which may well have the effect of shortening the act of dying. There is, also, vagueness as to the temporal limits of the "act of dying". . . .

*   *   *

It may be suggested that the most hopeful line of advance would be to bring forward a measure that does no more than give legislative blessing to the practice that the great weight of medical opinion approves. In other words, the reformers might be well advised, in their next proposal, to abandon all their cumbrous safeguards and to do as their opponents wish, giving the medical practitioner a wide discretion and trusting to his good sense.

*   *   *

. . . The essence of the bill would . . . be simple. It would provide that no medical practitioner should be guilty of an offence in respect of an act done intentionally to accelerate the death of a patient who is seriously ill, unless it is proved that the act was not done in good faith with the consent of the patient and for the purpose of saving him from severe pain in an illness believed to be of an incurable and fatal character. . . .

*   *   *

NOTES

NOTE 1.

GLANVILLE WILLIAMS
EUTHANASIA*

Why is murder a crime? I know that some will give a religious answer, or a mystical answer. They will say that life is a gift of God, and only God can take it away; or they will say that murder is absolutely wrong and must be punished for that reason alone. But most of us now agree that purely religious or metaphysical views are

* 63 *Proceedings of the Royal Society of Medicine* 663–667 (1970). Reprinted by permission.

not a sufficient basis for the criminal law. We have to find mundane justifications, and in this instance they come readily to mind. The reasons underlying the law of murder are particular applications of the reasons underlying the whole of our secular morality: utilitarianism and empathy.

The utilitarian reason for the crime of murder is that if murder were allowed there would be a general sense of fear and insecurity, which would not only be evil in itself but would in its consequences work disaster for civilization. . . .

The second reason for forbidding murder is empathy, or sympathetic identification with the victim. . . .

* * *

Now, neither of these two secular reasons for the law of murder stands in the way of mercy killing. To accelerate the death of a patient at his request for merciful reasons does not increase the sum of human suffering, but diminishes it. Sympathy, so far from requiring us to refrain from killing, may in exceptional circumstances compel us to do so.

[T]he question of mercy killing or euthanasia is not specifically a medical question. It affects doctors, but it is a general moral problem, and it is intimately connected with the right of suicide.

* * *

. . . We now acknowledge, as a society, that the patient may commit suicide without offending against the law. Why, then, should not his parent, spouse or doctor be allowed to help him? And if the doctor is allowed to give the patient tablets to take, why cannot he inject the lethal dose into the patient if that course appears preferable?/Morally, there is no difference between assisting suicide and killing another person with his consent.

I have tried to show that this is a general question relating to the proper limits of the criminal law, not specifically a medical question. But legislation aimed to alter the present law as a practical matter naturally concentrates on the doctors, because it is they who have the knowledge and ability to perform mercy killing in a humane manner. . . .

* * *

[W]e are told that no legislation is necessary because doctors can in fact speed their patient's passage, quite morally and legitimately, by the double effect of morphine. The morphine is given in increasing doses to overcome habituation, and these doses may eventually build up to one that produces respiratory failure. The doctor pretends to himself that he is only relieving pain, but he well knows that the result is to speed the end. He may even deliberately accelerate the doses for this purpose, secure in the knowledge that no one can prove his real motive. That, at least, has been the position. But it was always a precarious solution, dependent upon the accidental fact that morphine, the medically preferred analgesic, carried this side-effect of depressing respiration. There was always the possibility that the doctor's opportunity for benevolent hypocrisy would be ended by the development of an effective analgesic which did not produce respiratory depression; and claims have been made that drugs like dextromoramide and dihydrocodeine already fit this bill. Whether or not it has already happened, the time will surely come when the doctor who administers pure morphine in steadily mounting doses will be seen by the present law for a murderer, because the drug will have ceased to be medically justified. . . .

* * *

What, then, is the legislative proposal? My own proposal would be a simple one: but I must emphasize that it applies only to patients who are suffering severe distress without prospect of relief. In these cases it should not be murder for a doctor, acting at the patient's request and with the concurrence of another doctor, to accelerate the patient's death in good faith and for his benefit. Apart from some small formalities relating to the request I would not put in any other restrictions, leaving those, if any are required, to medical practice. As a layman, I have every confidence that members of your profession will exercise the permission I would give you wisely and humanely. I think it very unlikely that the permission would be over-used: look at the fight you are putting up against being entrusted with an explicit permission at all! The permissive law would much more likely be under-used. If any feared dangers did materialize the law could easily be repealed because no vested interests would be created by it.

* * *

There is only one argument against voluntary euthanasia in these cases worthy of serious consideration, and that is the fear that a change in the law would put a distressing pressure on some old or dying people to accelerate their end out of consideration for their relatives and those who are looking after them. Although this is a serious argument, my own view is that it does not weigh against the other considerations. It is true that under my measure a patient may ask for euthanasia and through his insistence succeed in getting it because he does not want to continue to be a burden, perhaps for his young daughter who is looking after him. One hears sometimes of persons suffering from severe disability who commit suicide for this noble reason. Lord Soper in the Lords' debate on the recent Euthanasia Bill referred with admiration to the suicide of Captain Oates, whose object was to disembarass Scott of his presence; and a cripple who commits suicide in order to set free his young wife or daughter may be just as deserving of our esteem. I should like to think that I myself would have the courage to do this in such circumstances, though I would certainly not blame anyone for not sacrificing himself. I do not believe that this question of consideration for one's family can be settled by rule, one way or the other. It is an immensely difficult human problem, and is surely best left to be settled by the patient himself, as one of the factors influencing his decision, but subject to the advice and support of his doctors which one knows would be forthcoming.

NOTE 2.

ROYAL SOCIETY OF MEDICINE DISCUSSION ON EUTHANASIA*

Sir Geoffrey Organe thought Professor Glanville Williams had been confused over one point, that voluntary euthanasia was practised now. He was quite certain that formal debate did not take place between doctor and patient leading to a formal decision to execute the patient. What happened was that if the patient was suffering more than the doctor thought he should suffer, he was helped on his way. Whether this was a good thing or not he did not know.

. . . He thought that if euthanasia became more formal than it was now, and if affidavits had to be sworn before solicitors or magistrates with the consent of relatives, that there would be much more resistance on the part of doctors than there was at the moment.

*   *   *

Professor Glanville Williams: As to the distinction between voluntary and involuntary euthanasia, he knew that medical men did not want to tell their patients that they were dying. They did not want to ask for explicit consent. He was very happy to leave the doctor, if he was willing to take the responsibility, to dispatch the patient without asking him, doing what it was extremely likely that the patient would desire if he knew the truth of the situation, but he knew that this could not be put into legislation. He knew, therefore, that legislation could not do very much, but at least it could do something in the voluntary field and he saw no danger whatsoever that legislation for voluntary euthanasia would ever be extended to allow killing otherwise than to relieve suffering. . . .

[ii]
Vincent J. Collins
Limits of Medical Responsibility in Prolonging Life*

In the unconscious or hopelessly ill patient requiring resuscitation, there are three courses of action: (1) active treatment, i.e., prolonged dying vs reanimation; (2) active intervention to end life, i.e., euthanasia; (3) passive management, i.e., shortening the dying process. The first problem that requires serious examination is that of prolonging life, in reality a problem of therapy. Second, in contrast, is euthanasia. This is a problem of a deliberate decision to actively end life; it is not a dilemma. The prolonging of life is the lengthening of life. Euthanasia has as its objective the shortening of life, and this contrasts with passive management, in which the objective is to shorten the dying process.

A physician's approach toward the inevitable ending of life may be either passive or active. Death could occur by actively interceding or by passively discontinuing therapy. In the first instance, one directly causes life to end by an overt act, whereas, by discontinuing therapy, one permits death to occur by omitting an act and permitting nature to take its course.

Euthanasia.—When one actively intercedes, one is, in fact, causing harm to the individual, even though this harm may apparently have a good intent; here man is acting. This course of action is abhorrent and prohibited. Here also there is the dilemma of motives. Behind every good deed is a motive. Motives can be colored. When man is the direct instrument to a

* 63 *Proceedings of the Royal Society of Medicine* 669–670 (1970). Reprinted by permission.

* 206 *Journal of the American Medical Association* 389, 390–391 (1968). Reprinted by permission.

death, the law has historically related this to his intention. The motive may be malice or mercy, but regardless of the intent, whether malice or mercy, the end is murder.

We should now dispose of this question immediately: Shall we perform a deliberate act to positively end a life? That is euthanasia. From the legal standpoint, from the moral codes, and from the guidelines of ethical practice, we find applied the general law that no one is permitted to actively kill, regardless of the intent.

Aspects of Prolonging Life.—The more complicated question is that of *prolonging life*. Can our scientific decisions to prolong life or let a patient die be reconciled with our ethics and morality? Yes! But we must continue to distinguish clearly between letting a patient die and euthanasia.

Every physician is liable for his actions, but every action of a physician requires medical judgment. In saving a life, in preventing death, and then in prolonging the life, the question must repeatedly be asked as to whether the end result is inevitable or irrevocable. Is the end result death, or is the end result of the sustained immediate life mere organic existence?

When one permits death by not continuing therapy, the harm that is done is done by nature acting. This is passive management based on reason and judgment—and shortening the act of dying. It is rational. Therapy is discontinued when the efforts to maintain sound life are manifestly ineffective.

Thus, the problem is a challenge in therapy. It is possible for the physician to support life artificially, at least the traditional vital functions of respiration and circulation. He must know what to do, when to do it, and when to stop. In his therapeutic approach, he will use both simple or ordinary means and extraordinary means to support life.

Ordinary and Extraordinary Means.—A definition of ordinary and extraordinary means is required. Ordinary measures of patient care are recognized as elements of essential care. They represent obligatory, proven, and justified therapies and procedures. They are denoted by the fact that the patient himself can obtain them and put them to his own use. They further represent measures which he can reasonably undergo with only minimal or moderate danger and maximal effectiveness. Such measures are also not an impossible or excessive burden.

Extraordinary measures, on the other hand, are complicated methods. They are impossible for the patient to use or apply by himself and present a costly and difficult burden. In addition, they represent a high level of danger, and the results expected are not predictable, i.e., the effectiveness is minimal or moderate while the dangers are maximal.

Extraordinary measures sustain life artificially at the level it is found. If, at this point in time, there is no organic deterioration, the measures of resuscitation may then arrest the lethal process. The aim is to gain time in order for natural restorative processes to operate.

Effectiveness of Therapy.—On the basis of medical facts and good judgment, the physician does those things in any situation which will benefit his patient. He must do those things which predictably result in improvement of his patient. The techniques of reanimation are proven, sound, and legitimate. They can and do prolong life, *but* it must be determined that the nature of the resultant life is not mere biological existence of several organs but totally integrated functional existence at a rational human level. To continue an act or proceed with therapy which produces no improvement, which does not achieve or have the potential to achieve "full human life," and which is demonstrably ineffective in its objectives, *is* imprudent, illogical, and irrational. This *is* the essence of medical practice.

When a physician and his team bring together all the knowledge and skill related to sustaining life processes and treating patients with disease, they do so rationally. The effectiveness of therapeutic skill must be constantly assessed. In artificially maintaining life or in arresting a disease process, the physician buys time. By his assistance he provides time for the patient's natural recovery processes to act, to allow natural restoration of functional organization and return of the individual to a spontaneous, personal full life.

If after some time all measures are obviously not effective and are not reversing the dying process, then the measures are failing. Deterioration may be observed. To persist may produce the appearance of life, but this is most often technical or mechanical life. The final decision will then be made in the face of a late phase or a second endpoint, namely, that of biological life. It is the physician's obligation to cease efforts early when they are determined to be ineffective in the total reanimation process and objectives. The patient should then be allowed to die. He has this right; he should not be cheated of a peaceful death when the physician is powerless to restore consciousness. A vegetating patient, hopeless and irresponsive, and showing no spontaneous activity, should be allowed to die peacefully. Physicians should make the dying process dignified.

*   *   *

NOTES

NOTE 1.

SAMUEL B. WOODWARD
MEDICAL ETHICS*

*   *   *

. . . When your patient is dying from old age, or is in the last stages of cancer, or tubercular infection, unable to swallow food, shall you give nutritive enemata, withhold morphine or by any other means endeavor to postpone the inevitable? There may be reasons for desperate efforts in that direction to enable, for instance, a son, daughter, husband or wife to reach a beloved relative before the end, but in the absence of such or similar motives I hold it to be your duty to smooth as much as possible the pathway to the grave even if life be somewhat shortened. Nor is it necessary to talk it over with friends and relations, nor need you expect them to formally countenance either neglect or expedition. Let that be your affair settled with your own conscience. I have no sympathy with the man who would shorten the death agony of a dog but prolong that of a human being.

*   *   *

NOTE 2.

KURT R. EISSLER
THE PSYCHIATRIST AND THE DYING PATIENT†

*   *   *

Actually some of those physicians who uncompromisingly deny patients the beneficence of euthanasia are not superior to their contemporaries in their general ethics, and it is quite possible that this moral stringency is often a concealed manifestation of their sadism. I hasten to add that this is by no means meant as a rule and that in turn one definitely can find among physicians practicing euthanasia fantasies of omnipotence and a deep-seated ambivalence. Euthanasia is not always born out of charity but may mean to the

physician's unconscious the gratification of a murderous impulse.

*   *   *

NOTE 3.

R. J. V. PULVERTAFT
THE INDIVIDUAL AND THE GROUP
IN MODERN MEDICINE*

*   *   *

The patient meets his doctor with a very wide mandate. He is anxious, and seeks peace of mind; he is in pain, and seeks relief; with the prospect of death, he asks reprieve. But the mandate goes further, and always there is in his mind the unspoken request: "Some time I must die. As a layman, I cannot tell the choice, if choice there be, of my path; but I trust your greater knowledge to see me through in the kindest way."

It is in the management of malignant disease that, to my mind, surgeons and radiotherapists of today are at times wrongly orientated. There is too much emphasis on the remote chance of "cure," too little on the mitigation of the reasonably certain course of the disease. There is some modern surgery which merely ensures that the patient's remaining days will be spent in convalescence from the operation. And there remains always the distressing fact that a patient or his relatives, faced on the one hand by an honest and correct statement that recovery is impossible and on the other by a statement that it may be ensured in certain especially skilled and expensive hands, will sometimes choose a road that is sadly against his interest. The final degradation of medicine is to become the blackmail of the dying with the fear of death.

*   *   *

NOTE 4.

THE FIFTH DEATH OF LEV LANDAU†

Six years ago, an auto accident "took the life" of Dr. Lev Davidovitch Landau, one of the world's most brilliant theoretical physicists. But through the determined efforts of medical specialists called to Moscow from as far away as Montreal, the Soviet scientist not only came back from apparent clinical death on four separate occasions, but he learned again to function and to work.

* 202 *New England Journal of Medicine* 843, 846 (1930). Reprinted by permission.
† New York: International Universities Press 118 (1955). Reprinted by permission of the International Universities Press, Inc., New York.

* 2 *The Lancet* 839, 842 (1952). Reprinted by permission.
† *Medical World News* 37 (April 19, 1968). Copyright 1968, McGraw-Hill, Inc. Reprinted by permission.

708 LIMITATIONS IMPOSED ON INFORMED CONSENT

When his battered body was examined shortly after a truck demolished his car on an icy Moscow highway on January 7, 1962, Czech neurologist Sdenek Kunz grimly announced that "the traumas sustained are incompatible with life." The international team of physicians gathered at Dr. Landau's bedside could find no reason to disagree.

Dr. Landau had multiple injuries, any one of which could have been fatal. The base of his skull was fractured, the fornix cerebri was lacerated, and there were contusions of the frontal and temporal lobes. Doctors counted nine broken ribs and also diagnosed pneumothorax and a dextral hemothorax, rupture of the pubic symphysis; fractures of the os pubis, ischium, ilium, and left femoral neck; severe contusions of the abdominal cavity, and rupture of the urinary bladder. In addition, the patient had paralysis of the left arm, paresis of the right arm and both legs, and steadily increasing respiratory and circulatory distress.

The brilliant scientist was deaf, blind, and speechless, and he showed no reflexes. For two months, he remained unconscious and unresponsive. Despite the seeming hopelessness of the situation, the team of more than 100 physicians who had come to Moscow refused to give up.

Four days after the accident, the Soviet physicist appeared to succumb. His pulse disappeared, blood pressure fell to zero, and the EEG tracing flattened out. Clinically, Dr. Landau was dead. But the persistent physicians at his side refused to turn off the respirator. They opened his left radial artery and infused blood. They gave him intravenous injections of epinephrine, strophantin, and other analeptics. Gradually life came back. During the next week, death had to be repelled three more times. The prognosis was gloomy at best.

Five weeks later, Dr. Landau's fractures began to ossify, but he was still unconscious, and his extremities remained paralyzed. Then, while an international team of neurologists . . . were consulting on the next step, a close friend and collaborator of the patient . . . burst into the room. "He recognized me. He really did!"

Eleven months after the accident—while Dr. Landau was still tortuously relearning the normal functions of memory, speech, hearing, and muscle control—he was able to sit up in bed and smilingly accept his Nobel Prize from the Swedish ambassador. The prize honored his pioneering work in low-temperature physics.

Recalling the medical "miracle" performed in bringing the physicist back to life, Dr. Boris Yegorov, director of the Neurosurgery Institute of the Soviet Academy of Sciences, noted that "the patient's brain had been in a state of near-anabiosis for more than 100 days. It was held previously that oxygen deficiency of the brain cells leads to their destruction. The Landau case compels us to reconsider the whole of accumulated medical experience." But another Soviet expert, Dr. V. A. Negovsky, injected a note of controversy into the case when he asserted that Dr. Landau had never been in a state of clinical death.

Dr. Landau returned to the Moscow Institute for Experimental Physics and participated in weekly seminars, but he never fully recovered. He suffered violent gastric and limb pains and had difficulties with his memory that prevented him from continuing his research.

This month, six years after his "fatal" auto accident, the famed Soviet physicist finally succumbed. . . .

[iii]
Renée C. Fox
A Sociological Perspective on
*Organ Transplantation and Hemodialysis**

*   *   *

Chronic hemodialysis can present the physician with still other troubling, sometimes tragic aspects of his ethical obligation to have a patient's continuing consent for maintenance on the artificial kidney machine. It has been written that ". . . submission, with the reaper smiling grimly behind every movement, knowing that his turn will come, does not lead to a placid temperament and easy acceptance. To the contrary, the person who lives successfully with hemodialysis lives in a state of suppressed inner turmoil, from which there can never be an escape except in death. . . ." The psychological, social, and economic, as well as physical, stresses of being kept alive by intermittent hemodialysis may become too burdensome for a patient. Consciously or unconsciously, he may decide that he does not wish to go on living "on borrowed time," tied by cannulas to an at once "miraculous" and "monstrous" machine. Physicians have noted that under these conditions, certain patients begin to have what appear to be motivated cannula failures: for example, they cease to take care of their cannulas by keeping them clean, or too vigorously exercise the arm or the leg in which they are in-

* 169 *Annals of the New York Academy of Sciences* 416–417 (1970). Reprinted by permission.

serted. Other patients no longer abide by the strict dietary regulations that are requisite for this treatment to be effective, and may go on eating "binges." Occasional patients have explicitly asked the physician to remove them from the chronic dialysis program without offering them a kidney transplantation as an alternative method of definitive treatment. In all these cases, it can be said that the patient has withdrawn his full and free consent to undergo hemodialysis. The agonizing question for the physician is whether or not it is moral and humane to try to persuade such patients that it is worthwhile to continue on the artificial kidney machine, rather than succumb to their endstage renal disease. It overlaps with the more familiar issue of when, if ever, the physician is justified in no longer employing extraordinary means to keep a dying patient alive.

* * *

NOTES

NOTE 1.

W. St.C. Symmers, Sr.
Not Allowed to Die*

A doctor aged 68 was admitted to an overseas hospital after a barium meal had shown a large carcinoma of the stomach. He had retired from practice five years earlier, after severe myocardial infarction had left his exercise tolerance considerably reduced. The early symptoms of the carcinoma were mistakenly thought to be due to myocardial ischaemia. By the time when the possibility of carcinoma was first considered the disease was already far advanced; laparotomy showed extensive metastatic involvement of the abdominal lymph nodes and liver. Palliative gastrectomy was performed with the object of preventing perforation of the primary tumour into the peritoneal cavity, which appeared to the surgeon to be imminent. Histological examination showed the growth to be an anaplastic primary adenocarcinoma. There was clinical and radiological evidence of secondary deposits in the lower thoracic and lumbar vertebrae.

The patient was told of the findings and fully understood their import. In spite of increasingly large doses of pethidine, and of morphine at night, he suffered constantly with severe abdominal pain and pain resulting from compression of spinal nerves by tumour deposits.

On the tenth day after the gastrectomy the patient collapsed with classic manifestation of

---

* 1 *British Medical Journal* 442 (1968). Reprinted by permission.

massive pulmonary embolism. Pulmonary embolectomy was successfully performed in the ward by a registrar. When the patient had recovered sufficiently he expressed his appreciation of the good intentions and skill of his young colleague. At the same time he asked that if he had a further cardiovascular collapse no steps should be taken to prolong his life, for the pain of his cancer was now more than he would needlessly continue to endure. He himself wrote a note to this effect in his case records, and the staff of the hospital knew his feelings.

His wish notwithstanding, when the patient collapsed again, two weeks after the embolectomy—this time with acute myocardial infarction and cardiac arrest—he was revived by the hospital's emergency resuscitation team. His heart stopped on four further occasions during that night and each time was restarted artificially. The body then recovered sufficiently to linger for three more weeks, but in a decerebrate state, punctuated by episodes of projectile vomiting accompanied by generalized convulsions. Intravenous nourishment was carefully combined with blood transfusion and measures necessary to maintain electrolyte and fluid balance. In addition, antibacterial and antifungal antibiotics were given as prophylaxis against infection, particularly pneumonia complicating the tracheotomy that had been performed to ensure a clear airway. On the last day of the illness preparations were being made for the work of the failing respiratory centre to be given over to an artificial respirator, but the heart finally stopped before this endeavour could be realized.

This case report is submitted for publication without commentary or conclusions, which are left for those who may read it to provide for themselves.

NOTE 2.

Erickson v. Dilgard
44 Misc.2d 27, 252 N.Y.S.2d 705
(Sup. Ct. 1962)

Bernard S. Meyer, Justice.

This is an application by the Superintendent of the County Hospital for an order authorizing administration of a blood transfusion to Jacob Dilgard, Sr. Testimony adduced by the petitioner shows that Jacob Delgard, Sr., was voluntarily admitted to the hospital and that a diagnosis of upper gastro-intestinal bleeding was made. It was suggested to the patient that he submit to an operation, including blood transfusion to replace lost blood. The patient declined to submit to a blood transfusion, but did indicate a willingness to submit to the operation without a blood transfusion. His son who is a party respondent in this proceeding also refused to give permission for a transfusion, but was willing to authorize the operation without blood transfusion. Petitioner testified that an operation was necessary to tie off the bleeding site, that in order to offer the best chance of recovery a transfusion of blood was necessary, and that there was a very great chance that the patient would have little opportunity to recover without the blood. He further testified that the patient was completely competent and capable of making decisions on his own behalf, that he had explained to the patient the increased risk of having the operation without the transfusion, and that refusal of a transfusion represented the patient's calculated decision.

The County argues that it is in violation of the Penal Law to take one's own life and that as a practical matter the patient's decision not to accept blood is just about the taking of his own life. The Court cannot agree with that argument because it is always a question of judgment whether the medical decision is correct. Without in any sense impugning Dr. Erickson's opinion, the Court concludes that it is the individual who is the subject of a medical decision who has the final say and that this must necessarily be so in a system of government which gives the greatest possible protection to the individual in the furtherance of his own desires.

The court knows of no precedent relating to adult patients. There are cases in which it has been held that a court will step in as the guardian of an infant or an incompetent and make the decision for the infant or incompetent. In this case, however, there is no question that the patient has been completely competent at all times while being presented with the decision that he had to make and in the making of the decision that he did. That being so, the court declines to make any order directing that blood be administered. The application is denied.

NOTE 3.

JOHN F. KENNEDY HOSPITAL v. HESTON
58 N.J. 576, 279 A.2D 670 (1971)

WEINTRAUB, C. J.

Dolores Heston, age 22 and unmarried, was severely injured in an automobile accident. She was taken to the plaintiff hospital where it was determined that she would expire unless operated upon for a ruptured spleen and that if operated upon she would expire unless whole blood was administered. Miss Heston and her parents are Jehovah's Witnesses and a tenet of their faith forbids blood transfusions. . . .

Death being imminent, plaintiff on notice to the mother made application at 1:30 a.m. to a judge of the Superior Court for the appointment of a guardian for Miss Heston with directions to consent to transfusions as needed to save her life . . . The court appointed a guardian with authority to consent to blood transfusions "for the preservation of the life of Dolores Heston." Surgery was performed at 4:00 a.m. the same morning. Blood was administered. Miss Heston survived.

* * *

The controversy is moot. Miss Heston is well and no longer in plaintiff's hospital. The prospect of her return at some future day in like circumstances is too remote to warrant a declaratory judgment as between the parties. Nonetheless, the public interest warrants a resolution of the cause, and for that reason we accept the issue.

* * *

It seems correct to say there is no constitutional right to choose to die. Attempted suicide was a crime at common law and was held to be a crime under N.J.S.A. 2A:85–1. It is now denounced as a disorderly persons offense. N.J.S.A. 2A:170–25.6. Ordinarily nothing would be gained by a prosecution, and hence the offense is rarely charged. Nonetheless the Constitution does not deny the state an interest in the subject. It is commonplace for the police and other citizens, often at great risk to themselves, to use force or stratagem to defeat efforts at suicide, and it could hardly be said that thus to save someone from himself violated a right of his under the Constitution subjecting the rescuer to civil or penal consequences.

Nor is constitutional right established by adding that one's religious faith ordains his death. Religious beliefs are absolute, but conduct in pursuance of religious beliefs is not wholly immune from governmental restraint. . . .

Complicating the subject of suicide is the difficulty of knowing whether a decision to die is firmly held. Psychiatrists may find that beneath it all a person bent on self-destruction is hoping to be rescued, and most who are rescued do not repeat the attempt, at least not at once. Then, too, there is the question whether in any event the person was and continues to be competent (a difficult concept in this area) to choose to die. And of course there is no opportunity for a trial of these questions in advance of intervention by the State or a citizen.

Appellant suggests there is a difference between passively submitting to death and actively seeking it. The distinction may be merely verbal, as it would be if an adult sought death by starvation instead of a drug. If the State may interrupt one mode of self-destruction, it may with equal authority interfere with the other. It is arguably different when an individual, overtaken by illness, decides to let it run a fatal course. But unless the medical option itself is laden with the risk of death or of serious infirmity, the State's interest in sustaining life in such circumstances is hardly distinguishable from its interest in the case of suicide.

* * *

Hospitals exist to aid the sick and the injured. The medical and nursing professions are consecrated to preserving life. That is their professional creed. To them, a failure to use a simple, established procedure in the circumstances of this case would be malpractice, however the law may characterize that failure because of the patient's private convictions. A surgeon should not be asked to operate under the strain of knowing that a transfusion may not be administered even though medically required to save his patient. The hospital and its staff should not be required to decide whether the patient is or continues to be competent to make a judgment upon the subject, or whether the release tendered by the patient or a member of his family will protect them from civil responsibility. The hospital could hardly avoid the problem by compelling the removal of a dying patient, and Miss Heston's family made no effort to take her elsewhere.

When the hospital and staff are thus involuntary hosts and their interests are pitted against the belief of the patient, we think it reasonable to resolve the problem by permitting the hospital and its staff to pursue their functions according to their professional standards. The solution sides with life, the conservation of which is, we think, a matter of State interest. A prior application to a court is appropriate if time permits it, although in the nature of the emergency the only question that can be explored satisfactorily is whether death will probably ensue if medical procedures are not followed. If a court finds, as

the trial court did, that death will likely follow unless a transfusion is administered, the hospital and the physician should be permitted to follow that medical procedure.

* * *

[Affirmed.]

[iv]
Petition of Nemser
51 Misc.2d 616, 273 N.Y.S.2d 624
(Sup. Ct. 1966)

JACOB MARKOWITZ, JUSTICE.

On September 9, 1966, a preliminary hearing was held by this court on petitioners' application to be appointed the temporary legal representatives of their mother, for the specific and limited purpose of executing a consent in her behalf to a transmalleolar amputation of her right ankle and foot.

As a result of such preliminary hearing, the court appointed a guardian ad litem for the respondent, Sadie Nemser, and subsequently requested an eminent psychiatrist to examine her for the purpose of obtaining competent medical opinion as to her capacity to execute a consent in the form required by the hospital and the attending physicians. In addition, petitioners were directed to join both the hospital and the physician (or physicians) in charge of the care of Mrs. Nemser as parties-respondents, so that all proper parties to this proceeding would be before the court on the continued and subsequent hearings.

[P]etitioners are two of three sons of respondent, Sadie Nemser. A third son, a practicing physician in the City of New York, has refused to consent to the surgical procedure recommended by his mother's attending physicians but, while duly served with the moving papers, he did not appear in court on the return day of the motion, either personally or by counsel, to state his reason for such refusal. At the continued hearing on September 13, 1966, however, he did appear before the court, pro se, and, together with each of his brothers, was afforded an opportunity to set forth fully his position with regard to the instant application.

It appears from the papers before the court that Mrs. Nemser, a widow, eighty years of age, had been a resident of the Jewish Home and Hospital for the Aged in this city from May 1964 to August 22, 1966. She has a history of arteriosclerotic heart disease, has suffered at least three strokes and an equal number of attacks of pneumonia. On August 22, in a medical emergency, she was moved and admitted to Beth Israel Hospital, where she has since then continuously remained. Her physical condition, in substance, was diagnosed as "diabetic and arteriosclerotic gangrene . . . with infection; . . . extensive gangrene of the right foot and heel with inflammatory reaction about both areas. . . ." While recommending an above-knee amputation, in view of their patient's general condition, the attending physicians of Beth Israel Hospital suggested Mrs. Nemser undergo a transmalleolar amputation (above the ankle). It appears, however, that if the present local infection extends any higher in the front to the leg, it will militate against the transmalleolar procedure. Moreover, Dr. George Lowen, under whose care Mrs. Nemser was admitted to the hospital, has expressed the opinion that "If delay ensues, further physical deterioration will surely occur. . . . If the deterioration is allowed to progress, death will follow." In a supplemental affidavit, dated September 12, 1966, Dr. Lowen still maintains that "The recommended operation is distinctly a matter of the difference between life and death for Mrs. Nemser." However, as more fully discussed hereinafter, Dr. Lowen's prognosis as to the urgency and immediate necessity of the recommended surgical procedure is not supported by any of the other competent medical evidence and opinion before the court.

In view of the fact that an attending psychiatrist of the staff of Beth Israel Hospital, after an examination of Mrs. Nemser, reported that she "is not capable of understanding the nature of any permit for surgery that she might be asked to sign," neither the hospital nor the surgeon will proceed with the recommended operation unless consent thereto is obtained from their patient's next of kin. Upon the physician-son's refusal to consent, as above noted, these legal proceedings were then instituted by petitioners.

It is noteworthy . . . that Beth Israel Hospital's staff psychiatrist does not categorically state that Mrs. Nemser is mentally incompetent for all purposes. Rather, as noted, he limits his opinion to the belief that she is not competent to consent to the operation which is advised by her attending surgeon.

Both Richard G. Green, Esq., the guardian ad litem, and Dr. Abraham N. Franzblau, the court-designated psychiatrist, after painstaking investigation and thorough examination, have submitted detailed reports to the court. Both conclude that Mrs. Nemser is not capable of making for herself an informed judgment of whether the subject operation should be performed. Both, however, recommend that under the circumstances recited in their respective reports, intervention by the court is not warranted.

Dr. Franzblau, after setting forth the facts concerning Mrs. Nemser's advanced age, her medical history and present physical condition, indicates that he has spoken with Drs. Friedman and Schwartz, Mrs. Nemser's two medical consultants, with the patient herself, her two sons (one of the petitioners and respondent Dr. Harold S. Nemser) and with the court-appointed Guardian. Dr. Franzblau's report succinctly states:

1. Some difference of opinion exists as to:
a) whether the proposed operation is essential to prolong or save Mrs. Nemser's life;
b) the prognosis if it is done or, on the other hand, not done; and
c) whether the patient's mental status is such that she can understand the proposed procedure, and the significance of any consent that she might give.

2. Both of Mrs. Nemser's sons whom I interviewed appear to be motivated by love for their mother and a wish to see her life prolonged, free of pain and discomfort. Norman, the lawyer is influenced by the opinions of the medical consultants who he has brought in that a transmalleolar amputation would arrest the spread of the infection and gangrene, and prolong his mother's life. Harold, the physician, is doubtful of his mother's ability to tolerate anesthesia and surgery, and hopes that, treated conservatively and kept "clean," the gangrenous parts would slough off through auto-amputation. The disagreement between the brothers appears to be further clouded by long-standing familial differences over the support and management of their mother, and over the question of the adequacy of her medical care up to the present episode.

3. There appears to be no disagreement among Drs. Friedman and Schwartz, that:
a) The recommended procedure as proposed is not a life-saving measure, nor is it a medical emergency
b) Its effectiveness is by no means assured
c) The same condition may recur in the stump, after surgery, since such wounds heal notoriously poorly in diabetics
d) there is no likelihood of ever applying a prosthesis or achieving ambulation in this patient
e) there is very little possibility of proceeding ultimately to do the mid-thigh amputation, which is considered as a second and ultimately beneficial stage, in such cases
4. The patient is clearly unable to understand the situation or to render informed consent. (I agree

completely with the opinion of Dr. Weiss as to her mental status.) However, she is aware of her bodily integrity and wants no amputation of any part of her. She wants both to live and to retain her limb, and is not clearly aware of the conflict implicit in these alternatives. Pressed to make a decision, she would be willing to leave it to the doctors, but she would not do so with clear mind or perception. Her consciousness of pain is mercifully diminished by the partial oblivion which has intervened in her condition.

Accordingly, I do not believe that intervention on the part of the Court is indicated.

In substance, the perceptive and detailed report of Mr. Green is the same and, as above noted, terminates in a similar conclusion.

Thus, it becomes apparent that this proceeding, where responsible members of a family, including a physician-son, unfortunately cannot agree on what is medically necessary or proper for their aged and infirm mother, presents an example of a grave dilemma which confronts those who engage in the healing arts and, on the other hand, some basic and fundamental issues on the nature and scope of judicial power and the wisdom or propriety of judicial intervention.

There can be no doubt at all that the Court, Mrs. Nemser's children, and the doctors are most desirous of prolonging the life of Mrs. Nemser without undue pain and suffering. The sympathetic feelings of the Court, however, are, by themselves, hardly enough to clothe it with the right to authorize the surgical procedure or to entertain favorably the within application, particularly in light of the recommendations of the guardian ad litem, the report, and conclusion of the Court-designated psychiatrist and his noted medical opinions of Drs. Friedman and Schwartz. The Court cannot overlook the fact that petitioners rely solely on the opinion and prognosis of *one* physician, whose "life and death" position is neither supported nor corroborated by any of the other medical evidence in the record. Moreover, regardless of their personal differences, I am certain petitioners will agree that their physician-brother-respondent Dr. Harold S. Nemser has the best interests of their mother at heart. It is, therefore, most significant to note that Dr. Nemser categorically stated in open court he believed "assaultive surgery in a terminal case in the name of emergency is cruelty beyond description." He pointed out that while his mother is "foggy" at times, she is, nevertheless, aware of her body and does not want her foot amputated. Dr. Nemser stressed the fact that the recommended operation is not curative, nor is it a mat-

ter of life or death, as suggested by Dr. Lowen alone. Significantly, Drs. Friedman and Schwartz concur in the opinion that the suggested operation, because of Mrs. Nemser's diabetic condition, will not heal. On the contrary, it appears that such surgical procedure may open new areas of infection.

Dr. Nemser also pointed out to the Court that his mother's condition, without the operation, had vastly improved; so much so, that since September 8, 1966 (for at least the immediate five days prior to the continued hearing) she had not required any antibiotics nor was there present any new infection. He feared that his mother's heart condition, her past history of congestive lung failure (not caused by the gangrene) and the traumatic effect of the contemplated operation, if she survived it, would hasten her demise rather than prolong her life.

*   *   *

[I]t is apparent that this proceeding was necessitated only because of the current practice of members of the medical profession and their associated hospitals of shifting the burden of their responsibilities to the courts, to determine, in effect, whether doctors should proceed with certain medical procedures definitively found necessary or deemed advisable for the health, welfare, and perhaps even the life of a patient who is either unwilling or unable to consent thereto. Thus, petitioners upon the hearing, indicated their concern that if the pending application were to be denied at this time, their mother's attending physicians and the respondent hospital, in the absence of written consent by the next of kin or prior judicial approval, would still refuse necessary surgical treatment if a sudden reversal of her present improved condition mandated it as a real "life or death" solution.

It seems incongruous in light of the physicians' oath that they even seek legal immunity prior to action necessary to sustain life. As the Court has had previous occasion to note, how legalistic minded our society has become, and what an ultra-legalistic maze we have created to the extent that society and the individual have become enmeshed and paralyzed by its unrealistic entanglements! Certainly, if medical procedures are of an emergency nature or are required suddenly to save the life of a human being, neither a physician nor a hospital should be deterred from the exercise of sound medical judgment with respect to necessary treatment merely by threat of possible legal action. Emergency requirements, if, in fact, they are such, should not be delayed nor the responsibility therefor shirked while fearful physicians and hospitals first seek judicial sanction for a determination which, at the end, must, in any event, be a medical decision rather than a legal one.

The history and triumphs of medicine are replete with the names of "medical giants" whose experimentations, medical procedures, techniques, miracle drugs and other discoveries became a boon to humanity. Men and women such as Semmelweis, Jenner, Curie, Sanger, Salk, Walter Reed, Lister, Pasteur and Wasserman would not be deterred by the mere fear of possible legal consequences of their acts. Many of them risked martyrdom to perpetuate the principles and ideals of the Hippocratic oath. . . .

* * *

Here, we have the consent of two of the three responsible members of the immediate family of the hospitalized patient, yet, without judicial approbation the doctors and hospital refuse to go forward with recommended surgical treatment; this, despite the fact that at least one of the attending physicians (Dr. Lowen) believes that if his patient's condition deteriorates, death will ultimately result. Should this or similar emergency conditions actually arise, are the courts prepared to continue to condone the medical practice of requiring written consent or judicial approval first, or is it time that hospitals and physicians are compelled to shoulder this responsibility of making a medical decision? If there were five, ten or more children or members of a patient's family, will the hospital and physician wait to perform a needed operation which they are morally obligated to perform until and unless *all* consent thereto? Is the court to be made the arbiter in all family disputes as to the wisdom or necessity of medical treatment, or is that, in reality, a medical problem to be resolved by the physician, his patient, where possible, and the family, if necessary?

* * *

It is regrettable that the court here is placed in the position of refusing, or what to many may seem the refusal, to act in order to save a life or to ameliorate suffering. The contrary is the fact. It is because of the court's deep concern for Mrs. Nemser's life and well-being that it is reminding those whose responsibility it actually is, to act appropriately, not arbitrarily, and without fear. The court, likewise, is not unmindful that whatever course is followed by those persons who

are ultimately responsible here, it may prove fatal. Similarly, the court is aware that on occasions where other agencies of government or society fail to act, it must intervene for the common good. . . .

* * *

. . . I am constrained to hold that the application to be appointed her temporary legal representatives for the specific and limited purpose of executing a consent to a transmalleolar amputation is denied and the petition is dismissed.

NOTES

NOTE 1.

E. E. MENEFEE
THE RIGHT TO LIVE AND THE RIGHT TO DIE*

* * *

The decision as to when it is best to push ahead with all resources or best to withhold or even draw back slightly is one that should not and cannot be made by the physician alone. The immediate and responsible family members must make the decision, but with the guidance, advice and help of the physician. . . .

Let me give you an illustration. I have a brilliant professional man as a patient. He has bronchogenic carcinoma with metastases to the skeletal system. It was severe pain that first took him to his personal physician. Full doses of radiation therapy have given only enough relief to make life bearable provided he lies perfectly still. The slightest motion precipitates paroxysms of excruciating pain. Neuro-surgical procedures have failed to give relief. Chemotherapy has made him symptomatically worse. For eight long weeks we have struggled along. I believe that, with intravenous feedings, oxygen therapy, constant nursing care, antibiotics, attention to correction of electrolytes, et cetera, we may be able to extend his span for two or three months. Should we? I have never thought of doing or giving anything that would shorten his life, but as a physician I wonder how determined I should be in extending a hopeless situation. If the patient had his full faculties, would he choose two months of pain? Would he prefer his financial resources to be spent on two more months of hospital and medical care, or would he think it better to use them to complete the college education of his children? Twice, when he has begun to develop pneumonia, we have checked his rapid

* 95 *Medical Times* 1171, 1178–1179 (1967). Reprinted by permission.

downhill course with antibiotics. If the same situation arises the third time, should I again start intensive drug therapy, and use oxygen and fluids and transfusions, or should I let him slip rapidly away? . . . If I were the patient, I think I should prefer comfort and solace to science. Nevertheless, key members of the family feel we should continue to put forth our maximum effort. We shall do so unless they change their minds. I feel it my duty to let them have the full facts, to let them see the situation as it is, but it is not my duty to try to persuade them. They have confidence in me and I am sure they will feel free to come to me and say, "This is enough," if they reach that decision.

In another instance, we were faced some years ago with a very personal problem when a loved member of our family developed a hopeless and painful disease. After she recovered enough from her second operation—pinning a pathological fracture—we decided to bring her home. We did not give fluid by hypodermoclysis nor did we insist she eat when it was agony to do so. We did not gavage her, nor did we give oxygen or blood or antibiotics. We did give love and support and care, and enough drugs so that she could get some rest and be relatively free from pain. She died in peace and in dignity, with only her family in attendance. I have never regretted that decision.

There is another aspect of prolonged hospital care and terminal illness which must be considered. This, in brief, is the question of whether, with the shortage of hospital rooms and personnel which exists now and perhaps for the foreseeable future, we as physicians have a right to tie up space that might otherwise be utilized for actually saving lives. The Federal Government has recognized this problem in its Medicare laws by requiring careful review of patients' records to make certain not only that they are receiving the best medical care but that hospitalization is necessary. As a member of the Utilization Review Committee in my hospital, I am aware of certain patients who have been maintained actually for years. This is certainly a tribute to medical science, hospital facilities, and devoted nursing care. On the other hand, the utilization of hospital space and personnel in this manner has meant that at least 200 other patients have been denied admission. There are not enough beds to admit everyone. Is it correct and is it proper that we should prolong life by using the hospital facilities and at the same time refuse other patients a chance which might mean not only the difference between life and death but

perhaps, as well, a complete recovery and return to a useful place in society?

NOTE 2.

Frank J. Ayd, Jr.
Voluntary Euthanasia—The Right to be Killed*

* * *

All ill people are obligated to use ordinary means to preserve life, but they are not bound to seek extraordinary treatment except in unusual circumstances. As one moralist puts it: "At times one may be bound in charity to one's dependents or to one's fellow citizens to employ extraordinary means to preserve one's life. In order that such an obligation be present, two conditions must be fulfilled: (1) One is necessary to one's family or fellowmen. (2) The success of the extraordinary means is very probable."

An ill person is not obligated to do what is physically or morally impossible. Hence, he can validly refuse treatment which would entail great suffering, which would overtax the will power and courage of the normal person, or which would financially impoverish his survivors, especially if the anticipated benefits would be of limited value and brief duration. Likewise, a physician, with the patient's consent, may licitly desist from administering treatments that are demonstrably ineffective and be satisfied with alleviating the patient's suffering. No one is required to do what is practically useless. A doctor is not under compulsion to make every effort to prolong every patient's life. Hence, what physicians call negative euthanasia in certain circumstances is not only morally permissible but can be obligatory. In fact, this is not euthanasia and should not be called even negative euthanasia.

* * *

There should be no need for positive euthanasia and there would be no demand for it if doctors acknowledge that it is neither scientific nor humane to use artificial life-sustainers when death is imminent and inevitable and realistic hope of recovery has evaporated. Also there should be no need or demand for positive euthanasia if physicians unhesitatingly administer whatever amount of pain-relieving drugs a dying patient needs. The medical profession already has the power to make any demand for legalized euthanasia seem pointless, or even mischievous.

* *Medical Counterpoint* 12, 20–22 (June 1970). Reprinted by permission.

All doctors have to do is apply their skills prudently, as they are morally and legally empowered to do. . . .

No one has the right to be killed and physicians should oppose strenuously any proposal to legalize euthanasia. There are many reasons for this. It would be very dangerous indeed to empower doctors to kill, on demand, the patients they cannot cure. For the conscientious doctor it would be a most difficult and strainful task to decide at what stage of an illness a patient would qualify for euthanasia. It also would be extremely difficult for such a doctor to be sure that the patient knew what he was doing when he requested euthanasia. (For the unscrupulous doctor, and there are such, there would have to be very rigorous safeguards against loopholes for murder.) And even with the conscientious doctor there would be patients at risk, for none of us are 100 per cent psychologically and morally sound and perversions could creep into the practice of legalized euthanasia. It is better for the community to tie the hands of a good doctor by refusing to legalize voluntary euthanasia, in order to restrain an unscrupulous one from violating the rights of the individual.

*   *   *

If voluntary euthanasia were legal, there would be a standing risk of a person consenting to his extinction on an erroneous calculation of his prospects. If it were to become an acknowledged function of the medical profession to end life prematurely, could patients place themselves with complete trust in the care of physicians? A patient's trust in his doctor is important both for his peace of mind and for his recovery.

*   *   *

NOTE 3.

JOSEPH FLETCHER
VOLUNTARY EUTHANASIA—
THE NEW SHAPE OF DEATH*

*   *   *

[T]here are four distinguishable and different forms of death as chosen rather than coming willy-nilly or perforce. This typology is based on the formal categories of ethics and moral theology.

First, there is euthanasia as a *direct voluntary;* that is, the patient chooses to end it all,

_____
* *Medical Counterpoint* 13, 17–23 (June 1970). Reprinted by permission.

whether it is done with or without medical help. . . .

Second, there is euthanasia as an *indirect voluntary;* that is, the patient gives others the discretion to end it all as the situation requires—especially if the patient is too comatose to decide. . . .

Third, there is euthanasia as an *indirect involuntary;* that is, the incompetent patient's wishes are not known and others have to choose for him. This is, of course, the most common case. It happens in thousands of hospitals every day. . . .

*   *   *

Fourth, there is euthanasia as a *direct involuntary;* that is, the simple "mercy killing" of another, with or without his present or past request—as when an idiot is given a fatal dose or a man trapped inextricably in a blazing fire is shot to end his suffering.

*   *   *

For a while in the past it seemed worthwhile to use the term "euthanasia" for only the direct form, and to call the indirect form ("letting the patient go") by the cumbersome neologism "anti-dysthanasia." But subsequent thought and experience has shown this to be a mistake. The problem of a good death is at stake in every and all forms. Nothing is won by playing the word game, and those who are locked in and committed to opposing euthanasia are not really being helped by linguistic escape hatches. . . . They might well quote Pascal's observation: "Since men have not succeeded in eliminating death, they have decided not to think of it."

In our investigation of the problem of elective death we should give very serious consideration to the distinction between merely biological life and truly human life. If it is a valid and important distinction, as this writer thinks, then it may provide some cross-illumination of our problems at both ends of the life spectrum. "When is life gone?" if seriously asked, becomes the question "When is *human* life gone?" whether biological life continues or not. . . .

*   *   *

In absolutistic and divine-natural law ethics some things, like euthanasia, are never open to responsible decision and choice (i.e., they are removed from the forum of conscience and morality); but in situation ethics all things (including birth and death) are subject to responsible decision. What is not open to choice is unmoral or non-moral, outside the range of ethical problems. . . .

Years ago at a meeting of the American Cancer Society the essence of medical objections to euthanasia in *any* of its forms was expressed by Dr. David Karnoffsky, whose work at the Sloan-Kettering Institute was a great step forward in research. He said that physicians are duty bound to do anything and everything they can to keep life as long as is technically possible. Like so many earnest and able people in medicine, Karnoffsky was saying in effect that *biological* life, not human life, is the first-order value, the highest good or *summum bonum* to which, if necessary, all other values should be subordinated. This is what philosophers call ethical vitalism, and it is opposed by all those who prize *human* life—such as dignity and self-possession and rationality—more than the sheer or mere facts of respiration, digestion or (alas) incontinent excretion! Humanism or personalism, rather than vitalism, is by far a better faith-foundation for medicine. As I have put it in another essay, "Doctors who will not respirate monsters at birth—the start of life—will not much longer have any part in turning people into monsters at the end of life."

I used to think that the physicians' Hippocratic Oath contradicted itself because it promised both to preserve life and to relieve suffering, while in some situations one or the other must be chosen. Further examination of the best texts of the Oath, however, have made it clear that it contains no such logical error. The Oath says nothing at all about preserving life. It says that "so far as power and discernment shall be mine, I will carry out regimen for the benefit of the sick and will keep them from harm and wrong." Whether we find any reason ever for euthanasia depends upon how we understand "benefit of the sick" and "harm" and "wrong." Dehumanized biological life is sometimes real harm and the opposite of benefit, and to refuse to welcome or even introduce death would be quite wrong.

The day will come when people will be able to carry a card, notarized and legally executed, which explains that they do not want to be kept alive beyond the *humanum* point, and authorizing the ending of their lives in *extremis* by any of the distinguishable methods which seems appropriate. . . .

In the same vein Dr. Charles Hofling of the Medical School at Washington University (St. Louis) says, "Hospitals of the future will have 'death boards' . . . to discontinue the artificial measures by which life is being maintained" to act upon a patient's request or a next-of-kin's or a physician's. Such proposals at least have the merit of rising above a lot of the present-day dishonesty and sub-rosa euthanasia, even though many physicians prefer to keep the under-the-rose policy because it gives them sole control. . . .

NOTE 4.

ARVAL A. MORRIS
VOLUNTARY EUTHANASIA*

* * *

. . . Voluntary euthanasia can be justified by reference to three basic values of western civilization: (1) prevention of cruelty; (2) allowance of liberty; and (3) the enhancement of human dignity, an ultimate goal which is achieved by adhering to the first two values.

All civilized men will agree that cruelty is an evil to be avoided. But few people acknowledge the cruelty of our present laws which require a man be kept alive against his will, while denying his pleas for merciful release after all the dignity, beauty, promise and meaning of life have vanished, and he can only linger for weeks or months in the last stages of agony, weakness and decay. In addition, the fact that many people, as they die, are fully conscious of their tragic state of deterioration greatly magnifies the cruelty inherent in forcing them to endure this loss of dignity against their will. . . .

Beyond such direct cruelties, our current law also indirectly results in other cruelties as well, and these must all be weighed in the balance. For example, it seems exceedingly cruel to compel the spouse and children of a dying man to witness the ever-worsening stages of his disease, and to watch the slow, agonizing death of their loved one, degenerating before their eyes, being transformed from a vital and robust parent and spouse into a pathetic and humiliated creature, devoid of human dignity. The psychological trauma that comes from witnessing such a spectacle may deeply affect, or permanently impair, the mental and physical health of both children and spouse. Finally, we cannot ignore the residual, indirect cruelty which survives the death of the afflicted person, and burdens the surviving family with the costs incurred in the treatment of the prolonged illness. Enormous medical debts can impair or destroy a child's educational opportunities, for example, and recogni-

---

* 45 *Washington Law Review* 239, 251–255 (1970). Reprinted by permission.

tion of such gloomy prospects will undoubtedly prey heavily on the mind of the terminally ill parent or relative, adding to the pain and suffering which he already endures.

*   *   *

The second social value which supports the case for voluntary euthanasia, and promotes the cause of human dignity, is that of liberty. In this context, our law has got the shoe on the wrong foot from the very beginning. Why does our law provide that when a person participates in voluntary euthanasia it constitutes the crime of murder? To have fidelity to liberty, the question should be reversed. We should start from the assumption that all voluntary acts are permissible, and, in the absence of some legitimate reason to deny it, we would presume that a doctor and a patient are free to act as they wish. The question should not be: "Why should people have a legal right to voluntary euthanasia?" but rather, the appropriate question should be: "Why should our criminal law restrain the liberty of the doctor and the patient, denying them from doing what they want?" In a free society it is the restraint on liberty that must be justified, not the possession of liberty. The criminal law should not be called upon to repress an individual's conduct unless such repression is demonstrably necessary on social grounds. Further, in the case of voluntary euthanasia, this demonstrably compelling interest must be secular, not religious. Yet it is entirely unclear what secular social interest is so compelling that it justifies preventing the incurably ill sufferer from exercising his liberty of choice to accelerate death by a few hours, days, or even months; or what interest justifies the application of criminal deterrents to a voluntary euthanasia case.

. . . Why should the law deny a man the ultimate decision about what to do with his life? In the final analysis, control over one's own death is a matter of human dignity, and it should not be denied without some very compelling reasons.

*   *   *

B.
In Society's Interests?

1.

Overruling Consent to Prevent "Harm"

a.

Alexander M. Kidd
Limits of the Right of a Person to
Consent to Experimentation on Himself*

*   *   *

[Consider] the question of experimentation on persons—with their consent—not for any disease and not for any direct benefit to the patient, but solely for the advancement of science. How far can one consent to serious injury to himself? The analogies are not close. Abortion, except for therapeutic reasons, is a crime, and the consent of the woman is no defense for the doctor. A person cannot legally consent to his own death; it is murder by the person who kills him. Societies in England and the United States are trying to legalize euthanasia for those suffering from incurable disease, and juries have sometimes acquitted a parent who has put a suffering child out of his misery. If it had been his dog instead of his child, he would have been punished for not killing it. In the case of the birth of monstrosities the doctor may perform the killing and no one be any the wiser, but legally it is murder. A person may not consent to a serious injury amounting to a maim. The classical case was the man who cut off his hand to make himself a more successful beggar. Injuries inflicted to avoid military service are not unknown, and are criminal.

Sterilization presents a more difficult problem. The late Lord Riddell seemed to condemn it without exception but, in the same volume, approved it for the feeble-minded. Statutes concerning the feeble-minded have been sustained. In this country what little authority there is seems to permit sterilization where death, insanity, or serious disability would result from pregnancy. Economic considerations based on the number of children are a doubtful basis, and it probably would not be sanctioned simply to avoid the possibility of having children.

These situations all involve serious injury inflicted by consent for the direct advantage of the one permitting it. The motive of the advancement of science presents a different case.

---

* 117 *Science* 211, 212 (1953). Reprinted by permission.

. . . No prosecution seems to have followed where antivaccinationists have been encouraged to receive smallpox germs, or religious fanatics to submit to snake bites. Although there are no cases, it could not be considered a crime of the experimenter where the highest public praise is accorded to those incurable who offer themselves for experimental purposes in order that persons may not have to suffer in the future as they have. The airmen who have died in pressure experiments to make air travel possible for others, the Walter Reeds who have risked disease germs to determine causation where animal experimentation has failed, and other martyrs to science who have missed success except in a negative way so that that particular experiment need not be repeated, are heroes.

* * *

NOTES

NOTE 1.

MATTHEW V. OLLERTON
90 ENG. REP. 438, COMBERBACK 218 (1693)

. . . If I licence a man to beat me, such licence is void.

CURIA. The defendant may refer to the plaintiff himself, if he will; but licence to beat me is void, because 'tis against the peace. . . .

NOTE 2.

BRAVERY V. BRAVERY
[1954] 3 ALL E. R. 59

* * *

DENNING, L. J.:

* * *

. . . An ordinary surgical operation, which is done for the sake of a man's health, with his consent, is, of course, perfectly lawful because there is just cause for it. If, however, there is no just cause or excuse for an operation, it is unlawful even though the man consents to it. . . .

. . . Take a case where a sterilisation operation is done so as to enable a man to have the pleasure of sexual intercourse without shouldering the responsibilities attaching to it. The operation then is plainly injurious to the public interest. It is degrading to the man himself. It is injurious to his wife and to any woman whom he may marry, to say nothing of the way it opens to licentiousness; and, unlike contraceptives, it allows no room for a change of mind on either side. It is illegal, even though the man consents to it, for it comes within the principle stated by

STEPHEN, J. (who was a great authority on criminal law), in R. v. *Coney* (2) (8 Q.B.D. 549):

The principle as to consent seems to me to be this: When one person is indicated for inflicting personal injury upon another, the consent of the person who sustains the injury is no defence to the person who inflicts the injury, if the injury is of such a nature, or is inflicted under such circumstances, that its infliction is injurious to the public as well as to the person injured.

* * *

NOTE 3.

H. L. ROXBURGH
EXPERIMENTS ON HUMAN SUBJECTS*

* * *

In England there is no statute which specifically controls the conditions under which experiments can be done. . . .

A civil action might arise as a result of an accusation of assault, or trespass to the person, in the absence of injury. This is unlikely to be successful provided that a valid consent has been obtained, on the principle of *volenti non fit injuria*. Should it be alleged, however, that a subject had suffered injury or death as a result of an experiment, the matter seems not so simple. Judgment would depend in large part on, in Ladimer's phrase, "How the investigator proceeded and how he checked himself." Courts might well construe any evidence in favour of the plaintiff if doubt existed, and it is useful to analyse this phrase in some detail. . . .

That a subject is a volunteer is not alone sufficient and, although he might weaken any case by volunteering, this would have to be decided in the courts, and he would still have the remedy in law against any negligence that had been committed. Suppose, however, there has been no negligence and an experimental procedure by its nature must have an unknown outcome, what is then the position if death or injury results? Obviously a consent valid in law is a prime essential. The subject must comprehend the nature and extent of the risks involved, and no element of force, fraud, duress or coercion may be used. . . .

Regarding criminal aspects, the following principles of English law appear to have relevance.

(a) No one has the right to consent to the infliction upon himself of death or of

---

* 3 *Medicine, Science and the Law* 132, 134–136 (1963). Reprinted by permission.

any injury likely to cause death, except for necessary surgical purposes.

(b) It is uncertain to what extent any person has the right to consent to his being put in danger of death or bodily harm by an act of another.

As distinct from civil actions, the question of consent is of little relevance, for if the experiment be itself criminal, agreement of the subject is immaterial. Justification of the experiment would not be recognised as a valid defence in law for any criminal action, though it might be accepted in mitigation of the gravity of an offence. The justification might change from time to time, for example in time of war the moral justification for any procedure might be increased by the urgent national need to gather data quickly.

Considerations of public policy may have significance in connection with experimental work for the general benefit of the state and its subjects, and exceptions to the general legal rules may have application. Well established exceptions do not, however, include any situation directly parallel to that under consideration. For example, the case of those who "cause injury in recreations for a trial of skill or manhood or for improvement in the use of their weapons" is quoted as an exception because "bodily harm was not the motive on either side" (*R.* v. *Donovan* [1934] 2 K.B. 498). Whether a court would, in fact, accept this as analogous cannot be stated with certainty. . . .

* * *

b.

Spead v. Tomlinson
73 N.H. 46, 59 A. 376 (1904)

* * *

Case to recover for damages alleged to have been suffered by the plaintiff at the hands of the defendant, who is a Christian Science healer. . . . In April, 1898, the plaintiff, who was then about 55 years old, suffered from an attack of appendicitis, employed a medical practitioner for several months, and learned in a general way the course pursued by physicians in the treatment of that disease. During the summer of 1899 she became interested in the doctrines of Christian Science, and attended meetings where the defendant told of wonderful cures he had performed. November 13, 1899, the plaintiff noticed symptoms similar to those which had ushered in the previous attack of appendicitis, visited the defendant at his home, informed him of the nature of her trouble and her dread of a

surgical operation, and employed him to treat her. The defendant told her that a surgical operation was not necessary, that she was not to take any medicine, and that he could and would cure her if she continued his treatment. He directed her to read "Science and Health," to continue her usual diet of solids, and to take her accustomed exercise. He also read to her extracts from "Science and Health," and administered treatment by sitting in front of her in an attitude of prayer. The plaintiff employed the defendant for several days, and during this time her illness increased. She finally placed herself in the hands of physicians, submitted to a surgical operation, and was cured. There was evidence tending to show that the defendant's treatment was injurious to the plaintiff, and that, if it had been persisted in, a cure would have been impossible. . . .

On Rehearing

* * *

Young, J.

By "public policy" is intended the policy of the state as evidenced by its laws. . . . If the plaintiff is to recover on the ground of public policy, she must establish (1) that it was illegal for the defendant to give her such treatment; (2) that the duty of not giving it was imposed on him for her benefit; and (3) that no illegal act of hers contributed to cause her injuries. It is the general rule that the plaintiff in an action sounding in negligence must show that the defendant failed to perform a duty owed him, and that his own failure to perform a duty owed the defendant did not contribute to cause his injury; or, in other words, he must show the defendant's fault and his own freedom from fault. Assuming (without deciding) that such treatment is forbidden by the provisions of section 8, c. 278, Pub. St. 1891, which makes the killing of a human being by culpable negligence manslaughter, or by the provision of the common law which makes it unlawful for any one to do what is liable to endanger the life or health of others, and that the duty of not doing what is forbidden by either provision was imposed on the defendant for the plaintiff's benefit, the question still remains whether the plaintiff's own wrong contributed to cause her injuries. It is elementary that, if it was illegal for the defendant to treat the plaintiff as he did, it was equally illegal for her either to knowingly employ him to give her such treatment, or to consent to be so treated. So far as the evidence goes, her knowledge in respect to the disease from which she was suffering and the treatment prescribed for it by regular physicians in good standing, and in respect to the way the defendant proposed to treat her, was at least equal to his.

It does not follow, as a matter of law, from the fact that the plaintiff cannot recover in this action on the count in negligence, that the defendant would not have been guilty of manslaughter if the plaintiff had died from the effects of his treatment. If he had been indicted under the provisions of section 8, c. 278, Pub. St. 1891, the state would base its right of action on his failure to perform a duty the law imposed on him for its benefit. The state has a direct interest in the lives and health of all its citizens. Every one who has to do with the lives and health of others not only owes the individuals with whom he comes in contact a legal duty, but also owes the state the duty of using ordinary care to do nothing which will endanger their lives or health. In an action by the state it would be no answer to show that, if the deceased had used ordinary care to avoid being injured, he would not have died; for the defendant is not indicted for his failure to perform a duty the law imposed on him for the deceased's benefit, but for his failure to perform one imposed on him for the benefit of the state. . . .

*   *   *

. . . The plaintiff fails because of the insufficiency of her evidence to prove the facts necessary to maintain her case.

Exceptions overruled.

c.

Edmond Cahn
Drug Experiments and the Public Conscience*

*   *   *

[S]ometimes a consent will be unacceptable because of extrinsic circumstances that convert it into an exploitation of sickness or need, for example, the consents to irreversible sterilization that certain states in India have been purchasing from untouchables for small sums of money. At other times, a consent is unacceptable because of intrinsic circumstances, that is, circumstances having to do with the prospective consequences of the experiment and their relation to human dignity. One can conceive conditions un-

der which a consent might be acceptable even where the experiment might involve a serious risk of death. Where however the experiment involves a serious risk of permanent physical or psychic mutilation, the consent should not be accepted. For example, a consent would be unacceptable if the experiment involved a serious risk of converting a subject who was mentally normal into a psychotic. On the other hand, as every physician knows, there are psychiatric conditions grievous or critical enough to warrant even the risk of psychic mutilation, but in such conditions the justification for taking the risk must be found in the possible benefit to the ailing subject, not alone in his consent or in possible increment of scientific knowledge.

*   *   *

[A]s I see it, it is not primarily a question of what a subject can consent to, for under sufficiently extreme circumstances he may insist that he can consent to almost anything, and who has the right to contradict him without having had personal experience of just such circumstances? The moral impossibility is on the other side, *our* side. It is we who *cannot accept* certain consents that are ostensibly free and voluntary; it is we who are unable to accept a profit from human sacrifice. The ceiling price that we impose on scientific progress is the product of our own moral self-image, our enduring convictions and our social conscience.

*   *   *

2.

Demanding Consent to Prevent "Harm"

a.

Louis L. Jaffe
Law as a System of Control*

*   *   *

[N]either in law nor in practice is the process of consent a single, clearly defined entity. Consent is a function of the relation between experimenter and subject and is modulated by the degree of risk, the alternative treatments (in a therapeutic situation), and the value of the experiment. There is wide range of opinion as to

---

* Paul Talalay, ed.: *Drugs in Our Society*. Baltimore: The Johns Hopkins Press 255, 264–265 (1964). Reprinted by permission.

* 98 *Daedalus* 406, 420–422 (1969). Reprinted by permission of Daedalus, Journal of the American Academy of Arts and Sciences, Boston, Massachusetts.

the significance of consent. Dr. Louis Lasagna has said:

I want to take issue with Dr. [Jay] Katz's notion that consent is the pre-eminent question. Consent is primarily important in the abstract and appeals to those who are interested in civil libertarian problems. The major protection of the patient, however, comes from the review of protocols by peer and non-peer groups, from the competence of the investigator, and all the ancillary facilities at his disposal, and from monitoring the performance of experiments.

Such an opinion may reflect two quite different and opposed attitudes: the angry and contemptuous attitude of the investigator who finds his project complicated by requirements of consent so elaborate that his experiment is impeded; and, on the other hand, the attitude, if you accept Dr. Lasagna's epithet, of "the civil libertarian" who is afraid that the will of the subject may be easily overborne or even disregarded, and who may take refuge from his concern in the hope that other safeguards will protect the subject.

   The common law sets a high value on consent to physical invasions that threaten the health or psychic integrity of the individual. The law rightly recognizes that the body is his fortress. Nevertheless, the inviolability of the body is not absolute. . . .

   . . . Consider the case of *O'Brien* v. *The Cunard Steamship Lines* . . . 28 N.E. 266 (1891), which had to do with an immigrant who was being brought into the port of Boston. All the immigrants were lined up rather ignominiously to be vaccinated. When she passed by the vaccinating physician, Mrs. O'Brien said that she had already been vaccinated. Nevertheless, the doctor told her to hold up her arm and she was punctured. She later claimed that she did not consent. The Court held that her actual state of mind was irrelevant; that the consent should be looked at from the point of view of the defendant. Had the plaintiff in this situation been submitting to serious risk, the Court would not have focused on the defendant alone, though as pointed out by Professor Calabresi there is a risk (though slight?) of encephalitis. There were, of course, great pressures on her to accede to vaccination that in another situation would be held to negate completely the idea of consent. (Her only alternative was to turn around and go home or perhaps into quarantine.) But given the kind of relationship, the

interests of the state, the interests of getting the vaccinations done effectively and quickly, the law was prepared to take a cavalier attitude toward the claims of Mrs. O'Brien's personality. This case exemplifies the notion that in any situation, as should be true whether or not the medical personnel are public officers, the law will look at the structure of the situation to see what is demanded in terms of the interest of society, on the one hand, and the interests of the individual, on the other.

* * *

NOTES

NOTE 1.

JACOBSON V. MASSACHUSETTS
197 U.S. 11 (1904)

Mr. JUSTICE HARLAN delivered the opinion of the court:

* * *

   . . . The defendant insists that his liberty is invaded when the state subjects him to fine or imprisonment for neglecting or refusing to submit to vaccination; that a compulsory vaccination law is unreasonable, arbitrary, and oppressive, and, therefore, hostile to the inherent right of every freeman to care for his own body and health in such way as to him seems best; and that the execution of such a law against one who objects to vaccination, no matter for what reason, is nothing short of an assault upon his person. But the liberty secured by the Constitution of the United States to every person within its jurisdiction does not import an absolute right in each person to be, at all times and in all circumstances, wholly freed from restraint. There are manifold restraints to which every person is necessarily subject for the common good. On any other basis organized society could not exist with safety to its members. Society based on the rule that each one is a law unto himself would soon be confronted with disorder and anarchy. Real liberty for all could not exist under the operation of a principle which recognizes the right of each individual person to use his own, whether in respect of his person or his property, regardless of the injury that may be done to others. This court has more than once recognized it as a fundamental principle that "persons and property are subjected to all kinds of restraints and burdens in order to secure the general comfort, health, and prosperity of the state; of the perfect right of the legislature to do which no question ever was, or upon acknowledged general principles ever can be, made, so far as natural persons are concerned." *Hannibal & St.J. R. Co.* v. *Husen, 95 U.S. 465, 471,* . . . In *Crowley* v. *Christensen, 137 U.S. 86, 89* . . . we said: "The possession and enjoyment of all rights are subject to such reasonable conditions as may be deemed by the governing authority of the country essential to the safety, health, peace, good order, and morals of the community. Even liberty itself, the greatest of all rights, is not unrestricted license to act according to one's own will. It is only freedom from restraint under conditions essential to the equal enjoyment of the same right by others. It is, then, liberty regulated by law". . . .

* * *

NOTE 2.

COMMITTEE FOR SAFEGUARDING HUMAN
DIGNITY
COMPULSORY POST-MORTEM
OPERATIONS IN ISRAEL*

* * *

The [autopsy] law in effect [in Israel] at present is the Anatomy-Pathology Law of 1953. Paragraph six of this law states:

A doctor may dissect a body in order to determine the cause of death, or to use parts of the body for healing purposes, if three authorized doctors sign a certificate attesting to the fact that the postmortem operation will serve one of these purposes. (Sefer Hachukim 184, 4.8.1953).

Neither the deceased nor his family are mentioned in or recognized by this law. They have been denied the right to make the decision on a matter in which they are vitally involved, and, in their stead, three doctors, who *need not even consult* the family, have been given the power to authorize a dissection.

* * *

NOTE 3.

R. A. MCCANCE
THE PRACTICE OF EXPERIMENTAL MEDICINE†

* * *

. . . I would feel happier, however, for the future, if patients could be made more aware

that at some hospitals—the best hospitals—experimental work is carried out not only for the benefit of the immediate sufferers, but also for the benefit of mankind, and that they themselves owe incalculable advantages to work of this kind which has already been done on others; furthermore, that if they or their children are privileged to be admitted to these hospitals, they may be expected to co-operate. In the form given to patients on admission to one hospital I know, there is a small paragraph and the addition of a few words to it illustrates the sort of thing I have in mind. The additions proposed are in italics. "The hospital staff seeks your assistance in carrying out the hospital's duty to the community in the *investigation of disease and in the* training of doctors and nurses; if a member of the staff wishes to *make a special study of your condition or to* explain it to a medical student, doctor or nurse, it is hoped that we may have your co-operation."

* * *

NOTE 4.

WALTER MODELL
THE ETHICAL OBLIGATIONS TO THE
NONSUBJECT*

The problem of the obligations of the experimenter to his human subject is generally recognized as a highly charged one. . . . It seems, to me, however, that the forgotten man is the innocent bystander, the patient whose medication will depend on the outcome of experiments on other men, the nonsubject whose apparent nonparticipation is only temporary since he will ultimately participate by virtue of the medication he is given. Eventually, collectively, the nonsubject is an interested party, albeit a late comer. It is he who, sooner or later, will suffer or benefit from experiments or from the failure to perform the right ones. . . .

* * *

b.
**Oscar M. Ruebhausen and Orville G. Brim, Jr.
Privacy and Behavioral Research†**

* * *

While the knowledgeable, freely given consent of a participant should be a basic ground

* Jerusalem: The Committee for Safeguarding Human Dignity (1968).
† 44 *Proceedings of the Royal Society of Medicine* 188, 194 (1950). Reprinted by permission.

* 1 *Clinical Pharmacology and Therapeutics* 137 (1960). Reprinted by permission.
† 65 *Columbia Law Review* 1184, 1201–1202 (1965). Reprinted by permission.

rule for all behavioral research, there is, of course, a need for exceptions. There must be, indeed, a fundamental exception to cover the many instances where society will accept the invasion of privacy as permissible and reasonable. Thus, when the general welfare requires it and due process is observed, our society permits the taking of private property without consent. There is no reason to doubt that, under similar circumstances, society will permit at least a limited invasion, or taking, of private personality. Circumstances under which the community tolerates the probing into private areas without the consent, and, if necessary, without the knowledge of the examinee do, in fact, exist. A number of examples can be easily found in law enforcement, in selection for military service, in social welfare work, in the protection of the public health, in the national census, and in the selection of employees for the Central Intelligence Agency or as airline pilots.

A public trial may also invade the privacy of the individuals involved in the litigation. Yet since our society is persuaded that a public hearing is essential to a fair trial and to social order, it finds entirely reasonable that the individual claim to privacy must yield in this instance. even here, however, the equilibrium between the competing values is sensitively preserved and there are occasions when the court is cleared, or the testimony sealed.

Even where the public interest may warrant the taking of private property or of private personality, no absolute license is justified. The taking should be reasonable, it should be conducted with due process, and it should be limited to no more than what is necessary for the fullfillment of the public purpose which, in fact, warranted the invasion.

*   *   *

PART FOUR

The Authority of Professional and Public Institutions

This Part explores the role of professional and public institutions in formulating, administering, and reviewing the human experimentation process. The preceding analysis of the authority of the investigator and the subject disclosed the limits of their capacity to make "acceptable" and "informed" decisions and indicated that society has an interest in encouraging or discouraging certain investigations. We now inquire whether, despite these considerations, the human experimentation process should nevertheless be left to the initiative of investigators and to the arrangements they make with their subjects because the participation of other decisionmakers would impose greater burdens than benefits on the process. If, on the other hand, the private ordering between investigators and subjects is found wanting, we must scrutinize how and to what extent it should be supplemented by other mechanisms of guidance and control exercised by the professions (*e.g.*, hospital committees, professional associations, and editorial boards), the state (*e.g.*, administrative agencies, courts, and legislatures), and other public or private groups (*e.g.*, the press, public interest organizations, and private litigants).

We have previously spoken of "subjects" as a group without taking into account differences among them. This reflects in part the lack of consensus about the ambit of experimentation and in part the lack of agreement on who is a fit subject for research. We now introduce a distinction between volunteers* (subjects who are not patients at the

---

* We have been unable to coin a better term for this group of subjects. The more precise term "nonpatient-subject" seems too cumbersome, and the simpler label "subject" is better suited as a generic term for all subjects be they patients or nonpatients. However, the use of the label "volunteer" must not foreclose a searching inquiry into the voluntariness of all subjects' participation.

725

initiation of a research project) and patient-subjects (subjects who are also patients at the initiation of the research project). This distinction should alert the student that the label "volunteer" has been employed all too indiscriminately to include, among others, "healthy" individuals and patients who undergo experimental manipulation; "healthy" individuals and patients who serve as controls for investigations; and incompetent individuals who are "volunteered" by others as subjects for investigation.

The distinctions between volunteers and patients suggest that differences in status among subjects require analysis. The examination of consent in Part Three has already uncovered major limitations on the capacity of some subjects, particularly when they are also patients, to give meaningful, informed consent. In light of such considerations, the framework of the chapters in this Part is built around a division of subjects into several groups. Chapter Eleven is primarily concerned with the general subject population who are considered capable of giving consent and who participate in research either as volunteers or as patients. In the three chapters which follow, the focus shifts to investigations with uncomprehending, captive, and dying persons, respectively. The division of subjects into these groups is based on the assumption—which must be carefully examined—that there are distinctions among these groups which require the development of special rules and mechanisms to reflect and respond to the varying capacity of the individuals in each group to participate understandingly in the experimentation process. Moreover, examining each of these groups separately highlights difficulties common to the human experimentation process as a whole; for example, the analysis of the special problems raised by investigations with prisoners illuminates the impact of external pressures which, though often not as clearly perceived, affect non-captive subjects as well.

The case studies which precede the analytic sections of these chapters are designed to provide data for the analysis of the interactions between the professions and state and the different groups of volunteers and patient-subjects. In addition, many of the case studies presented in the earlier chapters may bear re-examination. They have already suggested the need for professional and state participation in decisionmaking; they may now contribute further data for the ultimate task of this volume—analyzing the role of all participants in the human experimentation process.

Throughout we ask:

1. What persons and institutions should have the authority to formulate, administer, and review the human experimentation process?

2. Should the authority of these persons and institutions differ at each decisionmaking stage?

3. To what extent should this authority be modified once subjects are labeled "volunteer," "normal," "diseased," "competent," "uncomprehending," "captive," or "dying"?

CHAPTER ELEVEN

Experimentation with Volunteers and Patient-Subjects

As a prologue to the subsequent analysis, this chapter opens with an expression of views by a governmental commission, a theologian, a physcian, a judge, a lawyer, and a philosopher on the competing interests of science, society, and the individual. Their common quest is for a balancing of society's interests which at one and the same time will protect the individual's well-being and right to self-determination and encourage the acquisition of knowledge through scientific investigation.

The case studies in this chapter on the discovery of a reliable oral contraceptive pill and the search for an effective surgical treatment of mitral stenosis focus on the role assumed by professional and public institutions in experimentation with subjects who are sufficiently "competent" to participate in the decisionmaking process. Both investigations involved risktaking with only an approximate idea of the relative benefit and harm to individuals and to society.

Distinctions have traditionally been drawn between research conducted by investigators on "normal volunteers" in purely experimental settings and by therapist-investigators on "patients" in treatment settings. It has generally been assumed that more stringent controls should be placed on investigators whose actions are designed to gain knowledge rather than to promote the subject's "best interests." Yet in most situations it is difficult to draw lines between "normal volunteers," "patient-subjects," and "patients." Moreover, the "therapeutic" setting may be the one which deserves the closer scrutiny. While a volunteering subject can be alert to protect his own self-interest, a patient-subject's need for treatment may cause him to overrate the benefits and underestimate the risks of a research technique.

Thus, an important question to be explored in this chapter is the extent to which additional safeguards should be imposed on experimentation-with-therapy lest investigators, even unwittingly, expose "consenting" patient-subjects to "unreasonable" risks.

In examining the two case studies, consider the following questions:

1. For what purposes and to what extent should professional and public institutions intervene in the private interactions between investigators and subjects?

2. How and to what extent should the authority of each participant in the human experimentation process be affected by:

    a. the likelihood of immediate benefits to patient-subjects?

    b. the possibility of future benefits to patient-subjects?

    c. the degree of certainty with which known and speculative risks can be predicted?

    d. the availability of alternative procedures?

3. How should the authority of each participant in the human experimentation process be affected when:

    a. an investigation is conducted for the benefit of future patients or of society?

    b. an investigation, though conducted for the benefit of subjects, is also designed to test the efficacy of a new procedure for society at large?

A.
Balancing the Interests of Science, Society, and the Individual

1.

Office of Science and Technology
Privacy and Behavioral Research*

*   *   *

[T]here exists an important conflict between two values, both of which are strongly held in American society.

The individual has an inalienable right to dignity, self-respect, and freedom to determine his own thoughts and actions within the broad limits set by the requirements of society. The essential element in privacy and self-determination is the privilege of making one's own decision as to the extent to which one will reveal thoughts, feelings, and actions. When a person consents freely and fully to share himself with others— with a scientist, an employer, or credit investigator—there is no invasion of privacy, regardless of the quality or nature of the information revealed.

Behavioral science is representative of another value vigorously championed by most American citizens, the right to know anything that may be known or discovered about any part of the universe. Man is part of this universe, and the extent of the Federal Government's financial support of human behavioral research (on the order of $300 million in 1966) testifies to the importance placed on the study of human behavior by the American people. In the past, there have been conflicts between theological beliefs and the theoretical analyses of the physical sciences. These conflicts have largely subsided, but the behavioral sciences seem to have inherited the conflict that arises when strongly held beliefs or moral attitudes—whether theologically, economically, or politically based—are subjected to the free-ranging process of scientific inquiry. If society is to exercise its right to know, it must free its behavioral scientists as much as possible from unnecessary restraints. Yet behavioral scientists, in turn, must accept the constructive restraints that society imposes in order to establish that level of dignity, freedom, and personal fulfillment that men treasure virtually above all else in life.

* Washington, D.C.: U.S. Government Printing Office 3–5, 9–10, 14–17 (1967).

The root of the conflict between the individual's right to privacy and society's right of discovery is the research process. Behavioral science seeks to assess and to measure many qualities of man's mind, feelings, and actions. In the absence of informed consent on the part of the subject, these measurements represent invasion of privacy. The scientist must therefore obtain the consent of his subject.

To obtain truly informed consent is often difficult. In the first place, the nature of the inquiry sometimes cannot be explained adequately because it involves complex variables that the nonscientist does not understand. Examples are the personality variables measured by questionnaires, and the qualities of cognitive processes measured by creativity tests. Secondly, the validity of an experiment is sometimes destroyed if the subject knows all the details of its conduct. [I]f behavioral research is to be effective, some modification of the traditional concept of informed consent is needed.

Such a change in no sense voids the general proposition that the performance of human behavioral research is the product of a partnership between the scientist and his subjects. Consent to participate in a study must be the norm before any subject embarks on the enterprise. Since consent must sometimes be given despite an admittedly inadequate understanding of the scientific purposes of the research procedures, the right to discontinue participation at any point must be stipulated in clear terms. In the meantime, when full information is not available to him and when no alternative procedures to minimize the privacy problem are available, the relationship between the subject and the scientist (as well as with the institution sponsoring the scientist) must be based upon trust. . . .

Occasionally, even this degree of consent cannot be obtained. Naturalistic observations of group behavior must sometimes be made unbeknownst to the subjects. In such cases, as well as in all others, the scientist has the obligation to insure full confidentiality of the research records. Only by doing so, and by making certain that published reports contain no identifying reference to a given subject, can the invasion of privacy be minimized.

Basically then, the protection of privacy in research is assured first by securing the informed consent of the subject. When the subject cannot be completely informed, the consent must be based on trust in the scientist and in the institution sponsoring him. In any case the scientist and his sponsoring institution must insure privacy by the maintenance of confidentiality.

In the end, the fact must be accepted that human behavioral research will at times produce discomfort to some subjects, and will entail a partial invasion of their privacy. Neither the principle of privacy nor the need to discover new knowledge can supervene universally. As with other conflicting values in our society, there must be constant adjustment and compromise, with the decision as to which value is to govern in a given instance to be determined by a weighing of the costs and the gains—the cost in privacy, the gain in knowledge. The decision cannot be made solely by the investigator, who normally has a vested interest in his own research program, but must be a positive concern of his scientific peers and the institution which sponsors his work. Our society has grown strong on the principle of minimizing costs and maximizing gains and, when warmly held values are in conflict, there must be a thoughtful evaluation of the specific case. In particular, we do not believe that detailed governmental controls of research methods or instruments can substitute for the more effective procedures which are available and which carry less risk of damage to the scientific enterprise.

*   *   *

Science has made its contributions to human welfare by virtue of its freedom to inquire. The investigator pursuing knowledge, whether his subject is man or some other aspect of the natural world, must not feel constrained to limit his study to those things which have current social approval. Freedom of inquiry is a part of the general concept of intellectual freedom and has been built into the value structure of every university.

Behavioral science is obligated to explore all aspects of human behavior to the degree that such inquiry contributes to improved understanding of the nature of man and his society. The study of human behavior is challenging and difficult. When the scientist seeks to develop a meaningful and consistent set of concepts about some aspect of man's relations to others, he uses and must be free to use every means at his disposal to gain knowledge. In his search for truth he is less likely to think of social consequences of his work than he is of scientific consequences. In fact, most scientists in any discipline take the position that the search for truth should seek to replace myths, prejudices, and misconceptions, and hence they view with great suspicion any limitation on their endeavors.

*   *   *

The values held by an individual or by a society are, and must be, in competition since no single value can be absolute. Even the right to life is supervened by a society seeking to protect itself from criminal behavior. Thus the conflict between the claim of the individual to his privacy and the needs of society to become better aware of human characteristics is no rare or isolated phenomenon.

In each instance of conflict, the decision must rest on the totality of all the relevant issues and the result will vary from one occasion to another, and from one setting to another depending on the context within which the issue arises and the process by which a conclusion is reached. No general rule can be formulated to apply in each situation; rather, persons desiring to uphold our society's diverse values must make judgments. The strength of our society lies in pluralism and diversity. The shifting tensions among our values and in the relative primacy accorded them provide strong assurance for the continuance of the diversity on which much of our freedom and our growth are built.

*   *   *

Even the rights to bodily integrity and privacy of property, which are recognized within our system of law and accepted generally as inalienable, are not really absolute. Every highway that is built involves personal and social cost, especially for those who are displaced or diminished by the construction. Indeed, there is hardly a social act that does not involve some social or human cost. There is no escape from the fact that limits exist for every basic value. Failure to limit any single one inevitably circumscribes another. In summary, it is a logical impossibility to have freedom without limits or values without qualification.

*   *   *

The decision concerning proposed behavioral research therefore must be a balancing process without arbitrariness, rigidity, or absolutes. If both privacy and the pursuit of knowledge are to be accorded their due, no choice between them can be made without considering the circumstances of a particular case.

In this balancing process many factors must be considered and weighed.

One factor is the proposed research. Is it desirable? Has it been done before? If so, is it worth repeating? Is it well designed and strongly staffed? Has the privacy issue been taken into account? Is it possible to redesign the experiment so as to avoid offense to privacy and obtain the same knowledge?

In weighing the benefits expected from an experiment, the value of the knowledge it is hoped to obtain and the probability of obtaining it must be taken into account. This value judgment must be made both in terms of social utility and in terms of the likely contribution to our general understanding of human behavior. Although a stronger weight is given to knowledge which is expected to yield social benefits, our society attaches worth to pure knowledge, recognizing that pure knowledge often develops unexpected utility.

In practice, we deal with specific proposals, designed to answer specific questions through the use of specific research techniques. When a proposal involves a conflict between protection of privacy and pursuit of knowledge, a technical issue must be resolved at the outset. This issue is whether the investigator's experimental design minimizes the conflict or whether it can be reduced by redesigning the study. Since conflicts between privacy and the pursuit of knowledge can, in many cases, be reduced by the proper design of studies, it is essential that reviewers of research proposals examine this question first. Only after the research has been designed to assure that the knowledge will be obtained at minimum cost in terms of privacy, need the basic issues posed by conflicting values be examined.

If an invasion of privacy cannot be avoided, the extent and character of the invasion must be scrutinized. Is it actual or theoretical, real or technical? Is there potential harm to the subject? If so, is the harm substantial or insignificant, lasting or fleeting? Is the invasion minimal? For example, surveillance (by one-way mirror, camera, or monitoring devices) challenges directly and fundamentally the claim to privacy when the focus is on an individual. The challenge is drastically reduced if the focus is not on an individual but on social interactions; for example, at a bus stop or a street light.

*   *   *

While the community at large has an important stake in the outcome of this balancing process, it cannot play an effective role in most of the review. Few laymen can be effective critics of a research design and few scientists are willing to submit to a review by laymen. Review of a research proposal only by scientists in the same field as the investigator, however, fails to assure adequate representation of the values of the whole community. How to solve this dilemma without making the review process arbitrary, capricious, or irrelevant is a difficult problem which will require continuing experimentation and study.

This discussion of the balancing and decisional process has emphasized that the claim to privacy is not an automatic barrier to research. Nor is every intrusion on privacy automatically unreasonable. A wise and discriminating society has found, and will continue to find, that many invasions of privacy are tolerable and necessary for the health of the community.

*   *   *

2.

His Holiness, Pope Pius XII
The Moral Limits of Medical Research and Treatment*

*   *   *

Is there any moral limit to the "medical interests of the community" in content or extension? Are there "full powers" over the living man in every serious medical case? Does it raise barriers that are still valid in the interests of science or the individual? Or, stated differently: Can public authority, on which rests responsibility for the common good, give the doctor the power to experiment on the individual in the interests of science and the community in order to discover and try out new methods and procedures when these experiments transgress the right of the individual to dispose of himself? In the interests of the community, can public authority really limit or even suppress the right of the individual over his body and life, his bodily and psychic integrity?

To forestall an objection, We assume that it is a question of serious research, of honest efforts to promote the theory and practice of medicine, not of a maneuver serving as a scientific pretext to mask other ends and achieve them with impunity.

* 44 *Acta Apostolica Sedis* 779, 784–789 (1952); Rome: 3 *Proceedings of the First International Congress of Neuropathology* 713, 719–725 (1952). (Translated from the French by the N.C.W.C. News Service). Reprinted by permission.

In regard to these questions many people have been of the opinion and are still of the opinion today, that the answer must be in the affirmative. To give weight to their contention they cite the fact that the individual is subordinated to the community, that the good of the individual must give way to the common good and be sacrificed to it. They add that the sacrifice of an individual for purposes of research and scientific investigation profits the individual in the long run.

The great postwar trials brought to light a terrifying number of documents testifying to the sacrifice of the individual in the "medical interests of the community." In the minutes of these trials one finds testimony and reports showing how, with the consent and, at times, even under the formal order of public authority, certain research centers systematically demanded to be furnished with persons from concentration camps for their medical experiments. One finds how they were delivered to such centers, so many men, so many women, so many for one experiment, so many for another. There are reports on the conduct and the results of such experiments, of the subjective and objective symptoms observed during the different phases of the experiments. One cannot read these reports without feeling a profound compassion for the victims, many of whom went to their deaths, and without being frightened by such an aberration of the human mind and heart. But We can also add that those responsible for these atrocious deeds did no more than to reply in the affirmative to the question We have asked and to accept the practical consequences of their affirmation.

At this point is the interest of the individual subordinated to the community's medical interests, or is there here a transgression, perhaps in good faith, against the most elementary demands of the natural law, a transgression that permits no medical research?

One would have to shut one's eyes to reality to believe that at the present time one could find no one in the medical world to hold and defend the ideas that gave rise to the facts We have cited. It is enough to follow for a short time the reports on medical efforts and experiments to convince oneself of the contrary. Involuntarily one asks oneself what has authorized, and what could ever authorize, any doctor's daring to try such an experiment. The experiment is described in all its stages and effects with calm objectivity. What is verified and what is not is noted. But there is not a word on its moral legality. Nevertheless, this question exists, and one cannot suppress it by passing it over in silence.

In the above mentioned cases, insofar as the moral justification of the experiments rests on the mandate of public authority, and therefore on the subordination of the individual to the community, of the individual's welfare to the common welfare, it is based on an erroneous explanation of this principle. It must be noted that, in his personal being, man is not finally ordered to usefulness to society. On the contrary, the community exists for man.

The community is the great means intended by nature and God to regulate the exchange of mutual needs and to aid each man to develop his personality fully according to his individual and social abilities. Considered as a whole, the community is not a physical unity subsisting in itself and its individual members are not integral parts of it. Considered as a whole, the physical organism of living beings, of plants, animals or man, has a unity subsisting in itself. Each of the members, for example, the hand, the foot, the heart, the eye, is an integral part destined by all its being to be inserted in the whole organism. Outside the organism it has not, by its very nature, any sense, any finality. It is wholly absorbed by the totality of the organism to which it is attached.

In the moral community and in every organism of a purely moral character, it is an entirely different story. Here the whole has no unity subsisting in itself, but a simple unity of finality and action. In the community individuals are merely collaborators and instruments for the realization of the common end.

What results as far as the physical organism is concerned? The master and user of this organism, which possesses a subsisting unity, can dispose directly and immediately of integral parts, members and organs within the scope of their natural finality. He can also intervene, as often as and to the extent that the good of the whole demands, to paralyze, destroy, mutilate and separate the members. But, on the contrary, when the whole has only a unity of finality and action, its head—in the present case, the public authority—doubtlessly holds direct authority and the right to make demands upon the activities of the parts, but in no case can it dispose of its physical being. Indeed, every direct attempt upon its essence constitutes an abuse of the power of authority.

Now medical experiments—the subject We are discussing here—immediately and directly affect the physical being, either of the whole or of the several organs, of the human organism. But, by virtue of the principle We have cited, public authority has no power in this sphere. It cannot, therefore, pass it on to research workers and doctors. It is from the State, however, that the doctor must receive authorization when he acts upon the organism of the individual in the "interests of the community." For then he does not act as a private individual, but as a mandatory of the public power. The latter cannot, however, pass on a right that it does not possess, save in the case already mentioned when it acts as a deputy, as the legal representative of a minor for as long as he cannot make his own decisions, of a person of feeble mind or of a lunatic.

*　　*　　*

In the domain of your science it is an obvious law that the application of new methods to living men must be proceeded by research on cadavers or the model of study and experimentation on animals. Sometimes, however, this procedure is found to be impossible, insufficient or not feasible from a practical point of view. In this case, medical research will try to work on its immediate object, the living man, in the interests of science, in the interests of the patient and in the interests of the community. Such a procedure is not to be rejected without further consideration. But you must stop at the limits laid down by the moral principles We have explained.

Without doubt, before giving moral authorization to the use of new methods, one cannot ask that any danger or any risk be excluded. That would exceed human possibilities, paralyze all serious scientific research and very frequently be to the detriment of the patient. In these cases the weighing of the danger must be left to the judgment of the tried and competent doctor. Nevertheless, as Our explanation has shown, there is a degree of danger that morality cannot allow. In doubtful cases, when means already known have failed, it may happen that a new method still insufficiently tried offers, together with very dangerous elements, appreciable chances of success. If the patient gives his consent, the use of the procedure in question is licit. But this way of acting cannot be upheld as a line of conduct in normal cases.

People will perhaps object that the ideas set forth here present a serious obstacle to scientific research and work. Nevertheless, the limits We have outlined are not by definition an obstacle to progress. The field of medicine cannot be different in this respect from other fields of man's research, investigations and work. The great moral demands force the impetuous flow of human thought and will to flow, like water from the mountains, into certain channels. They contain the flow to increase its efficiency and usefulness. They dam it so that it does not overflow and cause ravages that can never be compensated for by the special good it seeks. In appearance, moral demands are a brake. In fact, they contribute to the best and most beautiful of what man has produced for science, the individual and the community.

*   *   *

3.

Andrew C. Ivy
Cross-Examination before the
Nuernberg Military Tribunal—
June 13, 1947*

*   *   *

DR. SERVATIUS: Witness, take the following case. You are in a city in which the plague is raging. You, as a doctor, have a drug that you could use to combat the plague. However, you must test it on somebody. The commander, or let us say the mayor of the city, comes to you and says, "Here is a criminal condemned to death. Save us by carrying out the experiment on this man." Would you refuse to do so, or would you do it?

Witness Dr. IVY: I would refuse to do so, because I do not believe that duress of that sort warrants the breaking of ethical and moral principles. That is why the Hague Convention and Geneva Convention were formulated, to make war, a barbaric enterprise, a little more humane.

Q: Do you believe that the population of a city would have any understanding for your action?

A: They have understanding for the importance of the maintenance of the principles of medical ethics which apply over a long period of years, rather than a short period of years. Physicians and medical scientists should do nothing with the idea of temporarily doing good which,

2 *Trials of War Criminals before the Nuernberg Military Tribunals* (*The Medical Case*). Washington, D.C.: U.S. Government Printing Office 42–44 (1948).

when carried out repeatedly over a period of time, would debase and jeopardize a method for doing good. If a medical scientist breaks the code of medical ethics and says, "Kill the person," in order to do what he thinks may be good, in the course of time that will grow and will cause a loss of faith of the public in the medical profession, and hence destroy the capacity of the medical profession to do its good for society. The reason that we must be very careful in the use of human beings as subjects in medical experiments is in order not to debase and jeopardize this method for doing great good by causing the public to react against it.

Q: Witness, do you not believe that your ideal attitude here is more or less that of a single person standing against the body of public opinion?

A: No I do not. That is why I read out the principles of medical ethics yesterday, and that is why the American Medical Association has agreed essentially to those principles. That is why the principles, the ethical principles for the use of human beings in medical experiments, have been quite uniform throughout the world in the past.

Q: Then you do not believe that the urgency, the necessity of this city would make a revision of this attitude necessary?

A: No, not if they were in danger of killing people in the course of testing out the new drug or remedy. There is no justification in killing five people in order to save the lives of five hundred.

Q: Then you are of the opinion that the life of the one prisoner must be preserved even if the whole city perishes?

A: In order to maintain intact the method of doing good, yes.

*   *   *

Q: You then, despite the order, would not carry out the order, and would prefer to be executed as a martyr?

A: That is correct, and I know there are thousands of people in the United States who would have to do likewise.

Q: And do you not also believe that in thousands of cities the population would kill the doctor who found himself in the position?

A: I do not believe so because they would not know. How would they know whether the doctor had a drug that would or would not relieve? The doctor would not know himself, because he would have to experiment first.

Q: Witness, I put a hypothetical case to you. If we are to turn to reality other questions would arise. I simply want to hear now your general attitude to this problem. You are then of the opinion that a doctor should not carry out the order. Are you also of the opinion that the politician should not give such an order?

A: Yes. I believe he should not give such an order.

Q: Is this not a purely political decision which must be left to the discretion of the political leader?

A: Not necessarily. He should seek the best advice that he can obtain.

Q: If he is informed that this one experiment on this one prisoner would save the whole city, he may give the order despite the fact that the doctor does not wish to carry it out, is that what you think?

A: He could then give the order, but if the doctor still believed that it was contrary to his moral responsibilities, then the doctor should not carry out the order.

Q: That is another question, whether or not he carries it out, but in such cases you consider it is permissible to give that order, is that what I understood you to say?

A: After he has obtained the best advice on the subject which he can obtain.

Q: Then he can give the order. Yes or no?

A: Yes.

*   *   *

4.

Warren E. Burger
Reflections on Law and
Experimental Medicine*

*   *   *

Science unrestrained would be somewhat like an absolute monarch—a great servant, but a terrible master. Law is inherently restraint; it is a restraint on science as it is a restraint on kings, congresses, and presidents, and none of them really likes it very much. Those who become impatient with the slow pace of the law's response to the needs of science must remember that the history of Western philosophy shows

---

* 15 *UCLA Law Review* 436, 441–442 (1968). Reprinted by permission.

that we cherish many values above scientific advances; science must function within this framework.

Theologians, philosophers, and lawgivers must be receptive and alert to these new and changing problems. Experimental medicine presents a wide range of problems for which no unitary attitude or approach can provide a universal guide. Organ transplants and use of mechanical devices to preserve life present one kind of problem. But planned or controlled genetics presents quite another, for there one deals largely with future beings. The lay mind cannot avoid a feeling or intuitive reaction that some of those who speak in terms of "managing" the development of a better strain of human beings may at best be confusing genetics with animal husbandry and at worst talking about plans for a "master race." Obviously there are certain genetic drawbacks to letting people reproduce themselves indiscriminately, but absent some specific disqualification where medicine can predict certain tragic consequences of a union between certain genetic types, ordinary mortals will continue to mate on an emotional rather than a scientific plane. Others will see some disturbing portents in any "planned propagation" however socially desirable and notwithstanding the benefit of breeding a disease-resistant race. It was one thing for Henry Wallace to make better and richer corn or for wealthy folk to breed better horses and dogs, but quite another to tinker with the human race. Perhaps some of the prize fight and professional football managers would like to pick mates for their stables of athletes and I am willing to assume they could propagate some superb gladiators. Perhaps no one could restrain willing participation in a program to breed better athletes, but one must shudder at the prospect of governmental intervention in this area of private choice.

*   *   *

One of the great episodes in legal history is that in which Lord Coke, as Lord Chancellor of England, first announced what was then a radical, indeed treasonable doctrine of English jurisprudence: Even the King was not above the law. Catherine Drinker Bowen relates that Lord Coke threw himself prostrate in front of the throne symbolically acknowledging that he was below the Crown just as he insisted the King was below the law.

Science and medicine, like kings, presidents,

and parliaments must remain below, but let us hope not immobilized by, law.

NOTE

PAUL FREUND
ETHICAL PROBLEMS IN HUMAN
EXPERIMENTATION*

*   *   *

[I]f the law is conservative, it is also creative and responsive. As the law has raised up a right of privacy, a creative, innovating doctrine, so it may come to recognize a right of experimentation on human beings. Social interests and expectations, if they are in fact justified, can expect eventually to be reflected in the law. For example, the duty of corporate directors to their stockholders, a duty that was long thought to be the single-minded obligation to provide the maximum profits to the shareholders, has not prevented recognition of a privilege to contribute corporate earnings to educational and charitable causes, a doctrine for which the medical schools and the hospitals have reason to be grateful. The social responsibility of the corporation has thus qualified the single-minded duty of the directors to their shareholders in the light of social concerns and social pressures.

*   *   *

The law has indeed yielded in its absolutes where some worthy risk has pressed for acceptance. . . . The crux of the matter is to find the inner checks or other safeguards that will mitigate and justify the risks.

*   *   *

5.

Hans Jonas
Philosophical Reflections on
Experimenting with Human Subjects†

*   *   *

[W]e must face the somber truth that the *ultima ratio* of communal life is and has always

* 273 *New England Journal of Medicine* 687 (1965). Reprinted by permission.
† 98 *Daedalus* 219, 223–224 (1969). Reprinted by permission of Daedalus, Journal of the American Academy of Arts and Sciences, Boston, Massachusetts.

been the compulsory, vicarious sacrifice of individual lives. The primordial sacrificial situation is that of outright human sacrifices in early communities. These were not acts of blood-lust or gleeful savagery; they were the solemn execution of a supreme, sacral necessity. One of the fellowship of men had to die so that all could live, the earth be fertile, the cycle of nature renewed. The victim often was not a captured enemy, but a select member of the group: "The king must die." If there was cruelty here, it was not that of men, but that of the gods, or rather of the stern order of things, which was believed to exact that price for the bounty of life. To assure it for the community, and to assure it ever again, the awesome *quid pro quo* had to be paid ever again.

Far be it from me, and far should it be from us, to belittle from the height of our enlightened knowledge the majesty of the underlying conception. The particular *causal* views that prompted our ancestors have long since been relegated to the realm of superstition. But in moments of national danger we still send the flower of our young manhood to offer their lives for the continued life of the community, and, if it is a just war, we see them go forth as consecrated and strangely ennobled by a sacrificial role. Nor do we make their going forth depend on their own will and consent, much as we may desire and foster these: We conscript them according to law. We conscript the best and feel morally disturbed if the draft, either by design or in effect, works so that mainly the disadvantaged, socially less useful, more expendable, make up those whose lives are to buy ours. No rational persuasion of the pragmatic necessity here at work can do away with the feeling, mixed of gratitude and guilt, that the sphere of the sacred is touched with the vicarious offering of life for life. Quite apart from these dramatic occasions, there is, it appears, a persistent and constitutive aspect of human immolation to the very being and prospering of human society—an immolation in terms of life and happiness, imposed or voluntary, of few for many. . . . We can never rest comfortably in the belief that the soil from which our satisfactions sprout is not watered with the blood of martyrs. But a troubled conscience compels us, the undeserving beneficiaries, to ask: Who is to be martyred? in the service of what cause? and by whose choice?

*   *   *

B.

Medical Innovation and the State—A Case Study of Oral Contraception

1.

Experimentation, Therapy, and Success— The First Phase (1951–1960)

a.

Gregory Pincus
The Control of Fertility*

*   *   *

In 1937, Makepeace, Weinstein, and Friedman noted the effectiveness of progesterone as an ovulation inhibitor in the rabbit, but the logical extension of this observation into a more intensive study of the nature of the progesterone action as well as the action of certain derivatives and putative metabolites were not reported by us until 1953.

Why this "logical extension" occurred after a latent period of approximately 16 years is a question concerning which we have raised some speculation. Certainly, judging by publications, there was a period during which our own activities in this field fell to a minimum, both absolutely and relatively. An examination of the bibliography of any book concerned with reproductive phenomena discloses similarly a minimum number of publications during the period 1942–1945, and a significant rise in output from 1950 on. In our own case, the special demands of "war" research accounted for a shift of interest to studies of adrenocortical function, particularly in relation to physical and mental stress, and this interest has continued to a greater or lesser degree. Indeed, World War II probably accounts for the lapse observed generally. In our case, the increase of activity as indicated by publications from 1950 on has been due to two overtly ascertainable factors: (a) a visit from Mrs. Margaret Sanger in 1951 and (b) the emergence of the appreciation of the importance of the "population explosion."

At the time of her visit, Mrs. Sanger's interest in the world-wide dissemination of information on birth control was at high tide. Her experience as President of the International Planned Parenthood Federation had made her aware of the deficiencies of conventional con-

traceptive methods, particularly in underdeveloped areas of the world. Her hope, expressed to us, was that a relatively simple and fool-proof method might be developed through laboratory research. Drs. Chang and Pirie and I had already had some experience with hyaluronidase inhibitors in the rabbit but we had found that such potent inhibitors could act only on direct contact with sperm and that there was no possibility of an effect by parenteral administration. Although some preliminary experiments by the late Dr. Abraham Stone had indicated that at least one of these inhibitors might be quite active as the component of an intravaginal preparation in the human, the limitations to its use still appeared to be rather formidable. Accordingly, Dr. Chang and I drew up a modest project proposal that received support under a grant from the Planned Parenthood Federation of America. Work under this grant resulted in the paper on the rabbits mentioned above and in the finding that the compounds that we found to be potent as ovulation inhibitors in the rabbit were also quite active as antifertility agents in the rat.

The impetus to research, particularly on the physiology of reproduction, given by the recognition of the population explosion has been described a number of times. Although the physiologist has generally been called upon to undertake research which might lead to easily effective and acceptable means of birth control, his role is indeed a much wider one. The modern-day investigator cannot be satisfied with the invention of a "cunning device." The present accumulated knowledge concerning reproductive processes indicates that the production of gametes, their transport and mating, their fusion, and the fate of the fertilized egg involves an intricate and delicately balanced set of sequential events. Interfering with this sequence at any of a large number of stages may have physiologic consequences that are not apparent on the surface. The research worker is therefore compellingly motivated to arrive at as complete an understanding as possible of the processes involved in the great act of reproduction. Furthermore, the understanding which the physiologist seeks must be imparted to others. Often both the nature and the degree of information that must be imparted for thorough understanding may be highly technical and even abtruse to professionals such as

---

* New York: Academic Press 5–8 (1965). Copyright 1965 Academic Press. Reprinted by permission.

physicians in family planning clinics and public health workers.

Under the ivory tower conception of scientific research, much of the foregoing is irrelevant. More simply stated, the job of the scientist is to undertake experimentation and to publish the results of such experimentation. What happens thereafter is allegedly not his business. This concept has been dealt demoralizing blows, particularly during and since World War II. The rapid transition from the research laboratory to the world-wide application of significant discovery has demanded the attention of the scientist to [the] . . . consequences of his activity. . . .

Although in the opinion of many the population problem facing the community of men is as important as the problem of the development of atomic energy, the biological scientist has thus far not been vigorously communicative. . . . The physiological research worker thus far has for the most part confined his publication to scientific journals, and the publications by members of the medical profession have been chiefly concerned with medical practice in relation to birth control. The call-for-action programs have largely passed over the research laboratory.

I suspect that the working physiologist is not too unhappy about being neglected by the "pointing-with-alarmers." It is not merely the residue of ivory-tower psychology that animates him. It is primarily his feeling that so much remains to be learned about the basic processes of reproduction, let alone practical control measures. . . .

*   *   *

NOTES

NOTE 1.

GREGORY PINCUS
SOME EFFECTS OF PROGESTERONE AND RELATED COMPOUNDS UPON REPRODUCTION AND EARLY DEVELOPMENT IN MAMMALS*

In several publications we have indicated the rather remarkable role that progesterone, the characteristic corpus luteum hormone, plays in mammalian reproduction. Consider that progesterone: (a) is a significant conditioning substance for normal mating reflexes in a number of animals; (b) has its special effect upon both tubal and uterine contraction while the eggs and sperm

---

* *Report of the Proceedings of the Fifth International Conference on Planned Parenthood.* London: International Planned Parenthood Federation 175–182 (1955). Reprinted by permission.

are travelling through the oviducts; (c) may in certain dosages act as an inhibitor of fertilization in vivo, perhaps because of its effect on oviductal contractility; (d) is essential for ovum implantation, the maintenance of the fetus, and of normal uterine tone during pregnancy; (e) inhibits ovulation during normal pregnancy, and can do so on administration to preovulatory animals; and (f) plays a role in parturition. Therefore, any experimental alteration of its normal action or abnormal intensification of certain of its effects may be expected to interfere with reproduction in the female. Experimental studies may take two courses: they may seek to antagonize or inhibit effects of progesterones, *e.g.*, by estrogens or specific progesterone antimetabolites, or they may be designed to induce progesterone effects at critical stages, *e.g.*, ovulation inhibition, during the follicular phase of the cycle by progesterone or other progestins.

Our efforts have largely been directed to the latter objectives. There have been a number of reasons for this. First of all the progestational phenomena are physiologically normal and unlikely to be accompanied by untoward and unwanted side-effects. Thus progesterone is a nontoxic steroid tolerated in large dose and in fact secreted endogenously in large amount during pregnancy. The human use of progesterone has long been established as a safe and efficacious procedure in a variety of conditions and diseases, and its effectiveness by oral, parenteral or intravaginal routes has been demonstrated. Finally, since our interest has been in the control of the early stages of the reproductive process, *i.e.*, ovulation, fertilization, ovum development and implantation, the use of a compound having established effects during these stages seemed advantageous.

*   *   *

Basing our initial investigations upon the known effects of progesterone as an inhibitor of ovulation in rabbits, rats and other mammals, *i.e.*, guinea pigs, mice, sheep and cow, we have observed that this inhibitory effect is proportional to dosage in the rabbit (by subcutaneous injection). In these two species also progesterone administered orally is a significant inhibitor of ovulation. This led us to examine the effects of oral progesterone upon the human menstrual cycle. Using a standard dosage (300 mgm. per day) and regime of administration (from days 5 to 20 of the menstrual cycle), we have observed a significant suppression of the usual signs of ovulation, *i.e.*, the characteristic basal temperature rise, the typical secretory endometrium and the "ovulation" flush of vaginal cornification. Since these indirect signs of ovulation are normally the result of the secretion of progesterone by the corpus luteum, the suppressive effect of oral progesterone would appear to involve an inhibition of endogenous corpus luteum hormone production with, in certain instances at any rate, little or no progestational effect of the administered hormone. There is some suggestion in our data of a somewhat greater inhibitory action of progesterone in successive cycles of administration. This is supported by our findings on direct inspection of ovaries in ten cases at laparotomy; these were examined from days 20 to 26 of the first cycle in which they received oral progesterone; five of the ten patients had no corpora lutea and an indication of abnormal corpora was had in three others. We may therefore conclude that progesterone taken by mouth during the follicular phase of the cycle tends to suppress ovulation in the human female. One undesirable feature of our data is the exhibition of escape bleeding during progesterone medication in approximately 18 per cent of the cycles.

There is a suggestion in our data that in women exogenous oral progesterone may act as an antifertility agent for reasons other than its ovulation-inhibiting action. The frequent occurrence of atypical endometria and . . . indication of suppressive action on endogenous progestin suggest possible effects on ovum and sperm transport and implantation. The fact that in 71 cycles of progesterone treatment there were no pregnancies, whereas in 44 cycles following its discontinuance four pregnancies occurred would tend to support this notion, particularly since our follow-up studies indicated prompt restoration of ovulation and normal cycle lengths in post-medication cycles.

We have described our studies with a series of steroid compounds administered to rabbits and rats. Some 15 compounds have acted as ovulation inhibitors in the rabbit, and three of these proved to be clearly more potent than progesterone on a dosage basis. One of these three, 17-a-methyl progesterone, was highly effective by the parenteral route but lacked effectiveness when administered orally. Two, 19-nor ethinyl testosterone (XIII) and 17-ethinyl estraeneolone (XIV), were much more effective than progesterone by either route. This same relationship was observed in the rat. XIII and XIV have been administered orally in low dosage to a lim-

ited number of patients. Each gave notable indication of ovulation inhibition not only by our indirect indices, but most strikingly by an almost complete prevention of pregnanediol excretion. With neither thus far has there been any escape bleeding.

. . . We cannot on the basis of our observations thus far designate the ideal antifertility agent, nor the ideal mode of administration. But a foundation has been laid for the useful exploitation of the problem on an objective basis. The delicately balanced sequential processes involved in normal mammalian reproduction are clearly attackable. Our objective is to disrupt them in such a way that no physiological cost to the organism is involved. That objective will undoubtedly be attained by careful scientific investigation.

* * *

NOTE 2.

SIR SOLLY ZUCKERMAN
SUMMING UP RESEARCH INTO BIOLOGICAL
METHODS OF CONTROLLING FERTILITY*

* * *

Promising though they may have appeared at first sight, I think it is also fair to conclude that the observations reported by Dr. Pincus do not bring us as close as we should like to the goal of our researches. We can all agree with him that progesterone is capable of inhibiting ovulation in rabbits, and the results which he has reported for rats are also best interpreted on this hypothesis. We are in difficulties, however, about the conclusion that progesterone, when taken by mouth, can also inhibit ovulation in women. This view was not shared by Dr. Masaomi Ishikawa, who, however, thought it possible that the treatment could prevent fertilization through changes induced by the hormone in the cervical epithelium; nor by Dr. Abraham Stone, who, too, has experimented with this form of treatment. When considering the results of all this work we need, however, to remind ourselves that we have little in the way of direct observation to go on. Dr. Pincus inferred the suppression of ovulation from a variety of indirect signs, as diagnosed for him by Dr. Rock: for example, changes in the basal body temperature; the character of the endometrium as revealed by biopsy; and the nature of the vaginal smear. But if we

* *Report of the Proceedings of the Fifth International Conference on Planned Parenthood.* London: International Planned Parenthood Federation 212 (1955). Reprinted by permission.

accept the views of other authorities, these indices are by no means 100 per cent certain; nor are they made more so by the few observations we have of ovaries at laparotomy, or by observations on pregnanediol excretion. Not until we have very many more fertility records of the kind to which Dr. Pincus has also referred will it, in fact, be possible to draw conclusions about the effectiveness of the oral administration of progesterone; or, indeed, about the more promising but smaller number of results which Dr. Pincus has reported about the use of 19-nor-17-ethinyl-testosterone and 17-ethinyl estraeneolone.

* * *

b.

**Hale H. Cook, Clarence J. Gamble, and
Adaline P. Satterthwaite
Oral Contraception by Norethynodrel—
A 3-Year Field Study***

In the many areas of the world where the standard of living is at subsistence level, each specific improvement in death control serves to depress that standard. As the living standard goes down, malnutrition grows, ill health increases, and the death rate rises. Furthermore, such low income levels leave little money available for public health activities. In these areas widespread provision of effective and acceptable methods of pregnancy spacing is essential to further health improvement. It is encouraging that statesmen in many countries are now becoming aware of this problem.

Methods of contraception have been available for years. Most of them involve some interference with the normal pattern of sexual intercourse, its prelude or postlude; others are of questionable reversibility (vasectomy and salpingectomy) or are considered dangerous (intrauterine and intracervical devices). Experience has shown that contraception can be widely effective when made available to all and promoted with enthusiasm. Yet, because of the disadvantages of present methods, the wish is commonly expressed for an oral contraceptive, preferably long lasting, and certainly easy to take.

The observation that certain western American Indians ate the leaves of *Lithospermum ruderale* to prevent conception suggested that oral contraception might be practical. Pharmacologists found that this and related plants contain substances that inactivate pituitary gonadotro-

pins in vitro and in vivo with failure of the gonads to develop in immature animals and reversible cessation of the estrous cycle in those already mature. Preliminary trials in humans were disappointing.

The observation by Nag that rats fed field peas (*Pisum sativum*) were less fertile stimulated Sanyal to isolate metaxylohydroquinone as the active substance. He reported that this apparently nontoxic and inexpensive substance reduced the pregnancy rate of women by 50 to 75 per cent. Such incomplete effectiveness inhibits widespread patient acceptance; the method has not gained general approval.

Antihyaluronidases are reported to be effective contraceptives when used as vaginal suppositories. Most investigations testing them by mouth have not shown any significant effect. Also recently under trial are cirantin, an oil extract of orange skins, and rottlerin, an extract of a Philippine milkweed. Mode of action and clinical effectiveness are under preliminary investigation.

Progesterone in pregnancy blocks ovulation and so prevents a superimposed pregnancy. Simulating this hormonal balance characteristic of pregnancy should thus be a form of contraception approximating normal physiology. Progesterone itself has been tried, but for oral use 300 mg. daily is required. This is expensive for general use. Several progestin-like synthetic steroids have been developed within the last 10 years. Tests by Pincus and associates show these effectively suppressed ovulation when given by mouth to animals and to women. Three of these compounds have reached commercial production: 17a-ethinyl-19-nortestosterone, 17a-ethyl-19-nortestosterone, and 17a-ethinyl-5(10)-estraeneolone, known as norethynodrel.

The ideal contraceptive must be effective in preventing conception, safe for the persons using it, psychologically and economically acceptable, and reliably reversible. Although no present method is ideal on all counts, the preliminary work with norethynodrel suggested that it might closely approach this ideal. Therefore, in 1957 we decided to test this product in the field.

Method

A region in which population pressure is a public health problem was sought—one which has a high birth rate, low death rate, and low per capita income. Puerto Rico has a birth rate which averaged 41 per 1,000 population from 1946 to 1950 and declined to 35 by 1956. The death rate dropped steadily from 1935 to 1955 and is now between 7 and 8 per 1,000 population. The an-

* 82 *American Journal of Obstetrics and Gynecology* 437–442, 444, 445 (1961). Reprinted by permission.

nual income per person rose rapidly in the last 10 years; it reached $410 in 1955. That for continental United States in the same year was $1,866. The population doubled during the last 50 years despite a net loss by migration of half a million people. The island contains 675 people for each of its 3,435 square miles, although half the land is steep and noncultivable. Population density is comparable to the flat and fertile Ganges River Valley and the Malabar Coast of India.

Headquarters for field work was Humacao, the twelfth largest municipality in Puerto Rico, population 35,000 in 1950, and demographically typical of the island. The study was under the auspices of the Ryder Memorial Hospital. Its gynecologist and obstetrician (A.P.S.) had medical supervision of the study, made the physical examinations, and arranged for social service workers to distribute the contraceptive materials and instructions, keep records, and visit patients as necessary. The data were analyzed at the Harvard School of Public Health after field visits to organize the plan of investigation and to collect the needed details.

*   *   *

The present report concerns two groups of women. Work with the R series started in April, 1957. Each family in three crowded urban areas was paid a home visit by a social worker. In the first two of these areas 1,107 persons were found living in one-story houses on 7 acres of land. This is five times the density for the city as a whole. Subsequently, one rural and one suburban area were surveyed; here poor families live on government land allotted to them for housing. All women living with their husbands, having at least 2 children, not then pregnant, and aged 40 years or less, were invited to use the contraceptive pills which the social worker offered to bring them, without charge, every month.

The second group, called the P series, was recruited, starting in May, 1957, from women who came to the Ryder Memorial Hospital Outpatient Clinic for contraceptive aid, met the R series requirements, and chose to try this method. Alternative methods offered were the diaphragm, vaginal jelly or foam, and condoms. Most of the early P cases were recruited from women coming for postpartum examinations; to these women contraception is regularly offered. As word spread that the pills were available, without charge other than the initial $2 clinic registration fee, increasing numbers came specifically to secure norethynodrel.

All women in both groups were given an initial pelvic and general physical examination. Each was provided a bottle of 20 tablets and instructed as follows:

Take one pill each day with your evening meal. Begin on the fourth day after the day on which menses start. Stop when your bottle of 20 pills is empty. Wait until your next menses and secure another bottle of pills. Start the pills again on the fifth menstrual day. If, by any chance, you do not have a period within 10 days of stopping, get a new bottle and start taking the pills that evening. If you wait longer than 10 days you may become pregnant.

If you begin to bleed while still taking the pills, take 2 pills every day until the bleeding stops, then one pill daily until the bottle is empty. If anything prevents you from getting the next bottle of pills until later than the fifth day of menstruation, start again by taking 2 pills each day for as many days as you started late, after the fifth day, then one pill every day.

Those with postpartum amenorrhea were directed to begin the pills immediately.

After their initial visit, women in the R series were given supplies each month in their homes while those of the P series were instructed to return to the hospital for further supplies when menstruation had begun. A record was made at each visit of the date of starting the tablets, the date, character, and duration of the menses, frequency of intercourse, and any symptoms or difficulties noted during the preceding interval. Women who had used the method regularly for several months without difficulty were given 2 months' supply. Those who did not return were followed up by a personal visit from one of the social workers or by letter if they lived too far away. Care was taken to find out why they had stopped using norethynodrel but no effort was made to influence them to resume the program.

Information available in 1957 suggested that 9.85 mg. of norethynodrel combined with 0.15 mg. of the synthetic estrin, ethynylestradiol-3-methyl ether, was the optimal daily dosage. Subsequent experience suggested that a smaller dose was equally effective and less apt to give certain unpleasant symptoms; therefore early in 1959 we began giving half the previous daily dose, tablets containing 5.0 mg. of norethynodrel with 0.075 mg. of ethynylestradiol-3-methyl ether.*

. . . Our report is based on all recorded experience of the first 150 R cases and the first 400 P cases through February, 1960. All women us-

---

* The 10 mg. and 5 mg. tablets, known as Enovid, have been supplied by G. D. Searle and Company.

ing the method, plus all who had discontinued it and could be located within 20 miles of the hospital, were interviewed beginning in November, 1959; a comprehensive questionnaire was filled out, and, on those who could come to the hospital, a pelvic and general physical examination was made. . . .

Results

During the 518 woman-years of experience with norethynodrel accumulated by the 550 women in this study 11 pregnancies occurred. Of these, 4 had started before norethynodrel was begun. Three occurred when the women waited more than the prescribed 10 days for the return of menses (one woman waiting 15, one 20, and one 30 days). The other 4 followed failure of the women to take the tablets daily; trustworthy details as to number and sequence of omissions could not be secured.

Tietze has defined three measures of the effectiveness of contraceptive methods: *physiologic* effectiveness is that measured when a given method is used according to instructions on every occasion of need; *clinical* effectiveness when in the hands of users under actual use conditions; and *demographic* effectiveness by the reduction of the birth rate of an entire population who have been instructed in the given method and to whom materials are available whether the individuals are using them or not.

No woman who followed instructions has become pregnant during 518 woman-years of use. Norethynodrel is thus physiologically completely effective. If the 11 pregnancies are attributed to faults in the method, the pregnancy rate for all users is 2.1 conceptions per 100 years of exposure. In Puerto Rico the fertility rate is approximately constant from age 20 years to age 30, after which it decreases. Our population, married an average of 8.7 years, was aged 27.5 years at the beginning of this trial. The rate of 2.1 thus contrasts directly with their pre-instruction rate of 110 pregnancies per 100 years of exposure.* Preceding attempts at contraception had not affected fertility; the 176 women reporting previous experience with one or more contraceptive methods had a rate of 106 pregnancies per 100 years of exposure, while the 328 reporting no such experience had a rate of 110.

---

* "Years of exposure" are the total years married less 10 months for each full-term delivery and 4 months for each abortion. Time of living separately, though appreciable for a few families, was not enough for the whole to warrant consideration in the calculation.

Considering the population of those who at any time tried norethynodrel one can compare the "community" preinstruction pregnancy rate . . . for all women who could be followed up, combining active and discontinued cases, of 17 per 100 years of exposure. The rate after stopping for all women who stopped was 91 pregnancies per 100 years of exposure. These results demonstrate that *physiological* effectiveness is complete, *clinical* effectiveness is great, and *demographic* effectiveness, though reduced by the continued fertility of those who have discontinued the method, is marked.

No method of pregnancy spacing, even though highly effective, is justifiable if it endangers life or health. Only 2 women have died while using this method, one from burns and one from chronic hypertension with congestive heart failure. Another woman developed pulmonary tuberculosis, controlled by therapy. None of these effects could in any way be attributed to norethynodrel. Hemoglobin levels of 137 women were determined after an average of 14 months of use; these women showed an average of 10.4 ± 0.11 (standard error) Gm. per cent as compared with 10.6 ± 0.13 Gm. per cent for 79 women of comparable age (28.6 years) and parity (3.7 pregnancies) attending the Ryder Memorial Hospital Outpatient Clinic but not using norethynodrel. Blood pressure was neither raised nor lowered significantly as shown by observations on 179 users (average 13 months' use) compared with 85 controls. Biochemical studies made on 300 users by Pincus and associates showed no evidence of hidden toxicity after as many as 33 months of use. Psychological effects . . . have not been detected.

Popular rumor had it that this procedure caused cancer. A definitive answer is impossible within 3 years and with as small a sample as now available. Careful watch has been kept for suggestive indications, especially during the final physical examinations. During 698 woman-years of observation (518 woman-years of use and 180 woman-years of post-use experience), no signs of cancer, other than cervical, have been noted.

Cervical biopsies were taken on 40 women and were examined histologically by Rock and Garcia at the Free Hospital for Women, Brookline, Massachusetts. Carcinoma in situ was reported once, in a woman 33 years old, after 6 months' use of norethynodrel. Eight months after this biopsy she discontinued the method. At that time and also 6 months later biopsies were negative. Lee found by biopsy of 3,149 healthy Puerto

Rican women that 25, or 0.79 per cent, had carcinoma in situ. After 3 years' observation without treatment none had invasive carcinoma. Other studies showed 28 per cent invasive after 5 years and 33 per cent invasive after 9 years, without treatment.

Epidermoid carcinoma, Grade II, was found in another woman. On starting the method she had normal pelvic findings. A vaginal smear 18 months later was reported suggestive of cancer. A cervical biopsy was made after 21 months' experience, carcinoma found, norethynodrel stopped, and radiation treatment begun. To be allowed to enter the series, this patient first gave her age as 36; actually she was 46 years old. The rate for cervical cancer in the 45 year age group in Puerto Rico is now 1.18 per 1,000 women per year, though only 0.25 at the average age for our group. Two cases during 698 woman-years of experience is well within the limits of what may be expected from chance alone.

Epigastric distress, nausea, and vomiting; headaches and dizziness; changes in accustomed menstrual pattern, including premenstrual tension and nervousness; pelvic pain; chloasma; and changes in weight and appetite were the more common side effects noted.

Some complaint was recorded in 18 per cent of the cycles; of the 550 users, 388 or 71 per cent voiced such complaints at least once. Symptoms were most common during the first 3 months of use, but could occur at any time, even after 30 months of trouble-free use. Withdrawals from the study because of side effects were at the rate of 6 per cent of cases in the first month of experience, 4 per cent in the second, 3 per cent in the third, and 1 per cent each month thereafter. Women of the R series and those in the P series receiving 5 mg. dosage from the outset have shown only two thirds the average withdrawal rate. Users described most symptoms as likely to be more severe when starting a medication cycle or in the interval between the twentieth tablet and the following menses, that is, during a change of the hormonal level of the body. For 121 persons, 22 per cent of all users, side effects were so unpleasant that the method was discarded. The other 267 complainers, finding the reactions could be tolerated until they disappeared, continued the method, at least until some other reason for stopping occurred.

Many of the changes observed are commonly associated with early pregnancy, for example, nausea, vomiting, dizziness, headache, increased vaginal discharge, and chloasma. Pa-

tients frequently volunteered that they felt pregnant. Softening and bluing of the cervix occasionally led other doctors examining these women to make a diagnosis of early pregnancy whereupon contraceptive treatment was stopped and the women did become pregnant.

* * *

The ratio of observed to expected pregnancies is a measure of the effectiveness of the program. In their preceding married lives during which their average age was 24 years, the users of norethynodrel had had 59 pregnancies per 100 woman-years. The first significant drop in fertility in Puerto Rico occurs after age 30 years, a greater age than the average for women of this series at the end of the study. The preceding rate thus may be used as a base for comparison. During 518 woman-years of experience 316 pregnancies would be expected, and 90 per cent or 284 would have resulted in live births. Only 11 children were born. Use of norethynodrel by the 550 women has apparently prevented the birth of 273 unwanted children.

* * *

Norethynodrel has proved in this field trial an effective, safe, reversible, and fairly acceptable method for the spacing of births. Its suitability in public health programs, applicable to a community within the usual resources of funds, physicians, and the habits of people remains to be tested.

NOTES

NOTE 1.

EDRIS RICE-WRAY
FIELD STUDY WITH ENOVID AS A
CONTRACEPTIVE AGENT*

* * *

The angle I have taken will interest anyone who is interested in Enovid as a contraceptive and also those who are interested in doing a field study because this is a report of an actual field study. There are many things you have to learn by trial and error, such as how to handle the patients, how you present the project and what you say to them so they take it. . . .

. . . Puerto Rico is one of the most densely populated countries in the world. We are all in-

* *Proceedings of a Symposium on 19-Nor Progestational Steroids.* Chicago: G. D. Searle & Co. 78–82, 92–93 (1957). Reprinted by permission.

terested in finding some reliable contraceptive which is cheap, acceptable to the people, easy to take and something the people themselves would be interested in taking. We are happy to say they have liked the oral tablet method very much.

Selection of Subjects

The women chosen for this (field) study were from the low income population living in a housing development project in a slum clearance area. They were chosen because of accessibility and because the stability of such a housing development population is greater than that of others.

Our objective was to have a case load of 100 subjects but, since some of them kept dropping out for various reasons which will be discussed later, we had to keep adding new subjects to keep from falling below 100.

Before starting the program, we interviewed the superintendent of the housing development to get his cooperation and to make sure that he would not oppose our work. We found him to be a very intelligent man with much enthusiasm for the work of reducing the birth rate in Puerto Rico. We were gratified to have him promise his wholehearted cooperation. He made available to us the records of the families living in the housing development and requested that his staff give us the cooperation necessary. The social worker on this program formerly worked with the housing authority and was already acquainted with a fair number of the people living in the area. She studied the records in the files of the housing development and selected names of families in which the mother was less than 40 and had one or more children. These were then visited in order to pick out 100 who were suitable for the program. Many of them were automatically unsuitable because they had been sterilized or were pregnant. Others had moved away.

Preliminary Interview

The worker introduced herself as the executive secretary of the Family Planning Association of Puerto Rico. She explained that it was a private agency such as the "National Foundation for Infantile Paralysis" or the "Cancer League" and had no connection with the government of Puerto Rico. It was made clear that the objective of this association was to help mothers and fathers to plan their families so that they do not have more children than they can properly take care of, and also so that they can have their children when they want them.

Of the group that was visited, only one did not accept because of religion. In one instance the husband was opposed to using any method. The rest were very receptive to the idea of avoiding pregnancies by a method so simple as that of taking tablets.

The control group was chosen the same way. The worker explained to these women that she was making a survey of families to learn something of the size of the families in the housing development. There were 125 in this control group, so as to allow for those who would move away or those who would not match with the study group. (They were being matched as to age of mother, number of children, number of pregnancies and years married.) All the people in this area are similar in their economic status and educational level. These women were questioned as to the number of children, the ages of their children, whether they used any contraceptive or not and, if so, since when.

We began giving the medication early in April. These women were advised to start taking the tablets five days after the start of the menses, whether they were bleeding or not. They were told to take one tablet daily for twenty days and then stop. They were told that during the period when they have finished the twenty tablets and are waiting for the menses, they may have intercourse without fear of pregnancy. They were made to understand that two or three days after stopping the medication they would have the menses. It was explained to them that it is necessary to use the method properly if they want to succeed or do not want to have escape bleeding during the month. They were told that if they were to stop the tablet one day the next day they would probably have bleeding. If this occurred they were instructed to double the dose for two days and, if it did not stop then, to take three for one day. In our experience, this always stopped bleeding.

A few weeks later, a reporter of Puerto Rico's "yellow sheet" called on the Secretary of Health and questioned him concerning a program of giving contraceptive tablets to people in Rio Piedras. He claimed that public health nurses were working in the program. The Secretary of Health called the writer, who was the director of the public health services in Rio Piedras, to find out about it. He was told that such a program was in progress and that the writer was directing it, but was doing so on her own time, apart from her public health duties. He replied that it was difficult to see how the two could be separated, whereupon he was told that since this is a democracy, the writer felt that any government employee had the right to spend his spare time as he pleased. He asked numerous questions concerning the project and, finally, when he was assured that none of these patients was being examined in the Health Department, nor were public health personnel working on the project on government time, he answered the reporter accordingly and apparently dropped the matter.

The next day an article appeared in the newspaper stating that Dr. Rice-Wray had "confessed" to directing the project and quoting Dr. Pons as saying that he did not consider it proper for government employees to engage in neo-Malthusian activities, and that he did not approve of the Department being used as "bait" for such a project.

Whether Dr. Pons actually said these things or not is uncertain because this newspaper is most unreliable. However, the very fact that the article did appear caused momentary harm to the program and prompted some of the patients to withdraw.

Problems Encountered

The first two months of the study the worker gave the patient just one bottle of twenty tablets. It was felt that this would make it easier for the patient to know when to stop the medication. Later it was decided to leave her two bottles of twenty tablets each, for two months. This was done because it was often found difficult to interview the patients at the proper time. A list was made of dates to visit the patients. The idea was to visit each one within a few days after she stopped the medication. This did not work out very well. . . .

*　　*　　*

However, it was found that when two bottles of tablets were left with the patients, 1 or 2 per cent kept on taking them without stopping the five days for the menses. In the beginning, several patients came to the office in a state of great excitement when the tablets were used up and the worker had not come to give them more. In spite of the careful instructions given, they thought that they were going to get pregnant if they did not take the tablets every day. This showed us the necessity of having to repeat and repeat the instructions given to these women. We cannot assume that having given the instructions once, or even twice, that they will be understood completely. To eliminate this prob-

lem, we supplied the patients with some printed instructions so that they could refer to them after the worker was gone. Most of these women can read and write, but for those who cannot there is always a school child in the family or a neighbor who can read them to them.

Sometimes people say to the patients: "How do you know what this is? It might be dangerous." This does not bother most of those who can reply: "I have been taking it eight or nine months and I am happy and I don't get pregnant." In the beginning, because of the newspaper article, some patients became afraid when hearing such remarks and stopped taking the tablets.

Analysis of Results of Study, Up to December 31, 1956

The total number of subjects who have taken the tablets is 221.

Adding the number of months of those patients who have been taking Enovid more than two months, we have a total of forty-seven patient years. During this time we have not had one single pregnancy that could be attributed to method failure. There was one woman who thought she only had to take the tablets when her husband was home. He traveled and she said: "I didn't take them when he was away. I took them only when he was here, of course." That is one of the women with whom we had a problem. She got pregnant.

There were seventeen pregnancies due to patient failure because they stopped the medication. Eight stopped it because of reaction, six because of carelessness (they forgot to take it), two because of fear of the medication already referred to, and one because she thought she had to take it only when her husband was home (his work caused him to be away often a week at a time). It was found that although the patients were often careless and forgot to take their tablets, they did not always get pregnant. . . .

*　　*　　*

Discussion

DR. [WARREN O.] NELSON: If I may, I should like to make a few remarks relevant to the use of this compound as a contraceptive measure. If it should be used in this capacity I believe there are certain considerations of importance.

*　　*　　*

I think there are at least two reasons for shortening the period of administration. Firstly, the matter of economy in countries where people really need an antifertility measure such as this compound might be. Secondly, the question of eliminating the need to administer so much drug for so long a time.

The latter consideration deserves attention since many people regard with concern the use of steroids or related substances over long periods of time. In the present instance, it is reasonable to suppose that a woman marrying at the age of 18 would begin to use the compound then. At that age she would have twenty-five to thirty years of reproductive expectancy. If we allow her four, five or six years off the drug while she has her planned family of two, three or four children, she still would be taking it for as long as twenty-five years. What would be the effect of this or any related compound over such a period of time? Obviously that question cannot be answered until such a study is actually made.

*   *   *

NOTE 2.

GREGORY PINCUS, JOHN ROCK, AND
CELSO R. GARCIA
FIELD TRIALS WITH NORETHYNODREL AS AN ORAL
CONTRACEPTIVE*

*   *   *

In the earliest report of the San Juan study Rice-Wray recorded the occurrence of unpleasant reactions . . . in approximately 17 per cent of the subjects. These side effects included occasional occurrence of nausea, dizziness, vomiting, headache, and gastralgia. We have noted previously that these reactions preponderate in the first few cycles of medication and that they are usually readily relieved by the administration of an antacid or of a placebo tablet consisting of lactose. . . . Again, it is suggestive that the frequency of occurrence is highest in the groups at the highest economic levels and lowest in the groups at the lowest economic levels. We have suspected a psychogenic element in these reactions since, on the initiation of each project, each subject was told she was to undertake a new type of contraception and that she should note the occurrence of special symptoms.

In Puerto Rico we have tested the possibility of a psychogenic element by studying two groups of women. In the first group were 15 women liv-

* Report of the Proceedings of the Sixth International Conference on Planned Parenthood. London: International Planned Parenthood Federation 216, 220–224 (1959). Reprinted by permission.

ing in a slum clearance area in a town quite distant from San Juan. They were offered the medication as a tried contraceptive, and no suggestion of the occurrence of side effects was made. The second group consisted of 28 women using other contraceptives who were told to continue with their accustomed method but to take the tablets for a few months to see if they were suited to continue with the new method later. To 15 of these women coded placebos were given, and to 13 coded true medication. The social workers distributing the tablets did not know which was which. . . . The percentage of reactions was lowest in the "no admonition" group, next highest in the group on placebos, and highest in the group receiving the true medication. The difference between the latter two groups is not significant statistically, and that between the "no admonition" group and the true medication group is marginally significant. The higher frequency of breakthrough bleeding in the true medication group is probably attributable to the medication . . . and is reflected in the lower mean cycle length. The amenorrhea incidence appears to be a matter of chance; but it is interesting to note that breakthrough and amenorrhea characterize the placebo group, the former doubtless representing the frequency of natural occurrence of short cycles. In brief, a psychogenic element in reaction rate is clearly indicated by these data, and it certainly accounts for the majority of the reactions.

*   *   *

[A] number of these subjects were given physical examinations from time to time. These examinations ordinarily involved a simple physical check-up, a thorough pelvic examination, and the taking of an endometrial biopsy. In the San Juan project there were 138 such examinations made during medication and 17 following cessation of medication [out of 438 subjects]; in the Humacao-R project there have been 13 examinations during medication [out of 117 subjects]; and in the Haiti project 19 in medication cycles and four post-medication [out of 149 subjects]. In the Humacao-P project practically every subject was given a pelvic examination before medication was initiated, and a little less than half the subjects were similarly examined at least once during medication. No obvious pathology was detected in the patients in the San Juan series except for a few conditions (e.g., a vaginal herniation, a few cervical infections, uterine fibroma) either antedating the medication or ascribable to acute events irrelevant to the medication. Similar unremarkable observations were made of the Haiti and Humacao-R subjects.

[T]he pre-medication and post-medication notes on the pelvic examinations . . . indicate: (a) that in the course of medication a large proportion of the small, involuted uteri tend to return to normal size but not to hypertrophy, (b) that cervical lesions tend to increase in frequency with increasing cycles of medication, and (c) that no significant change is observable in the adnexa. The apparent increase in cervical erosions may be ascribed to closer observation in the medication cycles, as only grossly observable lesions were recorded in the pre-medication examinations. Since in several instances erosions observed in one examination in fact declined in the next, this may indeed be a question of close observation. Also, the pre-medication and post-medication examinations were not always made by the same individual.

In the San Juan project, 16 individuals have been examined in early medication cycles and then considerably later. . . . It is obvious that there is no consistent trend in the state of the organs and tissue examined. The latter appears to respond typically to the medication in cycle after cycle. Generally, the state of the reproductive organs appears to be unaltered after many months of medication, with the previously noted tendency for a mild uterine growth response being exhibited in a small proportion of the subjects. The lack of systematic change in the cervical surface (except perhaps for a slight trend to improvement of erosions) suggests that the changes observed are a function of individual hygiene and practice.

NOTE 3.
INTERNATIONAL PLANNED PARENTHOOD
FEDERATION
DISCUSSION OF ORAL METHODS
OF FERTILITY CONTROL*

*   *   *

[DR. EDWARD T. TYLER]: The issue that I would like to present at the moment is the question of whether, when dealing with these com-

___
* *Report of the Proceedings of the Sixth International Conference on Planned Parenthood.* London: International Planned Parenthood Federation 231–232, 234, 235 (1959). Reprinted by permission.

pounds, we are getting the major antigonadotrophic effects from the estrogen or from the progestin. This, again, is more than just an academic question. Progestin is the really expensive part of the compound, so far as I know, whereas estrogen is relatively cheap. If, for example, these compounds can contain a sufficient amount of estrogen and a minimal amount of progestin, they may be able to reach large masses of people a great deal sooner, assuming that they are safe.

To carry this one step further. Why haven't estrogens been employed for this purpose and why are doctors reluctant about this? I think the answer may be somewhat simple. For many years there has been a feeling among physicians that the use of estrogens in some patients, at least those who have had a tendency towards malignancy in the family, should be limited. Whether this is reasonable or not I am not in a position to say, but I am in a position to say that many physicians are concerned about this possibility.

In my opinion it is doubtful whether we need be concerned about cancer-producing effects at this dosage level. We have not tried to run routine Papanicolaou stains on our patients and it isn't because we haven't been interested in doing this. But there is a problem in connection with it, and that is the simple one that if you run routine Papanicolaou smears among large numbers of patients you are bound to get suspicious ones regardless of whether they are taking medication or not. Once you get something suspicious-looking, you are bound to follow it further and you get into a problem where you are in the situation of performing gynecologic therapy, or at least involving yourself in diagnosis and treatment of patients when you shouldn't be. This has been our attitude until recently. However, we feel that our study has progressed far enough now for it to be necessary to get more involved in the matter of doing Papanicolaou smears routinely.

*   *   *

[DR. PINCUS]: The other questions which I will deal with very briefly are concerned with how we manage to get the women to take these pills with the regularity that they allege they take them. One of the things that I forgot to mention is that we distribute a calendar to the women. We ask them to mark the calendar daily, and most important are the visits of the social worker. The social worker is extremely important in this whole business. I cannot say more than that right now, but with an alert, careful, highly motivated social worker, the results are excellent. The lowest rate of withdrawal, you remember, was in one of the Humacao projects. Here the social worker was extremely faithful. She had the women under her control in almost every sense psychologically and she certainly did her job well. . . . Why Dr. Tyler is less successful than we in having this faithful continuance is probably a sociological problem rather than a biological one. It may be that women in continental United States are somewhat more temperamental.

*   *   *

[DR. WARREN O. NELSON]: Dr. Rock, may I direct this question to you? What happens if women swallow several tablets at once, as villagers might well do?

DR. JOHN ROCK: I haven't the slightest idea. One patient took three tablets and telephoned to find out if it would do her any harm. I assured her, without much background, that it wouldn't and it didn't. I cannot imagine it doing any harm. Hormones don't cause generalised disturbances. They are used up.

*   *   *

NOTE 4.
    P. ECKSTEIN, J. A. H. WATERHOUSE,
GLENYS M. BOND, W. G. MILLS, DOROTHY M.
SANDILANDS, AND D. MARGARET SHOTTON

THE BIRMINGHAM ORAL CONTRACEPTIVE TRIAL*

In March, 1960, the Birmingham Family Planning Association embarked on its first oral contraceptive trial. Its objects were twofold. First, in view of the existing widespread dissatisfaction with conventional techniques of birth control, it seemed desirable to assess the efficacy and acceptability of the method among British women. Second, while the ability of relatively large doses of oral contraceptives to control fertility had been adequately established, there was next to no information about the effect of lower doses with regard to both the suppression of ovulation and the incidence and severity of side-effects. With these aims in mind—and that of reducing the substantial cost of the larger dosage—the Executive Council of the Birmingham F.P.A. decided to conduct a trial on a reasonably large

_____
* 2 *British Medical Journal* 1172–1173, 1178 (Supplement, 1961). Reprinted by permission.

scale and under carefully controlled conditions laid down and supervised by a specially enlisted Medical Advisory Committee.

Messrs. G. D. Searle and Co. Ltd. agreed to support the trial both financially and by supplying adequate quantities of the test material (norethynodrel) to the Medical Advisory Committee.

*   *   *

All volunteers . . . were asked to agree to remain in the trial for a minimum of six months, and during that time to use no other form of contraceptive. It was explained to them that the efficacy of the method could not be guaranteed, and all accepted the possibility of another pregnancy in the event of failure of the tablets. In addition, each woman was required to return a consent form signed by both her husband and herself; her medical practitioner was also informed.

*   *   *

The compound selected was norethynodrel . . . 2.5 mg. with 0.05 mg. of the highly potent oestrogen, ethinyloestradiol-3-methyl ether (EO-3-ME). Subsequent chemical analysis carried out in the manufacturer's laboratories in the United States revealed, however, that the oestrogen content of the batch of tablets actually used in the trial was less, and amounted to 0.036 mg.; the concentration of norethynodrel proved to be approximately correct (2.3 mg.). The tablets supplied during the 2 OC trials contained 5 mg. of norethynodrel and 0.075 mg. of EO-3-ME.

*   *   *

The tablets were generally acceptable, but, although taken in strict conformity with instructions, failed to control fertility.

Of 48 subjects enrolled, 14 (29%) conceived, resulting in 11 pregnancies and three miscarriages. Ten single babies and one pair of twins have been born; all were healthy and there were no signs of virilization of females or other noticeable abnormalities among them.

The remaining 34 volunteers who had not conceived before the trial was closed were changed over to tablets containing 5 mg. of norethynodrel and 0.075 mg. of oestrogen. No pregnancies have occurred in the women who continued to take this dosage as instructed.

During the trial side-effects such as headache, nausea, tender breasts, and abdominal pain were relatively frequent but were usually slight and tended to diminish with time; the same was true of changes in weight. No participants withdrew because of these effects.

The tablets, however, caused derangement of the cycle, as a rule towards prolongation, short cycles (or breakthrough bleeding) being unexpectedly rare.

The results obtained are compared with those of similar trials reported in the literature.

It is suggested that with doses of norethynodrel as low as 2.5 mg. the concentration of oestrogen becomes critical and, if below it, may reduce or abolish the contraceptive activity of the compound, probably by delaying ovulation rather than completely inhibiting it.

*   *   *

2.

Therapy, Complications, and Experimentation— The Second Phase (1960–Present)

a.

Ad Hoc Committee for the Evaluation of a Possible Etiologic Relation with Thromboembolic Conditions Final Report on Enovid*

For centuries man has been interested in mechanisms and factors affecting the normal menstrual cycle, as well as those believed to be effective in either increasing or decreasing fertility. The artifacts of many civilizations attest to this. Therefore it should arouse no surprise that when a preparation which suppresses ovulation became available in tablet form it should be rapidly accepted and widely used. Such a tablet consisting of norethynodrel with ethinylestradiol 3-methyl ether (Enovid) has now been used by well over 1.5 million women for either contraception or for the treatment of disturbances of gynecologic endocrinology. It is believed that this substance acts by inhibiting the synthesis of gonadotropin by the anterior pituitary gland and in this manner suppresses ovulation in a high percentage of users.

It was soon recognized that Enovid produced a variety of side effects, including nausea and vomiting (sufficient to require discontinuation of the treatment in about 25 per cent of the cases) and there have been reports of edema,

weight gain, changes in thyroid or adrenal function, thyroiditis or toxicosis, hair loss or growth, dermatitis, cholestatic jaundice, chloasma, toxemia or pregnancy-like syndromes and others. Except for nausea and vomiting the proof that these have been a direct result of the use of Enovid is in most instances open to question and is not within the scope of this report.

Beginning in 1961 reports began to appear from numerous sources of thromboembolic conditions, including thrombophlebitis and pulmonary embolism, occurring in women who had taken or were taking Enovid. Some of these patients died. While the index of suspicion was raised it was also recognized by the scientific community that a very large number of young and middleaged females were involved, that such conditions do occur with and without obvious explanation, and that the coincidental factors involved in such situations are not necessarily etiological. One solution would have been to scrutinize carefully each case history in detail, select those which appeared to be idiopathic in all other aspects, but who had the common denominator of exposure to Enovid, and compare these with a proper sampling from the population as a whole to determine whether there was evidence of an increase in the incidence of thromboembolism and deaths in the exposed series. Unfortunately, the incidence of thromboembolism in the United States in this or any other population group is not known despite efforts in a few areas to obtain such figures. This type of condition is not reportable so that most of the patients which are not hospitalized are never recorded at all or the records remain in the physician's files. Once the attention of the medical profession and the general population was drawn to a possible relationship with Enovid, reporting of all types and severity of thromboembolic conditions in patients who had taken this drug was inevitably accentuated and comparable statistics became even more difficult. The death rate from thromboembolism in females of a comparable age group during the same period was not known, although this was obtained in the course of the present investigation.

In January of 1963 the Commissioner of the Food and Drug Administration, of the Department of Health, Education and Welfare established an ad hoc committee to review and analyze this situation and to determine if the use of Enovid resulted in an increase in the incidence of death from thromboembolic conditions. This constitutes a report of the efforts of the commit-

---

* I. S. Wright, M.D., Chairman. Washington, D.C.: Food and Drug Administration 1–15 (September 12, 1963).

tee to resolve the questions involved. The committee was composed of representatives with broad interests but especially experienced in the fields of gynecology and obstetrics, vascular diseases, thromboembolism, hematology (especially coagulation), and statistics, and epidemiology.

The committee has not been unmindful of the complexity of the overall considerations involved in this area. These include not only the medical implications but also those involving the biological, psychological, social, philosophical and religious aspects. The relationship of all of these to the population explosion must be of interest to all intelligent citizens. Nevertheless these factors were not permitted at any time to cloud the immediate issues which constituted the commission of the committee.

Background material was obtained from the Food and Drug Administration and G. D. Searle and Company. The representatives of both organizations were completely co-operative throughout this study. More than 350 case reports of both thromboembolism and death from the files of both sources were reviewed by the members of the committee together with much additional data. After this it was concluded that, because of the impossibility of obtaining solid comparable statistics regarding thromboembolic complications as they occur in the usual population groups, it was essential to concentrate on deaths where the documentation is more complete and valid.

*   *   *

The committee reviewed and evaluated the clinical records, the autopsy reports, the death certificates and other pertinent material of each patient alleged to have died from thromboembolic disease who had taken or was taking Enovid. From the records a list was developed consisting of those patients who were considered to have died of idiopathic thromboembolism. . . . There were 10 cases which were unanimously agreed upon as idiopathic. These cases plus two additional cases about which there was lack of unanimous agreement were accepted for the statistical analysis. . . .

*   *   *

From the beginning of the committee's deliberation, it was very apparent that an assessment of the true quantitative values for morbidity from thrombophlebitis would be fraught with great uncertainties. As suggested above such factors as the broad spectrum of the severity of the disease and hence the seeking of medical care for diagnosis with obvious variation in reporting, diagnostic acumen, geographic differences in occurrence, and the number of unhospitalized and medically untreated cases could contribute in a differential way between groups of Enovid users and non-Enovid users and hence create artifactual differences which did not in reality exist.

*   *   *

. . . The incidence of deaths among all Enovid users was 12.1 per million users. It will be noted that the unadjusted rate for the general population is 7.9 deaths per million. On adjustment of the general population for the age distribution of the Enovid user population this rate becomes 8.4. In either case the difference between the Enovid and population rates is not statistically significant (p = .14) utilizing Poisson probability for small expected rates. . . .

Inasmuch as the population number for Enovid users estimated from available data is not an exact figure, but based on drug distribution figures, some attempts were made to determine the effects of a 50 per cent decrease and a 10 per cent decrease in the estimated population of white users to see what effect this might have on the mortality rates among Enovid users and the significance of any difference from those in the general population.

Any increase in this estimate of users would obviously reduce the user death rates and these rates would approach those in the general population. This would be particularly true if we deducted too many as Negro users, a possibility which remains. A 50 per cent decrease in the estimate of users would double the Enovid rates. This would make the overall rate as well as the rates in the 20–24 and 40–44 year age groups very significantly greater. A 50 per cent decrease in the population estimate represents an extreme possibility rather than a probable estimate and is deemed highly unlikely. A 10 per cent decrease in our user-population estimate (which might represent a reasonable error) would, however, *not* yield Enovid-user death rates significantly different from the general population rates (total and individual 5-year age groups) at the level of p = 0.05.

In summary, on the basis of the available data and if the above outlined assumptions are reasonably correct, no significant increase in the risk of thromboembolic death from the use of Enovid in this population group has been demonstrated.

There is a need for comprehensive and critical studies regarding the possible effects of Enovid on the coagulation balance and related production of thromboembolic conditions. Pending the development of such conclusive data and on the basis of present experience this latter relationship should be regarded as neither established nor excluded.

Although a detailed study is not within the scope of this report it is recognized that in judging the overall risk from and the values of the use of Enovid, data concerning the risks of pregnancy and induced abortion in each age group would be extremely important.

Any firm reliance on the risks as calculated is tempered by the assumptions made. This committee recommends that a carefully planned and controlled prospective study be initiated with the objective of obtaining more conclusive data regarding the incidence of thromboembolism and death from such conditions in both untreated females and those under treatment of this type among the pertinent age groups.

NOTES

NOTE 1.

LETTER FROM THE FOOD AND DRUG
ADMINISTRATION TO SENATOR GAYLORD
NELSON—JUNE 3, 1970*

. . . The information requested for the record during Commissioner Charles C. Edwards' testimony on March 4, 1970, before the Senate Select Committee on Small Business, Subcommittee on Monopoly is herewith submitted:

*   *   *

Senator McIntyre requested that we comment on the quality of the data submitted in support of the first oral contraceptive approved for sale in this country on June 23, 1960.

Much of the data submitted in support of this oral contraceptive seem to be rather super-

---

* Except as otherwise indicated, all materials in the NOTES in this section are reprinted from *Hearings on the Present Status of Competition in the Pharmaceutical Industry before the Subcommittee on Monopoly of the Senate Select Committee on Small Business,* 91st Congress, 2d Session. Washington: U.S. Government Printing Office (1970). Members of the Subcommittee were Senators Nelson (Chairman), Sparkman, Long, McIntyre, Bible, Hatfield, Dole, Cook, and Javits. Benjamin Gordon served as staff economist, and James P. Duffy, III, was minority counsel.

ficial in content in the light of our present state of knowledge regarding oral contraceptives. Some of the data are little more than testimonial or opinionative in character. Many areas of investigation that would now be required were either not carried out or were not evaluated to an acceptable extent. The studies conducted were certainly not of as high a quality as we now demand, based in part on our hindsight.

The material submitted appears to have been deficient with regards to data relative to 1) carbohydrate and lipid metabolism, 2) ophthalmological evaluation, 3) follow-up on newborns (resulting either subsequent to method discontinuance or as a result of method or patient failure) for anomalies or genetic defects, 4) cervical cytological studies, conducted before, during, and after medication, 5) renal function studies, 6) cardiovascular evaluation, 7) thorough physical examinations including breast examinations, prior to, during, and after termination of drug use, 8) adequate liver function studies, 9) long term efficacy studies, 10) animal studies, 11) coagulation and other clinical pathology studies.

Senator McIntyre asked how soon after the approval of the original new drug application for an oral contraceptive did the first report of thromboembolism side effects come to the Agency's attention.

A report in our files indicates that a number of reports of thromboembolic episodes associated with the use of oral contraceptives appeared in the literature in 1961. One report was in *The Lancet* on November 18, 1961. While we do not believe that it is possible to determine from our files when the first report of this effect first came to the attention of the FDA, we certainly aware of them when they appeared in the literature.

*   *   *

NOTE 2.

EDWIN J. DeCOSTA, M.D.
BIRTH-CONTROL PILLS—
HAVE THEY SIDE EFFECTS?—
AN AUTHORITATIVE ANSWER TO A QUESTION
MANY WOMEN ARE ASKING*

"But doctor, are they really safe?" No wonder that after the thalidomide tragedy many patients worry about the possible harm from taking the new birth-control pills. And there have been a few medical reports—plus many rumors—of

---

* *This Week Magazine* 13 (July 12, 1964). Reprinted by permission of the author.

dangerous side effects. Without considering the controversial social or religious aspects of birth control, let us take a look at the medical facts about this important discovery.

First, no other method of birth control is as simple. The small hormone pills are taken at bedtime for 20 days each month. Apparently they work by suggesting to the body's master gland, the pituitary, that the woman is already pregnant, so the pituitary doesn't instruct the ovaries to produce an egg that month. When the patient stops taking pills after 20 days the lining of the uterus is sloughed and bleeding follows. Then the pills are started again for the next cycle. This simple method approaches 100 per cent effectiveness.

But . . . and there is always a but . . . there may also be undesirable effects when the pills are used. Generally, these effects are not serious—only nuisances similar to those experienced by some women during early pregnancy. They may become, for reasons we can't explain, bloated or nauseated, have fullness and soreness of the breasts, suffer from headaches or even changes in their personality. Some women also gain weight rapidly, some have disturbance of their menstrual flow. Rarely, the menses do not return for some time after the pills are discontinued—which, of course, makes the patient fear she is pregnant.

Fortunately, in most instances these complaints disappear within a couple of months, as in pregnancy. But not always. At times, the weight gain, bleeding and personality changes may be sufficiently disconcerting to warrant discontinuance of the pills.

But these are just nuisance factors. What about the reports of more serious problems? I have heard oral contraceptives accused of masculinizing female babies if taken inadvertently during early pregnancy, of interfering with future fertility, of causing uterine fibroids or even cancer. Most of these charges are palpable nonsense—there is no evidence to support any of them. Indeed, many patients report getting both physical and psychological benefits from the pills.

There is, however, one other widely reported problem connected with oral contraceptives. From time to time women taking them have developed blood clots (thrombosis) in the veins of their pelvis or legs. This can be serious—even fatal—but studies do not indicate that pills cause the clots. Thrombosis also occurs in men, and in women who are not taking contraceptive pills.

I am reminded of a recent medical meeting where a doctor reported several instances of leg clots occurring in patients taking the pills. Another doctor promptly rose. His patient too had been given a prescription for the pills, and had developed leg clots. But she had forgotten to have the prescription filled!

Do I myself prescribe the pills? I do, whenever I think they are indicated. But to avoid even the most remote risk, I would not prescribe them to women who have had blood clots, varicose veins, heart or kidney disease, or malignancy.

To sum up, my own answer to anxious patients is yes, there is good reason to believe that oral contraceptives are safe for normal women under their physicians' supervision.

NOTE 3.

MORTON MINTZ
ARE BIRTH CONTROL PILLS SAFE?—
SOME DOCTORS DOUBT THAT THE DRUG
HAS BEEN TESTED WELL ENOUGH FOR
POSSIBLE SIDE EFFECTS*

A small but growing number of physicians, including some in key research posts, have been expressing concern about the scientific quality of the testing done to establish that oral contraceptives do not seriously endanger the women who use them.

One of these physicians is Dr. James A. Shannon, director of the National Institutes of Health. When the matter came up at a hearing of a House Appropriations subcommittee last Feb. 17, Rep. John E. Fogarty (D–R.I.) remarked, "So people are really taking a chance" (in using them).

"I believe so," Dr. Shannon replied. "There are a great many studies on experimental animals that indicate that they can be taken without hazard, but there has not been adequate human exploration to be certain."

*   *   *

[T]he millions [of women] who have turned to birth control pills . . . have had an almost unquestioning trust that the pills pose no serious dangers.

Necessarily, their trust reflects the confidence of a majority—probably the great majority—of the medical profession, because the oral contraceptives are prescription drugs.

---

* The Washington Post E 1, col. 1, E 5, col. 1 (December 19, 1965). © 1965, The Washington Post. Reprinted by permission.

The physicians' confidence, in turn, has been furthered by assurances such as these:

"If the instructions of the physician are followed in taking : . . . the pills, I can imagine no danger whatsoever. . . . I can think of no condition in which these pills would not be safe to take."—Dr. Joseph W. Goldzieher, a consultant to Eli Lilly & Co., in an interview recorded last November 6 by "This Hour Has Seven Days," a Canadian Broadcasting Corp. program.

"The effects of birth control pills have been studied possibly more thoroughly and for a longer continuous time on the same persons than any other drug."—G. D. Searle & Co., manufacturer of Enovid, the first oral contraceptive.

Among critics, there is a growing belief that the confidence of most of the medical profession in the pills is, at least in part, a result of inadequate information, wishful thinking and questionable scientific and statistical analysis.

In the Searle statement, for example, critics say the word "possibly" automatically raises questions about the quality of the testing.

They also make a more serious objection. Because the pill studies have not been controlled, the data are less meaningful than that from scientific investigations made of other drugs in fewer people over shorter periods.

*   *   *

The advocates contend that the incidence of harmful effects is extremely low. But the fact remains that they have not established that the rate is low, or that it is even as low as they say it is, or that it is not actually many times higher than they say it is.

In addition, there is a widespread, resentful, "don't rock the boat" attitude in the medical profession.

Recently, one manufacturer said that if warnings about the pills are widely circulated, "literally *millions* of American women could be thrown into panic regarding the safety for *all* oral contraceptives."

Dr. Gregory Pincus, co-developer of the pill with Dr. John Rock, says it has yet "to be proved that there is a cause-and-effect relationship" between use of the pill and subsequent ill effects suffered by some.

*   *   *

Scientists recognize, however . . . that evidence is in a gray area, that it is relative, that it boils down to sufficient data on relative risks. This is the kind of data on which persons charged with protecting the public health must judge the relative safety of all drugs. With a small chance of being wrong, they must decide whether the occurrence of adverse reactions is significantly more than would have arisen under normal conditions.

To insist upon certainty rather than compelling evidence of lack of safety is to risk the public health.

Dr. LeRoy E. Burney, while Surgeon General of the Public Health Service, has said that to wait for "proof" is "to invite disaster, or at least to suffer unnecessarily through long periods of time."

*   *   *

Has FDA been adequately protecting the public health—has it been reverent of life and scientifically responsible—in taking the position that it must wait in such problems as clots and strokes for the kind of proof of a "cause-and-effect relationship" that is available for migraine?

In the labeling of oral contraceptives, has FDA promptly given physicians full information about all of the known factors in the benefit/risk ratio so they can make informed, intelligent decisions about whether to prescribe the pills?

*   *   *

Last Oct. 25, the *Journal of the American Medical Association* published a report on all methods for AMA's eight-member Committee on Human Reproduction.

None of the authors was an endocrinologist, although the oral contraceptives involve the endocrine system. And the article makes no clear, specific mention of the possibility of strokes in pill users.

Dr. Lasagna, asked for comment, said he believed the article, "in its concern for the benefits to be obtained from effective contraception, neglects what I consider to be all too definite warning signals on the horizon in regard to the ability of the oral contraceptives to cause vascular catastrophe."

Vascular catastrophe includes serious or fatal clots in the bloodways. Those that block brain arteries are called strokes. Those that reach the lungs are called pulmonary embolisms.

In a recent interview, the chairman of the AMA Committee, Dr. Raymond T. Holden of Washington, said frankly of the article, "Maybe it wasn't strong enough. . . . It's possible we didn't stress the side effects," although "we thought we were being emphatic."

Relying on the theory that the safety of the pills, if used as directed under medical supervision, has been assured by FDA, the article emphasizes their effectiveness ("virtually 100 percent") and says that their acceptability is "of prime importance."

*   *   *

While the kind of faith put in FDA by the AMA Committee has been commonplace in organized medicine, it has not been held by the chairman of congressional committees that have investigated the agency's performance.

Last summer, Rep. L. H. Fountain (D–N.C.) was so disturbed by the findings turned up during his inquiries that he felt impelled to remind top FDA officials that their responsibility is "not to the drug companies, not to the doctors, but to the consuming public that may live or die as a result of your decisions."

*   *   *

The Wright committee was convened after FDA and the manufacturer of Enovid had received, by late December, 1962, reports of thrombophlebitis—an inflammatory vein-clotting condition—in 272 women who had taken the pills. Thirty died after pieces of the clots broke loose and reached the lungs. By July 1963, the reported total had increased to 400 cases, with 40 deaths.

For the moment, the major point about the Wright committee is that it did *not* eliminate the possibility of a relation between the use of Enovid and the occurrence of clots in the legs, pelvis and lungs.

The committee felt that the data it had to work with required it to be cautious in drawing conclusions. In the 27 months since the committee made its report, its restraint has not always been mirrored by others, who have tended to assume that there is no reason for worry about a possible relation. Such an assumption has been nurtured in many places.

In March, 1964, for example, Dr. Robert Kistner, a Harvard gynecologist, said that "scrutiny of the available data by experts . . . has completely exonerated the drug" as the causative factor.

This defies an axiom followed by expert statisticians: that no data ever warrant a declaration that a drug has been "completely exonerated." They say that the most that can ever properly be said is that the data permit a cautious conclusion: that there is a high or low *probability* of a causal relation.

*   *   *

A few weeks ago, FDA said that a computer was "memorizing" more than 10,000 instances of "adverse experiences" with oral contraceptives. The agency said it had a "crash program" to catalogue every scrap of information connected with the pills.

Perhaps inadvertently, the agency thus acknowledged that, despite the gravity of the problems involved, its surveillance of adverse effects had to be strengthened by a crash program.

In explaining the program, FDA said it was about to convene a special Advisory Committee on Obstetrics and Gynecology "to look at broad, overall problems of adverse experiences with all contraceptive drugs," including discrepancies in labeling of identical and similar products that the committee is expected to ask be made uniform.

In its initial meeting Nov. 22–23, the committee said that its preliminary review "finds no evidence of a cause-effect relationship" between the pills and reports of eye damage, strokes and other injuries associated with blood clotting.

The committee did not include in its statement the usually expected counterbalance: that it has no evidence that a causal relation does *not* exist. Yet by adopting a resolution endorsing FDA's request for an interim eye-damage warning in the labeling, the committee clearly indicated that a causal relation might indeed exist.

The committee is scheduled to meet again Jan. 20–21 and to issue its final report after a third meeting next March. Its chairman is Dr. Louis M. Hellman of the State University of New York College of Medicine.

*   *   *

Today's concern is most intense not about nausea and other such effects associated with pill-induced pseudo-pregnancy, but about afflictions involving the circulatory system: fatal clots, disabling clots, eye damage. There are, however, other concerns, including a feared possible relation between pill use over several years and cancer.

Although his warnings about such a possible relation have been hotly and widely challenged, Dr. Roy Hertz, former chief endocrinologist of the National Cancer Institute, said in an interview that the estrogenic substances used in the pills are known to induce a wide variety of tumors in numerous species of animals.

"It is, therefore, imperative that their generalized distribution to women of child-bearing age for protracted periods of time be preceded by appropriately comprehensive epidemiologic studies to ascertain whether such effects are to be anticipated in man," he said.

* * *

b.
FDA Advisory Committee on Obstetrics and Gynecology Report on the Oral Contraceptives*

The oral contraceptives present society with problems unique in the history of human therapeutics. Never will so many people have taken such potent drugs voluntarily over such a protracted period for an objective other than for the control of disease. These compounds, furthermore, furnish almost completely effective contraception, for the first time available to the medically indigent as well as the socially privileged. These factors render the usual standards for safety and surveillance inadequate. Their necessary revision must be carefully planned and tested, lest the health and social benefits derived from these contraceptives be seriously reduced. Probably no substance, even common table salt, and certainly no effective drug can be taken over a long period of time without some risk, albeit minimal. There will always be a sensitive individual who may react adversely to any drug, and the oral contraceptives cannot be made free of such adverse potentials, which must be recognized and kept under continual surveillance. The potential dangers must also be carefully balanced against the health and social benefits that effective contraceptives provide for the individual woman and society.

The oral contraceptives currently in use are probably not those that will be employed 10 or even 5 years hence. Drugs with even less potentially adverse effect, utilizable in smaller dosage, will undoubtedly be developed through continuing research. At present several such promising compounds are under investigation. The research essential to the development and testing of these compounds is carried out by the drug industry working in close cooperation with the medical profession. It would be indeed unfortunate were such research and testing to be stifled by unnecessarily complicated, unscientifically harsh, and inelastic administrative procedures. It is axiomatic that all drugs must be carefully tested on several species of laboratory animals under comparable conditions before they can be given to human volunteers. It is equally important that the results of such experimentation be appropriately interpreted in extending their application to human beings. Particularly in reproductive functions man differs from experimental animals and other primates. To deprive a population of drugs of great benefit by overattention to adverse effects based on animal data without due consideration of clinical experience is unjustifiable. Throughout this report various types of adverse experience will be discussed. Most of them, however, occur naturally, with a definite though low incidence in our population. The data necessary to demonstrate an increase in these naturally occurring phenomena among users of oral contraceptives are not available. Most adverse reactions, including deaths, have been reported as individual cases or small series. Except in carefully controlled studies, neither the total number of people exposed to the oral contraceptives nor the number of adverse reactions in any locality is known. The crucial data are the numerator (adverse reactions) and the denominator (users) and a control made up of nonusers having the same or a different number of adverse reactions. The difficulty of obtaining such data for the oral contraceptives makes unreliable any assumption regarding a cause and effect relationship of drug and adverse reaction.

There are, however, several epidemiological approaches which can shed light on the problem. The simplest and most obvious method is a system of surveillance leading to the reporting by physicians of suspicious illness in their patients who are taking the drug. Such a system is essential because it can give the earliest warning of trouble in a situation where quick action may be imperative. It should, however, be recognized that when the physician reports a suspected adverse reaction to a drug he usually cannot know with any certainty that what he has seen is in fact an adverse reaction and not a coincidental happening. The major deficiencies of this system are:

(a) Incomplete reporting by physicians of adverse experience for medico-legal reasons, inertia, and lack of interest or awareness of the value of such data.

(b) Selective or biased reporting of incidents which may reflect fashions in medical interest rather than the magnitude of a possible hazard.

(c) The lack of a denominator population to evaluate the incidence of a possible adverse reaction.

(d) The lack of control populations not exposed to the oral contraceptives to permit comparison of the incidence of possible complications in

---

* Louis M. Hellman, M.D., Chairman. Washington, D.C.: Food and Drug Administration 1–13 (August 1, 1966).

users and nonusers, to see if, in fact, any excess risks occurs in users.

(e) The inability to detect potential long-term effects which might first appear after discontinuation of the oral contraceptives or even in the progeny of users.

Of the more formal and reliable epidemiologic methods, the one selected should depend upon the type of suspected complication and its temporal relation to the use of the drugs. Prospective studies of users and nonusers are capable of testing for each type of complication; however, they are extremely difficult and costly to perform if the suspected complication is thought to be of rare occurrence or if it is expected to occur after a latent period of many years. The prospective method has the advantages that it permits simultaneous study of all possible complications, including those which are initially unsuspected, and that certain biases are avoided. However, it does not reduce the problem that the inferences must be based on observation rather than experiment; i.e., that differences in disease frequency between the groups of users and nonusers may result from differences in their initial composition dependent on whatever determines the employment of contraceptive methods.

*   *   *

Utilization

The pharmaceutical industry has estimated the numbers of women taking oral contraceptives, based on the numbers of tablets distributed in the United States. The approach is straightforward: Since each user takes 20 tablets per cycle and the average woman has 13 cycles per year, the number of tablets sold, divided by 260, gives the average numbers of users during the year. The following estimates have been prepared by this method for the period 1961–65:

1961	408,000
1962	1,187,000
1963	2,235,000
1964	3,950,000
1965	5,000,000

*   *   *

Thromboembolic Disease

*   *   *

Of . . . concern are the deaths from thromboembolic disease. The deaths from idiopathic pulmonary embolism in women aged 15 to 44 in the United States appear to be of the order of 12 per million per year. The average annual

death rate for women of the same age group from cerebral embolism and thrombosis is about 5 per million. From these data one might expect that, of the 5 million women estimated to be taking the oral contraceptives in 1965, there should be about 85 deaths from idiopathic thromboembolic disease. Kohl's report . . . disclosed 20 such cases from all causes, only 13 of which were idiopathic. There are two possible explanations for this apparent discrepancy: (1) The oral contraceptives are protective against thromboembolic disease; (2) there has been gross underreporting. The second possibility seems to be the logical explanation, for the reported deaths fail to show the increment expected with the fivefold increase in use of the oral contraceptives from 1962 to 1965.

The present system of reporting deaths and adverse reactions relies on either the cooperation of physicians or the haphazard filtering of rumors to detail men. The latter route is patently unreliable, and the former not much better. Physicians are becoming increasingly fearful of reporting deaths or adverse drug reactions because of possible legal reprisal.

The data derived from mortality statistics are not adequate to confirm or refute the role of oral contraceptives in thromboembolic disease. They do, however, suggest that if oral contraceptives act as a cause, they do so very infrequently relative to the number of users. The committee believes, accordingly, that the only way this important question can be answered is through large, carefully designed epidemiologic studies.

Carcinogenic Potential

*   *   *

It is to be emphasized that all known human carcinogens require a latent period of approximately one decade. Hence any valid conclusion must await accurate data on a much larger group of women studied for at least 10 years. Furthermore, there is not sufficient evidence to support the contention that contraceptive pills may protect against the development of carcinoma of the cervix.

*   *   *

Sex steroids, particularly estrogens, have been shown to produce malignant lesions and to affect adversely the existing tumors in the mouse, rat, rabbit, hamster, and dog. These neoplasms have occurred in various organs, such as the cervix, endometrium, ovary, breast, testicle, pituitary, kidney, and bone marrow. The observations in animals given progesterone and the newer progestogens have been contradictory; however, these agents alone and in combination with other sex steroids have promoted neoplasia or metastatic growth in a few instances. A recent example is a 52-week study of six dogs that received massive doses of a combination of mestranol and ethyneron (MK-665, an experimental progestogen). Four of the dogs developed mammary lesions; one was a carcinoma in situ with early invasion; the second was a carcinoma in situ; the third represented atypical hyperplasia; and the fourth was a benign intraductal papilloma. Animal studies, in which certain susceptible strains and species are used and in which the dosage is excessive and continuous, cannot be directly transferred to human beings. There is, nevertheless, a warning that an altered endocrine environment in human tissues might result in an abnormal expression or potentiation of growth, as in experimental animals. In fact, there has always been the suspicion that experimental animal and human tissues follow the same biological laws in this regard, but conclusive data are not available. A great difficulty in obtaining a reliable answer involves the prolonged period of latency in human beings exposed to known carcinogens. Further epidemiologic studies must take full recognition of this fact.

* * *

Endocrine and Metabolic Effects

A considerable number of studies indicate that the oral contraceptives inhibit ovulation by a block at the pituitary level, specifically by inhibition of synthesis or release of LH. During such inhibition, the ovaries tend to become smaller, and changes suggestive of cortical stronal fibrosis have been described. After cessation of the medication recovery is usually prompt, with ovulation resuming in 4 to 8 weeks in most cases. Occasionally, the reappearance of cyclic ovulation may be delayed for several months. Fertility appears to be normal immediately after cessation of the oral contraceptives although a small but unknown number of patients remain amenorrheic. The outcome of pregnancy has been reported to be about the same as in the untreated population with regard to abortion, prematurity, abnormality, and anomaly. There are, however, no prolonged followup studies to ascertain the growth and development of infants born after cessation of therapy. There is no evidence that prolonged suppression of ovulation in nulliparas or multiparas will impair future fertility. The effects of

prolonged suppression of ovulation, however, are unknown and require further investigation.

* * *

Increased thyroxin-binding globulin has been noted in the majority of women on oral contraceptives. Most, but not all, investigators report a rise in PBI and a decreased T_3-RBC uptake. . . . The level of PBI may be in the hyperthyroid range but there is no clinical evidence of hyperthyroidism. If TSH is blocked at the pituitary level, it may be masked by increased protein binding. No precise data are available on this point.

Data regarding effects on carbohydrate metabolism in experimental animals and in women are contradictory. Recent studies in women taking oral contraceptives suggest a possible diabetogenic effect of these medications. Abnormal glucose tolerance tests have been observed in as many as 40 percent of women taking oral contraceptives; in women with diabetic family histories, abnormal tests were even more frequent. . . . Whether oral contraceptives can induce diabetes in normal women or even in those predisposed is not known, nor is it clear to what extent the induced changes in carbohydrate tolerance are reversible.

Liver Function

Many women on oral contraceptives show abnormalities of some liver function tests, especially the BSP and transaminase. A few develop clinical jaundice and evidence of mild hepatic damage, demonstrated by biopsy. . . .

Effect on Lactation

Oral contraceptives in high doses (5 and 10 mg. of progestogen) tend to decrease or stop lactation in many women in the first or second cycle of use. These compounds appear in breast milk but in minimal amounts (0.004–0.1 percent of the administered dose). Despite the small quantities of the steroids appearing in breast milk, mammary enlargement may occur in nursing infants. Administration of the androgenic steroids to newborn experimental animals at crucial periods can affect sex differentiation and behavior and result in sterility. No data on human beings are available.

Masculinization

Oral contraceptives have not produced serious masculinization in women taking these agents although all large series have reported some individuals with mild masculinizing symptoms. The 19-nor-compounds appear to have somewhat more masculinizing effect than other synthetic progestogens. These effects are mild, including acne and hirsutism. These changes regress with cessation of medication. The effect on the fetus is of greater importance. Synthetic progestogens, in doses used in the treatment of threatened or habitual abortion, may produce superficial masculinization of the genitals of the female fetus. These anatomic abnormalities are correctable, but the effect upon subsequent reproductive functions and psychosexual development is unknown.

Efficacy

*   *   *

The efficacy of the combined agents is exceptionally high. The more recently introduced sequential regimens are also highly effective in controlling fertility, although to a slightly lesser degree. Present evidence indicates that the frequency of pregnancies occurring with the patients on sequential medication remained unchanged over the 2½-year period, thus supporting the contention that tolerance to or escape from the medication probably does not occur.

The efficacy of oral contraceptives in the treatment of amenorrhea could not be readily ascertained from the material available to the committee because of the endpoint used. . . .

The comments pertaining to efficacy of the drugs in the management of patients with dysmenorrhea were similar to those cited in the previous paragraph. . . . Statistically, the submitted material was considered unsatisfactory because of the small number of patients in the individual series. It was surprising to find that a very small sample had been utilized in the study of such a common phenomenon. The members were aware of the difficulties in designing controlled studies, since placebos do not provide contraception, a fact that cannot remain undisclosed to the patient.

*   *   *

The committee found no data to indicate that any of the oral contraceptives are effective in altering the natural history of patients with habitual abortion. . . .

*   *   *

Recommendations

In making the following recommendations, the committee has given careful consideration to

this problem, which is unique because of the large number of healthy women taking the oral contraceptives over very long periods of time, the low incidence of serious side effects, the metabolic changes induced, the paucity of requisite statistical and scientific data, and, finally, the health and social benefits to be derived. These factors have imposed the requirement for unprecedented standards of safety; they have demanded the detection of sequelae that are often remote and infrequent; they have opened to question the existing methods of surveillance and retrieval of data: and they have required the design of highly refined epidemiological experiments.

As our case is new and unique in the history of therapeutics, so have we had to think anew in framing these recommendations.

I. A large case-control (retrospective) study of the possible relation of oral contraceptives to thromboembolism.

*   *   *

II. Continuation and support of studies such as the ones being carried out by the Kaiser Permanente group in California and the University of Pittsburgh group in Lawrence County, Pa.

III. Support of additional controlled population-based prospective studies utilizing groups of subjects that are especially amenable to long-term follow-up, such as married female employees of certain large industries and graduate nurses.

*   *   *

IV. Continuation and strengthening of the present surveillance system of the FDA.

V. Review of the mechanism of storage, retrieval, and analysis of surveillance data.

*   *   *

VI. A conference be held between FDA and the respective drug firms concerning uniformity and increased efficiency of reporting.

*   *   *

VII. Priority be given to support laboratory investigations concerning all aspects of the hormonal contraceptive compounds.

VIII. Uniformity in labeling of contraceptive drugs.

IX. Discontinuance of time limitation of administration of contraceptive drugs.

*   *   *

X. Simplification of administrative procedures to allow reduction in dosage of already approved compounds. Once safety has been established, reduction in dosage should require only minimal proof of efficacy, say 3,000–4,000 cycles without a pregnancy.

Conclusion

The foregoing considerations have been brought together to direct the attention of the medical profession and the Food and Drug Administration to those aspects of our knowledge, as well as our ignorance, that seem pertinent to our evaluation of the safety and risks involved in the use of these compounds.

The committee finds no adequate scientific data, at this time, proving these compounds unsafe for human use. It has nevertheless taken full cognizance of certain very infrequent but serious side effects and of possible theoretic risks suggested by animal experimental data and by some of the metabolic changes in human beings.

In the final analysis, each physician must evaluate the advantages and the risks of this method of contraception in comparison with other available methods or with no contraception at all. He can do this wisely only when there is presented to him dispassionate scientific knowledge of the available data.

NOTES

NOTE 1.

TESTIMONY OF DR. LOUIS M. HELLMAN, CHAIRMAN, DEPARTMENT OF OBSTETRICS AND GYNECOLOGY, STATE UNIVERSITY OF NEW YORK, DOWNSTATE MEDICAL CENTER, BROOKLYN, N.Y.—JANUARY 22, 1970

* * *

Adverse reaction reporting has a lot of pitfalls. In the first place, at that time, there was no uniform reporting sheet from the drug houses. This has been corrected. The method of data retrieval in FDA was deficient. You could not get quickly the information that you needed. Some of it was computerized, some of it was not. There have been efforts in FDA to correct this. I think the system still needs a good, hard look and some correction if correction is possible.

The chief difficulty with adverse reaction reporting, both in the United States and Great Britain, comes from the reluctance of the physicians themselves to report to anybody an adverse reaction. In this country it is easy to understand, because the physician does, to a certain extent, incur some liability, legal liability, in reporting an adverse reaction to anybody, and he is often very hesistant to do this.

Second, it is very difficult for a physician to tell whether what he actually sees in the patient is related to some event like taking the oral contraceptive or something entirely different. . . .

* * *

NOTE 2.

TESTIMONY OF FDA COMMISSIONER CHARLES C. EDWARDS—MARCH 4, 1970

* * *

SENATOR NELSON: We have had witnesses over the past 3 years, distinguished physicians, who deplored the state of reporting on various diseases as being wholly inadequate.

* * *

This is from a statement of William R. Best, chief, Midwest Research Support Center, Veterans Administration, Edward Hines, Jr. Hospital, Hines, Ill. He said:

* * *

I know that in a recent study in Philadelphia, for example, five of the medical school affiliated hospitals tried to set up their own reporting system to catch all the adverse reactions occurring in all of these hospitals. People being people, the way they are, when they went back to check and see how complete their reporting system was, even though the chief of every service told all of his residents and internes to report every case that came through, I think they reported somewhere in the neighborhood of 5 percent. About 95 percent still did not get reported, even though this was the rule of the particular hospital.

* * *

Do you think in your experience, in your judgment, that figure is anywhere near in the ball park of any kind of voluntary reporting the FDA gets on side effects?

DR. EDWARDS: I do not think I am in a position to give you an absolute figure. I would say without any hesitation our reporting system is poor. As long as we continue to have a reporting system that is voluntary, as it is right now, where we have very little access to the medical records in both hospitals and in doctors' offices, I think the likelihood of our establishing a really accurate, up to date reporting system is not going to be very encouraging.

*   *   *

SENATOR NELSON: I bring this up just to make the point that if the Philadelphia study and the five hospitals with the chiefs of all the services cooperating produced only a 5 percent reporting result, all of your reports on the incidence of deaths and other side effects from the pill, would have to be multiplied by 20 to get an accurate figure.

DR. EDWARDS: I have some reservations as to whether this is an accurate figure. I would add if I were chief of the service in a major teaching hospital and if I could not get my residents and internes to do better than that, I think that maybe I would look at myself, not my staff.

*   *   *

NOTE 3.

TESTIMONY OF FDA GENERAL COUNSEL WILLIAM W. GOODRICH—MARCH 4, 1970

SENATOR MCINTYRE: . . . You quoted the September 12, 1963, report of the Wright Committee to the effect that "No significant increases in the risk of thromboembolic disease had been demonstrated."

Did FDA not, in fact, issue two different versions of the Wright Committee report?

*   *   *

MR. GOODRICH: There was a first report which was found by Dr. Wright to have some statistical errors in it and those errors were corrected.

SENATOR MCINTYRE: How did the finding of the August 4, 1963, version differ from the one you quoted, from the September 12, 1963, version?

MR. GOODRICH: The first report of the Wright Committee indicated that on the basis of the statistical figures, the statistical calculations made, that there was an increased risk of thromboembolic disorder in ladies, as I remember, age 35 or older. I would have to go back to the record, but the problem there was that statisticians that looked at the information concluded that the incidence of thromboembolic disorders in nonusers, the data on which the comparison had been made, were inadequate and therefore there was no basis on which they could find a statistically significant difference in the appearance of thromboembolic disorders in these age groups.

Dr. Wright wrote to the Commissioner almost immediately to say that the statistical error had been discovered. The first report had been sent to the *Journal of the American Medical Association,* and the error was corrected.

But the problem was identified as a statistical error by the calculation of the normal risk based on the nonuser experience.

SENATOR MCINTYRE: Well, the reason for the change was based on the lack of what was considered to be sufficiently definite statistical information on the occurrence of thromboembolic disease in nonusers?

MR. GOODRICH: Yes.

*   *   *

SENATOR MCINTYRE: Because of these deficiencies in the available information, the Wright Committee recommended:

That a carefully planned and controlled prospective study be initiated with the objective of obtaining more conclusive data regarding the incidence of thromboembolism and death from such conditions in both untreated females and those under treatment of this type among the pertinent age groups.

What actions were taken by FDA to implement this recommendation in the 3-year period between the issuance of the Wright Committee report and the first report of the Advisory Committee on Obstetrics and Gynecology in August of 1966?

MR. GOODRICH: Dr. Wright did make that recommendation in the report. He also sent a letter to the Commissioner with it, in which he recognized that the preparation and execution of a prospective study would be difficult, if not impossible. . . .

Nonetheless, the problem there was that in order to do a meaningful prospective study involved thousands of ladies, under carefully controlled circumstances, by that I mean having a number of patients in the order of 10,000 examined at intervals of about 6 months, which was simply beyond our capability of financing, and the conclusion was reached about the time of the first Hellman report that the quickest and most effective way of obtaining information—reliable information about thromboembolic episodes—was to do a controlled retrospective study. That retrospective study was financed and completed.

We, in the meantime, got the retrospective experience from England. Even today, it is not possible for us within the resources Dr. Edwards has explained here, to mount a prospective study with the numbers of patients that would be necessary. We think a prospective study is no longer necessary with respect to thromboembolic episodes, but a prospective study may very well be meaningful in some other parameters.

SENATOR MCINTYRE: [T]he Commissioner's statement . . . list[s] eight recommendations contained in the 1966 report of the Hellman Committee, and describes efforts made by FDA to implement six of them. However, you make no mention of efforts to implement the other two. One of these was the restatement of the Wright Committee recommendation to support prospective studies utilizing groups of subjects especially amenable to long-term follow-ups.

Now, your answer, I suppose, covers it, but I want to ask it for the record: has FDA as yet undertaken or caused to be undertaken studies such as these, and if so, when?

MR. GOODRICH: Again, the prospective study recommended by the Hellman Committee in 1966 was not undertaken. Instead, the retrospective study was planned and executed. . . . Dr. Edwards' statement . . . describes a prospective study at the University of Miami. I believe there is also one underway at Temple University, and the Walnut [Creek] Study.

SENATOR MCINTYRE: That is a carbohydrate metabolism study?

MR. GOODRICH: These are parameters: I thought I made it clear we had enough data from the retrospective studies to say that a cause and effect had been established for thromboembolic disorders. We have now tied the proof to that effect. These other issues are the issues that have been identified to us, which do need a prospective study, and we are trying to fund those within the limits of our resources.

*   *   *

SENATOR MCINTYRE: You are telling us what FDA is doing now. My question was directed at what were you doing in 1965 and 1966 to support these programs and studies that we now have knowledge of by virtue of witnesses that have been here?

DR. SCHROGIE [of the FDA]: These studies were started at different points in time since 1966. It was in 1966 that as a result of the Advisory Committee report that additional funding was given to FDA to initiate such studies.

The Sartwell study was initiated at that time, the study on carbohydrate metabolism was initiated during 1967, and a feasibility study relating to a prospective study on carcinogenesis was also undertaken at that time. The other studies were phased in during 1968 and 1969, as they could be developed and as funds became available to support them. So the program developed in an orderly fashion over the space of 3 or 4 years.

*   *   *

Dr. Spellacy has been under support from the Food and Drug Administration since 1967. . . .

*   *   *

Dr. Wynn is funded by the National Institute of Child Health and Human Development. I would add in terms of timing, both Dr. Wynn's study of carbohydrate metabolism and lipid metabolism, and also the prospective multiphasic study of oral contraceptive users being conducted at the Kaiser Permanente Foundation at Walnut Creek, Calif., were initiated by NIH around 1966.

SENATOR MCINTYRE: You have now described to me all of the studies that FDA has supported among the witnesses who have appeared here and described their studies for this committee.

DR. SCHROGIE: To the best of my present recollection, yes.

SENATOR MCINTYRE: Well, to me anyway— I may be wrong, in 1960, the drug went on the market. And FDA seems to be getting into the act by 1966, in a concerted way by starting some of these studies. . . .

*   *   *

Mr. Chairman, at what now appears to be the conclusion of these hearings, I would like to say I am both surprised and disappointed to find that the Food and Drug Administration, which has legal responsibility for assuring the safety of all drugs on the market, after allowing the birth control pill to come on the market on the basis of questionable evidence, has also failed to take the lead in seeing that adequate studies are being done to answer the questions which have been raised about the safety of these drugs since they came on the market.

Instead, FDA's posture has consistently been one of reacting to studies done elsewhere, and in many instances, in other countries. I think these hearings have made it quite clear that there are a number of still unresolved questions about the safety of the birth control pill. I hope that in the future FDA will be more aggressive and will take the lead in seeing that adequate research is undertaken to answer these questions.

* * *

NOTE 4.

SYNTEX LABORATORIES, INC.
"DEAR DOCTOR" LETTER—JANUARY 22, 1968*

The Food and Drug Administration has asked us to call your attention to the fact that certain statements in recent advertising for our oral contraceptives, NORQUEN® and NORINYL®–1, may be misleading.

In the NORQUEN advertisement, the paragraph headed "Low incidence of side effects" emphasizes the low incidence of certain less serious side effects such as spotting, breakthrough bleeding, nausea, vomiting and other gastrointestinal disturbances, but fails to give adequate emphasis to the more serious known side effects such as cholestatic jaundice, rise in blood pressure in susceptible individuals, and mental depression which also occur in low incidence. Further, although a cause and effect relationship has neither been established nor disproved, the advertisement does not give adequate emphasis to the possible occurrence of thrombophlebitis, pulmonary embolism, and neuro-ocular lesions which have been observed in users of oral contraceptives.

The advertisements for both NORQUEN and NORINYL–1 state that "careful observation and caution are required for patients with symptoms or history of . . . cerebrovascular accident, psychic depression. . . ." The ads should have been more specific in stating:

Oral contraceptives should be used with caution in patients with a history of cerebrovascular accident and should be discontinued if there is a sudden partial or complete loss of vision, or if there is a sudden onset of proptosis, diplopia, or migraine, or if examination reveals papilledema or retinal vascular lesions, since these may be symptoms of cerebrovascular accident.

The advertisements disclose that careful observation and caution are required for patients with symptoms or history of psychic depression but do not specifically state that oral contraceptives should be discontinued if psychic depression recurs to a serious degree. Also, the ads fail to disclose that a decrease in glucose tolerance has been observed in a small percentage of patients on oral contraceptives.

We are modifying all future advertising to reflect these changes.

c.

FDA Advisory Committee on Obstetrics and Gynecology
Second Report on the Oral Contraceptives*

Since the publication of the last Report on the Oral Contraceptives in 1966, scientific as well as public interest in this method of family planning has remained high. The reservations of the first report appear to have been justified. Concern about the immediate and long-range side effects of the hormonal contraceptives has increased as scientific investigations have uncovered a host of diverse biologic effects, and as the drugs have become available to increasingly large segments of the world's population.

Adverse reactions are continually reported in the scientific literature and the lay press. Since the vast majority of the reported adverse experiences are conditions which occur spontaneously in women of reproductive age, identification of an etiologic relation has been difficult and slow.

An increased risk of thromboembolic disease attributable to the use of hormonal contraceptives has now been defined in both Great Britain and the United States. Other risks, such as those of hypertension, liver disease and reduced tolerance to carbohydrates, have not been quantitated with the same precision. Some of the risks have been recognized by isolated clinical observations, whereas others have been predicted on the basis of experiments with animals or merely on theoretical grounds.

Controversy has centered about two areas: the scientific data required to establish an etiologic relation and the balance between acceptable risk and potential benefit. The voluntary submission of reports by individual doctors to scientific journals, to the pharmaceutical industry, or directly to the Food and Drug Administration is fragmentary at best. Since the data on the natural incidence of the disorders in question are not available, it is impossible to ascertain whether the

* This is an example of letters sent by drug companies to physicians throughout the United States to correct prior advertisement. It is not taken from the Nelson hearings.

* Louis M. Hellman, M.D., Chairman. Washington, D.C.: Food and Drug Administration 1–9 (August 1, 1969).

haphazard voluntary reporting of an adverse reaction in fact represents an increase in the suspected complication. The limitations as well as the value of a voluntary reporting system for providing an initial warning of serious complications have been noted frequently. There is no easy escape from this dilemma. The current aggregate pharmacological experience with the oral contraceptives is unique, however, in that large numbers of healthy young women are using potent drugs for a purpose other than the control of disease. An improvement in national reporting of some of the alleged complications is therefore merited. If the annual national rates of incidence of the various complications thought to be associated with hormonal contraceptives were known, trends presently unsuspected might be quickly uncovered.

This pharmacological experience is unique also in the attention it has received by the press throughout the world. Particularly in Great Britain and the United States the press has attempted to keep the public informed of each discovery and each reported difficulty. Such reporting is the quickest way to satisfy the public's right to know.

* * *

The risk of thromboembolism associated with the oral contraceptives has been compared with that from pregnancy, cigarette smoking, and automobile accidents. Such comparisons are probably irrelevant, contributing little to evaluation of the relative risk. The task of balancing the risk against the benefit to the individual and to society must eventually be met. As contraceptive practices spread to all segments of our society, it becomes virtually essential that the requirements of effectiveness and safety, and the desirability of inexpensiveness and lack of association with coitus be satisfied. Oral contraceptives have proved to be highly acceptable to many couples who had found other methods inconvenient or impractical.

* * *

All available evidence indicates that the continuation rates of oral contraceptives are higher than those of traditional methods of contraception, such as the diaphragm, and lower than those of intrauterine devices. In its previous report the committee indicated an anticipated use of 6 million cycles monthly in the United States in 1970. If the present estimate of 8.5 million cy-

cles is correct, the committee's projections were conservative.

Efficacy

The theoretical effectiveness of the combined hormonal contraceptives is reflected in a pregnancy rate of approximately 0.1 per hundred women per year. The theoretical effectiveness of the sequential oral contraceptives appears to be somewhat lower as indicated by a pregnancy rate of 0.5 per hundred women per year. The usually given pregnancy rates, reflecting "use-effectiveness," average 0.7 per hundred women per year for the combined regimen, and 1.4 per hundred women per year for the sequential regimen.

Effectiveness, judged by the total number of pregnancies, is significantly higher with oral contraceptives, combined or sequential, than with intrauterine devices or any of the traditional methods. The pregnancy rates among users of diaphragms with contraceptive paste thus appear to be 10 to 30 times higher than those among users of oral contraceptives; those among users of intrauterine devices are 2 to 4 times higher.

Methods under evaluation

Since the committee's last report, pharmaceutical firms have continued to investigate synthetic progestins and estrogens in an effort to reduce side effects while maintaining maximal efficacy. For example, the most recently approved combination product contains one-third the dose of estrogen and about one-tenth the dose of progestin as was present in the original contraceptive. Steroids that are stored in and slowly released from adipose tissue after oral ingestion are currently under study with the aim of creating a pill that may require administration only once a month. Unpredictable uterine bleeding remains a problem, however.

Intramuscularly injected steroids with a prolonged effect that may last for one or more months have been widely studied. Although these compounds may suppress ovulation, uterine bleeding is often an unpredictable complication. The delay before resumption of ovulatory cycles often lasts from 12 to 21 months. There is considerable variation among patients. To regulate the uterine bleeding some investigators have administered oral or parenteral estrogen. Doing so, however, detracts from the simplicity of this purely progestational regimen.

Low-dose continuous progestin therapy has been investigated in several countries. Drugs of this kind exert their contraceptive effect without the addition of estrogen and without the inhibition of ovulation. The pregnancy rate appears to be approximately 2 per hundred women per year. Approximately two-thirds of the women studied have some cycle irregularity.

*   *   *

Thromboembolic disorders

An etiologic relation between oral contraceptives and an increase in some thromboembolic disorders has been disclosed by several groups of investigators using retrospective methods of inquiry and studies of mortality trends. In 1967 the Royal College of General Practitioners in Great Britain undertook interviews of young women with vascular disease. By comparing patients with superficial thrombophlebitis with a suitably matched series of controls, it could be shown that the risk of developing thrombophlebitis was tripled in women who used oral contraceptives. In a second study, Vessey and Doll investigated young women admitted to several hospitals in the northwest of London with a diagnosis of idiopathic thrombophlebitis. These patients also were matched with suitable controls. A third study involved all the deaths that occurred in England, Wales, and Northern Ireland during 1966 in women between the ages of 20 and 44 whose death certificates referred to thrombosis or embolism of the pulmonary, cerebral or coronary vessels. . . .

According to these British investigators, in the absence of other predisposing causes the risk of developing deep vein thrombosis, pulmonary embolism, or cerebral thrombosis is increased about eight times by the use of oral contraceptives, while the risk of developing coronary thrombosis is apparently unchanged. The results of these three studies led the Food and Drug Administration to order the following change of labeling for the oral contraceptives:

The physicians should be alert to the earliest manifestations of thrombotic disorders (thrombophlebitis, cerebrovascular disorders, pulmonary embolism, and retinal thrombosis). Should any of these occur or be suspected, the drug should be discontinued immediately.

Studies conducted in Great Britain and reported in April, 1968 estimate there is a seven to tenfold increase in mortality and morbidity due to thromboembolic diseases in women taking oral contraceptives. . . .

The conclusions reached in the studies are summarized in the table [which follows]:

Comparison of Mortality and Hospitalization Rates Due to Thromboembolic Disease in Users and Non-Users of Oral Contraceptives in Britain

| Category | Mortality rates | | Hospitalization rates (morbidity) |
	Age 20–34	Age 35–44	Age 20–44
Users of oral contraceptives	1.5/100,000	3.9/100,000	47/100,000
Nonusers	0.2/100,000	0.5/100,000	5/100,000

No comparable studies are yet available in the United States. The British data, especially as they indicate the magnitude of the increased risk to the individual patient, cannot be directly applied to women in other countries in which the incidences of spontaneously occurring thromboembolic disease may be different.

Since that time Vessey and Doll have continued their retrospective study to include a larger group of patients matched with controls. The results of this study confirm the findings of the previous investigation.

*   *   *

Carcinogenesis

Much indirect evidence suggests that steroid hormones, particularly estrogen may be carcinogenic in man. These data are derived from experiments on laboratory animals in which long-term administration of estrogen resulted in cancer in five species. Although all physical and chemical agents that are carcinogenic in man produce malignant tumors in experimental animals also, evidence of the carcinogenicity of estrogen in other species cannot be transposed directly to man. Suspicion lingers, however, that the results in laboratory animals may be pertinent to man. Many difficulties arise in the epidemiological elucidation of this suspected relation. The principal obstacle is the long latent period between the administration of a known carcinogen and the development of cancer in man. Thus far, no properly devised prospective or retrospective studies have provided an adequate solution to this problem.

The committee has focused its attention on three target organs: cervix, endometrium, and breast. Estrogens may produce a variety of epithelial changes in the human cervix of uncertain prognostic significance. A study of women attending the Planned Parenthood Clinics in New York City has revealed a higher prevalence of epithelial abnormalities that the investigators considered to be carcinoma in situ among women using oral contraceptives than in those who use the diaphragm. The committee believes that this study does not prove or disprove an etiologic relation between the oral contraceptives and these cervical changes. . . .

Although estrogen causes epithelial changes in the human breast, its carcinogenic effect on that organ has never been proved. Even in women with frank mammary carcinoma, estrogen produces variable changes in the clinical course of the disease. For example, ovariectomy leads to regression of metastatic breast carcinoma in approximately half of premenopausal women. Exogenous estrogens cause either regression or stimulation of similar tumors in menstruating women but induce regression in about half of post-menopausal women. The reasons for these paradoxical effects of estrogen on breast cancer are not clear.

In accordance with suggestions in the last report, the Food and Drug Administration has required mandatory testing for all currently licensed and investigational hormonal contraceptives on monkeys throughout their lifetimes and on dogs for 7 years. Thus far the presently licensed compounds have not produced tumors in these two groups of laboratory animals. Two estrogen-progestin combinations have, however, induced mammary tumors in beagles. Because these two compounds offered no clear therapeutic advantage over previously available hormonal contraceptives, clinical investigation was discontinued. This decision still leaves unresolved the question of similarity in hormonal induction of mammary tumors in a highly susceptible canine strain and in man. Continued testing of the presently available drugs is indicated.

Currently available data on death rates from genital and mammary cancer in women in the United States do not clarify the problem of association between steroids and carcinoma. The long latent period of action of known carcinogens (10 years) and the length of time between diagnosis and death eliminate vital statistics as a source of information about this association until the mid-1970's or later.

The massive program of prophylaxis launched against cervical cancer in this country has accomplished a steady decline in deaths from the disease. The common practice of repeating cervical smears, annually or semi-annually, in women taking oral contraceptives has contributed to the decline, but it has clouded the question of the effect of oral contraceptives on cervical cancer.

Since there is no method of early detection of mammary carcinoma comparable in efficacy to that of the cervical Papanicolaou smear, the problem of the possible carcinogenic effect of oral contraceptives on the breast remains unresolved. . . .

Lacking conclusive information about the applicability of existing animal data to women and sufficient observations of human disease, the committee concludes that potential carcinogenicity of the oral contraceptives can be neither affirmed nor excluded at this time. Clinical surveillance of all women taking oral contraceptives must be continued. A major effort to resolve the questions about steroid-induced neoplasia in human beings should be undertaken.

Metabolic effects

Hormonal contraceptives produce numerous effects on many organs, for example, the liver, the thyroid, and the adrenal. They also affect some of the body's homeostatic mechanisms; for example, they produce changes in salt and water metabolism and occasionally induce hypertension. Recently morphologic changes in blood vessels have been described. In many areas where alteration in function or structure has been noted, basic information is lacking. Little is known, for example, about the effects of the oral contraceptives on water metabolism or renal function.

Observations that large doses of estrogen hasten epiphyseal closure in girls has created fear that oral contraceptives may limit growth. Such concern is unjustified, however, because these drugs are usually prescribed only after the growth spurt and in doses far smaller than those required to stunt growth.

There is no evidence at this time that any of these drug-induced metabolic alterations pose serious hazards to health. The systemic effects of the drugs are so fundamental and widespread, however, that continued medical surveillance and investigation is required.

*   *   *

Conclusion

Although the Kefauver-Harris Amendments of 1962 indicate that the term "safe" has reference to health of man, nowhere do they define safety. Discussing this subject before the Sub-committee of the Committee on Government Operations of the House of Representatives, the Commissioner of FDA pointed out that no effective drug can be absolutely safe. Therefore, evaluation of safety of a drug requires weighing benefit against risk.

The Advisory Committee on Obstetrics and Gynecology has continued to assess the risk of oral contraceptives in this light, weighing knowledge of potential hazards against benefit. It has periodically reviewed the labeling of these compounds, repeatedly advocated strict surveillance by physicians, and recommended the accumulation of additional information about biological action and clinical effects. This report states the benefits of these compounds compared with those of other contraceptives.

Specific risks as well as requisite practices for follow-up of patients have been detailed in the labeling of all hormonal contraceptives. When these potential hazards and the value of the drugs are balanced, the committee finds the ratio of benefit to risk sufficiently high to justify the designation safe within the intent of the legislation.

NOTES

NOTE 1.

TESTIMONY OF DR. LOUIS M. HELLMAN—
JANUARY 22, 1970

* * *

In the first report [in 1966] we had to make some statement about safety. This was at the request of the Commissioner, and as you know, he is charged with both the efficacy and safety of drugs. It is quite apparent, if you read the report, even the first report, that the committee recognized certain very serious problems with oral contraceptives. They, however, were unwilling, and rightly, I believe, to say these things ought to come off the market. And they were faced with the dilemma, you have to make the statement.

Now, the statement we made in the first report said that these compounds are not unsafe for human consumption, which may not be the exact words, but that is what was said. That is a cute statement, more than a good statement, because we use the double negative to imply doubt. I never was very happy with that statement. I think it is kind of like the Delphic Oracle. You ask him what did you say, we did not understand it, and it is just about like that.

I always, in discussing that, said what this means is there [is] a yellow light of caution being exhibited by this committee.

Now, in discussing the . . . second report with the committee, I said to them that a more forthright statement has to be made. We cannot just hide behind rhetoric. We are going to have to say something. And we had options. "These are not safe," and then the Commissioner might have to take them off the market if he believed us. We can say "these are safe," and our scientific data did not really permit that kind of statement.

I took it upon myself to look into, as I am sure you have, the Kefauver-Harris amendments that regulate the actions of the Food and Drug Administration at the present time. As I indicated here, although those amendments are specific when they talk about food additives and were made much more specific by the Delaney amendment, which talks to this point. When they talk about safety of drugs, they face the same kind of dilemma that the committee faced.

* * *

. . . I take full responsibility for writing the sentence, "Safe within the intent of the legislation." But I did have consultation in writing that sentence. I did not just dream it up sitting up in Maryland. It was read to the committee and discussed. They approved it. . . .

* * *

I do not know anything other that I could have said about the oral contraceptives. I think it implied that there are problems with these drugs. And if you read this report, you cannot escape the fact that there are problems. I think, though, that you have to look at benefits.

Now, benefits are of two kinds when you are discussing a drug. There are benefits to the population as a whole. I do not want to go into the population problem, but I will say that the introduction of modern contraceptive methods has made the problem of population control immeasurably easier. With the traditional methods of contraception, it is very difficult, as you must have seen in India, to get any response out of the impoverished people. They have neither the time nor the privacy nor the motivation to use diaphragms, condoms, or whatever you will.

* * *

SENATOR NELSON: This question of what the word "safe" means in the 1962 act is a difficult one, and I do not know the answer to it. But I wonder if, in talking about weighing the risks versus the benefits, the word "safe" in the statute contemplated that the benefit of general population control was contemplated. I would guess, it would seem to me you would come up with risk-benefit vis-à-vis that particular patient. I would doubt whether anybody contemplated that you could put on the balance side on the scale the question of the fact that the control of the population is a benefit to that patient in any direct way. I think the rapid growth of the world population is disastrous. But it seems to me, and I raised this question the other day, that when we talk about risk, we are concerned about safety of an individual patient.

*   *   *

DR. HELLMAN: I think you put it very well, and it is quite unlikely that the hearings in 1963, or whenever they were, really considered population as a threat.

*   *   *

Then the argument comes up, do you really have at this moment a satisfactory alternative to these compounds for the number of people you have to treat and the actual conditions for which you are treating them? And I think I would say to you, and this is a judgment statement and not a factual statement, that we really do not.

You can argue about the effectiveness of the diaphragm and you can argue about intrauterine devices, but when you treat the people that I am treating, and these are the economically deprived individuals, you have a problem of quite considerable magnitude over what you can give them that will work for what they want to do.

SENATOR NELSON: I would remind you of your statement that many of the people you are treating, 55 percent are on the IUD and 40 percent are on the pill.

DR. HELLMAN: I think that here again, you can not expect a governmental regulatory agency to act as "big brother" to the physicians in the United States. . . .

*   *   *

NOTE 2.
TESTIMONY OF FDA COMMISSIONER
CHARLES C. EDWARDS AND FDA GENERAL
COUNSEL WILLIAM W. GOODRICH—
MARCH 4, 1970

*   *   *

DR. EDWARDS: . . . In categorizing this drug as safe, I do not want to imply, by any stretch of

the imagination, that this is an innocuous drug. It is a very potent drug, and when arriving at this decision to call it a safe drug we had to utilize the same standards we use for all other drugs.

As you well know, most of the other "safe" drugs, the powerful drugs, have certain contraindications. There are certain dangers in taking any drug, and they have to be taken under the conditions which are stated very clearly in the labeling.

So again, I would like to emphasize that in establishing this classification, we applied the same standards for the oral contraceptives as we have for all other drugs in categorizing them as safe.

SENATOR NELSON: The use in this context, then, was not in the ordinary dictionary use of the word—

DR. EDWARDS: It certainly was not. It was a Food and Drug Administration description of the word "safe," which really is "safe under the conditions of labeling," and which perhaps is a more accurate definition.

SENATOR NELSON: . . . If it had been my responsibility, I might have come to the same conclusion, but it does raise a question about the intent of the law and its meaning.

In 1938 Congress passed the statute requiring that, to market a drug, proof of safety must be submitted, adequate proof of safety or proof of safety acceptable to the FDA must be presented.

I would just like to ask Mr. Goodrich what he thinks was intended at that time. Let me state it this way:

In 1938 there were no oral contraceptives. In 1938, I would assume that the Congress was thinking of a drug for treatment of a specific target organism in a specific disease situation. In fact, it was in response to a particular safety problem that arose at that time respecting sulfanilamide, and maybe Mr. Goodrich will have a different view—and correct me if you do—that Congress was thinking then of a drug in which the issue was, is it safe for the particular disease situation which it is being used for, that is, the drug does have side effects, we are well aware of that; however, under the circumstance the illness of the patient indicates that on balance the risks of the side effects from the use of the drug are far outweighed by the benefits that the patient would get from the use of the drug for the particular disease situation that exists.

*   *   *

MR. GOODRICH: Yes. My understanding is

that all safety decisions have to be made in the context of the conditions for which the drug is prescribed, recommended or suggested.

Now, going back to what Congress had in mind in 1938 when they focused on an acute episode of poisoning, it happened to be due to the vehicle and not the drug itself. But as soon as we began passing on safety from the very first drug, the sulfanilamides, that were involved there, those drugs were not safe in any absolute sense of the term but they were quite safe treating infectious disease at that time, because many of those were life threatening.

Now, in that class of drugs, of course, it is relatively easy to balance benefit to risk, which is the test here. But there are other types of drugs that we have had to deal with over the years, drugs used for prophylaxis, or that type of drug, and in each instance it is essential that the agency balance benefit to risk, because there are very few drugs that have no side effects whatever, if they do anything.

* * *

SENATOR NELSON: Let me ask this question, though. Is it not correct when using the word "safe" that you do not mean safe in general, you mean safe for this particular patient who has a particular disease situation which the doctor decides that this drug will effectively treat, that is, target organism is subject to control by this drug, and on balance it is better that the patient risk whatever side effect this drug has rather than risk letting the disease run its course untreated by any drug.

It is an individual case, an individual disease, an individual prescription under an individual circumstance; is that not what we mean by "safe"?

MR. GOODRICH: That is the decision for the individual prescriber, but the decision for the Food and Drug Administration has to take into account different circumstances in which the drug will be used, some in private practice, others in university medical centers.

It has to take into account the total experience with the drug in the total prescribing population, and make a judgment there on all of these circumstances, this drug will be reasonably safe, that is, its benefits outweigh its risk under the circumstances in which it enters the market.

There have been a few instances in which drugs were allowed to enter the market only for use in university-type hospital settings, but in others the drug is permitted for widespread prescribing in most instances. But the Food and Drug

decision has to take into account all of these circumstances in reaching a safety decision.

SENATOR NELSON: Maybe I am not making myself clear. When you say "safe within the meaning of the law" are you not saying that we mean safe for the appropriate use of that drug under an appropriate circumstance in a specific disease situation?

MR. GOODRICH: Certainly.

SENATOR NELSON: Now, then, how do we bring the word "safe" to bear in the circumstance here of the oral contraceptive when: (1) there are alternative methods; (2) when, let us say, you are dealing with an intelligent, healthy well-motivated prospective user? How does the word "safe" apply in that respect?

The person has available medical care and a good hospital, has a good physician, has all of the facilities of the medical profession available as contrasted with the situation in which the patient has diabetes, or the patient has a history of high blood pressure, or carcinoma in the immediate family, something like that. How do you evaluate that specific case, the healthy patient with the finest medical facilities available with respect to the phrase "safe within the intent of the law"?

MR. GOODRICH: As you pointed out, that individual evaluation is for the prescriber, but as I approach it, as I see the responsibility of the Food and Drug Administration, it is to make sure that that prescriber has before him the information that is necessary for the safe, effective use of this drug.

* * *

The issue balancing benefit to risk in reaching a safety decision came to the Food and Drug Administration very shortly after the enactment of the first new drug provision in 1938. We could never have approved a number of classes of drugs, such as the corticosteroids, without balancing benefit to risk.

When Dr. Hellman called me, he asked if there was in the legislative development anywhere that I knew of a discussion of this point. It happened that there had been a very comprehensive discussion of this before the Intergovernmental Relations Subcommittee of the House and before the Committee on Interstate and Foreign Commerce and before the Antitrust Subcommittee at the time of the enactment of the 1962 Drug Amendments.

* * *

SENATOR MCINTYRE: . . . Actually, in 1938,

the law was just absent of any legislative history explaining the intent with respect to the statutory meaning of the word "safe."

MR. GOODRICH: And the reason was that the revision of the Federal Food, Drug and Cosmetic Act started in 1933. It was practically at the end point in 1937. The bill, indeed, had passed both Houses of Congress, when the elixir sulfanilamide episode occurred. This focused on the need for new drug provisions.

These provisions were proposed as separate legislation and were added on to that legislation at the very end, and there was no real discussion of the legislative intent there, other than to be sure that we protected the public from episodes of acute poisoning, which was what had been involved in the elixir sulfanilamide case.

*   *   *

NOTE 3.

TESTIMONY OF DR. VICTOR WYNN—
JANUARY 22, 1970

I appreciate particularly the fact that you have invited me here to give testimony, because I come from another country, Great Britain. As I am sure you are aware, far more women are taking oral contraceptive medications abroad than are taking them in this country, and they are doing so in imitation of the American woman, and they are doing so with the confidence which is inspired by the very high standard not only of American medicine, but also of the American regulating agencies, and especially the Food and Drug Administration.

*   *   *

In this book [a *Textbook of Contraceptive Practice* published in 1969, and acclaimed by members of the Family Planning and International Planned Parenthood Federations as being an extremely good textbook] a statement appears that under certain circumstances oral contraceptive medication would be acceptable, if they had several hundred times greater mortality than that which is already understood to be the case with this medication.

This implies that in certain communities at any rate according to these authors, and they are intelligent men, dedicated men, men who have the interests of the world at heart, but according to this statement, the oral contraceptive medication would still be acceptable if something like two out of every hundred women were to die every year of its use, and scores of others to be admitted to hospitals every year of its use,

leaving the surviving women to care for those who were hospitalized.

*   *   *

Now, it is my purpose merely to try and draw attention to some of those chemical changes which occur as the result of the use of these compounds. At least in this field we do have data. At least in this field we need not speculate. We can present evidence which one can inspect, and we have done so.

What we still cannot do with any degree of certainty is to interpret the evidence to you. We cannot tell you in what precise way, in how many years, and in what numbers women are going to have their health impaired by these metabolic changes, if indeed they are going to suffer such disadvantages, but it has always been and it still is and it must remain a condition of medical practice that medication must not be used unless it can be proved to be safe, and that the onus of proof is not on those who are investigating the medication. The onus of proof is on those who wish the medication to be used.

*   *   *

The first point I would like to make is this. That when contraceptive medication was introduced, the possibility that the biochemistry, the chemistry of the body, would be modified in very many ways was not fully understood.

Now, it is all very well for doctors to say "Of course we understood it. We anticipated it. Pregnancy does the same thing." This is not true. I refer to Dr. Gregory Pincus' book published in 1965 and called *The Control of Fertility*.

Dr. Pincus, as you know, was a very great man, a great experimenter, endocrinologist, and the originator with others of this form of fertility control. But in his book, which is very comprehensive he barely refers to the metabolic effects of the contraceptive medication.

Why is this? It is because when the book was published the metabolic effects were either inadequately understood or not understood at all. Now Dr. Doar and I had the opportunity of discussing this point in great detail with Dr. Pincus in the following year. He visited us in our laboratory, and we discussed the metabolic findings which we had made, and it was apparent to us that Dr. Pincus was unaware of a wide-ranging nature of metabolic intervention which follows and which must follow from the use of this type of chemical.

When I say these changes occur, I mean

they occur in everybody, more in some than in others, but no person entirely escapes from the metabolic influence of these compounds. It is merely that some manifest the changes more obviously than others.

* * *

. . . The glucose tolerance of the women taking the pill was impaired. And using criteria which are generally acceptable, using the criteria of the British Diabetic Association and the criteria of the American Diabetic Association, we came to the conclusion that in about 15 to 18 percent of women using this medication, the degree of impairment was such as to justify the term "chemical diabetes."

Now, what do we mean by chemical diabetes? Do we mean diabetes? The answer is "No, we do not." Chemical diabetes is defined as an abnormal glucose tolerance, and nothing else. Diabetes implies that there is also a clinical manifestation of this abnormality in the terms of, let us say, weight loss, or thirst, or passing a lot of urine, and so forth. The difference probably resides in the fact that diabetes is a more severe form of disorder than chemical diabetes, but is chemical diabetes insignificant? It is not.

* * *

Abnormalities of glucose tolerance, impairment of glucose tolerance, and elevation in lipid value and an alternation toward the male pattern lead one to suppose that there may be a risk of the development or the accelerated development of hardening of the arteries or atherosclerosis as it is more correctly known.

The studies we carried out were called cross-sectional in the sense that we had a group of women who were users and another group of women who were nonusers. We decided to repeat these studies using the same women as the controls. We investigated them before they started taking the medication, and then at intervals after the medication had been administered.

* * *

To be brief, what we found was that the impairment of glucose tolerance, which we had observed before, was reproduced in these women, and in addition we found that the insulin levels, the hormone which normally controls glucose metabolism, that the insulin values were higher in these women than when they were users.

Insulin-glucose interrelationships and their interrelationships with fat metabolism and the

relationships of these three to the accelerated development of atherosclerosis are one of the main medical topics of our time.

* * *

I do not know what the significance of the data is. I repeat this, that I am concerned, and every reasonable physician that I have spoken to on the subject is concerned. The Food and Drug Administration and the experts at the National Institutes of Health are equally concerned. We are not alarmed, and there is no reason why women should be alarmed at the results of my pronouncements.

We have to examine this situation. I listened very carefully to your words yesterday, when you were looking at the same proposition: Should we in fact be sitting here, with television cameras, and the world press, to discuss such an important subject?

I have had to ask myself this question, and I have no doubt that you have also seriously asked yourself this question, and I have no doubt about the answer, and the answer is this: We must discuss it. We must discuss it as rational, intelligent beings, as unemotionally as we can, and we must examine the evidence.

If the evidence is there, let us examine the evidence. If the evidence is not there, let us do everything we can to obtain the evidence. But on no account can we put this subject completely behind not an Iron Curtain but something which is substantially much worse.

* * *

It gives me no pleasure to give such an account on this subject. I derive no satisfaction from having to give a detailed description of events which we all would prefer not to be occurring in women, but it is my duty to do so.

The metabolic changes are there. It is necessary that those with responsibility examine the health of women in such a way that they can detect in good time whether these changes are deleterious or not, and if so what is the order of magnitude of the risks, but there is no time to be lost. Far too much time has already gone by without these relevant studies having been carried out.

* * *

SENATOR MCINTYRE: Dr. Wynn, the statement has been made here several times that the British findings regarding increased risk of thromboembolic disease with use of the pill cannot be applied directly to women in other countries including the United States. In fact, a statement to this effect was allowed in the official labeling of the oral contraceptives by FDA in 1968.

Moreover, the Sartwell study did come up with a different finding regarding the magnitude of the increased risk in the United States as opposed to Great Britain.

Do you know, Doctor, of any reasons why the British and the American female population should be any different with respect to the increased risk of thromboembolic disease resulting from use of oral contraceptives?

DR. WYNN: Taking the women by and large, I think the answer to that question is no. I would not expect there would be substantial differences between British and American women so far as risk of thromboembolism is concerned.

What the data reveal is the very great difficulty of carrying out epidemiological studies. You see, you take the Sartwell study. It was not identical to the British study.

They identified over 2,500 cases—I am speaking from memory—2,500 cases of thromboembolism, but they excluded all but a small fraction, 176, for one reason or another. Now some of the reasons for exclusion were in my view unreasonable.

They excluded women with varicose veins and family histories of diabetes, and so on. Now in conversation with Dr. Sartwell, he has agreed with me that some of the reasons for exclusion were not really those which he would advocate at the present time. Be that as it may, it merely gives some indication of the great difficulties in this type of study.

*   *   *

NOTE 4.

TESTIMONY OF DR. HUGH J. DAVIS,
ASSISTANT PROFESSOR OF OBSTETRICS AND
GYNECOLOGY, THE JOHNS HOPKINS
UNIVERSITY SCHOOL OF MEDICINE—
JANUARY 14, 1970

*   *   *

The fundamental problem with the oral contraceptives can be readily understood by anyone: It is medically unsound to administer such powerful synthetic hormones in order to achieve birth control objectives which can be reached by simple means of greater safety. This view was expressed by prominent gynecologic endocrinolo-gists prior to the approval of the pill for contraception 10 years ago, and subsequent history has shown that it is even more true today.

Meanwhile, 9 million women are consuming these compounds almost automatically and without much information about the hazards. The impression has been given the public that the oral contraceptives are nothing more than innocent natural female hormones. Yet milligram for milligram the synthetic chemicals used in these pills are 20 to 40 times as potent as the natural estrogenic substances. To think of them as natural is comforting but quite false.

The synthetic chemicals in the pills are quite unnatural with respect to their manufacture and with respect to their behavior once they are introduced into the human body. In using these agents, we are in fact embarked on a massive endocrinologic experiment with millions of healthy women.

*   *   *

One can argue that this is an acceptable risk since it is safer to take the pill than for 1 million women to become pregnant, but I do not believe this is relevant since there are safer alternatives available for either spacing pregnancies or for permanent contraception, and even if 1 million women commenced taking the pill, experience has shown they will not achieve the 100 percent protection they are often promised.

The effectiveness of the pill has been greatly overrated. Between 20 percent and 50 percent of women who start the pill abandon the method by the end of the year. Whether they abandon the method because of side effects or because of human failure to get their prescriptions renewed is, in my view, irrelevant. The fact is that failure to take the pill, just as surely as failure to insert a diaphragm, results in pregnancies. But these failures never appear in the glowing reports about the efficacy of the steroid hormones. . . .

Even among the patients who continue using the pill for birth control, pregnancies occur in between 1 and 3 percent, either because of omission of one or two tablets—that is human error—or because the method itself failed. It is very difficult to discriminate between these types of failure.

In our experience, some modern intrauterine devices provide a 99 percent protection against pregnancy and can be successfully worn by 94 percent of women, to cite but one alternative. Very similar results can be obtained with a properly used diaphragm in a well motivated population.

It is especially tragic that for the individual who needs birth control the most—the poor, the disadvantaged, and the ghetto-dwelling black— the oral contraceptives carry a particularly high hazard of pregnancy, as compared with methods requiring less motivation. The pill is less than ideal as a contraceptive among these women for precisely the same reason that the diaphragm often leads to unwanted pregnancy—both methods require a sustained repetitive act for continued protection. For many women, the diaphragm is too messy and inconvenient and the pill too complicated. Yet these women, who desperately need birth control services the most, are frequently offered the pill as if it were the only effective contraceptive. Because of these factors, it is the suburban middle class woman who has become the chronic user of the oral contraceptives in the United States in the past decade, getting her prescription renewed month after month and year after year without missing a single tablet.

*   *   *

Public policy with respect to oral contraceptives has been unsound in other respects. Is the consumer—the woman—aware of, or even capable of fully understanding all of these complex questions which have puzzled and concerned some of the best brains in medicine for the past decade? Again, as Senator Nelson has brought out, I think certainly little attempt has been made either to inform her or to protect her. In many clinics, the pill has been served up as if it were no more hazardous than chewing gum. The colorful brochures, movies, and pamphlets which are used to instruct women about the pill say next to nothing about possible serious complications. The same can be said for the veritable flood of articles in popular magazines and books which have convinced many women that there are few satisfactory alternatives to these steroids and that careful studies have proved that there is little risk to life or health in the pill.

Does the woman receive the same warnings and information about contraindications to the pill as the doctor? She does not. Is she privy to the fact that her risk of thromboembolism is greatly increased if she is taking the pill and is also over the age of 30? She is not. Is she aware that prolonged use of these compounds entails a completely unknown hazard of diabetes, harden-

ing of the arteries, and possible breast cancer? Not if she must depend on the brochures prepared for her information by the drug companies.

*   *   *

[I]f the oral contraceptives were an article of food there would be sufficient evidence on the basis of the animal experiments to consider seriously removing them from the market. We are in a curious situation with the oral contraceptives because they are classified as a drug although they are taken chronically by many people almost as if they were an article of diet. It is chronic use beyond 2 to 3 years that is particularly disturbing from a long range point of view. The numbers of women involved, and the unknown nature of the hazard, and the very disturbing evidence we have from the animal experiment, all of these things taken together, I think, should incline us all to be extremely cautious about long-term use of these agents.

*   *   *

SENATOR NELSON: I noticed that Dr. Kistner states in his book that a user of the pill should have a physical examination, in his judgment, every 6 months and that, therefore, he did not give a prescription that would exceed that period so that the user would have to come back to him, at which time Pap smears and various appropriate examinations would be made.

*   *   *

The estimate is that there are 9 million women using the pill in this country, is that right?

DR. DAVIS: The Food and Drug Administration estimate was approximately 8½ million women at this time.

SENATOR NELSON: Supposing that figure was doubled, supposing it was 20 million, are we prepared, from a laboratory standpoint and from the standpoint of availability of the physician, in fact, to examine 20 million women every 6 months, in addition to all other demands upon the laboratories and physicians?

DR. DAVIS: It would be a pretty massive undertaking. Let's hope it doesn't happen. I think there are other reasons for wishing it not to happen, but it surely would tax the capacity of the existing facilities if you double the patient load with the existing medical manpower situation. I think it could partly be overcome by using paramedical personnel for taking blood pressures and streamlining some of our rather archaic practices in handling people.

*   *   *

NOTE 5.

TESTIMONY OF J. HAROLD WILLIAMS,
M.D., LL.B., BERKELEY, CALIFORNIA—
JANUARY 22, 1970

*   *   *

We all recognize that drugs are essential to modern medicine, but the power of the doctor's prescription prerogative sometimes is a serious intrusion into the doctor-patient relationship. Indeed, that power is so awesome that I fear many physicians do not fully comprehend its ramifications when they put pen to pad.

Sometimes the physician is unsuspectingly caught in the middle, between his conscientious desire to serve his patients and intensive promotional pressure by drug manufacturers. The sad saga of the pill is one of the most phenomenal examples of such an entrapment of our medical profession.

*   *   *

As I point out some of the things that have happened in the advertising and promotion of the pill, please bear in mind that the average practicing physician relies upon the drug companies for much, if not all, of his information about the drugs. He may read some of the articles in medical journals which report adverse reactions to certain drugs, but by and large he does not have time, nor is he motivated, to read all journals, to sift the poor articles from the good, and to correlate all the information.

Obviously, he cannot repeat the research that has been done on drugs in his own practice. Usually he looks to the most convenient central source of information, the *Physicians Desk Reference*, a compendium of drug company advertising. Most of us here in this room, I think, understand that the PDR is no more than a compendium of drug company advertising. The doctor assumes that the drug companies are honest and that the FDA has been a vigilant watchdog to protect him and his patients. This is true sometimes; sometimes it is not.

*   *   *

Advertising of the pill to the medical profession has been characterized by many statements that tend to be misleading. . . .

*   *   *

. . . In Enovid *Bulletin No. 20,* published in 1964, under a section headlined "The responsibility of leadership" is this statement:

". . . [F]ew drugs in any category have ever been subjected to clinical tests as exhaustive as those already undergone by Enovid."

The reader was expected, no doubt, to understand that statement as applying to safety as well as to efficacy. I think much of the testimony that has been heard before this committee in the last 2 weeks underscores the fact that research as to safety has been a long time in coming and that it had not been exhaustive by 1964 and certainly has not been exhaustive even today.

*   *   *

Ambiguous language has been employed many times to take away the sting from information which should have had a warning impact on the physician. For example, in *Physicians' Product Brochure No. 62,* printed March 16, 1964:

"There is no direct evidence that Enovid alters the diabetic state. However, in a few instances some degree of difficulty in the management of diabetic patients has been reported in connection with Enovid therapy. . . . They may be expected to return to their pretreatment manageability on discontinuance of the drug."

It does not alter the diabetic state but they return to their pretreatment manageability on discontinuance of the drug.

*   *   *

Obsolescence of statements in advertising, amounting to untruthful misrepresentation, has occurred from time to time, as newer knowledge superseded older. Such were not restricted to the early days of aggressiveness, however, an outstanding example of this practice appeared in the past year. This was at a time when past events and warnings should have made everyone, everyone on the side of promotion, more vigilant than ever to be promptly forthright with physicians and their patients. This relates to the British statistical data, first published in 1967 as preliminary findings on thromboembolism then in 1968 as firm conclusions, about the increased risk of thromboembolism in pill users.

In May 1968 those data were added to the labeling on the pill, all brands, as an emergency measure by the FDA. However, the manufacturers successfully persuaded the FDA to allow a neutralizer in the material.

*   *   *

"No comparable studies are yet available in the United States. The British data, especially as they indicate the magnitude of the increased risk to the individual patient, can not be applied directly to women in other countries in which the incidences of spontaneously occurring thromboembolic disease may differ."

*   *   *

In November 1968, Drs. Markush and Siegal of NIH disclosed that their study of mortality rate "indicate[s] an association of oral contraceptives with an increase in mortality from diseases of the veins. . . ." Although that study was not comparable in technique, it was certainly comparable in conclusion—it did indeed exist. It seems to me it may not have been included up to the present time because it would have helped debunk sooner than this January some of the language quoted in this "no comparable studies" paragraph.

The results of the Sartwell study, reported in the Second Report on Oral Contraceptives by the Advisory Committee, were known in the spring of 1969, if in fact not sooner, were circulated widely in mimeographed form in August, released to the press in September, but as late as the issue of JAMA for December 29, 1969—which was the last issue I got before I left home—had not been incorporated in the labeling.

This "no comparable studies in the United States" was still there for doctors to read and get whatever reassurance they could get out of it.

. . . At the very least, this represents a 5-month delay in disseminating the new information. I submit, gentlemen, it does not take that long to revise the wording or do the new printing required in the advertising for the *Journal of the American Medical Association.*

The tone of much of the advertising has been to suggest to the doctor that he is indeed in a supreme position to order and manipulate life with his prescription pad.

Let me show you what I mean. On a number of occasions in the *Journal of the American Medical Association* has appeared this ad for Enovid–E. A photograph of a beautiful child on the lefthand side, and on the righthand side in big bold letters "Just what the doctor ordered."

Now, how God-like can you get, gentlemen?

In smaller print, "And spaced just right in the family plan, worked out years before by the physician," and oh, yes, "the baby's parents."

. . . If the pill is as good as they say it is, and if it is as safe as they say it is, that kind of advertising would not be necessary.

*   *   *

NOTE 6.
TESTIMONY OF DR. ALAN F. GUTTMACHER, PRESIDENT, PLANNED PARENTHOOD/WORLD POPULATION—FEBRUARY 25, 1970

*   *   *

Now, I need not extol the competence of the Food and Drug Administration Advisory Committee, because I think you know full well that it was picked from the most representative and competent people in this whole area. It is made up of very respected physicians, other scientists, and statisticians, and no doubt you know, but I would like to emphasize once more, their final statement in their recent report, which says when these potential hazards and the value of the drugs are balanced, the committee finds the ratio of benefit to risk sufficiently high to justify the designation safe within the intent of the legislation.

In mid-January, the American College of Obstetricians and Gynecologists made the statement that it "considers that the oral contraceptives are accepted therapeutic methods," and they deplored the inaccurate and sensational reports concerning the drugs.

At the January 28th meeting of my own very distinguished medical committee, which forms the National Medical Committee of the Planned Parenthood Federation, our physicians went over the data and they came up with the report that the committee continues to recommend the prescription of oral contraceptives.

Of course, the reason I quote these authorities is not to whitewash the pill, but I have a compelling interest to place this matter in proper perspective, in the hope, which I am sure you will agree with, of stemming unwarranted and dangerous alarm.

The pill, in my opinion and that of my colleagues, is an important prophylaxis, perhaps the most important, against one of the gravest sociomedical illnesses extant. That, of course, is unwanted pregnancy.

I would like to tally the results of unwanted pregnancy, a condition which is tragically common in our country. First, experts estimate that between 200,000 and 1,000,000 illegal abortions are performed each year in this country, with a death rate estimated to be 100 per 100,000 illegal operations when performed by nonmedical persons.

*   *   *

I think that pregnancy, in good hands—that

means excellent facilities, in a well-nourished woman who has had excellent prenatal care—carries with it a relatively minimal risk. But I think that anyone would state that if you took a thousand women—you would have to take them in terms of 100,000 women—who were so fortunate as to have this type of care, this type of nutrition, I think you would find you have a higher maternal mortality of more than 3 per 100,000. It may not be the 20 that we find in our American white population; it may not be the 30 which we find in our American black population.

*   *   *

SENATOR NELSON: I . . . have a pamphlet that discusses a particular oral contraceptive. The cover says, "So Close to Nature," . . . it is the pamphlet of one of the drug companies, explaining the use of the drug. . . .

*   *   *

So close to your natural feminine pattern. Your doctor has prescribed this newest kind of fertility-control tablet for you. Unlike others available for the same purpose, this preparation follows the principles and system of nature itself. Its actions closely resemble those of your natural menstrual pattern, and it works without upsetting the delicate balance of your normal body function.

Would you agree with that statement?
DR. GUTTMACHER: No, sir; I do not.

*   *   *

SENATOR NELSON: Well, this is one of the reasons for the hearings, the fact that all the data included in the FDA-sponsored study have not been widely disseminated. Although they have been published, they do not go to the user. Instead, the information in this pamphlet is what goes to the user.

This is the sort of thing being widely run in women's magazines, with an exception or two. Now, do you think that the patient who gets this, or even the doctor, is aware of the Salhanick report on "Metabolic Effects," etc.; this is the one from the workshop sponsored by NIH. Do you think the women of America are aware of what is said there?

In fact, do you think that most of the doctors—I would like the answer to both of those questions—I mean doctors who are not professionals in this field, such as you are, the gynecologic phase of it—do you think doctors are aware of what this report says? I shall read to you from it.

Until recently the metabolic effects of the sex steroids have been inadequately investigated or ignored. These accumulated data and others suggest that no tissue or organ system is free from a biological, functional and/or morphological effect of contraceptive steroids. Many of these changes appear to be reversible after short periods of treatment, but it is impossible to form judgments on the reversibility of some of the changes resulting from prolonged administration. This question becomes more important daily for the many patients who have already had long-term contraceptive steroid treatment.

*   *   *

Nevertheless, the consistency of such reports on such findings reject the possibility that they are of no consequence and require that certain questions be answered.

Does the user of the pill in America know this?
DR. GUTTMACHER: No, sir; she would not get much if she read that, either. That is the difficulty. I have been in active practice for 25 years as a private practitioner, and in addition, a full-time chief of service for 10 years. I have had contact with thousands of patients in my long medical life. Unfortunately the physician has to make the decisions for patients. You may discuss this with the patient at considerable length, and usually, when the discussion is over and you are talking about a particular therapy or operation, the patient will look at you and say, "What shall I do?"

Now, I do not think that you are going to be able to educate the American woman as to what she should or should not do with regard to the pill. . . . I think that the average doctor certainly has not read this volume of Salhanick, and I think that much of the information which is in there might be new to the American physician.

I think on the other hand the American physician is a conscientious man. I do not think that he willfully threatens the life of his patient. I think he probably is so overwhelmed by his medical practice and the normal activities of making a living that he tries to get his medical information in capsule form and he is very likely to take the particular throwaway literature which comes across the desk, not seldom, from the pharmaceutical firms.

*   *   *

Now, I certainly feel that the more we can instruct the American physician about the intricacies of the birth control pill, the wiser the effort. My feeling is that when you attempt to instruct the American womanhood in this, which is a pure medical matter which I am afraid she has not the background to understand, you are creating in her simply a panic reaction without much intellectual background. And this is what I think has been unfortunate.

I do not accuse these hearings of any diabolical purpose, but I must say that the reaction of the American public, parading this across the news media, particularly with the news media picking out those portions which are inflammatory, has done a great deal of harm.

I think educating the American physician is absolutely commendable and important and necessary, and I think perhaps the American physician has been remiss in not trying to educate himself about the intricacies of the pill.

*   *   *

SENATOR DOLE: Doctor, we all recognize that you indicate it is difficult to inform the patient by setting forth a list of the possible risks involved. Is the pill in this respect different from any other medication?

Is there anything different about the pill and hundreds of other medications? Is there anything about oral contraceptives where the problem of communication is any greater?

DR. GUTTMACHER: I suppose not. Certainly, when it comes to aspirin, we know that we have gastric hemorrhages for aspirin. We have fatal cases of aspirin, even in people who are not taking a vast amount. But I feel that the pill probably is a pretty special kind of medicament.

Of course, other drugs have reactions. Certainly, we know of death from penicillin, one of the most widely used drugs, or virtually any drug you can name. Whether the rate from penicillin is higher than from the pill, I cannot answer; I do not know that.

On the other hand, as Senator Nelson has pointed out, this is a drug given to women who are in a state of good health. My reaction to those remarks is that this is a powerful combination of drugs given to women to prevent a most serious illness, and that is unwanted pregnancy. From my point of view, it is justified.

Now, you asked me whether special things should be done in, I suppose, packaging and la-

beling. I have the feeling that most patients do not read what is put into their pill packages or medicines, and, if they do, they have some difficulty understanding it.

Again, my thesis goes back to the fact that your target should be the education of the American physician and that he has to take the responsibility of whether or not to prescribe the pill for Mrs. A or Miss B. This has to be his judgment. I would like to give him, equip him, with all the knowledge possible so that he can make his judgment correctly and authoritatively.

I am all for educating the American medical profession. I have rather dim enthusiasm for attempting to educate the recipients of therapy. I think that the dispenser of the therapy is the person who must be educated and not the recipient.

*   *   *

SENATOR NELSON: I want to just finish the discussion of this pamphlet. One of the issues we are concerned about is informed consent. The question raised here is, as a matter of public policy, are we entitled to withold information that is known about a prescription drug which gets the stamp of approval of the Federal agency under a statute passed by Congress? . . .

*   *   *

. . . Do we have a right not to have public hearings and not to make the information available on the ground that all the press may not carry it the way some people think they ought to carry it? Or that it is too complicated for the public to understand? Is this the kind of decision that we have a right to make, to withold knowledge developed by the Federal government itself through research and studies and conferences like the NIH, or should these matters be made a matter of public knowledge, counting, as it seems we always have to do, upon the ultimate good judgment of the public to come to a reasonable conclusion?

*   *   *

Now, let us assume that when the FDA report came out, the findings in that report had been put on the front page of the papers? Would not your reaction have been about the same as it is now?

DR. GUTTMACHER: I think people would have read it and then come to the final conclusion, which I admit is framed in verbiage which is difficult to define. But at least it is verbiage which does create a certain sense of complacency in the user. I think that if this committee has the power and the wisdom to perhaps issue a statement at the end of the hearings to put this whole thing in proper perspective, to grant the fact that the pill has magnificent and necessary use for many segments of the population, that there are other birth control methods for some which may be substituted with equally good effect, perhaps this will help a great deal.

I think that the American public is leaning on this committee for guidance. My hope is that if you agree with me that there has been a lot of material which perhaps has been misinterpreted and has become inflammatory, you will attempt in an honest and perhaps even cautious way to undo this, I think it would be a great service.

*   *   *

SENATOR NELSON: I at least do not have the qualifications to draw up a summary of what the experts have said and conclusions on it, and present it to the public as a valid position respecting the pill, its side effects, and its uses. I have no such qualifications. That is the reason we have called upon distinguished experts such as yourself and many others to state the case for the record.

DR. GUTTMACHER: . . . I have not attacked the hearings, sir. I do not think I have. I am unhappy about the results on our patients in my clinics. This distresses me because I do not think that anything has changed materially.

I think they could wait a little longer, but I think there has been a very sudden kind of stampede. This, of course, I regret.

Now, whether the hearings could have been differently tailored so that this was not the result, it is certainly not within my competence to tell you. You are much more experienced at this than I am.

I am not attacking the hearings. I believe in free speech. I believe everybody has a right to be heard. But unfortunately, when it comes to medical matters, the negative is so often more clearly understood than the positive by lay people. This is just the nature of the problem, sir. I have not the solutions to it.

*   *   *

The fact that our clinics have grown so magnificently since the pill was introduced, I am sure, is not due to the fact that other social factors have made deep impact. The fact that we now

have a product which is extraordinarily acceptable to our type of patient, and if we did not have this product and if we deny them this product or scare them to death from using it, unfortunately, we are going to revert back to situations which are most unhealthy in America.

SENATOR JAVITS: Has anything happened in the testimony or otherwise to change your view as an authority that this is a landmark and historic development in population control?

DR. GUTTMACHER: I think that the two methods, the pill and the intrauterine device, have been significant contributions. I think we are still in the horse-and-buggy day of effective contraception. I am optimistic in feeling that in 5 years, we shall have methods that are infinitely superior and safer than either.

*   *   *

I think the only influence we have not covered by question is the influence these hearings are leaving in their path throughout the world. I state in my testimony that Professor Alvarez from Montevideo and Professor LaVergne from Panama actually came to the United States because they are members of the Medical Committee of the International Planned Parenthood, to talk with me and others about these hearings because they are so terribly upset and because patients throughout Latin America are upset.

*   *   *

SENATOR NELSON: I am puzzled as to why they would come to the United States to find what was fact and what was fancy when you have testified that everything that was presented here was in the FDA Report. Did they not have that report?

DR. GUTTMACHER: I am not sure they have had it.

As a matter of fact, I received from London an editorial in one of the Pakistan papers, in which the editorial ends with the admonition that they should discontinue the pill in Pakistan. This, of course, is a very serious problem, because I know you, Senator Nelson, are among the great protagonists of world population control. Unfortunately, the pill is being depended upon more and more throughout the world for population control, and I feel that this setback has been most unfortunate.

Now, I am not blaming you. I think you are taking it for granted that I am trying to levy a certain amount of blame, and I am not blaming you at all. I just cannot help but decry that this has gotten so much adverse publicity in the press. I cannot help but say that nothing really has materially changed. Millions of people were on the pill before the hearings were held, and nothing has happened, really, to their knowledge about the pill.

Facts and conjectures have been ventilated to physicians who had less knowledge of the pill and ventilated to a lay public which is allergic to all kinds of scare propaganda. I feel our task is to try to put the thing in perspective so that people realize that the pill is still, to me, a magnificent therapeutic agent which has tremendous necessity, until, as Senator Javits says, this 5-year span can be passed and we have much better and safer methods.

Senator Nelson: There is no use going back into that. It is just a question of whether you believe the people of the United States should have all the facts or whether they should not. In my view, I think they should. Many people concerned about the question are concerned that the facts are out; some people may decide not to use the pill and therefore raise the problem about population control. I do not think we ought to use individual persons for sociological purposes.

Would you agree with the letter sent out by Dr. Edwards, Acting Commissioner of Food and Drug Administration, sent about the 18th of January . . . to 324,000 doctors. The last sentence reads:

In most cases, a full disclosure of the potential adverse effects of these products would seem advisable, thus permitting the participation of the patient in the assessment of the risk associated with this method.

Do you agree or disagree?

Dr. Guttmacher: I have not seen it, but we have discussed it before. I think it places a great burden on the patient. I think it is impractical, sir. I think the physician has to make the decision.

*　　　*　　　*

NOTE 7.

Testimony of Dr. Joseph W. Goldzieher, Director, Division of Clinical Sciences, Southwest Foundation for Research and Education, San Antonio, Texas—January 22, 1970

*　　　*　　　*

. . . Given the uncertain information about side effects, given the probable but certainly not unequivocal information regarding thromboembolic deaths, given the serious question of metabolic disorders (which in my opinion at the moment must remain within the realm of scientific inquiry and supervision, and not in the realm of decisionmaking), given these circumstances—how can one give women a proper set of facts so that they can make an intelligent decision as to whether to use the pill or not?

Human beings are generally not impersonal decisionmaking machines. Emotions tend to color thinking, especially when life or safety is at stake. There are innumerable sayings, like, "The doctor who treats himself has a fool for a patient." How coolly and objectively can a lay person, a woman or her husband, weigh information and make a sensible decision if they know that there is a risk of life or death, no matter how small, in the decision they make?

Aside from all emotion, making a sound decision requires having the necessary information and being able to evaluate this information correctly. It is certain that these hearings have produced one piece of information about which no one can quarrel: that even the experts on this subject disagree as to the interpretation of many of the available data. Literally centuries of experience have paraded before this committee, and there is no consensus. Is it then reasonable to suppose that a discussion between the physician and his patient, no matter how careful and well intentioned will, in 10 or 20 minutes, so well orient that individual so that she can now make a truly informed decision for herself?

On occasion I have had patients who have discussed with me the various methods of contraception and then came back with PDR in their hand, and quizzed me about the side effects of the pill like a trial attorney. Such a patient needs, and deserves, every bit of cooperation and information the physician can give her, so that she can make a psychologically and intellectually acceptable decision.

But how many women like this do you suppose there are? Many women have heard that the pill is the most reliable of all contraceptives, and they want to be certain as possible that they do not get pregnant, and that is all they are interested in. Is the doctor serving her best by trotting out a long list of statistical uncertainties, and making her anxious about a course of action she is already content to take?

There are other women, on or off the pill, who have been frightened by misinformation and distortion of facts. They deserve to have all the information they can understand and utilize. Unfortunately, few physicians have the power of communication, as well as the exact information, to carry out this task as well as one would wish.

Finally, we must recognize that there are vast numbers of women who simply do not have inquiring minds like those that fill this room, and do not have enough education to comprehend much more than the simplest facts of biology. A misguided effort to "inform" such women leads only to anxiety on their part, and loss of confidence in their physician. They did not come for a lecture on statistics; they came for help in not having the 10th baby. The doctor is the man who is supposed to know such things, and they want him to tell them what to do, not to confuse them by asking them to make decisions beyond their comprehension. The sound physician, by judicious questioning, can determine which contraceptive method is most likely to be acceptable and effective in that particular woman. This is the prime consideration. Then it remains to be determined if there are any medical contraindications to that particular method, and we have discussed this at great length. But the idea of informing such a woman is not possible. It depends on the woman herself. It depends on her socioeconomic status. It depends on her education. It depends on her cultural pattern.

One final point I would like to address myself to, and that is the question of who should give the information to the inquiring woman. To make this point briefly: I feel, as a practicing physician, that it is my responsibility and all other physicians' responsibility. If a doctor wishes to use teaching aids in the form of pharmaceutical pamphlets, charts, sketches he makes on his prescription pad, so long as he gets the message across, this is the important thing. In no way can that responsibility be delegated to anyone else.

*   *   *

NOTE 8.
AMERICAN ASSOCIATION FOR MATERNAL AND
CHILD HEALTH, INC.
PRESS RELEASE ON THE PILL*

*   *   *

Summarizing the responses, 3,240 (97 percent) physicians believe oral contraceptives are

_____
* Chicago: American Association for Maternal and Child Health, Inc. (April 29, 1970). Reprinted by permission.

medically acceptable; 61 (2 percent) believe they are not, and 51 (1 percent) are undecided. This vote of confidence for The Pill is the result of a careful balancing of the risks and benefits involved. The survey asked physicians to rank contraceptive modalities, considering pregnancy risk, general user health, and patient convenience. The results of the process appear below: oral contraceptives, with a ranking of 1.6 on a scale of 1 to 9 (where 1 indicates high desirability and 9 indicates low preference), are still the preferred method of birth control. Next, with a ranking of 2.7, was sterilization, followed by the intrauterine devices at 3.0.

Physician Rankings of Birth Control Methods

1—Medically most desirable
9—Medically least desirable

Though practicing physicians continue to endorse oral contraceptive use, many women have reacted to the recent publicity about the safety of The Pill. Obstetrician/gynecologists report that new patients asking for oral contraceptives have declined by 20 percent since the recent publicity. Further, established patients using oral contraceptives asking about safety tripled in the same period. Usually these patients are just seeking reassurance. After a discussion with their physician about the comparative risks and benefits of all the available birth control methods, 82 percent elect to remain on The Pill.

Despite current observations of a 20 percent drop in oral contraceptive use among new patients and 18 percent among especially concerned patients, these physicians report that when all patients under their supervision are considered, the decline in The Pill's use is much smaller. A year ago, 72 percent of their patients desiring contraception were using The Pill. Now they estimate this level at 65 percent, a drop of 7 percent.

*   *   *

NOTE 9.
TESTIMONY OF DR. ROBERT W. KISTNER, DEPARTMENT OF OBSTETRICS AND GYNECOLOGY, HARVARD MEDICAL SCHOOL—JANUARY 15, 1970

*   *   *

Although the pill was declared safe in 1969 by the advisory committee on obstetrics and gynecology to the Federal Food and Drug Administration, strangely divergent views continue in the medical and lay press. The pill is either blessed or damned; a valuable therapeutic tool or a potential killer. The medical profession seems to me to be undergoing a schism into "those for" and "those against" the pill. The proponents are largely clinicians who have used the pill day in and day out, over many years, in thousands of patients and have not been impressed by the newspaper scare stories. The opponents are usually physicians or investigators who have not, for one reason or another, been in contact with patients or who have chosen not to prescribe the pill even if they are. The year 1969 did not, unfortunately, bring forth a verdict; neither a winner nor a loser was chosen. Only one decision stands or stood: The pill is safe. Safer than what? Safer than pregnancy on the basis of mortality figures but not as safe as continence.

Almost without exception the consequences of contraception are beneficial and contribute significantly to the health and well-being of the community. In contrast, many societies permit drugs and other practices which are of questionable value or are demonstrably harmful. The ill effects of alcohol and tobacco, which are tolerated for no better reason than that they provide comfort and pleasure, add appreciably to the mortality and morbidity rates of many societies, but they are inadequately regulated by civil law and social custom and do not fall within the sphere of medical prescription. John Peel and Malcolm Potts, in their recently published book, *Textbook of Contraceptive Practice,* state:

Thirty thousand deaths from lung cancer occur yearly in Britain, the majority due to smoking. By the end of the century more British men will have died from smoking-induced cancer than in two world wars. For every pill-induced death in Britain there are at least 1,500 cigarette-induced deaths; based on the total sales of the two products during 1967 one cigarette is three times as dangerous to life as one pill.

MR. GORDON: Dr. Kistner, may I interrupt for just one moment? Since you compared the risks of smoking with that of the pill, do you know of any cases where smoking three packages of cigarettes has caused either serious illness or death? Three packages?

DR. KISTNER: Smoking three packages?

MR. GORDON: Right.

DR. KISTNER: Obviously the answer to that question is no.

MR. GORDON: I have here the proceedings of a conference held on September 10, 1962, at the headquarters of the American Medical Association sponsored by G. D. Searle and Co. In the back of that, appendix 3, there are case reports, and several reports where people have either died or have become seriously injured taking the pill for only 3 months, in other words, three packages of pills.

DR. KISTNER: Is there a cause and effect relationship demonstrated or proved?

MR. GORDON: Well, it just says "Case reports: Thrombosis and embolism in patients taking the pill."

DR. KISTNER: There is no cause and effect relationship so far as I understand.

MR. GORDON: They said the same thing about tobacco.

*   *   *

SENATOR MCINTYRE: . . . Doctor, I agree to a certain extent with your observation that the medical profession seems to be undergoing a schism into those for and those against the pill although none of those who have thus far testified about the danger of the pill have advocated that it be completely removed from the market. However, I am afraid that I cannot agree at all with your identification of the proponents as clinicians, who have used the pill daily, and the opponents as physicians or investigators who have not been in contact with patients or have chosen not to prescribe the pill.

Each of the four witnesses we had yesterday might be considered opponents of the pill to some extent. However, three of the four do have regular contact with patients and have prescribed the pill.

A more accurate description, I think, would be that the proponents are largely those who were involved in the development of the pill or in the promotion of its use or who have never observed a serious adverse reaction in their patients.

The opponents appear to be largely those who have observed potentially serious side effects either through research or medical practice. Do you agree?

DR. KISTNER: I will accept that.

*   *   *

SENATOR MCINTYRE: Dr. Kistner, the labeling of all oral contraceptives now contains a long list of side effects of varying severity and a listing of certain conditions under which the drug should not be used. In your own practice do you regularly inform a woman of these potential side effects and question her concerning any of these preexisting conditions before starting her on the pill?

DR. KISTNER: Yes.

*   *   *

MR. GORDON: Let me read from testimony that you gave [in a legal action for damages against a pill manufacturer].

*   *   *

You were asked the question "What do you tell them about Enovid when you prescribe it?" Then you said, "Well, my routine is and I hope I may be able to give my routine" and you talk about taking a thorough history, do a complete pelvic examination and so on and so forth, and then you say "in addition to this I will usually give her one of the prepared booklets that all of the pharmaceutical houses have in order to have her better understand exactly what is going on in the physiology, in her basic physiology. I like my patient to know what is going on and how the drug she has taken is effective in preventing pregnancy," and so on.

The question is then asked "To what extent do you go over with your patients the information contained in the package insert?" Your answer "I don't relate the package insert to the patient. The package insert is related to me"; then the next question, "When you give Enovid to your patients in the manner which you prescribe, do you discuss with them the reports that appear in the Searle literature?" And then "Did you tell your patients about the reports that appeared in the Searle literature in the package insert regarding the occurrence of thromboembolic phenomena of takers of Enovid?"

"[A:] Are you asking me whether I initiated the conversation?"

"Q: Yes, whether you told your patient about it," . . .

"[A:] Well as an initiation, no. I did not."

"[Q:] How would it come up if it came up?"

Your answer, "If the patient asked me that she had read there was some problem with blood clotting then I would reply to the question."

"Then what would you reply?" So on and so forth.

This was on direct examination. Then in the cross-examination the counsel asked "But you never tell your patient there is a risk of this oral contraceptive pill?" Your answer "No, I do not."

"Q: Isn't that correct?"

"A: That is correct.

You are asked later, then, "Why don't you tell them?" And you say "Well, they might get, if you tell them they have headaches then they have headaches," and so on and so forth.

Then the counsel asked, "Well, if you warn them they may get blood clots, would that warning induce them to get blood clots?"

This testimony indicates that you have not, at least as of that time, warned your patients of the risks.

*   *   *

DR. KISTNER: . . . But the testimony just read here has to do with complications. If you ask if I sit down and I take this out and I say "Now, I want you to know that you may die of blood clotting or you may get hepatitis or you may get this, that or the other thing," and besides that the only thing that has been said today as far as ipso facto evidence is that of blood clotting, then I would say no. I don't believe it is good medical practice with any medication to go through the list of possible complications.

If I prescribed this particular tranquilizer I wouldn't read off this list of complications. I would tell the patient, "Now, you may get dizzy from taking this. I don't want you to drive," but I wouldn't list to her the total list of complications, and the testimony was in regard to complications, and my direct reply to the interogator was that if the patient asked me about the risk then I would tell her about that.

*   *   *

NOTE 10.
TESTIMONY OF DR. HAROLD SCHULMAN,
ASSOCIATE PROFESSOR, DEPARTMENT OF
OBSTETRICS AND GYNECOLOGY,
ALBERT EINSTEIN COLLEGE
OF MEDICINE, NEW YORK, N.Y.—
MARCH 3, 1970

*   *   *

There is little doubt that the reporting of these hearings by the press, radio and television has created widespread alarm among women, and many have stopped taking oral contraceptives because of this. Tragically, it is once again the poor who are discriminated against in this type of situation, because they stop their method of birth control, and do not have easy access to a physician to obtain other methods.

We have already seen several women seeking abortion because of these developments. If hearings such as this are going to be held, I believe the committee must carefully plan and screen all individuals who are invited to testify as to the content of their testimony.

MR. GORDON [Committee Staff Economist]: Doctor, doesn't that sound something like censorship? Ar you saying that the testimony of a witness should be examined thoroughly before he be allowed to testify?

DR. SCHULMAN: No, I am certainly not advocating the suppression of minority opinion.

MR. GORDON: Or majority opinion? What kind of opinion are you referring to?

DR. SCHULMAN: I think opinion expressed in a responsible way, and I amplify this statement in the remaining paragraph.

MR. GORDON: Who would make the decision whether it is responsible or not?

DR. SCHULMAN: I think in years past, newspapers and magazines have hired science writers and deliberately trained them so they would have some ability to present information in a way which does not alarm the public, regardless of what the content might be.

MR. GORDON: You are saying that the committee must carefully plan and screen all individuals who are invited to testify, as to the contents of their testimony. Do you think that the content of the testimony of various witnesses should be screened before it is allowed to be presented to the public? Is that what you are saying?

DR. SCHULMAN: I think in an area such as this, I think that is necessary, yes. Because you screen it does not mean you would not allow it to be heard.

MR. GORDON: But the committee, you say, should determine what should be stated publicly?

DR. SCHULMAN: No, I think it should determine how it is said publicly.

MR. GORDON: You do not think that is a type of censorship?

DR. SCHULMAN: Well, I do not see it as a type of censorship. It is conceivable that it could be, but if a committee has broad representation, presumably there would be a majority opinion or at least another opinion expressed where it would not be censorship. The committee does

not have a uniform viewpoint towards this issue, either, I would presume.

MR. GORDON: Thank you very much.

SENATOR DOLE: Perhaps the hearings should have been held in executive session because of the somewhat sensational nature of the publicity they generated. If we were concerned only with the problem, we may have been able to explore it more quickly and perhaps have a more detailed examination of witnesses in executive session.

Certainly, no one here suggests censorship, but it does seem we are dealing with a very delicate medical problem, one we Senators are not at all well qualified to deal with. We can ask questions, we can enlist the witnesses, and we can listen to their statements, but we really do not understand the problem. We have had no experience at all with the problem, except in the work we have done—I cannot speak for Mr. Gordon, because he does have great knowledge in this area—that is in the record.

DR. SCHULMAN: Well, I am certainly not advocating censorship, but freedom also implies responsibility and I think the minority [opinion] should be responsibly expressed.

As I mentioned, reputable newspapers and magazines have employed science writers to ensure that the public gets accurate information without unduly alarming the public. Furthermore, the committee must use its legal skills to question and deliberately point out to witnesses and the public at the time of testimony when inflammatory statements such as "mass experiment," and a number of others that have been made today, are being used.

NOTE 11.

POLL ON THE PILL*

* * *

Largely because of all the recent publicity, 18 per cent of the 8.5 million U.S. women on the pill—nearly one in five—say they have stopped it altogether. In addition, 23 per cent say they are giving serious consideration to quitting.

What makes the proportion of women who are defecting even more remarkable is the fact that many of them also say that they have had entirely satisfactory experiences with the pill. Fully 76 per cent of users say they have been "very satisfied" with oral contraceptives, and another 11 per cent were "fairly satisfied." Moreover, two-thirds of U.S. users continue to believe

---

* *Newsweek* 52–53 (February 9, 1970). Copyright Newsweek Inc., 1970. Reprinted by permission.

that the advantages of oral contraceptives outweigh the risks. Forty-one per cent of the women say they have had no side effects or complications, and 38 per cent attribute their approval of oral contraceptives to their unquestioned effectiveness.

*   *   *

The influence of the recent bad news about the pill is easy to understand. An astonishing 87 per cent of American women have heard or read about the Senate pill hearings, a degree of awareness rare on public issues or events. And no matter what their own personal reaction, more than a third, on the basis of the reports, are prepared to believe that the pill is linked to cancer, blood-clotting problems, diabetes and heart trouble. There remain, however, a good many women who are not particularly frightened by what they have heard. Twenty per cent of the users believe that the relationship between the pill and cancer, or between the pill and blood clotting, has yet to be established, and another 14 per cent believe that conflicting testimony has made it impossible to reach positive conclusions about the hazards. "It seems to me most of the people who testified stressed the detrimental effects," said a wary housewife in Morristown, N.J. "You could die in childbirth just as easy as taking the pill," noted the wife of a Hastings, Neb., laborer.

One of the main purposes of the Nelson hearings was to determine whether women are being adequately informed by their doctors about the suspected dangers of oral contraceptives. And in the light of the survey, the sub-committee's concern was well founded. A startling two-thirds of pill-taking women say they have never been told about possible hazards by their physicians. On the other hand, only 16 per cent of women have taken the trouble themselves to discuss the dangers of the pill with their doctors as a result of the Senate investigation. Most of these were reassured by their physicians that the pill is safe and that they have prescribed it for a considerable time without noting serious side effects. An Omaha woman quoted her doctor as saying that he had prescribed the pill "long before they were called birth-control pills and never had any patient get cancer or anything else."

Less than 1 per cent of women have found their doctors to be totally against the pill. A Norfolk, Va., woman reported that her physician told her oral contraceptives were "not natural." And still other physicians seem evasive to their uneasy patients when asked about the risks of the pill. A 26-year-old Denver woman reported that

her physician "couldn't be tied down to an answer."

*   *   *

NOTE 12.

L. L. COLEMAN, M.D.
"PILL" SCARE STORIES*

A most terrifying article on birth control pills appeared in a ladies' magazine. It was filled with terrible tales of disabling injuries to the brain and the uterus. I am certain my doctor would never suggest that I take these drugs if they are as harmful as this article says they are. Are we really risking death or permanent injury by taking these pills?

—Mrs. C.W.T.

Dear Mrs. T.: I happened to see the article you referred to and am distressed by the unnecessary fears it highlighted. Unfortunately, some eager writers, with little or no scientific knowledge, find that the greatest impact can be made by emphasizing fear rather than hope in their writing. I disagree completely with this destructive attitude.

Before contraceptive pills were distributed to the general public, untold control studies were done to be sure of their safety. This is one of the great responsibilities of government health agencies which constantly protect the American people from the "overenthusiasm" for new drugs by their manufacturers.

All drugs may have some potential danger. Even the most innocuous drugs can call forth an unusual reaction in the highly sensitive or allergic person. It is with this understanding that your doctor prescribed the birth control pills. The advantages and disadvantages are carefully weighed in the choice of these pills. You can be certain that all these considerations were appreciated by him for you. There are some risks in everything we do. We must not permit ourselves to be terrified into believing that our health and lives are in jeopardy every time we read scare statistics that have no solid basis in scientific truth.

d.

Testimony of FDA Commissioner
Charles C. Edwards—March 4, 1970

*   *   *

Under the present system we try to keep the physician abreast of adverse reactions as we be-

---

* *The San Francisco Examiner* (June 12, 1969). Copyright 1969, King Features Syndicate. Reprinted by permission.

come aware of them. This is certainly true with regard to the oral contraceptives. There is no question that it is vitally important to communicate this information to the physician, but there is also corresponding need to keep the patient well informed. I believe that the patient should receive as much accurate information as is necessary for her to make certain decisions.

Let me examine for just a moment how women are currently being informed as regards the oral contraceptive.

They get a good deal of information and misinformation from sources other than the physician—through newspapers, pamphlets, books, television, and from discussion with others. This additional information is reaching a large number of people in a short period of time. While we can control the prescribing information which goes to the physician and any printed or graphic matter that may ultimately reach the patient through him, we have no such opportunity to see that other presentations are accurate, balanced, and properly informative.

I have come to the conclusion that the information being supplied to the patient in the case of the oral contraceptive is insufficient and that a reevaluation of our present policies is in order.

Accordingly, I have asked our Bureau of Drugs to examine this area of consumer information and to give me their recommendations.

I have with me today, which I will submit to you, a statement which we are going to publish in the *Federal Register* so that all interested parties will have an opportunity to comment on it. This statement is the proposed language for a reminder leaflet of uniform content which will be placed by the manufacturer into each package of oral contraceptives produced.

This leaflet is designed to reinforce the information provided the patient by her physician. I emphasize the word "reminder" as its purpose is to recall to the patient her discussion with the physician when she made her decision to begin taking an oral contraceptive.

*   *   *

What You Should Know About Birth Control Pills (Oral Contraceptive Products)

All of the oral contraceptive pills are highly effective for preventing pregnancy, when taken according to the approved directions. Your doctor has taken your medical history and has given you a careful physical examination. He has discussed with you the risks of oral contraceptives, and has decided that you can take this drug safely.

This leaflet is your reminder of what your doctor **has** told you. Keep it handy and talk to him if you think you are experiencing any of the conditions you find described.

A WARNING ABOUT "BLOOD CLOTS"

There is a definite association between blood-clotting disorders and the use of oral contraceptives. The risk of this complication is six times higher for users than for non-users. The majority of blood-clotting disorders are not fatal. The estimated death rate from blood-clotting in women *not* taking the pill is one in 200,000 each year; for users, the death rate is about six in 200,000. Women who have or who have had blood clots in the legs, lung, or brain should not take this drug. You should stop taking it and call your doctor immediately if you develop severe leg or chest pain, if you cough up blood, if you experience sudden and severe headaches, or if you cannot see clearly.

WHO SHOULD NOT TAKE BIRTH CONTROL PILLS

Besides women who have or who have had blood clots, other women who should not use oral contraceptives are those who have serious liver disease, cancer of the breast or certain other cancers, and vaginal bleeding of unknown cause.

SPECIAL PROBLEMS

If you have heart or kidney disease, asthma, high blood pressure, diabetes, epilepsy, fibroids of the uterus, migraine headaches, or if you have had any problems with mental depression, your doctor has indicated you need special supervision while taking oral contraceptives. Even if you don't have special problems, he will want to see you regularly to check your blood pressure, examine your breasts, and make certain other tests.

When you take the pill as directed, you should have your period each month. If you miss a period, and if you are sure you have been taking the pill as directed, continue your schedule. If you have not been taking the pill as directed and if you miss one period, stop taking it and call your doctor. If you miss two periods, see your doctor even though you have been taking the pill as directed. When you stop taking the pill, your periods may be irregular for some time. During this time you may have trouble becoming pregnant.

If you have had a baby which you are breast feeding, you should know that if you start taking the pill its hormones are in your milk. The pill may also cause a decrease in your milk flow. After you have had a baby, check with your doctor before starting to take oral contraceptives again.

WHAT TO EXPECT

Oral contraceptives normally produce certain reactions which are more frequent the first few weeks after you start taking them. You may notice unexpected bleeding or spotting and experience changes in your period. Your breasts may feel tender, look larger, and discharge slightly. Some women gain weight while others lose it. You may also have episodes of nausa and vomiting. You may notice a darkening of the skin in certain areas.

OTHER REACTIONS TO ORAL CONTRACEPTIVES

In addition to blood clots, other reactions produced by the pill may be serious. These include mental depression, swelling, skin rash, jaundice or yellow pigment in your eyes, increase in blood pressure, and increase in the sugar content of your blood similar to that seen in diabetes.

POSSIBLE REACTIONS

Women taking the pill have reported headaches, nervousness, dizziness, fatigue, and backache. Changes in appetite and sex drive, pain when urinating, growth of more body hair, loss of scalp hair, and nervousness and irritability before the period also have been reported. These reactions may or may not be directly related to the pill.

NOTE ABOUT CANCER

Scientists know the hormones in the pill (estrogen and progesterone) have caused cancer in animals, but they have no proof that the pill causes cancer in humans. Because your doctor knows this, he will want to examine you regularly.

REMEMBER

While you are taking ——————————, call your doctor promptly if you notice any unusual change in your health. Have regular checkups and your doctor's approval for a new prescription.

* * *

SENATOR NELSON: The figures that have been used frequently before the committee indicate that hospitalization from blood clotting occurs in 1 of every 2,000 users. Is there any reason for not using that figure in here?

* * *

DR. JENNINGS: . . . That was a hospitalization rate, which is one indication of morbidity. I think what we attempted to do here was not a literal translation of the information given to the physician, who is, after all, much more sophisticated and capable of handling these numbers, but to try in a simple fashion to alert the woman to the fact that there was an increased risk and then to give her some idea of the magnitude of this, especially in relation to the most important, that is, the fatality.

SENATOR NELSON: Well, all I say, as just a layman reading it, is that when you talk about the death rate being one in 200,000 for women not taking the pill and for users six in 200,000, those are very large figures. But when you get down to the more practical aspect in a higher incidence and talk about almost one in 2,000 being hospitalized, which is a very high incidence, it is a figure that is much easier to understand, and does not just talk about deaths, it talks about hospitalization rates.

* * *

DR. EDWARDS: I think your point is well taken, and I would emphasize that this is not the final package. This is for discussion purposes primarily, and we certainly anticipate making changes, as requested by groups such as your committee and others.

I think your particular point is a good one.

SENATOR DOLE: Dr. Edwards, this insert has been in the making for sometime; is that correct?

DR. EDWARDS: Right.

SENATOR DOLE: I am not certain whether the average person realizes there is any great risk if it is one out of 200,000 or six out of 200,000. We have had witnesses indicate we should not include a laundry list with medication, because to do so would confuse the patient.

I am not certain where you draw the line, whether you should indicate any numbers, whether you should indicate there is some risk. The question is how to best communicate with patients, but we do not want to frighten the few people left who are not frightened as a result of these hearings.

I would hope that we do not try to rewrite the memorandum in committee hearing.

SENATOR NELSON: I hope the Commissioner did not think I was trying to rewrite the memorandum; I was just asking the question for information purposes because I thought it was a good question. I would not think of trying to write the memorandum, but I would think it is within the province of a member of the committee or any citizen in America, and there are 200 million of them, to ask a question.

* * *

NOTES

NOTE 1.
F.D.A. RESTRICTING WARNING ON PILL— A DRAFT REVISION INDICATES ORIGINAL IS TONED DOWN*

The Food and Drug Administration is toning down its announced package warning for 8.5

—————
* *The New York Times* (March 24, 1970). © 1970 by the New York Times Company. Reprinted by permission.

million users of oral contraceptives after pressure from physicians, drug manufacturers, and high Government officials.

An F.D.A. spokesman and sources in the Department of Health, Education, and Welfare confirmed today that the 600-word leaflet announced earlier this month was being extensively reworded.

The original leaflet referred to such serious possible reactions to the pill as blood clots, mental depression, swelling, skin rash, jaundice, high blood pressure, and elevation of blood sugar levels. . . .

One draft revision runs less than 100 words, mentions only a single specific danger from oral contraceptive use, and deletes detailed suggestions on when women using the pill should see a physician.

"Any similarity between this draft and what the F.D.A. proposed is purely coincidental," said one knowledgeable Senate source.

Dr. Charles C. Edwards, F.D.A. commissioner, read to a Senate monopoly subcommittee on March 4 the leaflet's specific wording, which he said, "We are going to publish in *The Federal Register* so that all interested parties will have an opportunity to comment on it."

* * *

It is not unusual for an agency to revise a proposed regulation after publication and after receipt of comments. But it is unusual, informed sources said, for the regulation to be drastically reworded before publication and before formal comment is received.

* * *

Dr. Edwards ruffled bureaucratic feathers when he told the Senate subcommittee about the leaflet and its specific warning without first informing his superior, Dr. Roger O. Egeberg, Assistant Secretary of Health, Education, and Welfare.

The American Medical Association complained to Dr. Egeberg and the H.E.W. Secretary, Robert H. Finch, that the leaflet would interfere with the doctor-patient relationship and possibly could lead to malpractice suits.

The drug industry objected, contending that the leaflet overemphasized dangers and minimized benefits from oral contraceptives.

The revised draft leaflet has this to say about the pill's dangers:

"As with all effective drugs, they may cause side effects in some cases and should not be taken at all by some. Rare instances of blood clotting are the most important known complications of the oral contraceptives."

The original wording was much sharper on clots. It said:

"There is a definite association between blood-clotting disorders and the use of contraceptives. The risk of this complication is six times higher for users than for nonusers."

The original warning offered signpost symptoms requiring immediate medical attention. It also said:

"Your doctor has taken your medical history and has given you a careful physical examination."

The revised draft said the contraceptives "should be taken only under the supervision of a physician," and users should have "periodic examinations at intervals set by your doctors."

NOTE 2.

MORTON MINTZ
PILL ADVICE STILL UNCLEAR AS FDA
SPURNS NEW WORDING—AGENCY PREFERS
SHORT WARNING, DESPITE PROTESTS*

An entirely new warning to users of the Pill has been recommended to the Food and Drug Administration by its outside advisers on birth control.

At least temporarily, however, the FDA is rejecting the recommendation in favor of a proposal of its own.

Thus it was still unclear yesterday what advice an estimated 8.5 million women eventually will get with each package of oral contraceptive pills.

The recommended new warning resulted from a hitherto undisclosed development last Wednesday—the invasion by two members of the Women's Liberation Movement of a closed meeting of the Advisory Committee on Obstetrics and Gynecology at FDA headquarters in Rockville.

After hearing the Women's Liberation protests, Dr. Roy Hertz, a committee member, wrote this draft for a sticker to be affixed to every package of pills:

"Do not take these pills without your doctor's continued supervision. Contact him if you experience any unusual symptoms, particularly the following: 1. Severe headache. 2. Blurred vi-

---

* *The Washington Post* (April 6, 1970). © 1970, The Washington Post. Reprinted by permission.

sion. 3. Pain in the legs. 4. Pain in the chest or cough. 5. Irregular or missed periods."

All but "5" can be symptoms of blood-clotting diseases.

The committee suggested that the FDA publish the draft in the *Federal Register* and drop a 96-word agency proposal that would tell women about the Pill in general terms, with none of the committee's emphasis on symptoms and what to do about them. A Women's Liberation member denounced the 96-word statement as "worse than no warning at all."

However, Commissioner Charles C. Edwards told a reporter last week that if the Secretary of Health, Education, and Welfare approves, the FDA soon will publish the 96-word statement "without any change." At the end of a 30-day period for filing of comments, he said, the agency will consider modifications, giving "very top priority" to the advisory committee draft.

Dr. Edwards emphasized that he was not foreclosing the possibility that the statement ultimately adopted will be stronger than the 96-word version. His primary goal is to start the legal process by which a warning of some kind will go directly to users, he said.

*   *   *

NOTE 3.
HEW Publishes Warning on the Pill*

The Department of Health, Education, and Welfare settled yesterday on a fourth version of a warning to be enclosed in every package of birth control pills.

The language is not necessarily final. After publication today in the *Federal Register* comments can be filed for 30 days. Then this language or a modification will be ordered into effect, provided there is not a court challenge.

The fourth version, announced by HEW Secretary Robert H. Finch at the end of a press conference on civil rights, follows:

"The oral contraceptives are powerful, effective drugs. Do not take these drugs without your doctor's continued supervision. As with all effective drugs they may cause side effects in some cases and should not be taken at all by some. Rare instances of abnormal blood clotting are the most important known complications of the oral contraceptives. These points were discussed with you when you chose this method of contraception.

---
* *The Washington Post* (April 8, 1970). © 1970, The Washington Post. Reprinted by permission.

"While you are taking this drug, you should have periodic examinations at intervals set by your doctor. Tell your doctor if you notice any of the following: 1. Severe headache; 2. Blurred vision; 3. Pain in the legs; 4. Pain in the chest or unexplained cough; 5. Irregular or missed periods."

The portion of the warning dealing generally with the pill was taken from a 96-word proposal that Dr. Charles C. Edwards had wanted to publish and which, in turn, was a watered-down version of an 800-word warning he had endorsed on March 4 at a hearing before Sen. Gaylord Nelson (D–Wis.).

The second portion of the warning—advising women to be alert to possible symptoms of blood-clotting and gynecological disorders—had been recommended by the FDA's outside advisers on the pill.

HEW overrode Dr. Edwards, who had tentatively rejected the advice of the consultants. Secretary Finch acknowledged that he now has endorsed a compromise, which he called "a delicate balance." He said he believed the shorter statement is more likely to be read.

NOTE 4.
Food and Drug Administration
Statement of Policy Concerning Oral
Contraceptive Labeling Directed to
Users*

On April 10, 1970, there was published in the *Federal Register,* 35 F.R. 5962, a notice of proposed rule-making to establish new labeling which would assure that the user is provided information necessary for her safe use of these drugs.

The proposal was controversial and drew a substantial number of comments. . . .

*   *   *

[P]ursuant to the provisions of the Federal Food, Drug, and Cosmetic Act . . . the following new section is added to Subpart A of Part 130:

*   *   *

. . . The oral contraceptives are restricted to prescription sale, and their labeling is required to bear information under which practitioners licensed to administer the drugs can use them safely and for the purpose for which they are intended. In addition, in the case of oral contracep-

---
* 35 *Federal Register* 9001–9002 (June 11, 1970).

tive drugs, the Commissioner concludes that it is necessary in the best interests of users that the following printed information for patients be included in or with the package dispensed to the patient:

(Patient Package Information)

ORAL CONTRACEPTIVES

(Birth Control Pills)

Do Not Take This Drug Without Your Doctor's Continued Supervision.

The oral contraceptives are powerful and effective drugs which can cause side effects in some users and should not be used at all by some women. The most serious known side effect is abnormal blood clotting which can be fatal.

Safe use of this drug requires a careful discussion with your doctor. To assist him in providing you with the necessary information,—(Firm name)— has prepared a booklet (or other form) written in a style understandable to you as the drug user. This provides information on the effectiveness and known hazards of the drug including warnings, side effects, and who should not use it. Your doctor will give you this booklet (or other form) if you ask for it and he can answer any questions you may have about the use of this drug.

Notify your doctor if you notice any unusual physical disturbance or discomfort.

Providing the patient package information to users may be accomplished by including it in each package of the type intended for the user as follows:

(1) If such package includes additional printed materials for the patient (e.g., dosage schedules), the text . . . shall be an integral part of the printed material and be in boldface type set out in a box, preceding all other printed text.

(2) If such package does not include printed material for the patient, the text . . . shall be provided as a printed leaflet in boldface type.

(3) Include in each bulk package intended for multiple dispensing, a sufficient number of the patient package information leaflet, with instructions to the pharmacist to include one with each prescription dispensed.

Written, printed, or graphic materials on the use of a drug that are disseminated by or on behalf of the manufacturer, packager, or distributor and are intended to be made available to the patient are regarded as labeling. The commissioner also concludes that it is necessary that information in lay language, concerning effec-

tiveness, contraindications, warnings, precautions, and adverse reactions be incorporated prominently in the beginning of any such materials, and that such labeling must be made available to physicians for all patients who may request it. Such labeling shall be substantially as follows, based on the approved package insert for prescribers of the oral contraceptives, and shall include the following points:

(1) A statement that the drug should be taken only under continued supervision of a physician.

(2) A statement regarding the effectiveness of the product.

(3) A warning regarding the serious side effects with special attention to thromboembolic disorders and stating the estimated morbidity and mortality in users vs nonusers. Other serious side effects to be mentioned include mental depression, edema, rash, and jaundice. The possibility of infertility following discontinuation of the drug should be mentioned.

(4) A statement of contraindications.

(5) A statement of the need for special supervision of some patients including those with heart or kidney disease, asthma, high blood pressure, diabetes, epilepsy, fibroids of the uterus, migraine, mental depression or history thereof.

(6) A statement of the most frequently encountered side effects such as spotting, breast changes, weight changes, skin changes, and nausea and vomiting.

(7) A statement of the side effects frequently reported in association with the use of oral contraceptives, but not proved to be directly related such as nervousness, dizziness, changes in appetite, loss of scalp hair, increase in body hair, and increased or decreased libido.

(8) A statement regarding metabolic effects such as on blood sugar and cholesterol setting forth our current lack of knowledge regarding the long-term significance of these effects.

(9) Instructions in the event of missed menstrual periods.

(10) A statement cautioning the patient to consult her physician before resuming the use of the drug after childbirth, especially if she intends to breastfeed the baby, pointing out that the hormones in the drug are known to appear in the milk and may decrease the flow.

(11) A statement regarding production of cancer in certain animals. This may be coupled with a statement that there is no proof of such effect in human beings.

(12) A reminder to the patient to report

promptly to her physician any unusual change in her general physical condition and to have regular examinations.

Optionally, the booklet may also contain factual information on family planning, the usefulness and hazards of other available methods of contraception, and the hazards of pregnancy. The material shall be neither false nor misleading in any particular and shall follow the material presented above.

*   *   *

Existing stocks may be shipped without the package insert for a period of 90 days, provided the labeling booklet is prepared and disseminated as promptly as possible.

Effective date. This order shall become effective 30 days from the date of publication in the *Federal Register.*

NOTE 5.

VICTOR COHN
AMA PLEDGES ALL-OUT FIGHT AGAINST BIRTH-PILL WARNING*

The American Medical Association today promised a "legal and legislative battle" against a printed warning due soon in every package of birth control pills.

But Dr. Charles C. Edwards, commissioner of the Food and Drug administration, defended the warning as a kind of "insurance policy" in the patient's interest.

The warning—ordered by the FDA this month despite AMA and other medical opposition—would tell women of possible side effects such as increased risk of blood clotting and advise "careful discussion with your doctor."

"We must remember that we are long past the medicine man times when no patient knew anything about medicine except where it hurt," Edwards told a meeting here of the Pharmaceutical Advertising Club.

At almost the same hour, the AMA house of delegates voted to oppose "any requirement that interjects a federal agency between a physician and his patient."

The resolution listed these objections:

"The proposal to supply information on side effects . . . intrudes on the patient-physician relationship and compromises individual medical evaluation. . . . The proposed statement would confuse and alarm many patients. The package

_____
* *The Washington Post* (June 24, 1970). © 1970, The Washington Post. Reprinted by permission.

insert is an inappropriate means of providing a patient with information regarding any prescription drug; the most effective way to inform the patient is through the physician."

The resolution also stressed "the importance of making certain this FDA requirement not be extended to other prescription drugs."

*   *   *

NOTE 6.

TURNER V. EDWARDS
F.D. COSM. L. REP. ¶ 40, 422 (D.D.C. 1970)

GESELL, DISTRICT JUDGE: This cause came before the Court September 8, 1970 on plaintiff's motion for a preliminary injunction. On the basis of the pleadings, affidavits, and documents, and upon argument of counsel, the Court denied the motion, and herein sets forth its findings of fact and conclusions of law. . . .

Plaintiffs, individually and on behalf of all women who are presently taking or are considering taking oral contraceptives, seek a mandatory injunction directing the Food and Drug Administration to require that each package of oral contraceptives contain more detailed labeling with respect to the health hazards of the pill. The F.D.A. issued a regulation on June 11, 1970, effective September 9, 1970, requiring that a short warning accompany each package of oral contraceptives, stating certain health hazards of the pill and directing users to consult their physicians for further information. The regulation required that manufacturers prepare a pamphlet for distribution by all prescribing physicians, detailing more fully the potential side effects of oral contraceptives and the symptoms of adverse reactions. For the purposes of the motion for a preliminary injunction, the adequacy of the warnings contained in the pamphlet is not challenged. Plaintiffs seek only to have this longer pamphlet placed in packages of the drug, pending final resolution of this litigation.

Plaintiffs have not shown a substantial likelihood that they will ultimately prevail on the merits. The central issue in the case is whether the labeling required by the F.D.A. meets the statutory standards of the Food, Drug, & Cosmetic Act, 21 U.S.C. § 352. These provisions require essentially that labeling of a drug not be false or misleading, that it bear adequate instructions for use, and that it include adequate warnings of potential health hazards. Following elaborate rule-making procedures, the F.D.A. determined that the labeling required by its regulation of June 11 meets each of these standards. [P]laintiffs' claim that the agency's decision was arbitrary, irrational, or not in accordance with the relevant statute and the regulatory scheme governing other prescription drugs is not supported by the record. Upon final disposition of this case, it will be open to plaintiffs to question the premise that oral contraceptives are distributed through normal prescription channels; but such a finding is not now warranted.

[T]he Court does not believe that plaintiffs will suffer irreparable injury by the denial of the relief requested. That consumers should be informed of the dangers of oral contraceptives and adequately cautioned as to their use is unquestioned, but the Court is not persuaded that placing the longer pamphlet in packages of the drug, as opposed to the labeling scheme formulated by the Food and Drug Administration, is required to afford protection to the consumer. Indeed a preliminary injunction would delay regulated distribution of the warning pamphlets. These pamphlets at the time of hearing were in the hands of physicians for distribution, and all necessary steps had been taken to operate under the regulations effective the next day. Plaintiffs' requested injunction would change the status quo rather than preserve it pending final judgment. Only in unusually pressing circumstances, which the Court does not find present in this case, should such an injunction be issued. . . .

e.

Joyce Barrett
Product Liability and the Pill*

* * *

The lion's share of the oral contraceptive market belongs to G. D. Searle & Co.—"Where the Pill Began". . . . Litigation stemming from alleged Pill-caused side effects began at Searle too. The first of such cases to come to trial was *Simonait* v. *Searle,* which went to the jury on theories of negligence and breach of implied warranty. Plaintiff claimed that she had contracted thrombophlebitis (formation of blood clots within the veins) as a result of taking the defendant's oral contraceptive Enovid. She charged Searle with negligence in failing to warn of the possibility that Enovid might cause thrombotic disorders. Among the battery of doctors who testified for Searle were Victor A. Drill, who headed Searle's investigation of Enovid, and Celso-Ramon Garcia, who performed Searle's Puerto Rico field trials of Enovid. The doctors

---

* 19 *Cleveland State Law Review* 468–470, 472–478 (1970). Reprinted by permission.

testified that they believed plaintiff's condition was caused by her varicose veins and not by her use of Enovid. The jury agreed, and after a short deliberation brought back a defendant's verdict.

Black v. *Searle* came to trial on May 12, 1969, and went to the jury on May 20 on counts of negligence, breach of implied warranty, and strict liability. This was an action brought by Raymond Black, as administrator of the estate of his deceased wife, Elizabeth, who had died on September 18, 1965, at the age of twenty-nine, from a pulmonary embolism allegedly caused by Enovid. Plaintiff charged that Searle had failed to adequately warn in its instruction booklets given to doctors, and, in turn, to patients, that the Pill could cause thromboembolic phenomena (clotting). The issue of warning went to the state of knowledge chargeable to Searle as of the date of Mrs. Black's death. Plaintiff maintained that at the time there were approximately 600 reports of thromboembolic phenomena, including a number of deaths, among women using Enovid. The plaintiff had a difficult time, however, proving causation. . . .

* * *

From this conflicting testimony emerged a "qualified" defendant's verdict. The jury found for the defendant on all three counts, but appended this recommendation to their verdict:

Further, it is the recommendation of this jury that, effective immediately, G. D. Searle & Company, in instruction literature both to doctors and patients, advise the dangers of the possibility of phlebitis, thrombotic, and embolic phenomena.

Judge Robert Grant, however, advised the jury that their added directive would not be legally binding upon Searle.

* * *

Attorney Paul D. Rheingold is trustee of a seventy-member Birth Control Pill Group comprised of attorneys with Pill cases who have banded together to render mutual assistance. Most of the group members have one or two cases; a few have a half dozen or more. Mr. Rheingold thinks that many more suits are imminent and will probably be joint malpractice-product liability actions.

Such a suit is *Charles Gillette, Administrator of the Estate of Alinie Gillette* v. *Samuel L. Friedman, M.D., and G. D. Searle and Company.* Plaintiff's decedent was twenty-two years old, had two children, and a history of rheumatic heart disease, anemia, and pulmonary congestion. She had been using foam as a contraceptive when, in May of 1967, the defendant doctor started her on Searle's oral contraceptive Ovulen. During June and July Mrs. Gillette reported migraine headaches, menstrual frequency and irregularity, and small hairlike veins appearing on the lower extremities. She was hospitalized on August 27, 1967, and died two days later. The autopsy showed rheumatic heart disease, bilateral pulmonary congestion, edema, hemorrhage, and apparent obstruction of major bronchi.

The defendant doctor was charged with negligence in that he knew, or should have known, that oral contraceptives should not be prescribed for a patient with the medical history of plaintiff's decedent; that he assured her that Ovulen was safe; that thereafter he negligently examined, treated, and advised her and failed to observe and investigate the cause of certain warning symptoms and continued her on Ovulen until the date of the last treatment on August 5, 1967.

* * *

As regards the failure-to-warn count, the plaintiff must establish the state of medical knowledge of oral contraceptives as of and prior to August 29, 1967, the date of his wife's death. In the year 1966, the *Index Medicus,* for the first time under its general heading "Oral Contraceptives" listed a subheading called "Adverse Effects." Reports of vascular problems are prominent in this list. Numerous other medical articles reporting adverse Pill effects had been published prior to August 29, 1967. As early as 1964, the *Physician's Desk Reference,* the chief source of drug information that is available to physicians, reported "thromboembolic phenomena with some fatalities" among women on the Pill.

Was Searle disseminating information about these side effects to prescribers and/or users of Ovulen? The package insert in the Ovulen–21 Compack "warns" of the following "adverse effects":

1. Spotting or breakthrough bleeding.
   "Such irregular bleeding seldom occurs with Ovulen. . . ."
2. Nausea.
   "A mild nausea may come and go for several days of the first cycle or two. The vast majority of women never experience this."
3. Feeling of fullness and weight gain.
   "A few women, once they no longer fear pregnancy, feel better and actually eat more, which, of course, will result in weight gain."

Searle's final "warning" is: "Unusual changes in your health should be reported to your physician—just as they should if you were not on Ovulen."

Were Searle's detail men "bringing the warning home" to physicians about the Pill's harmful side effects? Searle's suggested presentation of Ovulen by detail men to doctors went like this:

Dr. _____:
Searle is happy to present a chemically new, clinically unique oral contraceptive—OVULEN—offering at the lowest dosage, positive prevention of pregnancy, with the lowest incidence of side effects—at the lowest price. The safety of OVULEN has been well established by world-wide experience including 4 million women's cycles. Ovulen has no additional contraindications or precautions to those that apply to all oral contraceptives.

* * *

[T]he chief roadblock to the argument for strict liability to the drug manufacturer is found in Comment *k* to §402A of the Second Restatement of Torts, which provides:

There are some products which, in the present state of human knowledge, are quite incapable of being safe for their intended and ordinary use. These are made *especially common in the field of drugs.* An outstanding example is the vaccine for the Pasteur treatment of rabies, which not uncommonly leads to very serious and damaging consequences when it is injected. *Since the disease itself invariably leads to a dreadful death, both the marketing and the use of the vaccine are fully justified,* notwithstanding the unavoidable degree of risk which they involve. Such a product, properly prepared and *accompanied by proper directions and warning,* is not defective, nor is it unreasonably dangerous. The same is true of many other drugs, vaccines, and the like, many of which for this very reason cannot legally be sold except to physicians, or under the prescription of a physician. It is also true in particular of many new or experimental drugs as to which, because of lack of time and opportunity for sufficient medical experience, there can be no assurance of safety, or perhaps even of purity of ingredients, but such experience as there is justifies the marketing and use of the drug notwithstanding a medically recognizable risk. The seller of such products, again with the qualification that they are properly prepared and marketed, and *proper warning is given,* where the situation calls for it, is not to be held to strict liability for unfortunate consequences attending their use, merely because he has undertaken to supply the public with an apparently useful and desirable product, attended with a known but apparently reasonable risk. (Emphasis added.)

The question then to be considered is what

constitutes a "defective condition." Comment *g* to § 402A defines it as a "condition not contemplated by the ultimate consumer, which will be unreasonably dangerous to him," and Comment *h* goes a step further by suggesting that where a defendant has reason to anticipate a possible danger from a particular use, and it fails to give adequate warning thereof, a product sold without such warning is in a defective condition.

* * *

. . . With the sword of legal responsibility for the Pill harm hanging over the prescribing physician's head as well as the manufacturer's, one insurance company, providing malpractice coverage for some 18,000 physicians, sent out on May 14, 1969, the following "Dear Doctor" letter:

Dear Doctor:
Contraceptive Pills
Because of the increasing awareness of potential complications from contraceptive pills, and because we are already handling lawsuits dealing with some of these complications, we are advising physicians to obtain signed statements from their patients which acknowledge requests for these pills despite awareness of the serious risks involved.
We offer the enclosed form which can be used in most instances.

Sincerely,

The suggested form:

CONTRACEPTIVE DRUGS
Read Carefully Before Signing!
The prescription for contraceptive drugs on this date and for every refill hereafter is at my request. In making this request, I am aware that such drugs can cause serious reactions and complications, both known and presently unknown.

Date: _____ Signature of patient: _____

The great social value of the Pill in this era of the population explosion has been stressed. As the simplest and most effective form of contraception available, the Pill has enjoyed a "diplomatic immunity" from criticism. However, in light of the Senate hearings into the Pill and other reports of its adverse effects, the Pill's halo is rapidly tarnishing. Also ending is the immunity from liability enjoyed by Pill manufacturers for the past five years.

On April 15, 1970, after a five-week trial, a Brooklyn, New York jury returned a $250,000.00 plaintiff's verdict in *Meinert* v. *Searle*. Mrs. Meinert developed a mesenteric thrombosis in 1962 after taking Enovid for eight months, necessitating an operation to remove

portions of her intestines. Plaintiff proceeded on the bases of express warranty, implied warranty, strict liability, and common-law negligence; the latter theory being subdivided into failure to properly test before marketing and failure to warn of dangers known or which should have been known. The court rejected the express warranty theory, but submitted the other three to the jury, along with interrogatories asking the jury to specify on which theory it made its findings. The jury brought back a verdict for the plaintiff on all three submitted counts.

Lightning struck again on April 24, 1970, when a Federal District Court jury in Detroit brought back a plaintiff's verdict in *Tobin* v. *Searle*. Mrs. Tobin was awarded $225,000.00 (her husband received $50,000.00 for the loss of her consortium) for clotting in the deep veins of her right leg following the use of Enovid. Plaintiff was hospitalized eight times from 1963 through 1965, and underwent surgery twice—once to sever a nerve in an attempt to end severe pain in her groin and right leg, and a second time to replace her destroyed long thigh bone with artificial tissue. Bolstering plaintiff's case was testimony from plaintiff's own prescribing physician that he had relied on data sent to him by Searle, which were incomplete, and some 350 case reports of other clotting incidents obtained from Searle by discovery.

* * *

f.
Placebo Stirs Pill "Side Effects"*

The least serious but most common problems associated with oral contraceptives are those discomforting side effects noted, discussed, and catalogued since the earliest pill trials. . . .

"What we've shown is that a vast majority of reported side effects can also be found in a placebo group, and may indeed reflect the symptomatology of everyday life," says Dr. Joseph Goldzieher of San Antonio's Southwest Foundation for Research and Education. In a randomized, double-blind study . . . he and his associates recorded, after the first treatment cycle, only small differences in the incidence of headache, nervousness, nausea, vomiting, depression, and breast tenderness in women taking oral contraceptives and those on a placebo pill.

The trial—sponsored by Syntex Labs and the Agency for International Development—in-

* *Medical World News* 18–19 (April 16, 1971). Copyright 1971 by McGraw-Hill, Inc. Reprinted by permission.

volved 398 women and a total of 1,523 cycles. Besides the placebo, it included a commercial high-estrogen sequential, a high-estrogen combination, a low-estrogen combination, and an investigative progestin preparation, chlormadinone acetate. . . .

[T]he San Antonio test subjects . . . were multiparous women, almost all of them Mexican-American and poor, who had come to the foundation's research clinic—which is associated with Planned Parenthood—seeking contraceptive assistance.

In a crossover procedure, the 76 women in the placebo group were switched to active agents after the first four cycles. The changeover came too late to entirely nullify the hazards of placebo use, though. Despite warnings about the need to apply vaginal cream, one major side effect showed up in ten women on the dummy pill, plus one on chlormadinone: They became pregnant.

Some of those randomly assigned the placebo may have been lax about the precaution, comments Dr. Goldzieher. But he also concedes that the pregnancy ratio turned up in his study is entirely consistent with results of trials with vaginal cream or foam. "It just doesn't always work all that well," he says.

* * *

Says Dr. Goldzieher: "The words 'dummy pill' were not mentioned to the women. However, they did have to agree [all of the placebo group and some of those on the pill] to use a vaginal cream 'until we're sure your pill is effective.' "

* * *

What about the 11 pregnancies? "We could have aborted them if the abortion statute here in Texas weren't in limbo right now," replies Dr. Goldzieher. "A court here overturned the law and the case is awaiting Supreme Court review. If we had a liberalized law, we'd abort them."

None of the women selected had used the pill before. All the capsules given out were identical in appearance and packaged in 28-day strips. Before the study was to be completed, the federal government—basing its action on studies in beagles—banned all further investigation with chlormadinone; since the Texas trial was double-blind, it had to be discontinued at that point —after only six cycles.

* * *

The investigator stresses that his findings in no way prove that any of the symptoms do not occur in association with oral contraceptives. But he feels they do indicate that "the true incidence is far less than generally supposed" and less than suggested by previous uncontrolled testing.

* * *

g.

Barry Kramer
Chemical Offers Hope for a New Approach to Population Control*

The claims sound like they're coming from a pitchman pushing his magic snake-oil elixir at an old medicine show: A "morning-after" contraceptive and yet also a cure for male infertility, a palliative for asthma and a treatment for ulcers and high blood pressure.

These claims aren't being made by hucksters, however. Rather, they're being discussed by medical researchers who are seriously studying the possibility of such future uses for a new family of chemicals into whose secrets they are now delving. Called prostaglandins, the substances are found in minute amounts in the body, where they perform an amazing variety of jobs.

The results of recent experiments are astonishing even the most skeptical researchers, and some scientists are classing the prostaglandins in the same "wonder-drug" category as antibiotics.

Considerable excitement has been generated over the use of prostaglandins in the whole field of fertility and birth control. Researchers know that prostaglandins are closely involved in the reproductive process, including the induction of labor. Thus, trials are under way on using the prostaglandins to bring on childbirth.

More intriguing, however, are the findings that if used earlier in pregnancy, prostaglandins cause abortions. Indeed, some early trials in women indicate that prostaglandins can end pregnancy only a few days after conception. Thus, there's promise of the frequently discussed morning-after birth-control drug.

* * *

"Much work remains to be done to establish the efficacy and safety of the prostaglandins and their therapeutic role," cautions a British scientist, Mostyn P. Embrey of the University of Oxford. Echoing other scientists, he says in a letter to the medical journal *Lancet* that extensive testing will have to be completed before prostaglandins can be safely used.

----
* *The Wall Street Journal* 1, col. 1, 21, col. 3 (December 11, 1970). Reprinted by permission of The Wall Street Journal.

And the research director of a major American pharmaceutical concern says that although the compound's ability to induce abortions and clear asthmatic lungs has been shown, "the rest of the uses haven't been proved yet."

Part of the excitement over prostaglandins' possible use in fertility control stems from research by a 35-year-old Ugandan, Sultan M.M. Karim. Last September he announced findings that could open the way for a birth-control method women could administer without clinical supervision. This is considered a must in lesser-developed countries, where present methods of birth control aren't denting population growth.

*   *   *

Several years ago Mr. Karim, who is a pharmacologist at Makere University in Kampala, Uganda, identified prostaglandins as the substance that clamps shut the severed umbilical cord, preventing newborn babies from bleeding to death. After noting that prostaglandins had an apparent role in labor, he reported in 1968 the first use of the compound, by intravenous infusion, to induce labor in several women when they were due.

Mr. Karim then went on to test the anti-fertility effects of prostaglandins on more than 1,000 women. Such tests wouldn't have been possible in the U.S., where the Government rigidly controls human experiments with new drugs. The Ugandan's work has probably shaved years off the development of the compound as a useful medical tool, some scientists believe.

Since Mr. Karim began his work, other researchers have used the compound on pregnant women to induce labor and abortion, refining dosages and methods of application. Drs. Marc Bygdeman and Nils Wiqvist of Sweden, for example, have experimentally induced abortions using intrauterine infusions.

Side effects have been limited to diarrhea, nausea and vomiting, not uncommon with abortifacients. Researchers say such effects can be ameliorated by using other prostaglandins and altering the method of administration and the amount used.

*   *   *

If prostaglandins prove effective, their use to control pregnancy will raise difficult moral and religious questions. The most obvious: Are prostaglandins contraceptives or abortifacients? No one knows for sure. One determinant is the debatable one of when pregnancy actually begins.

*   *   *

C.
Medical Innovation and the Profession—A Case Study of Mitral Valve Surgery*

1.
Therapy, Experimentation, and Failure— The First Phase (1902–1929)

a.
Sir Lauder Brunton
Preliminary Note on the Possibility of Treating Mitral Stenosis by Surgical Methods†

Mitral stenosis is not only one of the most distressing forms of cardiac disease, but in its severe forms it resists all treatment by medicine. On looking at the contracted mitral orifice in a severe case of this disease one is impressed by the hopelessness of ever finding a remedy which will enable the auricle to drive the blood in a sufficient stream through the small mitral orifice, and the wish unconsciously arises that one could divide the constriction as easily during life as one can after death. The risk which such an operation would entail naturally makes one shrink from it, but in some cases it might be well worth while for the patients to balance the risk of a shortened life against the certainty of a prolonged period of existence which could hardly be called life, as the only conditions under which it could be continued might to them be worse than death. I was much impressed by the case of a man under middle age whom I had under my care at St. Bartholomew's Hospital. For no fault

---

* Grateful acknowledge is made to Judith P. Swazey and Renée C. Fox whose article on "The Clinical Moratorium—A Case Study of Mitral Valve Surgery" was invaluable in identifying much of the original source material which appears in this section.

† 1 *The Lancet* 352 (1902). Reprinted by permission.

of his own, but simply because of his disease, this man was really exiled from his family and one might almost say imprisoned for life inasmuch as he could only live in a hospital ward or a workhouse infirmary. Whenever he left the hospital or infirmary with an amelioration of his distressing symptoms and returned home the exertion brought on an exacerbation and he had to leave home again in a few days to return to the hospital or infirmary. It occurred to me that it was worth while for such a patient to run a risk, and even a very grave risk, in order to obtain such improvement as might enable him at least to stay at home. But no one would be justified in attempting such a dangerous operation as dividing a mitral stenosis on a fellow-creature without having first tested its practicability and perfected its technique by previous trials on animals. Accordingly I obtained a licence and certificate a year ago in order to make the necessary experiments, but unfortunately other calls upon my time have not allowed me to do more than to make trial experiments of dividing stenosed valves in diseased hearts from the post-mortem theatre and on healthy valves in the hearts of cats, and also to try the proposed operation in the dead animal. It may be some months longer before I can get anything more done, and I therefore think that it may be worth while to write this preliminary note, especially as, after all, if the operation is to be done in man it will be surgeons who will do it, and they must, of course, make their own preliminary experiments, however fully the operation may be described by others, and each must find out for himself the method which he will employ in each particular case.

The first question that arises is whether the mitral orifice should be enlarged by elongating the natural opening or whether the valves should be cut through their middle at right angles to the normal opening. I think there can be little doubt that the former would be the better plan, but the latter is the more easily performed, and it might be sufficient to effect the desired purpose of facilitating the flow of blood from the auricle into the ventricle. The knives which I have used have been like tenotomy knives, but some which I have had made of ladies' bonnet pins were too thin and flexible for stenosed valves although they were sufficiently strong to divide the normal valves in the hearts of cats. The cutting edge of some of these was only a quarter of an inch, but this is too short and a cutting edge of one-half an inch to an inch is really required. The main part

of the valve can be divided with comparative ease, but the thickened edge is firm and it resists the knife. I have not yet decided on the best form of knife, and its form will depend to some extent upon whether the surgeon decides to operate from the auricle or from the ventricle. The latter is less likely to bleed as the knife need not be much thicker than a needle, and a needle wound of the ventricle rarely gives rise to any bleeding. . . .

*   *   *

The good results that have been obtained by surgical treatment of wounds in the heart emboldens one to hope that before very long similar good results may be obtained in cases of mitral stenosis.

NOTES

NOTE 1.

EDITORS OF THE LANCET
SURGICAL OPERATION FOR MITRAL STENOSIS*

A NOTE by Sir LAUDER BRUNTON published in our columns last week contains a sufficiently heroic therapeutic suggestion. It calls attention to the grave effects of stenosis of the mitral valve and to the possibility that relief might be obtained by a surgical division of the diseased valve. With an ambition to bring relief to these patients Sir LAUDER BRUNTON obtained a licence and certificates a year ago to enable him to test on animals the validity of his suggestion. We gather that he has proceeded no further than the table of the dead-house in making his investigation, and having many other claims upon his time he now publishes the suggestion in the hope that others will complete what he has begun. This is a somewhat unusual course to pursue and we think that Sir LAUDER BRUNTON would have been better advised to have himself completed his experiments, even at considerable inconvenience, rather than to incite others to pursue a path into the unknown which must be beset with very grave difficulties and responsibility. The experiments on animals which he advocates require considerable delicacy and skill on the part of the experimenter, and we have a strong feeling that the man with whom the idea originated is certainly the most fitted to cope with the initial difficulties and to bring the experiments to a satisfactory conclusion, if that be possible.

---

* 1 *The Lancet* 461–462 (1902). Reprinted by permission.

Having taken this preliminary objection to the form in which the proposal has been published, let us consider the proposal itself. As it is only a suggestion and the operation has never been performed we can only fall back upon *a priori* arguments. And we are all aware how fallacious such arguments are. How many of the great advances which have raised surgery to its present exalted position have been ruthlessly condemned on *a priori* grounds? The surgery of the brain, the stomach, the spleen, the liver, and the uterus has all been advanced and almost perfected in spite of weighty *a priori* reasons against the procedures which are now known to be useful. So that, as a general rule, we deprecate such a line of reasoning. Experiment and observation are the "weapons of our warfare," and the only ones in which we have much confidence. But Sir LAUDER BRUNTON's proposal challenges criticism in two directions—the difficulty of the operation and the doubt as to its efficacy, even if successfully carried out. On a dead and motionless heart the division of the mitral valve through a fine puncture in the ventricle is a difficult and very delicate step. But when the operation is complicated by the rapid movements of the auricle and ventricle and the respiratory movements of the chest it is plain that the operation is beset with very grave difficulties—difficulties that only the boldest surgeons, with the best-balanced sense of the limitations of their science, could for a moment face. We think that these difficulties have been under-estimated and that the very technique of the operation will prove fatal to its adoption. The introduction of a fine knife through the ventricular wall would have to be done rapidly, and then the manipulation of the knife into the orifice between the deformed cusps of the mitral valve and the section of the valve would also have to be accomplished very rapidly; and all this in conditions most embarrassing and most destructive of that entire self-control which is the chief secret of success in rapid and exact surgical manoeuvers. But were this difficulty overcome and the safety and feasibility of the operation established, a further doubt arises in our mind. If the narrowed valve is divided, what hope is there that the incision in the valve will heal without renewing the contraction? The incision in such a valve would show a great tendency to unite directly and the state of the valve would then be worse than before. . . . It has also to be borne in mind that the operation might convert the valvular lesion from a mitral stenosis into a mitral regurgitation with very

doubtful benefit to the patient. For the difficulties of the procedure must be enormous.

* * *

NOTE 2.

W. ARBUTHNOT LANE
SURGICAL OPERATIONS FOR MITRAL STENOSIS*

Referring to the preliminary note on the possibility of treating mitral stenosis by surgical methods by Sir Lauder Brunton . . . it may interest your readers to know that this suggestion was made by me to my colleague, Dr. Lauriston Shaw, some years ago. I then went into the matter fully, both as to the surgical measures to be adopted and the physical conditions of the valve which seemed most suitable for such interference, and was quite prepared to act as soon as Dr. Shaw succeeded in finding a case likely to derive benefit. It was entirely due to his perhaps wise caution that the operation has not yet been performed by me. The method by which I proposed to divide the contracted valve through the ventricle was practically identical with that described by Sir Lauder Brunton. Personally I believe that the operation is feasible and, under certain circumstances, justifiable.

NOTE 3.

THEODORE FISHER
SURGICAL OPERATIONS FOR MITRAL STENOSIS†

In your leading article upon the suggestion by Sir Lauder Brunton that it may be possible to operate upon some cases of mitral stenosis you give several reasons why such an operation is likely to fail. It seems to me that another may be added. Marked fibrosis of the cardiac muscle is found after death in many cases of mitral stenosis and it is probable that the prognosis in this variety of valvular disease depends as much upon the condition of the heart wall as upon the size of the mitral orifice. If the cardiac muscle remains healthy it is possible not only for life to be prolonged, but for the man or woman in whom the mitral orifice is narrowed to live an active life. For example, in an ostler, aged 64 years, who was busy at his work to within a few days of his death, which was caused by acute bronchitis, I found a mitral orifice which would only admit one finger.

---

* 1 *The Lancet* 547 (1902). Reprinted by permission.
† 1 *The Lancet* 547–548 (1902). Reprinted by permission.

NOTE 4.

LAURISTON E. SHAW
SURGICAL OPERATIONS FOR MITRAL STENOSIS*

In reference to the correspondence in your columns with regard to Sir Lauder Brunton's preliminary communication upon the above subject, I can corroborate Mr. Arbuthnot Lane's statement that he and I fully discussed the matter at least 12 years ago. Mr. Lane introduced the subject to my notice and satisfied me that he probably could without any immediately harmful result temporarily enlarge, by surgical means, the orifice of a constricted mitral valve. Lest however, it should appear from Mr. Lane's letter that I am still hoping to succeed "in finding a case likely to receive benefit" therefrom, I shall be obliged if you will allow me to state that the *a priori* arguments against the probability of any patient deriving benefit from this operation seemed to me so conclusive that I deliberately decided against regarding it as a justifiable therapeutic measure. These arguments are so clearly summarised in your leading article of Feb. 15th that your readers will, I think, agree with me that Sir Lauder Brunton's chief task is not to show his surgical colleagues that it is possible to enlarge the stenosed mitral orifice, but to persuade his medical colleagues that such a proceeding is useful. It is possible to do many things that are useless and some things that are harmful.

b.

Elliott C. Cutler and S. A. Levine
Cardiotomy and Valvulotomy for Mitral Stenosis—Experimental Observations and Clinical Notes Concerning an Operated Case with Recovery†

During the recent decennial celebration of the former and present members of the nursing and professional staff of the Peter Bent Brigham Hospital, we presented (May 24, 1923) a case of mitral stenosis upon which we had operated four days previously in an attempt to alleviate the condition by diminishing the degree of stenosis of the valve.

. . . So far as we can determine, this is the only case on record of such a surgical attack upon a mitral stenosis being completed. Doyen

previously attempted a similar case, but his patient did not survive the operation.

Ever since Sir Lauder Brunton in 1902 suggested the possibility of the surgical treatment of valvular disease of the heart, investigators have studied the experimental creation of valvular lesions. Papers by McCallum, Cushing and Branch, Bernheim, Schepelmann, and Carrel and Tuffier from 1906 to 1914 describe fully the experimental methods in use. All of these methods were only successful in creating defective valves resulting in regurgitation. The most successful methods consisted in inserting a knife-hook (valvulotome) into the apex or down the aorta and cutting or tearing out valve cusps. Carrel and Tuffier added a new method of creating an insufficiency by the use of an endothelial transplant over the region of valves, the ring at the base of the valve then being cut, thus permitting a bulging at that point. In 1922 Allen and Graham reported investigations of a similar nature with the addition that they used a cardioscope in which a small knife was carried, and by inserting the instrument *via* the left auricular appendage they were able to cut the mitral valve under direct vision.

For over two years we have sought to clear up by experimentation some of the points still left unanswered by all this work. The chief difficulty has always been to create a stenosis. Obviously until this can be produced further animal investigation will not tell us what benefits accrue when such a lesion is converted into an insufficiency. Temporary, but purely temporary, stenoses can be made by placing a thread in the ring about the base of the valves and tying it snugly. We attempted to improve on this by various methods of partial ventriculectomy, by plicating, and by plastic operations at the region of the valves. None of these methods proved successful in our hands. The experience gained, however, proved of great value, chiefly educating us in the ability of the heart muscle to stand trauma, in the methods of restoring an injured heart to renewed function, and in our ability to locate and "feel" valves in a writhing, pulsating organ.

We had reached a point where it appeared to us that further knowledge could only be gained by an attempt in an actual case, and, much as we feared the difficulties, our experimental work gave us the courage to carry out what must appear as a hazardous trial. Our experimental work with the cardioscope left us with the impression that the greater intricacy of the

---

* 1 *The Lancet* 619 (1902). Reprinted by permission.

† 188 *Boston Medical and Surgical Journal* 1023–1027 (1923). Reprinted by permission.

operation and the greater amount of time consumed with this method was such that it seemed wiser to use the simpler and more speedy route through the ventricular wall with the valvulotome in the first human case.

The opportunity arrived through the interest and vision of Dr. Maurice Fremont-Smith, who asked us to see in consultation with him a child in the Good Samaritan Hospital. The history is as follows:

The patient is a girl 12 years old, whose chief complaints are dyspnea and bloody sputum. . . .

* * *

During the past six months repeated attempts were made to get the patient out of bed, but each time the pulse would become rapid—120 to 140—and the dyspnea would increase. During this time there were frequent pulmonary hemorrhages. She would raise from 20 to 300 cc. of pure bright blood at a time and would seem desperately sick, so that for a while she was on the danger list.

On May 15, when we saw her, the patient presented the following picture: She was sitting up comfortably in bed, but could not lie flat. . . .

* * *

In general, the picture presented was one of mitral stenosis in a child who had no cardiac reserve. She could be fairly comfortable in bed except for the repeated attacks of severe hemoptysis. It proved to be impossible to get her out of bed. Our studies indicated that the heart muscle was still in fair condition and that the stenosis was sufficient to be an important factor from a purely mechanical point of view.

* * *

[The operation was performed on May 20, 1923.] Towards the end of her third postoperative day, the temperature and pulse and respiratory rates fell, the signs in the right apex rapidly cleared except for some sticky râles, and after a comfortable night the patient seemed in as good general condition as before operation.

Indeed, we felt so sanguine of her ultimate recovery that she was brought down to the large amphitheater and presented before the reunion group of doctors and nurses the fourth day after operation (May 24, 1923). From this time on her recovery was rapid, as it is in most children once the period of convalescence becomes well

established. Her appetite, spirits, strength, and general condition responded marvelously. . . .

* * *

At this stage of our observations we cannot with accuracy define just what has occurred nor what benefits may have accrued, if any. It is true that we do not feel very sanguine about the latter, although, should any improvement occur in the patient's vital capacity, that might be taken as a definite indication that some alleviation of the stenosis had resulted. The experience with this case, however, is of importance in that it does show that surgical intervention in cases of mitral stenosis bears no special risk, and should give us further courage and support in our desire to attempt to alleviate a chronic condition, for which there is now not only no treatment, but one which carries a terrible prognosis. Unquestionably further attempts will be made, and our own experience in this instance has shown us technical improvements that should render a subsequent attempt both less hazardous as well as more hopeful for success.

* * *

NOTE

THE EDITORS OF THE BRITISH MEDICAL JOURNAL
OPERATIVE TREATMENT OF MITRAL STENOSIS*

The ambitious efforts of surgery to remove conditions which physicians are unable to cure has been extraordinarily successful in the comparatively recent past, but hitherto valvular disease of the heart has remained outside the sphere of those who have been described as "physicians who can use their hands". . . .

A milestone has . . . been reached by the recent publication of a paper by Drs. E. C. Cutler and S. A. Levine. . . .

[T]he authors, who must be sincerely congratulated on this brilliant operation, are cautious in avoiding any statement as to the benefit that the patient has received, but they feel that the experience gained in this operation, now for the first time successfully accomplished, has provided technical improvements which should render any subsequent attempt both less dangerous and more likely to be followed by a satisfactory result.

---

* 2 *British Medical Journal* 530–531 (1923). Reprinted by permission of the editor of The British Medical Journal.

c.

Elliot C. Cutler, Samuel A. Levine, and Claude S. Beck
The Surgical Treatment of Mitral Stenosis— Experimental and Clinical Studies*

*   *   *

It is difficult to analyze at this time the stimuli that led us to begin this investigation in 1920. Certainly, we were increasingly impressed with the inadequacy of medical treatment in many cases of mitral stenosis. The suggestion of Sir Lauder Brunton had been brought to our attention. . . . The proposal and useful methods for its study were at hand, and the technical improvements in surgery had advanced to the stage in which difficulties from this aspect alone no longer assumed the dominant role. The cranial chamber having been successfully brought into the province of safe surgery, chiefly through the technical methods of Professor Cushing and his pupils, it appeared that the heart alone remained as a field for the almost unchallenged labors of the internists. That this state of affairs was not to continue long was evidenced by the developments already stated.

Fortunately, one of us had already conducted experimental studies involving exposure of the heart of the cat. In these experiments, levers had been sutured against the walls of the heart, and cannulas had been inserted into the various chambers without much disturbance of function, so that we began with no particular trepidation concerning the inability of the heart to withstand trauma and manipulation.

From the beginning, we set out to develop a surgical method for the treatment of mitral stenosis. It seemed to us . . . that the medical treatment of chronic cardiac valvular disease, and especially that of mitral stenosis, was inefficient. It was hoped and expected that the technical difficulties could be surmounted. This could only be accomplished by means of animal experimentation.

*   *   *

A series of experiments were conducted on cats and dogs, with the purpose of developing a technic to be used in the surgical treatment of certain heart affections in human beings.

---

* 9 *Archives of Surgery* 689, 712, 723–724, 769–770, 812, 814 (1924). Reprinted by permission.

It was learned that the heart could withstand considerable trauma and yet recover normally. The use of hot salt solution applied directly over the exposed heart, manual massage and epinephrin solution was found of great value in restoring proper cardiac contraction.

The entire circulation to and from the heart could be clamped off from two to eight minutes with recovery of a satisfactory circulation; but when the circulation was stopped in this way for more than two or three minutes, although the heart could be made to recover properly, the animals died in a few hours or a few days in opisthotonos or marked rigidity. It seemed that the cerebral centers, unlike the heart, could not tolerate the standstill in the circulation. Experiments were successfully performed in which the circulation was clamped; during this procedure, the left ventricle was opened and the mitral valve cut under direct inspection. This operation as a general procedure had to be given up because of the damage to the higher nervous centers.

An attempt was made to produce mechanical mitral stenosis by a puckering stitch in the heart in the region of the auriculoventricular ring, and by excising wedge-shaped portions of musculature in this region. These experiments failed because, although insufficiency of the valve lasting a few weeks would result, the valves would always return to a normal condition. Attempts to create stenosis were made by implanting radium emanation seeds about the base of the mitral valve.

An approach to the mitral valve through the left ventricle proved to be successful in cutting valve leaflets without clamping the circulation. Such animals could recover good health and manifest a mitral systolic murmur for many months. When finally examined, the hearts would show that the rent in the valve did not close up, and that there was no tendency to thrombus formation either at the site of the incision through the left ventricle or on the cut valves.

These experiments enabled us to feel that enough had been learned to warrant an attempt to relieve the obstruction in man.

*   *   *

[The] four cases constitute the first attempts to enlarge the stenosed mitral orifice in human patients. A preliminary report of Case 1 appeared in the *Boston Medical and Surgical Journal* of June 28, 1923, one month after the operation. . . .

These cases are not, however, the first attempts to operate on man for valvular disease. In 1912, Tuffier operated on a young man with a marked aortic stenosis. He states that he would have liked to attempt division of the valve, but that he thought that the experimental data justifying this were insufficient. Instead, he attempted to dilate the orifice by the insertion of his little finger. He reported that there was temporary improvement, and that in 1920 the man was still living. Tuffier also reported that Doyen attempted to operate on a patient considered to have mitral stenosis, but that the operation disclosed an interventricular communication. The patient did not recover.

. . . It seems best, however, to call to your attention at this point that the experimental and clinical work, except for the early investigations . . . were going on simultaneously. Thus, in the first three cases, the knife method was used in the dividing of the valves. However, after the postmortem examination in Case 2, we became convinced that this method would not prove satisfactory, and we began at once the development of the cardiovalvulotome. . . . The principle of excising a fragment of the valve had been in our minds for at least a year. The new and powerful valvulotome was actually sterilized and on the table in Case 3, but as this case was complicated by an adherent pericardium, we felt it unwise to use it when the opportunity to do so arrived. An hour's struggle with the pericardial adhesions had unfortunately dissipated much of our courage. The new instrument, however, was used in the last case and proved effective. With each clinical attempt, new questions arose which could only be answered by fresh laboratory investigation. The experience in such work enabled us to approach each new patient with both better instruments and an improved procedure. Carrel once stated that many of the questions put to him regarding the possibilities of the surgical treatment of valvular disease could only be answered by experience obtained in human cases. It is our hope that we have obtained as much benefit as our capacities enable us to obtain from the following attempts in human cases.

*   *   *

From such a limited experience no final deduction can be drawn either for or against the proposal or the procedure. We feel, however, that much has been learned that should be of value in the consideration of such cases and in subsequent operations. Certainly, there can be no

doubt that the method of exposure used is satisfactory, simple in execution and that it apparently produced no especially harmful effect on our patients. The fact that there were no operative deaths, or any indication that the procedure per se was a factor in the subsequent fatalities, is comforting.

A mortality of 75 percent is alarming, but to those who will analyze the full reports of the separate cases it may not appear so disastrous. The three fatalities seem fully explained by causes not inherent in the procedure itself, except in Case 3, in which the slight but continuous oozing from the divided cardiopericardial adhesions added to the burden of an already diseased heart. Death in Case 2 was obviously due to cardiac failure. We might in retrospect think that this type of case, in which fibrillation gave evidence of considerably advanced myocardial damage, was too poor a risk to be considered for such a procedure. But even our judgment here may be faulty because, if we could have produced in such a case a real decrease in the mechanical obstruction, great relief might have occurred. Of course we do not know how the diseased auricle would have borne the increased regurgitation, or how the damaged ventricle would have tolerated its increased amount of blood. In Case 4, a common, and often serious, pulmonary complication was apparently a factor in the fatal issue.

Indeed there are so many questions, obviously unanswered before the first and even after the last operation, that we feel that our mortality rate should be judged, if one wishes to use this as a criterion, only in comparison with figures obtained in the early surgery of other parts of the body, when similar important questions were still unanswered. May we recall the mortality figures in the early surgery of such a relatively simple field as that of the stomach, collected by Dr. W. W. Keen for his Cartwright lectures. Of the first twenty-eight gastrostomies, collected in 1875, all the patients died, and in a series of thirty-five gastroenterostomies in 1885 the operative mortality was 65.7 percent. Moreover, it took years for these figures to improve. In 1884, the mortality for gastrostomy was still 81.6 percent.

*   *   *

We feel that the proposal that certain cases of mitral stenosis may be relieved by surgery has not been contradicted by our experiences, and we hope that similar opportunities in other cases will prove that the proposition is well founded and desirable.

NOTE

J. S. GOODALL AND LAMBERT ROGERS
SOME SURGICAL PROBLEMS OF CARDIOLOGY—
TECHNIC OF MITRALOTOMY*

Disheartened by the distressing nature, the progressive character, and the frequent inefficacy of the medical treatment of certain cardiac lesions, enterprising workers have from time to time endeavored to develop a surgical aspect to the treatment of heart disease, their prevailing idea being not to supplant medical treatment by surgery but to introduce the latter in a more radical attempt to relieve pain or prolong life.

*   *   *

The tragic death of the young sufferer from mitral stenosis, whose systemic circulation is starved of oxygenated blood because of the obstruction at the mitral valve, is well known. "Desperate diseases need desperate remedies," and desperate though an attempt at relieving the obstruction by surgical means may seem, it would appear that in the hands of an operator who has developed and sufficiently practiced an efficient technic, the operation may afford a ray of hope for the future.

It has been well said that in order to decide upon the justification for operating, a surgeon should endeavor to put himself in his patient's place and imagine the operation applied to himself. With death imminent from mitral obstruction who of us would not clamor for something to be done, could we but place our faith in an operator and a technic sufficiently sound to give at least a chance of life?

It should be obvious in the first place that so highly a specialized technic as is required for any intracardiac operative procedure can be carried out only by the specialist who has devoted much time and patience to perfecting his methods of operating upon the heart, and however expert an operator a general surgeon may be, he would be quite unjustified in attempting such an operation without first developing this technic by experimenting upon the cadaver and upon animals.

*   *   *

* 38 *American Journal of Surgery* 108 (1924). Reprinted by permission.

d.

H. S. Souttar
The Surgical Treatment of Mitral Stenosis*

There can be no more fascinating problem in surgery than the relief of pathological conditions of the valves of the heart. Despite the consecutive changes to which these lesions may have given rise in the cardiac muscle, the relief of the lesions themselves would undoubtedly be of immense service to the patient and must be followed by marked improvement in his general condition. Expressed in these terms, the problem is to a large extent mechanical, and as such should already be within the scope of surgery, were it not for the extraordinary nature of the conditions under which the problem must be attacked. . . .

*   *   *

. . . I have been interested for some time in the development of a suitable technique for reaching this valve, and I owe to Dr. Otto Leyton the opportunity . . . for putting my ideas to the test. A description of the case itself will give the clearest indication of the method of approach I adopted and of the technique which I devised.

L. H., aged 15, was admitted to the London Hospital in January, 1921, suffering from chorea and mitral stenosis. Her subsequent history was one of many relapses, with steadily increasing failure of compensation. In September, 1924, she was admitted with haemoptysis, vomiting, and severe dyspnoea. She was cyanosed, her feet were swollen, and her liver was enlarged and tender. After three weeks in hospital she had greatly improved and was sent to a convalescent home, whence three weeks later she was discharged.

Early in March, 1925, she appeared at the London Hospital with cough, dyspnoea, and pain in the limbs. She was sent home to bed and given digitalis and aspirin, but she did not improve. After a severe attack of epistaxis and precordial pain she was again admitted as an inpatient.

*   *   *

In view of her many relapses it appeared that her heart was unable to establish compensation for the combined stenosis and regurgitation from which she suffered, and it was therefore

* 2 *British Medical Journal* 603–606 (1925). Reprinted by permission.

decided to attempt to relieve the stenosis by surgical means.

* * *

The auricular appendage was . . . drawn forward, a soft curved clamp was applied to its base, and it was incised in an antero-posterior direction with scissors. Into this opening the left forefinger was inserted, the clamp was withdrawn, and the appendage was drawn over the finger like a glove by means of the sutures. The whole of the inside of the left auricle could now be explored with facility. It was immediately evident from the rush of blood against the finger that gross regurgitation was taking place, but there was not so much thickening of the valves as had been expected. The finger was passed into the ventricle through the orifice of the mitral valve without encountering resistance, and the cusps of the valve could be easily felt and their condition estimated.

The finger was kept in the auricle for perhaps two minutes, and during that time, so long as it remained in the auricle, it appeared to produce no effect upon the heart beat or the pulse. The moment, however, that it passed into the orifice of the mitral valve the blood pressure fell to zero, although even then no change in the cardiac rhythm could be detected. The blood stream was simply cut off by the finger, which presumably just fitted the stenosed orifice. As, however, the stenosis was of such moderate degree, and was accompanied by so little thickening of the valves, it was decided not to carry out the valve section which had been arranged, but to limit intervention to such dilatation as could be carried out by the finger. It was felt that an actual section of the valve might only make matters worse by increasing the degree of regurgitation, while the breaking down of the adhesions by the finger might improve the condition as regards both regurgitation and stenosis.

It was now decided to withdraw the finger and close the appendage. . . .

* * *

She made an uninterrupted recovery, the freedom from pain or any disturbance which might have been expected to result from the operation being remarkable. Her general condition appeared to be greatly improved, but the physical signs showed little or no change. She was sent to the country and kept in bed for six weeks, but as at the end of that time her pulse rate had remained constant at about 90 she was gradually allowed to get up. At the end of three months she declared that she felt perfectly well, although she still became somewhat breathless on exertion.

I believe that this is the first occasion upon which an attempt has been made to reach the mitral valve by this route in the human being, or to subject the interior of the heart to digital examination. The value of the method cannot possibly be judged on a single case, but I think that I may claim to have shown that the method is practicable and that it is reasonably safe. Indeed, the features which most struck all who were present at the operation were the facility and the absolute safety of the whole procedure, while even on a first attempt the amount and precision of the information to be gained by digital exploration were very remarkable. I had intended to divide the aortic cusp by passing a thin hernia bistoury along my finger and thus to relieve the stenosis, and this could have been done with perfect facility had it been considered advisable.

* * *

It appears to me that the method of digital exploration through the auricular appendage cannot be surpassed for simplicity and directness. Not only is the mitral orifice directly to hand, but the aortic valve itself is almost certainly within reach, through the mitral orifice. Owing to the simplicity of the structures, and, oddly enough, to their constant and regular movement, the information given by the finger is exceedingly clear, and personally I felt an appreciation of the mechanical reality of stenosis and regurgitation which I never before possessed. To hear a murmur is a very different matter from feeling the blood itself pouring back over one's finger. I could not help being impressed by the mechanical nature of these lesions and by the practicability of their surgical relief.

NOTE

HARRINGTON SAINSBURY
THE SURGICAL TREATMENT OF MITRAL
STENOSIS*

I have read with the greatest interest Mr. Souttar's description of his operation for the relief of mitral stenosis. It shows triumphantly the accessibility of the interior of the left auricle, and

* 2 *British Medical Journal* 818 (1925). Reprinted by permission.

of its passage of communication with the ventricle, to surgical measures.

My object in writing is to draw attention to a danger which must attend an operation such as that described, but to which no reference is made. . . . The danger arises from the fact that these cases of pronounced mitral stenosis are so often the seat of recurrent attacks of acute endocarditis (Mr. Souttar's case was admitted with pain in the limbs, though the temperature is not recorded). In such cases fresh vegetations are a common pathological feature, and the risk of the detachment of these in passing the finger through the auriculoventricular orifice, with embolism as a necessary consequence, is plain. I need not dilate upon this peril, which even very delicate manipulation might involve. . . .

*　　*　　*

e.
Elliot C. Cutler and Claude S. Beck
The Present Status of the Surgical Procedures in Chronic Valvular Disease of the Heart—Final Report of All Surgical Cases*

[It] seems opportune to review the cases of valvular disease in which surgical treatment has been used. In summarizing these cases, we shall attempt to evaluate the general idea of subjecting such disorders to surgical therapy and we shall also attempt to emphasize the problems that must in the future be overcome to make surgical procedures on the cardiac valves useful and beneficial.

Operation has been performed in twelve cases of chronic valvular disease of the heart. . . .

*　　*　　*

[The cardiac abnormalities included] one case of pulmonic stenosis, one case of aortic stenosis and ten cases of mitral stenosis. We have not had any personal experience with pulmonic stenosis and aortic stenosis. It seems that mitral stenosis offers greater promise than do any other of the valvular lesions, and for this reason we shall confine discussion to the cases of mitral stenosis.

Of the ten patients with mitral stenosis who were operated on, only one is living, giving a mortality of 90 per cent. Eight of the ten patients died so soon after operation that the changes brought about in the mechanics of the circulation could not be adequately studied. One

patient lived four and a half years after the operation. It is difficult to say definitely whether in this case the enlargement effected in the mitral valve by the operation was followed by an improvement in the circulation. We believe, however, that there was an improvement in the patient's condition. If it be true that the mechanics of the circulation were improved by reduction of the stenosis, a definite advance in this subject has been brought about. It will require, however, a number of cases in which operation is successful to determine definitely whether an improvement in the circulation can be expected by enlarging the orifice in the stenosed valve. Such physiologic observations have not been produced in animals. Unfortunately, it seems that the basic idea underlying this development will have to be established by attempts on human patients.

If it be taken for granted that the mechanics of the circulation become more compatible with life when the degree of mitral obstruction is decreased, there remain the technical problems of the operation. . . .

*　　*　　*

[T]hree kinds of procedures were utilized in the attempts to enlarge the stenotic orifice. These methods were finger dilatation, incision of the stenotic valve and excision of a segment of the stenotic valve. We have not had any experience with dilation of the stenosis. We feel, however, that the method may be worthy of trial. A small instrument . . . could be devised, and this instrument could be inserted into the stenotic ring and the latter stretched and dilated. It will be seen that the only two patients of the series living are those on whom dilatation was done. Incision of the stenotic valve was carried out in four cases. From our experience in cases 5 and 6, we felt that the enlargement effected by a simple incision of the stenotic valve was inadequate. We then devised an instrument which could excise a segment from the valve and remove it from the blood stream. This instrument was used in five cases. In each of the four patients that we operated on, some difficulty was experienced in orientation within the heart. We feel at the present time that that is one of the most serious problems in cardiac surgery. The cardioscope devised by Allen and Graham affords a slight degree of visualization of the endocardium at the point of contact with the instrument. The examination that can be carried out with this instrument, however, is so slight that we have not used it in any human cases.

---

* 18 *Archives of Surgery* 403, 413–416 (1929). Reprinted by permission.

Finally, it may be that we already have the evidence that the success in the finger dilatation method and the success in our first case are due to the fact that only a slight change was made in the size of the orifice of the valve. It may be that the cardiovalvulotome with its actual removal of a piece of valve creates a too sudden change. We know that all the changes created by nature are slow and gradual; could we return a stenotic valve to the insufficient type by a gradual procedure, we might well achieve success. This question unfortunately cannot be answered until we can experimentally produce stenosis similar to what occurs in man, and then suddenly change this to an insufficiency. We have convinced ourselves that a simple knife cannot enlarge a typically stenosed, thickened and often calcareous valve; we do not know whether the actual removal of a piece of the valve by the powerful cardiovalvulotome is deleterious or not. And we have not yet available evidence as to what excision of a segment of a stenosed valve will result in when the operative procedure is simplified (as performed in our last case), and the post-operative course, therefore, less of a strain on the already lowered vitality.

It may seem that the information obtained from the twelve cases of chronic valvular disease in which operation was performed is so meager that further attempts are not justified. However, in view of the preceding discussion, we feel that a few more attempts are necessary in order to answer certain questions already mentioned. Should it be possible to produce experimental stenoses, these questions could be answered in the laboratory. Unfortunately, our own attempts for seven years along this line have been as unsuccessful as the attempts of other and more experienced investigators.

It is our conclusion that the mortality figures alone should not deter further investigation both clinical and experimental, since they are to be expected in the opening up of any new field for surgical endeavor.

NOTE

Elizabeth H. Thomson
Harvey Cushing—Surgeon, Author, Artist*

*   *   *

The story is told of Sir Victor Horsley by one of his graduate students, Dr. Ernest Sachs,

* New York: Henry Schuman 134 (1950). Reprinted by permission of Murnat Publications, Inc.

that he walked into the wards at the Queen Square Hospital one morning to see a patient at the request of Dr. Charles Beevor. He decided that the patient had a pituitary tumor and announced that he would operate the following Tuesday. Beevor, knowing the usual result of such attempts, protested, "But Victor, if you operate on that man, he will die." "Of course he will die," returned Horsley, "but if I don't operate on him, those who follow me won't know how to perform these operations."

This had to be the underlying philosophy of all who attempted surgery of the brain in the first discouraging years. . . .

*   *   *

2.

Experimentation and Moratorium—
The Second Phase (1929–1945)

From 1929 to 1949 no further reports on mitral valve surgery were published. At least insofar as publication was concerned, a complete moratorium on such interventions had been declared. However, work in the laboratory continued.

John H. Powers
Surgical Treatment of Mitral Stenosis*

The technical difficulties and hazards of an operative procedure on the heart are great. Medical therapy in chronic cardiac valvular disease offers nothing but supportive and palliative treatment without hope of permanent relief. Consequently the surgical treatment of mitral stenosis presents a most fascinating and interesting problem to both surgeon and physician.

The rationale for the procedure has been based on the assumption that mitral insufficiency is functionally a less damaging lesion than mitral stenosis. With this hypothesis as a major premise, the first operation of election on the mitral valve was performed by Dr. Elliott C. Cutler in May, 1923. A tenotome was inserted into the mitral orifice through the left ventricle, and an attempt was made to incise each segment of the obstructing ring. The patient recovered and was definitely improved until the onset of a terminal illness four and one-half years later.

After this first intrepid effort, Allen and Graham attempted a three-stage procedure with

* 25 *Archives of Surgery* 555–557, 568–569 (1932). Reprinted by permission.

an instrument carrying an optical system, by which they hoped to cut the valve under direct vision. The patient died on the operating table.

The experience gained in their first and two subsequent cases convinced Cutler and Beck of the impossibility of enlarging the mitral orifice sufficiently with a simple knife to obtain an adequate degree of regurgitation. Consequently the cardiovalvulotome was developed, a powerful cutting instrument by which a segment of the valve could be excised and removed from the circulation.

With one exception all subsequent operations have been performed with this instrument. The exceptional, and only successful, case is that reported by Souttar, in which the mitral orifice was dilated with the finger, introduced through the left auricular appendix. This patient is living and apparently improved.

In all, ten patients with mitral stenosis have been subjected to surgical treatment. The mortality has been 90 per cent. Except for Cutler's first case, death occurred from three hours to six days after operation, and in the majority of instances was due, not to operative shock, but to cardiac failure. The mechanical difficulties of the operation have been overcome, mitral insufficiency has been created both by incising the stenotic orifice and by excising a segment of the sclerosed valve, and yet the patients have died. The question presents itself therefore: Is valvulotomy or partial valvulotomy a feasible and justifiable operation in patients with mitral stenosis?

It is undeniably true that an insufficient valve is a more tolerable valve from the patient's standpoint than a stenotic one. Furthermore, Cutler and his collaborators showed experimentally that mitral regurgitation was well tolerated by normal dogs. One may reasonably assume, however, that the physiologic alterations that take place in the circulation after the excision of a segment of normal valve do not approximate those which obtain when a defect of similar degree is made in the thickened and sclerotic postrheumatic valve. The facts suggest that an embarrassed cardiac mechanism, laboring under the mechanical difficulties of a chronic mitral obstruction, is unable to tolerate the additional insult of a sudden, superimposed regurgitation and death occurs from cardiac failure.

The experiments presented here are offered in support of this contention.

Since the development of a method for creating chronic cardiac valvular disease in dogs,

certain phases of the problem, which previously were restricted to clinical impressions and observations on patients have become amenable to precise physiologic study in the laboratory. Four distinct procedures have been carried out:

1. Experimental stenosis of the mitral valve has been produced in dogs, a chronic, sclerosing lesion which, in its mechanical and gross pathologic aspects, is comparable with mitral stenosis in man.

2. Physiologic observations have been made on the circulation of these animals with experimental mitral stenosis.

3. The stenosis has been abruptly converted into insufficiency by partial valvulectomy with the cardiovalvulotome.

4. The physiologic observations have been repeated to determine what effect this procedure has on the mechanics of the circulation, and why the sudden transformation of chronic mitral stenosis into stenosis with insufficiency should be incompatible with life.

*   *   *

All five dogs with experimental mitral stenosis died after the removal of a portion of the obstructing valve. Postmortem examination of each animal disclosed tremendous dilatation and engorgement of the right side of the heart, acute pulmonary congestion and edema, pleural effusion, acute and chronic congestion of the liver with central necrosis and, in one case, ascites.

*   *   *

From [the] results, one must conclude that although mitral regurgitation may be created in normal dogs without clinical evidence of decompensation, the abrupt conversion of experimental chronic mitral stenosis into insufficiency produces such sudden and radical alterations in the mechanics of the circulation that cardiac decompensation and death ensue.

The canine lesion was comparable in its gross pathologic aspects to mitral stenosis of rheumatic origin in man. The instrument and the operative technic were similar to those which have been employed on human beings. It seems justifiable to assume, therefore, that the physiologic alterations in the circulation that account for death after partial valvulectomy on animals may explain the same result following a similar procedure on man.

Could mitral stenosis be relieved more gradually, either by repeated excision of tiny fragments of the valve, by multiple incisions into the obstructing segments or by dilatation of the stenotic orifice, the results might be more satisfactory. The only two cases in which the operation was not succeeded immediately by a fatal outcome were Cutler's first case, in which simple incision into the segments of the valve was performed, and Souttar's case, in which the mitral orifice was dilated with the finger. In both of these procedures only a slight change was produced in the size of the orifice. Souttar's patient is living five years after operation and presents the appearance observed in a well-compensated case of mitral stenosis.

* * *

3.

Therapy, Experimentation, and Success— The Third Phase (1945–Present)

a.

Charles P. Bailey
The Surgical Treatment of Mitral Stenosis (Mitral Commissurotomy)*

Stenosis of the mitral valve has long challenged the therapeutic ingenuity of the medical profession. It has seemed unreasonable that young persons in otherwise satisfactory health should be condemned to a life of invalidism and early death. Success in treating strictures and stenoses in other organs has suggested that such a simple mechanical defect should not present an insuperable problem.

However, fear of surgical attack upon the heart, discouraging results of early attempts, and a general lack of appreciation among the medical profession of the extreme seriousness of this disease, have greatly hampered those interested in the problem. Many internists, among whom are cardiologists, feel that with proper medical management and limited activity these patients may live a normal span of life. It is true that most older practitioners know of a case or two of mitral stenosis which has survived to an advanced age. Unfortunately, these men do not have any roughly accurate idea of the much larger number of cases which have died at an early age. It is also notable that these same older patients will admit that they have not especially enjoyed their prolonged life of limited activity.

_____
* 15 *Diseases of the Chest* 377–393 (1949). Reprinted by permission.

The author has recently been consulted by a woman of 58 and another of 62 who have been "successfully" treated medically for 25 and 28 years, respectively. They now, at their advanced age, being no more limited than they were 10 years ago, are futilely petitioning for a chance at surgical relief.

The serious prognosis of mitral stenosis can hardly be properly presented statistically, since cases vary in severity, and since death is often wrongly attributed to some other heart condition, to asthma, or to pulmonary tuberculosis with hemorrhage. This latter syndrome (mitral stenosis with serious hemoptysis) has been shown by Wolfe and Levine in 1941 to have a mortality of 66 per cent within 3 years. This has been brought home dramatically to the author, who recommended surgery in two such cases eight and six weeks ago, respectively. Both at first accepted surgery and then changed their minds because of the presumed risk. Both have already died of pulmonary hemorrhage.

With such a dismal outlook, it is time to take steps to differentiate those cases which are mild or non-progressive from those who will not have any useful existence. It then is incumbent upon the profession to learn how to alleviate the severe cases.

* * *

It is my belief that there are at least one million cases of mitral stenosis in the United States, one-quarter of which are suitable for surgery. . . .

* * *

A review of the reports in the literature by Cutler and Beck in 1929 of operations upon the aortic and mitral valves revealed that of the first 10 cases of mitral stenosis subjected to operation, one died during insertion of an instrument into the left auricular appendage, two were subjected to finger dilatation of the mitral valve after insertion through the left auricular appendage (both cases lived and were improved) three cases were treated by tenotome division of a valve cusp (one lived 4½ years and was much improved), and five cases were subjected to partial valvulectomy by the cardiovalvulotome (all died).

* * *

After 1929 no more surgical attempts were made until 1945. Both Dr. Dwight Harken and Dr. Horace Smithy, as well as the author, have made recent operative attempts to improve cases of mitral stenosis. Our clinical experience with the surgery of the mitral valve has been with five cases to date.

During the past eight years the author and his associates have performed diverse and repeated operations upon the mitral valve of some 60 mongrel dogs. Several conclusions have been reached: (1) The approach through the left auricular appendage is the most satisfactory one since there is less danger of arrhythmia, greater ease of entering the valve, and greater ease in controlling hemorrhage. . . . (2) Production of an appreciable degree of sudden mitral regurgitation is tolerated poorly by dogs. Thus extensive cutting of the anterior cusp of the mitral valve is nearly always attended by operative mortality. It would seem that regardless of the reported observation that clinical mitral regurgitation is less crippling than clinical mitral stenosis these sick human hearts will not tolerate the sudden production of a large mitral regurgitation very well. (3) The accurate placement of an instrument to divide a mitral valve depends upon actually palpating the valve and instrument from within the auricle at the time of operation. Thus, whether the cutting instrument is inserted through the ventricle or auricle, it is necessary that the right index finger be passed through an incision opening. These incisions should be extended well into the normal valve tissue margin. . . .

Case 1: Our first clinical case was W.S., a man of 37 years who had been severely incapacitated for 16 years and who had had several severe episodes of hemoptysis. On November 14, 1945 his left anterior chest was opened. . . . The patient died on the operating table of hemorrhage, no valvulotomy having been performed. We have ever since realized that the human auricular appendage in mitral stenosis is friable and entirely unlike that of a normal dog. We no longer permit a hemostat to be closed on an auricular appendage beyond the first tooth of the ratchet, and prefer not to actually close the ratchet.

Case 2: Our next case was W.S., a 29-year-old married female who had been a cardiac invalid for 11 years, and who had been in congestive failure on several previous occasions during the preceeding 7 years. On this occasion she failed to respond to the usual medical measures and remained in a precarious state with engorged liver and ascites in spite of digitalis and mercurial diuretics. Since she was deemed hopeless, her physicians felt that she might be subjected to valvulotomy. At operation on June 12, 1946 the

heart was approached through a left anterior thoracic incision. . . . Up to this point the blood pressure was approximately 60/50 mm. mercury, and the surgeon began to seek an honorable way of abandoning the procedure. However, the medical consultants stressed that she would undoubtedly die from the anesthesia and exploration unless some relief of the stenosis could be obtained. . . . The mitral valve was found to be a tiny slit which would not admit the tip of the index finger. There was considerable calcification about the valve mouth. This had been palpated by the instrument, but the actual orifice was too small to admit the punch (about the size of a small lead pencil). The valve was forcibly dilated digitally, so that the finger could be inserted into the orifice to the second phalangeal joint. Care was taken not to obstruct the opening for longer than three heart beats at a time. The valve appeared to tear open at both commissures. The thrill which was prominent prior to dilating the valve, immediately disappeared. The blood pressure promptly rse to 80 systolic and the patient's condition began to improve. Because of the improvement and the desperate nature of the risk, the finger was withdrawn and the auricular appendage ligated without any attempt at incising the valve.

The patient's condition continued to improve so that the blood pressure was 130 systolic at the conclusion of the procedure. . . . Improvement was continued for 30 hours. After that the condition began to deteriorate and she died rather quickly 48 hours after surgery. Autopsy revealed a greatly dilated heart. . . . The mitral valve showed evidence of having been torn open at both commissures, but the tears had not extended into the normal marginal valve tissue. The torn surfaces had therefore not separated much, and had become agglutinated by fibrin which accumulated in the orifice and gradually reduced the effective mitral opening to probably a smaller size than that existing at the time of operation. It was difficult to imagine any degree of regurgitation through that valve orifice. No anticoagulant therapy had been employed. As a result of the autopsy findings, the idea was conceived of performing what had been later termed "commissurotomy". . . .

Case 3: The next patient was W.W., a white male 38 years of age, who had been having episodes of severe hemoptysis over a period of 1½ years. In fact, he had had a segmental resection of the right lung performed for bronchiectasis one year previously, in the belief that his hemorrhages were of pulmonary origin. However, after 8 months his hemorrhages had returned in an exsanguinating form. Re-study then revealed that a marked enlargement of the heart had taken place during the interim and typical evidences of severe mitral stenosis were now evident. The patient was also showing early signs of decompensation. On March 22, 1948 at the Memorial Hospital in Wilmington, Delaware, the left 4th anterior rib was removed and the pericardium was opened. . . .

Because of the bitter experience with the previous patient, it was decided to use anticoagulant therapy. . . . The patient did reasonably well until the second postoperative day, when evidence of hemorrhage into the left pleura required repeated thoracenteses. Heparin therapy was discontinued. When the red blood count had dropped to 2,450,000 on the third postoperative day, it was felt necessary to transfuse him, and this was done, 2600 cc. blood being given. Unfortunately, there was a misunderstanding regarding orders pertaining to fluid balance, and a total of 7,400 cc. of fluid by mouth and parenterally on the fourth postoperative day, and 1,500 cc. on the fifth postoperative day was administered. As a result the patient became markedly edematous. At about 4 P.M. he suddenly developed pulmonary edema and expired. . . .

In reviewing this case, we considered that the following errors had been made: (1) Perhaps the use of the heparin therapy was unwise, since it had required the administration of a considerable volume of fluid, and since it undoubtedly played a major role in the secondary intrapleural bleeding. (2) The use of saline rather than glucose solution as a vehicle for the heparin. (3) Inadequate incision in the lateral commissure of the valve, partly due to the repeated disengaging of the knife blade on account of its shape. The medial commissure could not be cut because of the large calcification. (4) Unwise and excessive fluid therapy. (5) Perhaps accepting a case for surgery who had had diminished contralateral lung function from previous disease and partial lung resection. It was the consensus, however, of all physicians concerned that if we had just returned the patient to bed postoperatively, and not treated him, recovery would have followed.

Case 4: The next case was J.R., a 32-year-old white male who had had advanced mitral stenosis for 7 years. During the past 1½ years he

had been in chronic congestive failure, although ambulant much of the time. Digitalis and mercurial diuretics did not completely control the congestion. Since his prognosis was extremely grave without surgery, it was finally decided to attempt a commissurotomy. . . . The pericardium was incised. [T]he least touching of the heart, either ventricle or auricle, was followed by frequent extrasystoles and other irregularities. Because of this extreme irritability of the myocardium, no attempt at valvulotomy was made. The surgeon became worried and suggested abandoning the procedure at that time. The staff felt that this would be the last opportunity for surgery to be utilized in this man. Intravenous atropine did not relieve the myocardial irritability, nor did 50 mgm. doses of procaine intravenously. Intravenous quinidine was administered slowly by personnel experienced in its use. Before completion of the injection, the heart rate had become slow, so the quinidine was discontinued. The systoles became weaker and stopped.

Immediate manual massage restored regular contractions which ceased after a few minutes. Massage was repeated. After that, various stimulants, venesection, artificial respiration, etc., were used. After the heart had been revived by massage a number of times and had failed as many, it was suggested that he might improve if the left ventricular output was increased by opening the mitral valve. Since all was already lost, the auricular appendage was opened and the left index finger was inserted into a tight mitral orifice containing calcium deposits. It was widely dilated, and the finger withdrawn. No instruments were used. The auricular appendage was ligated. After massage had again reestablished a temporary heart beat, it was evident that the left ventricle had become considerably enlarged. However, in spite of repeated massage and all recognized forms of drug stimulation, no permanent restoration of cardiac function could be accomplished. . . .

*   *   *

We do not consider this a death attributable to mitral valve surgery, since death and an irreversible state had apparently become established well before a last ditch emergency dilation of the valve was performed. Undoubtedly this man was too bad a risk for mitral surgery. The pre-operative ballistocardiogram had revealed a poor cardiac output, increased only slightly on exercise.

Case 5: C.W., a 24-year-old white housewife, had been known to have a heart murmur for 17 years and mitral stenosis for 24 months. She had had gradual and progressive onset of dyspnea on exertion and had an attack of congestive failure in November 1947. Since that time she had been on extremely limited activity and received a daily maintenance dose of digitalis. [S]he was admitted to Episcopal Hospital in Philadelphia for study preliminary to a possible mitral commissurotomy. . . . Operation was performed on June 10, 1948. . . . The mitral valve was found to be small, just admitting the tip of the finger. It was not calcified and had a leathery feel, more like kid-skin than cow-hide. It was displaced high up anteriorly. The hooked knife was inserted through the valve orifice and engaged on the lateral commissure under direct digital guidance. The knife was then drawn backward an inch, widely dividing the commissure. The finger was now inserted through the cut valve and some fine remaining fibrous strands were broken up. The valve was now widely patent. The finger was withdrawn and the auricular appendage ligated. . . . The entire operation had taken 80 minutes. . . .

. . . . She was out of bed on the third day, and walking the fourth. Her greatest difficulty was inability to void for four days postoperatively. On the seventh postoperative day the patient had no cardiac murmur audible to the author. . . .

Because of her evident good condition she was transported without incident by train to a 1,000-mile-distant medical convention for presentation in person.

* * *

(February 1, 1949: Patient is continuing to do well 7½ months subsequent to surgery. She is now able to perform all her own housework. . . .)

* * *

February 1, 1949: Since this time, 5 additional patients have been subjected to this operation. Two are doing very well. One died 2½ months after surgery. One died of an error in technique at operation (cutting across a valve leaflet). One did very well for 6 days but died suddenly of a cerebral arterial embolus. Clotting had occurred in the sutured left auricular appendage. We now ligate the appendage at the base to prevent this.

* * *

NOTES

NOTE 1.
JUDITH P. SWAZEY AND RENÉE C. FOX
THE CLINICAL MORATORIUM—
A CASE STUDY OF MITRAL VALVE SURGERY*

* * *

Bailey's three operations had been performed at three different hospitals in the Philadelphia area, and he was informed that further intracardiac surgery would not be permitted at those institutions. Nevertheless, he scheduled two more cases of mitral surgery for June 10, 1948, at the last two Philadelphia hospitals where he still had operating privileges. Case four died during surgery in the morning, of cardiac arrest judged by Bailey to be unrelated to an attempted finger dilatation. Success finally came that afternoon, at Episcopal Hospital, when a 24-year-old housewife withstood her surgery. . . .

* * *

NOTE 2.
RICHARD A. MEADE
A HISTORY OF THORACIC SURGERY†

* * *

In 1945, Bailey operated on a patient with mitral stenosis expecting to bite out a piece of the mitral valve, but he tore the auricle and lost the patient from hemorrhage. In 1946, he operated on his next patient with the same object in view. He was planning to use a backward cutting instrument which he could pass through the left auricular appendage. During the operation, the stenosis was found to be so severe that he could not pass his instrument through the valve. Quoting from Bailey's letter to me,

At that moment my medical men became a great help to me because they urged me to go ahead, to make further efforts to relieve the valvular obstruction because the rapid deterioration of the patient on the operating room table augured ill for a survival from this exploratory operation unless something definitive could be accomplished. In desperation, remembering Souttar's report, I inserted my finger through the auricular appendage, palpated the valve and pushed my finger through the diminished slit. Although the leaflets were calcified, both commissures

* Paul A. Freund, ed.: *Experimentation with Human Subjects.* New York: George Braziller 315, 330 (1970). Reprinted by permission of the American Academy of Arts and Sciences.
† Springfield, Ill.: Charles C. Thomas 440–448 (1961). Reprinted by permission of Charles C. Thomas.

split well and I immediately appreciated three things. One was that there was now an opening many times larger than that which had existed previously. Second, the diastolic thrill, which in this particular case was very prominent in the region of the valvular structure itself, immediately disappeared. At the same time I was unable to recognize any regurgitant jet of blood from the valve. I was quite familiar with the digital feel of the regurgitant jet from my animal experimentation. I was, therefore, convinced that I had both relieved the stenosis and failed to produce any regurgitation. For about twenty-four hours postoperatively, the patient's condition improved remarkably and steadily. There was no clinical evidence of regurgitation. However, one day later, she suddenly collapsed and died. From the post-mortem examination it was clearly evident that both commissures had been split and considerable mobility of the leaflets had been accomplished. It was evident from the intact suspension of the valve leaflets that regurgitation had not been produced.

Before continuing the account of the progress of Bailey's work, it is well here to refer to the work done by Horace Smithy during 1948. In spite of his knowledge of the literature and especially of the experimental work of Powers, he revived the Cutler operation and carried out the procedure on seven patients with mitral stenosis. He differed from Cutler in that he used the auricular approach in four of the cases. One patient was operated on twice because at the first operation, when he attempted to pass the instrument through the auricular appendage, he tore the auricle and, after controlling the hemorrhage, he abandoned the procedure. Later, he used the ventricular approach with success. He concluded that the ventricular approach was the better of the two. Two of his patients died soon after operation, and one after ten months. One patient showed marked improvement during the year in which she was followed. The other three showed only slight improvement. The fact that five of the patients survived the operation was presumably due to the great improvements in anesthesia and surgical technique since the 1920's. These patients survived, and showed some improvement in spite of the regurgitation produced. . . .

* * *

[W]hile Bailey and Harken were working in this country on the problem of the surgical relief of mitral stenosis, Russell Brock in England was also planning an attack. Following his success in dividing a stenotic pulmonary valve, he decided that the same procedure could be used on the mitral valve. Remembering Souttar's article, he successfully carried out the Souttar opera-

tion on a patient with mitral stenosis in September, 1948. At this time he was not aware of the work done by Bailey and Harken. He became convinced that the operation was a sound one and carried it out on seven more patients before publishing his results in 1950. Two of his patients died after operation, but one of them died of hemorrhage, having been given heparin on the second postoperative day because of a cerebral embolus. One other patient developed a cerebral embolus but fully recovered. The other five patients had uneventful recoveries. Following this first report, he began operating on an increasingly large number of patients. He has used finger fracture in the great majority of his cases but occasionally resorts to the use of a knife to cut the commissure.

Following the reports of the work of Bailey, Glover, and O'Neil, and of Harken in this country, and of Brock in England, the operation became widely adopted. At first the mortality rates were high, but as the cardiologists changed their points of view and began referring better risk patients, the mortality rate fell. It soon became apparent that finger fracture was all that was needed in most of the cases but in some it was necessary to use a knife to open the commissures sufficiently. Harken in this country and Brock in England have made important contributions regarding the anatomy of the mitral valve, and have pointed out the relative importance of the major and minor leaflets.

* * *

Although the modern operation for relief of mitral stenosis differs very little from that done by Souttar in 1925, it is worth noting [one] . . . technical [advance], the use of special knives in those cases in which it is felt that complete splitting along the commissures has not been accomplished by the finger.

* * *

The one unexplained fact in the history of the development of an operation for mitral stenosis is the failure of other surgeons to repeat Souttar's operation until 1948. In retrospect, it seems incredible that he himself did not continue his work, and that the men in this country who had done so much work on surgery of the heart did not recognize its value.

The explanation for Souttar's failure to continue his work is simple. He had no more patients referred to him for operation. And yet, he was Director of Surgery of the London Hospital and one of the leading surgeons in England at the time. However, Sir James Mackenzie was the leading cardiologist at that time and had a profound influence over the other cardiologists in England and even in this country. He believed that the chief feature of mitral stenosis was the diseased myocardium, and that the stenosed valve was of secondary importance. So he was opposed to operation for relief of the stenosis. And this opposition prevented Souttar from continuing his work.

In this country, there was the same general opposition to surgery for mitral stenosis. Even Dr. Evarts Graham was unable to persuade his medical colleagues of the value of operation. In Boston, Dr. Samuel Levine stood out in opposition to Sir James, and was responsible for Cutler being able to operate on some seven patients with mitral stenosis. Why then, did not Cutler and Beck follow Souttar's lead? We shall never know why Cutler failed to do so, but Beck has stated, in a letter to me and in an article in the *Journal of the American Medical Association,* his reason for not adopting the operation. He believes that there has been a change in the character of the mitral valve as a result of the use of sulfonamides and antibiotics. The hearts he studied in the pathology laboratory in the 1920's had valves that were calcified and so tough that he does not believe finger fracture could have been used. In this connection, it must be remembered that in Souttar's case he did not fracture the valve with his finger. He merely placed his finger through the valve and was assured of its patency by doing so. He probably was not aware of the possibility of actually fracturing the valve, although he was sure that the stenosis could be corrected by passing his finger through it.

It is interesting to hear the comment of Dr. Samuel Levine who worked with Cutler and with him reported the first successful case of surgery for mitral stenosis. He wrote, "the fact that no further case reports or experiences were recorded indicated that nothing very much had been accomplished. I do recall that the criticism on the part of the leading authorities at that time, particularly Sir James Mackenzie, was that it was useless to attack the valve because that was not important. Mackenzie thought that the all-important part was the myocardium and that would not be altered by surgery of the valve. In fact, he wrote me just to that effect, after Cutler and I had published our first case. I was certain even then, and have felt the same way ever since, that the valvular defect was all-important in rheumatic heart disease." He also stated that he did

not believe there had been any change in the character of the valve. He felt that our surgery was just not sufficiently advanced at the time. When one recalls that lobectomy carried a mortality rate of around 45 percent at that time, his comment seems reasonable.

Another reason for the failure of American surgeons to adopt the Souttar operation has been well expressed by Dr. Evarts Graham. He wrote, "when I heard about Souttar's case, I was, of course, much interested but felt that his procedure would never amount to very much because it lacked precision and was a blind one. It had always been my feeling that, in surgery, one of the first rules is to have exposure so that you can see exactly what you are doing."

So, for one reason or another, twenty-three years passed after Souttar's operation before it was tried again, and then within a period of three months, in widely separated places in the world, his operation was revived. The time was not ripe in 1925. It was in 1948.

*   *   *

NOTE 3.

FRANCIS D. MOORE
REPORT OF THE SURGEON-IN-CHIEF*

A creative science defines problems worthy of solution, and seeks their solution by every effective method available. Both parts of this definition are important.

One of the duties of science is to define problems which should be solved. The Greek philosophers defined their problems very broadly; they wanted to understand the whole universe and the relationship of its parts. The scientist of today sometimes defines his problems in a much more narrow area, as one can see by reading over a list of thesis titles at Commencement. When a field of research ceases to describe problems, it ceases to be effective.

The second part of the definition, stating that the investigator must use any techniques whatsoever to attain his ends, is also important. All is fair in love, war and research. Many fields of science have developed methods which ultimately have come to dominate and sterilize the field; they must reach out for new techniques to revitalize their search for knowledge.

In many respects surgery is an art; it is also a creative science. Let us look at [an example].

*   *   *

* *37th Annual Report of the Peter Bent Brigham Hospital* (Boston) 48, 55–58 (1950). Reprinted by permission.

In 1940, Dr. Dwight Harken returned to Boston from his year in England with Mr. Tudor Edwards and took up a residency at the Boston City Hospital. During this time he spent many hours in the laboratory, and in August of 1942 published an article entitled "Experiments in Intracardiac Surgery." His original idea had been to invade the heart surgically through the auricular appendage to excise the vegetations of bacterial endocarditis. Again surgery had posed a question: "May we operate within the human heart and rectify major valvular disease?" Surgery also sought an answer. In this case the initial approach was to the experimental animal, that unsung hero whom a few agitators would like to remove from the scene!

During this work Dr. Harken found to his interest and surprise that the function of the two mitral valve leaflets was very different. The aortic, or major leaflet, had to be preserved intact. If it were destroyed, one wall of the aortic outflow tract was gone and the animal soon died of mitral regurgitation. This observation was of fundamental importance several years later when mitral surgery was being revitalized. It was a basic conceptual advance. Twenty years previously we had assumed mitral regurgitation to be the price of relieving mitral stenosis. Now Dr. Harken knew that stenosis could be relieved without adding such a burden to the already sick heart and lungs, providing the surgeon did not disturb the aortic leaflet.

The war intervened; the investigator found himself treating soldiers with wounds of the heart. Besides the development of operative techniques and personal facility with cardiac surgery, one further observation of fundamental interest was made. Dr. Harken saw that dislocation of the heart from its normal position in the thorax resulted in the development of sudden arrhythmias incompatible with life. If the heart were returned quickly to its position of optimum function, normal rhythm was quickly restored. Here was a guiding principle for further work and here was an explanation for some of Dr. Cutler's difficulties twenty years before: not only had he entered through the ventricular muscle—which in itself must carry some special hazard—but he had found it necessary to dislocate the rheumatic heart from its normal position, a dislocation that the hearts of well-conditioned soldiers could not tolerate.

With this background, Dr. Harken commenced his first clinical work with mitral stenosis in the spring of 1947. The basic premises were (1) to approach the mitral valve from above

rather than through the ventricle, (2) to operate on the heart without dislocating it from its normal position, (3) to remove only portions of the lesser leaflets, thus leaving the aortic outflow tract intact and avoiding regurgitation, and (4) to use the superior pulmonary vein as the port of entry.

The progress of knowledge often simplifies rather than complicates. This was true with the technique of valvular surgery. Many complex instruments were developed and used in these early operations. The results were disappointing; the instruments were hard to control. Several of the early patients failed to survive. All had been operated upon in a far advanced and hopeless stage of disease and approached their operation knowing fully its formative character and the hazards it entailed. We are apt to think of the long hours of work or difficult problems faced by the investigator. There are many occasions when we must also recognize the knowing sacrifice of those dangerously sick patients who are willing to take well-understood risks in the interest of more than personal benefit—in the assurance of benefit to others.

*   *   *

The problem then (early 1949) seemed to rest on the question of how to control the intracardiac manipulation which broke apart the fusion bridges of the valve. The surgeon's finger, endowed with a sense of feeling and position, was clearly more controllable than any other device. Instead of using a complicated instrument through the difficult approach of the superior pulmonary vein, the surgeon's finger was introduced through the auricle itself and the two fusion bridges were broken apart. Fracture is a good word for this procedure. The fused valve is rigid and the rigid area breaks where it is difficult or impossible to cut. With experience in a few more cases, it became apparent that the fracture of the valve made by the surgeon's finger through an opening in the auricle had made possible an entirely new evaluation of valvular surgery because it was done with a new order of accuracy.

The selection of cases was not easy. One possibility would have been to select patients who were not very ill, feeling that they might recover more easily. This would hardly yield information about the value of the procedure. A much more critical approach would be to select patients who were severely ill and whose outlook was very limited; this was the approach Dr. Harken selected. His selection was based on the studies of his medical colleagues in the cardiac laboratory.

As testimony that this selection was realistic, we must point out that of 16 patients selected for operation but who were not operated upon, 14 are now dead, 11 within six months of the time when surgery was advised.

Forty-two other patients in exactly the same sort of situation have now been operated upon; 29 are now alive and 24 are outstandingly successful results.

The surgery of mitral stenosis has now been through its "dark days," days when the surgeon, his medical colleagues and those with whom he sought counsel were tried as to whether or not the effort should be maintained through such difficulties. It is through those dark days and into a phase where its scope should be broadened. Recently a group of six patients who were *not* in the last stages of the disease have been operated upon. All of them have done well and have showed a gratifying return to normal heart function.

NOTE 4.
DWIGHT E. HARKEN, LAURENCE B. ELLIS, AND LEONA R. NORMAN
THE SURGICAL TREATMENT OF MITRAL STENOSIS*

* * *

Our experience with mitral stenosis now involves a study group of twenty-five patients, eight of whom have been treated surgically. There have been three surgical deaths. The operations have been as follows: Five valvuloplasties, two interatrial septal defects, and one denervation. The deaths were all in the valvuloplasty group. The first patient of the series was lost because we did not at that time appreciate the devastating effect of tachycardia. The second death was the fourth valvuloplasty. This death was on the operating table from uncontrolled blood loss. The third death was from pulmonary edema on the fifth postoperative day, and autopsy revealed that too little valvuloplastic incision had been made. This debilitated patient was therefore subjected to a very strenuous operation without the relief of adequate correction of the fundamental mechanical handicap.

The experience to date seems to indicate that essential knowledge of the technical difficulties and the indications for various surgical procedures is being gathered.

The possibility of practical surgical relief of

mitral stenosis calls for more complete understanding of the disease. Means must be sought to predict the probable clinical course of a given patient. Those who have a truly malignant form of valvular disease should be selected, if possible, before the pulmonary changes render the patient an inordinately serious risk for surgical intervention.

Objective evaluation before, during, and after operation must be conducted in order to determine which procedures are best tolerated and most beneficial. . . .

* * *

NOTE 5.
JUDITH P. SWAZEY AND RENÉE C. FOX
THE CLINICAL MORATORIUM—
A CASE STUDY OF MITRAL VALVE SURGERY*

* * *

. . . In the winter of 1948/49, six out of Harken's first nine patients died during or shortly after valvulotome surgery.

At this point I went home depressed and said "I quit." Some people suggested I should try my technique on better-risk patients, in order to help me get better results, so I wouldn't "ruin the reputation of cardiac surgery." But I wouldn't do that. After I lost my sixth patient, I had a call from Dr. Laurence Ellis [then President of the New England Cardiovascular Society]. I told him I wouldn't kill any more patients [through mitral valve surgery], and that no respectable referring physician would send me any more patients anyhow. Ellis asked me what I meant: didn't I realize that these patients surely would die if I didn't operate? He said he would still refer patients to me, and didn't I think he was a good cardiologist? This talk with Ellis was a turning point. I went back and operated and my patients suddenly started doing better. But I almost called a moratorium.

Early in 1949, Dr. Harken realized that he "couldn't do an operation successfully with the [valvulotome] and have the patient survive in a substantial number of cases." As he studied postmortem specimens of mitral stenosis, seeking to improve his procedure, he became convinced that the best way to open up the fused bridges of the valve's leaflets, without unduly damaging the valves themselves, was the simple technique Souttar had pioneered: finger dilatation through an auricular entry. After a few cases it "became apparent" that this method, which Harken aptly

---

* 19 *Journal of Thoracic Surgery* 1, 13–14 (1950). Reprinted by permission.

* Paul A. Freund, ed.: *Experimentation with Human Subjects.* New York: George Braziller 315, 331–332 (1970). Reprinted by permission of the American Academy of Arts and Sciences.

named finger-fracture valvuloplasty, "had made possible an entirely new evaluation of valvular surgery because it was done with a new order of accuracy."

Apart from some technical refinements, the operation done today for most cases of mitral stenosis differs little from that done by Souttar in 1925. . . .

* * *

NOTE 6.
    DWIGHT E. HARKEN, LEWIS DEXTER,
  LAURENCE B. ELLIS, ROBERT E. FARRAND,
    AND JAMES F. DICKSON, III
    THE SURGERY OF MITRAL STENOSIS*

* * *

The principal purpose of this publication is to present a simple surgical technic for converting . . . mitral stenosis into effective valves. It is important to realize that stenosis is not being corrected at the expense of producing mitral regurgitation. Contrariwise, minor degrees of regurgitation may be corrected by this maneuver. We have consistently found, by postoperative catheterization, that finger-fracture valvuloplasty can correct mitral stenosis without producing mitral regurgitation.

* * *

Once the exploring finger is in the auricle, the position of the stenotic funnel is determined, the character and type of stenosis is assessed. . . . Gentle pressure is then exerted in a posterolateral direction to effect fracture of the posterior fusion bridge. . . . Gentle anterolateral pressure will then effect fracture of the anterior fusion bridge with much less difficulty. . . . Having fractured the anterior and posterior fusion bridges, careful appraisal is made of the mobility of the major leaflet and of its competence in closing the mitral orifice in systole. Also, the size of the newly created orifice is determined. While every effort is made to conduct this intracardiac blunt dissection deliberately, the surgeon must avoid excessive periods of obstruction of the mitral orifice. . . .

. . . If . . . the elastic fusion bridge resists the simple efforts at fracture described above, the surgeon may then advance the exploring finger 2 or 3 cm. farther into the chamber of the ventricle, hook the finger posterior to the fused posterior chordae and then make a circular motion

from behind forward, in a counter-clockwise direction, in an effort to fracture the lesser leaflet. If this is effective, a similar maneuver will probably fracture the leaflet in the region of the anterior fusion bridge, this time catching the anterior chordae in front of the finger as it is rotated in a clockwise fashion. *Should this simple secondary attempt at fracture fail, the surgeon must not use force but, rather, gently retreat in order to resort to incisional valvuloplasty* (Bailey's "commissurotomy"). . . . On the basis of this exploration of the stenotic funnel, the surgeon is prepared to select the valvulotome best suited to the pathologic process at hand.

* * *

Initially, it was our feeling that it was morally right to accept only those patients who were dying of their disease. We felt that technical failures would inevitably account for the loss of a number of the earlier patients. We could not properly accept patients for surgery who had a reasonable chance of surviving until a better era of surgical technic emerged. That we did in fact select such a group of patients who were dying is attested by two control groups. The first control group was comprised of 19 patients who were either offered surgery or whom we considered proper candidates for surgery but who did not, for one reason or another, come to surgery (through refusal and fear on their part or their families' part or because of hospital admission details). *Seventeen of this self-selected control group of 19 patients were dead within one year and 15 of the 17 died within six months of the time that surgery was recommended.* We are dealing, therefore, with a malignant disease. Conversely, that we have not generally rejected patients because they were too ill for operation is attested by the fact that there were only six patients for whom operation was deferred because they were too ill for immediate surgical intervention. Four of the six died within two weeks and all six died within a month. They were all but moribund.

* * *

Eighty-six operations have been performed to relieve patients with mitral stenosis. There have been nine valvulotome valvuloplasties, two reservoir-shunt operations, two denervations of the heart, two interauricular septal defects and 71 finger-fracture valvuloplasties. This latter operation is vastly superior to the others. . . . Of this latter group, 20 are dead. Eighteen of the deaths were associated with the surgical proce-

* 134 *Annals of Surgery* 722, 726, 734, 737–740 (1951). Reprinted by permission.

dure and two were not related to the valvuloplasty.

In spite of the fact that we have described the original group as in a malignant phase and have confirmed this fact by the mortality rate in the control group, it is true that some were more desperately ill than others. Also, recently we have accepted patients who were even less critically ill and deserve a separate classification. It is very difficult to present an accurate, serviceable, clinical classification of a protean disease such as mitral stenosis. A preliminary effort at such a clinical classification will be made here and elaborated later.

GROUP I comprises patients whose present course is *benign*. They have auscultatory signs of mitral stenosis but few if any symptoms and minimal evidence of increase in pulmonary vascular pressure. We believe that there is no justification for operation on these patients at this time. Patients in this group may continue to run a benign course or they may develop an acceleration of their lesion which shifts them to one of the other groups.

GROUP II includes patients somewhat *handicapped* by a static degree of moderate dyspnea on effort or by infrequent attacks of acute dyspnea or other pulmonary symptoms usually provoked by an extrinsic cause such as unusual exertion, fatigue or by infection. Rarely they may have some peripheral edema but do not have evidence of right ventricular failure.

GROUP III includes patients whose disability is progressive either with increasing dyspnea on effort or with alarming and increasing and easily provoked attacks of hemoptysis, chest pain, pulmonary edema, etc. They suffer from palpitation, tachycardia, and distress over the liver on exertion. At any time they may slip into GROUP IV, or may die of an acute attack of pulmonary edema, or with peripheral or pulmonary infarctions. Their life expectancy under medical therapy is *hazardous*.

GROUP IV is a *terminal* group. They are completely incapacitated, usually with right ventricular failure manifested by chronically elevated venous pressure, considerably enlarged liver, and a marked tendency to congestion. Their pulmonary disability may or may not be greater than those in Group III. They often have poor liver function, evidence of decreased peripheral blood flow, and many have had emboli. Most of them are in auricular fibrillation.

*   *   *

With respect to these categories, it is particularly interesting to note that in Group III there have been 22 patients and but one death. This single death was due to a technical error incident to forcing hastily a Type II valve following cardiac arrest. Contrast this low Group III mortality with Group IV. There have been 34 patients and 16 of these have died, a mortality rate approaching 50 per cent. Furthermore, the clinical improvement of Group III is far more dramatic than Group IV. This is really not surprising in view of the fact that in Group IV the correction of the mitral stenosis follows irreversible changes in the lungs, the liver, and the heart muscle. Whereas in Group III the correction of the mechanical barrier was effected before severe or irreversible secondary damage occurred. Group III, therefore, gets more benefit and risks much less than Group IV.

*   *   *

With respect to future activities in this field, there would seem to be no argument about Group III. Surgery is easy and good. That we should now offer surgery to Group II has been suggested. Group IV demands further scrutiny. It is our feeling that we must continue to operate in this group if we can actually select patients who are dying. It does seem that we have been able to do this. These patients, who are suffering from a malignant disease and for whom life is a burden, do not always succumb for the same reason. Sometimes the cause is disturbed electrolyte balance; sometimes it is embolism; sometimes it is pulmonary failure. As long as there continue to be various causes for death in this group but there is salvage in life and comfort, we must continue to accept the acknowledged hazards of surgery and explore the possibilities of a reasonable method. This application of valvuloplasty to the desperate risk group must continue until such time as we have established conclusively which patients are benefited and, conversely, which patients have no salvage in life or comfort. This effort must continue until the above requirements have been fulfilled or, better still, until the time when the awareness of our medical colleagues to a useful, surgical technic brings the patient to surgical correction in an earlier phase and thereby eliminates this late and disappointing phase. The responsibility of the medical man has nowhere been more clearly defined nor the obligation of the surgeon more richly rewarding.

NOTE 7.
Dwight E. Harken, Laurence B. Ellis,
Lewis Dexter, Robert E. Farrand,
and James F. Dickson, III
The Responsibility of the Physician in
the Selection of Patients with Mitral
Stenosis for Surgical Treatment*

* * *

. . . Group II disability may justify waiting for improved surgery because the illness is static but if that static disability is unacceptable to the patient, it may constitute a reasonable justification for surgical intervention. To date, we have not felt that these patients should have operation now.

Those patients in group III are the ideal candidates for surgery now as the prognosis without intervention is bad and the risk of valvuloplasty is low (less than 10 per cent) considering the severity of the disease. . . .

* * *

Certain patients can be selected whose present course is benign (group I) but who of course may degenerate to one of the more serious categories at any time. If properly followed and observed, these patients should not have surgical intervention at this time. Some of these patients will never require surgical intervention. Furthermore, there is a real possibility that surgery can render this group a substantial disservice (a) incident to the risk and discomfort of an unnecessary operation, (b) incident to the valvular alteration itself, and (c) incident to the sacrifice of the auricular appendage in the event that subsequent operation should become necessary.

In group II, patients whose degree of disability is static, selection of cases for operation must be made on the basis of the discomfort and limitation in the individual case. The risk of operation in this group is not great; it can be carried below 5 per cent. The chance of relieving the handicap is good. On the other hand, if patients in this group are not materially discommoded by their illness, it is entirely possible that better valvuloplasty may be available within the next year or so. We have deferred surgery in this group, placing the patients on a waiting list and meanwhile insisting on careful clinical check lest they slip into group III.

Group III. The risk in this group is rela-

* 5 *Circulation* 349, 360–361 (1952). Reprinted by permission of the American Heart Association, Inc.

tively low, below 10 per cent in this series, whereas the benefits are considerable. These patients are usually restored to comfortable, useful lives. This is because they get good, functional valvuloplasty before there is irreversible damage in the lung, myocardium and liver. In short, they are treated before they have slipped into group IV or die. These patients in group III *constitute the ideal and urgent candidates for surgery at this time* . . . .

Group IV. This, like group II, again represents a borderline group but in quite another way. These patients are suffering from a malignant disease. During the early phases of this study we preferred to take our surgical candidates from the group of dying patients. A control group demonstrates how group IV patients fared without surgical intervention. The control group constituted patients in group IV acceptable for surgery but who did not have it for various reasons, such as refusal of surgery on the part of the patient or the patient's family. There were 19 of these patients and 17 died within one year, 15 within six months. Thus, it becomes apparent that it is fair to call this a terminal or malignant phase. There were 39 patients in group IV who were operated on and 14 died from this intervention. Of course, these results are far better than those in the control group and if we were discussing carcinoma of the stomach or liver we would be delighted with such salvage rates. However, in this malignant phase the results are being improved.

* * *

b.
**Laurence B. Ellis, Dwight E. Harken, and
Harrison Black
A Clinical Study of 1,000 Consecutive Cases
of Mitral Stenosis Two to Nine Years
after Mitral Valvuloplasty***

The present study is a report of the clinical results in 1,000 consecutive cases with a preoperative diagnosis of predominant mitral stenosis on whom mitral valvuloplasty was performed between the years 1949 and March 1956. . . .

* * *

. . . Because of the very small number of group-II patients in this series these have been included with group-III patients in the subsequent analyses, and whenever the expression "group

* 19 *Circulation* 803–820 (1959). Reprinted by permission of the American Heart Association, Inc.

III" is used, it denotes group II and III patients. There was 1 operative death in the group-II patients. For the purpose of this analysis "operative mortality" denotes death during the operation or during the period of the hospitalization when the operation was performed. [913 patients survived the operation.]

*   *   *

In spite of the great number of studies that have been made over the years on the survival of patients with mitral stenosis it is extremely difficult to obtain data on medically treated patients that are comparable to this series. Many studies are statistically invalid or are made on groups that are not easily comparable, or consider only the survival period of those who ultimately were known to be dead. . . .

[T]he series most comparable to ours which has been medically treated and followed is that by Olesen, who studied a group of patients first observed between the years of 1933 and 1949 in Copenhagen. . . . We have therefore utilized his data to compare our group-III patients with his male and female patients in class 3. . . . [I]ncluding an operative mortality of 3 per cent, 83 per cent of our group-III patients have survived over the period of observation up to 7 years, and 71 per cent to 9 years, although the numbers dealt with in the last 2 years are small. This survival is better than for the medically treated patients. In group IV 57 per cent have survived up to 9 years, which include an operative mortality of 24 per cent for the group as a whole. This survival is vastly better than for the medically treated patients of whom none was alive at 8 years. . . .

*   *   *

Ninety-five patients have died since operation. . . . Eleven died of conditions clearly unrelated to their heart disease. Two of these, however, were patients in which death might be considered related to the operative procedure, including 1 death 2½ months following surgery from hepatitis, which might have been homologous serum jaundice acquired from a transfusion at the time of surgery, and 1 death from a reaction occurring during the course of an intercostal block for treatment of residual intercostal pain. There were 4 sudden deaths that have been assumed to be cardiac in origin. Patients developing cerebral vascular accidents, whether fatal or not, following surgery have been considered to have had these on the basis of emboli dislodged from the heart, though some of these may have been due to independent vascular disease of the brain. In the calculation of the survival curves all deaths have been included, whether or not they were of cardiac origin.

*   *   *

Sixty-nine per cent of group-II and III patients and 55 per cent of the group-IV patients have improved. . . .

*   *   *

Two hundred twenty-eight of the patients in this study have become worse after having been significantly improved, that is "markedly" or "moderately," for at least 1 year after valvuloplasty. For the sake of this analysis, the definition of "deterioration" is that they have slipped by at least 1 class, according to the American Heart Association classification. Sixty-two of these patients slipped only from "markedly" to "moderately" improved, and hence would still be classed in the "improved" category. The remaining 166 deteriorated from either being originally "markedly" or "moderately" improved into the "unimproved" classification; that is, they are now either only "slightly" improved, their condition is unchanged as compared to the preoperative state, they are worse, or dead. Of these patients, 48 have died since operation, and 45 have been reoperated on for mitral valvular disease. These patients were not all personally observed by the authors at the time of their deterioration; evidence for their deterioration was obtained in some from their answers to annual questionnaires or from letters from their physicians.

*   *   *

NOTES

NOTE 1.
ANDREW LOGAN, CLIFTON P. LOWTHER,
AND RICHARD W. D. TURNER
REOPERATION FOR MITRAL STENOSIS*

After successful mitral valvotomy, improvement may last for several years; but thereafter many patients deteriorate. Experience has now shown that re-stenosis is the most frequent cause of this deterioration. It is also the most important cause, being the only one for which essentially satisfactory treatment is available. As soon as

_____

* 1 *The Lancet* 443 (1962). Reprinted by permission.

stenosis is believed to be again severe, a second operation would be advised.

*   *   *

Of 500 consecutive patients with severe stenosis treated by mitral valvotomy in the past eleven years, 264 survivors have now been followed for more than five years and can reasonably be regarded as having been "at risk" for a second operation. Experience has shown that symptoms from re-stenosis rarely become evident in less than four years. 80 patients have now had a second valvotomy at which an important degree of re-stenosis was found, while the remaining 184 have not deteriorated in this way. . . .

*   *   *

Varying opinions on the incidence of re-stenosis have been reviewed by Wilcken. Doubtless these are related to differences in selection of cases, efficacy of operation, and duration of subsequent observation. Earlier in our experience we thought that re-stenosis of the mitral valve was infrequent, because after five years few patients had apparently deteriorated for this reason. Similar views were held by other observers.

Wilcken reported re-stenosis in 10 per cent of 73 selected patients considered to have had an adequate valvotomy. . . . Harken et al. (1961) repeated valvotomy in 80 of 1000 cases (8 per cent) within nine years of the first operation.

In the present series there have been 80 operations for re-stenosis among 264 patients followed for more than five years after the first operation—an incidence of 30 per cent. The rate has increased steadily from 5 per cent for patients followed for only five years to 70 per cent in the small group who have been followed for ten years, and it may be expected to increase further. . . .

*   *   *

NOTE 2.

LAURENCE B. ELLIS AND DWIGHT E. HARKEN
CLOSED VALVULOPLASTY FOR MITRAL
STENOSIS—A TWELVE-YEAR FOLLOW-UP
STUDY OF 1571 PATIENTS*

*   *   *

The question whether or not operation for patients with symptomatic mitral stenosis is

* 270 *New England Journal of Medicine* 643, 648–649 (1964). Reprinted by permission.

worthwhile has now become academic. It is now generally agreed that it is a very useful procedure. The questions that remain are how long lasting and how good the results are and what conditions lead to deterioration.

*   *   *

Is there any way that mitral surgery can be improved so that longer lasting results can be obtained? Those who advocate routine open surgery for mitral stenosis contend that adequate visualization of the valve permits more accurate and careful fracture of the commissures and relief of subvalvular stenosis as well as debridement of calcium and the correction of any insufficiency that may be present. If required, prosthetic devices of various types, including total valve replacement, can be employed. It has been claimed that the immediate postoperative results are better as far as both clinical and hemodynamic findings are concerned. Long-term results, however, are not yet available in sufficiently large numbers to have any significance. Some authors have also failed to indicate how severely disabled the patients have been before surgery. This is a critical factor in the assessment of the mortality and postoperative results of any type of surgery.

The arguments of the advocates of open surgery for mitral stenosis have obvious appeal. However, some surgeons experienced in various technics of mitral surgery believe that it may be more difficult to assess mitral incompetence, either that occurring before surgery or that produced by surgery, unless the heart is turgid and functioning. One must also bear in mind the possibility that more late complications will follow open cardiac surgery, particularly if a prosthetic device has been inserted, than have taken place after closed mitral valvuloplasty. The two major complications of this type are late embolization and late infection, particularly bacterial endocarditis. We have previously shown, and have emphasized earlier in this paper, that postoperative emboli are infrequent after closed mitral valvuloplasty. Moreover, to our knowledge, there has not been a single case of bacterial endocarditis that has occurred in any of our patients undergoing closed mitral valvuloplasty within four months, or a time span that would make it unlikely that the operation was a factor in initiating the infection.

*   *   *

D.

Appraising the Role of the Participants

Throughout this volume we have suggested that the analysis of the role of the participants in the human experimentation process will be facilitated by focusing separately on the different stages in this process at which the authority of the participants may vary to a significant degree. We have distinguished three such stages, and the materials in this section accordingly divide the appraisal of the participants' roles into three parts. First, we are concerned with the *formulation* of policies which encompasses, most generally, the establishment of guides for decision for the entire process and, more specifically, such policy decisions as the qualifications of subjects and investigators, the determination of societal interests and priorities, and the establishment of criteria for harm and disclosure. We then turn to the *administration* of research and explore such issues as the allocation of authority to conduct and supervise ongoing investigations as well as the means and organizational structure by which the participants should arrive at their decisions. Finally, we examine mechanisms for after-the-fact *review* of the consequences of particular investigations and the entire experimentation process through congressional hearings, scholarly analysis, press coverage, or actions initiated by the government, public interest groups, the subject, or the investigator himself.

Though the focus in this section is on the professions, the state, and the public, the materials also touch on the roles of the other participants so as to facilitate the construction of a comprehensive theory of decisionmaking about experimentation. The task of the student of human experimentation is to identify those decisions which most adequately promote and protect the interests and values that he deems important. Nevertheless, concern with the ultimate outcome should not diminish the attention given to the participants and methods of decisionmaking for a number of reasons. First, the content of any decision is largely dependent on the people and institutions who make it and the procedures they follow. Since all the issues which deserve resolution cannot be anticipated, achieving "good" decisions requires designing a system which employs the means and participants most likely to advance the interests one favors. Second, the choice of decisionmakers and methods is itself a value choice which can have a greater impact, for better or worse, on the interests of science, subject, and society than that of any particular decision. Finally, the focus on "who" and "how" highlights the need to examine decisionmaking from the vantage points of both those who are given authority and those who give the authority.

In studying these materials, consider the following questions in addition to those posed at the beginning of the chapter:

1. What purposes should professional or state regulation of the human experimentation process serve?

   a. At what stages in the process would regulation by the professions, state, or public be most effective in protecting, rather than undermining, the interests of investigators, subjects, science and society?

   b. What specific decisions in this process should be formulated, administered, and reviewed by the professions, state or public?

c. What specific decisions at each stage in this process should be left to the investigator and subject?

2. What alternatives to present regulations of the human experimentation process by the professions, state, or public are better suited to promote the interests of all the participants?

a. Should the goal of any regulation be to encourage maximal self-regulation by the profession with minimal state and public intervention? If so, how can this be accomplished while still providing adequate safeguards for all the participants?

b. Should the goal of any regulation be to encourage maximal self-regulation by the investigator and subject with minimal interaction by the professions, the state, and the public? If so, how can this be accomplished while still providing adequate safeguards for all the participants?

1.

In Formulating Policy

a.

Deciding about Societal Interests and Priorities?

[i]
United States Congress
Joint Resolution to Provide for a Study
and Evaluation of the Ethical, Social, and
Legal Implications of Advances in
Biomedical Research and Technology*

*   *   *

Resolved by the Senate and House of Representatives of the United States of America in Congress assembled, That . . . .

SEC. 2. There is hereby established a National Advisory Commission on Health Science and Society (hereinafter referred to as the "Commission").

SEC. 3. (a) The Commission shall be composed of fifteen members to be appointed by the President from the general public and from individuals in the fields of medicine, law, theology, biological science, physical science, social science, philosophy, humanities, health administration, government, and public affairs.

*   *   *

SEC. 4. (a) The Commission shall undertake a comprehensive investigation and study of the ethical, social, and legal implications of ad-

---

* Senate Joint Resolution 75, 92d Congress, 1st Session, introduced on March 24, 1971, and adopted by the Senate as amended on December 2, 1971, 117 *Congressional Record* S20089–S20093 (1971). It is presently before the Subcommittee on Public Health and Environment of the House Committee on Interstate and Foreign Commerce.

vances in biomedical research and technology, which shall include, without being limited to—

(1) analysis and evaluation of scientific and technological advances in the biomedical sciences, past, current and projected;

(2) analysis and evaluation of the implications of such advances, both for individuals and for society;

(3) analysis and evaluation of laws, codes, and principles governing the use of technology in medical practice;

(4) analysis and evaluation, through the use of seminars and public hearings and other appropriate means, of public understanding of and attitudes toward such implications;

(5) analysis and evaluation of implications for public policy of such findings as are made with respect to the biomedical advances and public attitudes.

(b) The Commission shall make maximum feasible use of related investigations and studies conducted by public and private agents.

(c) The Commission shall transmit to the President and to the Congress one or more interim reports and, not later than two years after the first meeting of the Commission, one final report, containing detailed statements of the findings and conclusions of the Commission, together with its recommendations, including such recommendations for action by public and private bodies and individuals as it deems advisable.

*   *   *

SEC. 7. For the purpose of carrying out this joint resolution, there are authorized to be appropriated such sums as may be necessary, but not to exceed $1,000,000 for each of the two years during which the Commission shall serve.

*   *   *

NOTES

NOTE 1.

SENATOR WALTER F. MONDALE
HEALTH SCIENCE AND SOCIETY*

* * *

MR. MONDALE: Mr. President, I introduce for myself and Senators Bayh, Brooke, Case, Fong, Harris, Hart, Hughes, Humphrey, Javits, Kennedy, McGee, McGovern, Moss, Nelson, Pell, Randolph, and Schweiker for appropriate reference a joint resolution to create a National Advisory Commission on Health Science and Society.

Recent advances in biology and medicine make it increasingly clear that we are rapidly acquiring greater powers to modify and perhaps control the capacities and activities of men by direct intervention into and manipulation of their bodies and minds. Certain means are already in use or at hand—for example, organ transplantation, prenatal diagnosis of genetic defects, electrical stimulation of the brain. Others await the solution of relatively minor technical problems, while still others depend upon further basic research. All of these developments raise profound and difficult questions of theory and practice, for individuals and for society.

* * *

[T]hree years ago I introduced a joint resolution which was essentially the same as the one I am introducing today. At that time, heart transplants were a startling new medical breakthrough. Since then, several hundred heart transplants have been performed. When I reintroduced the resolution in the last Congress, the first successful test-tube fertilization of a human egg had just been reported. Now, just 2 months ago, Nobel Prize winner Dr. James D. Watson told the House Committee on Science and Astronautics that we will soon see the day when a baby will be conceived in a test tube and placed in a woman who will bear the child. As you may recall, Dr. Watson's reported prediction was that when such an implantation is successfully made, "All hell will break loose."

These brief comments indicate that the need for a sober and thoughtful analysis and evaluation of biomedical advance is even more urgent

---

* 117 *Congressional Record* S3708–S3709 (March 24, 1971).

now than it was 3 years ago when I first proposed this commission.

* * *

While holding forth the promise of continued improvements in medicine's abilities to cure disease and alleviate suffering, [recent] developments also pose profound questions and troublesome problems. There are questions about who shall benefit from and who shall pay for the use of new technologies. Shall a person be denied life simply because he does not have enough money for an organ transplant?

There will be questions about the use and abuse of power. When and under what circumstances can organs be removed for transplanting? Who should decide how long a person is to be kept alive by the use of a machine? . . .

There will be questions about our duties to future generations and about the limits on what we can and can not do to the unborn. Is it ethical for a man and wife, each carrying a gene for a serious hereditary disease, to procreate, knowing that their children have a significant chance of acquiring the disease? Should the law enjoin certain marriages or require sterilization for such eugenic consideration? What rights do unborn children have to protect them in experiments involving genetic engineering or test-tube fertilization? . . .

We shall face questions concerning the desirable limits of the voluntary manipulations of our own bodies and minds. Some have expressed concern over the possible dehumanizing consequences of increasing the laboratory control over human procreation or of the increasing use and abuse of drugs which alter states of consciousness.

We shall face questions about the impact of biomedical technology on our social institutions. What will be the effect of genetic manipulation or laboratory-based reproduction on the human family? If laboratory fertilization can produce children for sterile couples, what will be the consequences for those orphaned or abandoned children who might otherwise have been adopted by these couples? What will be the effect on the generation gap of any further increases in longevity?

We shall face serious questions of law and legal institutions. What will the predicted newfangled modes of reproduction do to the laws of paternity and inheritance? What would happen to the concept of legal responsibility if certain genetic diseases were shown to predispose to anti-social or criminal behavior? What would be done to those individuals with such traits?

We should expect that some people will try to have certain particularly frightening technologies banned by statute. Should this be done? Could such prohibition be effective?

Finally, we as legislators will face problems of public policy. We shall need to be informed of coming developments, of the promises they hold forth and the problems they present, and of public attitudes in these matters. We shall need to decide what avenues of research hold out the most promise for human progress. And we shall need to help devise the means for preventing undesirable consequences.

*   *   *

[W]e can ill afford to wait until the crush of events forces us to make hasty and often ill-considered decisions. We cannot again allow events to pass us by. We face an increasing number of new and far-reaching technological possibilities, touching the very nature of man. We face the need for some wise, deliberate, and sober decisions. These questions are not going to go away or answer themselves. They will become progressively more difficult as time goes on. As Dr. Watson said in his testimony:

"If we do not think about the matter now, the possibility of our having a free choice will one day suddenly be gone."

It would be foolish to expect the Commission to provide answers to all the questions we face, but we can expect that it will provide help in making some of our difficult decisions. The findings and considered judgments of excellent minds with a wide range of experience and training will be invaluable to individuals who must struggle with the awesome responsibility of coping with these new technologies.

*   *   *

NOTE 2.
ABRAM CHAYES AND JOSEPH GOLDSTEIN
LETTER OF INVITATION FOR THE SALK
INSTITUTE COMMISSION ON BIOLOGY, ETHICS,
AND THE LAW—SEPTEMBER 24, 1970*

We wish to invite you to become a member of the Commission on Biology, Ethics, and the Law.

---

* Printed by permission of the authors.

Concurrent with educating ourselves about the state of knowledge and potential developments in the life sciences, with your help, we plan to concentrate upon two major but more general problems:

First, the development of a framework for judging the occasions and the desirable extent of official intervention by local, state, national, and international decision-making bodies concerning the use and implementation of new biological knowledge and technique; and

Second, the design of procedures and agencies of decision for continuous evaluation of the significance of developments in the life sciences.

As to the first, it appears that major decisions about the dissemination and use of new knowledge and new procedures in the biological sciences, some of them having fundamental implications for the future of the human race, are, with certain important exceptions, made by private individuals—researchers, doctors, patients—without significant public intervention or regulation. It further appears that the general "set" of the decision-making apparatus is predisposed toward these laissez-faire premises. The Commission will attempt to verify these general impressions and to ask how far these premises ought to prevail. In particular, it will examine the possibility of a more aggressively "interventionist" approach. The Commission recognizes that one major form of intervention is public support of research. Because many other groups are now studying the appropriate criteria for public funding of scientific work, we will not place major emphasis on this question. Thus the Commission, working in the context of a governmental role in funding research, will attempt to set forth guides for decisions about the implementation and use of new knowledge and techniques.

The search for these criteria leads to the second and perhaps major concern of the Commission. This is the design of agencies and processes for decisions at local, state, national, and international levels in the area of technological and scientific assessment which may determine the need, if any, and methods of socially controlling the implementation of new techniques and knowledge. One of us, in a memo prepared for the Life Sciences and Social Policy Panel of the National Research Council, briefly posed that problem in this way:

What institutions and procedures exist or need to be established at local, state, national, and/or international levels for the purposes of (*i*) *identifying* and (*ii*) *assessing* on a continuing basis major developments in science and technology as well as for the purposes of (*iii*) *recommending* and (*iv*) *implementing* opportunities for action or nonaction (governmental and private) which will maximize gains for and minimize harm to preferred human values and arrangements?

In making assessments and recommendations to what extent can and should second-, third-, and more remote-order consequences for these values and arrangements be consciously considered or consciously left to chance?

How can private and public decision-making institutions and procedures, to the extent existing ones are inadequate, be established?

*   *   *

[*ii*]
President's Commission on Heart Disease,
Cancer, and Stroke
A National Program to Conquer Heart
*Disease, Cancer, and Stroke**

The conquest of heart disease, cancer, and stroke requires the continuation and expansion of our highly productive medical research effort in the years ahead.

Today's successes in detection, treatment, and cure sprang from yesterday's research. But many problems related to these three diseases remain beyond our scientific capability. Of these, a large number appear to be just outside our grasp. We stand on the threshold of further advances.

To cross this threshold as soon as possible— to take advantage of the tremendous momentum built up by our biomedical research enterprises in the recent past—certain new elements should be added to our existing scientific resources. In addition, current procedures need to be strengthened or modified to assure ever-increasing productivity of new life-saving knowledge.

The national network of regional centers, each primarily oriented toward the solution of a specific disease problem, will generate and verify a tremendous amount of new information on heart disease, cancer, and stroke.

But there is also the need for a more general research attack on the fundamental problems of human biology, to which all the sciences basic to medicine can contribute. In addition there is need for highly specialized

----
* Washington, D.C.: U.S. Government Printing Office 47–52 (1964).

avenues of research related to heart disease, cancer, and stroke.

*   *   *

Recommendation 13. The Commission recommends the establishment of 25 non-categorical biomedical research institutes at qualified institutions throughout the country.

*   *   *

The Commission recognizes the importance and promise of non-categorical biomedical research. Indeed, such research is essential to basic understanding of heart disease, cancer, and stroke. Clues of great significance, coming from such endeavors, can be used effectively by research groups investigating specific disease problems.

For example, through such research, we can hope to attain the more detailed understanding of the living cell which may reveal the nature of the delicate change in the balance of cellular activities which manifests itself as cancer. Hopefully, also, there may be an unraveling of the next layer of understanding—the manner in which highly specialized cells such as those of the brain, kidney, or heart perform the specific functions which, uniquely, they contribute to the total living organism.

*   *   *

Recommendation 14. The Commission recommends the establishment of Specialized Research Centers for intensive study of specific aspects of heart disease, cancer and stroke to supplement the research and training efforts of the regional centers previously described.

Specifically, at least 10 such centers in heart disease, 10 in cancer, and 10 in stroke should be established in various health and medical research facilities throughout the country over a 5-year period.

In addition, it is recommended that three Bioengineering Centers and three Rehabilitation Biomedical Engineering Research Centers be established over a 5-year period in order to take advantage of the potential offered by bioengineering research in heart disease, cancer, and stroke.

*   *   *

Recommendation 15. The Commission endorses the existing system of review of research project grants by study sections and advisory councils at the National Institutes of Health and recommends intensified and expanded support of research in heart disease, cancer, and stroke.

Specifically it recommends:

That a total of $40 million be appropriated to the National Heart Institute, $40 million to the National Cancer Institute, $15 million to the National Institute of General Medical Sciences, and $10 million to the National Institute of Neurological Diseases and Blindness in a 3-year period over and above current appropriations to these institutes for research project grants.

*　　*　　*

That several important areas of research be given special emphasis because of the valuable contribution in the past and their high potential for the future. For example, epidemiological studies provide evidence which may lead to the identification of factors causing a specific disease or condition.

Of vital importance is the strong support of broad clinical field trials of drugs and other methods of treatment. As we have emphasized a number of times, there is a critical lag between the research discovery of new medication and the rapid evaluation of its effectiveness against a particular form of disease. We must wait too long while individual investigators report their limited findings in technical publications which print articles 12 to 18 months after their submission.

*　　*　　*

Recommendation 17. The Commission recommends that the existing General Research Support Grants Program of the National Institutes of Health be expanded as rapidly as possible to a level of 15 percent of the total NIH research and training budget and that the program be altered to increase its effectiveness.

Specifically, the Commission recommends:

That graduate schools engaged in biomedical research, supported by grants from NIH, should be permitted to receive grants under the general research support program; and

That general research support grants should be awarded in two categories: (1) unrestricted funds to be devoted to research, as at present, and awarded on a formula basis; and (2) negotiated awards, based on documented applications to defray the direct and indirect costs of the supporting organization and services provided by each institution to facilitate the conduct of research and which are not ordinarily chargeable as indirect costs.

*　　*　　*

NOTES

NOTE 1.

FRANCIS D. MOORE
THERAPEUTIC INNOVATION—ETHICAL
BOUNDARIES IN THE INITIAL CLINICAL TRIALS OF
NEW DRUGS AND SURGICAL PROCEDURES*

*　　*　　*

[W]e should mention the present crisis in laboratory finance in the biomedical sphere. While the 1968 cutback is considered by the Congress in terms of budget savings, and by the scientific public as one of the highly undesirable consequences of our military involvement in Southeast Asia, the sudden withdrawal of large amounts of federal support for biomedical research is going to have an inevitable ethical consequence: The necessary preliminary laboratory work is going to be severely curtailed in the instance of many forthcoming therapeutic innovations.

During the past ten years, the expense of conducting laboratory experimental work has doubled as a result of inflationary spirals in all the goods and services concerned. Prior to 1967, the National Institutes of Health budget increases had barely kept pace with laboratory inflation, but these had been sufficiently large so that other sources of laboratory support (such as certain philanthropic foundations and industry) had tended to withdraw from the field. With the withdrawal of laboratory financial support due to the congressional policy of pursuing military action in Southeast Asia, we are greeted with an almost unsupportable situation in biological research. An ironic example will illustrate. A certain young man of excellent medical background had just completed two years of service as a military surgeon in Vietnam. Here he had been handsomely supported in one of the largest and most wasteful of military encounters, and had worked himself without stint and without surcease to assist in the care of the wounded. Returning to civilian life, he was to become a Research Fellow in our laboratories to study the transplantation of the liver (liver transplant being a potential help to babies born with bile duct anomalies, to individuals with liver tumors, and to soldiers with severe bullet wounds of the liver). On returning to civilian life, he

---

* 98 *Daedalus* 502, 512–513 (1969). Reprinted by permission of Daedalus, Journal of the American Academy of Arts and Sciences, Boston, Massachusetts.

was told by the government that although his name had been accorded one of the highest places in the priority list for Senior Research Fellowships, funds were not available to support him. In the Sunday supplements that week, there was an account of new research being done to make a lunar module perform in a high vacuum simulating the surface of the moon, a research expending more money each month than has ever been spent on any aspect of tissue transplantation. It is clear, then, that ethical considerations in preliminary laboratory trial go to the roots of our society and to the question of what we regard as suitable priorities for human effort at this time.

*   *   *

NOTE 2.

PAUL FREUND
ETHICAL PROBLEMS IN HUMAN EXPERIMENTATION*

*   *   *

The law on the whole subject of experimentation will be worked out in close reliance on the moral sensibilities of the community. It therefore behooves the medical profession to take the public into its confidence and to educate public opinion rather than to risk the shock and explosion of pent-up revulsion if the lid is pressed down on information and then blown up by some melodramatic case like that of the hospital for chronic diseases. The primary step is to recognize that difficult moral problems—indeed, moral dilemmas—do exist on which help and guidance may be sought from many sources.

*   *   *

NOTE 3.

H. S. CONRAD
CLEARANCE OF QUESTIONNAIRES WITH RESPECT TO "INVASION OF PRIVACY," PUBLIC SENSITIVITIES, ETHICAL STANDARDS, ETC.†

*   *   *

. . . Who makes the rules by which acceptability is judged? Who interprets and applies the rules? What are the checks and balances, if any, in the whole process?

In the last analysis, I suppose that in a de-

---

* 273 *New England Journal of Medicine* 687, 691 (1965). Reprinted by permission.

† 22 *American Psychologist* 358–59 (1967). Reprinted by permission.

mocracy it is the people who ultimately make the rules. By "people" I do not, of course, mean any abstract, homogeneous mass; but rather such forces as, first, custom and generally accepted ethics; second, the pressures of organized, interested, active groups; and third, the influence of Government officials (both legislative and administrative), from Congress on down to the local school superintendent and principal. Beyond these there are the two key persons in any study involving data-gathering instruments: namely, first, the individual researcher, whose sense of discretion and professional ethics can generally be relied on to recognize desirable restraints; and second, the individual respondent, who can always frustrate an inquiry simply by withholding or falsifying his answers.

*   *   *

. . . To leave the decision entirely to the individual researcher himself, or to a group of his colleagues, would seem to us to violate seriously what some political scientists term *the principle of shared or countervailing force.* The researcher and his colleagues represent a party at interest—the scientific party: And there is good reason to believe that any party at interest is likely, more often than not, to give himself the "benefit of the doubt." Whether he does or not, the public generally *thinks* or *suspects* that he does. And in our democracy, both theoretically and pragmatically, the views of the public must be recognized as of paramount importance.

As we see it, the role of Government . . . is to serve as an honest broker between the scientist who presses for scientific freedom, and the public which, generally speaking, places considerably greater emphasis on the value of personal privacy.

*   *   *

. . . *The ultimate authority rests with the people,* and with the legislators and administrators who respond to the will of the people. In bluntest terms, the Federal appropriation of millions of dollars for research cannot be expected to continue and grow, unless scientists pay reasonable respect to the wishes of the people and their elected representatives. There doubtless are some exceptions to this rule for a field like engineering, or for certain segments of medicine; but the rule appears to hold true with special force for the behavioral sciences.

. . . *Social science must not become identi-*

fied in the public mind with "*snooping*" and "*prying*"—i.e., with the unwarranted invasion of privacy. To this end, professional discretion in the preparation and use of questionnaires is essential; and—in the case of Government-supported research—appropriate regulations, reasonably enforced, are required. Such regulations, in practice, generally have only minimal (if any) effect on the quality and productivity of research. In any event, social scientists cannot expect to operate free from societal restraints. With reasonable adaptation to normal restraints, an increase in both budgetary and public support for the social sciences may be anticipated, and the future of the social sciences should be bright.

NOTE 4.

R. J. V. PULVERTAFT
THE INDIVIDUAL AND THE GROUP IN MODERN MEDICINE*

*   *   *

I recall an occasion in the late war when a very limited amount of typhus vaccine was made available by the American manufacturers for civilian distribution during a typhus epidemic. My own view was that it should be given to armament workers and other men of importance in the prosecution of the war; my American colleague insisted that it should be distributed without regard to age, sex, race, or occupation. He won. . . .

*   *   *

b.
Deciding about the Ambit of Experimentation?

[i]
R. A. McCance
The Practice of Experimental Medicine†

*   *   *

Let us start with the word experiment, which most biologists use very loosely to cover any investigation, however trifling, made to advance knowledge. The term generally implies some deliberate change of conditions without foreknowledge of the results but with subsequent observation of them. It may be used, however, even when the conditions are not being deliberately changed, when the term observation

* 2 *The Lancet* 841 (1952). Reprinted by permission.
† 44 *Proceedings of the Royal Society of Medicine* 189–194 (1950). Reprinted by permission.

would be more correct. Many doctors would not regard the attempt to cure an individual patient as an experiment, yet it undoubtedly may be, if the results are observed and followed up, for the essence of treatment is to do something positive to a patient, i.e., alter his condition, in the hope that the effect will be of benefit to him.

People who are sick are often apprehensive. They long for reassurance which they do not find in the word "experiment." Worse still, the word may conjure up alarming possibilities in their minds. . . .

There is one fundamental difference between the investigator and the physician. A good investigator may be as full of bedside charm and therapeutic ability as a good physician, but he must primarily be interested in his problem. The physician is interested first, last, and all the time in his patients. . . .

Patients provide the problems, and disease may produce conditions which could never have been achieved experimentally and which demand detailed investigation, but if the illness is acute and treatable it is usually unjustifiable to withhold the remedy for long enough to make all the observations desirable in a satisfactory experiment. . . .

*   *   *

We should, I think, for present purposes, regard anything done to a patient, which is not generally accepted as being for his direct therapeutic benefit or as contributing to the diagnosis of his disease, as constituting an experiment, and falling, therefore, within the scope of the term experimental medicine. The definition, however, should not include all those unplanned experiments which are inseparable from the admission of any child or adult to a hospital, and which are often attended with considerable physical and psychological dangers, nor should it include the administration of established prophylactic remedies, even though some of them, particularly the attenuated viruses, may involve risk. The experiment visualized may be one of omission and consist of withholding treatment from a "control," or it may be one of commission and consist of making some test on a patient for which there is no obvious and immediate need. Whatever the problem interesting the investigator, however, it is, of course, true to say that the results of such tests must always help to characterize the diseased state and when known may sometimes be of benefit to the patient on whom the tests have been made. There is a case to be made out for regarding all these tests as being "investigations" conducted in the sufferer's best interests and therefore not constituting an experiment made solely for the advancement of knowledge. Wassermann reactions [blood test for syphilis] are carried out on every patient admitted to some hospitals and every patient entering the Mayo Clinic is, I believe, subjected to an elaborate series of investigations. The real distinction is a subtle one and may depend upon the mental approach of the man who makes the tests. Nevertheless, I regard collecting an extra specimen of urine or taking an extra 5 cc. of blood from a vein puncture, made purely for established diagnostic or therapeutic purposes, as falling within the range of the term "experiment"; I would certainly regard weighing a baby "unnecessarily" as an experiment. Some people may think I am taking up a ridiculous attitude over this, but if an experiment is not defined in this way, where is the line to be drawn?

All experiments involve some risk. It may be an infinitesimally small one, but it is always there—you, or the nurse, may drop the baby, for instance. If the experiment involves special vein punctures, or perhaps infusions, the risk is considerably enhanced, but it still remains immeasurably small in the hands of an experienced operator. Nevertheless, I have myself seen and experienced the most alarming effects from pyrogens and I think it quite likely that the virus which gave me a mild attack of jaundice in 1939 reached me through a syringe. In assessing the risks involved in any experiment and therefore the justification for doing it, there are many factors which require consideration. The skill and experience of the investigator are important ones, but so is the place where the experiment is to be performed. A procedure which would be perfectly safe in a well-equipped and well-staffed establishment might be quite unjustifiable somewhere else. . . .

*   *   *

If an experiment is the first of a series it involves much more risk than one which has been made many times before by the same people out of the same bottles. I never worry at all, however, about trying out an unknown substance on man, for with a little patience one can work up the dose on oneself or other normal people so gradually that the risk can be reduced to vanishing point, but I do not think I would ever have had the temerity to carry out the first hepatic biopsy or cardiac catheteriza-

tion. Our pioneer studies of renal function in newborn infants were made on babies which had been born with inoperable meningomyelocoeles. Hundreds of these experiments have now been made on normal newborn and on premature infants in other countries—yet I am still hesitating about doing so.

The risk involved in any experiment depends very much on whether the investigator knows that he will always retain control of the situation. An experiment on salt deficiency or dehydration can be pushed till the subject is showing severe effects, because the remedy is available all the time. To inoculate someone with icterogenic serum is a risk that I personally would never take, nor would I ever have cared to take it even before the risks were so well known, for once the inoculation had been made, I would have lost control. Everyone working experimentally with normal human subjects or with patients must remember not only his responsibility to the subject or patient but also his responsibility to the discipline of experimental medicine. One irresponsible experimenter can do great harm to medical science.

*   *   *

NOTES

NOTE 1.

WALTER MODELL
LET EACH NEW PATIENT BE A COMPLETE EXPERIENCE*

*   *   *

. . . If meticulous observers do not execute a disciplined experiment with a drug in a limited number of carefully chosen and well-controlled subjects, there will inevitably be an undisciplined natural experiment with it on a much larger uncontrolled group of indiscriminately chosen patients—conducted by much less critical observers—which will take much longer to tell its gory or (less likely) glorious tale. One needs only to recall that, not so very long ago, when lithium chloride was used as a salt substitute, it caused several hundred disasters and deaths simply because it was introduced into medical practice without appropriate consideration of existing experimental information and without appropriate clinical trial. In this instance, it was actually the practicing physicians

---

* 174 *Journal of the American Medical Association* 1717 (1960). Reprinted by permission.

who unwittingly conducted the critical pharmacologic experiments on man. The potential for disaster in these natural experiments on large sections of the population is far greater than when a new drug is used in a circumscribed and well-controlled scientific experiment. Every practitioner who would not consciously deprive his patient of effective medication will, therefore, have done so unconsciously a thousand times over in haphazard, dangerous, and wasteful trials on his own patients if he does not rest his therapy on carefully thought out private investigations as well as carefully disciplined clinical evaluations. Moreover, his unwitting "subjects" will have been unwittingly tested by him for their responses to new drugs with something less than the minimal requirements for experimentation in man. . . .

NOTE 2.

JAY KATZ
THE EDUCATION OF THE
PHYSICIAN-INVESTIGATOR*

*   *   *

Experimentation in the practice of medicine is as old as medicine itself. Hippocrates tells us that while treating a boy whose cortex was exposed, he not only picked out the spicules of bone embedded in the brain, but also "gently scratched the surface of the cortex with his fingernail" and observed convulsions on the opposite side of the body. Physicians throughout history have seized similar opportunities to combine therapy with the quest for knowledge. But only during the last hundred years, since the age of Pasteur, has medicine become more aware of the need for deliberate and well-planned experimentation; at the same time it has realized how difficult it is to separate the practice of medicine from experimentation. The oft-made distinction that the physician is primarily concerned with the patient qua patient and the investigator with the research is not a useful one for the majority of medical situations, for most investigations occur in the context of "clinical research combined with professional care." As A. C. Ivy points out, "the therapy of disease is, and will always be, an experimental aspect of medicine." Moreover, in terms of consequences to the patient

and subject, distinctions between therapy and research contribute little. Louis Lasagna has observed, for example, that "the patient is, paradoxically, often better served by the restraint observed in therapeutic approach by the critical experimentalist." What is new in medicine is not experimentation on man, but the realization that experiment and therapy have much in common and that knowledge can only be acquired by experimentation, ultimately only by experiment on man.

Thus the recent increased concern about the ethics of medical experimentation extends to the ethics of therapeutic care. Contributing to the reluctance to examine these issues is the conscious or unconscious realization that any resolution of the problems posed by human experimentation cannot be limited to research settings, but instead has far-reaching consequences for medical practice. . . .

*   *   *

[ii]
Carmichael v. Reitz
17 Cal. App. 3d 958, 95 Cal. Rptr. 381 (1971)

*   *   *

AISO, ASSOCIATE JUSTICE:

Plaintiff Vira Dee Mae Carmichael . . . brought this action for damages against defendants James Reitz, M.D., J. G. Dahlquist, M.D., the Harriman-Jones Medical Clinic, and G. D. Searle & Company, a corporation (hereinafter "Searle"), for pulmonary embolisms and thrombophlebitis allegedly caused by Dr. Reitz's having prescribed the drug Enovid, manufactured and marketed by Searle, in treating plaintiff for endometriosis.

*   *   *

The trial was completed as to Searle, and the jury returned a verdict in its favor. Plaintiff . . . appeals from the judgment entered on the verdict.

*   *   *

Plaintiff first sought the professional services of Dr. Reitz, a specialist in obstetrics and gynecology, on July 10, 1963. She complained that she was experiencing pain in conjugal sexual intercourse, that she had a "dropped uterus," and that she had been married for a period of two and one-half years without becoming preg-

* 98 *Daedalus* 480, 481–482 (1969). Reprinted by permission of Daedalus, Journal of the American Academy of Arts and Sciences, Boston, Massachusetts.

nant. She also informed Dr. Reitz that she was having "a great deal of pain with her menstrual periods" and "had been passing formed blood clots" during these periods. . . .

During this visit, Dr. Reitz conducted a physical examination which, in addition to the pelvic area, encompassed the chest, head, neck, abdomen, rectum, and extremities. Percussion and auscultation examinations of the chest indicated no abnormality and no chest problems as of that time. An X-ray of the chest was also taken; it proved negative for abnormalities. . . .

Dr. Reitz diagnosed a minimal case of endometriosis. He recommended that plaintiff attempt to become pregnant and prescribed Cyclex, a combination diuretic and tranquilizer, for the abdominal bloating and personality changes (premenstrual tension) of which plaintiff complained. He advised her to return in a year. . . .

Plaintiff returned to Dr. Reitz's office on May 12, 1964. The doctor noted on this occasion that there had been no progression in her symptoms; in fact, they were slightly more favorable despite her having been unable to become pregnant since her July 10, 1963, visit. Plaintiff stated that she was desirous of becoming pregnant. . . . She informed the doctor that she had been suffering from "flu" for a few weeks prior to her visit.

On this May, 12, 1964, occasion plaintiff was not given a complete physical examination. Dr. Reitz examined her chest by percussion and auscultation; the indications were that it was then clear. No X-ray was taken as less than a year had elapsed since his taking of the X-ray in July 1963. Plaintiff stated that she was being seen elsewhere for her chest problem. Dr. Reitz relied upon the physician treating her for her "flu" to take X-rays if that doctor should feel it necessary. He also believed that X-rays had been taken in that other doctor's office. Plaintiff did not complain of any present chest pain on this second examination. On the basis of the July 10, 1963, chest X-ray and his current physical examination of the chest area, Dr. Reitz at that time ruled out any pulmonary embolisms up to that time. Consequently, he did not inquire further about any chest pains.

*   *   *

Dr. Reitz decided to prescribe Enovid, which he considered the drug of choice, for . . . treating the endometriosis (including pre-menstrual tension syndrome); treating the heavy ("characterized by the passage of clotted blood") and painful menstrual flow (dysmenorrhea); and assisting in achieving pregnancy.

Dr. Reitz testified that he advised plaintiff of the risks and hazards of breakthrough bleeding, nausea, and vomiting in taking Enovid, and instructed her that if she had problems with the medicine to contact him. Plaintiff testified that Dr. Reitz discussed endometriosis with her; that it caused blood cysts; that he informed her that in some instances Enovid might be helpful in treating endometriosis and that a purpose for prescribing Enovid was to treat the endometriosis.

Prior to his prescribing Enovid for plaintiff, Dr. Reitz knew of a statistical relationship between thromboembolic episodes and Enovid, but he did not believe that there was a causal relationship between the two. The *Physicians' Desk Reference* for the 1964 (copyrighted in 1963), which he used, indicated that no contraindications were known. . . .

The prescription was filled at a pharmacy on May 14, 1964. The directions on the label were: "One tablet daily for 14 days then one tablet 2 times a day." Plaintiff waited until May 25, 1964, before she started taking the pills. . . . By Friday, June 5, 1964, she was spitting up blood and experiencing chest pains and shortness of breath. . . .

Plaintiff was examined by Dr. Reitz on Monday, June 8, 1964, and was instructed to continue with the antibiotic as prescribed by Dr. Horvitch. Her pain continued to get worse, so she went to the clinic on Tuesday as soon as it opened. Dr. Reitz examined her again and then turned her over to Dr. Joseph G. Dahlquist (originally a codefendant, a partner of Dr. Reitz in the Harriman-Jones Medical Clinic, and a specialist in internal medicine) for further treatment. Dr. Dahlquist had plaintiff immediately hospitalized in the Long Beach Community Hospital. He took a detailed history from plaintiff at the time of her admission to the hospital on June 9, 1964. His diagnosis, as of this date, was pneumonia with possible pulmonary embolism originating from a pelvic thrombophlebitis.

On June 10, 1964, Dr. Dahlquist inquired into plaintiff's chemical exposure and learned that she had taken Enovid as prescribed by Dr. Reitz. He then made a notation of the "possibility of Enovid-induced embolism." Due to Dr. Dahlquist's absence from the city for the next four days, plaintiff was cared for during Dr. Dahlquist's absence by Dr. Martin, Dr. Dahlquist's associate and also a board-certified internal medicine specialist. Dr. Martin recorded on Thursday, June 11, 1964, that he had no doubt but that plaintiff had suffered a pulmonary embolism. Dr. Martin contacted Dr. Dahlquist by telephone just as soon as the latter returned . . . around 4 P.M. on Sunday, June 14, 1964, and informed Dr. Dahlquist that a venogram disclosed large clots in the inferior vena cava, and that "they" felt that immediate surgery to tie off the inferior vena cava should be performed to prevent further possibly massive and fatal pulmonary embolism. Following consent to the operation, a plication of the inferior vena cava was performed that day by Dr. Gaspar, a surgeon, who was "already scrubbing" when Dr. Dahlquist returned.

A D & T (diagnostic and therapeutic) conference was held at the Harriman-Jones Clinic following the operation. Prior to the conference, a more detailed history of the plaintiff was obtained. What plaintiff had characterized as "flu" consisted of "generalized chest pain and symptoms of coryza" (common cold). There were also revealed episodes in 1961 and 1963 wherein plaintiff had experienced a sudden onset of pain in the right chest with low-grade fever, along with coughing of blood in 1963. Dr. Dahlquist testified that these symptoms were consistent with thromboembolism; that low-grade fever would generally cause a doctor to suspect thromboembolism.

*   *   *

The plication of plaintiff's vena cava inferior performed on June 14, 1964, by Dr. Gaspar was successful. Postoperatively, plaintiff was placed on Coumadin, an anticoagulant drug, by Dr. Dahlquist, who further instructed plaintiff to wear elastic stockings. She remained under Dr. Dahlquist's care, notwithstanding the fact that she had named him as a defendant in this action filed on May 3, 1965. When Dr. Dahlquist saw her on March 1, 1966, plaintiff had made an excellent recovery from her 1964 problems. She was not on any anticoagulant, and was not wearing elastic stockings. He was informed by plaintiff that she was able to walk, hike, swim, and engage in similar activities, which he had encouraged her to undertake. He had interdicted only heavy lifting and the like. She had no varicose veins at that time. She was working full time.

On May 13, 1967, plaintiff suffered a thrombophlebitis of the right calf. She had ingested Enovid just prior to her admission to the Long Beach Community Hospital on June 10, 1964. It was almost one year after plaintiff had been completely taken off of anticoagulant therapy in July 1966. Plaintiff returned to Dr. Dahlquist for treatment; he again placed her upon Coumadin and a tranquilizer to minimize the risk of another pulmonary embolism.

While still under Dr. Dahlquist's treatment, plaintiff was referred by her attorneys in this action to Dr. Arthur Samuels for the purposes of his conducting a clinical experimental study on plaintiff involving the use of Enovid. He testified that because the May 13, 1967, thrombophlebitis was "spontaneous," there was some question as to its cause. One purpose of the study was to either prove or disprove a causal relationship between Enovid and plaintiff's thrombophlebitis and pulmonary embolism. He also knew that another purpose of the experiment was to enhance plaintiff's position in this action.

July 11, 1967. Dr. Samuels saw plaintiff for the first time. He took a detailed (some ten pages) history from her, but he, like Dr. Reitz, did not pick up plaintiff's chest ailments of 1961 and 1963 other than as "flu" and accepted that to be true. A large blood specimen was taken for laboratory test purposes. On this date, Mr. Wolfe, plaintiff's associate counsel who had referred plaintiff to Dr. Samuels, advised the latter to keep this hematological consultation private and to refrain from contacting Dr. Dahlquist until further notice from Mr. Wolfe.

July 12, 1967. Dr. Samuels examined plaintiff physically. Although he found a rather prominent pulmonary sound (P–2), an indication that something might be wrong with her pulmonary circulatory system, he concluded that plaintiff was "medically asymptomatic and in a reasonable state of clinical equilibrium while taking her daily anticoagulant and tranquilizer therapy."

July 18, 1967. Actual studies were commenced. Another blood specimen was taken and laboratory tests thereon performed. Plaintiff told Dr. Samuels that she was experiencing pain in the lower right side of her chest. At this time, Dr. Samuels attributed these pains to anxiety-imagination. In retrospect, Dr. Samuels diagnosed these complaints as indicative of "thrombi and emboli possibly to lung for two weeks prior to discontinuation of Coumadin," and that plaintiff had "presence of pulmonary emboli" on July 18.

July 24, 1967. Plaintiff stopped taking Coumadin upon Dr. Samuels' direction. Mr. Wolfe instructed Dr. Samuels that he would now be permitted to contact plaintiff's personal physician.

July 25, 1967. Although good clinical practice called for tapering off when taking a patient off of an anticoagulant Dr. Samuels in this instance suddenly stopped plaintiff's ingestion of Coumadin. He was aware of the hazard that thrombophlebitis could result from the "rebound" or "overshoot" reaction from suddenly stopping the taking of Coumadin. But he had advised plaintiff of this hazard as well as the hazard of having plaintiff take Enovid. In fact, this study on plaintiff was "a very hazardous life-threatening study." He testified that he informed both plaintiff and her husband of the risks involved. And according to him, plaintiff realized that to get her answers to her problems, "she might have to further submit herself to further hazards." Dr. Samuels had plaintiff execute a so-called written informed consent form on this date (July 25, 1967), which was witnessed by Dr. Samuels' office manager. Dr. Samuels phoned the Harriman-Jones Clinic on this date, but was informed that Dr. Dahlquist was out of town and would not be back for two weeks from the time he had left.

July 27, 1967. Plaintiff was still having pain in her mid-epigastrium and her lower chest.

July 28, 1967. Dr. Samuels noted an acceleration of blood clotting time in plaintiff after the discontinuance of the anticoagulant and tranquilizer. He also wrote a letter informing Dr. Dahlquist that he had "recommended" discontinuance of the anticoagulant therapy. He did not tell Dr. Dahlquist that it had in fact been discontinued, and that it had been discontinued abruptly. (Dr. Dahlquist testified that when he first heard of the sudden termination of the anticoagulant, his reaction was, "Oh, my God!") Dr. Samuels did not inform Dr. Dahlquist that one purpose of the study was to enhance plaintiff's position in this lawsuit against him. He did not inform Dr. Dahlquist of his intention of using Enovid in the study.

August 2, 1967. Dr. Samuels first talked to Dr. Dahlquist over the telephone.

August 3, 1967. Plaintiff was given one 10-milligram tablet of Enovid out of the 1964 container. No chemical assay of the tablets was made. Plaintiff also took one tablet daily on August 4, 5, 6, 7, 8, 9, 10, and 11, 1967.

August 7, 1967. Dr. Samuels noted the plaintiff reported to him as feeling nauseous and having abdominal pain. She was afraid. The pain did not resemble the pain of 1964, although the nausea did.

August 8, 1967. Dr. Samuels noted: patient reports symptoms of discomfort in the right calf. "Telephone conversation from Mr. Carmichael. Upset about lack of definiteness of effect of Enovid—patient not experiencing same effects—patient upset about not experiencing same effects—as two years ago and not producing results."

August 9, 1967. Dr. Samuels held a conference with Mr. Carmichael and Mr. Wolfe as to whether clinical study should be continued. Apparently, it was decided that it should be. Communication of the decision to plaintiff was left up to Mr. Carmichael.

August 10, 1967. Dr. Samuels noted: "Discomfort in right side of chest, particularly on deep breathing, particularly in back. Coughed up spot of blood in A.M. once. Tenderness in right calf." He testified that there was a Homan's sign, definitely showing thrombophlebitis and recurrent pulmonary emboli. He gave plaintiff the choice of taking or not taking the Enovid pill that day. Plaintiff chose to go ahead. She told him: "I am not getting the same reaction at all as before although I have a lot more fear."

August 11, 1967. Plaintiff took another Enovid pill. At this time Dr. Samuels had a thorough discussion with plaintiff; he warned her of the hazards of further continuing with the studies. At the same time he informed her that there were now good theoretical grounds on which "to expect that she might now demonstrate maximum sensitivity to Enovid." On this date she had thrombophlebitis in both legs. Plaintiff was re-started on her anticoagulant and tranquilizer therapy. She was given a maximum dose (4 tablets; 20 milligrams) of Coumadin and instructed to thereafter take 2 tablets (total of 10 milligrams) daily. Plaintiff turned out, however, to be "particularly resistant to anticoagulant therapy" so she was given 4 tablets for 3 days and 3 tablets per day for the balance of the week. She was given as much as 25 milligrams on one occasion. Dr. Samuels instructed her to return to Dr. Dahlquist on August 12 and then report back to him the following Monday.

In the meantime, diagnosis of endometriosis had been confirmed at the UCLA Medical Center. Dr. Samuels agreed that Enovid is a treatment for endometriosis.

August 17, 1967. Dr. Samuels received confirmation from Dr. Dan Simmons, a pulmonary expert, that Dr. Simmons' studies (which included a lung scan on August 17, 1967) were partially complete. The lung scan indicated "a far advanced degree of pulmonary disease particularly on the right, including lower base."

Plaintiff required a "ligation" operation as a result of her 1967 pulmonary embolisms, in which her inferior vena cava was entirely tied off. Dr. Samuels testified: "Very unexpectedly Mrs. Carmichael suffered a minimum of symptoms right after surgery, of which we were terribly delighted, and since that time has done extremely well." At the time she was examined by Dr. Joseph Boyle, an internist, on behalf of defendant Searle in 1969; plaintiff was working. He opined that plaintiff should be able to carry on life "in a completely normal fashion without any difficulty."

The question, whether Enovid caused plaintiff's thrombophlebitis and pulmonary embolism in 1964 or whether it was due to her idiosyncratic hypersensitivity resulting from her endometriosis and abnormal blood clotting time, was hotly disputed. On direct examination, Dr. Samuels stated: "I believe that Mrs. Carmichael was *uniquely sensitive* to Enovid and sustained an adverse effect on her blood-clotting mechanism as a result of that ingestion," which would make Enovid medically defective in her case. (Emphasis added.) On cross-examination he stated that he thought plaintiff's endometriosis was a substantial factor in causing her thromboembolism. The blood factor changes induced by taking Enovid would have no clinically significant effect on normal women. On redirect examination, however, he believed that Enovid rather than the endometriosis was the causative factor producing the 1964 pulmonary embolism. A biochemist, Laurence Pilgeram, Ph.D., and Dr. John D. Wilson, a board-certified general surgeon, testified in support of the theory that Enovid was the cause.

On behalf of Searle, Dr. Robert W. Kistner, board-certified in obstetrics and gynecology, testified that there was no cause-and-effect relationship between Enovid and intravascular clotting, thromboembolism, or pulmonary embolism. He did not think the studies introduced into evidence established any definitive causal relationship. The pulmonary embolism in this case was not due to the ingestion of Enovid; the two events were coincidental. Dr. Joseph Boyle, an internist specializing in heart and lung disease, testified that plaintiff's pulmonary embolism in 1964 was caused by a chronic pelvic thrombophlebitis which had existed over a period of years. He noted the possibility of endometriosis itself having caused the thrombophlebitis in this case. The sudden discontinuance of Coumadin in the course of Dr. Samuels' clinical experimental study aggravated the plaintiff's problems due to her 1967 right calf thrombophlebitis episode. Dr. Herbert S. Sise, an internist specializing in cardiology and thrombosis, had no opinion as to the cause of the 1964 thromboembolism. His own studies performed in 1964 disclosed no really significant changes in the blood of women who took Enovid. He criticized Dr. Samuels' study as inadequate for lack of proper control data. Gerard Lanchantin, Ph.D., a biochemist, testified showing wherein biochemist Pilgeram's study was inadequate.

*   *   *

Plaintiff complains of the giving of the instruction which stated that Searle had the burden of proving that plaintiff and Dr. Samuels were aware of any dangers in the use of Enovid by plaintiff in August 1967 and that they "nevertheless proceeded to make use of Enovid despite such knowledge." She strenuously argues that the concept of assumption of risk properly belongs to a negligence theory of recovery and has no place in strict liability, detailing the requirements for invoking "assumption of risk" in negligence cases. We have already seen that a special type of "contributory negligence" or "assumption of risk" has its place as a defense to a claim of strict liability. . . . If a user or a consumer discovers a defect in the article and is aware of the dangers of such defect, but nevertheless proceeds to unreasonably make use of the product and suffers injury by it, he may not recover.

Here, plaintiff was seeking damages not only for the pulmonary episode of June 1964, but also for episodes following the experimental studies Dr. Samuels conducted on plaintiff by having her ingest Enovid for nine days in August 1967, at a time when he knew that plaintiff had previously suffered thrombophlebitis, when he had the benefit of her previous history, when the extent of available medical literature was much more extensive than in 1964, and when the need for prescribing Enovid, by his own admission, was not overwhelming. Consequently, this contention of error lacks merit.

*   *   *

c.

Deciding about Harm?

[i]

*Ninety-first Congress, Second Session
Comprehensive Drug Abuse Prevention and
Control Act of 1970**

SEC. 101. The Congress makes the following findings and declarations:

(1) Many of the drugs included within this title have a useful and legitimate medical purpose and are necessary to maintain the health and general welfare of the American people.

(2) The illegal importation, manufacture, distribution, and possession and improper use of controlled substances have a substantial and detrimental effect on the health and general welfare of the American people.

*   *   *

SEC. 502. (a) The Attorney General is authorized to carry out educational and research programs directly related to enforcement of the laws under his jurisdiction concerning drugs or other substances which are or may be subject to control under this title. Such programs may include—

(1) educational and training programs on drug abuse and controlled substances law enforcement for local, State, and Federal personnel;

(2) studies or special projects designed to compare the deterrent effects of various enforcement strategies on drug use and abuse;

(3) studies or special projects designed to assess and detect accurately the presence in the human body of drugs or other substances which are or may be subject to control under this title, including the development of rapid field identification methods which would enable agents to detect microquantities of such drugs or other substances;

(4) studies or special projects designed to evaluate the nature and sources of the supply of illegal drugs throughout the country;

(5) studies or special projects to develop more effective methods to prevent diversion of controlled substances into illegal channels; and

(6) studies or special projects to develop information necessary to carry out his functions under section 201 of this title.

(b) The Attorney General may enter into contracts for such educational and research activities without performance bonds and without regard to section 3709 of the Revised Statutes (41 U.S.C. 5).

(c) The Attorney General may authorize persons engaged in research to withhold the names and other identifying characteristics of persons who are the subjects of such research. Persons who obtain this authorization may not be compelled in any Federal, State, or local civil, criminal, administrative, legislative, or other proceeding to identify the subjects of research for which such authorization was obtained.

(d) The Attorney General, on his own motion or at the request of the Secretary, may authorize the possession, distribution, and dispensing of controlled substances by persons engaged in research. Persons who obtain this authorization shall be exempt from State or Federal prosecution for possession, distribution, and dispensing of controlled substances to the extent authorized by the Attorney General.

*   *   *

SEC. 601. (a) There is established a commission to be known as the Commission on Marihuana and Drug Abuse (hereafter in this section referred to as the "Commission"). The Commission shall be composed of—

(1) two members of the Senate appointed by the President of the Senate;

(2) two members of the House of Representatives appointed by the Speaker of the House of Representatives; and

(3) nine members appointed by the President of the United States.

*   *   *

(d) (1) The Commission shall conduct a study of marihuana including, but not limited to, the following areas:

(A) the extent of use of marihuana in the United States to include its various sources, the number of users, number of arrests, number of convictions, amount of marihuana seized, type of user, nature of use;

(B) an evaluation of the efficacy of existing marihuana laws;

(C) a study of the pharmacology of

---

* Act of October 27, 1970, Pub. Law No. 91–513, 84 Stat. 1271, 1280–1281.

marihuana and its immediate and long-term effects, both physiological and psychological;

　　(D) the relationship of marihuana use to aggressive behavior and crime;

　　(E) the relationship between marihuana and the use of other drugs; and

　　(F) the international control of marihuana.

(2) Within one year after the date on which funds first become available to carry out this section, the Commission shall submit to the President and the Congress a comprehensive report on its study and investigation under this subsection which shall include its recommendations and such proposals for legislation and administrative action as may be necessary to carry out its recommendations.

(e) The Commission shall conduct a comprehensive study and investigation of the causes of drug abuse and their relative significance. The Commission shall submit to the President and the Congress such interim reports as it deems advisable and shall within two years after the date on which funds first become available to carry out this section submit to the President and the Congress a final report which shall contain a detailed statement of its findings and conclusions and also such recommendations for legislation and administrative actions as it deems appropriate. The Commission shall cease to exist sixty days after the final report is submitted under this subsection.

(f) Total expenditures of the Commission shall not exceed $1,000,000.

　　　　*　　*　　*

NOTES

NOTE 1.

JONATHAN O. COLE
DANGERS IN THE DRUG-ABUSE BILL*

My review of the version of the Administration's drug-abuse bill which has come out of the Senate leads me to believe that the section dealing with penalties is a modest improvement over the bill originally filed by Senator Dirksen and a substantial improvement over existing statutes governing opiates and marijuana.

The regulatory sections which would affect scientists doing research on dangerous drugs

---

* 4 *Hospital Tribune* 1, 9 (February 23, 1970). Reprinted by courtesy of *Hospital Tribune*.

are, unfortunately, very vague and leave a great deal to the Attorney General and the Department of Justice in determining how research work with these drugs will be encouraged, regulated, or hindered. The very vagueness—it is not even clear how a Ph.D. scientist doing work with these drugs would be licensed or registered and how he would obtain the drugs—makes it possible to take either an optimistic or a pessimistic view of the bill's effect on research on drugs liable to abuse.

An *optimist* who assumes there will always be a benign and science-oriented Attorney General and a sensitive, flexible, research-oriented staff of the Bureau of Narcotics and Dangerous Drugs would paint the following picture:

Two excellent sections in the bill give the Attorney General the right to assure investigators full confidentiality for their research data involving human subjects and permit him to enable investigators to do research with controlled drugs even in states where law might prevent this. The provisions would enable the Attorney General to improve substantially the status of both sociologic and pharmacologic research on drugs of abuse. The staff of the Department of Justice could ensure that all investigators were registered to use appropriate drugs for research rapidly and with a minimum of red tape and could ensure that adequate quantities of drugs not currently used for medical purposes were made available for research. Given an adequate budget, the bill would even permit the Department of Justice to support a good deal of research on drugs of abuse under the contract mechanism.

A *pessimist* would paint the following picture:

The Department of Justice, which has absorbed the Bureau of Narcotics (*not* widely known for its permissiveness in the research area), could essentially stifle research in drugs of abuse by denying registration to qualified investigators on the grounds that their research was not in the public interest.

The public interest is so broadly defined as to make almost anyone's research capable of being suppressed. The Attorney General can suppress all research with drugs such as heroin, marijuana, and LSD by simply preventing their manufacture or preparation. He designates the amounts of such drugs which can be made; the amount can, obviously, be zero. Such projects as were allowed to proceed could be harassed by frequent inspections of all records. The Attorney

General would even have the right, with a court's acquiescence, to break and enter the investigator's premises to make sure that no drugs were being diverted illicitly. All in all, the bill provides power by which most research could be brought to a screeching halt.

Unenthusiastic administration of mildly restrictive regulations could in itself discourage a good many investigators from working in this area. Further, the red tape and bureaucratic harassment could extend to drugs such as the amphetamines and minor tranquilizers not currently covered in any such restrictive manner under existing laws.

In short, the bill has potentialities for both considerable good and great harm to research. This makes me very apprehensive. I would like to see it rewritten in such a way that an unbiased group of nongovernmental scientists selected in a manner outside the control of the Department of Justice had the major say in all matters dealing with research on these drugs. Such controls would be best set up under the Department of Health, Education, and Welfare, an agency likely to be more responsive to the needs of the medical and scientific community than the Department of Justice. I would also like to see the section giving the Attorney General the power to support contract research in the area of drug abuse more tightly written, so that only research directly applicable to his enforcement mission was authorized. I would also like to see built into that part of the law a provision that outside scientific review groups be used in screening such contract proposals in a manner similar to that currently employed at the National Institutes of Health.

*   *   *

... I view with real alarm the vesting in the Department of Justice of such major power over medical research and medical practice. I know of no evidence that either area is responsible for more than an infinitesimal fraction of the current drug-abuse problem. An enforcement mission focused on major illicit sales of really dangerous drugs seems to me to be the legitimate mission of a Department of Justice. Medical and research issues belong in the Department of Health, Education, and Welfare. The major need for much more research on drug abuse makes it necessary that research with drugs of abuse not be discouraged by bureaucratic systems.

NOTE 2.

DANIEL X. FREEDMAN
THE COST OF SILENCE NOW*

In December, 1968, the American Psychiatric Association publicly warned of dangers lurking in the early drafts of the Administration's drug-abuse control bill. That statement urged increased support to provide skills and programs to combat epidemics of drug abuse and stated that the separation of needed enforcement measures from health-related research and education was imperative.

The statement also noted that research and education conducted under the direction of the Bureau of Narcotics and Dangerous Drugs would not be likely to compel confidence or belief. Education and *not* propaganda, facts and *not* distortions, are the powerful and credible means of assessing the dangers of drugs and dealing with the anguish and confusion of parents and youth.

What provoked the 1968 statement? It was not the commendable effort of the Narcotics Bureau to coordinate drug law enforcement. It was, I think, the bureaucratic impulse to extend the stranglehold of former Commissioner Anslinger on "narcotics" to many other drugs—an approach of wielding vague threat and legal authority—which for 40 years stifled and distorted research, information, and innovative medical treatment.

What began in the summer of 1968 as an attempt of Justice Department agents to merely codify complex drug regulations has—after a year and a half—revealed a history of bureaucratic intransigence if not slyness. In the process the BNDD has documented its contempt for relevant advice and expertise while endowing itself with sweeping powers.

These new powers are not simply the authority to prosecute drug abusers and traffickers. Rather, there is *new* power to initially and finally decide—to judge—with respect to a wide range of commonly used and therapeutically valuable drugs: (1) acceptable medical practice; (2) acceptable medical research; (3) who is competent to conduct this. The essential new power is to adjudicate the abuse potential and medical usefulness not only of old but of newly discovered substances and the conditions under which they may be used—not only in everyday medical

* 4 *Hospital Tribune* 7 (March 9, 1970). Reprinted by courtesy of *Hospital Tribune*.

practice, but for any conceivable kind of scientific investigation.

*   *   *

The unwritten tale of the consequences of the Administration bill should be heard. If passed, it *will* be! The fact that 35 per cent or more of legal prescriptions are for the drugs covered in this bill indicates the extent to which legitimate medical practice is covered. With the vague wording and legal twists and turns in the bill, potential dangers do indeed exist. The fact that a patient's confidential records can be available for inspection, even though his pill may be a mild tranquilizer or sedative, should alert all patients and physicians. The bathroom cabinet as well as the street are in the scenario in which we can see future action!

*   *   *

What is tragic, then, is that apparently a large segment of the practice of medicine and the advancement of badly needed knowledge is being politicized. In fact, we should strive to keep matters of public health in sane focus, to use the best instruments with which Western civilization has endowed us to arrive at informal decisions.

Health professionals, pharmaceutical specialists, and experts in drug-abuse education should have been brought together with experts in governmental administration, regulatory practices, and law enforcement to review the entire complex issue of the manufacture and distribution of medicinals and the appropriate measures to combat illicit diversion and criminal use. It is clear that this will eventually have to be done— perhaps by the National Academy of Sciences.

*   *   *

[ii]
United Nations
Draft Covenant on Civil and Political Rights*

*   *   *

3. Article 7 of the draft Covenant on Civil and Political Rights, as submitted by the Commission on Human Rights reads as follows:

No one shall be subjected to torture or to cruel, inhuman or degrading treatment or punishment. In particular, no one

---

* Report of the Third Committee, Doc. A/4045.
13 *United Nations General Assembly Official Records*, Annexes, Agenda Item No. 32 (1958).

shall be subjected without his free consent to medical or scientific experimentation involving risk, where such is not required by his state of physical or mental health.

*   *   *

Amendments Submitted

*   *   *

6. The amendment of the Netherlands called for the deletion of the words: "involving risk, where such is not required by his state of physical or mental health" from the second sentence.

7. The amendment of Pakistan consisted in replacing the full stop after the words "treatment or punishment" by a comma and in replacing the words "In particular, no one shall be" by the words "or even." At the 854th meeting, the representative of Pakistan withdrew the amendment.

8. The Philippine amendment called for the insertion of the word "unusual" between the words "inhuman" and "or degrading" in the first sentence. The representative of the Philippines withdrew this amendment at the 853rd meeting.

9. The Ecuadorian amendment consisted in the deletion of the words "involving risk" from the second sentence. The representative of Ecuador withdrew this amendment at the 853rd meeting, on the understanding that a separate vote would be taken on the words "involving risk" in the Netherlands amendment.

10. The amendments of Guatemala called for:

(1) The amendment of article 7 to read as follows:

No person shall be subjected to torture or to cruel, inhuman or degrading treatment or punishment.

(2) The insertion of an additional article reading as follows:

Article 8. No person shall be subjected without his free and spontaneous consent to medical or scientific experimentation. Medical experimentation shall not be permitted in the case of a person who is incapable of giving his free and spontaneous consent, unless the main and essential purpose of the experimentation is the restoration of the physical and mental health of the said person and in that case the consent shall be obtained from those persons who in accordance with the law of the country concerned are the legal representatives of the person who is incapacitated from giving his consent.

The subsequent articles were to be renumbered accordingly.

At the 853rd meeting, the representative of Guatemala withdrew these amendments.

11. The Australian amendment called for the replacement of the full stop after the word "punishment" by a comma and the replacement of the text thereafter by the following words: "and in particular no one shall be subjected to such treatment in the form of medical or scientific experimentation."

12. The revised amendment of Greece and Italy called for the replacement of the second sentence by the following: "No one shall, *inter alia*, be subjected without his free consent to medical or scientific experimentation."

13. Canada submitted a sub-amendment to the revised amendment of Greece and Italy replacing the words "No one shall, *inter alia*, be subjected" by the following: "*Inter alia*, no one shall be made to undergo any form of torture or cruel treatment by being subjected." The representative of Canada accepted a suggestion by the representative of Ireland to the effect that the words "inhuman or degrading" should be inserted between the words "cruel" and "treatment."

14. The representative of Mexico re-introduced the original amendment of Greece and Italy submitting it as a sub-amendment to the revised text. The original Greek-Italian amendment consisted in the replacement of the second sentence of the article by the following text:

No one shall be made to undergo any other form of torture or cruel treatment by being subjected without his free consent to medical or scientific experimentation when such experimentation is not required by his state of physical or mental health.

At the 855th meeting, the Mexican representative withdrew this sub-amendment.

15. The word "unusual" proposed in the Philippine amendment gave rise to some discussion. It was argued that while cruel, degrading and inhuman treatment or punishment might be "unusual," the converse was not necessarily true. The amendment was supported by some representatives who felt that it might be applicable to certain actual practices which, although not intentionally cruel, inhuman or degrading, nevertheless affected the physical or moral integrity of the human person. On the other hand, it was objected that the term "unusual" was vague. What was "unusual" in one country might not be so in other countries.

16. Most of the discussion centered on the second sentence. Some felt that the sentence was unnecessary, since what it sought to prohibit was already covered by the first sentence. Moreover, it weakened the article in that it directed attention to only one of the many forms of cruel, inhuman or degrading treatment, thereby lessening the importance of the general prohibition laid down in the first sentence. On the other hand, most representatives attached special importance to the second sentence which, they pointed out, was intended to prevent the recurrence of atrocities such as those which had been committed in Nazi concentration camps during the Second World War. In their view the second sentence, far from being superfluous, seemed to complement the provisions of the first.

17. Several suggestions were made with a view to meeting the objection that the second part of the article was emphasized at the expense of the first. One was to replace the words "in particular" in the second sentence by the words "*inter alia,*" as proposed by Greece and Italy. Others thought that the substance of the second sentence might be embodied in a separate paragraph or, as proposed by Guatemala, in a separate article. However, these proposals were opposed by those who regarded the first and second sentences as closely linked and wished, therefore, to preserve the unity of the article. The amendment of Pakistan sought to resolve the difficulty by combining the two clauses of the article in a single sentence, thereby making the act covered in the second clause an addition to that covered in the first. The main objection to this amendment was that it weakened the second clause. As the debate developed, it became apparent that there was wide agreement that the second sentence should be retained. Some representatives, however, felt that, as drafted, it lacked precision and clarity. The main problem was how to find a formulation which, while outlawing criminal experimentation, would not hinder legitimate scientific or medical practices. There was general agreement that the Covenant should not attempt to lay down rules concerning medical treatment, as that was a matter which should be left to national legislation and the medical profession.

18. One approach to the problem, exemplified by the Australian amendment was to limit explicitly the scope of the provision to scientific and medical experimentation which constituted

torture or cruel, inhuman or degrading treatment. However, the Australian proposal was opposed on the grounds that, by not referring to "free consent," it failed to provide a satisfactory criterion for determining whether a given experiment was of the prohibited type or not. It was also pointed out that the proposed text sought to cover only experiments of a cruel, inhuman or degrading nature, while permitting other experiments conducted without the consent, or even the knowledge, of the subject.

19. Another approach, proposed by the Netherlands, was simply to eliminate from the text any references to legitimate medical practices. It was pointed out that the term "experimentation" did not cover medical treatment required in the interest of the patient's health. Hence, the clause "where such is not required by his state of physical or mental health" should be deleted, as it only served to confuse the meaning and intent of the provision by implying that medical or scientific practices having the welfare of the patient in view came within its scope. A similar approach was proposed by Greece and Italy in their revised amendment, except that the words "in particular" were to be replaced by "inter alia." However, several representatives preferred the term "in particular," since it linked the second sentence to the first more closely, making it clear that what was referred to was medical or scientific experimentation which amounted to torture or cruel, inhuman or degrading treatment.

20. Some doubts were raised as to the desirability of retaining the words "without his free consent" if the intention of the provision was solely to prohibit criminal experimentation. It was argued that the words were not only redundant, but might open the door to abuses in that it would be possible to justify experimentation of a criminal nature on the pretext that the subject had given his "consent." Such practices should be forbidden even if undertaken with the free consent of the subject. In reply, it was argued that consent given under pressure could never be regarded as "free" consent. It was unthinkable that anyone would freely submit himself to torture or cruel, inhuman or degrading practices. The introduction of the notion of "free consent" provided not only a safeguard, but also a criterion for determining whether an experiment was legitimate or not. Certain kinds of treatment became cruel, inhuman or degrading only because they were administered without the subject's free consent.

*　　*　　*

Text as Adopted

22. Article 7, as adopted by the Committee, reads as follows:

No one shall be subjected to torture or to cruel, inhuman or degrading treatment or punishment. In particular, no one shall be subjected without his free consent to medical or scientific experimentation.

NOTE

WALTER MODELL
HAZARDS OF NEW DRUGS*

No drug, no matter how thoroughly tested by time or trial, is absolutely safe. The size of the problem is indicated by a report in the *Journal of the American Medical Association* that one of every 20 patients admitted to a large hospital in New York City was there because of adverse reaction to treatment. Serious reactions occur with all therapies—the safe as well as the hazardous, the useful as well as the useless, the old as well as the new, the folk remedy as well as the modern miracle drug. What seems an innocent therapeutic procedure may have serious unanticipated effects. . . . Nothing must be accepted at face value in modern medicine; modern proof by modern standards is essential. The thoroughgoing scientific experiment and the scientific attitude are the only safeguards against the specter of drug disaster.

The aim with all new therapies is to establish a more favorable ratio between probable adverse effect of treatment and probable adverse effect of untreated disease. Testing new drugs involves developing and pursuing the most effective methods for determining therapeutic effectiveness and reaction hazard. Only with tested drugs is there an index of danger of adverse reaction and of potential for therapeutic usefulness. If the information is substantial, one can elect to use the drug on the basis of a calculable risk; without such information one has no way of knowing whether the clinical use of the new drug is defensible.

*　　*　　*

Obviously, testing should be conducted with minimum risk to the subject, but since there is no drug without hazard, there can be no testing of new drugs without risk. The justification for

* 139 *Science* 1180 (1963). Copyright 1963 by the American Association for the Advancement of Science. Reprinted by permission.

taking this risk is that without it there can be no reasonable basis for introducing and using new drugs, and that the danger involved in using them clinically without such testing would be greater than the danger involved in preclinical testing. Therefore, society must recognize that in its demand for new drugs there is clearly implicit a license for qualified individuals to take calculable risks in using them clinically. Medical science is obligated to keep these risks within reasonable limits. But both the medical profession and society in general must be fully aware of the potentiality of drugs to produce disaster.

[iii]
Ninety-first Congress, Second Session
An Act to Promote Public Health and
Welfare by Expanding, Improving, and
Better Coordinating the Family Planning Services
and Population Research Activities of the
Federal Government, and for Other Purposes**

*   *   *

SEC. 2. It is the purpose of this Act—
(1) to assist in making comprehensive voluntary family planning services readily available to all persons desiring such services;
(2) To coordinate domestic population and family planning research with the present and future needs of family planning programs. . . .

*   *   *

(8) to establish an Office of Population Affairs in the Department of Health, Education, and Welfare as a primary focus within the Federal Government on matters pertaining to population research and family planning, through which the Secretary of Health, Education, and Welfare (hereafter in this Act referred to as the "Secretary") shall carry out the purposes of this Act.

*   *   *

SEC. 6. . . .
(c) The Public Health Service Act is . . . amended by adding after title IX the following new title:

TITLE X—POPULATION RESEARCH AND VOLUNTARY FAMILY PLANNING PROGRAMS

Project Grants and Contracts for Family Planning Services

SEC. 1001. (a) The Secretary is authorized to make grants to and enter into contracts with public or nonprofit private entities to assist in the establishment and operation of voluntary family planning projects.
(b) In making grants and contracts under this section the Secretary shall take into account the number of patients to be served, the extent to which family planning services are needed locally, the relative need of the applicant, and its capacity to make rapid and effective use of such assistance.
(c) For the purpose of making grants and contracts under this section, there are authorized to be appropriated $30,000,000 for the fiscal year ending June 30, 1971; $60,000,000 for the fiscal year ending June 30, 1972; and $90,000,000 for the fiscal year ending June 30, 1973.

*   *   *

SEC. 1004. (a) In order to promote research in the biomedical, contraceptive development, behavioral, and program implementation fields related to family planning and population, the Secretary is authorized to make grants to public or nonprofit private entities and to enter into contracts with public or private entities and individuals for projects for research and research training in such fields.
(b) For the purpose of making payments pursuant to grants and contracts under this section, there are authorized to be appropriated $30,000,000 for the fiscal year ending June 30, 1971; $50,000,000 for the fiscal year ending June 30, 1972; and $65,000,000 for the fiscal year ending June 30, 1973.

*   *   *

SEC. 1007. The acceptance by any individual of family planning services or family planning or population growth information (including educational materials) provided through financial assistance under this title (whether by grant or contract) shall be voluntary and shall not be a prerequisite to eligibility for or receipt of any other service or assistance from, or to participation in, any other program of the entity or individual that provided such service or information.
SEC. 1008. None of the funds appropriated under this title shall be used in programs where abortion is a method of family planning.

---

* Act of December 24, 1970, Pub. Law No. 91–572, 84 Stat. 1504; *see* 42 U.S.C. § 201 (1971).

NOTES

NOTE 1.

MARTI MUELLER
ORAL CONTRACEPTIVES—
GOVERNMENT-SUPPORTED PROGRAMS
ARE QUESTIONED*

Last year a VISTA volunteer in Alaska watched in dismay as an Eskimo woman being treated in a federally financed birth-control center was handed a sack of oral contraceptives, given no counseling on how to take them, and told to come back in a year.

At a time when questions are being raised about the safety of the pill, the federal government has become one of the major distributors of the oral contraceptive in family-planning programs for the poor. Some doubts have been expressed about how safely these programs are administered. Officials within the Food and Drug Administration (FDA) have suggested in the past, for example, that its parent, the Department of Health, Education, and Welfare (HEW) has been lenient in monitoring side effects and adverse reactions to the pill and in supervising general medical health standards in its own programs. One reason for such shortcomings, if they exist, may be that, while HEW programs are federally financed, many are administered on the local level by states, cities, and private organizations, and, as former HEW Assistant Secretary Philip Lee has said, "in many cases we are buying into the existing program."

Lee also commented to *Science* that the quality of care for the poor in the United States is well below what it should be. "We thought we were doing much better than we are doing," Lee said. "The poor were not getting adequate care, either therapeutic or diagnostic." Lee . . . estimates there are 5 million women of childbearing age at or below the poverty level in the United States. He told *Science* that giving medically supervised family-planning guidance to the entire 5 million would cost about $30 per woman, or about $150 million in all. (This year Congress appropriated about $50 million for birth control programs for the poor, which now serve about a million women.) . . .

* * *

HEW officials deny that a physician has any direct responsibility to HEW to submit a report on adverse drug reactions. Lee sees the problem as a jurisdictional one. He feels, in effect, responsibility for monitoring medical practices belongs to the American Medical Association; Lee, a physician, says HEW must rely on the built-in systems of peer review to ensure that physicians practice medicine responsibly. Others feel this is an uncertain means of ensuring safety, particularly in governmented-supported family planning. . . .

* * *

NOTE 2.
USSR PICKS IUD OVER THE PILL*

Spurred by a spiraling abortion rate and by citizens' demands for modern contraceptives, the Soviet Union has launched a major birth control program. Soviet health leaders have given their official blessing to intrauterine devices as the basis of the new effort. Other methods will also be made available, though free choice of contraceptives is not being encouraged.

More than 300,000 IUDs have already been produced in the Soviet Union, reports Dr. Boris Petrovsky, Minister of Public Health. He estimates that the total output this year will reach one million. Among the Soviet Union's population of 230 million are about 55 million women of childbearing age.

* * *

Until now, abortions, legal since 1955 and costing the equivalent of $5.50, have been the most common method of preventing unwanted births. But assembly-line abortions have been widely criticized for medical and psychological reasons.

Up to now, Soviet couples have also been able to obtain three types of contraceptives from Soviet pharmacies: a condom, a spermicidal jelly, and a suppository—all of limited effectiveness.

Dr. Petrovsky said his government's decision to mass-produce IUDs was based on experience gained from other countries—and on their own three-year comparative studies of the IUD and the pill. These were conducted by the Soviet Academy of Medicine's Scientific Research Institute of Obstetrics and Gynecology and the Public Health Ministry's All-Union Scientific Research Institute of Obstetrics and Gynecology.

---

* 163 *Science* 553–554 (1969). Copyright 1969 by the American Association for the Advancement of Science. Reprinted by permission.

* *Medical World News* 16–18 (January 10, 1969). Copyright 1969, McGraw-Hill, Inc. Reprinted by permission.

Dr. Leonid Persiyaninov, director of the Academy of Medicine's ob-gyn institute, called the IUD the "lesser of two evils." Soviet research showed that both methods were more than 90 percent effective, Dr. Persiyaninov said, so that the decision to mass-produce IUDs over pills was based primarily on differences in side effects.

*   *   *

Despite judgment against the pill, research on it and limited clinical trials will be carried out in the Soviet Union. The Russians plan to continue importing from Hungary a hormonal preparation called *Infecundin*. And they are reportedly tooling up for production of a progestogen-estrogen preparation similar to a U.S. brand.

[T]he recent Soviet decision to mass-produce IUDs fits in with their generally conservative approach to medicine. "They favor a mechanical device over a chemical one because its effects are limited to the uterus. But they do not want to miss out on something that might prove to be better, so they are proceeding cautiously in many directions. Meanwhile, the Western world is their guinea pig for the pill."

*   *   *

Dr. George Langmuir, medical director of Planned Parenthood, sees another factor behind the Soviet choice of the IUD over the pill. Abortion is legal in the Soviet Union, he emphasizes, so a contraceptive need not be 100 percent effective. The Russian approach to contraception may parallel what has occurred in Sweden, he suggests. Both countries practice conservative medicine and sanction abortions, though far fewer are performed in Sweden. Swedes use mechanical means of contraception most often, and only a small number of prescriptions are filled for the pill.

*   *   *

[iv]
United States Congress
A Bill to Provide for Humane Treatment of Animals Used in Experiment and Research by Recipients of Grants from the United States, and by Agencies and Instrumentalities of the United States, and for Other Purposes*

[I]t is declared to be the policy of the United States that animals used in experiments, tests, the teaching of scientific methods and techniques, and

* H.R. 3036; 111 *Congressional Record* 831 (1965).

the production of medical and pharmaceutical materials shall be spared avoidable pain, stress, discomfort, and fear, that they shall be used only when no other feasible and satisfactory method can be used to obtain necessary scientific information for the cure of disease, alleviation of suffering, prolongation of life, or for military requirements, that the number of animals used for these purposes shall be reduced as far as possible, and that all animals so used shall be comfortably housed, well fed, and humanely treated.

SEC. 2. As used in this Act—
(1) The term "animal" means any living creature of any vertebrate species;
(2) The term "stress" means the effect of any condition of housing, diet, climate, confinement, care or use unsuitable to the species or to the particular animal, or differing from its ordinary and normal mode of life, to a degree which produces physical deterioration in any respect or markedly a typical conduct or reaction, or which, if prolonged, would have a tendency to produce either of the above aberrations from normal condition or reaction;
(3) The term "pain" means any sensation which, if felt by a human being, a competent and conscientious physician would ordinarily take steps to relieve, by anesthesia, sedation, nursing care, or otherwise;
(4) The term "substitution" means the use in any research project, test, demonstration, or production procedure of a less highly developed species of animal for species more highly developed, the development to be evaluated on the basis of the brain and nervous system of the species, in terms of its elaboration and sensitivity to pain;
(5) The term "reduction" means the use of a reduced number of animals, by means of the application of statistical techniques, use of insentient material or models, or any other method;

*   *   *

SEC. 3. There is hereby established in the Department of Justice of the United States an Agency for Laboratory Animal Control (hereinafter in this Act referred to as the "Agency"). The Agency shall be headed by a Commissioner of Laboratory Animal Control, who shall be appointed by the President of the United States, by and with the advice and consent of the Senate. To be eligible for appointment as Commissioner, a person must be an attorney eligible for admission to practice before the Supreme Court of the United States.

SEC. 4. After the one hundred and eightieth day following the date of enactment of this Act, no agency or instrumentality of the United States shall use any animal for research, experiments, tests, training in scientific or technical procedures, or production of materials unless the agency or instrumentality has been granted a certificate of compliance with this Act, issued by the Commissioner for Laboratory Animal Control.

* * *

SEC. 8. No certificate of compliance shall be issued by the Commissioner unless the laboratory applying for such certificate shall have agreed, in writing, that authorized representatives of the Commissioner and law enforcement officers of the State in which the laboratory operates shall be given access at any time to the animals, premises, and records of the laboratory, for the purpose of obtaining information relevant to the administration and enforcement of this Act; except that no laboratory shall be required to permit access to any person not duly cleared for such access with respect to any materials or area which is restricted pursuant to any law of the United States relating to the national security.

SEC. 9. No use of animals shall be undertaken by any holder of a certificate of compliance with this Act until a project plan has been filed with the Agency in such form as the Commissioner shall prescribe, describing the nature and purposes of the proposed use of animals, and the project plan has been approved by the Commissioner. The Commissioner shall refuse to approve a project plan that would not comply with this Act and the policies enunciated herein.

SEC. 10. The Commissioner shall upon application issue a letter of qualification to use animals in research to persons having all of the following qualifications:

(1) the applicant has been awarded a doctoral degree in medicine, veterinary medicine, physiology, psychology, or zoological science by an accredited university or college;

(2) the applicant has never been convicted of cruelty to animals or been found by the Commissioner to have participated knowingly in a violation of this Act;

* * *

SEC. 12. Every laboratory holding a certificate of compliance, and every agency or instrumentality of the United States that uses animals in research, experiments, tests, training in scientific procedures, or technique, or the production of materials, shall comply with the following requirements:

(1) all projects shall be designed and executed so as to obtain maximum reduction and substitution;

(2) animals used in any way that would cause pain shall be anesthetized so as to prevent the animals from feeling pain during the experiment or procedure, except that the Commissioner may waive this requirement for a specified project if the Commissioner, with the concurrence of the Surgeon General, finds that anesthesia would frustrate the purpose of the project;

(3) no unanesthetized animal shall be burned, scalded, or subjected to major surgery or to any similarly acutely painful procedure;

(4) regardless of the nature or purpose of any experiment or procedure, animals that would suffer prolonged pain or stress as a result of an experiment or procedure shall be painlessly killed immediately after the procedure causing pain or stress is completed, whether or not the objective of the experiment or procedure has been attained;

(5) animals used in surgery or other procedures causing pain or stress shall be given pain-relieving care and convalescence conditions substantially equal to those customarily or usually given to human patients before, during, and after similar procedures;

* * *

(9) all premises where animals are kept shall provide a comfortable resting place, adequate space and facilities for exercise normal to the species, sanitary and comfortable cleanliness, and lighting, temperature, humidity, and ventilation appropriate to the species;

(10) animals shall receive food and water adequate to maintain health and comfort and shall not be permitted to suffer pain or stress through neglect or mishandling;

(11) an accurate record shall be maintained of all experiments and procedures performed and the records shall be in such form as to make possible the identification of animals subjected to specified experiments and tests, and a record shall be kept of the disposition of all animals;

(12) all cages or enclosures containing animals shall at all times be identified by cards stating the nature of the experiment or test in progress and identifying the project approved by the Commissioner;

(13) an annual report and such additional reports or information as the Commissioner may require by regulation or individual request shall be submitted to the Commissioner. The annual report shall specify, for each project plan previously filed and approved, the number and species of animals used, the procedure employed, the sources from which all animals were acquired, and such matters as the Commissioner may prescribe, and shall include a copy of any published work prepared or sponsored by the reporting person or laboratory, involving the use of animals;

* * *

SEC. 14. The Commissioner shall suspend or revoke any certificate of compliance or any letter of compliance issued pursuant to this Act upon a determination on the record after opportunity for an agency hearing of failure to comply with any provision of this Act or the policy stated herein or for refusal to permit inspection or to produce records pursuant to the agreement required in section 8. . . .

d.
Deciding about Choice of Subjects?

[i]
United States Congress
A Bill for the Regulation of Scientific Experiments upon Human Beings in the District of Columbia*

SEC. 1. [No] physician, surgeon, pathologist, student of medicine or of science, or any other person shall make or perform upon the body of any human being, in any hospital, asylum, retreat, or infirmary established for the treatment of the sick, or in any other place in the District of Columbia, any scientific experiment involving pain, distress, or risk to life and health, whether by administration of poisonous drugs for the purpose of ascertaining their toxicity, by inoculating the germs of disease, by grafting cancerous tumors into healthy tissues, or by performance of any surgical operation for any other object than

---

* S. 3424; 33 *Congressional Record* 2460 (1900).

the amelioration of the patient, except subject to the restrictions and regulations hereinafter prescribed. Any person performing, advising, or assisting in the performance of any such experiment upon any newborn babe, pregnant woman, lunatic, idiot, or patient, in any public or private hospital, in any infants' home, hospital asylum, or private house, or upon any other person whatsoever, shall be deemed guilty of the crime of human vivisection, and upon conviction shall be liable to a fine of not less than one thousand dollars or imprisonment for not less than one year, or both. If any such experiment shall be followed within forty-eight hours by the death of the person thus operated upon, or if it shall appear that death was accelerated in any way by such experiment, the performance of any such experiment shall be deemed manslaughter or murder, as the circumstances of the case shall determine; and all persons taking part therein shall be liable to the penalties prescribed for such crime.

SEC. 2. That any physician or surgeon duly qualified to practice medicine in the District of Columbia, or any medical student, who shall perform any such scientific experiment, or who by his advice or presence shall in any way assist, aid, or abet the performance of any such experiment, shall, upon conviction, be forever disqualified from the practice of medicine in the District of Columbia. Any person engaged in any capacity in the service of the United States Government or in any of its departments who shall perform, or by his presence, suggestion, or advice, aid or abet the performance of any such experiment upon a human being, shall, upon conviction, in addition to other penalties herein provided, be forthwith dismissed from Government service and be forever disqualified therefor.

SEC. 3. That any description or account of any such experiment upon a human being, printed or published in any scientific or medical periodical or book, or in any reputable newspaper, shall be deemed evidence demanding immediate inquiry into all the circumstances of the alleged crime, and, if corroborated by further evidence, shall be accepted as testimony in regard to the offense.

SEC. 4. That an experiment performed upon a human being with a view to the advancement by new discovery of physiological or pathological knowledge shall, if it involves pain or distress, be permitted only under the following restrictions:

(a) The experiment must be performed only by a duly qualified physician or surgeon holding such special license from the Commissioners of the District of Columbia as in this Act mentioned; and

(b) The subject of such experiment must be not less than twenty years of age and in full and complete possession of all his or her reasoning faculties. No scientific experiment of any kind liable to cause pain or distress shall be permissible upon any newborn babe, infant, child, or youth; nor upon any woman during pregnancy nor within a year after her confinement, nor upon any aged, infirm, epileptic, insane, or feeble-minded person under any circumstances whatever.

(c) The physician or surgeon proposing to make any such experiment or series of experiments shall, at least one week in advance, apply to the Commissioners of the District of Columbia for license permitting such experiment or experiments to be performed. Such application shall fully state the objects and methods of the proposed experiments, and shall be accompanied with the written permission of the subject of the proposed experimentation, agreeing thereto, signed in presence of two witnesses and duly acknowledged before a public notary under seal.

(d) Upon receipt of such application, the Commissioners of the District of Columbia shall cause investigation to be made; and if it shall appear that the experiments involve no risk to human life; that the person offering himself or herself for experimentation is of requisite age, in full possession of all his or her reasoning faculties, and fully aware of the nature of the proposed experiment, and desires that it be made, then the Commissioners may issue a license authorizing such scientific experiment or series of experiments as desired; but

(e) No such experiment shall at any time be continued against the expressed will of the person experimented upon.

(f) The Commissioners of the District of Columbia shall require a report to be made to them of the methods employed and the results attained of each experiment or series of experiments thus made. Such report need not be made public until after six months from the beginning of the experimentation, in order to permit the investigator to present the results of his work in his own way. But in the event of any untoward circumstance attending any such experimentation, the full details shall immediately be reported and printed.

SEC. 5. That nothing in this Act contained shall be construed to prohibit or interfere with any properly conducted method of medical treatment or surgical operation, whether experimental or otherwise, having for its demonstrable end and object the amelioration of suffering or recovery of the patient thus treated or operated upon.

SEC. 6. That nothing in this Act contained shall be construed to prohibit or interfere with any experiments whatsoever made by medical students, physicians, surgeons, physiologists, or pathologists upon one another.

[ii]
Sir John Eccles
Animal Experimentation versus
*Human Experimentation**

. . . It has been traditional that quite a lot of the experimentation related to medicine is done with human subjects. As we become more and more expert in applying experimental procedures to animals, in finding the right animals, and in carrying out these procedures under the appropriate scientific conditions, there will be progressively less necessity for human experimentation. We must try to diminish human experimentation as far as possible by substituting animal experimentation.

I think that no serious and hazardous experimental procedure should be done on humans unless it is quite impossible to carry them out on animals. Such a statement severely limits human experimentation. Furthermore, experimenting on humans in any way that involves risk, should be preceded by experiments on animals by which the technical procedures can be developed.

*   *   *

[W]e must plan to minimize human experimentation and maximize animal experimentation, and we must define quite rigorously the conditions under which human experimentation can be carried out. This is something that the societies concerned with animals, animal care, and animal experimentation should understand. They should recognize, moreover, how important animals are and how significant they are in mimimizing human experimentation. The more effec-

* *Defining the Laboratory Animal.* Washington, D.C.: National Academy of Sciences 285–292 (1971). Publication ISBN 0-309-01862-5, International Committee on Laboratory Animals and The Institute of Laboratory Animal Resources, National Academy of Sciences-National Research Council, Washington, D.C. Reprinted by permission.

tive animal research centers can become and the more facilities they can provide, the more they will be able to eliminate the really dangerous and damaging forms of human experimentation.

Let us also consider allowable forms of human experimentation. Many such experiments are quite without risk. For example, during the final three terms of physiology, which I taught from 1944 to 1951 at the medical school of the University of Otago, New Zealand, the students performed 85 percent of the total experiments on themselves. I had three three-hour courses on the systematic study of pain—muscle pain, skin pain, all kinds of inflammatory pains, and periosteal pain. Of course, a great many procedures like this can be performed on human subjects without any danger and with little discomfort. I designed these courses originally because we were so short of animals, and I discovered that it was far better to use the students as subjects. They investigated their own muscle contractions, stimulated their nerves and tested their reflexes. This experimentation can be effectively and appropriately done by medical students on themselves in order to give them some feeling for their eventual work in neurology. Similarly, excellent experiments on respiration and urinary secretion can be carried out on human subjects.

* * *

There are also advanced levels of experimentation that require human subjects. . . . a friend of mine subjected some volunteer medical students to an aseptic operation in which small cutaneous nerves in the forearm were dissected down until there was only a single fiber left. He was then able to test their sensory perceptions aroused by stimulating these single fibers in cutaneous nerves. I think this is about the limit to which one can ask students to participate!

* * *

In California today, Libet is doing most ethical and careful work on the sensations evoked in human subjects by varying the parameters of gentle electrical stimulation of the somesthetic area of the cerebral cortex. This work relates to some most interesting philosophical problems about how man actually derives conscious sensations from the complex patterned impulse transmission in the neural machinery of his brain. It is much more complicated than anybody had imagined. This type of investigation has to be done on human subjects who can report what they feel. But this is done only on volunteers whose brains are exposed for the purpose of a therapeutic operation, for example in a patient suffering from Parkinsonism. It is explained to the patient that the experiment has nothing whatsoever to do with the therapeutic procedures. Nevertheless, almost all volunteer under those conditions to give half an hour of their time on the operating table unanesthetized.

* * *

There are, however, several problems relative to unethical human experimentation. For the most part such experiments are carried out by people who are loathe to use primates or by people who do not have the cost structure for primate investigations and are unwilling to ask for it. One such experiment involves chronically implanted electrodes in the human brain. In animals this is a marvelous technique. It is being employed at the National Institutes of Health with monkeys in which electrodes have been implanted in the various parts of the cerebral cortex and the cerebellum. With microelectrode recording the investigators study the responses of single nerve cells in the cerebrum and cerebellum while the animals carry out trained procedures of various kinds. It is beautiful work and can lead to new levels of understanding of the mode of action of the brain.

It does, however, require an immense cooperative effort, because the people involved must ensure that highly trained animals will be kept under the best conditions and be well nurtured. Under ideal conditions the animals can go on for many weeks or months learning and being experimented on. Animals can learn only when they are comfortable and happy, so such investigations demand highly skilled experimenters and technicians.

The value of this kind of work in understanding the nervous system is becoming more and more apparent. The more perfect animal experimentation can become, the more obvious it will be that no one should subject human beings to chronically implanted electrodes. Surprisingly, it is cheaper to do the experiment on human subjects. Patients come along with some kind of psychosis or neurosis, and the doctors say "Yes, now we have to study your brain more. We will have to drill some holes and put some things in." A cap is placed over the assemblage of implanted electrodes, and these people go about their work at home and so on, and come in every now and then for recordings from these electrodes.

I regard this work as quite unethical. Because of these buried implanted electrodes, the brain will never be the same and many people will suffer from epileptic seizures. Because this procedure is destructive, and not at all therapeutic, it is unethical. I do not countenance any destruction or damage to the brain under conditions that are not related to the therapeutic treatment of the patient. This kind of human experimentation should be stopped completely, and to remove the need for it, we must establish primate centers. The centers we have in this country are very good ones, but we need more facilities in primate centers, so no one will be tempted to do these unethical human experiments.

*   *   *

[T]he task facing the laboratory animal researcher is a tremendous one. It is one that will become greater in the future. It will become necessary to provide a much wider variety of animals for specific purposes. Certain problems in living organisms are best investigated with invertebrates, like the nerve impulse and synapse in squid or the ganglia of aplysia. So a wide variety of animals, an almost zoological collection, must be made available for research. This will provide a tremendous service not only in advancing biological and medical science, but also in saving humans from suffering the risks and the travail that come when unethical experiments are done upon them.

*   *   *

NOTE

Dwight E. Harken
Heart Transplantation—
A Boston Perspective*

*   *   *

Why . . . are human heart transplants *not* being performed at the Peter Bent Brigham? . . .

. . . In spite of extensive experience with the relatively reproducible surgical technics contributed by Shumway and Hanlon and others to make orthotopic transplants realistic, the vast majority of our animals die within 24 hours, often of unexplained causes, including atelectasis. Furthermore, although laboratories throughout the world have conducted *thousands of animal heart transplants,* there have been, to our knowl-

edge, but a trivial number of long-term survivors. Indeed, the most successful among these is Kantrowitz's puppy recipient of a littermate donor heart. This animal matured and bore puppies. Probably fewer than a dozen recipients of non-littermate canine transplants have survived for one year.

It becomes urgent that we have a clearer knowledge of the *incidence of survival* in cases of canine (and other) unselected orthotopic homotransplants; it is not enough simply to know that there can be long-term survival in animals of undetermined genetic constitution.

Experience with heart-lung machines taught us that *canine survival is not necessarily a prerequisite to human experiment.* However, much useful information could be obtained if we could achieve a significant number of long-term survivors, which is not consistently possible now. This fact becomes even more significant if we accept the likelihood that the rejection mechanisms are similar in dogs, rats and man.

*   *   *

[iii]
American Medical Association
Ethical Guidelines for Clinical Investigation*

*   *   *

The following guidelines are intended to aid physicians in fulfilling their ethical responsibilities when they engage in the clinical investigation of new drugs and procedures.

(1) A physician may participate in clinical investigation only to the extent that his activities are a part of a systematic program competently designed, under accepted standards of scientific research, to produce data which are scientifically valid and significant.

(2) In conducting clinical investigation, the investigator should demonstrate the same concern and caution for the welfare, safety, and comfort of the person involved as is required of a physician who is furnishing medical care to a patient independent of any clinical investigation.

(3) In clinical investigation *primarily for treatment*—

A. The physician must recognize that the physician-patient relationship exists and that he is expected to exercise his pro-

---

* 22 *American Journal of Cardiology* 449–450 (1968). Copyright 1968 by the Reuben H. Donnelley Corp. Reprinted by permission.

* *Opinions and Reports of the Judicial Council.* Chicago: American Medical Association 9–11 (1969). Reprinted by permission.

fessional judgment and skill in the best interest of the patient.

B. Voluntary consent must be obtained from the patient, or from his legally authorized representative if the patient lacks the capacity to consent, following: (a) disclosure that the physician intends to use an investigational drug or experimental procedure, (b) a reasonable explanation of the nature of the drug or procedure to be used, risks to be expected, and possible therapeutic benefits, (c) an offer to answer any inquiries concerning the drug or procedure, and (d) a disclosure of alternative drugs or procedures that may be available.

   i. In exceptional circumstances and to the extent that disclosure of information concerning the nature of the drug or experimental procedure or risks would be expected to materially affect the health of the patient and would be detrimental to his best interests, such information may be withheld from the patient. In such circumstances such information shall be disclosed to a responsible relative or friend of the patient where possible.

   ii. Ordinarily, consent should be in writing, except where the physician deems it necessary to rely upon consent in other than written form because of the physical or emotional state of the patient.

   iii. Where emergency treatment is necessary and the patient is incapable of giving consent and no one is available who has authority to act on his behalf, consent is assumed.

(4) In clinical investigation *primarily for the accumulation of scientific knowledge*—

A. Adequate safeguards must be provided for the welfare, safety, and comfort of the subject.

B. Consent, in writing, should be obtained from the subject, or from his legally authorized representative if the subject lacks the capacity to consent, following: (a) a disclosure of the fact that an investigational drug or procedure is to be used, (b) a reasonable explanation of the nature of the procedure to be used and risks to be expected, and (c) an offer to answer any inquiries concerning the drug or procedure.

C. Minors or mentally incompetent persons may be used as subjects only if:

   i. The nature of the investigation is such that mentally competent adults would not be suitable subjects.

   ii. Consent, in writing, is given by a legally authorized representative of the subject under circumstances in which an informed and prudent adult would reasonably be expected to volunteer himself or his child as a subject.

D. No person may be used as a subject against his will.

*   *   *

NOTES

NOTE 1.

DANIEL C. MARTIN, JOHN D. ARNOLD,
T. F. ZIMMERMAN, AND ROBERT H. RICHART
HUMAN SUBJECTS IN CLINICAL RESEARCH*

*   *   *

[This] study dealt with general opinions about volunteerism. Who should assume the risk as the experimental subject? This may well be the most pressing of all questions related to clinical research. Subjects from a wide range of socio-economic positions (154 in number) were asked their feelings about the human subject in medical research. These people were allowed to phrase their own answers without help from the interviewer. Their responses were subsequently arranged into classes and tabulated. The results are shown in Table 4.

The most pervasive tendency to be noted is the apparent reluctance of people from many socio-economic classes to suggest the use of the sick or dying as subjects in clinical research. Since this particular question was not pursued further, we do not know whether this set of answers might be altered if specific qualifications were appended to the original question. For instance, would the use of the sick or dying in chemotherapeutic research on cancer be more acceptable to respondents than our generalized proposal for "medical research"?

Although the scale of risks used in the previous . . . studies encompasses the majority of those to be encountered in human experimentation, it omits one of the extremes. We believe this extreme is presently represented by the problem of the single-organ transplant. . . .

---

* 279 *New England Journal of Medicine* 1426, 1429–1430 (1968). Reprinted by permission.

TABLE 4
Preferred Source of Volunteers

Source	Frequency of Selection	Rank of Acceptability
Anybody who is willing to volunteer	60	1
Prisoners	44	2
Don't know	17	3
People involved doing research	15	4
Institutions—mental, custodial, juvenile etc.	6	5
Sick or dying	6	5
Paid unemployed (welfare)	6	5
Total respondents	154	

The heart transplant requires the participation of two human experimental subjects. One subject must give up his heart. The other accepts the donated heart and its potential benefits. The once abstract, philosophical and academic considerations of "life" and "death" have become real.

The person who becomes the donor of a heart faces not a risk but a certainty—death, if this has not already occurred. How should this extreme "risk" be distributed in society? The other experimental partner receives potential benefit from the transplant procedure. How should this benefit be distributed in society? The investigators took these two questions to the community, using standard survey procedures.

*   *   *

It is obviously the donor who takes the extreme risk in the heart-transplant procedure. The results of this study indicate that the community continues to support the principle of voluntary participation. Seventy per cent of the respondents rank volunteers as the most preferred source of experimental donors. The sample population expressed once again the expectation that prisoners might become a prime source for experimental subjects. Prisoners about to be executed were specifically mentioned by a number of respondents who were given this as one of a number of possible choices. There appeared little enthusiasm in our in-depth interviews for use of the sick and dying as donors, although this may be the only large practical source of single organs for transplant. The sample population tended to consider factors outside the medical sphere in selecting both donors and recipients.

*   *   *

NOTE 2.
BRITISH MEDICAL RESEARCH COUNCIL
MEMORANDUM ON CLINICAL INVESTIGATIONS*

*   *   *

To obtain the consent of the patient to a proposed investigation is not in itself enough. Owing to the special relationship of trust which exists between a patient and his doctor, most patients will consent to any proposal that is made. Further, the considerations involved are nearly always so technical as to prevent their being adequately understood by one who is not himself an expert. It must, therefore, be frankly recognized that, for practical purposes, an inescapable responsibility for determining what investigations are, or are not, undertaken on a particular patient will rest with the doctor concerned. Nearly always his judgment will be accepted by the patient as decisive.

Even in the routine case, where no question of special investigation arises, judgment may not be easy. At the frontiers of medical knowledge,

* Memorandum M.R.C. 53/649 (October 16, 1953). Reprinted by permission. In issuing their memorandum, members of the M.R.C. stated that "having recently undertaken wide responsibilities for the development of clinical research in this country . . . it would be opportune if they gave an indication of their attitude towards the considerations involved in carrying out investigations on patients. They are, therefore, circulating this memorandum to medical members of their staff and research workers in receipt of grants from the Council. Further, as this matter must be of concern to all responsible for the promotion of clinical research, the memorandum is also being sent, for information, to the Deans of Medical Faculties and Medical Schools, to the Secretaries of the Medical Scientific Societies, and to the Editors of the relevant scientific journals."

where many procedures are novel and their value to the individual patient may often be problematical, judgment is always difficult and decisions can be open to question. It is in these circumstances that doubt may be felt and views differ and that, inevitably, responsibility bears heavily on the clinical investigator.

* * *

NOTE 3.

KING HEALTH CENTER
YOUR RIGHTS AS A PATIENT*

The patient has a right to consent to, or refuse, any treatment.

The patient has a right to have things explained clearly. (For example, any possible side effects of medicines.)

* * *

You have a right to refuse to participate in or be interviewed for research purposes. You have the right to full explanation of purposes and uses of the information if you do participate.

* * *

You have a right to know what's going on. Always ask questions about anything that you do not understand or that is worrying you.

* * *

e.

Deciding about Qualifications of Investigators?

Henry K. Beecher
Tentative Statement Outlining the Philosophy and Ethical Principles Governing the Conduct of Research on Human Beings at the Harvard Medical School†

* * *

All of the so-called codes as guides to human experimentation emphasize the necessity that the experimenter be well trained and adequate as a scientist to undertake the study proposed. Medical research, when it involves treatment of any physical procedures beyond the simplest, requires that the investigator or his close associate be a qualified physician. No other pro-

fession gives such prerogatives and no other profession, probably, presents such a generally high level of unselfishness and compassion in directly caring for the sick or in planning procedures for the future. Of the qualities of the investigators, unselfishness is the most important for subject and project alike. Imagination, objectivity and the power to generalize soundly are all essential. In the forefront of the qualities which lead to protection of subject and patient in investigation is a deep sense of responsibility on the part of the investigator, coupled with unselfishness and a keen and well-trained intelligence. . . .

* * *

After some years of careful study of the available codes of the past which have been established to guide the medical investigator and after earnest attempts to write down a comprehensive code, the writer has had to conclude that it is not possible to lay down very many "rules" in terms of a code which can govern experimentation in man. In most cases these are more likely to do harm than good. Rules will not curb the unscrupulous.

* * *

It is the writer's point of view that the best approach concerns the character, wisdom, experience, honesty, imaginativeness and sense of responsibility of the investigator who, in all cases of doubt or where serious consequences might remotely occur, will call in his peers and get the benefit of their counsel. Rigid rules will jeopardize the research establishments of this country where experimentation in man is essential.

NOTES

NOTE 1.

NEW YORK EDUCATION LAWS (1970)

* * *

§ 6501. *Definitions.* . . . . 4. The practice of medicine is defined as follows: A person practices medicine within the meaning of this article, except as hereinafter stated, who holds himself out as being able to diagnose, treat, operate or prescribe for any human disease, pain, injury, deformity or physical condition, and who shall either offer or undertake, by any means or method, to diagnose, treat, operate or prescribe for any human disease, pain, injury, deformity or physical condition.

* * *

* Bronx, N.Y.: Dr. Martin Luther King, Jr. Health Center 3–7 (1970). Reprinted by permission of Mr. Liery Wynn, Community Health Advocacy Office, Montefiore Hospital.
† Unpublished manuscript (undated). Printed by permission of the author who retains all rights.

§ 6502. *Qualification for practice.* No person shall practice medicine . . . unless licensed by the department and registered as required by this article. No person shall practice osteopathy or physiotherapy, unless licensed by the department and registered as required by this article. No person shall be licensed to practice under this article who has ever been convicted of a felony by any court, or whose authority to practice is suspended or revoked by the department. The conviction of felony shall be the conviction of any offense which if committed within the state of New York woudl constitute a felony under the laws thereof. If a person convicted of a felony is subsequently pardoned by the governor of the state where such conviction was had, or by the president of the United States, or if such a person shall receive a certificate of good conduct granted by the board of parole pursuant to the provisions of the executive law to remove the disability under this section because of such conviction, the regents may, in their discretion, on application of such person, and on the submission to them of satisfactory evidence, restore to such person the right to practice medicine, osteopathy or physiotherapy in this state.

*   *   *

§ 6506. *Admission to examination.* The department shall admit to examination any candidate who pays a fee of thirty dollars and submits evidence, verified by oath, and satisfactory to the department, that he: 1. Is more than Twenty-one years of age and a citizen of the United States or has declared his intention of becoming such citizen.

2. Is of good moral character.

3. Had prior to beginning the first year of medical study the preliminary general education required by the rules of the department, except where the application is for a license to practice osteopathy, in which case he must have had the general education required by the rules of the department preliminary to receiving the degree of doctor of osteopathy.

4. Has completed not less than four satisfactory courses of at least eight months each in a medical school in this country or Canada registered as maintaining at the time a standard satisfactory to the department, or in a medical school in a foreign country maintaining a standard not lower than that prescribed for medical schools in this state.

5. Has received the degree of bachelor or doctor of medicine from a medical school in this country or Canada, registered as maintaining at the time a standard satisfactory to the department. . . .

*   *   *

NOTE 2.

CALIFORNIA HEALTH AND SAFETY CODE (1970)

§ 1700. *Legislative findings.* The effective diagnosis, care, treatment, or cure of persons suffering from cancer is of paramount public importance. Vital statistics indicate that approximately 16 percent of the total deaths in the United States annually result from one or another of the forms of cancer. It is established that accurate and early diagnosis of many forms of cancer, followed by prompt application of methods of treatment which are scientifically proven, either materially reduces the likelihood of death from cancer or may materially prolong the useful life of individuals suffering therefrom.

Despite intensive campaigns of public education, there is a lack of adequate and accurate information among the public with respect to presently proven methods for the diagnosis, treatment, and cure of cancer. Various persons in this State have represented and continue to represent themselves as possessing medicines, methods, techniques, skills, or devices for the effective diagnosis, treatment, or cure of cancer, which representations are misleading to the public, with the result that large numbers of the public, relying on such representations, needlessly die of cancer, and substantial amounts of the savings of individuals and families relying on such representations are needlessly wasted.

It is, therefore, in the public interest that the public be afforded full and accurate knowledge as to the facilities and methods for the diagnosis, treatment, and cure of cancer available in this State and that to that end there be provided means for testing and investigating the value or lack thereof of alleged cancer remedies, devices, drugs, or compounds, and informing the public of the facts found, and protecting the public from misrepresentation in such matters.

The importance of continuing scientific research to determine the cause or cure of cancer is recognized, and the department shall administer this chapter with due regard for the importance of bona fide scientific research and the clinical testing in hospitals, clinics, or similar institutions of new drugs or compounds.

*   *   *

§ 1704. *Powers and duties of department of public health.* The department shall:

(a) Prescribe reasonable rules and regulations with respect to the administration of this chapter.

(b) Investigate violations of the provisions of this chapter, and report such violations to the appropriate enforcement authority.

(c) Secure the investigation and testing of the content, method of preparation, efficacy, or use of drugs, medicines, compounds, or devices proposed to be used, or used, by any individual, person, firm, association, or other entity in the state for the diagnosis, treatment, or cure of cancer, prescribe reasonable regulations with respect to such investigation and testing, and make findings of fact and recommendations upon completion of any such investigation and testing.

(d) Adopt a regulation prohibiting the prescription, administration, sale, or other distribution of any drug, substance, or device found to be harmful or of no value in the diagnosis, prevention, or treatment of cancer.

* * *

§ 1706. *Necessity of license for treatment of cancer by use of drugs, surgery, or radiation.* No person may undertake to treat or alleviate cancer by use of drugs, surgery, or radiation unless such person holds a license issued under a law of this State expressly authorizing the diagnosis and treatment of disease by use of drugs, surgery, or radiation.

* * *

§ 1708. *Exemptions from chapter.* This chapter shall not apply to the use of any drug, medicine, compound, or device intended solely for legitimate and bona fide investigational purposes by experts qualified by scientific training and experience to investigate the safety and therapeutic value thereof unless the department shall find that such drug, medicine, compound, or device is being used in diagnosis or treatment for compensation and profit. In order to qualify for an exemption under this section there shall be on file with the Federal Department of Health, Education, and Welfare a current and unrevoked investigational new drug application issued pursuant to Section 5051 of the Federal Food, Drug, and Cosmetics Act, or the following conditions shall be complied with:

(a) The label of the drug, medicine, compound, or device shall bear the statement "Caution: New drug (or medicine or compound or

device). Use-in the diagnosis, treatment, alleviation, or cure of cancer limited by law to investigational use."

(b) The drug, medicine, compound, or device has had adequate testing on appropriate experimental animals to demonstrate a lack of toxicity and hazard sufficient to permit its use in or on human beings and to establish with clarity the margins of safety ordinarily recognized by experts qualified by scientific training and experience to investigate the safety and effectiveness of such drugs, substances or devices.

(c) The drug, medicine, compound, or device is to be used solely for investigational use by, or under the direction of, an expert qualified by scientific training and experience to investigate the safety and effectiveness of such drug, medicine, compound, or device.

(d) A written statement signed by the expert has been filed with the board. The statement shall show what facilities the expert will use for the investigation to be conducted by him, and that the drug, medicine, compound, or device will be used solely by him or under his direction for the investigation. The statement shall contain information identifying any assistant or agent of the expert who uses the drug, medicine, compound, or device under the direction of the expert.

(e) Complete records of the investigation shall be kept by the expert and all records shall be made available by the expert for inspection upon the request of any agent of the board at any reasonable hour as long as the expert desires exemption.

(f) The expert shall inform any persons who participate in the investigation as patients, that such drug, medicine, compound, or device is being used for investigational purposes and shall obtain the consent of such persons or their representatives.

NOTE 3.

RENÉE C. FOX
EXPERIMENT PERILOUS*

* * *

The facts that the hormones with which the Metabolic Group was experimenting had unanticipated negative side effects on patients and that they were proving to be ameliorative rather

---

than curative, along with their difficulties in keeping alive and managing the clinical course of patients who had undergone radical experimental surgery, account for many of the stressful problems which these research physicians faced at the time this study was made.

"Viewed from a few years later, we seem rather sophomoric," a member of the Metabolic Group commented when he read this book in manuscript. "In fact, we *were* young," he went on to say, "relatively inexperienced and enthusiastic, with less good judgment and more immediate goals than are probably ideal for clinical investigation". . . .

[T]he members of the Group were young. The oldest among them was thirty-four years of age, the youngest twenty-eight, and the majority (seven) between the ages of thirty and thirty-one.

The members of the Group were not only young chronologically. They were also in a relatively early phase of their professional careers. All had completed their internships and served as residents. Two members of the Group had Ph.D. degrees (one in Pharmacology, the other in Biochemistry). All had done some teaching, some research (for the most part, basic rather than clinical research), and (with the exception of one physician) each had published several articles before joining the Group. (Eight members of the Group had published two articles; one had published four; and the physician with a Ph.D. in Pharmacology had published twelve articles.) Only one member of the Group had spent any time in practice (one and a half years).

These physicians were all seriously interested in having a career in academic medicine which would combine "work with patients, teaching, and clinical research." However, although committed to an academic career in this general sense, they were less decisive about some of its more specific aspects. They did not know exactly what kind of balance between caring for patients, teaching, and research they wished to strike permanently; and they were not yet sure about the kinds of metabolic-endocrine problems they would most like to investigate. In fact, without exception, these young physicians looked upon their affiliation with the Group as an opportunity to "get excellent fundamental training, in a very stimulating environment, in the field of metabolic-endocrine disease . . . to learn how to do clinical research in this area . . . to see how [they] would like this sort of research . . . [and] on that basis to definitely decide how much of

[their] professional career [they] would devote to it."

One final distinguishing characteristic of the Group as a whole was that they were exceptionally competent, select young physicians who had been carefully chosen by the Professor of Medicine who was their Chief on the basis of their demonstrated and potential abilities as clinicians and investigators.

* * *

f.

Deciding about Delegation of Authority to Control, Review, and Reformulate the Process?

[*i*]
New York Assembly
A Bill to Amend the Education Law, in
Relation to Scientific Research on Human
Subjects, to Provide for the Advancement
of Such Research through the Protection
of its Subjects, and to Establish a State
Board on Human Research*

* * *

Section 7801. *Legislative findings and declaration of purpose.* 1. It is hereby found that research and experimentation that employs human subjects, properly planned and conducted, is essential to the progress of medicine, psychology, and other sciences related to human health and contentment. Accompanying the progress of such sciences has been an unprecedented increase in the number of researches and experimentation that employ human subjects. The protection of the subject of such research and experimentation is found to be wholly consistent with the progress of scientific investigation, and a system of regulation that advances both is found to be in the public interest.

2. It is the purpose of this article to provide for the establishment and continuing development of regulations to govern the conduct of research and experimentation employing human subjects, in accordance with legislative guidelines, and to protect the human subject by regular review committees established by the several research institutions in the state, and by the establishment of a state board on human research to exercise general supervisory control over and to regulate research and experimentation using

---

* A. 1837, introduced January 13, 1971, by Assemblyman Leonard P. Stavisky.

human subjects, to such an extent as may be necessary.

*   *   *

§ 7803. *Definitions.* 1. Board means the state board on human research established by this article.

2. Institutional committee means the institution research review committee established by this article.

3. Research institution means any corporation, association, or other organization, including but not limited to a hospital, university, laboratory, and institute, that conducts or is responsible for conducting, or on whose premises there is conducted any human experimentation or research.

4. Human experimentation or research means the physical, medical, or psychological manipulation of human subjects for the purpose of observation and collection of data, unrelated to the furnishing of medical or psychological services, including diagnosis or therapy, to such subjects.

5. Investigator means the person directing or supervising human experimentation or research.

6. Subject or human subject means a human individual who is subjected to manipulation in human experimentation or research.

§ 7804. *Scope.* This act shall regulate all human experimentation or research conducted in this State. No investigator or research institution shall conduct any human experimentation or research without compliance with the provisions of this act.

§ 7805. *State board on human research.* 1. There is established within the department of education a state board on human research, to consist of nine members appointed by the governor with the advice of the board of regents. The membership of the board shall include five members who are licensed physicians and psychologists or other professiona persons with experience in human experimentation or research, and four members who include persons from non-scientific professional fields, such as social workers, teachers, and lawyers.* Members of the

_____
* The original draft of this bill, which was prepared by Prof. Frank Grad of Columbia University, included "representatives of the general public" as board members. *See* 169 *Annals of the New York Academy of Sciences* 542 (1970).

board shall serve overlapping terms of three years; of the members first appointed, however one-third shall serve for terms of one, two, and three years respectively. The governor shall designate the chairman.

2. The board shall meet at least once every three months and as often as necessary. A majority of the members shall constitute a quorum for the conduct of the board's business. The board shall keep a record of its proceedings. I shall make rules of procedure for its own conduct and for the calling of regular and special meetings upon notice.

3. Members of the board shall receive a per diem compensation of one hundred dollars and shall be reimbursed for actual and necessary expenses incurred in the performance of their duties.

4. The Board shall employ a staff director and, subject to applicable provision of the civil service law, a staff to assist it in the performance of its duties.

§ 7806. *State board on human research regulations; guidelines for human experimentation or research.* The board shall make rules and regulations, and at its discretion amend or repeal the same, for the conduct of human experimentation and research, and for the operation of institutional research review committees. In making rules and regulations, the board may make reasonable classifications and may differentiate in the applicability of its rules and regulations between different kinds of human experimentation or research, and may make separate rules and regulations for different kinds of psychological, medical or other scientific investigation as it may deem appropriate. All of the rules and regulations made by the board shall, however, be guided by and be consistent with the following standards:

a) The informed consent of the human subject or his guardian or representative as specified hereinafter is essential. This means that the person providing consent must have the legal capacity or authority to give consent; must be so situated as to be able to exercise free power of choice, without the intervention of any element of force, fraud, deceit, duress, overreaching, or other ulterior form of constraint or coercion; and must have sufficient knowledge and comprehension of the elements of the subject matter involved as to enable him to make an understanding and enlightened decision. This latter element requires that before the acceptance of an ffirmative decision by the subject or other person having authority to consent there shall be made known to him the nature, duration, and purpose of the experiment; the method and means by which it is to be conducted; all inconveniences and hazards reasonably to be expected; and the effects upon his health or person which may possibly result from the participation in the experiment.

b) The experiment should be such as to yield fruitful results for the good of society, unprocurable by other methods or means of study, and not random and unnecessary in nature.

c) The experiment should be so designed and based whenever feasible or appropriate on the results of animal experimentation and a knowledge of the natural history of the disease or other problem under study that the anticipated results will justify the performance of the experiment.

d) The experiment should be so conducted as to avoid all unnecessary physical and mental suffering and injury.

e) No experiment should be conducted where there is a prior reason to believe that death or disabling injury may occur.

f) The degree of risk taken should never exceed that determined by the humanitarian importance of the problem to be solved by the experiment.

g) Proper preparations should be made and adequate facilities provided to protect the subject against even the most remote possibilities of injury, disability, or death.

h) The experiment should be conducted only by scientifically qualified persons.

i) Procedures should be established to allow the subject to terminate the experiment at any time if he feels that he has reached the physical or mental state where continuation of the experiment seems to him to be impossible.

j) The experimenter should be prepared to terminate the experiment at any stage, if he has probable cause to believe, in the exercise of good faith, superior skill, and careful judgment that a continuation of the experiment is likely to result in injury, disability, or death to the subject.

§ 7807 *State board on human research; powers.* The board shall have jurisdiction over all human experimentation and research within the state. In pursuance of its jurisdiction, it shall have the following powers:

a) To review institutional rules for the conduct of human experimentation and research submitted to it by institutional committees, and to require changes or modifications in such rules;

b) To look into the conduct of any human experimentation and research, and to require the change or modification of the research design, or the suspension or termination of the human experimentation or research whenever the same fails to comply with the rules of the institutional committee, the rules and regulations of the board, or with the provisions of state or federal law or regulation, or when such research otherwise endangers the health and safety of the subjects.

c) To hold public hearings, conduct investigations, issue subpoenas and compel the attendance of witnesses; inspect research institutions; require the maintenance of adequate records by all investigators and research institutions, and to inspect and copy such records at all reasonable times in accordance with applicable legal provision governing such inspections.

d) To issue cease and desist orders for the protection of subjects and to take other measures to enforce the requirements of law and regulations, in accordance with the provisions of section 7809.

e) To issue advisory opinions with respect to proposed projects of human experimentation and research, or with respect to rules proposed by an institutional committee whenever requested to do so.

§ 7808 *Institutional research review committees; membership; powers and duties.* a) The chief administrative officer of a research institution shall establish an institutional research review committee to consist of no fewer than five and no more than fifteen members, to serve for fixed terms of not less than one year. The membership shall include at least two persons who are not scientists who engage in human experimentation or research, and such other persons as the board may require by rule or regulation. The committee shall take no action without the affirmative vote of a majority of its members. Each committee shall adopt its own rules of procedure.

b) Each institutional committee shall make rules for the conduct of human experimentation and research at the research institution. Such rules shall comply with the rules and regulations of the board and the requirements of law. The committee shall submit its rules to the board for review, but the research institute may operate pursuant to such rules until the board has ordered that they be modified or changed.

c) Each institutional committee shall review all proposals for human experimentation and research at the research institution for compliance with its own rules, with the rules and regulations of the board, and with the requirements of law, and no human experimentation or research shall be undertaken at any research institute unless it has been approved by its institutional committee. The institutional committee should not review a proposal unless it has been submitted in writing, in such form as may be required. The committee may require a modification of the research design and may require an opportunity to review the actual conduct of human experimentation and research as a condition of its approval. The committee may also request an advisory opinion from the board before giving its approval.

d) The committee shall maintain full records of its proceedings and deliberations, and of all proposals, reports, and other papers submitted to it, which shall be open to inspection by the board at all reasonable times.

e) No member of an institutional committee shall review a proposal in which he is the investigator.

§ 7809 *Enforcement; review.* a) When a research institution, institutional committee, or an investigator violates any provision of this article or of any rule or regulation made pursuant thereto, the board may serve a written notice of complaint specifying the nature of the violation upon the violator, and setting a reasonable time for compliance. If the respondent fails to comply, the board shall require him upon proper notice to answer the complaint at a hearing before the board, or before any designated committee or hearing officer of the board. The respondent may file an answer, appear with counsel, and submit testimony, and may request the board to exercise its power of subpoena to compel the attendance of witnesses with the production of papers on his behalf. The board may also apply to the supreme court for its assistance in the appearance of witnesses and the production of evidence. Testimony taken at hearings before the board shall be under oath and shall be recorded. After hearing and considering all of the evidence offered, or upon default of the appearance of the respondent, the board shall make such a final determination or order as it may deem appropriate to assure the respondent's future compliance with law and regulations.

b) Any final determination or order of the board shall be subject to review pursuant to article seventy-eight of the civil practice law and rules.

c) The board may bring an action for an injunction to compel compliance with its orders. In any such action for injunction, any determination of the board shall be *prima facie* evidence of the facts found therein.

d) In an emergency situation, the board may issue cease and desist and other appropriate orders in advance of employing the procedures provided in this section.

e) Nothing contained in this section shall prevent the board from seeking to obtain compliance by such informal and non-coercive means as it may deem appropriate.

§ 7810 *Subject's consent; strict liability.* a) No person's consent to become a subject shall be valid when there is a reasonable possibility that the particular human experimentation or research will result in death, serious injury, permanent or temporary physical impairment, or psychological injury.

b) Valid consent for an incompetent to become a subject may be given by his legal guardian if the human experimentation or research bears directly upon such incompetent's condition or disability.

c) Valid consent for a person under the age of eighteen years may be given by his parent or legal guardian only if there is no reason to believe that the human experimentation or research will result in physical or psychological injury or harm.

d) A written, witnessed statement is required for each subject as evidence of his consent. The statement shall include a written statement of the purposes of the experiment, the techniques to be employed, and the possible risks to the subject. Such statements are not conclusive evidence of consent and may be rebutted by other evidence or testimony of witnesses.*

*   *   *

---

* The draft bill further provided that: "e) Notwithstanding the valid and informed consent of a subject, the investigator and the research institution shall be absolutely liable, severally and jointly, for any damages resulting from any physical or psychological injury suffered by the subject in consequence of his participation in human experimentation or research." *See* 169 *Annals of the New York Academy of Sciences* 545 (1970).

[ii]
United States Public Health Service
Clinical Research and Investigation
Involving Human Beings*

Expanding Public Health Service support of clinical research and investigation involving human beings emphasizes the need for more formal attention to the critical issues raised by such research.

In December 1965 the National Advisory Health Council, after study of these critical issues, made certain recommendations to me which I have now formulated as the following Public Health Service grant policy:

No new, renewal, or continuation research or research training grant in support of clinical research and investigation involving human beings shall be awarded by the Public Health Service unless the grantee has indicated in the application the manner in which the grantee institution will provide prior review of the judgment of the principal investigator or program director by a committee of his institutional associates. This review should assure an independent determination: (1) of the rights and welfare of the individual or individuals involved, (2) of the appropriateness of the methods used to secure informed consent, and (3) of the risks and potential medical benefits of the investigation. A description of the committee of the associates who will provide the review shall be included in the application.

Effective immediately, this policy will be included in all future statements of Public Health Service research and research training grant policy. The wisdom and sound professional judgment of you and your staff will determine what constitutes the rights and welfare of human subjects in research, what constitutes informed consent, and what constitutes the risks and potential medical benefits of a particular investigation.

I wish to define more explicitly, however, what is meant by a committee of his institutional associates to assure an independent determination because the policy requires that the application include a description of the associates who will provide the review. The committee would need to be made up of staff of, or consultants to, your institution who are at the same time acquainted with the investigator under review, free to assess his judgment without placing in jeopardy their own goals, and sufficiently mature

and competent to make the necessary assessment. It is important that some of the members be drawn from different disciplines or interests that do not overlap those of the investigator under review.

The policy does not ask for the names of the members of the committee. It does ask for a description of its composition; e.g., the number of members and the professional or public interests they reflect.

I have directed all my staff who administer the initial review of applications for grants for clinical research and investigation involving human beings—regardless of whether these applications are for new, supplemental, renewal, or continuation support—to ascertain that each application includes the information required by this policy and to obtain this information, whenever necessary, in a document signed by both the principal investigator or program director and the official for the institution.

I know that you are as deeply concerned with this issue as are any of us in the Public Health Service. I urgently request that you give my staff your cooperation in making this policy an effective instrument for the good of the public and science.

NOTE

GUIDO CALABRESI
REFLECTIONS ON MEDICAL
EXPERIMENTATION IN HUMANS*

* * *

. . . No one has purposefully chosen the market method of controlling accidents, and no one, in our society, has the clear responsibility for making radical changes in the method. These facts happily leave us with the feeling that no one is directly responsible for any specific life taken and that neither as individuals nor as a society do we choose against lives in order to save money. Yet it remains true that we are unlikely to want to scrap the system of control that luckily has come into being. And to say this is precisely to say that a method which gives *satisfactory* control of the choice between lives and cost is operating without anyone bearing the onus of having purposefully chosen the method, let alone the onus of seeming to destroy individual lives

* Memorandum of Surgeon General William H. Stewart to the Heads of Institutions Conducting Research with Public Health Grants (February 8, 1966).

* 98 *Daedalus* 387, 393–394 (1969). Reprinted by permission of Daedalus, Journal of the American Academy of Arts and Sciences, Boston, Massachusetts.

for the sake of money. Since no adequate control system over medical experiments has arisen by itself, we cannot avoid the onus of working purposefully toward establishing a control system. This indicates that we will not end with so psychologically satisfactory a result as we have in the field of accidents. But, if anything, this fact heightens the need for establishing a system in which the actual choice over the taking of lives is as diffuse as possible.

Thus, the question remains as to whether or not we can find a control system in the medical experiment field that affords an adequate balancing of present against future lives and is still sufficiently indirect and self-enforcing as to avoid clear and purposive choices to kill individuals for the collective good. It is not my purpose in this article to suggest any complete control system for medical experiments. That task—even if feasible—would require an intimate knowledge of medicine. A few of the problems involved in establishing a control system and a few suggestions leading toward such a system can, however, be mentioned.

In the first place, a direct collective societal control—like approval of research plans by a qualified government agency—is not the answer. Not only is such a device likely to be too cumbersome but, perhaps more importantly, it seems to place the whole society in the position of openly approving the taking of individual lives. Analogy to accident law suggests that this situation is to be avoided if possible, and that the best role for the government is that of watchdog to step in and demand higher standards in specific situations where a general control system, independent of the government, has failed to work adequately.

Leaving the choice to the individual doctor might be all right were there some way to insure that such a choice would tend to coincide with the choice between present and future lives that society wants. No exact correspondence is needed (any more than we require the market to bring about a perfect correspondence between accidents and costs of avoiding them). But there must be the assurance that, on the whole, the individual choice will approach what society would choose. Unfortunately, there is no such assurance today. Some doctors will be too concerned with the individual patient and thereby sacrifice too many future lives by cutting off an experiment too soon. Others will be too concerned with the unassailability of their result and, therefore, continue an experiment beyond the point at

which society's interest in future lives is met. We cannot, moreover, rely on individual consciences to reduce these errors, because individual doctors do not and cannot know the degree to which our society wants present risks to be taken for future benefits. And the best a conscience can do is make individuals adhere to society's wants as these are made known by society. In contrast, the beauty of the accident system, with all its faults, is that through the market it conveys to individual deciders what society more or less wants without requiring an identifiable societal statement. (Furthermore it relies on self-interest rather than conscience to effectuate even this decision.)

*   *   *

2.
In Administering Research

a.

Who Should Participate, within What Structure, in State Regulation?

[i]

*Eighty-seventh Congress, Second Session
An Act to Protect the Public Health by
Amending the Federal Food, Drug, and
Cosmetic Act to Assure the Safety,
Effectiveness, and Reliability of Drugs . . .
and for Other Purposes**

§ 355. New drugs—Necessity of effective approval of application.

(a) No person shall introduce or deliver for introduction into interstate commerce any new drug, unless an approval of an application filed pursuant to subsection (b) of this section is effective with respect to such drug.

Filing application; contents

(b) Any person may file with the Secretary an application with respect to any drug subject to the provisions of subsection (a) of this section. Such person shall submit to the Secretary as a part of the application (1) full reports of investigations which have been made to show whether or not such drug is safe for use and whether such drug is effective in use; (2) a full list of the arti-

---
* Act of October 10, 1962, Pub. Law No. 87–781, §§ 102(b)–(d), 103(a)–(b), 104(a)–(d2), 76 Stat. 781–785; *see* 21 U.S.C. § 355 (1964).

cles used as components of such drug; (3) a full statement of the composition of such drug; (4) a full description of the methods used in, and the facilities and controls used for, the manufacture, processing, and packing of such drug; (5) such samples of such drug and of the articles used as components thereof as the Secretary may require; and (6) specimens of the labeling proposed to be used for such drug.

Period for approval of application; period for, notice, and expedition of hearing; period for issuance of order

(c) Within one hundred and eighty days after the filing of an application under this subsection, or such additional period as may be agreed upon by the Secretary and the applicant, the Secretary shall either—

(1) approve the application if he then finds that none of the grounds for denying approval specified in subsection (d) of this section applies, or

(2) give the applicant notice of an opportunity for a hearing before the Secretary under subsection (d) of this section on the question whether such application is approvable. If the applicant elects to accept the opportunity for hearing by written request within thirty days after such notice, such hearing shall commence not more than ninety days after the expiration of such thirty days unless the Secretary and the applicant otherwise agree. Any such hearing shall thereafter be conducted on an expedited basis and the Secretary's order thereon shall be issued within ninety days after the date fixed by the Secretary for filing final briefs.

Grounds for refusing application; approval of application; "substantial evidence" defined

(d) If the Secretary finds, after due notice to the applicant in accordance with subsection (c) of this section and giving him an opportunity for a hearing, in accordance with said subsection, that (1) the investigations, reports of which are required to be submitted to the Secretary pursuant to subsection (b) of this section, do not include adequate tests by all methods reasonably applicable to show whether or not such drug is safe for use under the conditions prescribed, recommended, or suggested in the proposed labeling thereof; (2) the results of such tests show that such drug is unsafe for use under such conditions or do not show that such drug is safe for

use under such conditions; (3) the methods used in, and the facilities and controls used for, the manufacture, processing, and packing of such drug are inadequate to preserve its identity, strength, quality, and purity; (4) upon the basis of the information submitted to him as part of the application, or upon the basis of any other information before him with respect to such drug, he has insufficient information to determine whether such drug is safe for use under such conditions; or (5) evaluated on the basis of the information submitted to him as part of the application and any other information before him with respect to such drug, there is a lack of substantial evidence that the drug will have the effect it purports or is represented to have under the conditions of use prescribed, recommended, or suggested in the proposed labeling thereof; or (6) based on a fair evaluation of all material facts, such labeling is false or misleading in any particular; he shall issue an order refusing to approve the application. If, after such notice and opportunity for hearing, the Secretary finds that clauses (1) through (6) do not apply, he shall issue an order approving the application. As used in this subsection and subsection (e) of this section, the term "substantial evidence" means evidence consisting of adequate and well-controlled investigations, including clinical investigations, by experts qualified by scientific training and experience to evaluate the effectiveness of the drug involved, on the basis of which it could fairly and responsibly be concluded by such experts that the drug will have the effect it purports or is represented to have under the conditions of use prescribed, recommended, or suggested in the labeling or proposed labeling thereof.

Withdrawal of approval; grounds; immediate suspension upon finding imminent hazard to public health

(e) The Secretary shall, after due notice and opportunity for hearing to the applicant, withdraw approval of an application with respect to any drug under this section if the Secretary finds (1) that clinical or other experience, tests, or other scientific data show that such drug is unsafe for use under the conditions of use upon the basis of which the application was approved; (2) that new evidence of clinical experience, not contained in such application or not available to the Secretary until after such application was approved, or tests by new methods, or tests by methods not deemed reasonably applicable when such application was approved, evaluated together with the evidence available to the Secretary when the application was approved, shows that such drug is not shown to be safe for use under the conditions of use upon the basis of which the application was approved; or (3) on the basis of new information before him with respect to such drug, evaluated together with the evidence available to him when the application was approved, that there is a lack of substantial evidence that the drug will have the effect it purports or is represented to have under the conditions of use prescribed, recommended, or suggested in the labeling thereof; or (4) that the application contains any untrue statement of a material fact: *Provided,* That if the Secretary (or in his absence the officer acting as Secretary) finds that there is an imminent hazard to the public health, he may suspend the approval of such application immediately, and give the applicant prompt notice of his action and afford the applicant the opportunity for an expedited hearing under this subsection; but the authority conferred by this proviso to suspend the approval of an application shall not be delegated. The Secretary may also, after due notice and opportunity for hearing to the applicant, withdraw the approval of an application with respect to any drug under this section if the Secretary finds (1) that the applicant has failed to establish a system for maintaining required records, or has repeatedly or deliberately failed to maintain such records or to make required reports, in accordance with a regulation or order under subsection (j) of this section, or the applicant has refused to permit access to, or copying or verification of, such records as required by paragraph (2) of such subsection; or (2) that on the basis of new information before him, evaluated together with the evidence before him when the application was approved, the methods used in, or the facilities and controls used for, the manufacture, processing, and packing of such drug are inadequate to assure and preserve its identity, strength, quality, and purity and were not made adequate within a reasonable time after receipt of written notice from the Secretary specifying the matter complained of; or (3) that on the basis of new information before him, evaluated together with the evidence before him when the application was approved, the labeling of such drug, based on a fair evaluation of all material facts, is false or misleading in any particular and was not corrected within a reasonable time after receipt of written notice from the Secretary specifying the matter complained of. Any order under this subsection shall state the findings upon which it is based.

Revocation of order refusing, withdrawing, or suspending approval of application

(f) Whenever the Secretary finds that the facts so require, he shall revoke any previous order under subsection (d) or (e) of this section refusing, withdrawing, or suspending approval of an application and shall approve such application or reinstate such approval, as may be appropriate.

* * *

Appeal from order

(h) An appeal may be taken by the applicant from an order of the Secretary refusing or withdrawing approval of an application under this section. Such appeal shall be taken by filing in the United States court of appeals for the circuit wherein such applicant resides or has his principal place of business, or in the United States Court of Appeals for the District of Columbia Circuit, within sixty days after the entry of such order, a written petition praying that the order of the Secretary be set aside. . . .

Exemptions of drugs for research; discretionary and mandatory conditions; direct reports to Secretary

(i) The Secretary shall promulgate regulations for exempting from the operation of the foregoing subsections of this section drugs intended solely for investigational use by experts qualified by scientific training and experience to investigate the safety and effectiveness of drugs. Such regulations may, within the discretion of the Secretary, among other conditions relating to the protection of the public health, provide for conditioning such exemption upon—

(1) the submission to the Secretary, before any clinical testing of a new drug is undertaken, of reports, by the manufacturer or the sponsor of the investigation of such drug, or preclinical tests (including tests on animals) of such drug adequate to justify the proposed clinical testing;

(2) the manufacturer or the sponsor of the investigation of a new drug proposed to be distributed to investigators for clinical testing obtaining a signed agreement from each of such investigators that patients to whom the drug is administered will be under his personal supervision, or under the supervision of investigators responsible to

him, and that he will not supply such drug to any other investigator, or to clinics, for administration to human beings; and

(3) the establishment and maintenance of such records, and the making of such reports to the Secretary, by the manufacturer or the sponsor of the investigation of such drug, of data (including but not limited to analytical reports by investigators) obtained as the result of such investigational use of such drug, as the Secretary finds will enable him to evaluate the safety and effectiveness of such drug in the event of the filing of an application pursuant to subsection (b) of this section.

Such regulations shall provide that such exemption shall be conditioned upon the manufacturer, or the sponsor of the investigation, requiring that experts using such drugs for investigational purposes certify to such manufacturer or sponsor that they will inform any human beings to whom such drugs, or any controls used in connection therewith, are being administered, or their representatives, that such drugs are being used for investigational purposes and will obtain the consent of such human beings or their representatives, except where they deem it not feasible or, in their professional judgment, contrary to the best interests of such human beings. Nothing in this subsection shall be construed to require any clinical investigator to submit directly to the Secretary reports on the investigational use of drugs.

Records and reports; required information; regulations and orders; access to records

(j) (1) In the case of any drug for which an approval of an application filed pursuant to this section is in effect, the applicant shall establish and maintain such records, and make such reports to the Secretary, of data relating to clinical experience and other data or information, received or otherwise obtained by such applicant with respect to such drug, as the Secretary may by general regulation, or by order with respect to such application, prescribe on the basis of a finding that such records and reports are necessary in order to enable the Secretary to determine, or facilitate a determination, whether there is or may be ground for invoking subsection (e) of this section: *Provided, however,* That regulations and orders issued under this subsection and under subsection (i) of this section shall have due regard for the professional ethics of the medical profession and the interests of patients and

shall provide, where the Secretary deems it to be appropriate, for the examination, upon request, by the persons to whom such regulations or orders are applicable, of similar information received or otherwise by the Secretary.

(2) Every person required under this section to maintain records, and every person in charge or custody thereof, shall, upon request of an officer or employee designated by the Secretary, permit such officer or employee at all reasonable times to have access to and copy and verify such records. . . .

*   *   *

NOTES

NOTE 1.

ALFRED GILMAN
RESPONSIBILITIES OF THE ACADEMIC
MEDICAL SCIENCES AND THE PROFESSION IN
THE EVALUATION OF DRUGS*

*   *   *

[In 1962] there were no statutes in the United States that required the proof of efficacy of drugs. All that was demanded was the proof of safety and these demands were not very stringent. At this time, the Kefauver Committee of the United States Senate was investigating the drug industry—not in terms of the efficacy and safety of drugs but rather in terms of the economics of the industrial profits. By a rare coincidence, the time of these hearings coincided with the dramatic and explosive disclosure of the convincing evidence of the teratogenicity of thalidomide. Profit motives became a secondary issue and safety and efficacy of drugs primary. The result of this unique juxtaposition of events was the passage of the Kefauver-Harris amendment to the U.S. Pure Food and Drug Laws, the first such amendment since 1938. . . . A major feature of the amendment required proof of efficacy as well as safety of a drug. Extensive toxicity data in animals and the submission of an Investigation of a New Drug application were required before a drug could be tested in man. Detailed protocols for the testing of the efficacy of a drug in man were outlined. Toxicity tests in animals were made much more stringent before a New Drug Application could be approved. Mechanisms for reporting the untoward effects

---

* *Evaluation of Drugs: Whose Responsibility?* Liége: Council for International Organizations of Medical Sciences 15–18 (1970). Reprinted by permission.

of new drugs as well as those already on the market also were made more stringent.

No one could take serious exception to these logical demands, and though it meant greatly increased research and development costs to the drug industry, insofar as I know it did not in any way diminish research activities. However, a federal agency was given the full responsibility of assessing the adequacy of the data submitted by the pharmaceutical industry with respect to the safety as well as the efficacy of a drug. Needless to say, the lines of battle were quickly drawn. New drug applications were returned by the score with comments from the Commissioner of the Food and Drug Administration that pharmaceutical research by industry was poorly conducted, inadequately controlled and directed toward selfish interests. The response from the industry was predictable. The research efforts of their eminent scientists and outstanding clinical investigators were being judged by a group of individuals whose background and training were inadequate for their responsibilities.

[A] second provision of the Kefauver-Harris amendments of 1962 . . . stated that all drugs marketed under a New Drug Application between years 1938 and 1962 be reevaluated by the Food and Drug Administration for the newly required proof of efficacy as well as the former requirement relating only to safety. If efficacy was questionable, the drug was to be withdrawn from the market. . . . A physician who is deprived of a new drug by a federal dictate, a drug that he has never had occasion to use— or one of whose potential or existence he may be unaware—will have little or no reaction if a governmental agency denies a New Drug Application. On the other hand, if he is deprived of a drug that he has used in his own practice for a period up to thirty years, what will be his reaction when this decision for revocation has been made by a government agency?

It is little wonder that the Food and Drug Administration, overwhelmed by their new responsibilities as a result of the Kefauver-Harris amendments, chose to procrastinate on implementing its retroactive features. But Congress was not to be denied. Therefore in 1966, Commissioner Goddard of the Food and Drug Administration addressed a memorandum to President Seitz of the National Academy of Sciences, requesting the Academy to act as an advisory body to the Food and Drug Administration to ascertain the efficacy of all drugs introduced into therapy between the years 1938 and 1962. I need

not emphasize . . . the enormity of this task. These were golden years of pharmacotherapy, spanning the time from the early sulfonamide days to the very recent past. Close to 4,000 drugs were involved, single entities and combinations, requiring more than 10,000 decisions of efficacy because many drugs made several therapeutic claims.

*   *   *

To make a long story short, the request of Dr. Goddard was approved by the subcommittee and later by the Governing Board of the National Academy of Sciences, since the Academy is advisory to government agencies and this was a request for a single, albeit an enormous advisory, task but not one of a continuing nature.

The implementation of the Efficacy Review can be summarized briefly. Thirty panels, the members of which were experts in all representative areas of drug therapy, were designated. Each panel consisted of a chairman and five members. Nominations for chairmen and membership of the panels were received from their peers, usually from professional societies, and the selection was made by an Advisory Board to the Drug Efficacy Study. Almost invariably the panel members were academicians. . . . The organizational arrangements were achieved within a period of three months and at the present time, just two years later, practically all efficacy decisions have been made and most are already in the hands of the Food and Drug Administration.

*   *   *

Why did Commissioner Goddard and other administrative officials of the Food and Drug Administration request the advisory help from the National Academy of Sciences? They could have set up advisory panels under their own supervision.

Did they feel that outstanding academicians would perform their arduous task at the request of the National Academy of Sciences and refuse to serve in a similar capacity for the Food and Drug Administration, a federal bureau?

Did they feel that the strict conflict of interest regulations of governmental agencies precluded the possibility of enlisting the best minds in academic medicine—many of whom consult for pharmaceutical industries?

Did they anticipate unfavorable decisions with respect to the efficacy of drugs in current use that would largely absolve the Food and

Drug Administration from further conflict with organized medicine and pharmaceutical industry?

Did they feel that standards of academic medicine would be equally or more demanding than those of the Food and Drug Administration although based upon somewhat different criteria?

Were they truly concerned with raising the level of drug therapy, and therefore sought the knowledge and prestige of the National Academy?

Was this purely a device to placate the Congress and allow the Food and Drug Administration to catch up with a large backlog of unfinished business, since all future decisions as to efficacy would be in their hands?

Do they have any intention to involve academic medicine in future decisions of drug efficacy?

*   *   *

[T]he review in my mind has been an unqualified success. The panels have worked diligently, and interest of the participants in general has been high. In many instances panels, in addition to their evaluation of individual drugs, have written comprehensive reports outlining the criteria for good therapeutic practices in their particular field. Some contemplate similar reviews to be published in the open literature. In brief, in my opinion, the study has been a great academic success. However, not all panel chairmen were equally enthusiastic about their responsibilities. In fact, one wrote to me that it was a particularly arduous and unrewarding task.

It must be borne in mind that this was a single, non-continuing review. Evaluations of efficacy were based on the published literature and the panel's background of experience. No one was evaluating drugs outside of the area of his own particular interests. What would be the reaction of the panel members if asked to continue these reviews indefinitely and base their evaluations on the volumes of data submitted by the pharmaceutical industry relating both to animal and clinical experimentation, the latter largely in the form of individual case reports? I doubt that many of these busy academicians would accept an invitation for continuous consultant activity to the Food and Drug Administration, and I doubt if the responses would be much more enthusiastic if the National Academy of Sciences were still involved.

*   *   *

NOTE 2.

FREEMAN H. QUIMBY
MEDICAL EXPERIMENTATION ON
HUMAN BEINGS*

*   *   *

The chart below shows a marked reduction in the production of new pharmaceutical specialties since 1959. This includes all forms of new products as well as new single chemical drugs.

	New Single Chemicals	Total Number of New Products Marketed
1955	31	403
1956	42	401
1957	51	400
1958	44	370
1959	63	315
1960	45	311
1961	41	265
1962	28	255
1963	18	213
1964	17	162
1965	23	119
1966	13	82

These data may reflect the now slower process of obtaining approved New Drug Applications from FDA since the enactment of the 1962 amendments, or they may not. Since the downtrend predates the amendments, it is difficult to point to the amendments as the cause of any effect except possibly the continuation of the trend since 1962. The low number of new single chemicals marketed in 1966 (13) and the total number of new products (82) is a bit on the alarming side in view of the nation's overall competence in organic and pharmaceutical chemistry and in view of the large amounts of funds invested by government and industry for developing new drugs. Research and Development spending by both government and drug firms has been especially high in recent years in the areas of cancer chemotherapy, psychopharmicals, vaccines, and antibiotics. It is unlikely that the 1966 data in the above chart reflect the July 1, 1966, policies from Bethesda or the August 24, 1966, "patient consent in writing" policy of FDA.

---

* Washington, D.C.: Library of Congress Reference Service 80–81 (1967). Reprinted by permission.

The low number of new drugs in some categories probably indicates industrial efforts to concentrate research on more original and effective drugs and perhaps on newer methods of comparative physiology and chemical testing. The purpose of these new methods is to "signal" the promise, or lack of it, of a new chemical without the risk and expense of human trials. Fewer products and the extensive technical information required by FDA, of course, increase the cost per product. The Pharmaceutical Manufacturers Association now estimates the average cost of a single fundamental new drug entity at $5 million. DuPont's "Symmetril" cost $8 million dollars. . . .

*   *   *

NOTE 3.

CODE OF FEDERAL REGULATIONS
TITLE 21—FOOD AND DRUGS (1971)

§ *130.3. New drugs for investigational use in human beings; exemptions from section 505*(a).*

(a) A shipment or other delivery of a new drug shall be exempt from section 505(a) of the act if all the following conditions are met:

(1) The label of such drug bears the statement "Caution: New drug—Limited by Federal (or United States) law to investigational use."

(2) The person claiming the exemption has filed with the Food and Drug Administration a completed and signed "Notice of Claimed Investigational Exemption for a New Drug" in triplicate–with the information shown below in form FD 1571; and not less than 30 days have elapsed following the date of receipt of the notice by the Food and Drug Administration; and the Food and Drug Administration has not, prior to expiration of such 30-day interval, requested that the sponsor continue to withhold or to restrict use of the drug in human subjects. The 30-day delay requirement may be waived by the Food and Drug Administration upon a showing of good reason for such waiver.

[Form FD–1571 appears on the pages which follow.]

Provided, however, That where a new drug limited to investigational use is proposed for shipment to a foreign country and the circumstances are such that the submission of the "Notice of

---

* Section 505 refers to the numbering of 21 U.S.C. § 355 as it appeared in the Federal Food, Drug, and Cosmetic Act of June 25, 1938, 52 Stat. 1040, as amended.

Claimed Investigational Exemption for a New Drug" (Form FD 1571) is not feasible, the Commissioner may authorize the shipment of the drug if he receives, through the U.S. Department of State, a formal request to allow such shipment from the government of the country to which the drug is proposed to be shipped. This request should specify that said government has adequate information about the drug and its proposed use and is satisfied that the drug may legally be used by the intended consignee in that country.

(3) Each shipment or delivery is made in accordance with the commitments in the "Notice of claimed investigational exemption for a new drug."

(4) The sponsor maintains adequate records showing the investigator to whom shipped, date, quantity, and batch or code mark of each such shipment and delivery, until 2 years after a new-drug application is approved for the drug; *or,* if an application is not approved, until 2 years after shipment and delivery of the drug for investigational use is discontinued and the Food and Drug Administration has been so notified. Upon the request of a scientifically trained and properly authorized employee of the Department at reasonable times, the sponsor makes the records referred to in this subparagraph and in subparagraph (2) of this paragraph available for inspection, and upon written request submits such records or copies of them to the Food and Drug Administration.

(5) The sponsor monitors the progress of the investigations and currently evaluates the evidence relating to the safety and effectiveness of the drug as it is obtained from the investigators. Accurate progress reports of the investigations and significant findings, together with any significant changes in the informational material supplied to investigators, shall be submitted to the Food and Drug Administration at reasonable intervals, not exceeding 1 year. All reports of the investigation shall be retained until 2 years after a new-drug application is approved for the drug; or, if an application is not approved, until 2 years after shipment and delivery of the drug for investigational use is discontinued and the Food and Drug Administration so notified. Upon request of a scientifically trained and properly authorized employee of the Department, at reasonable times, these reports shall be made available for inspection, and on written request copies of these reports shall be submitted to the Food and Drug Administration.

DEPARTMENT OF HEALTH, EDUCATION, AND WELFARE
PUBLIC HEALTH SERVICE
FOOD AND DRUG ADMINISTRATION

Form Approved
OMB No. 57-R0030

NOTICE OF
CLAIMED INVESTIGATIONAL EXEMPTION
FOR A NEW DRUG

Name of Sponsor_____

Address _____

Date _____

Name of Investigational Drug _____

Commissioner
Food and Drug Administration
Bureau of Drugs (BD-26)
5600 Fishers Lane
Rockville, Maryland 20852

Dear Sir:

The sponsor, _____ , submits
this notice of claimed investigational exemption for a new drug under the provisions of section 505(i) of the
Federal Food, Drug, and Cosmetic Act and §130.3 of Title 21 of the Code of Federal Regulations.

Attached hereto, in triplicate, are:

1. The best available descriptive name of the drug, including to the extent known the chemical name and structure of any new-drug substance, and a statement of how it is to be administered. (If the drug has only a code name, enough information should be supplied to identify the drug.)

2. Complete list of components of the drug, including any reasonable alternates for inactive components.

3. Complete statement of quantitative composition of drug, including reasonable variations that may be expected during the investigational stage.

4. Description of source and preparation of, any new-drug substances used as components, including the name and address of each supplier or processor, other than the sponsor of each new-drug substance.

5. A statement of the methods, facilities, and controls used for the manufacturing, processing, and packing of the new drug to establish and maintain appropriate standards of identity, strength, quality, and purity as needed for safety and to give significance to clinical investigations made with the drug.

6. A statement covering all information available to the sponsor derived from preclinical investigations and any clinical studies and experience with the drug as follows:

a. Adequate information about the preclinical investigations, including studies made on laboratory animals, on the basis of which the sponsor has concluded that it is reasonably safe to initiate clinical investigations with the drug: Such information should include identification of the person who conducted each investigation; identification and qualifications of the individuals who evaluated the results and concluded that it is reasonably safe to initiate clinical investigations with the drug and a statement of where the investigations were conducted and where the records are available for inspection; and enough details about the investigations to permit scientific review. The preclinical investigations shall not be considered adequate to justify clinical testing unless they give proper attention to the conditions of the proposed clinical testing. When this information, the outline of the plan of clinical pharmacology, or any progress report on the clinical pharmacology, indicates a need for full review of the preclinical data before a clinical trial is undertaken, the Department will notify the sponsor to submit the complete preclinical data and to withhold clinical trials until the review is completed and the sponsor notified. The Food and Drug Administration will be prepared to confer with the sponsor concerning this action.

b. If the drug has been marketed commercially or investigated (e.g. outside the United States), complete information about such distribution or investigation shall be submitted, along with a complete bibliography of any publications about the drug.

c. If the drug is a combination of previously investigated or marketed drugs, an adequate summary of pre-existing information from preclinical and clinical investigations and experience with its components, including all reports available to the sponsor suggesting side-effects, contraindications, and ineffectiveness in use of such components: Such summary should include an adequate bibliography of publications about the components and may incorporate by reference any information concerning such components previously submitted by the sponsor to the Food and Drug Administration. Include a statement of the expected pharmacological effects of the combination.

7. A total of three copies of all informational material, including label and labeling, which is to be supplied to each investigator: This shall include an accurate description of the prior investigations and experience and their results pertinent to the safety and possible usefulness of the drug under the conditions of the investigation. It shall not represent that the safety or usefulness of the drug has been established for the purposes to be investigated. It shall describe all relevant hazards, contraindications, side-effects, and precautions suggested by prior investigations and experience with the drug under investigation and related drugs for the information of clinical investigators.

8. The scientific training and experience considered appropriate by the sponsor to qualify the investigators as suitable experts to investigate the safety of the drug, bearing in mind what is known about the pharmacological action of the drug and the phase of the investigational program that is to be undertaken.

9. The names and a summary of the training and experience of each investigator and of the individual charged with monitoring the progress of the investigation and evaluating the evidence of safety and effectiveness of the drug as it is received from the investigators, together with a statement that the sponsor has obtained from each investigator a completed and signed form, as provided in subparagraph (12) or (13) of this paragraph, and that the investigator is qualified by scientific training and experience as an appropriate expert to undertake the phase of the investigation outlined in section 10 of the "Notice of Claimed Investigational Exemption| for a New Drug." (In crucial situations, phase 3 investigators may be added and this form supplemented by rapid communication methods, and the signed form FD 1573 shall be obtained promptly thereafter.)

10. An outline of any phase or phases of the planned investigations and a description of the institutional review committee, as follows:

a. Clinical pharmacology. This is ordinarily divided into two phases: Phase 1 starts when the new drug is first introduced into man--only animal and in vitro data are available--with the purpose of determining human toxicity, metabolism, absorption, elimination, and other pharmacological action, preferred route of administration, and safe dosage range; phase 2 covers the initial trials on a limited number of patients for specific disease control or prophylaxis purposes. A general outline of these phases shall be submitted, identifying the investigator or investigators, the hospitals or research facilities where the clinical pharmacology will be undertaken, any expert committees or panels to be utilized, the maximum number of subjects to be involved, and the estimated duration of these early phases of investigation. Modification of the experimental design on the basis of experience gained need be reported only in the progress reports on these early phases, or in the development of the plan for the clinical trial, phase 3. The first two phases may overlap and, when indicated, may require additional animal data before these phases can be completed or phase 3 can be undertaken. Such animal tests shall be designed to take into account the expected duration of administration of the drug to human beings, the age groups and physical status, as for example, infants, pregnant women, premenopausal women, of those human beings to whom the drug may be administered, unless this has already been done in the original animal studies.

b. Clinical trial. This phase 3 provides the assessment of the drug's safety and effectiveness and optimum dosage schedules in the diagnosis, treatment, or prophylaxis of groups of subjects involving a given disease or condition. A reasonable protocol is developed on the basis of the facts accumulated in the earlier phases, including completed and submitted animal studies. This phase is conducted by separate groups following the same protocol (with reasonable variations and alternatives permitted by the plan) to produce well-controlled clinical data. For this phase, the following data shall be submitted:

i. The names and addresses of the investigators. (Additional investigators may be added.)

ii. The specific nature of the investigations to be conducted, together with information or case report forms to show the scope and detail of the planned clinical observations and the clinical laboratory tests to be made and reported.

iii. The approximate number of subjects (a reasonable range of subjects is permissible and additions may be made), and criteria proposed for subject selection by age, sex, and condition.

iv. The estimated duration of the clinical trial and the intervals, not exceeding 1 year, at which progress reports showing the results of the investigations will be submitted to the Food and Drug Administration.

(The notice of claimed investigational exemption may be limited to any one or more phases, provided the outline of the additional phase or phases is submitted before such additional phases begin. This does not preclude continuing a subject on the drug from phase 2 to phase 3 without interruption while the plan for phase 3 is being developed.)

Ordinarily, a plan for clinical trial will not be regarded as reasonable unless, among other things, it provides for more than one independent competent investigator to maintain adequate case histories of an adequate number of subjects, designed to record observations and permit evaluation of any and all discernible effects attributable to the drug in each individual treated, and comparable records on any individuals employed as controls. These records shall be individual records for each subject maintained to include adequate information pertaining to each, including age, sex, conditions treated, dosage, frequency of administration of the drug, results of all relevant clinical observations and laboratory examinations made, adequate information concerning any other treatment given and a full statement of any adverse effects and useful results observed, together with an opinion as to whether such effects or results are attributable to the drug under investigation.

c. Institutional review committee. If the phases of clinical study as described under 10a and b above are conducted on institutionalized subjects or are conducted by an individual affiliated with an institution which agrees to assume responsibility for the study, assurance must be given that an institutional review committee is responsible for initial and continuing review and approval of the proposed clinical study. The membership must be comprised of sufficient members of varying background, that is, lawyers, clergymen, or laymen as well as scientists, to assure complete and adequate review of the research project. The membership must possess not only broad competence to comprehend the nature of the project, but also other competencies necessary to judge the acceptability of the project or activity in terms of institutional regulations, relevant law, standards of professional practice, and community acceptance. Assurance must be presented that neither the sponsor nor the investigator has participated in selection of committee members; that the review committee does not allow participation in its review and conclusions by any individual involved in the conduct of the research activity under review (except to provide information to the committee); that the investigator will report to the committee for review any emergent problems, serious adverse reactions, or proposed procedural changes which may affect the status of the investigation and that no such change will be made without committee approval except where necessary to eliminate apparent immediate hazards; that reviews of the study will be conducted by the review committee at intervals appropriate to the degree of risk, but not exceeding 1 year, to assure that the research project is being conducted in compliance with the committee's understanding and recommendations: that the review committee is provided all the information on the research project necessary for its complete review of the project; and that the review committee maintains adequate documentation of its activities and develops adequate procedures for reporting its findings to the institution. The documents maintained by the committee are to include the names and qualifications of committee members, records of information provided to subjects in obtaining informed consent, committee discussion on substantive issues and their resolution, committee recommendations, and dated reports of successive reviews as they are performed. Copies of all documents are to be retained for a period of 3 years past the completion or discontinuance of the study and are to be made available upon request to duly authorized representatives of the Food and Drug Administration. (Favorable recommendations by the committee are subject to further appropriate review and rejection by institution officials. Unfavorable recommendations, restrictions, or conditions may not be overruled by the institution officials.) Procedures for the organization and operation of institutional review committees are contained in guidelines issued pursuant to Chapter 1-40 of the Grants Administration Manual of the U.S. Department of Health, Education, and Welfare, available from the U.S. Government Printing Office. It is recommended that these guidelines be followed in establishing institutional review committees and that the committees function according to the procedures described therein. A signing of the Form FD 1571 will be regarded as providing the above necessary assurances. If the institution, however, has on file with the Department of Health, Education, and Welfare, Division of Research Grants, National Institutes of Health, an "accepted general assurance," and the same committee is to review the proposed study using the same procedures, this is acceptable in lieu of the above assurances and a statement to this effect should be provided with the signed FD 1571. (In addition to sponsor's continuing responsibility to monitor the study, the Food and Drug Administration will undertake investiga-

tions in institutions periodically to determine whether the committees are operating in accord with the assurances given by the sponsor.)

11. It is understood that the sponsor will notify the Food and Drug Administration if the investigation is discontinued, and the reason therefor.

12. It is understood that the sponsor will notify each investigator if a new-drug application is approved, or if the investigation is discontinued.

13. If the drug is to be sold, a full explanation why sale is required and should not be regarded as the commercialization of a new drug for which an application is not approved.

14. A statement that the sponsor assures that clinical studies in humans will not be initiated prior to 30 days after the date of receipt of the notice by the Food and Drug Administration and that he will continue to withold or to restrict clinical studies if requested to do so by the Food and Drug Administration prior to the expiration of such 30 days. If such request is made, the sponsor will be provided specific information as to the deficiencies and will be afforded a conference on request. The 30-day delay may be waived by the Food and Drug Administration upon a showing of good reason for such waiver; and for investigations subject to institutional review committee approval as described in item 10c above, an additional statement assuring that the investigation will not be initiated prior to approval of the study by such committee.

Very truly yours,

SPONSOR	PER
	INDICATE AUTHORITY

(This notice may be amended or supplemented from time to time on the basis of the experience gained with the new drug. Progress reports may be used to update the notice.)

ALL NOTICES AND CORRESPONDENCE SHOULD BE SUBMITTED IN TRIPLICATE.

(6) The sponsor shall promptly investigate and report to the Food and Drug Administration and to all investigators any findings associated with use of the drug that may suggest significant hazards, contraindications, side effects, and precautions pertinent to the safety of the drug. If the finding is alarming, it shall be reported immediately and the clinical investigation discontinued until the finding is adequately evaluated and a decision reached that it is safe to proceed.

(7) If the investigations adduce facts showing that there is substantial doubt that they may be continued safely in relation to the drug's potential therapeutic effects, the sponsor shall promptly discontinue the investigation, notify all investigators and the Food and Drug Administration, recall all stocks of the drug outstanding, and furnish the Food and Drug Administration with a full report of the reason for discontinuing the investigation. The Food and Drug Administration will be prepared to confer with the sponsor on the need to discontinue the investigation.

(8) The sponsor shall discontinue shipments or deliveries of the new drug to any investigator who has repeatedly or deliberately failed to maintain or make available his records or reports of his investigations.

(9) The sponsor shall not unduly prolong distribution of the drug for investigational use but shall submit an application for the drug pursuant to section 505(b) of the act (or give reasons for not submitting such application, or a statement that the investigation has been discontinued and the reasons therefor):

(i) With reasonable promptness after finding that the results of such investigation appear to establish the safety and effectiveness of the drug; or

(ii) Within 60 days after receipt of a written request for such an application from the Commissioner.

(10) Neither the sponsor nor any person acting for or on behalf of the sponsor shall disseminate any promotional material representing that the drug being distributed interstate for investigational use is safe or useful for the purposes for which it is under investigation. This regulation is not intended to restrict the full exchange of scientific information concerning the drug, including dissemination of scientific findings in scientific or lay communications media; its sole intent is to restrict promotional claims of safety or effectiveness by the sponsor while the drug is under investigation to establish its safety or effectiveness.

(11) The sponsor shall not commercially distribute nor test-market the drug until a new-drug application is approved pursuant to section 505(b) of the act.

(12) The sponsor shall obtain from each investigator involved in clinical pharmacology a signed statement in the following form:

[Form FD–1572 appears on the pages which follow.]

(13) The sponsor shall obtain from each investigator involved in clinical trials a signed statement in the following form:

[Form FD–1573 appears on the pages which follow.]

*   *   *

(c) (1) Whenever the Food and Drug Administration has information indicating that an investigator has repeatedly or deliberately failed to comply with the conditions of these exempting regulations outlined in Form FD–1572 or FD–1573 . . . or has submitted to the sponsor of the investigation false information in his Form FD–1572 or FD–1573 or in any required report, the Director of the Bureau of Medicine will furnish the investigator written notice of the matter complained of in general terms and offer him an opportunity to explain the matter in an informal conference and/or in writing. If an explanation is offered but not accepted by the Bureau of Medicine, the Commissioner will provide the investigator an opportunity for an informal hearing on the question of whether the investigator is entitled to receive investigational-use drugs, if the hearing is requested within 10 days after receipt of notification that the explanation is not acceptable.

(2) After evaluating all available information, including any explanation and assurance presented by the investigator, if the Commissioner determines that the investigator has repeatedly or deliberately failed to comply with the conditions of the exempting regulations in this section or has repeatedly or deliberatedly submitted false information to the sponsor of an investigation and has failed to furnish adequate assurance that the conditions of the exemption will be met, the Commissioner will notify the investigator and the sponsor of any investigation in which he has been named as a participant that the investigator is not entitled to receive investigational-use drugs with a statement of the basis for such determination.

DEPARTMENT OF HEALTH, EDUCATION, AND WELFARE
PUBLIC HEALTH SERVICE
FOOD AND DRUG ADMINISTRATION
5600 FISHERS LANE
ROCKVILLE, MARYLAND 20852

STATEMENT OF INVESTIGATOR
(Clinical Pharmacology)

Form Approved
OMB No. 57-R0031

TO: SUPPLIER OF THE DRUG *(Name and address, include Zip Code)*

NAME OF INVESTIGATOR *(Print or Type)*

DATE

NAME OF DRUG

Dear Sir:

The undersigned, _____ ,
submits this statement as required by section 505(i) of the Federal Food, Drug, and Cosmetic Act and §130.3 of Title 21 of the Code of Federal Regulations as a condition for receiving and conducting clinical pharmacology with a new drug limited by Federal (or United States) law to investigational use.

1. STATE THE EDUCATION AND TRAINING YOU HAVE HAD THAT QUALIFIES YOU FOR CLINICAL PHARMACOLOGY

2. GIVE NAME AND ADDRESS OF THE MEDICAL SCHOOL, HOSPITAL, OR OTHER RESEARCH FACILITY WHERE THE CLINICAL PHARMACOLOGY WILL BE CONDUCTED

3. If the experimental project is to be conducted on institutionalized subjects or is conducted by an individual affiliated with an institution which agrees to assume responsibility for the study, assurance must be given that an institutional review committee is responsible for initial and continuing review and approval of the proposed clinical study. The membership must be comprised of sufficient members of varying background, that is, lawyers, clergymen, or laymen as well as scientists, to assure complete and adequate review of the research project. The membership must possess not only broad competence to comprehend the nature of the project, but also other competencies necessary to judge the acceptability of the project or activity in terms of institutional regulations, relevant law, standards of professional practice, and community acceptance. Assurance must be presented that the investigator has not participated in the selection of committee members; that the review committee does not allow participation in its review and conclusions by any individual involved in the conduct of the research activity under review (except to provide information to the committee); that the investigator will report to the committee for review any emergent problems, serious adverse reactions, or proposed procedural changes which may affect the status of the investigation and that no such change will be made without committee approval except where necessary to eliminate apparent immediate hazards; that reviews of the study will be conducted by the review committee at intervals appropriate to the degree of risk, but not exceeding 1 year, to assure that the research project is being conducted in compliance with the committee's understanding and recommendations; that the review committee is provided all the information on the research project; and that the review committee maintains adequate documentation of its activities and develops adequate procedures for reporting its findings to the institution. The documents maintained by the committee are to include the names and qualifications of committee members, records of information provided to subjects in obtaining informed consent, committee discussion on substantive issues and their resolution, committee recommendations, and dated reports of successive reviews as they are performed. Copies of all documents are to be retained for a period of 3 years past the completion or discontinuance of the study and are to be made available upon request to duly authorized representatives of the Food and Drug Administration. (Favorable recommendations by the committee are subject to further appropriate review and rejection by institution officials. Unfavorable recommendations, restrictions, or conditions may not be overruled by the institution officials.) Procedures for the organization and operation of institutional review committees are contained in guidelines issued pursuant to Chapter 1-40 of the Grants Administration Manual of the U.S. Department of Health, Education, and Welfare, available from the U.S. Government Printing Office. It is recommended that these guidelines be followed in establishing institutional review committees and that the committees function according to the procedures described therein. A signing of the Form FD 1572 will be regarded as providing the above necessary assurance; however, if the institution has on file with the Department of Health, Education, and Welfare, Division of Research Grants, National Institutes of Health, an "accepted general assurance," and the same committee is to review the proposed study using the same procedures, this is acceptable in lieu of the above assurances and a statement to this effect should be provided with the signed FD 1572. (In addition to sponsor's continuing responsibility to monitor the study, the Food and Drug Administration will undertake investigations in institutions periodically to determine whether the committees are operating in accord with the assurances given by the sponsor.)

FD FORM 1572 (5/71)   PREVIOUS EDITION MAY BE USED UNTIL SUPPLY IS EXHAUSTED.

4. ESTIMATE DURATION OF THE PROJECT AND INDICATE THE MAXIMUM NUMBER OF SUBJECTS THAT WILL BE INVOLVED

5. GENERAL OUTLINE OF THE PROJECT TO BE UNDERTAKEN *(Modification is permitted on the basis of experience gained without advance submission of amendments to the general outline, but with the approval of the review·committee and upon notification of the sponsor.)*

6. THE UNDERSIGNED UNDERSTANDS THAT THE FOLLOWING CONDITIONS GENERALLY APPLICABLE TO NEW DRUGS FOR INVESTIGATIONAL USE GOVERN HIS RECEIPT AND USE OF THIS INVESTIGATIONAL DRUG

a. The sponsor is required to supply the investigator with full information concerning the preclinical investigation that justifies clinical pharmacology.

b. The investigator is required to maintain adequate records of the disposition of all receipts of the drug, including dates, quantity, and use by subjects, and if the clinical pharmacology is suspended or terminated to return to the sponsor any unused supply of the drug.

c. The investigator is required to prepare and maintain adequate case histories designed to record all observations and other data pertinent to the clinical pharmacology.

d. The investigator is required to furnish his reports to the sponsor who is responsible for collecting and evaluating the results, and presenting progress reports to the Food and Drug Administration at appropriate intervals, not exceeding 1 year. Any adverse effect which may reasonably be regarded as caused by, or is probably caused by, the new-drug shall be reported to the sponsor promptly; and if the adverse effect is alarming it shall be reported immediately. An adequate report of the clinical pharmacology should be furnished to the sponsor shortly after completion.

e. The investigator shall maintain the records of disposition of the drug and the case reports described above for a period of 2 years following the date the new-drug application is approved for the drug; or if no application is to be filed or is approved until 2 years after the investigation is discontinued and the Food and Drug Administration so notified. Upon the request of a scientifically trained and specifically authorized employee of the Department, at reasonable times, the investigator will make such records available for inspection and copying. The names of the subjects need not be divulged unless the records of the particular subjects require a more detailed study of the cases, or unless there is reason to believe that the records do not represent actual studies or do not represent actual results obtained.

f. The investigator certifies that the drug will be administered only to subjects under his personal supervision or under the supervision of the following investigators responsible to him,

_____

_____

_____

_____

and that the drug will not be supplied to any other investigator or to any clinic for administration to subjects.

g. The investigator certifies that he will inform any patients or any persons used as controls, or their representatives, that drugs are being used for investigational purposes, and will obtain the consent of the subjects, or their representatives, except where this is not feasible or, in the investigator's professional judgment, is contrary to the best interests of the subjects.

h. The investigator is required to assure the sponsor that for investigations involving institutionalized subjects the studies will not be initiated until the institutional review committee has reviewed and approved the study. (The organization and procedure requirements for such a committee should be explained to the investigator by the sponsor as set forth in Form FD 1571, division 10, unit c.)

Very truly yours,

_____
(Name of Investigator)

_____
(Address)

_____

DEPARTMENT OF HEALTH, EDUCATION, AND WELFARE PUBLIC HEALTH SERVICE FOOD AND DRUG ADMINISTRATION 5600 FISHERS LANE ROCKVILLE, MARYLAND 20852	STATEMENT OF INVESTIGATOR	Form Approved OMB No. 57-R0029

TO: SUPPLIER OF DRUG *(Name and address, include Zip Code)*	NAME OF INVESTIGATOR *(Print or Type)*
	DATE
	NAME OF DRUG

Dear Sir:

The undersigned, _____,
submits this statement as required by section 505(i) of the Federal Food, Drug, and Cosmetic Act and $130.3 of Title 21
of the Code of Federal Regulations as a condition for receiving and conducting clinical investigations with a new drug
limited by Federal (or United States) law to investigational use.

1.   STATEMENT OF EDUCATION AND EXPERIENCE

a. COLLEGES, UNIVERSITIES, AND MEDICAL OR OTHER PROFESSIONAL SCHOOLS ATTENDED, WITH DATES OF ATTENDANCE, DEGREES, AND DATES DEGREES WERE AWARDED

b. POSTGRADUATE MEDICAL OR OTHER PROFESSIONAL TRAINING *(Indicate dates, names of institutions, and nature of training)*

c. TEACHING OR RESEARCH EXPERIENCE *(Indicate dates, institutions, and brief description of experience)*

d. EXPERIENCE IN MEDICAL PRACTICE OR OTHER PROFESSIONAL EXPERIENCE *(Indicate dates, institutional affiliations, nature of practice, or other professional experience)*

e. REPRESENTIVE LIST OF PERTINENT MEDICAL OR OTHER SCIENTIFIC PUBLICATIONS *(Indicate titles of articles, names of publications and volume, page number, and date)*

FD FORM 1573 (4/71)   PREVIOUS EDITION MAY BE USED UNTIL SUPPLY IS EXHAUSTED.

2a. If the investigation is to be conducted on institutionalized subjects or is conducted by an individual affiliated with an institution which agrees to assume responsibility for the study, assurance must be given that an institutional review committee is responsible for initial and continuing review and approval of the proposed clinical study. The membership must be comprised of sufficient members of varying background, that is, lawyers, clergymen, or laymen as well as scientists, to assure complete and adequate review of the research project. The membership must possess not only broad competence to comprehend the nature of the project, but also other competencies necessary to judge the acceptability of the project or activity in terms of institutional regulations, relevant law, standards of professional practice and community acceptance. Assurance must be presented that the investigator has not participated in the selection of committee members; that the review committee does not allow participation in its review and conclusions by any individual involved in the conduct of the research activity under review (except to provide information to the committee) that the investigator will report to the committee for review any emergent problems, serious adverse reactions, or proposed procedural changes which may affect the status of the investigation and that no such change will be made without committee approval except where necessary to eliminate apparent immediate hazards; that reviews of the study will be conducted by the review committee at intervals appropriate to the degree of risk, but not exceeding 1 year. to assure that the research project is being conducted in compliance with the committee's understanding and recommendations; that the review committee is provided all the information on the research project necessary for its complete review of the project; and that the review committee maintains adequate documentation of its activities and develops adequate procedures for reporting its findings to the institution. The documents maintained by the committee are to include the names and qualifications of committee members, records of information provided to subjects in obtaining informed consent, committee discussion on substantive issues and their resolution, committee recommendations, and dated reports of successive reviews as they are performed. Copies of all documents are to be retained for a period of 3 years past the completion or discontinuance of the study and are to be made available upon request to duly authorized representatives of the Food and Drug Administration. (Favorable recommendations by the committee are subject to further appropriate review and rejection by institution officials. Unfavorable recommendations, restrictions, or conditions may not be overruled by the institution officials.) Procedures for the organization and operation of institutional review committees are contained in guidelines issued pursuant to Chapter 140 of the Grants Administration Manual of the U.S. Department of Health, Education, and Welfare, available from the U.S. Government Printing Office. It is recommended that these guidelines be followed in establishing institutional review committees and that the committees function according to the procedures described therein. A signing of the Form FD 1573 will be regarded as providing the above necessary assurances; however, if the institution has on file with the Department of Health, Education, and Welfare, Division of Research Grants, National Institutes of Health, an "accepted general assurance," and the same committee is to review the proposed study using the same procedures, this is acceptable in lieu of the above assurances and a statement to this effect should be provided with the signed FD 1573. (In addition to sponsor's continuing responsibility to monitor the study, the Food and Drug Administration will undertake investigations in institutions periodically to determine whether the committees are operating in accord with the assurances given by the sponsor.)

b. A description of any clinical laboratory facilities that will be used. (If this information has been submitted to the sponsor and reported by him on Form FD 1571, reference to the previous submission will be adequate).

3. OUTLINE THE PLAN OF INVESTIGATION (Include approximation of the number of subjects to be treated with the drug and the number to be employed as controls, if any; clinical uses to be investigated; characteristics of subjects by age, sex and condition; the kind of clinical observations and laboratory tests to be undertaken prior to, during, and after administration of the drug; the estimated duration of the investigation; and a description or copies of report forms to be used to maintain an adequate record of the observations and tests results obtained. This plan may include reasonable alternates and variations and should be supplemented or amended when any significant change in direction or scope of the investigation is undertaken.)

4. THE UNDERSIGNED UNDERSTANDS THAT THE FOLLOWING CONDITIONS, GENERALLY APPLICABLE TO NEW DRUGS FOR INVESTIGATIONAL USE, GOVERN HIS RECEIPT AND USE OF THIS INVESTIGATIONAL DRUG

a. The sponsor is required to supply the investigator with full information concerning the preclinical investigations that justify clinical trials, together with fully informative material describing any prior investigations and experience and any possible hazards, contraindications, side-effects, and precautions to be taken into account in the course of the investigation.

b. The investigator is required to maintain adequate records of the disposition of all receipts of the drug, including dates, quantities, and use by subjects, and if the investigation is terminated to return to the sponsor any unused supply of the drug.

c. The investigator is required to prepare and maintain adequate and accurate case histories designed to record all observations and other data pertinent to the investigation on each individual treated with the drug or employed as a control in the investigation.

d. The investigator is required to furnish his reports to the sponsor of the drug who is responsible for collecting and evaluating the results obtained by various investigators. The sponsor is required to present progress reports to the Food and Drug Administration at appropriate intervals not exceeding 1 year. Any adverse effect that may reasonably be regarded as caused by, or probably caused by, the new drug shall be reported to the sponsor promptly, and if the adverse effect is alarming, it shall be reported immediately. An adequate report of the investigation should be furnished to the sponsor shortly after completion of the investigation.

e. The investigator shall maintain the records of disposition of the drug and the case histories described above for a period of 2 years following the date a new-drug application is approved for the drug; or if the application is not approved, until 2 years after the investigation

is discontinued. Upon the request of a scientifically trained and properly authorized employee of the Department, at reasonable times, the investigator will make such records available for inspection and copying. The subjects' names need not be divulged unless the records of particular individuals require a more detailed study of the cases, or unless there is reason to believe that the records do not represent actual cases studied, or do not represent actual results obtained.

f. The investigator certifies that the drug will be administered only to subjects under his personal supervision or under the supervision of the following investigators responsible to him,

_____

_____

_____

and that the drug will not be supplied to any other investigator or to any clinic for administration to subjects.

g. The investigator certifies that he will inform any subjects, including subjects used as controls, or their representatives, that drugs are being used for investigational purposes, and will obtain the consent of the subjects, or their representatives, except where this is not feasible or, in the investigator's professional judgement, is contrary to the best interests of the subjects.

h. The investigator is required to assure the sponsor that for investigations involving institutionalized subjects, the studies will not be initiated until the institutional review committee has reviewed and approved the study. (The organization and procedure requirements for such a committee should be explained to the investigator by the sponsor as set forth in form FD 1571, division 10, unit c.)

Very truly yours,

_____

(Name of Investigator)

_____

(Address)

_____

(This form should be supplemented or amended from time to time if new subjects are added or if significant changes are made in the plan of investigation.)

(3) Each "Notice of Claimed Investigational Exemption for a New Drug" [Form FD 1571] and each approved new-drug application containing data reported by an investigator who has been determined to be ineligible to receive investigational-use drugs will be examined to determine whether he has submitted unreliable data that are essential to the approval of any new-drug application.

(4) If the Commissioner determines after the unreliable data submitted by the investigator are eliminated from consideration that the data remaining are inadequate to support a conclusion that it is reasonably safe to continue the investigation, he will notify the sponsor and provide him with an opportunity for a conference and an informal hearing in accordance with paragraph (d) of this section. If an imminent hazard to the public health exists, however, he shall terminate the exemption forthwith and notify the sponsor of the termination. In such event the Commissioner, on request, will afford the sponsor an opportunity for an informal hearing on the question of whether the exemption should be reinstated.

(5) If the Commissioner determines after the unreliable data submitted by the investigator are eliminated from consideration that the data remaining are such that a new-drug application would not have been approved, he will proceed to withdraw approval of the application in accordance with section 505(e) of the act.

(6) An investigator who has been determined to be ineligible may be reinstated as eligible to receive investigational-use drugs when the Commissioner determines that he has presented adequate assurance that he will employ such drugs solely in compliance with the exempting regulations in this section for investigational-use drugs.

(d) If the Commissioner of Food and Drugs finds that:

(1) The submitted "Notice of claimed investigational exemption for a new drug" contains an untrue statement of a material fact or omits material information required by said notice; or

(2) The results of prior investigations made with the drug are inadequate to support a conclusion that it is reasonably safe to initiate or continue the intended clinical investigations with the drug; or

(3) There is substantial evidence to show that the drug is unsafe for the purposes and in the manner for which it is offered for investigational use; or

(4) There is convincing evidence that the drug is ineffective for the purposes for which it is offered for investigational use; or

(5) The methods, facilities, and controls used for the manufacturing, processing, and packing of the investigational drug are inadequate to establish and maintain appropriate standards of identity, strength, quality, and purity as needed for safety and to give significance to clinical investigations made with the drug; or

(6) The plan for clinical investigations of the drugs described under section 10 of the "Notice of claimed investigational exemption for a new drug" is not a reasonable plan in whole or in part, solely for a bona fide scientific investigation to determine whether or not the drug is safe and effective for use; or

(7) The clinical investigations are not being conducted in accordance with the plan submitted in the "Notice of claimed investigational exemption for a new drug"; or

(8) The drug is not intended solely for investigational use, since it is being or is to be sold or otherwise distributed for commercial purposes not justified by the requirements of the investigation; or

(9) The labeling or other informational material submitted for the drug as required by section 7 of the "Notice of claimed investigational exemption for a new drug" or any other labeling of the drug disseminated within the United States by or on behalf of the sponsor fails to contain an accurate description of prior investigations or experience and their results pertinent to the safety and possible usefulness of the drug, including all relevant hazards, contraindications, side effects, and precautions; or any promotional material disseminated within the United States by or on behalf of the sponsor contains any representation or suggestion that the drug is safe or that its usefulness has been established for the purposes for which it is offered for investigations; or

(10) The sponsor fails to submit accurate reports of the progress of the investigations with significant findings at intervals not exceeding 1 year; or

(11) The sponsor fails promptly to investigate and inform the Food and Drug Administration and all investigators of newly found serious or potentially serious hazards, contraindications, side effects, and precautions pertinent to the safety of the new drug;

he shall notify the sponsor and invite his immediate correction or explanation. A conference will be arranged with the Bureau of Medicine if requested. If the Bureau of Medicine does not accept the explanation and/or the correction submitted by the sponsor, the Commissioner will provide the sponsor an opportunity for an informal hearing on the question of whether his exemption should be terminated, if the hearing is requested within 10 days after receipt of notification that the explanation or correction is not acceptable. After evaluating all the available information including any explanation and/or correction submitted by the sponsor, if the Commissioner determines that the exemption should be terminated he shall notify the sponsor of the termination of the exemption and the sponsor shall recall unused supplies of the drug. If at any time the Commissioner concludes that continuation of the investigation presents an imminent hazard to the public health, he shall terminate the exemption forthwith and notify the sponsor of the termination. The Commissioner will inform the sponsor that the exemption is subject to reinstatement on the basis of additional submissions that eliminate such hazard(s) and will afford the sponsor an opportunity for an informal hearing, on request, on the question of whether the exemption should be reinstated. The sponsor shall recall the unused supplies of the drug upon notification of the termination.

*   *   *

§ *130.3a. New drugs for investigational use in animals; exemptions from section 505(a).*

(a) *New drugs for tests in vitro and in laboratory research animals.* (1) A shipment or other delivery of a new drug intended solely for tests in vitro or in animals used only for laboratory research purposes shall be exempt from section 505(a) of the act if it is labeled as follows:

Caution—Contains a new drug for investigational use only in laboratory research animals, or for tests in vitro. Not for use in humans.

*   *   *

§ *130.4 Applications.*

(a) Applications to be filed under the provisions of section 505(b) of the act shall be submitted in the form described in paragraph (c) of this section. . . .

(b) Pertinent information may be incorporated in, and will be considered as part of, an application on the basis of specific reference to such information, including information submitted under the provisions of § 130.3, in the

files of the Food and Drug Administration; however, any reference to information furnished by a person other than the applicant may not be considered unless use of such information is authorized in a written statement signed by the person who submitted it.

(c) Applications for drugs for human use shall be assembled and submitted in the manner prescribed by paragraph (e) of this section. Applications for human and veterinary drugs shall be submitted in one of the following appropriate forms. . . .

[Form FD–356H appears on the pages which follow.]

*   *   *

§ *130.6 Comment on applications.*

(a) After the application has been studied, the applicant will be furnished comment on any apparent deficiencies in the data submitted or on the need for any additional data or changes in the application to facilitate its consideration.

(b) When the description of the methods used in, and the facilities and controls used for, the manufacture, processing, and packing of such drug appears adequate on its face, but it is not feasible to reach a conclusion as to the safety and effectiveness of the drug solely from consideration of this description, the applicant may be notified that an inspection is required to verify their adequacy.

(c) Withdrawal of an application may be suggested when it is found that additional evidence is required to support a finding that the drug is safe or effective or that the methods, facilities, and controls used in manufacturing, processing, and packing the drug are adequate.

(d) On the basis of preliminary consideration of an application or supplemental application containing typewritten or other draft labeling in lieu of final printed labeling, an applicant may be informed that such application is approvable when satisfactory final printed labeling identical in content to such draft copy is submitted.

§ *130.7 Amended applications.*

The applicant may submit an amendment to an application that is pending, but in the case of a substantive amendment, the unamended application may be considered as withdrawn and the amended application may be considered resubmitted on the date on which the amendment is received by the Food and Drug Administration. The applicant will be notified of such date.

DEPARTMENT OF HEALTH, EDUCATION, AND WELFARE
PUBLIC HEALTH SERVICE
FOOD AND DRUG ADMINISTRATION
ROCKVILLE, MARYLAND 20852

Form Approved
OMB No. 57-R0003

NEW DRUG APPLICATION *(DRUGS FOR HUMAN USE)*
(Title 21, Code of Federal Regulations, § 130.4)

Name of applicant _____

Address _____

Date _____

Name of new drug_____

☐ Original application (regulation § 130.4).

☐ Amendment to original, unapproved application (regulation § 130.7).

☐ Abbreviated application (regulation § 130.4(f)).

☐ Amendment to abbreviated, unapproved application (regulation § 130.7).

☐ Supplement to an approved application (regulation § 130.9).

☐ Amendment to supplement to an approved application.

The undersigned submits this application for a new drug pursuant to section 505(b) of the Federal Food, Drug, and Cosmetic Act. It is understood that when this application is approved, the labeling and advertising for the drug will prescribe, recommend, or suggest its use only under the conditions stated in the labeling which is part of this application; and if the article is a prescription drug, it is understood that any labeling which furnishes or purports to furnish information for use or which prescribes, recommends, or suggests a dosage use of the drug will contain the same information for its use, including indications, effects, dosages, routes, methods, and frequency and duration of administration, any relevant warnings, hazards, contraindications, side effects, and precautions, as that contained in the labeling which is part of this application in accord with §1.106(b) (21 CFR 1.106(b)). It is understood that all representations in this application apply to the drug produced until an approved supplement to the application provides for a change or the change is made in conformance with other provisions of §130.9 of the new-drug regulations.

Attached hereto, submitted in the form described in §130.4(e) of the new-drug regulations, and constituting a part of this application are the following:

1. Table of contents. The table of contents should specify the volume number and the page number in which the complete and detailed item is located and the volume number and the page number in which the summary of that item is located (if any).

2. Summary. A summary demonstrating that the application is well-organized, adequately tabulated, statistically analyzed (where appropriate), and coherent and that it presents a sound basis for the approval requested. The summary should include the following information: (In lieu of the outline described below and the evaluation described in Item 3, an expanded summary and evaluation as outlined in §130.4(d) of the new-drug regulations may be submitted to facilitate the review of this application.)

   a. Chemistry.
   i. Chemical structural formula or description for any new-drug substance.
   ii. Relationship to other chemically or pharmacologically related drugs.
   iii. Description of dosage form and quantitative composition.
   b. Scientific rationale and purpose the drug is to serve.
   c. Reference number of the investigational drug notice(s) under which this drug was investigated and of any notice, new-drug application, or master file of which any contents are being incorporated by reference to support this application.
   d. Preclinical studies. (Present all findings including all adverse experiences which may be interpreted as incidental or not drug-related. Refer to date and page number of the investigational drug notice(s) or the volume and page number of this application where complete data and reports appear.)
   i. Pharmacology (pharmacodynamics, endocrinology, metabolism, etc.).
   ii. Toxicology and pathology: Acute toxicity studies; subacute and chronic toxicity studies; reproduction and teratology studies; miscellaneous studies.
   e. Clinical studies. (All material should refer specifically to each clinical investigator and to the volume and page number in the application and any documents incorporated by reference where the complete data and reports may be found.)
   i. Special studies not described elsewhere.
   ii. Dose-range studies.
   iii. Controlled clinical studies.
   iv. Other clinical studies (for example, uncontrolled or incompletely controlled studies).
   v. Clinical laboratory studies related to effectiveness.
   vi. Clinical laboratory studies related to safety.
   vii. Summary of literature and unpublished reports available to the applicant.

3. Evaluation of safety and effectiveness. a. Summarize separately the favorable and unfavorable evidence for each claim in the package labeling. Include references to the volume and page number in the application and in any documents incorporated by reference where the complete data and reports may be found.
   b. Include tabulation of all side effects or adverse experience, by age, sex, and dosage formulation, whether or not considered to be significant, showing whether administration of the drug was stopped and showing the investigator's name with a reference to the volume and page number in the application and any documents incorporated by reference where the complete data and reports may be found. Indicate those side effects or adverse experiences considered to be drug-related.

4. Copies of the label and all other labeling to be used for the drug (a total of 12 copies if in final printed form, 4 copies if in draft form):

FD FORM 356H (4/71)

PREVIOUS EDITION MAY BE USED UNTIL SUPPLY IS EXHAUSTED.

a. Each label, or other labeling, should be clearly identified to show its position on, or the manner in which it accompanies, the market package.

b. If the drug is to be offered over the counter, labeling on or within the retail package should include adequate directions for use by the layman under all the conditions for which the drug is intended for lay use or is to be prescribed, recommended, or suggested in any labeling or advertising sponsored by or on behalf of the applicant and directed to the layman. If the drug is intended or offered for uses under the professional supervision of a practitioner licensed by law to administer it, the application should also contain labeling that includes adequate information for all such uses, including all the purposes for which the over-the-counter drug is to be advertised to, or represented for use by, physicians.

c. If the drug is limited in its labeling to use under the professional supervision of a practitioner licensed by law to administer it, its labeling should bear information for use under which such practitioners can use the drug for the purposes for which it is intended, including all the purposes for which it is to be advertised or represented, in accord with §1.106(b) (21 CFR 1.106(b)). The application should include any labeling for the drug intended to be made available to the layman.

d. If no established name exists for a new-drug substance, the application shall propose a nonproprietary name for use as the established name for the substance.

e. Typewritten or other draft labeling copy may be submitted for preliminary consideration of an application. An application will not ordinarily be approved prior to the submission of the final printed label and labeling of the drug.

f. No application may be approved if the labeling is false or misleading in any particular. (When mailing pieces, any other labeling, or advertising copy are devised for promotion of the new drug, samples shall be submitted at the time of initial dissemination of such labeling and at the time of initial placement of any such advertising for a prescription drug (see §130.13 of the new-drug regulations). Approval of a supplemental new-drug application is required prior to use of any promotional claims not covered by the approved application.)

5. A statement as to whether the drug is (or is not) limited in its labeling and by this application to use under the professional supervision of a practitioner licensed by law to administer it.

6. A full list of the articles used as components of the drug. This list should include all substances used in the synthesis, extraction, or other method of preparation of any new-drug substance, and in the preparation of the finished dosage form, regardless of whether they undergo chemical change or are removed in the process. Each substance should be identified by its established name, if any, or complete chemical name, using structural formulas when necessary for specific identification. If any proprietary preparation is used as a component, the proprietary name should be followed by a complete quantitative statement of composition. Reasonable alternatives for any listed substance may be specified.

7. A full statement of the composition of the drug. The statement shall set forth the name and amount of each ingredient, whether active or not, contained in a stated quantity of the drug in the form in which it is to be distributed (for example, amount per tablet or per milliliter) and a batch formula representative of that to be employed for the manufacture of the finished dosage form. All components should be included in the batch formula regardless of whether they appear in the finished product. Any calculated excess of an ingredient over the label declaration should be designated as such and percent excess shown. Reasonable variations may be specified.

8. A full description of the methods used in, and the facilities and controls used for, the manufacture, processing, and packing of the drug. Included in this description should be full information with respect to any new-drug substance and to the new-drug dosage form, as follows, in sufficient detail to permit evaluation of the adequacy of the described methods of manufacture, processing, and packing and the described facilities and controls to determine and preserve the identity, strength, quality, and purity of the drug:

a. A description of the physical facilities including building and equipment used in manufacturing, processing, packaging, labeling, storage, and control operations.

b. A description of the qualifications, including educational background and experience, of the technical and professional personnel who are responsible for assuring that the drug has the safety, identity, strength, quality, and purity it purports or is represented to possess, and a statement of their responsibilities.

c. The methods used in the synthesis, extraction, isolation, or purification of any new-drug substance. When the specifications and controls applied to such substance are inadequate in themselves to determine its identity, strength, quality, and purity, the methods should be described in sufficient detail, including quantities used, times, temperatures, pH, solvents, etc., to determine these characteristics. Alternative methods or variations in methods within reasonable limits that do not affect such characteristics of the substance may be specified.

d. Precautions to assure proper identity, strength, quality, and purity of the raw materials, whether active or not, including the specifications for acceptance and methods of testing for each lot of raw material.

e. Whether or not each lot of raw materials is given a serial number to identify it, and the use made of such numbers in subsequent plant operations.

f. If the applicant does not himself perform all the manufacturing, processing, packaging, labeling, and control operations for any new-drug substance or the new-drug dosage form, his statement identifying each person who will perform any part of such operations and designating the part; and a signed statement from each such person fully describing, directly or by reference, the methods, facilities, and controls in his part of the operation.

g. Method of preparation of the master formula records and individual batch records and manner in which these records are used.

h. The instructions used in the manufacturing, processing, packaging, and labeling of each dosage form of the new drug, including any special precautions observed in the operations.

i. Adequate information with respect to the characteristics of and the test methods employed for the container, closure, or other component parts of the drug package to assure their suitability for the intended use.

j. Number of individuals checking weight or volume of each individual ingredient entering into each batch of the drug.

k. Whether or not the total weight or volume of each batch is determined at any stage of the manufacturing process subsequent to making up a batch according to the formula card and, if so, at what stage and by whom it is done.

l. Precautions to check the actual package yield produced from a batch of the drug with the theoretical yield. This should include a description of the accounting for such items as discards, breakage, etc., and the criteria used in accepting or rejecting batches of drugs in the event of an unexplained discrepancy.

m. Precautions to assure that each lot of the drug is packaged with the proper label and labeling, including provisions for labeling storage and inventory control.

2

n. The analytical controls used during the various stages of the manufacturing, processing, packaging, and labeling of the drug, including a detailed description of the collection of samples and the analytical procedures to which they are subjected.   The analytical procedures should be capable of determining the active components within a reasonable degree of accuracy and of assuring the identity of such components.   If the article is one that is represented to be sterile, the same information with regard to the manufacturing, processing, packaging, and the collection of samples of the drug should be given for sterility controls.   Include the standards used for acceptance of each lot of the finished drug.

o. An explanation of the exact significance of the batch control numbers used in the manufacturing, processing, packaging, and labeling of the drug, including the control numbers that appear on the label of the finished article.   State whether these numbers enable determination of the complete manufacturing history of the product. Describe any methods used to permit determination of the distribution of any batch if its recall is required.

p. A complete description of, and data derived from, studies of the stability of the drug, including information showing the suitability of the analytical methods used. Describe any additional stability studies underway or contemplated.   Stability data should be submitted for any new-drug substance, for the finished dosage form of the drug in the container in which it is to be marketed, including any proposed multiple-dose container, and if it is to be put into solution at the time of dispensing, for the solution prepared as directed.   State the expiration date(s) that will be used on the label to preserve the identity, strength, quality, and purity of the drug until it is used. (If no expiration date is proposed, the applicant must justify its absence.)

q. Additional procedures employed which are designed to prevent contamination and otherwise assure proper control of the product.
(An application may be refused unless it includes adequate information showing that the methods used in, and the facilities and controls used for, the manufacturing, processing, and packaging of the drug are adequate to preserve its identity, strength, quality, and purity in conformity with good manufacturing practice and identifies each establishment, showing the location of the plant conducting these operations.)

9. Samples of the drug and articles used as components, as follows: a. The following samples shall be submitted with the application or as soon thereafter as they become available.   Each sample shall consist of four identical, separately packaged subdivisions, each containing at least three times the amount required to perform the laboratory test procedures described in the application to determine compliance with its control specifications for identity and assays:

i. A representative sample or samples of the finished dosage form(s) proposed in the application and employed in the clinical investigations and a representative sample or samples of each new-drug substance, as defined in §130.1(g), from the batch(es) employed in the production of such dosage form(s).

ii. A representative sample or samples of finished market packages of each dosage form of the drug prepared for initial marketing and, if any such sample is not from a commercial-scale production batch, such a sample from a representative commercial-scale production batch; and a representative sample or samples of each new-drug substance as defined in §130.1(g), from the batch(es) employed in the production of such dosage form(s).

iii. A sample or samples of any reference standard and blank used in the procedures described in the application for assaying each new-drug substance and other assayed

components of the finished drug: *Provided, however,* **That** samples of reference standards recognized in the official U.S. Pharmacopeia or The National Formulary need not be submitted unless requested.

b. Additional samples shall be submitted on request.

c. Each of the samples submitted shall be appropriately packaged and labeled to preserve its characteristics, to identify the material and the quantity in each subdivision of the sample, and to identify each subdivision with the name of the applicant and the new-drug application to which it relates.

d. There shall be included a full list of the samples submitted pursuant to Item 9a; a statement of the additional samples that will be submitted as soon as available; and, with respect to each sample submitted, full information with respect to its identity, the origin of any new-drug substance contained therein (including in the case of new-drug substances, a statement whether it was produced on a laboratory, pilot-plant, or full-production scale) and detailed results of all laboratory tests made to determine the identity, strength, quality, and purity of the batch represented by the sample, including assays. Include for any reference standard a complete description of its preparation and the results of all laboratory tests on it.   If the test methods used differed from those described in the application, full details of the methods employed in obtaining the reported results shall be submitted.

e. The requirements of Item 9a may be waived in whole or in part on request of the applicant or otherwise when any such samples are not necessary.

f. If samples of the drug are sent under separate cover, they should be addressed to the attention of the Bureau of Medicine and identified on the outside of the shipping carton with the name of the applicant and the name of the drug as shown on the application.

10. Full reports of preclinical investigations that have been made to show whether or not the drug is safe for use and effective in use. a. An application may be refused unless it contains full reports of adequate preclinical tests by all methods reasonably applicable to a determination of the safety and effectiveness of the drug under the conditions of use suggested in the proposed labeling.

b. Detailed reports of the preclinical investigations, including all studies made on laboratory animals, the methods used, and the results obtained, should be clearly set forth.   Such information should include identification of the person who conducted each investigation, a statement of where the investigations were conducted, and where the underlying data are available for inspection. The animal studies may not be considered adequate unless they give proper attention to the conditions of use recommended in the proposed labeling for the drug such as, for example, whether the drug is for short- or long-term administration or whether it is to be used in infants, children, pregnant women, or women of child-bearing potential.

c. Detailed reports of any pertinent microbiological and *in vitro* studies.

d. Summarize and provide a list of literature references (if available) to all other preclinical information known to the applicant, whether published or unpublished, that is pertinent to an evaluation of the safety or effectiveness of the drug.

11. List of investigators.   a. A complete list of all investigators supplied with the drug including the name and post office address of each investigator and, following each name, the volume and page references to the investigator's report(s) in this application and in any documents incorporated by reference, or the explanation of the omission of any reports.

b. The unexplained omission of any reports of investigations made with the new drug by the applicant, or

3

submitted to him by an investigator, or the unexplained omission of any pertinent reports of investigations or clinical experience received or otherwise obtained by the applicant from published literature or other sources, whether or not it would bias an evaluation of the safety of the drug or its effectiveness in use, may constitute grounds for the refusal or withdrawal of the approval of an application.

12. Full reports of clinical investigations that have been made to show whether or not the drug is safe for use and effective in use. a. An application may be refused unless it contains full reports of adequate tests by all methods reasonably applicable to show whether or not the drug is safe and effective for use as suggested in the labeling.

b. An application may be refused unless it includes substantial evidence consisting of adequate and well-controlled investigations, including clinical investigations, by experts qualified by scientific training and experience to evaluate the effectiveness of the drug involved, on the basis of which it could fairly and responsibly be concluded by such experts that the drug will have the effect it purports or is represented to have under the conditions of use prescribed, recommended, or suggested in the proposed labeling.

c. Reports of all clinical tests sponsored by the applicant or received or otherwise obtained by the applicant should be attached. These reports should include adequate information concerning each subject treated with the drug or employed as a control, including age, sex, conditions treated, dosage, frequency of administration of the drug, results of all relevant clinical observations and laboratory examinations made, full information concerning any other treatment given previously or concurrently, and a full statement of adverse effects and useful results observed, together with an opinion as to whether such effects or results are attributable to the drug under investigation and a statement of where the underlying data are available for inspection. Ordinarily, the reports of clinical studies will not be regarded as adequate unless they include reports from more than one independent, competent investigator who maintains adequate case histories of an adequate number of subjects, designed to record observations and permit evaluation of any and all discernible effects attributable to the drug in each individual treated and comparable records on any individuals employed as controls. An application for a combination drug may be refused unless there is substantial evidence that each ingredient designated as active makes a contribution to the total effect claimed for the drug combination. Except when the disease for which the drug is being tested occurs with such infrequency in the United States as to make testing impractical, some of the investigations should be performed by competent investigators within the United States.

d. Attach as a separate section a completed Form FD-1639, Drug Experience Report (obtainable, with instructions, on request from the Department of HEW. Food and Drug Administration. Bureau of Drugs (BD-200) Rockville, Maryland 20852), for each adverse experience or, if feasible, for each subject or patient experiencing one or more adverse effects, described in Item 12c, whether or not full information is available. Form FD-1639 should be prepared by the applicant if the adverse experience was not reported in such form by the investigator. The Drug Experience Report should be cross-referenced to any narrative description included in Item 12c. In lieu of a FD Form 1639, a computer-generated report may be submitted if equivalent in all elements of information with the identical enumerated sequence of events and methods of completion; all formats proposed for such use will require initial review and approval by the Food and Drug Administration.

e. All information pertinent to an evaluation of the safety and effectiveness of the drug received or otherwise obtained by the applicant from any source, including information derived from other investigations or commerical marketing (for example, outside the United States), or reports in the scientific literature, involving the drug that is the subject of the application and related drugs. An adequate summary may be acceptable in lieu of a reprint of a published report which only supports other data submitted. Reprints are not required of reports in designated journals, listed in §130.38 of the new-drug regulations, about related drugs; a bibliography will suffice. Include any evaluation of the safety or effectiveness of the drug that has been made by the applicant's medical department, expert committee, or consultants.

f. If the drug is a combination of previously investigated or marketed drugs, an adequate summary of pre-existing information from preclinical and clinical investigation and experience with its components, including all reports received or otherwise obtained by the applicant suggesting side effects, contraindications, and ineffectiveness in use of such components. Such summary should include an adequate bibliography of publications about the components and may incorporate by reference information concerning such components previously submitted by the applicant to the Food and Drug Administration.

g. The complete composition and/or method of manufacture of the new drug used in each submitted report of investigation should be shown to the extent necessary to establish its identity, strength, quality, and purity if it differs from the description in Item 6, 7, or 8 of the application.

13. If this is a supplemental application, full information on each proposed change concerning any statement made in the approved application. Observe the provisions of §130.9 of the new-drug regulations concerning supplemental applications.

_____
(Applicant)

Per _____
(Responsible official or agent)

_____
(Indicate authority)

(Warning: A willfully false statement is a criminal offense. U.S.C. Title 18, sec. 1001.)

NOTE: This application must be signed by the applicant or by an authorized attorney, agent, or official. If the applicant or such authorized representative does not reside or have a place of business within the United States, the application must also furnish the name and post office address of and must be countersigned by an authorized attorney, agent, or official residing or maintaining a place of business within the United States.

§ 130.8 Withdrawal of applications without prejudice.

The applicant may at any time withdraw his pending application from consideration as a new-drug application upon written notification to the Food and Drug Administration. Such withdrawal may be made without prejudice to a future filing. Upon resubmission, the time limitation will begin to run from the date the resubmission is received by the Food and Drug Administration. The application itself will be retained by the Food and Drug Administration although it is considered withdrawn, but the applicant shall be furnished a copy at cost, on request.

*   *   *

§ 130.10 Notification of applicant of approval of application.

If the Commissioner determines that none of the grounds for denying approval specified in section 505(d) of the act applies, the applicant shall be notified in writing that the application is approved and the application shall be approved on the date of the notification.

*   *   *

§ 130.12 Refusal to approve the application.

(a) If the Commissioner determines upon the basis of the application, or upon the basis of other information before him with respect to the new drug, that:

(1) The investigations, reports of which are required to be submitted pursuant to section 505(b) of the act, do not include adequate tests by all methods reasonably applicable to show whether or not such drug is safe for use under the conditions prescribed, recommended, or suggested in the proposed labeling thereof; or

(2) The results of such tests show that such drug is unsafe for use under such conditions or do not show that such drug is safe for use under such conditions; or

(3) The methods used in, and the facilities and controls used for, the manufacture, processing, and packing of such drug are inadequate to preserve its identity, strength, quality, and purity; or

(4) Upon the basis of the information submitted to the Food and Drug Administration as part of the application, or upon the basis of any other information before it with respect to such drug, it has insufficient information to determine whether such drug is safe for use under such conditions; or

(5) (i) Evaluated on the basis of information submitted as part of the application and any other information before the Food and Drug Administration with respect to such drug, there is lack of substantial evidence consisting of adequate and well-controlled investigations, including clinical investigations, by experts qualified by scientific training and experience to evaluate the effectiveness of the drug involved, on the basis of which it could fairly and responsibly be concluded by such experts that the drug will have the effect it purports or is represented to have under the conditions of use prescribed, recommended, or suggested in the proposed labeling.

(ii) The following principles have been developed over a period of years and are recognized by the scientific community as the essentials of adequate and well-controlled clinical investigations. They provide the basis for the determination whether there is "substantial evidence" to support the claims of effectiveness for "new drugs" and antibiotic drugs.

(a) The plan or protocol for the study and the report of the results of the effectiveness study must include the following:

(1) A clear statement of the objectives of the study.

(2) A method of selection of the subjects that—

(i) Provides adequate assurance that they are suitable for the purposes of the study, diagnostic criteria of the condition to be treated or diagnosed, confirmatory laboratory tests where appropriate, and, in the case of prophylactic agents, evidence of susceptibility and exposure to the condition against which prophylaxis is desired.

(ii) Assigns the subjects to test groups in such a way as to minimize bias.

(iii) Assures comparability in test and control groups of pertinent variables, such as age, sex, severity, or duration of disease, and use of drugs other than the test drug.

(3) Explains the methods of observation and recording of results, including the variables measured, quantitation, assessment of any subjective response, and steps taken to minimize bias on the part of the subject and observer.

(4) Provides a comparison of the results of treatment or diagnosis with a control in such a fashion as to permit quantitative evaluation. The precise nature of the control must be stated and an explanation given of the methods used to minimize bias on the part of the observers and

the analysts of the data. Level and methods of "blinding," if used, are to be documented. Generally, four types of comparison are recognized:

(*i*) No treatment: Where objective measurements of effectiveness are available and placebo effect is negligible, comparison of the objective results in comparable groups of treated and untreated patients.

(*ii*) Placebo control: Comparison of the results of use of the new drug entity with an inactive preparation designed to resemble the test drug as far as possible.

(*iii*) Active treatment control: An effective regimen of therapy may be used for comparison, e.g., where the condition treated is such that no treatment or administration of a placebo would be contrary to the interest of the patient.

(*iv*) Historical control: In certain circumstances, such as those involving diseases with high and predictable mortality (acute leukemia of childhood), with signs and symptoms of predictable duration or severity (fever in certain infections), or, in case of prophylaxis, where morbidity is predictable, the results of use of a new drug entity may be compared quantitatively with prior experience historically derived from the adequately documented natural history of the disease or condition in comparable patients or populations with no treatment or with a regimen (therapeutic, diagnostic, prophylactic) the effectiveness of which is established.

(5) A summary of the methods of analysis and an evaluation of data derived from the study, including any appropriate statistical methods. *Provided, however,* That any of the above criteria may be waived in whole or in part, either prior to the investigation or in the evaluation of a completed study, by the Director of the Bureau of Drugs with respect to a specific clinical investigation; a petition for such a waiver may be filed by any person who would be adversely affected by the application of the criteria to a particular clinical investigation; the petition should show that some or all of the criteria are not reasonably applicable to the investigation and that alternative procedures can be, or have been followed, the results of which will or have yielded data that can and should be accepted as substantial evidence of the drug's effectiveness. A petition for a waiver shall set forth clearly and concisely the specific provision or provisions in the criteria from which waiver is sought, why the criteria are not reasonably applicable to the particular clinical investigation, what alternative procedures, if

any, are to be, or have been, employed, what results have been obtained, and the basis on which it can be, or has been, concluded that the clinical investigation will or has yielded substantial evidence of effectiveness, notwithstanding nonconformance with the criteria for which waiver is requested.

(*b*) For such an investigation to be considered adequate for approval of a new drug, it is required that the test drug be standardized as to identity, strength, quality, purity, and dosage form to give significance to the results of the investigation.

(*c*) Uncontrolled studies or partially controlled studies are not acceptable as the sole basis for the approval of claims of effectiveness. Such studies, carefully conducted and documented, may provide corroborative support of well-controlled studies regarding efficacy and may yield valuable data regarding safety of the test drug. Such studies will be considered on their merits in the light of the principles listed here, with the exception of the requirement for the comparison of the treated subjects with controls. Isolated case reports, random experience, and reports lacking the details which permit scientific evaluation will not be considered.

(6) Based on a fair evaluation of all material facts, such labeling is false or misleading in any particular;

the Commissioner shall within 180 days after the filing of the application inform the applicant in writing of his intention to issue a notice of hearing on a proposal to refuse to approve the application.

(b) Unless by the 30th day following the date of issuance of the letter informing the applicant of the intention to issue a notice of hearing, the applicant:

(1) Withdraws the application; or

(2) Waives the opportunity for a hearing; or

(3) Agrees with the Commissioner on an additional period to precede issuance of such notice of hearing,

the Commissioner shall expeditiously notify the applicant of an opportunity for a hearing on the question of whether such application is approvable as provided in §130.14.

§ 130.13 *Records and reports concerning experience on drugs for which an approval is in effect.*

(a) On receiving notification that an application for a new drug is approved, the applicant shall establish and maintain records and make reports that are necessary to facilitate a determination whether there may be grounds for invoking section 505(e) of the act to suspend or withdraw approval of the application, including adequately organized and indexed files containing full reports of any of the following kinds of information, pertinent to the safety or effectiveness of the drug or the adequacy of the methods used in, or the facilities and controls used for, the manufacture, processing, and packing of the drug to assure and preserve its identity, strength, quality, and purity, that has not previously been submitted as part of his application for the drug and which is received or otherwise obtained by him from any source:

(1) Unpublished reports of clinical experience, studies, investigations, and tests conducted by the applicant or reported to him by any person involving the drug that is the subject of the application and related drugs, and reports in the scientific literature involving the drug that is the subject of application. An adequate summary and bibliography of reports in the scientific literature will ordinarily suffice. (The applicant must identify at the time of each report submission each drug he considers related to the subject drug.)

(2) Unpublished reports of animal experience, studies, investigations, and tests conducted by the applicant or reported to him by any person involving the drug that is the subject of the application and related drugs, and reports in the scientific literature involving the drug that is the subject of the application. An adequate summary and bibliography of reports in the scientific literature will ordinarily suffice. (The applicant must identify at the time of each report submission each drug he considers related to the subject drug.)

(3) Experience, investigations, studies, or tests involving the chemical or physical properties or any other properties of the drug; such as, its behavior or properties in relation to micro-organisms, including both the effects of the drug on micro-organisms and the effects of micro-organisms on the drug.

(4) The information required by this section shall include, when known, adequate identification of its source, including the name and post office address of the person who furnished such information.

(5) Copies of all mailing pieces and other labeling, and if it is a prescription drug all advertising, other than that contained in the application, used in promoting the drug; and copies of the currently used package labeling that gives full information for use of the drug, whether or not such labeling is contained in the application.

(6) Information concerning the quantity of the drug distributed, in a manner and form that facilitates estimates of the incidence of any adverse effects reported to be associated with the use of the drug. This does not require disclosure of financial or pricing data.

(7) Information concerning any previously unreported changes from the conditions described in an application. . . .

(b) The applicant shall submit to the Food and Drug Administration copies of the records and reports described in paragraph (a) of this section (except routine assay and control records) appropriately identified with the new-drug application(s) to which they relate as follows. . . .

(1) Immediately upon receipt by the applicant, complete records or reports covering information of the following kinds:

(i) Information concerning any mixup in the drug or its labeling with another article.

(ii) Information concerning any bacteriological, or any significant chemical, physical, or other change or deterioration in the drug, or any failure of one or more distributed batches of the drug to meet the specifications established for it in the new-drug application.

(2) As soon as possible, and in any event within 15 working days of its receipt by the applicant, complete records or reports concerning any information of the following kinds:

(i) Information concerning any unexpected side effect, injury, toxicity, or sensitivity reaction, or any unexpected incidence or severity thereof associated with clinical uses, studies, investigations, or tests, whether or not determined to be attributable to the drug, except that this requirement shall not apply to the submission of information described in a written communication to the applicant from the Food and Drug Administration as types of information that may be submitted at other designated intervals. "Unexpected" as used in this subdivision refers to conditions or developments not previously submitted as part of the new-drug application or not encountered during clinical trials of the drugs, or conditions or developments occurring at a rate higher than shown by information previously submitted as part of the new-drug application, or than encountered during such clinical trials.

(ii) Information concerning any unusual failure of the drug to exhibit its expected pharmacological activity.

* * *

(c) The reports submitted under the provisions of this section are not required to furnish the names and addresses of individual patients unless the applicant is notified in writing by the Food and Drug Administration that individual patient identification is required with respect to designated reports in order to permit further investigation or because there is reason to believe that such reports do not represent actual results obtained.

(d) The applicant shall upon request of any properly authorized officer or employee of the Department, at reasonable times, permit such officers to have access to and copy and verify any records and reports established and maintained under the provisions of this section.

(e) If the Food and Drug Administration finds that the applicant has failed to establish a system for maintaining required records, or has repeatedly or deliberately failed to maintain such records or to make required reports, in accordance with the provisions of this section, or that the applicant has refused to permit access to, or copying, or verification of such records or reports, the Commissioner shall give the applicant due notice and opportunity for a hearing on the question of whether to withdraw the approval of the application. . . .

* * *

§ 130.14 Contents of notice of hearing.

(a) The notice to the applicant of opportunity for a hearing on a proposal by the Commissioner to refuse to approve an application or to withdraw the approval of an application will specify the grounds upon which he proposes to issue his order. On request of the applicant, the Commissioner will explain the reasons for his action. The notice of hearing will be published in the Federal Register and will specify that the applicant has 30 days after issuance of the notice within which he is required to file a written appearance electing whether:

(1) To avail himself of the opportunity for a hearing at the place specified in the notice of hearing; or

(2) Not to avail himself of the opportunity for a hearing.

(b) If the applicant elects to avail himself of the opportunity for a hearing, he is required to file a written appearance requesting the hearing within 30 days after the publication of the notice and giving the reason why the application should not be refused or should not be withdrawn, together with a well-organized and full-factual analysis of the clinical and other investigational data he is prepared to prove in support of his opposition to the notice of opportunity for a hearing. A request for a hearing may not rest upon mere allegations or denials, but must set forth specific facts showing that there is a genuine and substantial issue of fact that requires a hearing. When it clearly appears from the data in the application and from the reasons and factual analysis in the request for the hearing that there is no genuine and substantial issue of fact which precludes the refusal to approve the application or the withdrawal of approval of the application, e.g., no adequate and well-controlled clinical investigations to support the claims of effectiveness have been identified, the Commissioner will enter an order on these data, making findings and conclusions on such data. If a hearing is requested and is justified by the applicant's response to the notice of hearing, the issues will be defined, a hearing examiner will be named, and he shall issue a written notice of the time and place at which the hearing will commence, not more than 90 days after the expiration of such 30 days unless the hearing examiner and the applicant otherwise agree in the case of denial of approval, and as soon as practicable in the case of withdrawal of approval.

(c) The hearing will be open to the public: Provided, however, That if the Commissioner finds that portions of the application which serve as a basis for the hearing contain information concerning a method or process which as a trade secret is entitled to protection, the part of the hearing that involves such portions will not be public unless the respondent so specifies in his appearance.

* * *

§ 130.17 Hearing examiner.

The hearing will be conducted by a hearing examiner appointed as provided in the Administrative Procedure Act and designated for conducting the hearing. Any such designation may be made or revoked by the Commissioner at any time. Hearings will be conducted in an informal but orderly manner in accordance with these regulations and the requirements of the Administrative Procedure Act. The hearing examiner will have the power to administer oaths and affirmations, to rule upon offers of proof and the admissibility of evidence, to receive relevant evidence, to examine witnesses, to regulate the course of the hearing, to hold conferences for the simplification of the issues, and to dispose of procedural requests, but will not have the power to decide any motion that involves final determination of the merits of the proceeding.

*   *   *

§ *130.24 Tentative order.*

The hearing examiner, within a reasonable time, shall prepare tentative findings of fact and a tentative order, which shall be served upon the applicant and the Food and Drug Administration or sent to them by certified mail. If no exceptions are taken to the tentative order within 20 days or such other time specified in such order, that order shall become final.

*   *   *

§ *130.26 Issuance of final order.*

Within a reasonable time after the filing of exceptions, or after oral argument (if such argument is requested), the Commissioner shall issue the final order in the proceeding. The order will include the findings of fact upon which it is based.

§ *130.27 Withdrawal of approval of an application.*

The Commissioner shall, in writing, notify the person holding an approved new-drug application and afford an opportunity for a hearing on a proposal to withdraw approval of the application as provided in section 505(e) of the act and in accordance with the procedure in §§130.14 to 130.26, inclusive, if:

(a) The Secretary has suspended the approval of such application on a finding that there is an imminent hazard to the public health; or

(b) The Commissioner finds:

(1) That clinical or other experience, tests, or other scientific data show that the drug is unsafe for use under the conditions of use upon the basis of which the application was approved; or

(2) That new evidence of clinical experience, not contained in the application or not available to the Food and Drug Administration until after the application was approved, or tests by new methods, or tests by methods not deemed reasonably applicable when the application was approved, evaluated together with the evidence available when the application was approved, reveal that the drug is not shown to be safe for use under the conditions of use upon the basis of which the application was approved; or

(3) Upon the basis of new information before the Food and Drug Administration with respect to the drug, evaluated together with the evidence available when the application was approved, that there is a lack of substantial evidence that the drug will have the effect it purports or is represented to have under the conditions of use prescribed, recommended, or suggested in the labeling thereof (the provisions of §130.12(a) (5) apply to the meaning of "substantial evidence" as used in this subparagraph); or

(4) That the application contains any untrue statement of a material fact; or

(c) The Commissioner finds:

(1) That the applicant has failed to establish a system for maintaining required records, or has repeatedly or deliberately failed to maintain such records or to make required reports, in accordance with a regulation or order under section 505(j) of the act and of § 130.13, or that the applicant has refused to permit access to, or copying or verification of, such records as required; or

(2) That on the basis of new information before the Food and Drug Administration, evaluated together with the evidence available when the application was approved, the methods used in, or the facilities and controls used for, the manufacture, processing, and packing of the drug are inadequate to assure and preserve its identity, strength, quality, and purity; or

(3) That on the basis of new information before the Food and Drug Administration, evaluated together with the evidence available when the application was approved, the labeling of the drug, based on a fair evaluation of all material facts, is false or misleading in any particular; and that the matter complained of was not corrected by the applicant within a reasonable time after his receipt of written notice from the Commissioner specifying the matter complained of.

(d) Any hearing following summary suspension on a finding of imminent hazard to health shall be afforded promptly and shall proceed on an expedited basis.

*   *   *

[ii]
United States Code
Title 42—Public Health and Welfare (1971)

§ 218. *National Advisory Councils; composition, qualifications; appointment and tenure; duties.* (a) The National Advisory Health Council . . . shall . . . consist of the Surgeon General, who shall be chairman, the chief medical officer of the Veterans' Administration or his representative, and a medical officer designated by the Secretary of Defense, who shall be ex officio members; and twelve members appointed without regard to the civil-service laws by the Surgeon General with the approval of the Secretary of Health, Education, and Welfare. The twelve appointed members of . . . such council shall be leaders in the fields of fundamental sciences, medical sciences, or public affairs, and six of such twelve shall be selected from among leading medical or scientific authorities who . . . are skilled in the sciences related to health. . . . Each appointed member of each such council shall hold office for a term of four years. . . .

(b) The National Advisory Health Council · shall advise, consult with, and make recommendations to, the Surgeon General on matters relating to health activities and functions of the Service. . . .

*   *   *

§ 241. *Research and investigations generally.* The Surgeon General shall conduct in the Service, and encourage, cooperate with, and render assistance to other appropriate public authorities, and scientific institutions, and scientists in the conduct of, and promote the coordination of, research, investigations, experiments, demonstrations, and studies relating to the causes, diagnosis, treatment, control, and prevention of physical and mental diseases and impairments of man, including water purification, sewage treatment, and pollution of lakes and streams. In carrying out the foregoing the Surgeon General is authorized to—

*   *   *

(d) Make grants-in-aid to universities, hospitals, laboratories, and other public or private institutions, and to individuals for such research or research training projects as are recommended by the National Advisory Health Council . . . and make, upon recommendation of the National Advisory Health Council, grants-in-aid to public or nonprofit universities, hospitals, laboratories, and other institutions for the general

support of their research and research training programs. . . .

*   *   *

(i) Adopt, upon recommendation of the National Advisory Health Council . . . such additional means as he deems necessary or appropriate to carry out the purposes of this section.

*   *   *

NOTE

HYPOTHETICAL CASES REVIEWED BY THE
NATIONAL ADVISORY HEALTH COUNCIL (1971)

[*All functions of the Public Health Service, including those of the Surgeon General and the Advisory Councils, were transferred to the Secretary of Health, Education, and Welfare by the President's 1966 Reorganization Plan No. 3, 31 Federal Register 8855 (1966). Suppose, however, that the National Advisory Health Council (NAHC) were again reviewing protocols submitted to the Federal government for funding. The following hypothetical cases suggest the way in which the NAHC might respond to the actions of local review committees. In studying these cases, consider the appropriateness of review and of the decisions made as well as the nature and extent of the functions such a national body should assume.*]

I. Patients with a diagnosis of primary myocardial disease (PMD) were to be subjected to bilateral percutaneous cardiac biopsy using a modified Vim-Silverman needle. Samples were to be divided to permit routine histological studies, some histochemical analyses, and standard bacteriological tests. The principal investigator noted that it had not yet been established that PMD is a pathologic entity. In addition, there is no rational etiology for the condition, other than that derived from its frequent association with chronic alcoholism.

The reviewers of the National Advisory Health Council (NAHC) asked the investigator's institutional committee to provide its estimate of the possible risk to the subject through the use of closed chest cardiac biopsy. The committe replied that no such assessment had been made since the individuals involved were patients, not subjects, and the study was intended for diagnostic benefit of the patients. Under these circumstances, they did not feel that the review required by the NAHC was necessary, nor was a special form of consent required. The NAHC then asked if closed chest biopsy was an accepted diagnostic procedure in the institution. The reply, which arrived too late to influence initial review, was negative.

NAHC noted that the mere fact that persons are admitted as "patients" does not place them in a separate category from "subjects;" that the procedure to be used here was not standard or accepted and constituted a research procedure; and that the proposed procedure was associated with a high mortality rate in experimental animals. In addition, accidental cardiac biopsies, sometimes resulting from improperly performed sternal marrow punctures, were extremely hazardous. They recommended that the project be disapproved.

II. An entomologist at Meridian Hill College proposed a series of studies on microclimate adaptive mechanisms in Anopheles mosquitoes. In the course of a visit to the laboratory, NAHC consultants were critical of the arrangements for containing and controlling the mosquito population. When a revised protocol showed no proposed improvement in these arrangements, the advisory group concerned asked if the project had been reviewed and accepted by the institution's committee. The institution's administration replied that no human subjects were involved, only mosquitoes. In reply NAHC staff pointed out that this genus is a potential vector for malaria and that the institution was located in an area heavily populated by recent immigrants from Puerto Rico, Cuba, and other Latin American countries, and that a substantial pool of active and latent malaria undoubtedly existed in these groups. Failure to control the mosquito population could, at least during the summer months, permit spread of malaria within the local population.

III. The investigators proposed a study using both conventional histologic techniques and electron microscopy, on human ova to be obtained from normal women at relatively short intervals after ovulation. Women presenting themselves for post-partum sterilization, would be asked to forego tubal ligation, to become pregnant, and then to undergo bilateral salpingectomy. The excised uterine tubes would be flushed to recover the ovum. Married women would become pregnant in the usual manner. Unmarried women would be asked to accept A.I.D. The NAHC reviewers rejected this proposal on several counts.

Though the proposed written consent document was complete in its description of the potential benefits of the procedure, its efficacy, possible complications, and associated morbidity, the NAHC committee stated that the investigator could not ask for consent since salpingectomy, while standard and accepted, carried with it a higher rate of risk than the procedure of choice, tubal ligation, but no additional benefits. In the committee's opinion, in the absence of the needs of the research project, there would be no indication for salpingectomy in these cases.

The committee also expressed serious doubts that the investigator would be justified in arguing that the risks of the project could be justified "in the interests of humanity" since the scientific return from straightforward cytological and histological studies would be small.

Finally, the committee noted a minority opinion from three members pointing out that the proposal to subject women to A.I.D. solely for the purposes of the project was morally repugnant and unacceptable.

IV. An application received from a physiologist at Mideastern University involved studies of absorption from doubly perfused 20 cm. lengths of human intestine. Inquiries by the NAHC as to the review status of this project brought a reply that no human subjects were involved, only materials obtained at surgery from the Marimar Hospital. In reply the NAHC noted that use of such materials did require review of the circumstances under which the materials were obtained but that this review could be carried out in cooperation with the hospital. Copies of the correspondence were forwarded to the Marimar.

The next letter arrived from the chairman of the committee at Marimar. Their policy required that all requests for surgical materials be cleared through the Chairman of the Department of Pathology, and that patient consent be obtained for other than diagnostic use of these materials. Neither of these steps had been followed. The entire project had now been reviewed in a joint meeting of the university and hospital committees.

Review had disclosed that the investigator had approached the Chief of the Gastrointestinal Service directly to obtain 40 cm. lengths of normal intestine. The surgeon had already provided several sections for pilot studies, mostly obtained from resections performed in treating regional ileitis. While some of these had been removed together with two adjacent diseased areas, most had been obtained by extending the area resected into normal areas. The surgeon argued that the difficulty in defining the area justified some extension of the region to be excised and that, in his judgment, this did not involve any additional risk to the patient.

The committees granted the project contingent approval. Specific written prior permission was to be obtained from each candidate patient for the use of surgically removed intestine. The consent statement proposed by the committee indicated that the material was to be used for research purposes and that removal would "cut down the length of the intestine through which food could be taken into your body. Also, since the operation will be longer and the tissues which support the intestines in your body will be more disturbed than is usually the case, there is some small but additional chance of complications." In addition, the decision as to the extent of ileotomy in each case was to be made by the attendant surgeon in agreement with one of three associates named by the committee. The attendant surgeon rejected the contingency on the grounds that this constitutes an unwarranted intrusion by the hospital into the doctor-patient relationship. The hospital committee pointed out that this relationship did not, in its opinion, include the conduct of research. No agreement being reached, permission to carry out the project was not granted.

V. The applicant proposed a study of fetal body composition to be based on therapeutic abortion material. Fetuses obtained by dilatation and curettage during the first trimester would be subjected to total body analysis. Fetuses obtained during the second and third trimesters would be delivered by cesarean section, dissected, and subjected to organ by organ analysis plus total analysis of the undissected tissues. Fetal material was to be obtained from a collaborating hospital licensed by the state to perform therapeutic abortions. Since the great majority of abortions performed in the institution were done in the first trimester, the collaborating physicians would "encourage" some participants to delay abortion until the second trimester.

The sponsoring institution objected to establishing initial and continuing review procedures since: 1) under the laws of the state no "human subjects" were involved, only fetuses which are "legal non-persons," 2) procurement of the fetal material was under the control of

another institution, and 3) the procedures proposed were customary medical practice in this state.

The reactions of the reviewers for the NAHC were: 1) despite the fact that the fetus had no legal status in this jurisdiction, the mothers did, 2) responsibility for initial and continuing review always stays with the sponsoring institution, and 3) the protocol clearly showed that choice of a procedure or timing of a procedure were to be altered to meet the requirements of the project.

The institution instituted its own review and subsequently withdrew the application without explanation.

VI. In a study involving premature infants born with respiratory distress syndrome (RDS), patients were to be exposed to either 80 percent or 90 percent oxygen therapy on a random basis. Since high tension oxygen therapy is considered "standard," the investigator suggested that no specific parental consent to an infant's participation in the project was necessary. He also pointed out that problems involved in locating the parents and explaining the project's purposes might delay treatment.

The institution's committee concurred, noting that application of "standard" procedures did not constitute research.

The NAHC questioned this decision, holding that a comparison of two accepted procedures constituted research, particularly when assignment of patients to treatment modalities was based on statistical rather than medical criteria. The NAHC cited a legal opinion that: "an informed written consent should be obtained from both, or at least one parent, prior to participation of the infant in the study even though both procedures involved are currently 'standard' and that generally, medical judgment dictates neither the one or the other."

VII. Response contingent reinforcement of infant vocal behavior was to be attempted using a variety of visual stimuli in a controlled environment. Stimuli were to be drawn from the infant's immediate world but were to center around the mother. Initially, reinforcement would be attempted using videotape of the mother moving about the room and approaching the child. The videotape would be started in the absence of vocal activity. If normal vocal activity were interrupted by crying or other "non-responsive" behavior, the tape would be shut off for varying periods. Healthy subjects were to be introduced into the program at the age of 3 months and continued at intervals over a period of 3 years.

The consent statement to be presented to the parents or legal guardians stressed the benefits of early vocal competence and mentioned the possible hazards of temporary isolation (1-hour periods) and adjustment to companions with lesser vocal abilities.

The NAHC raised questions with regard to possible deleterious effects of such a program on the maternal-child relationship, pointing out that crying usually reflected need on the part of the child. Systematic withdrawal of the "mother image" seemed ill-advised. The investigator emphasized that volunteers had already been obtained. The committee pointed out that not all possible hazards had been explained and that the consents could not be considered informed. After some negotiation and pretesting of alternate consent statements, the project was withdrawn by mutual agreement of the investigator and the committee.

VIII. The investigator had proposed a study of the lymphatic drainage of the thoracic cavity and its relation to the route of metastases in mammary carcinoma. The initial several months of the study had coincided with an exceptionally high incidence of appropriate cases coming to autopsy, and the initial aims of the project were rapidly accomplished. The investigator proceeded to a logical second step, the cannulation of the thoracic duct and study of circulating tumor cells in the lymph of mammary cancer patients as well as studies on tumor cells in the blood.

Review by the NAHC of a renewal application led to questions as to the morbidity associated with the procedure and as to the circumstances under which consent was being obtained from cancer patients and "normal" patients. The investigator quite frankly admitted that the morbidity rate approached 25 percent, some of it serious, and that both groups of patients were being told that the procedure was necessary for diagnostic purposes. Since the cancer patients had already been diagnosed, and the criterion for selection of the "normal" group was an absence of lymphatic involvement, the patients were clearly being misinformed. The reviewers asked the institution for an explanation of its apparent approval of deliberate misinformation of patients. The institution replied, "Surely, you do not expect us to question a decision by the Chief of Surgery." The project was disapproved.

b.

Who Should Participate, within What Structure, in Professional Regulation?

[i]
*United States Public Health Service Protection of the Individual as a Research Subject**

Safeguarding the rights and welfare of human subjects involved in research supported by the Public Health Service is the responsibility of the institution to which support is awarded. It is the policy of the Public Health Service that no grant, award, or contract for the support of research involving human subjects shall be made unless the research is given initial and continuing review and approval by an appropriate committee of the applicant institution. This review shall assure that (a) the rights and welfare of the individuals involved are adequately protected, (b) the methods used to obtain informed consent are adequate and appropriate, and (c) the risks to the individual are outweighed by the potential benefit to him or by the importance of the knowledge to be gained.

The institution must provide written assurance to the Public Health Service that it will abide by this policy for all research involving human subjects supported by the Public Health Service. This assurance shall consist of a written statement of compliance with the requirements regarding initial and continuing review of research involving human subjects and a description of the institution's review committee structure, its review procedures, and the facilities and personnel available to protect the health and safety of human subjects. In addition to providing the assurance, the institution must also certify to the Public Health Service for each proposal involving human subjects that its committee has reviewed and approved the proposed research before an award may be made.

Since the welfare of the subject is a matter of concern to the Public Health Service as well as to the institution, PHS advisory groups, consultants, and staff will independently review all research involving human subjects, recommending unfavorable action on grants, contracts, or awards if the research presents unacceptable hazards.

Similarly, the institution should be prepared at all times to question the conduct of research,

* Washington, D.C.: U.S. Department of Health, Education, and Welfare (1969).

even though previously approved by both the institution and the Public Health Service. The safety and welfare of the subject are paramount.

If any conflict exists between institutional policy, PHS policy, or State or local laws, the more restrictive requirements will be followed.

Research subjects.

A subject is considered to be any human being exposed to any research procedure as the result of the availability of Public Health Service funds, whether provided through research, training, or other types of grants, awards, or contracts. Subjects may include, therefore, persons involved in behavioral science studies; normal volunteers; donors of services; inpatients and outpatients; living donors of body fluids, organs, and tissues; and members of the general population who may be involved in environmental or epidemiological studies or similar activities.

An individual should generally be accepted as a research subject only after he, or his legally authorized guardian or next of kin, has consented to his participation in the research. Such consent is valid, however, only if the individual is first given a fair explanation of the procedures to be followed, their possible benefits and attendant hazards and discomforts, and the reasons for pursuing the research and its general objectives.

The subject does not abdicate his rights by consenting to participate in a research project. He may withdraw his consent at any time. Further, he has the right to be secure in his person, to receive proper professional care, to enjoy privacy and confidentiality in the use of information about himself, and to be free from undue embarrassment, discomfort, and harassment.

Applicability.

This policy applies to all projects which go beyond the diagnostic and therapeutic needs of the subject, as determined by his attending professional and the institutional committee. Such projects may involve the procurement of human materials or services and may be supported by a variety of mechanisms, e.g., research training, or demonstration grants; general research support grants; and fellowship, traineeship, or contract awards.

The applicability of this policy is most obvious in medical and behavioral science research involving procedures that may induce a potentially harmful altered state or condition. Surgical procedures; the removal of organs or tissues for biopsy, transplantation, or banking; the administration of drugs or radiation; the use of indwelling catheters or electrodes; the requirement of strenuous physical exertion; subjection to deceit, public embarrassment, and humiliation are all examples of procedures which require thorough scrutiny by institutional committees.

There is a wide range of medical, social, and behavioral research in which no immediate physical risk to the subject is involved. However, some of these may impose varying degrees of discomfort, irritation, and harassment. In addition, there may be substantial potential injury to the subject's rights if attention is not given to maintenance of the confidentiality of information obtained from the subject and the protection of the subject from misuse of findings.

There is also research concerned solely with discarded human materials obtained at surgery or in the course of diagnosis or treatment. The use of these materials involves no possible element of risk to the subject. In such instances application of the policy requires only review of the circumstances under which the materials are to be procured.

* * *

Minimum requirements for an acceptable assurance.

An acceptable assurance consists of two parts:

Formal statement.

A formal statement of compliance with Public Health Service policy must be signed by an appropriate institution official. . . .

Implementing guidelines.

The institution's description of its own procedures should embody the three headings listed below. The explanatory paragraphs following each heading indicate the type of information which should be supplied.

Statement of principles concerning the treatment of human subjects.

It is necessary that the guidelines make reference to the principles the institution will apply in its review of research involving human subjects. The institution may adopt an already existing statement of principles (e.g., the Nuremberg Code, the Declaration of Helsinki, the Statement of Ethical Standards in Research of the American Psychological Association) or it may develop its own statement.

Description of the review committee

The committee must be composed of sufficient members with varying backgrounds to assure complete and adequate review of the research. The committee may be an existing one, or one especially appointed for the purpose. Institutions may utilize subcommittees to represent major administrative components in those instances where establishment of a single committee is impractical or inadvisable. The institution may utilize staff, consultants, or both. The membership should possess not only broad specific competence to comprehend the nature of the research, but also other competencies necessary in the judgment as to acceptability of the research in terms of institutional regulations, relevant law, standards of professional practice, and community acceptance. The committee's maturity and experience should be such as to justify respect for its advice and counsel.

No individual involved in the conduct of the research activity shall participate in its review, except to provide information to the committee.

Committee members should be identified in the assurance to the Public Health Service in terms of position, earned degrees, board certifications, licensures, memberships, and other indications of experience and competence. Names need not be given.

Description of the initial and continuing review procedures to be followed by the committee.

Timing of review.
Research described in applications and contract proposals should, whenever possible, be given institutional review and approval prior to submission to the Public Health Service. Where review prior to Public Health Service submission is not possible, the review must be made prior to issuance of the award by the Public Health Service. Review of initial applications by institutions which have not previously filed acceptable assurances must be performed after acceptance of the assurance by the Public Health Service.

There may be occasions when a second review by the committee will be required before the research is initiated. For example, a long interval has elapsed between committee review and initiation, or the investigator proposes changes in protocol after the application has been reviewed by the committee but before the research is initiated. Perhaps the investigator has proposed research in a rapidly moving scientific area. The second review, in this case, would determine if changing standards of practice indicate a hazardous procedure unrecognized as such during the initial review (e.g., reduction of acceptable radiation levels).

Adequacy of the protection of the rights and welfare of the subjects involved.
Institutional committees should carefully examine the research plan to arrive at an independent determination of possible hazards. The committee must be alert to the possibility that investigators, program directors, or contractors may, quite unintentionally, introduce unnecessary or unacceptable hazards, or fail to provide adequate safeguards. This is particularly true of research that crosses disciplinary lines. The committees should consider the research plan as a whole in order to determine that normally minor and acceptable risks are not aggravated by the way it is designed. The severity of the risk from a procedure may vary with the circumstances under which it is carried out. Age, development, size, maturity, intercurrent disease, and other factors with respect to the subject may adversely affect the acceptability of a procedure. Simultaneous or consecutive performance of several minor tests or procedures may add up to a substantial risk. The committees must assure themselves that proper precautions will be taken to deal with emergencies that may develop even in the course of routine procedures.

Relevant to the decision of the committees are those rights of the subject that are defined by law, particuarly those concerned with the rights of children and unborn infants; the termination of pregnancy; the use of prisoners, institutionalized, and military personnel; and the donation of tissues and organs.

Methods used to obtain adequate, appropriate, informed consent.

*   *   *

Consent should be obtained, whenever possible, from the subjects themselves. When the subjects are not legally or physically capable of giving informed consent, because of age, mental incapacity, or inability to communicate, or when the attending professional believes that the giving of full information would be contrary to the best interests of the subject, the review committee may consider the validity of consent by next of kin, legal guardians, or by other responsible third parties who are representative of the subject's interests. In the latter instances, careful consideration should be given by the committee not only to the third parties' depth of interest and concern with the subjects' rights and welfare, but also to whether the third parties are authorized to expose the subjects to the risks involved. A parent, for example, may have no authority to expose his child to risk, except for the child's own benefit.

The review committee should determine if the consent, whether secured as a written document or given orally, or whether the consent is implicit in voluntary participation in a well-advertised activity, is adequate in the light of the risks to the subject and the circumstances of the research. The review committee should also determine if the information to be given to the subject or to qualified third parties, orally or in writing, is a fair explanation of the procedure, its possible benefits, and its attendant hazards. Where debriefing procedures are considered as a necessary part of the research plan, the committee should ascertain that these will be complete and prompt.

When the sponsoring institution routinely obtains a generalized form of consent for treatment or care, the committee shall determine whether these routine procedures provide an adequate basis for the subject's informed consent to the research procedures involved.

Relative weights of risks versus benefits.
Even though informed consent has been obtained or can be anticipated, the committee shall carefully consider the relative weights of the risks and benefits of the procedures to the subjects. If a procedure may confer a substantial benefit to the subjects, the committee may be justified in permitting them to accept an equally substantial or lesser risk. Where the potential benefits to the subjects are negligible, or nonexistent, as in some cases of normal volunteers, the committee may be justified in permitting subjects to accept a risk in the interests of humanity. In all instances, careful consideration must be given by the committee to the subjects' motivation in accepting them.

*   *   *

Continuing review of research.
The committee shall require the project or program director to report to the committee for review any emergent problems or proposed procedural changes which may affect the status of the research with regard to the institution's review criteria. No such changes, except those necessary to eliminate apparent immediate hazards, should be made without prior approval by the committee.

In addition, the committee shall carry out interim review of the conduct of all research in such a manner and at appropriate intervals in the light of apparent risks, existing administrative and supervisory organization, and other factors as to assure itself that its advice is being followed.

The facilities available to protect the health and safety of human subjects.
The assurance should describe in general terms the

facilities and personnel available to protect the health and safety of human subjects, particularly those requiring emergency care.

*   *   *

Records and reports.
The institution is required to keep informative records of group reviews and decisions on the use of human subjects, and to obtain and keep documentary evidence of informed consent relating to research carried out with the assistance of Public Health Service financial support. At a minimum these records should include a summary of the factors leading to the group decision. Documentary evidence of informed consent may consist of a record of the decision of the committee as to the type of consent which it considers acceptable. Copies of the information statement, if any, to be given to the subject, where signed consent statements are required, should be retained in institution files. Where oral or implied consents are obtained, notations should be made on official records.

*   *   *

NOTES

NOTE 1.

LOUIS G. WELT
REFLECTIONS ON THE PROBLEMS OF HUMAN EXPERIMENTATION*

*   *   *

A letter was written to every university department of medicine in the country seeking answers to the following questions:
1. Does your department or school have a procedural document dealing with problems of human experimentation?
2. What are your personal views concerning the principles which may serve to guide the clinical investigation?
3. What criteria should be satisfied in the creation of the experimental design to assure appropriate attention to the moral and ethical problems involved?
4. Do you think a committee of disinterested faculty should review the experimental design to insure maximum protection for the subject?

Responses were received from 66 departments. Of these only eight have a procedural document and only 24 have or favor a commit-

* 25 *Connecticut Medicine* 75 (1961). Reprinted by permission of *Connecticut Medicine*.

tee to review problems in human experimentation. The discussions of the second and third questions have been interesting and helpful. Since there was no true consensus an attempt will be made to express some of the more prevalent views.

1. Many felt that a procedural document might be a poor idea. This stemmed, for the most part, because it was anticipated that no one can prepare a document which can hope to be more useful than hindering. It was felt by some that a document of rules would place obstacles in the path of legitimate research by responsible investigators, and would provide little or no protection from the irresponsible. Many would agree, perhaps, that if a document is deemed necessary it would be more reasonable to prepare a statement of general principles that would serve to guide rather than rule.

2. There is division on the question of the value of a committee to review experimental protocols. Some favor it and others see this as either useless or harmful. The latter argue that a committee cannot take responsibility, that this must always be in the hands of the individual investigators and should be shared by his department chairman who is, in fact, ultimately responsible for all that goes on within his department. The departmental chairman will seek consultation and advice when he feels this is necessary. In this fashion the valuable consultative features of the committee are available, but there is emphasis on the fact that the legal and moral responsibilities return to their rightful place in the minds and hearts of the investigators.

The other view emphasizes the more certain assurances of safety and the improvements in design that may accrue from a careful and responsible review by a committee of peers.

* * *

NOTE 2.
BERNARD BARBER, JOHN LALLY,
JULIA MAKARUSHKA, AND DANIEL SULLIVAN
THE STRUCTURE AND PROCESSES OF
PEER GROUP REVIEW*

* * *

Many people had predicted widespread opposition to the "imposition" of P.H.S. guide-

* A preliminary version (1970) of *Experimenting With Humans: Problems and Processes of Social Control in the Bio-Medical Research Community.* New York: Russell Sage Foundation (forthcoming). Printed by permission of the authors who retain all rights.

lines when they were put into effect in 1966. In fact, as our data show, the guidelines and their mandated committees have been fairly well received. In 52.5 percent of the institutions in our sample, our respondents reported that the work of the committee was "very well received." In another 36.8 percent, the committee was "fairly well received, no opposition." In only 10.7 percent of the institutions did our respondents report any opposition to the work of the committee. Assuming that our respondents have accurately estimated the response of their colleagues to the P.H.S.-initiated control over their research, what can account for this perhaps unexpectedly favorable reception to a restrictive social innovation? . . .

First . . . there was less opposition to the P.H.S.-mandated peer review committees in those institutions which already had a review procedure of their own. Though the differences . . . are small, they are significant. Further . . . if the P.H.S. guidelines required changes in the existing review procedure, the new procedures were less likely to be "very well received."

Neither of the above two findings is unexpected. Somewhat unexpected, however, is our next finding, namely, that in institutions which required that all research be reviewed, the committee was more likely to have been "very well received". . . . This seems to indicate that though researchers prefer less rather than more restrictions on their work, they react favorably when local institutional policy, restrictive or not, is applied universalistically. The finding seems to imply that researchers think it more fair if no researcher is exempt just because his research is funded by some other agency than the P.H.S.

* * *

By far the largest determinant of the acceptance of peer review, however, was whether the committees actually did anything which infringed on the independence of the researchers. Where review committees rejected one or more proposals, required some revisions, or where one or more researchers withdrew proposals before the committee made a formal decision, then the P.H.S.-mandated committees were much more likely to run into some opposition. . . .

Thus, it seems fairly clear that the amount of opposition to this social innovation was as small as it was because slightly more than one-third of the review committees that were set up have never done anything but approve the research proposals that were submitted.

[ii]
*Yale Medical School Clinical Investigation
Committee
Instructions Regarding Medical Research
Involving Human Subjects* (1968)*

The Clinical Investigation Committee is charged with the responsibility of reviewing protocols for *all research involving human subjects* by the faculty of the Yale University School of Medicine. The Committee is not only concerned with the safety of the experimental subjects but also the suitability of the study and the legal protection of each investigator. There are few hard and fast rules, but certain minimum requirements are essential.

Most research protocols submitted to the Committee are well designed and do not involve unreasonable risk, but final approval for many has been delayed because of lack of certain critical information. In order to expedite the mechanism for obtaining Committee approval and the coordination of activities in the clinical research centers new forms and new procedures have been developed. A *single form* now is used as the protocol for both the Clinical Investigation Committee and either of the clinical research centers. The following instructions and comments may be helpful:

1. *The Research Protocol—for each study 5 copies of the Research Protocol are prepared by the investigator, signed by his departmental chairman and returned to . . . (Dr. Finch).* (Protocols for multi-departmental projects should be signed by the chairman of each department.) One copy of each protocol is sent to each member of the Clinical Investigation Committee for study. Committee meetings usually are held the last Friday of each month. At that time protocols previously circularized to Committee members are reviewed. The *deadline* for protocol consideration by the Clinical Investigation Committee is one week before the monthly meeting. If the Chairman of the Clinical Investigation Committee anticipates problems concerning a particular project he may request that the senior investigator be present at the meeting. If approved, either 4 or 5 copies of the protocol are signed by the Chairman; one copy is returned to the principal investigator, one copy is retained in the files of the Clinical Investigation Committee, and two copies are for-

warded to the Dean's Office for appropriate university distribution. If the investigator requested use of a clinical research center the fifth copy of the protocol is sent to the director of the appropriate clinical research center for his records.

If clearance for *single patient* study in a *clinical research center* is needed the investigator should submit completed protocols in triplicate to the director of the clinical research center. He will promptly review the project protocol for the Clinical Research Committee. One copy of the approved protocol is retained by the director of the clinical research center, one copy is inserted in the patient's clinical record, and one copy is forwarded to the Chairman of the Clinical Investigation Committee. All single-patient protocols will be brought to the attention of the members of the CIC at their monthly meetings.

The *Research Protocol* should provide a concise, yet explicit description of the research procedure along with information concerning known or potential side effects, risks, or hazards. Background material, research objectives, and design are much less important than is information concerning the actual experimental procedure and its potential dangers. Information concerning the uses of *new drugs and new uses for old drugs* frequently is insufficient. The human administration of new drugs or foods, even in tracer amounts, requires FDA approval. If there is any question about the human use of a compound (or food) as described in the protocol, prior FDA (Bureau of Medicine, Office of New Drugs) opinion or clearance is essential.

2. *Guidelines concerning patient consent—* The Clinical Investigation Committee endorses the position taken concerning informed consent in the "AMA Ethical Guidelines for Clinical Investigation" (*Annals of Internal Medicine.* 67: Supplement 7, pp. 76–77, September, 1967). In general, the Committee will require that consent be obtained from the subject or his legal guardian in writing on a standard form (supplied by the Committee) unless, in the opinion of the investigator, written consent is inappropriate. Reasons for not requiring written consent must be clearly stated. It would be helpful in these instances if a specific exclusion from the AMA Ethical Guidelines could be cited in the research protocol.

The Committee wishes to remind investigators that in some studies, involving either new foods or drugs or new applications of established drugs, some of the options stated in the AMA

* S. C. Finch, M.D., chairman. Reprinted by permission.

Ethical Guidelines do not apply. It is the responsibility of the investigator to find out whether or not his study is covered by FDA regulations; if in doubt, he can check with the FDA; Bureau of Medicine, Office of New Drugs. In studies of new drugs, ordinarily there will be institutional sponsorship (e.g., a drug company); it is the responsibility of the sponsor to file Statement of Investigator forms with the FDA; these forms specify requirements for informed consent for each type of study. Filing an Investigational New Drug Application with the FDA is so formidable a procedure that the Committee doubts that any individual investigator would wish to proceed without institutional sponsorship. The FDA has summarized its policy regarding *drug testing* in a publication entitled *FDA Papers* dated March 1967 in an article entitled "Clinical Testing: Synopsis of the New Drug Regulations."

3. *Consent Form—If written consent is to be obtained 5 copies of a completed form must accompany each research protocol.* They are processed along with the research protocols in the same fashion. The upper portion of the consent form should contain a clear description of the program in words that are understandable to the patient. (Describe purpose, type of research and major potential hazards or side effects.) It should be emphasized to all investigators that a signed consent form provides little actual legal protection, but without such a form signed by the experimental subject, his parent, or legal guardian, the investigator's position is much less secure. The most important aspect of informed consent is to certify that the experimental subject is willing to participate in a study with full knowledge of the objectives and all major risks. . . .

* * *

NOTE

YALE MEDICAL SCHOOL CLINICAL INVESTIGATION COMMITTEE GUIDELINES FOR PREPARATION OF PROTOCOLS (1971)*

* * *

The most common reason for delay of approval of a protocol is an improperly prepared consent form. The consent form should be a

---

* Draft Memorandum prepared by Drs. Robert J. Levine, Chairman, Clinical Investigation Committee, and George Lister. Reprinted by permission.

statement addressed to the patient and should read as such. Ordinarily, it is best to word it in the second person. It should not repeat what is stated in Section 6 on the protocol but rather should describe in language that the average layman can be expected to understand the general nature, intent, and design of the experiment with particular attention to those aspects of it in which the subject must participate. The following points must be covered:

1. The subject should understand why he has been selected for participation in the study. Ordinarily this is because of a specific disease or condition that he or one of his relatives might have.

2. Ordinarily, the study is being done not for the benefit of the subject but rather for purposes of deriving information which may in the future be of benefit to others; this should be made clear on the consent form.

3. It must be clearly stated that agreement to participate in the study bears some risk of either hazards or—at least—inconveniences.

4. When appropriate it should be stated that the subject is free to refuse to participate and that such refusal will not adversely prejudice his future treatment. Further, it should indicate that the subject is free to withdraw from the study unless the investigation, once commenced, precludes this.

5. In cases where consent will be obtained by persons other than the investigating physician this should be indicated in the lower left corner of the consent form by either replacing or adding to the word "physician."

* * *

Subjects should be invited to raise questions about anything in the consent form that they feel requires clarification. It is further recommended that subjects be given a copy of the signed consent form.

In some studies it may be appropriate to secure consent orally rather than in writing. Ordinarily such studies involve minor manipulations such as a single drawing of a small volume of blood. If the investigator feels that oral consent is appropriate for his study he should put on the consent form the information he plans to present to the subject for purposes of securing oral consent. Also on the consent form there should be a request that the CIC waive the requirement of securing consent in writing.

[iii]
The Massachusetts General Hospital
Human Studies—Guiding Principles and
Procedures*

*   *   *

Procedure in Cases of Research Involving
Human Subjects—General Hospital Division

Whenever an investigative project is planned
which will involve one or more human subjects,
the investigator concerned shall first consult with
the Chief of Service or Department as to the
character of the project. The investigative plan
shall then be referred to the Committee on Research and its Subcommittee on Human Studies
for review and advice. In all instances, not only
will such a review be conducted prior to and at
the same time as close as possible to the initiation of the studies involved, but also all research
projects will be so reviewed to assure the Committee on Research and the Board of Trustees
that other projects do not in fact include studies
of human subjects. . . .

In its review, after establishing that a given
proposal involves human subjects, the Subcommittee on Human Studies shall carefully examine the research plan for its conformance to the
"Guiding Principles" and render its advice and
recommendations to the Executive Committee
of the Research Committee. The Executive
Committee shall forward its advice and recommendations to the Committee on Research
which in turn will report its recommendations
to the Chief of Service and the General Director. In the event that the Subcommittee decides
that the research plan does not ensure adequately
the rights and welfare of the human subject (as
outlined in the "Guiding Principles"), the Committee on Research shall report its advice to the
Chief of Service or Department and the General Director. Any corrective action recommended by the Committee on Research and its
Subcommittee on Human Studies shall be carried
out by the Chief of Service or Department.

It is the responsibility of the Chief of Service to decide whether to accept the advice of the
Committee on Research or to refer the matter to
the General Director and the Trustees for a
definitive decision. The Trustees may seek the
advice of its Advisory Committee on Research

and the Individual* in the unlikely event of
disagreement among those concerned.

In addition, it shall be the Chief's responsibility to know when any significant change is
contemplated or has been made in a project on
his Service that involves human subjects which
would then require further review.

A record will be made in the Research
Office as to the actions taken with regard to any
project.

The chart shows diagrammatically the decision-making process [see following page].

NOTES

NOTE 1.
OFFICE OF SCIENCE AND TECHNOLOGY
PRIVACY AND BEHAVIORAL RESEARCH†

*   *   *

Responsibility for monitoring the propriety
of behavioral research must be shared by the
entire community of colleagues of the investigator in his home institution. The investigator
may be too deeply involved in his hoped-for outcomes, as may colleagues in his own discipline;
responsibility for reviewing matters of propriety

---

* Boston: The Massachusetts General Hospital
13–14 (2nd ed., 1970). Reprinted by permission.

* Trustees' Advisory Committee on Research
and the Individual, 1970: The Right Reverend Henry
Knox Sherrill, *Chairman;* Henry K. Beecher, M.D.,
*Henry Isaiah Dorr Professor of Research and Teach-
ing in Anaesthetics and Anaesthesia, Emeritus,
Harvard University;* Mary I. Bunting, Ph.D., *Presi-
dent, Radcliffe College;* William J. Curran, LL.M.,
S. M. Hyg., *Frances Glessner Lee Professor of Legal
Medicine, Harvard University;* Daniel D. Federman,
M.D., *Associate Professor of Medicine, Harvard
University, Physician, Massachusetts General Hos-
pital, Ex officio as Chairman of the Subcommittee
on Human Studies of the Committee on Research,
Massachusetts General Hospital;* Paul A. Freund,
S.J.D., *Carl M. Loeb University Professor, Harvard
University;* Franz J. Ingelfinger, M.D., *Clinical Pro-
fessor of Medicine, Boston University, Editor, New
England Journal of Medicine;* John H. Knowles,
M.D., *Professor of Medicine, Harvard University,
Ex officio as General Director, Massachusetts Gen-
eral Hospital;* Charles P. Price, Th.D., *Plummer Pro-
fessor of Christian Morals, Harvard University;*
Francis O. Schmitt, Ph.D., *Institute Professor, Mas-
sachusetts Institute of Technology, Trustee, Massa-
chusetts General Hospital;* Ralph G. Meader, Ph.D.,
*Deputy Director (Research Administration) and
Executive Secretary, Committee on Research, Massachusetts General Hospital.*

† Washington, D.C.: U.S. Government Printing
Office 23–24 (1967).

894

Procedure in Cases of Research Involving Human Subjects
General Hospital Division

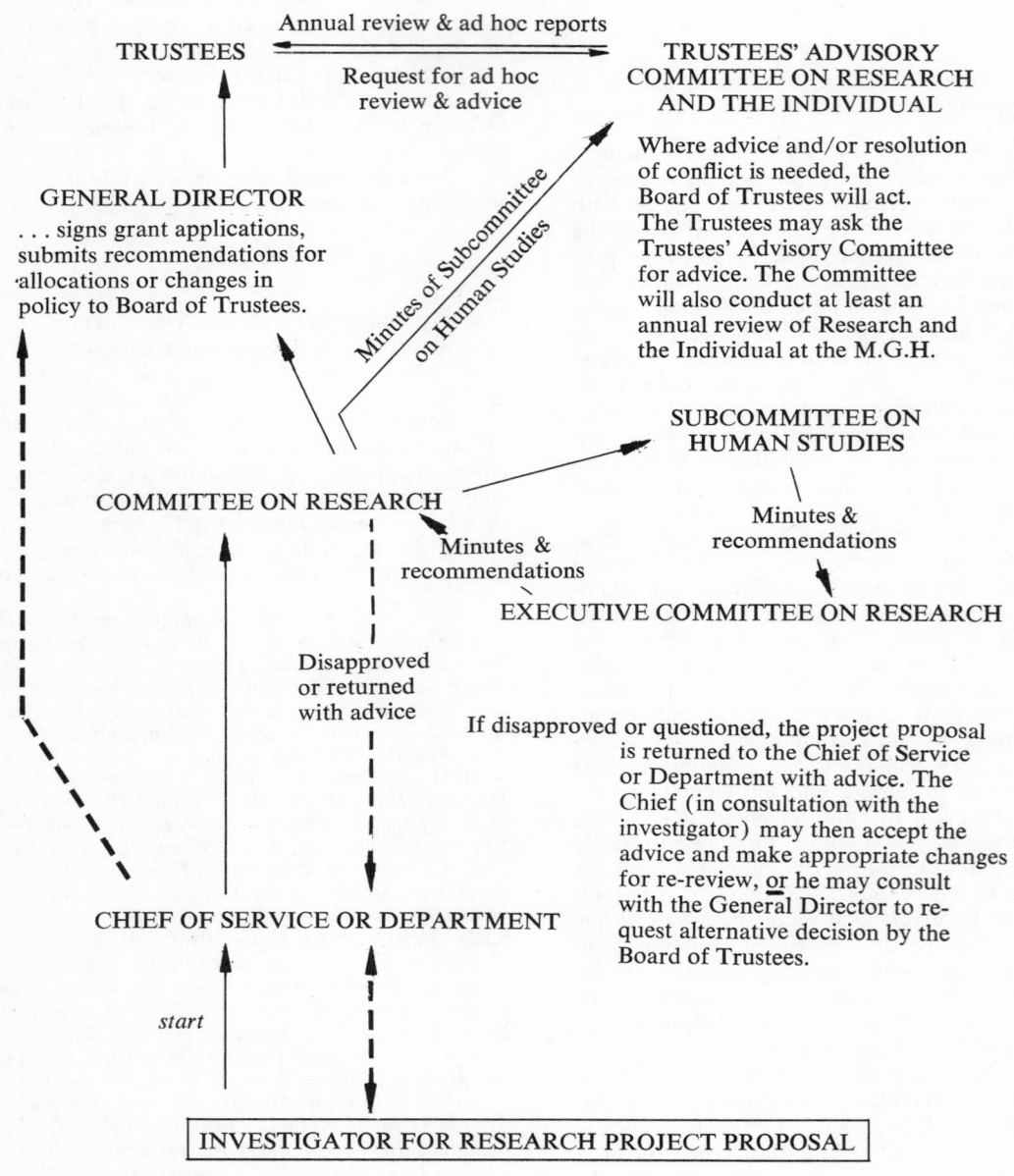

must therefore be shared with less-concerned but well-informed associates. When the investigator is a member of the faculty of a university, there will be scientists and scholars in his own and in unrelated fields who can provide independent judgments about the quality of his research and the appropriateness of the methods he plans to use. In Government agencies and laboratories and, in fact, in almost every institution, similar peer groups can be established.

The individual investigator must accept the obligation for consulting with appropriate colleagues and senior associates about his work. In addition, the institution itself must accept the responsibility for insuring that the work is done by methods which it is willing to defend, and by investigators whose judgment it is willing to defend. The universities, especially those which have substantial research programs, can provide patterns that will serve as models for other institutions that sponsor research.

Beyond this, the universities, as the chief educators of the next generation of research workers, must accept the obligation to imbue their students with the highest standards in the conduct of research.

A university sometimes finds it difficult to play the role that it would be willing to accept since the individual investigator often establishes his primary relationship with the financing agency. The financial implications of this independence of the investigator and of his relationships with the funding agency have already been referred to in the report of the Wooldridge Committee. The same considerations that apply to fiscal responsibility apply to the propriety of research. When an agency of the Federal Government awards a grant to an investigator, it should assign to the institution where he works the continuing responsibility for insuring that the investigation is carried out in accordance with the highest standards of conduct.

The Public Health Service has recently moved to place this responsibility upon the sponsoring institution. The procedures instituted and the instructions issued should have the very desirable effect of increasing the responsible review of research proposals by institutions. A further benefit of the new procedures used by the Public Health Service is the decentralization of supervision and review from agencies in Washington to institutional representatives who can play a more effective role on a continuing basis.

*   *   *

NOTE 2.

HAROLD J. LASKI
THE LIMITATIONS OF THE EXPERT*

*   *   *

[I]t is one thing to urge the need for expert consultation at every stage in making policy; it is another thing, and a very different thing, to insist that the expert's judgment must be final. For special knowledge and the highly trained mind produce their own limitations which, in the realm of statesmanship, are of decisive importance. *Expertise*, it may be argued, sacrifices the insight of common sense to intensity of experience. It breeds an inability to accept new views from the very depth of its preoccupation with its own conclusions. It too often fails to see round its subject. It sees its results out of perspective by making them the centre of relevance to which all other results must be related. Too often, also, it lacks humility; and this breeds in its possessors a failure in proportion which makes them fail to see the obvious which is before their very noses. It has, also, a certain caste-spirit about it, so that experts tend to neglect all evidence which does not come from those who belong to their own ranks. Above all, perhaps, and this most urgently where human problems are concerned, the expert fails to see that every judgment he makes not purely factual in nature brings with it a scheme of values which has no special validity about it. He tends to confuse the importance of his facts with the importance of what he proposes to do about them.

*   *   *

. . . However much we may rely upon the expert in formulating the materials for decision, what ultimately matters is the judgment passed upon the results of policy by those who are to live by them. Things done by government must not only appear right to the expert; their consequences must seem right to the plain and average man. And there is no way known of discovering his judgment save by deliberately seeking it. This, after all, is the really final test of government; for, at least over any considerable period, we cannot maintain a social policy which runs counter to the wishes of the multitude.

It is not the least of our dangers that we tend, from our sense of the complexity of affairs,

* London: The Fabian Society 4, 12 (1931). Reprinted by permission.

to underestimate both the relevance and the significance of those wishes. We are so impressed by the plain man's ignorance that we tend to think his views may be put aside as unimportant. . . . But the inference from a knowledge that the plain man is ignorant of technical detail and, broadly speaking, uninterested in the methods by which its results are attained, is certainly not the conclusion that the expert can be left to make his own decisions.

*   *   *

NOTE 3.

LEO SZILARD
THE VOICE OF THE DOLPHINS*

*   *   *

"[W]hy not do something about the retardation of scientific progress?"

"That I would very much like to do," Mark Gable said, "but how do I go about it?"

"Well," I said, "I think that shouldn't be very difficult. As a matter of fact, I think it would be quite easy. You could set up a foundation, with an annual endowment of thirty million dollars. Research workers in need of funds could apply for grants, if they could make out a convincing case. Have ten committees, each composed of twelve scientists, appointed to pass on these applications. Take the most active scientists out of the laboratory and make them members of these committees. And the very best men in the field should be appointed as chairmen at salaries of fifty thousand dollars each. Also have about twenty prizes of one hundred thousand dollars each for the best scientific papers of the year. This is just about all you would have to do. Your lawyers could easily prepare a charter for the foundation. As a matter of fact, any of the National Science Foundation bills which were introduced in the Seventy-ninth and Eightieth Congresses could perfectly well serve as a model."

"I think you had better explain to Mr. Gable why this foundation would in fact retard the progress of science," said a bespectacled young man sitting at the far end of the table, whose name I didn't get at the time of introduction.

"It should be obvious," I said. "First of all, the best scientists would be removed from their laboratories and kept busy on committees passing on applications for funds. Secondly, the scientific workers in need of funds would concentrate on problems which were considered promising and were pretty certain to lead to publishable results. For a few years there might be a great increase in scientific output; but by going after the obvious, pretty soon science would dry out. Science would become something like a parlor game. Some things would be considered interesting, others not. There would be fashions. Those who followed the fashion would get grants. Those who wouldn't would not, and pretty soon they would learn to follow the fashion, too."

*   *   *

NOTE 4.

FRANCIS D. MOORE
THERAPEUTIC INNOVATION—ETHICAL
BOUNDARIES IN THE INITIAL CLINICAL
TRIALS OF NEW DRUGS AND
SURGICAL PROCEDURES*

*   *   *

There can be little question that personal ambition, usually for career advancement or public acclaim, underlies much intense motivation in research work and in the trial of new ideas, drugs, operations, or treatment. Such personal ambition is usually well hidden under the sophisticated affect of the dedicated clinical scientist and, far from being remiss, is the sign of a healthy society. While social convention requires its disguise in the masquerade of scientific intercourse, this ambition is not a thing to be ashamed of. Personal ambition for advance and recognition is a far better motive for the work of difficult or protracted clinical investigation than is the seeking of political advancement or financial reward. No matter how deep the urge for pure knowledge, few scientists have not derived some excitement from a general acceptance of their ideas or procedures, particularly if these were of potential social benefit. The possibility of such acceptance provides a more stimulating environment for scientific work than the even temper of an apathetic society where, because of the heavy system of penalties placed upon failure, there is neither a channel for innovation nor an interest in departure from tradition.

But ambition, no matter how praiseworthy,

---

* New York: Simon and Schuster 100–101 (1961). Copyright © 1961 by Leo Szilard. Reprinted by permission.

* 98 *Daedalus* 502, 518–519 (1969). Reprinted by permission of Daedalus, Journal of the American Academy of Arts and Sciences, Boston, Massachusetts.

can certainly lead individuals astray. A common example is found in the premature publication of scientific results. Personal ambition for recognition has clearly outstripped the cooler judgment of awaiting more definitive data. The active collaboration of scientists provides the best way of harnessing these fine qualities of excitement and ambition so as to maintain their force for forward motion and yet prevent them from running wild. For this reason, a collaborative group with open discussion, avoidance of secrecy, and frequent review of plans and policies seems far more important than the short-term arbitrary review of some one drug or operation by a formal panel with a strictly *ad hoc* mission. Such formal panels are usually composed of individuals who know little of the work contemplated, and they may even come to include individuals who for reasons of jealousy or ignorance would rather not see the old order challenged anyway. The ethical acceptability of therapeutic innovation documented in a research application, for example, is far better attested by the nature of the scientific consultants working on the project than it is by the nature of the hospital panel that is to review each case.

* * *

NOTE 5.

IRVING L. JANIS
PROFESSIONAL ROLES, NORMS, AND ETHICS—
A SOCIAL PSYCHOLOGICAL VIEWPOINT*

* * *

. . . I have heard some informal discussions in which a team of research workers puts forth a simple formula that all of them agree upon as an adequate justification, absolving themselves of responsibility for any potentially untoward effects of their human experiments: e.g., "You can't do scientific research on important human problems without taking risks." Research teams, like any other face-to-face work group, seem to be quite capable of developing shared rationalizations that give the members moral support in carrying out questionable actions—actions that, in any other social context, each individual would be inclined to forego. In extreme instances, a cohesive local group develops an informal code of its own that deviates from the norms of the superordinate organization and the community at large.

One major factor that must be taken into account in this connection is the attitude conveyed by the local leaders. Obviously, when a group of psychologists has a strong department chairman or clinical director who openly opposes the norms of the professional organization, the chances are greater that the group working under him will develop an informal code that deviates from the professional organization's norms. . . .

* * *

NOTE 6.

BERNARD BARBER
SOME "NEW MEN OF POWER"—THE CASE
OF BIOMEDICAL RESEARCH SCIENTISTS*

* * *

[T]he matter of outsiders is one that I consider particularly important. One of the possible defects of formal review committees is that even they, like informal groups, are too ingrown, too particularistic, too narrow in their perspectives, to function as well as they might. In view of these possibilities, I should like to see two kinds of outsiders mandated as members of all review committees. One kind is relevant biomedical research experts from institutions other than the one where the review committee functions. Such expert outsiders would carry from Harvard to Texas, or from Kansas to Cornell, for instance, a different perspective and an impersonal objectivity that is harder to provide from the inside. A second kind of outsider should be the sociological-legal-ethical expert, fairly knowledgeable about biomedical research, but, rather, an expert in such problems as the nature of social norms, the problems of fair or judicial procedure, and the relevance of public feelings, values, and knowledge to the ethical matter in hand. Indeed, with this kind of outsider in mind, I foresee a whole new social role, one in which people with various kinds of social science and legal training undergo further formal and on-the-job training to qualify themselves to serve on ethical review committees in biomedical research institutions. It is not sufficient to have a slightly trained person in this role. Some members of the clergy can fill it, but not all, and even those who are suited should have further training. Some members of the general public might fill it,

* 6a *The Canadian Psychologist* 143, 148 (1965). Reprinted by permission.

* 169 *Annals of the New York Academy of Sciences* 519, 521 (1970). Reprinted by permission.

but, once again, only if they have special socio-logical-legal skills and further training.

* * *

NOTE 7.
KENNETH L. MELMON, MICHAEL GROSSMAN,
AND R. CURTIS MORRIS, JR.
EMERGING ASSETS AND LIABILITIES OF A
COMMITTEE ON HUMAN WELFARE
AND EXPERIMENTATION*

* * *

The Committee [on Human Welfare and Experimentation of the University of California at San Francisco] realized that the number of applications, the diversity of subject matter and the seriousness of the task would preclude meaningful review of consistent and high quality by a small fixed group. Therefore, the Committee established itself as parent group to three-man ad hoc review committees it appointed for each submitted protocol. Members of the parent committee could review some applications and take "administrative action," or they could serve on ad hoc committees. Members of the ad hoc groups were chosen by the Committee on Human Welfare and Experimentation from the faculty at large. Each member was chosen for his objectivity, morality, expertise in some area related to the research protocol, ability to communicate critical information to the investigator and lack of personal involvement in the research project.

* * *

The chairmen of ad hoc committees were asked to file a written report to the parent committee within 10 days of its assignment to the ad hoc committee. Disagreement by any member on any of the six points used for review was interpreted as a potential disapproval and required that the parent committee transmit recommendations for revision to the investigator. Re-examination of the revised protocol by the parent committee could then result in approval. If the ad hoc group disapproved unanimously of any of the six points, revision became mandatory, and the protocol could be accepted only with the unanimous approval of the ad hoc committee. In response to disapproval, an investigator could withdraw the request, alter the protocol to comply with recommendations or request an-

---

* 282 *New England Journal of Medicine* 427, 428–431 (1970). Reprinted by permission.

other ad hoc committee that would review the protocol de novo. No more than two ad hoc committees could review an unaltered protocol.

Administrative approval was given by the chairman of the Committee on Human Welfare and Experimentation under two circumstances. When an unanticipated opportunity for research arose and required immediate response, the investigator could submit a written request for a single study. The permission for such a study could be granted without committee action, but additional studies could not be done before formal approval by an ad hoc committee. Administrative approval could also be granted for studies involving routine tests or minimal risk. The great majority of such requests were for venous-blood sampling totaling less than 50 ml from nonanemic volunteers or patients. No protocols could be finally rejected by administrative action alone.

The first-year and second-year experiences were compared on the basis of the following criteria: Was there compliance with the questions listed above? Could evolutionary patterns of committee function be appreciated? Did aspects of protocol procedure affect an ad hoc committee's action? What were the judgments or philosophies of the reviewers on the ad hoc committees, and were changing or unanticipated factors operating in decision making?

Difficulties are many and perhaps obvious in such an evaluation. Protocols vary widely in the care with which they are prepared, reviewers may be internally inconsistent, and various reviewers approach the evaluation with different standards. In view of such considerations, it is perhaps surprising that useful information could be gleaned from the review of the data.

* * *

New applications averaged greater than three per week and the number in the second year was greater than in the first. This trend has continued. In the first six months of the third academic year of committee function, 265 applications have been received for a projected total of greater than 500 for the third year. In each of the first two years, the number of applications assigned to ad hoc committees remained approximately the same, but initial rejections increased from 12 to 20 and final rejections tripled (from four to 13) in the second year. An increasing seriousness of approach to review by the ad hoc committees can be inferred from the increased percentage of unqualified dissensions in the second year. Similarly, the standards of the ad hoc committees approximated more closely those of the representatives of the parent committee (and of the entire parent committee, whose members have not changed). Inconsistencies were fewer in the second year than in the first. Literature citations were more carefully selected, and greater care was taken to explain the objectives and methods in both the protocol and the consent form. During the second year, progressively more disagreement arose within ad hoc committees regarding the appropriateness of the way in which consent was secured and risk described.

All 17 rejected protocols were reviewed by at least two ad hoc committees. A striking finding is that each protocol rejected initially was rejected by a second committee that was unaware it was reexamining a previously rejected protocol. Seven protocols were rejected because risk benefit could not be assessed from the description of objectives and methods. None of the seven decisions were contested. Eight protocols were rejected because of inadequate precautions, and the remaining two rejections were because of unacceptable risk.

When a sample of seven rejected protocols was compared to acceptable proposals by the same authors, striking differences were apparent in the care of preparation of the protocol (including length, number of references, number of misspelled words and uncorrected typographical errors). Although this was a subjective appraisal, there seemed little doubt that investigators had given considerably less thought and care to the protocols that were rejected than to those approved.

Most of the reviewers interviewed believed that protocols should be submitted anonymously; some admitted that they were swayed by the academic status of the investigator. A distinct minority admitted that incomplete protocols were more likely to be passed if submitted by a full professor with a "good reputation" than if submitted by a younger, "less established" faculty member. Of note was the fact that all rejected protocols were submitted by University of California tenure faculty members. The majority (58 per cent) of total applications were submitted by nontenure faculty.

The majority of reviewers, who also serve as referees or editors to scientific journals or members of National Institutes of Health study sections, observed that time expended on an average review during the second year was considerably greater than during the first; the average time necessary for a review of a protocol for the ad hoc committee was greater than that spent on an average paper reviewed for a journal. The reviewers all suggested a larger pool of reviewers, but only one preferred not to continue.

None of the reviewers interviewed knew of flagrant violations of committee policy (investigators who had proceeded without approval from the committee), and yet two probable violations were discovered during the second year. Neither violation was detected as a result of policing, but each became evident upon casual observation by faculty either previously involved in evaluations or concerned with standards of human experimentation. Such an observation may imply that formal policing may not be necessary as long as a broad spectrum of faculty participates in reviewing protocols. There is a clear division of opinion over whether policing should be instituted, but many agree that a high-level administrator should be apprised of all detected violations. Such a policy might influence the quality of applications by some and the adherence to regulations by others. Now, infractions of policy are brought to the attention of the involved department chairman and sent to a research policy committee of the school in which the infraction has been involved. Action by this committee is not included in the files of the Committee on Human Welfare and Experimentation. Although preliminary investigation can be undertaken by the parent committee, it is convinced that definitive decisions on punitive action should not be within its purview. Such judicial action could severely and unduly prejudice future reviews of projects proposed by the same investigator, would be unrelated to measures taken after other violations of campus policy, and could alter the focus of the function of the Committee on Human Welfare and Experimentation.

*   *   *

The most difficult tasks for the Committee on Human Welfare and Experimentation were as follows: to disseminate convincing information that there is a legal as well as a moral obligation for investigators with any affiliation to the University of California to submit protocols on investigations in human beings for peer-group evaluation; to establish a guide for investigators that clearly stated that objectives of peer-group review and the requirements of an actual application; to emphasize the importance of specific criteria by which the risk-benefit ratio could be assessed; to help create useful written consent forms; to be certain that fail-safe methods were provided to reverse or terminate an experimental procedure; and to educate the investigators to recognize when new or old investigational drugs were being used. We think that such problems have been overcome to a large degree.

A majority liability lies in the long-term consistency and beneficial evolution in policy. We believe that slow rotation of the membership of the Committee on Human Welfare and Experimentation, slow progress of a member to chairmanship and overlapping terms of service will provide consistency in policy. We strongly endorse the ad hoc committee concept both for its flexibility in providing the best reviewers for each situation and for continuously and painlessly expanding the number of faculty informed on and concerned with policy on investigation in human beings. Broadening of the base of faculty awareness of the needs for high standards in human experimentation should also obviate the need for specific policing procedures.

Committee function has evolved steadily and has led to alterations of policy and suggestions for the future. We believe that ad hoc committees of experts should be selected on a randomized basis to evaluate each protocol. Such randomization of reviewer selection can be accomplished by the following steps: establishing separate categories requiring expert evaluation; listing eligible qualified reviewers recommended by department chairmen; determining categories from which reviewers should be picked; having the secretary of the committee draw names from each category as designated by the chairman; and establishing a rotation for reviewers. In addition, an attempt should be made to ensure anonymity of the investigator by coding protocols.

NOTE 8.

BERNARD BARBER, JOHN LALLY,
JULIA MAKARUSHKA, AND DANIEL SULLIVAN
THE STRUCTURE AND PROCESSES OF
PEER GROUP REVIEW*

*   *   *

Evidence from our interviewing of bio-medical researchers at University Hospital and Research Center and at Community and Teaching

* A preliminary version (1970) of *Experimenting with Humans: Problems and Processes of Social Control in the Bio-Medical Research Community.* New York: Russell Sage Foundation (forthcoming). Printed by permission of the authors who retain all rights.

Hospital indicates that even in institutions where there is a peer review committee presumably reviewing *all* research, there is another perhaps important minority of research activities which is not submitted to peer review. In these two institutions where we interviewed researchers, 9 percent of them *volunteered* the information that one or more of their investigations using human subjects had not been reviewed by the peer review committee. A few more informed us that they knew of what they called "ad hoc" or "nonsystematic" human research by others which was not reviewed by the committee.

Those who volunteered this information about unreviewed research by themselves or others suggested two structured sources for such bypassing of the review committee. First, what is considered "delay" in the reviewing process may generate evasion techniques. At University Hospital and Research Center, it takes about a month from the time a protocol is submitted to the time it is considered by the review committee. Researchers racing to establish priority of discovery or those who feel that some case or situation presents them with "now or never" opportunities to do research both may feel that this is an unacceptably long time to wait. Instead of waiting, they go ahead without submitting a protocol for review at all or, alternatively, submit a protocol but go ahead before it is approved. . . . Procedures for especially speedy review where the researchers were afraid of undue delay would probably be necessary only in a minority of cases and would cut down the evasion that is caused by these exigencies in bio-medical research.

A second structural source of evasion of, or indifference to, peer review procedures arises from the genuine and not infrequent ambiguity regarding what is "research" and what is a small, everyday variation on standard medical or surgical procedures. Evidence on this ambiguity is available in the responses to a question we asked in our national sample survey. We asked our respondents whether the following definition of research was "personally acceptable to you without addition or deletion?"—

Clinical Research or Investigation: Anything done to a person which is as yet not established, by clinical experience or scientific research, as being for his direct therapeutic benefit or as contributing to the diagnosis of his disease. (What is done may eventually, of course, be for the person's own direct or indirect therapeutic benefit and/or for the eventual therapeutic benefit of the population at large.) Investigations which involve the analysis of human substances collected as a by-product of established diagnostic or other procedures should be included here as clinical research.

While 75.2 percent (299) of our respondents agreed with this definition, 24.8 percent did not. Those who disagreed with our definition suggested alternative definitions. Some were more inclusive than ours, and some were more exclusive. Until definitional ambiguities are reduced, it is inevitable that a certain amount of research may not be defined as such and may be carried out without peer review.

*   *   *

As might be expected from the recency of its development, and as the data from our national sample survey of bio-medical research institutions indeed confirm, the peer review committee in its typical structure is still not highly differentiated or specialized. . . . 68 percent of the respondents said their peer review committees were not specialized in any way. 15 percent indicated that there were other review committees in their institutions, either at some higher or lower level of the structure or at some affiliated institution. Only 9 percent report specialization into subcommittees, and only 5 percent report specialized departmental committees. Only 8 percent of the institutions have executive committees for their peer review groups. Only 5 percent of the institutions claim that they have any members at all who spend "full time" in the activities of the peer review committee, and in every instance these "full-time" people were clerical.

As might be further expected from such relatively undifferentiated groups, the number of members is typically small: 27 percent of the institutions reported 1–5 members; another 48 percent reported 6–10; and 25 percent report 11–40.

A further indication of the lack of differentiation in peer review committee structure is the admixture of other functions besides that of ethical review. In 22 percent of the responding institutions, for example, the peer review committee also allocates the institution's research funds to its clinical investigators. In about two-thirds of our sample, the peer review committee also evaluates the scientific merit of proposed clinical research. Since scientific merit (e.g., representativeness and size of sample) is often related to ethical issues (e.g., too small a sample merely puts subjects at risk unnecessarily, too

large a sample may put too many subjects at risk), it is often not desirable to separate the reviewing of ethical and scientific issues. But insofar as a committee is not relating scientific merit to ethical concerns, its lack of differentiation may reduce its competence with either one of these two issues. One respondent even informed us that his peer review committee reviewed the cost-effectiveness of all proposed researches. While again this may sometimes be related to ethical matters, it is often quite another and related issue which should be left to other committees.

As to rank of peer review committee members in the formal hierarchy of their institutions, here again the typical structure seems to be less differentiated than it might be. Four-fifths of the institutions report that most of the members of their peer review committees come from the highest level of the formal institutional hierarchy, including the clinical, administrative, and academic. In the other institutions, the majority of the peer review members are from the intermediate level. Nowhere is a majority from the lower levels. A different mixture of members from different levels might give the peer review committees a more differentiated set of viewpoints on the ethical issues they are required to screen.

Finally, the relative lack of differentiation of the structure of review committees is manifest in the categories of types of activities, specialties, and occupational roles that their members are selected from. There is a heavy emphasis on members with experience in clinical research, as there of course needs to be, though perhaps somewhat too much so at the expense of other types of members who have other knowledge and viewpoints to bring to the decisions of the committee. 15 percent of the responding institutions report that they have only persons who engage in clinical research on their peer review committees. Overall, 91 percent of the institutions report members from among those who actually engage in clinical investigations. 27 percent report M.D. members who do not do clinical research. 43 percent report that they have pathologists either as members or as consultants. 59 percent report administrators as members, probably in recognition of the administrative responsibility of the institution for complying with P.H.S. regulations. 18 percent say that nurses are members. And then there is a scattering from other types of roles: 10 percent use lawyers employed by the institution, 8 percent have members of the board of trustees as members, 9 percent use basic scientists, 9 percent use social scientists (a term which includes social workers and psychologists), and 2 percent have pharmacologists or pharmacists as members.

As for outsiders of various kinds, that is, outsiders who are either clinical research specialists in other institutions or outsiders who have non-medical roles in the larger community, the typical peer review committee has small place for them. 9 percent of the responding institutions said they had members on their peer review committees from other institutions who do clinical research in the general areas in which members of the institution do research and 9 percent also use M.D.'s from other institutions who do no clinical research in the institution's areas of specialization. Only 4 percent use outside lawyers; only 4 percent use outside social scientists; and only 4 percent use clergymen. Only one institution has a patient sitting on its peer review committee. Thus, very few peer review committees use outsiders as regular members either to bring them kinds of expertise they might want or to provide what is probably even more important, namely, the universalistic standards that may often be hard for members of a particular institution to apply to one another just because they are caught up inevitably in a web of personal and particularistic relationships with many of their colleagues. Some institutions do use outside consultants on an irregular basis, but we do not have data on this practice.

. . . We were interested . . . in the intensiveness of the review process, so we asked if there were any kinds of pre-review before the whole committee met and we also asked if indeed the whole committee did meet. 77 percent of the respondents reported some kind of pre-review, that is, by all the individual members, or by a few of them, or by at least one. This procedure is obviously a more intensive kind of review than that engaged in by the 15 percent of our respondents who indicated that there was no pre-review at all before the committee met as a whole. 8 percent of our respondents, further, indicate that the committee does not meet as a body. Instead, one or more individual members perform the review and a decision is reached after communication among the chairman and the members by phone or mail only. In such cases, the degree of intensiveness of consideration which might come from face-to-face interaction among the members of the peer review committee is obviously lacking.

In that large majority (92 percent) of the responding institutions where the committee does meet as a body, either with or without pre-review, a varying number of meetings is required to handle the work-load. 56 percent of these committees that meet as a body come together 1–10 times a year; 37 percent meet 11 times or more; and 7 percent are indefinite, indicating only that they come together "as required." Of the committees meeting as a body, 37 percent report an average of no more than one proposal considered per meeting; 39 percent indicate 2–3 proposals; and 24 percent report 4 or more proposals.

. . . 41 percent of the responding institutions said their procedures required unanimity; 25 percent, a simple majority; 6 percent, a two-thirds majority; and 27 percent, no specific proportion stipulated in their procedure. These data show some considerable tendency toward that large degree of consensus, even toward unanimity, that we expected from groups that define themselves as "collegial," that is, as a company of near-equals sharing a single set of values, rather than as "political," that is, a group of unequals with divergent values and interests. In the former type of group, there would be a greater tendency to unanimity; in the latter, a simple majority would tend to be adequate for deciding among somewhat different interests and values.

* * *

. . . In well-differentiated systems for making adjudicatory decisions, there is some mechanism for those whose cases are being adjudicated to make an appeal from what they consider erroneous decisions. In this respect, again, we find that the review committee system has not moved all the way toward adequate functional differentiation. In response to our question on this matter, only 47 percent of the responding institutions reported that they have any formal procedure by which a negative decision can be appealed from the review committee to some other body.

* * *

[R]espondents were slightly more likely to say the committee at their institution was less than "very effective" if there were no additional controls over the ethical aspects of research at that institution. (It will be remembered that these additional controls were approval by department chairmen, board of trustees, or some other person or group.) This finding supplements our earlier finding that, in institutions where there were no additional controls, the peer review committee was less likely to request revisions or make rejections of research proposals. Our respondents' estimates seem to coincide with the facts about actual decisions. . . .

We also found . . . that our respondents viewed their committees as less effective when it was not committee policy to review all research as opposed to just that research funded by P.H.S. Once again . . . these estimates coincide with the facts about decisions.

The presence of continuing review is also connected with respondents' estimates of effectiveness. [R]espondents who considered their committees less than very effective were more likely to be from institutions without continuing formal or informal review.

* * *

NOTE 9.
OSCAR D. RATNOFF AND MARION F. RATNOFF
ETHICAL RESPONSIBILITIES IN
CLINICAL INVESTIGATION*

* * *

The urge for [human experimentation] is fostered, too, by the practical needs of academic life. Despite miles of verbiage about the need to recognize fine clinical teachers, the route to promotion is all too often dependent upon the production and publication of experimental results. Even disregarding promotion, the economic well-being of the member of a clinical department may be inextricably hitched to his ability to carry out experimental work. In a period of gradual inflation, the proportion of a departmental budget which is in the form of "hard money" is inevitably, shrinking. The beleaguered departmental director must apply pressure upon his colleagues to include substantial portions of their salaries in their applications for research grants. "You are expected to generate a portion of your own salary," is the euphemism in a letter offering one of our colleagues an otherwise fine position. Research, it would seem, must be conducted not only for its own sake but to gain both salary and advancement. No wonder the desire for short cuts to attractive answers blunts the investigator's judgment about what is and what is not appropriate.

* * *

* 11 *Perspectives in Biology and Medicine* 82, 84 (1967). Copyright 1967 by the University of Chicago. Reprinted by permission.

[iv]
*Food and Drug Administration Institutional Committee Review of Clinical Investigations of New Drugs in Human Beings**

In the *Federal Register* of August 22, 1969. . . . a notice was published in which the Commissioner of Food and Drugs proposed that § 130.3 be amended to assure that clinical investigations of new drugs on institutionalized human subjects are appropriately supervised in and approved by such institutions and to assure adequate safeguards for the health, safety, and welfare of the human subjects during all phases of clinical studies of new drugs. . . .

Comments were received from more than 20 representatives of the drug industry and from interested individuals. . . .

* * *

C. The National Academy of Sciences—National Research Council, Drug Review Board, suggests that:

* * *

2. Changes in protocol are often required as a given investigation proceeds; however, the present peer group proposal does not make clear under what circumstances these changes would require a rereview by the peer group. It is clear that only substantial changes in protocol ought to require this additional review.

3. If foreign investigators conduct studies in other countries under IND's, they should be required to follow the procedure set forth for investigators in the United States.

4. The Code of Helsinki ought to be a minimum basis for the decisions reached by the peer committees.

D. An individual physician suggests that:

1. Peer group committees must not set themselves up as censoring groups except insofar as they function to safeguard patients or volunteers from irresponsible and careless investigators.

2. Some of the suggestions made for expanding the activities of these committees are not realistic in terms of how much work is involved and what the effect may be on the performance of research.

3. A 1-day meeting be held of lawyers,

* Charles C. Edwards, Commissioner of Food and Drugs. 36 *Federal Register* 5037–5038 (1971).

judges, consumer group representatives, the FDA, the drug industry, etc., to bring out all the ramifications and complexities and to develop a workable, realistic program that will protect the public without needlessly hamstringing researchers.

E. The American Society of Hospital Pharmacists, Washington, D.C., suggests that the regulation be changed to indicate that there be pharmacy representation in the peer committees and to provide for the designation of pharmacy and therapeutics committees as peer group committees.

The Commissioner of Food and Drugs, having considered the comments, finds that:

1. To achieve a balanced review of a study that will take into consideration the nature of the research as well as the acceptability of the research in terms of relevant law and community acceptance, varying backgrounds of committee members are essential. The need for broad considerations of the ethical and moral aspects of research in humans, in addition to the scientific justification, is too important to limit review of such proposals to individuals with the same areas of interests, training, and background.

2. In view of the need for committee members with varying backgrounds, referring to the review committee as a "peer committee" is inappropriate. The designation "institutional review committee" is more appropriate.

3. The approval or disapproval of a study is the committee's responsibility. The review by the Food and Drug Administration is in addition to the committee review for those studies that are approved by the committee.

4. The requirement for institutional committee review applies to all three phases of clinical studies on institutionalized human subjects and to studies conducted by an individual investigator affiliated with an institution which agrees to assume responsibility for the study to assure adequate protection of the patient's or subject's interests. The requirements of the regulation as amended below do not extend to clinical studies conducted by an individual investigator independent of any institution. . . .

* * *

Therefore, pursuant to provisions of the Federal Food, Drug, and Cosmetic Act . . . and under authority delegated to the Commissioner § 130.3 *New drugs for investigational use in human beings; exemptions from section 505(a)* is amended. . . .*

* * *

NOTES

NOTE 1.
COUNCIL OF HEALTH ORGANIZATIONS
COMMENTS ON PROPOSAL FOR PEER GROUP
COMMITTEE REVIEW OF CLINICAL
INVESTIGATIONS OF NEW DRUGS ON
HUMAN BEINGS (1969)†

* * *

[S]ignificant questions are raised by the FDA's use of the Public Health Service peer group committee model, since those committees are specifically designed for the universities, research institutions, and hospitals which do research with NIH funds. There is reason to doubt that the same model without modification would suit the prisons, orphanages, or homes for the aged where new drugs are often tested. The NIH-PHS program is grounded on the assumption that all members of the hospital community share a professional concern about experimentation with human subjects. As a result, the staff has the competence and motivation to make certain that the hospital selects a knowledgeable, concerned, and objective review committee. There is no evidence that any similar widespread concern and competence exists in other kinds of institutions. As a result, an investigator operating in a prison or orphanage might have inordinate influence in choosing the members of the committee. Furthermore, if the committee members come from within the institutions—as the NIH-PHS committee members often do—there is little likelihood that they would have either the requisite interest or competence. It is unclear who on the staff of a prison, for example, is a "peer" of the investigator. In our view, to speak of a "peer group" in a prison is a non sequitur.

* * *

Commissioner Ley suggested in his testimony before Senator Nelson's Subcommittee on Monopoly of the Select Committee on Small Business on August 12 that the review committees would . . . provide a check on a test's scientific adequacy and necessity. This aspect of the review committee's role is totally ambiguous in the FDA proposal. The scientific quality of new drug testing badly needs to be improved, and

---

* The text of Section 130.3, as amended, is set forth at pp. 862–873 *supra.*

† Reprinted by permission of Paul Lowinger, M.D., Chairman.

some consideration of the scientific adequacy and necessity of a new drug test is essential to a consideration of the rights and welfare of test subjects.

* * *

[A]ssessment of the relative benefits against risks also calls for some scientific expertise and understanding of the particular area of medicine in which the experimentation is taking place.*

The review committees will have to be especially vigilant to insure that . . . "adequate and appropriate" methods are "used to obtain informed consent." Major problems were left unresolved by the FDA regulations adopted in 1967 (section 130.37) concerning consent by test subjects. For example, obtaining the consent of children in orphanages and the senile in homes for the elderly is a delicate matter at best. Often their legal guardian is the state. Members of such groups would benefit from a review committee acting in their interest to make sure that the state safeguards their rights. . . .

* * *

The most glaring omission of the proposed regulation is the failure of the FDA to deal with phase 3 testing problems or to provide a review mechanism for noninstitutional tests of new drugs. Any comprehensive scheme adopted by the FDA to safeguard the rights of human subjects on whom new drugs are tested must deal with phase 3 problems as well as phase 1 and phase 2. In addition, the FDA should devise a method of bringing noninstitutional investigators under the surveillance of a review committee, perhaps through regional review committees.

* * *

NOTE 2.

HOFFMANN-LA ROCHE, INC.
COMMENTS ON NOTICE OF PROPOSED
RULEMAKING (1969)†

* * *

The August 22 notice applies the peer group concept to Phase III studies. . . . We believe that

* The Council believes that it can never be ethical to ask a person to take the risks associated with new drug testing if the tests themselves are unnecessary or will not, because of their design, yield significant results. Hence, any committee charged with protecting the rights and safety of test subjects must have the capacity to review the scientific aspects of the tests.
† Reprinted by permission of E. B. Anderson, Vice–President.

the peer group concept should not be applied to Phase III studies for the following reasons:

First, Phase III studies are less hazardous than Phase I and Phase II studies. By the time the drug reaches Phase III, considerably more is known about its toxicology, pharmacology, and safety.

The question of whether a drug can be allowed to proceed to Phase III testing is reviewed and answered before such testing starts. It should be noted that normally the FDA must be supplied with a protocol before Phase III studies begin. Also, while Phase III studies are in progress, progress reports must be submitted to the FDA at not more than yearly intervals.

The sponsor is also required to submit immediately to the FDA any alarming findings received from investigators relative to the safety of the drug.

Second, peer group committees would not have enough time to monitor all Phase III studies. As an investigational drug moves from one phase to another, the number of investigators involved pyramids. In comparison to the number of investigators involved in Phase I and Phase II studies, the number of Phase III investigators is quite large. We do not believe that institutions would be able to impose the administrative burdens required by the proposed regulation on their expert committees. As a consequence, many institutions would not accept Phase III work which . . . would be detrimental to drug research.

* * *

[T]he proposed regulation speaks in terms of committee members of "varying backgrounds." This language is indefinite as to whether it refers only to persons with scientific backgrounds, e.g., pharmacologists, internists, physiologists, etc., or whether the committee is also to be composed of persons from non-scientific pursuits, e.g., clergymen, lawyers, etc.

The primary concern of a peer group committee, as we understand it, is to supervise investigational drug work to help insure that the risks to the patient will be minimized as much as possible. This supervision should be based primarily on the scientific aspects of the studies being conducted at the institution. Such supervision, we believe can be handled only by persons trained in the type of work involved, e.g., physicians, pharmacologists, physiologists, etc.

A committee composed of persons particularly suited for such supervision could ask clergymen and lawyers for advice on any moral and legal issues which might arise. However, whether the study should proceed should be governed basically by scientific issues and only persons trained in scientific fields should have voting power in deciding whether a study should be conducted.

Therefore, we suggest that the proposed regulations be amended to reflect that the committee need only be composed of persons qualified in areas directly related to drug research.

* * *

[W]e believe that the August 22 notice should be revised in regard to the relationship of the investigator with the committee. . . .

. . . Oftentimes, the investigator conducting the study is the most expert person at the institution relative to the study being conducted, or he is at least as expert as the members of the committee.

To relegate an investigator to being a mere conduit of information demeans the investigator's position as an expert.

His opinions are as vital to an investigation as those of the committee members inasmuch as the investigator has a closer relationship to persons involved in the study and to the data that the study are constantly developing.

We believe that the investigator involved in the study must be a member of the peer group committee. Since an investigator may be prominent enough to exert influence on the committee, we suggest that in order that undue influence by the investigator be avoided, the investigator be a non-voting member of the committee. In any event, the investigator's comments and opinions, as well as information regarding the study, are vital to any decision made by a peer group committee.

* * *

NOTE 3.
FOOD AND DRUG RESEARCH LABORATORIES, INC.
PEER GROUP COMMITTEE REVIEW
OF CLINICAL INVESTIGATIONS OF NEW
DRUGS IN HUMAN BEINGS (1969)*

* * *

The proposals developed by the FDA . . . seem to be an unnecessarily complicated and time-consuming approach to the problem and likely to act as a bottleneck in the development of drug research. As a more workable approach

* Reprinted by permission of John E. Silson, M.D., Vice–President.

to the problem, I would suggest devising a means for rapidly reviewing by computer the Forms 1571 as they are received, and that submission of Forms 1572 and 1573 be required for a similar review. This would enable the FDA to quickly evaluate the qualifications of every proposed investigator and to decide whether sufficient safeguards have been incorporated in the study design.

Furthermore, routine computerized cross-tabulations would pinpoint those investigators who had run into difficulties in the past or who were undertaking too many clinical studies to supervise them all adequately, probably a major factor contributing to the poor quality of some investigations. Such a procedure, coupled with the requirement for reporting immediately any unexpected untoward reactions, would, in my opinion, provide more efficient control of the quality and safety of clinical investigation than review by peer committees.

* * *

c.
Should Research Design and Scientific Merits Be Evaluated?

[i]
David D. Rutstein
The Ethical Design of Human Experiments*

* * *

It may be accepted as a maxim that a poorly or improperly designed study involving human subjects—one that could not possibly yield scientific facts (that is, reproducible observations) relevant to the question under study—is by definition unethical. Moreover, when a study is in itself scientifically invalid, all other ethical considerations become irrelevant. There is no point in obtaining "informed consent" to perform a useless study. A worthless study cannot possibly benefit anyone, least of all the experimental subject himself. Any risk to the patient, however small, cannot be justified. In essence, the scientific validity of a study on human beings is in itself an ethical principle.

How, then, can the experimental human subject be protected from incompetent investigators so that he will not become a victim in feckless studies? There are two lines of defense. The

* 98 *Daedalus* 523, 524, 527–528 (1969). Reprinted by permission of Daedalus, Journal of the American Academy of Arts and Sciences, Boston, Massachusetts.

research committee of a medical school, institution, or hospital must be concerned with the ethical principles as well as the scientific validity of the proposals placed before them. To perform this task effectively, every committee must have among its membership a biostatistician to insure scientific validity and an expert (for whom there is as yet no name) who is concerned with the ethical aspects of human experimentation. The biostatistician can assist the committee in evaluating the scientific quality of the proposed investigation and make recommendations for improvement of the scientific aspects of the study design. Experiments on human beings must not be performed without a carefully drawn protocol, which in turn can best be prepared in consultation with experts in study design. In the same way, experts in the ethical aspects of human experimentation should assist the committee in passing on the ethical issues of proposed studies and in recommending modifications that might make the studies ethically acceptable.

*   *   *

The design of an experiment depends at first on the question asked by the investigator. Some questions are in themselves unethical. One cannot ask whether plague bacilli are more virulent in human beings when injected into the bloodstream than when they are sprayed into the throat. One may obtain hints as to the answer to such a question by epidemiologic comparison of the spread of pneumonic plague (spread from the lungs into the air) and bubonic plague (spread by insect bite). Anecdotal information on the spread of plague can also be obtained through the study of laboratory accidents. But a deliberate experiment to answer this question cannot be performed.

The human experiments performed by the Nazis during World War II horrified the world because they were designed to answer unethical questions. "How long can a human being survive in ice cold water?" will, it is to be hoped, never again be a question to be answered by a scientific experiment. Thus, as a first step in the design of any human experiment, we must first be sure that the question itself is an ethical one.

Moreover, an unethical experiment can sometimes be converted into an ethical one by rephrasing the question. In drug testing, for example, it is not ethical to design an experiment to answer the question: "Is treatment of the disease with the new drug more effective than no treatment at all?" In answering such a question, the patients in the control group would literally have to receive "no treatment" and that is completely unacceptable. Instead, if the patients in the control group are given the best possible current treatment of the disease, we may now ask an ethical question: "Is treatment with the new drug more effective than the generally accepted treatment for this particular disease?"

We faced this problem in the design of the United States–United Kingdom Cooperative Rheumatic Fever Study, which was concerned with measuring the relative effectiveness of cortisone and ACTH in the treatment of that disease. We could not give rheumatic fever patients in the control group "no treatment." We would have had to go so far as to prohibit bed rest, which in itself may be helpful to rheumatic fever patients, because patients in bed have a slower heart rate. Instead, we asked the question: "Is treatment with ACTH or cortisone better, worse, or the same as the best generally accepted drug treatment for this disease?"

*   * .   *

[ii]
John R. Platt
The Step to Man*

Scientists tend to keep up a polite fiction that all science is equal. Outside of the misguided opponent whose work we happen to be refuting at the time, we speak as though every scientist's field and methods of study are as good as every other scientist's, and perhaps a little better. This keeps us all cordial when it comes to recommending each other for government grants.

But I think anyone who looks at the matter closely will agree that some fields of science are moving forward very much faster than others. . . .

Why should there be such rapid advances in some fields rather than others? I think the usual explanations that we tend to think of—such as the tractability of the subject, or the quality or education of the men drawn into it, or the size of research contracts—are important but inadequate. I have begun to believe that the primary factor in scientific advance is an intellectual one. These rapidly moving fields are fields where a particular method of doing scientific research is systematically used and taught, an accumulative

* New York: John Wiley & Sons 19–20, 23–24, 35–36 (1966). Copyright 1966. Reprinted by permission of John Wiley & Sons, Inc.

method of inductive inference that is so effective that I think it should be given the name of "strong inference". . . .

In its separate elements, strong inference is just the simple and old-fashioned method of inductive inference that goes back to Francis Bacon. The steps are familiar to every college student and are practiced, off and on, by every scientist. The difference comes in their systematic application. *Strong inference consists of applying the following steps to every problem in science, formally and explicitly and regularly:*

(1) *devising alternative hypotheses;*

(2) *devising a crucial experiment* (or several of them), *with alternative possible outcomes,* each of which will, as nearly as possible, *exclude one or more of the hypotheses;*

(3) *carrying out the experiment* so as to get a clean result; and

(1') *recycling* the procedure, making sub-hypotheses or sequential hypotheses to refine the possibilities that remain; and so on.

* * *

This analytical approach to biology has sometimes become almost a crusade, because it arouses so much resistance in many scientists who have grown up in a more relaxed and diffuse tradition. At the 1958 Conference on Biophysics at Boulder, there was a dramatic confrontation between the two points of view. Leo Szilard said: "The problems of how enzymes are induced, of how proteins are synthesized, of how antibodies are formed, are closer to solution than is generally believed. If you do stupid experiments, and finish one a year, it can take 50 years. But if you stop doing experiments for a little while and *think* how proteins can possibly be synthesized, there are only about 5 different ways, not 50! And it will take only a few experiments to distinguish these."

One of the young men added: "It is essentially the old question: How *small* and *elegant* an experiment can you perform?"

These comments upset a number of those present. An electron microscopist said, "Gentlemen, this is off the track. This is philosophy of science."

Szilard retorted, "I was not quarreling with third-rate scientists: I was quarreling with first-rate scientists."

A physical chemist hurriedly asked, "Are we going to take the official photograph before lunch or after lunch?"

But this did not deflect the dispute. A distinguished cell biologist rose and said, "No two cells give the same properties. Biology is the science of heterogeneous systems. . . ." And he added privately, "You know there are *scientists;* and there are people in science who are just working with these oversimplified model systems —DNA chains and *in vitro* systems—who are not doing science at all. We need their auxiliary work: They build apparatus, they make minor studies, but they are not scientists."

To which Cy Levinthal of M.I.T. said: "Well, there are two kinds of biologist, those who are looking to see if there is one thing that can be understood, and those who keep saying it is very complicated and that nothing can be understood. . . . You must study the *simplest* system you think has the properties you are interested in."

As they were leaving the meeting, one man could be heard muttering, "What does Szilard expect me to do—shoot myself?"

* * *

. . . I will mention one severe but useful private test—a touchstone of strong inference—that removes the necessity for third-person criticism, because it is a test that anyone can learn to carry with him for use as needed. It is our old friend the Baconian "exclusion," but I call it "The Question." Obviously it should be applied to one's own thinking as much as or more than to others'. It consists of asking in your own mind, on hearing any scientific explanation or theory put forward:

"But sir, what experiment could *disprove* your hypothesis?" Or on hearing a scientific experiment described:

"But sir, what hypothesis does your experiment *disprove?*"

This goes straight to the heart of the matter. It forces everyone to refocus on the central question of whether there is a testable scientific step forward or not.

If such a question were asked aloud, many a supposedly great scientist would sputter and turn livid and would want to throw the questioner out, as a hostile witness! Such a man is less than he appears, for he is obviously not accustomed to think in terms of alternative hypotheses and crucial experiments for himself; and one might also wonder about the state of science in the field he is in. But who knows, the question might educate him, and the field too!

On the other hand, I think that throughout most of molecular biology and nuclear physics, the response to The Question would be to outline immediately not one, but several tests to disprove the hypothesis!—and it would turn out that the speaker already had two or three graduate students working on them!

I almost think that government agencies could make use of this kind of touchstone. It is not true that all science is equal, or that we cannot justly compare the effectiveness of scientists by any method except by a mutual-recommendation system. The man to watch, the man to put your money on, is not the man who wants "to make a survey" or a "more detailed study," but the man . . . with the alternative hypotheses and the crucial experiments; the man who knows how to answer your question of disproof, and is already working on it.

*   *   *

NOTES

NOTE 1.

ROBERT H. GIFFORD AND ALVAN R. FEINSTEIN
A CRITIQUE OF METHODOLOGY IN
STUDIES OF ANTICOAGULANT THERAPY
FOR ACUTE MYOCARDIAL INFARCTION*

Despite two decades of statistical studies, anticoagulant therapy for acute myocardial infarction remains a controversial issue. The persistence of controversy can be explained either by the claim that nature is inscrutable or by the suspicion that man's best efforts to understand it have not been very good. A particular focus of suspicion is that the existing statistics were obtained without adequate attention to fundamental principles of clinical science. The work reported here was done to test that suspicion.

We used three criteria in selecting papers for review in this study: to simplify the language problem, we examined only papers that had been English . . . we confined our attention to reports of anticoagulant therapy for the acute phase of myocardial infarction; and to assess the validity of "control" groups, we chose only investigations in which a specific comparison had been made between different modes of therapy—either one type of anticoagulant vs another or anticoagulants vs no anticoagulants.

From the literature published between 1948 and 1966, we found 32 reports that fulfilled these three criteria. In the first 27 reports patients

* 280 *New England Journal of Medicine* 351–357 (1969). Reprinted by permission.

treated with anticoagulants were compared with a "control" group not receiving anticoagulants; and in the last five reports, one type of anticoagulant treatment was compared with another type.

. . . We . . . established a series of eight methodologic standards that would be generally regarded as scientific necessities for ensuring comparability of treated patients in a clinical investigation of therapy. . . .

Diagnostic criteria for myocardial infarction. The first scientific requirement in any investigation of therapy is a clear, precise statement of diagnostic criteria for the disease under study. . . .

. . . Our sole concern was for the authors to state their interpretational criteria clearly enough so that another investigator could use them with scientific reproducibility.

*   *   *

[O]nly eight (25 per cent) of the 32 reports contained a satisfactory statement of the evidence used for making a clinical diagnosis of acute myocardial infarction. In 13 papers, the criteria were described equivocally, and in 11 (34 per cent), no criteria were stated.

*   *   *

Concurrent controls. If treatment is to be compared in two groups of patients who have not been studied experimentally, they should have been treated during approximately the same years in the calendar. If patients from one era are compared, in a survey, with those from another, the group treated later may have better results not because of the improved therapeutic agents but because of improvements, with advancing time, in methods of diagnosis and of ancillary therapy. . . . Thus, if anticoagulant-treated patients are compared with "controls" taken from medical records of the earlier era before anticoagulant therapy, the better results of the later group may have little or nothing to do with the anticoagulant therapy.

*   *   *

[O]nly 72 per cent of the investigators rigorously observed the principle of concurrent controls.

Hospital coordination. Comparisons of treatment should preferably be concurrent not only in time, but also in space. If the comparison extends to patients managed in more than one hospital, the ancillary treatment used at the different hospitals should be co-ordinated so that elastic stockings, chair rest, early ambulation, tactics in nursing care and other nonpharmaceutical therapeutic maneuvers are carried out in a comparable way for all patients. . . .

In 24 of the 32 investigations reviewed here, the work was "coordinated" because it was all done at a single hospital. The other eight reports combined data from different hospitals, often widely separated geographically. . . .

*   *   *

Random allocation. The next principle deals with the random allocation of treatment, which is intended to ensure against bias when the modes of therapy are assigned in a trial. Unless this principle is observed, the investigator's conscious or unconscious bias may affect the assignment of treatment so that patients with a milder form of the disease and a better prognosis receive one mode of therapy, and the other agent is given to a more severely ill or "poor-risk" group.

*   *   *

[O]nly four of the 32 reports in this review used a strictly random method of allocating treatment. These four reports constitute 31 per cent of the 13 investigations that were performed as experimental clinical trials.

*   *   *

Diagnostic criteria for thromboembolism. If anticoagulants are being used to prevent thromboembolic phenomena, an investigator should specify the way the phenomena were diagnosed. A thromboembolism can be manifested by symptoms or signs in a leg, by certain clinical findings in the chest or brain, by roentgenographic silhouettes or by various other items of evidence. These findings can be given such diagnostic names as "pulmonary embolus," "thrombophlebitis," "cerebrovascular accident" or "mural thrombus," but each such diagnosis requires criteria to state the prerequisite evidence. . . .

. . . In the 32 reviewed reports, thromboembolic phenomena had not been assessed in eight. . . . We searched the remaining 24 reports for statements of their diagnostic criteria for thromboembolism [but] none of the investigators made a specific statement. . . .

Double-blind procedure. In a double-blind procedure, neither the patient nor the doctor knows which drug is being given. The double-blind procedure helps eliminate the bias in selection of cases that may occur if treatment is assigned by someone who knows the identity of the therapeutic agents. After a trial is under way, the double-blind procedure helps preserve the objectivity of the investigator when he evaluates clinical and other evidence for such diagnoses as thromboembolism, particularly if precisely defined criteria are not used for those diagnoses.

*   *   *

[O]nly one of the 32 investigations cited here was done with a double-blind procedure.

*   *   *

Therapeutic conclusions. [W]e have cited the therapeutic conclusions reached in each of the 32 reports; we listed the anticoagulants as "significantly better" only when the authors had expressed this conclusion. In the last five reports, the comparison was either between strict and nonstrict methods of anticoagulant regulation, or between oral and parenteral methods. Since so much controversy has developed about the issue of anticoagulants vs nothing, the remainder of our analysis is confined to the 27 reports in which such a comparison was performed.

Of these 27 reports, 14 concluded that anticoagulants were superior, and 13 did not. To examine this issue in greater detail, we correlated the therapeutic conclusions of each investigation with the methodologic standards that had been used in that investigation. [F]or each of the cited methodologic standards, anticoagulant therapy was found superior to no treatment more often in the reports that did *not* observe the standard than in those that did. Moreover, the differences are particularly striking for the standards that are most likely to eliminate bias in comparability of cases—random allocation, stratified prognostic correlation and double-blind procedure.

*   *   *

Our purpose in this review is not to single out any investigations for adverse criticism, and we apologize to any investigators whose methods we may have misinterpreted. . . . Instead, we want to call attention to certain clinical and scientific principles that are the basis for sound statistical appraisals of treatment. The violation of these principles seems to be the source of the current controversy about anticoagulant therapy. . . .

. . . As clinicians and statisticians collaborate in planning future research projects, an important point to be recognized is that treatment is an act of clinical medicine, and that valid statistical inferences must be based on this clinical context; accordingly, the critical features of scientific design for therapeutic experiments must be clinical and not merely statistical. Among the needed improvements are better clinical methods for selecting, classifying, specifying and comparing the patients who are the "experimental material."

NOTE 2.

YALE REPORTS
ETHICS AND MEDICINE—
CONTROL OF HUMAN EXPERIMENTATION*

* * *

MR. CALABRESI: [T]he first thing that [the review committee should] look at is whether the plan of research is adequate and whether experiments on animals have been made beforehand. . . . After that, you study the question of whether consent was adequately sought, and beyond that you impose a kind of control which is supposed to be a judgment essentially by other physicians as to whether this experiment, involving the risks it does, is in the interest of society at large. Now, it is this last part which is most interesting to me because it says: consent is not enough, we have to have another judgment. What is interesting to me is that this other judgment is made by physicians for society, they are the ones who are asked to represent the decision, if you want, between future lives and present lives. I can perfectly well see that it would not be desirable to have some kind of central governmental group making this decision, but is it really sensible to think that physicians, and especially physicians in the same institution who have so many relationships with the experimenter, are the best suited to make this kind of judgment? Would it not be better if, at least as a start, one had physicians from other institutions who had no particular interest or relationship with the experimenter and perhaps people from other disciplines involved in such a committee?

* * *

* A weekly broadcast review presented by Yale University and *WTIC*, March 3, 1968. Participating were Guido Calabresi, Professor of Law; Morton Kligerman, Chairman, Department of Radiology, Yale Medical School; and Jay Katz, Professor (Adjunct) of Law and Psychiatry. Reprinted by permission.

DR. KLIGERMAN: . . . As you indicated, those of us who are involved professionally in doing a certain job, although we are experts in the ability to do this job (to make judgments about the manner in which the job is being done), hopefully, we are experts in making decisions on how to improve the teaching and the execution of our specialities. When it comes to making a decision as to what is good for society, the very fact that we say: "What is good for society" takes it out of our hands and must put society, that is the non-specialists, in. I think in this instance the specialist becomes the adviser to society's representatives. He is an expert witness, but he alone probably often is not the best one to make the decision about whether something should be done. It would be burdensome, I think, if one had a committee which decided on scientific merits, and then the question would be sent to another committee to have a decision as to whether society can tolerate the experiment at all.

I think that the way to do this is similar to the way the National Institutes of Health have solved the problem of their advisory councils. For instance, the National Advisory Cancer Council does not have solely scientists on its board; there are physicians, there are biologists, and other scientists, but then there are lay people on it. I would, therefore, like to suggest that a committee which reviews proposals for clinical investigation have community representatives in addition to scientists on its board.

MR. CALABRESI: I think that you would probably find that such a committee would be, if anything, more lenient with experiments than one made up only of physicians because sometimes I think that physicians are concerned with not hurting the profession, and, therefore, are more careful than society's interest might dictate.

DR. KATZ: I am not certain whether our committee should evaluate the design of the experiment. [As yet] we have not delegated to members of the committee the specific task of evaluating either the merits or the design of the experiment. Perhaps, this should be done. We do have one additional safeguard; before an experiment is submitted to us, it has to be reviewed by the Department Chairman, and we hope that the Department Chairman will pay some attention to that particular problem.

[I]n the light of a year's experience, I have been impressed by the fact that we have not received an experiment which raises the question should this experiment be done? Is it, for example, so risky that we have to evaluate societal interests? If we had in addition to our committee, another committee which has a much broader representation (including people from the community, law, sociology, etc.) that would address itself to these issues, maybe then experimenters would feel much freer to think about doing these kinds of experiments [and] submit them [for review] to such a group. It may be that the absence of such a group precludes experimenters from even considering such experimentation.

MR. CALABRESI: I think so. And especially I think it would be useful if there were someone who could pass on such things as [the] design [of the] experiment. I frankly was a little bit worried by your comment that that is one of the things you don't examine and you leave it up to the Department Chairman. The Department Chairman is not the ideal person for making this decision. After all, he has made his own way by making experiments. He feels a great many qualms about keeping back his able men in a situation where some really significant experiment might be made, especially where someone in another medical center may get permission to do it. A whole series of pressures come on him so that I would rather have it be scientists in the same general area who are not so related to this particular experiment.

*   *   *

DR. KLIGERMAN: I agree with Guido and I think there would be a very easy mechanism to do that. You would simply select two other individuals, even from within our school, because I do feel that people will, when asked to put on paper their reasons for support or non-support of a subject, be very, very careful to do the right thing. By the way, even if they didn't have to sign it, they would want to do the right thing anyway. No one wants to see his colleague do the wrong thing; no one wants to see a patient harmed. And I think then that your committee should select two people who would be, (shall we call them primary reviewers?) in a field of relevance. By the way, I am certain that on some occasions, it would include a member of your committee, and that they would then present their opinion at least about the scientific merits of the situation to your committee which then could look at the other aspects that you are charged with.

*   *   *

NOTE 3.

BRITISH MEDICAL RESEARCH COUNCIL
MEMORANDUM ON CLINICAL INVESTIGATION*

*   *   *

. . . In such a diverse and rapidly expanding subject as clinical research it is impossible to frame a code of general advice which would adequately cover the ever changing circumstances which arise. In any particular case—so specialised has medical knowledge become—only a small group of experienced investigators, who have devoted themselves to this branch of medicine, are likely to be competent to pass an opinion on the advisability of undertaking any particular investigation. But in every branch of medicine such a group of investigators exists. It is upon them, and the specialised scientific societies to which they belong, that the medical profession must mainly rely for the creation of the body of precedents and the climate of opinion which shall guide investigators in clinical research. Hitherto no deliberate attempt to provide guidance in this way has been made: but it is important that it should be. The Medical Research Council feel, therefore, that they must clearly express their belief that it is incumbent upon the medical scientific societies to accept this responsibility and, by encouraging critical discussion on the communications presented to them, help to resolve doubts and to form a body of opinion of what is necessary, desirable and justifiable to guide investigators in their field.

*   *   *

NOTE 4.

RENÉ TATON
REASON AND CHANCE IN SCIENTIFIC DISCOVERY†

*   *   *

One of the saddest examples of a scientist falling a victim to his own discovery is that of the Hungarian physician Ignaz-Philipp Semmelweiss (1818–1865), who, after having discovered the cause of puerperal infection, tried, but unfortunately without success, to introduce the general use of antiseptics. The factors surrounding his discovery give a clear illustration of his scientific rigour, and thus merit our attention.

---

* Memorandum M.R.C. 53/649 (October 16, 1953). Reprinted by permission. See p. 847 supra.

† Translated by A. J. Pomerans. New York: Philosophical Library 153–154 (1957). Reprinted by permission.

In the middle of the nineteenth century puerperal fever was so rampant in maternity hospitals that women in labour were truly terrified. At the time speculations on its causes were fantastic rather than scientific; we need but mention the assumed influence of some food-stuffs and even of scents. During the autopsy of a laboratory assistant, who had died of an infection that he had contracted during a dissection, Semmelweiss noticed that some anatomical and pathological symptoms were similar to those observed in women who had died of puerperal fever. From this he concluded that both diseases had similar origins, and he was confirmed in this idea by his discovery that deaths from puerperal fever were much more common in clinics where students did their obstetrics without taking any of the precautions that today are a matter of routine. He immediately communicated his observations and ideas to the Medical Council of Vienna, and stated that puerperal fever was due to blood poisoning caused by the absence of antiseptic precautions. The rapid drop in mortality which followed upon the implementation of his advice that all who came into contact with women in labour should take care to wash their hands, and that wards should be disinfected by chlorination, was a remarkable justification of Semmelweiss's point of view.

However, the leading obstetricians of Vienna fought so bitterly against this thesis that Semmelweiss had to leave the hospital where he practised. In 1855 he was appointed professor at the University of Budapest, where he continued propounding his ideas. In 1861 he published his *On the etiology, the pathology, and the prophylaxis of puerperal fever,* in which these ideas were developed further and based on new observations. Refusing to accept clearly established facts, his adversaries redoubled the violence of their attacks to such a point that Semmelweiss had to abandon his Chair. Broken by such obstinacy and by the most vicious abuse, the Hungarian doctor some years later died a sad death in a lunatic asylum.

However, the work of Pasteur and the unquestionable triumph of the great English surgeon, Joseph Lister (1827–1912), slowly overcame the obstinacy of those who opposed antisepsis in the prevention of infectious diseases, and some twenty years later the correctness of the ideas of Semmelweiss was finally recognized and antiseptic methods were applied successfully to the prevention of puerperal fever. The statue that the city of Budapest erected in 1894 in honour of the great Hungarian physician, pioneer and genius, and martyr to his own discovery, unfortunately does not erase the memory of his tragic death, and of the thousands of innocent victims who had to pay with their lives for the blind obstinacy of orthodox medicine of the time.

*   *   *

NOTE 5.

FIORENTINO v. WENGER
19 N.Y.2D 407, 227 N.E.2D 296 (1967)

BREITEL, JUDGE:

*   *   *

It should be evident that a hospital generally cannot be held liable, other than derivatively, for another's malpractice. Thus, where, as here, there is no vicarious liability, the plaintiff must establish that the hospital, through its own agents, was guilty of malpractice or other tort concurring in causing the harm. Where a hospital's alleged misconduct involves an omission to act, the hospital will not be held responsible unless it had reason to know that it should have acted within the duty it concededly had. . . . More particularly, in the context of the present case, a hospital will not be held liable for an act of malpractice performed by an independently retained healer, unless it had reason to know that the act of malpractice would take place. . . . As Mr. Justice Lazansky noted, dissenting in the Appellate Division in *Hendrickson* [v. *Hodkin*], "[A hospital] is not required to pass upon the efficacy of treatment; it may not decide for a doctor whether an operation is necessary, or, if one be necessary, the nature thereof; but it owes to every patient whom it admits the duty of saving him from an illegal operation or false, fraudulent, or fictitious medical treatment." (250 App. Div., p. 621, 294 N.Y.S., p. 984.)

To be sure, Dr. Wenger stands responsible for proven acts of malpractice on this record, but not because a spinal-jack operation is per se an act of malpractice. Hence, the mere fact that the hospital knew the surgeon was to perform a spinal-jack operation does not charge it with a tort. The surgeon's responsibility stemmed from his failure to obtain an informed consent from the boy's parents, and perhaps for some of the incidents of the operation about which proof was made with the contention that he had been negligent. But none of these acts or omissions are chargeable to the hospital. Only if, because of the nature of the operation, the hospital was required to obtain a further consent from the patient or his parents or to verify in some other way that the surgeon had done his duty in that respect could liability attach to the hospital.

Moreover, it would not be just for a court, having the benefit of hindsight, to impose liability on a hospital for its failure to intervene in the independent physician-patient relationship. That relationship is always one of great delicacy. And it is perhaps the most delicate matter, often with fluctuating indications, from time to time with the same patient, whether a physician should advise the patient (or his family), more or less, about a proposed procedure, the gruesome details, and the available alternatives. Such a decision is particularly one calling for the exercise of medical judgment. . . .

In the exercise of that discretion, involving as it does grave risks to the patient, a third party should not ordinarily meddle. . . .

* * *

[iii]
*Ninety-first Congress, Second Session
An Act to Amend the Act of August 24, 1966,
Relating to the Care of Certain Animals Used
for Purposes of Research, Experimentation,
Exhibition, or Held for Sale as Pets**

* * *

SEC. 14. Section 13 of such Act† is amended to read as follows:

"SEC. 13. The Secretary [of Agriculture] shall promulgate standards to govern the humane handling, care, treatment, and transportation of animals by dealers, research facilities, and exhibitors. Such standards shall include minimum requirements with respect to handling, housing, feeding, watering, sanitation, ventilation, shelter from extremes of weather and temperatures, adequate veterinary care, including the appropriate use of anesthetic, analgesic or tranquilizing drugs, when such use would be proper in the opinion of the attending veterinarian of such research facilities, and separation

---

* Act of December 24, 1970, Pub. Law No. 91–579, 84 Stat. 1560; *see* 7 U.S.C. § 2143 (1971).

† The regulation of laboratory animals' care and handling was the subject of a number of bills in the Eighty-ninth Congress. One of these (H.R. 3036), which was not adopted, is set forth at pp. 840–842 *supra;* another (H.R. 13881) was enacted on August 24, 1966, as Public Law No. 89–544, which is incorporated in 7 U.S.C. §§ 2131 *et seq.* (1971).

by species when the Secretary finds such separation necessary for the humane handling, care, or treatment of animals. In promulgating and enforcing standards established pursuant to this section, the Secretary is authorized and directed to consult experts, including outside consultants where indicated. Nothing in this Act shall be construed as authorizing the Secretary to promulgate rules, regulations, or orders with regard to design, outlines, guidelines, or performance of actual research or experimentation by a research facility as determined by such research facility: *Provided,* That the Secretary shall require, at least annually, every research facility to show that professionally acceptable standards governing the care, treatment, and use of animals, including appropriate use of anesthetic, analgesic, and tranquilizing drugs, during experimentation are being followed by the research facility during actual research or experimentation."

* * *

d.

Should Consent Be Supervised?

[i]
Louis Loss
The Role of Government in the Protection of Investors*

[S]ecurities are, in a phrase used by a committee of our Congress in 1934, "intricate merchandise." Although one cannot imagine a system of private capital without them, it is a regrettable fact that their very nature makes them a ready device by which people of questionable morals may prey upon the unsophisticated and the gullible. An English historian named John Francis, who wrote on the Bank of England in 1862, claimed to have seen with his own eyes a prospectus issued in 1825 by a company formed "to drain the Red Sea in search of the gold and jewels left by the Egyptians in their passage after the Israelites." A spiritual descendant of those promoters was convicted in one of our federal courts just a few years ago on a charge that he had obtained more than $100,000 from persons in several midwestern states and Canadian provinces by means of a fraudulent scheme which was no less fantastic. . . .

* * *

. . . If the period 1890–1914 which produced our two great anti-monopoly statutes had

---

* Address Delivered at the Mexico Stock Exchange 3–4, 8–13 (1957). Reprinted by permission.

THE ROLE OF THE PARTICIPANTS IN ADMINISTRATION   915

also seen the promulgation of federal controls over securities, there might never have been any substantial state legislation in this area. But federal regulation of securities—like the federal social legislation and much of the federal labor legislation now on the books—dates only from President Roosevelt's New Deal in 1933. Indeed, although there had been agitation for securities legislation from the turn of the century, this much at least of the New Deal might never have eventuated except for the stock market crash of 1929.

This left the states free to act in the first third of the century, and they did. Actually there was sporadic state legislation much earlier. But it applied only to railroads and public utilities. . . .

General securities legislation at the state level dates from the second decade of this century. Some of the frauds practiced by promoters in those days were so brazen that someone said they would sell building lots in the blue sky. The state securities statutes thus became popularly known as "blue sky laws." And the fashion soon spread to the point where blue sky laws of one kind or another were found in every one of our forty-eight states except Delaware and Nevada, as well as in Hawaii and every one of the ten Canadian provinces.

Except in a handful of states, these statutes went considerably beyond the philosophy of the English Companies Act. . . . The English philosophy is one of disclosure. There is no government agency comparable to the securities commissions of our countries. Prospectuses are merely filed with the Registrar of Companies in the Board of Trade. They are not examined. It is a criminal offense to fail to give a prospectus to a person who is asked to purchase shares or debentures. But there are no criminal or administrative sanctions for misstatements in the prospectus. The sanction is a civil liability which is imposed upon every director or promotor individually and the liability is to pay the buyer any damage sustained by reason of an untrue statement included in the prospectus.

The theory, in short, is that government should not attempt to dictate which securities may and which may not be offered to the public. It should merely see to it that full and fair disclosure is made to those who are asked to buy. Then, if a prospective investor does not take the trouble to inform himself before risking his money, he has no one to blame but himself. If government were to do more in this area, the

Lord Davey Committee said in 1895, "It would be an attempt to throw what ought to be the responsibility of the individual on the shoulders of the State, and would give a fictitious and unreal sense of security to the investor, and might also lead to grave abuses."

There is a simple grandeur about this philosophy. It has an aura of Plato's *Republic* and of what we in my country like to call Jeffersonian democracy. "All men are created equal," and "The truth shall make you free." But, of course, if all men have an inalienable right to equality before the law, they are not endowed by their Creator with equal wisdom. The question remains whether the ordinary investor will take the trouble to study a modern corporate prospectus, down to the vital footnotes to the financial statements, or will be able to understand what he reads in any event. The typical prospectus does not make light bedtime reading.

With few exceptions, the state legislatures decided that their citizens needed something more than mere disclosure. The forty-seven statutes vary greatly in their terms. But they do embody three general philosophies. The first is the so-called "fraud" approach: the attorney-general or the securities administrator is given broad authority to investigate frauds, to sue in the courts for injunctions, and to prosecute criminally. The second approach requires the registration of brokers and dealers, as well as investment advisers more recently. The third approach requires the issuing corporation or an interested dealer to register the securities themselves—not on the basis of a simple disclosure test, but under various substantive standards. That is to say, the securities administrator is directed by the legislature to examine the registration statement and to permit it to become effective only if he finds that the offering "would not tend to work a fraud," or that the terms of the offering and the proposed plan of business are "fair, just and equitable," or that it is not proposed to issue an excessive amount of securities in payment for physical property or intangible assets such as good will. There are many similar standards, which vary from state to state. In a few states there is a broad standard which simply speaks in terms of "public interest."

These three regulatory philosophies—the fraud approach, registration of dealers, and registration of securities—are not mutually exclusive. Most states follow all three. This is not to say that the blue sky laws and their enforcement are equally stringent in their application throughout most of the country. . . .

*   *   *

When Congress finally entered the scene in 1933, it decided that federal legislation was essential because the state statutes were inadequate for what had become very largely an interstate economy. The first major decision which Congress faced was whether to follow the disclosure philosophy of the English statute or the more stringent regulatory philosophy of the states. . . . The latter choice would clearly have been more consistent with the idea of a planned economy which underlay the National Industrial Recovery Act, with its codes for various industries. But philosophical consistency is not an outstanding characteristic of legislation in a democracy. At any rate, Congress chose the milder disclosure philosophy of Great Britain rather than the substantive controls of the state blue sky laws.

The man who was perhaps most responsible for this choice was the great Supreme Court Justice, Louis D. Brandeis. . . . In *Other People's Money,* published in 1914, he had strongly urged publicity as a remedy for social and industrial disease generally, and excessive underwriters' charges specifically: "Sunlight is said to be the best of disinfectants; electric light the most efficient policeman." At the same time, the law should not try to keep investors from making bad bargains; it should not even undertake (except incidentally in connection with railroads and public-service corporations) to fix bankers' profits. He cited the Pure Food Law as an example: it does not guarantee quality or prices, but it does help the consumer to judge quality by requiring the disclosure of ingredients.

*   *   *

. . . Brandeis . . . cautioned in [*New State Ice Company* v. *Liebmann,* 285 U.S. 262 (1932)]: "Denial of the right to experiment may be fraught with serious consequences to the Nation. It is one of the happy incidents of the federal system that a single courageous State may, if its citizens choose, serve as a laboratory; and try novel social and economic experiments without risk to the rest of the country." Whether out of this spirit of federalism to which both our countries are attached or out of considerations of political feasibility—perhaps it was a little of both—Congress did not interfere with the more drastic blue sky laws of the states.

The Brandeisian philosophy which prevailed at the federal level was not without its critics. The present Justice Douglas, who was destined to become Chairman of the Securities and Exchange Commission and then to succeed Brandeis on the Supreme Court, wrote as a Yale law professor in 1934 that the Securities Act of 1933 was "superficial." It was essentially, he said, a "nineteenth-century piece of legislation" which unrealistically envisaged a return to the simpler days of small business units. Douglas did not favor a federal statute of the "blue sky" type either. That type of control on a nationwide basis, he thought, would be far too complex. What he advocated was a philosophy which would combine self-regulation by industry with supervision by government—something, in short, like the then current industrial codes under the National Recovery Administration, which was soon to be declared unconstitutional by the Supreme Court.

*   *   *

. . . I shudder at the thought of giving a federal agency life-and-death power over virtually the entire industry of the country by subjecting all public financing to such vague tests as "fair, just, and equitable" or "sound business principles." Although the disclosure philosophy has its inadequacies, it has turned out to be considerably more potent than many people anticipated. It may be permissible in theory for a company to offer shares in a venture which is nothing nore than "a hole in the ground," or to pay promoters exorbitant amounts of stock for good will or promotional services. But the practicality of doing this sort of thing on the basis of the disclosure which the Commission requires is another matter. And, if not too many investors read or could understand prospectuses, the information on file in Washington seeps down to them through their advisers and the financial publications. . . .

*   *   *

Our Securities Act of 1933, with certain exceptions, requires the federal registration of all new issues of securities which are offered to the public by use of the mails or any instrumentality of interstate or foreign commerce. . . . The registration requirement also applies to secondary distributions of outstanding securities by persons who are in a relationship of control with the issuer. And a prospectus containing the basic information in the registration statement must be given to each buyer.

The Act includes a civil liability provision which was largely modeled on the English Companies Act. But it also contains administrative machinery which is not found in England. The prospectus and various other documents, which are collectively called the registration statement, are carefully examined by the Securities and Exchange Commission. The Commission has no power to pass on the merits of securities, and it is a criminal offense to represent that it does. But it may issue a so-called stop order, subject to judicial review in a federal appellate court, upon a finding that the registration statement is incomplete or misleading. Since this administrative power exists, it seldom has to be exercised. An informal procedure has been developed whereby the registration statement is examined by a group of financial analysts, accountants, lawyers, and engineers on the Commission's staff and then amended to repair any deficiencies which are thus found. This detailed examination, if it frequently proves annoying to registrants and their lawyers, is essentially welcomed by the financial and legal communities as a cheap form of insurance against what might otherwise be disastrous civil judgments.

The Securities Act of 1933 was the first, but by no means the last, of the federal statutes. Almost annually for the next seven years Congress added a new statute, until there are now seven under which the SEC functions.

The Securities Exchange Act of 1934, the second statute in the series, is concerned with trading in securities already issued rather than the process of capital formation. Every stock exchange must be registered with the Commission, which has certain supervisory functions with respect to their rules. Every security which is listed for trading on a stock exchange must likewise be registered. Annual and other periodic reports must be filed to keep the registration data current. The Commission has a quasi-legislative power to adopt rules regulating the solicitation of proxies. Directors, officers and ten-percent stockholders must file monthly reports of their holdings, and must surrender to the corporation any profits they make from trading in their corporation's securities within any period of six months.

These several provisions apply only to securities listed on exchanges. So far as the over-the-counter market is concerned, the securities themselves are not registered unless they are the subject of a distribution which falls within the 1933 statute, but brokers and dealers in the over-the-counter market must be registered and file annual financial statements. Moreover, the Commission has very broad powers to define fraudulent practices by rule; to enforce the statute and the regulations by investigation, injunction, and criminal prosecution; to control various stock exchange practices such as short selling, stabilization, floor trading, and the hypothecation of customers' securities; and to suspend or expel stock exchange members, as well as to revoke the registration of over-the-counter brokers and dealers, for illegal conduct.

All this regulation is supplemented on an ethical plane by the National Association of Securities Dealers, an organization of over-the-counter brokers and dealers which has semi-official status. And the 1934 statute also attempts to control the amount of the nation's credit which is channeled into the securities markets by authorizing the Board of Governors of the Federal Reserve System to promulgate margin rules, which are enforced by the Commission.

*   *   *

[ii]
Kenneth L. Melmon, Michael Grossman, and R. Curtis Morris, Jr.
*Emerging Assets and Liabilities of a Committee on Human Welfare and Experimentation**

*   *   *

. . . This report examines the operations of the Committee on Human Welfare and Experimentation of the University of California at San Francisco in the first two years of its existence and attempts to evaluate the Committee's past and current effectiveness.

*   *   *

Acceptability of the protocol was at first judged on a number of points, the first being the question, *Will the rights and welfare of the subject be protected?* Attempts were made to assess the manner in which subjects were sought, the enticement offered, the explanation of means by which the subject could withdraw from the study, the manner in which studies were to be monitored, the expressed provisions protecting the subjects from potential harm, the feasibility relating to time factors, drug doses and availability of antidote, the expressed clinical criteria

---

* 282 *New England Journal of Medicine* 427–428 (1970). Reprinted by permission.

for termination of an experimental procedure, the degree of experience and sophistication of an investigator in the area to be studied, and the applicability of the cited references to the substance of the proposal as an index of the care and seriousness of the exposition of the protocol. As a second point, the question was asked, *Are the methods used to obtain a subject's informed consent appropriate?* Are subjects approached only by physicians involved in the experimental procedure? If so, there could be no guarantee that an objective and unbiased explanation of the protocol would be made to the patient. Therefore, some specific mention is required of the presence of an impartial but knowledgeable witness to judge the suitability of the explanation to the subject of the experimental procedures. Such witnesses are also required to sign the consent form. Are subjects fully informed of their rights to withdraw and realistically told of the risks? Are subjects told which of the agents or procedures are experimental and what experience with these the principal investigators have had? The third question was, *Are the potential scientific benefits of the procedure proportionate to the risks involved?* This question is perhaps the most difficult to answer. All would agree that the risk-benefit ratio is low if only 10 ml of venous blood needs to be withdrawn from a single normal volunteer and results of experimentation would reveal a cure of an otherwise fatal disease. The question of risk benefit is usually considerably less clear. However, protocols were rarely rejected because of unacceptable risk.

After the first year, three additional questions were considered necessary because unanticipated inconsistencies arose in the judgment made by the parent committee as opposed to ad hoc committees. *Is the informed patient consent form to be used appropriate for the type of patients involved?* The question became necessary because of discrepancies between the subject's understanding of the experimental procedure and its realities. *Are the risks described completely and in reasonable language? If not, why? Does the project require the use of investigational or new drugs?* Eight of 80 randomly selected protocols in the second year elicited partial, and two complete, disagreement on whether a drug to be used was new. Yet, in the first year, the question was not put because the parent committee did not anticipate serious difficulties in an investigator's ability to identify new drugs. . . .

*   *   *

NOTES

NOTE 1.

T. T. BRÜCKE
CLINICAL RESEARCH IN AUSTRIA*

*   *   *

In Austria therapeutic experiments are permitted in university clinics, but the law forbids them in other hospitals. Thus the patient admitted to a university hospital knows that new procedures not yet in current use may be used for his benefit. This being the case, it is unnecessary to inform him fully; nor is it possible when a new procedure is being utilized. In any case the surgeons, even in current practice, do not tell their patients that an accident occurs in every 10,000 cases. It is undesirable that the patient should know everything, and that is indeed the problem involved in his being informed of a trial to be carried out on him.

NOTE 2.

OTTO GUTTENTAG
THE PROBLEM OF EXPERIMENTATION WITH HUMAN BEINGS†

*   *   *

Present types of experimentation on the sick clearly challenge tremendously the basic concepts of the original patient-physician relationship. . . .

Perhaps a glance at the way the legal profession meets the moral and technical demands of society and the individual when a conflict arises between the two will offer a clue to a solution of our problem. As we all know, that profession provides each of the two with a representative of equal stature: there, the prosecuting attorney and, here, the defense attorney. Similar arrangements may have to be developed in the field of human experimentation, performed not for the good of the individual patient but made to confirm or disprove a doubtful or suggested biological generalization. Research and care would not be pursued by the same doctor for the same person, but would be kept distinct, the physician-friend and the physician-experimenter would be two different persons as far as a single

* V. Fattorusso, ed.: *Biomedical Science and the Dilemma of Human Experimentation.* Paris: Council for International Organizations of Medical Sciences 38 (1968). Reprinted by permission.
† 117 *Science* 205 (1953). Reprinted by permission.

patient is concerned—for instance, my patients would become research objects for someone else, and I would be permitted to experiment only with the patients of another physician. The responsibility for the patient would rest, during the experimental period, with the physician-friend, unless the patient decided differently. Retaining his original physician as personal adviser, the patient would at least be under less conflict than he is at present when the question of experimentation arises.

* * *

. . . A given situation may demand that the attitude of the physician-experimenter and that of the physician-friend be embodied in one person. Unless we recognize the basic differences of the two attitudes, each will suffer, as demonstrated by the confused concept of the "hopelessly incurable"; or one will be needlessly neglected, as demonstrated by our failure to supplement forms requesting consent from a patient with some corresponding affirmation of utmost concern for his welfare on the part of the attending physician.

e.
Should Ongoing Research Be Monitored?

[i]
Senate Committee on Government Operations Interagency Drug Coordination*

* * *

The tragedy of thalidomide was not that a drug caused a deformity, but that it continued for so long to cause deformities in the thousands before notice was taken and the cause tracked down.

Recording and evaluation of birth defects was inadequate in the countries where the epidemic first occurred; months went by before significant suspicion was aroused. This was despite the fact that the pattern of malformations was so rare that it should have promptly evoked strong curiosity.

As early as October 1960 the first two cases of "grossly deformed" babies with *seal-like deformities* were presented in a medical exhibit in West Germany.

These cases were described in a later article by Helen B. Taussig, M.D., School of Medicine, Johns Hopkins University. Dr. Taussig is

* Senate Report No. 1153, 89th Congress, 2d Session 8–25 (1966).

the distinguished American physician who, on hearing of the early defects from a German colleague, journeyed to West Germany to study the problem at first hand. It was Dr. Taussig who, on return, alerted the United States to the drug's danger.

Later, Dr. Taussig wrote of the two initial cases in the medical exhibit of October 1960:

Photographs and X-ray pictures showed that the long bones of the infants' arms had almost completely failed to grow; their arms were so short that their hands extended almost directly from their shoulders. Their legs were less affected but showed signs of a similar distortion of growth.

* * *

But over a year was to elapse before the cause of what had become an epidemic was traced.

* * *

Like so many other drugs with a strong market potential, Thalidomide naturally became available in a number of countries through a system of licensing, export of bulk supplies, and other arrangements. The news of side effects of the drug did not, however, proceed through systematic channels between the interested companies of the various nations.

* * *

Many months after the first report on peripheral neuritis, the news of an infinitely more serious nature came. Thalidomide had been withdrawn from the market in West Germany on November 25 because the drug was suspected of responsibility for deformity of babies.

The news from West Germany broke the "dam." A full flood of similar news began to break in country after country. Doctors reported scores and hundreds of deformed babies.

But no intergovernmental action ensued. No international resource, such as the World Health Organization, was informed, consulted, or used so as to minimize the disaster.

* * *

Exchange of information was (and is) handicapped by the fact that a single drug may be called by any one of five or more types of names—by a code name, a chemical name, a generic, an official, and a proprietary name. Within the single "proprietary" category, a drug may be known by dozens or scores of brand names in any one country and by hundreds of such names in many countries. Thalidomide was the generic non-brand name. A physician, reacting to news about the danger of "thalidomide," might unwittingly continue to prescribe the very same chemical ingredient under any one of dozens of trade names.

*   *   *

The international practice of identifying *prescription* drugs to laymen by *number,* not by name, lowered the chance of the public getting rid of the drug, once its hazards became known.

Dr. Taussig wrote in her July 1963 article:

Some pills which were prescribed in good faith by physicians, are now tucked away in many a medicine closet, with *only a prescription* number and no name. The serious consequence of this well-established custom of filling prescriptions *by number* is illustrated by one unfortunate woman who, because the bottle was *unlabeled,* unwittingly took Distaval (a trade name for thalidomide in Great Britain—ed.), during two successive pregnancies and has two children with phocomelia.

The New England Journal of Medicine editorialized:

Dr. Taussig carries her reasoned apprehension beyond the matter of proprietary versus generic names and raises the question whether physicians' prescriptions, which usually bear on the label no other identification than a number, should not also carry the name of the drug or drugs embodied in them. After all, *the less secrecy with which the business of administering medicines can be surrounded, the safer it will become.*

Upon her return from studying the deformities in Western Germany, Dr. Taussig sought to report her findings promptly to American physicians. Her report did not, however, appear in any medical journal until 3½ months after the investigational use in the United States had ended.

A memo by Dr. [Frances] Kelsey to the file discussed her interview later on with Dr. Taussig:

Dr. Taussig mentioned that since she wished authentic information concerning the hazard of this drug to reach the practicing physician as rapidly as possible, she submitted a letter to the AMA for publication shortly after her return from Europe in the late winter. She was told that inasmuch as *Time Magazine* had already run an item on the drug, they would not be interested in publishing such a letter. They are however publishing an article but this inevitably entails a considerable delay.

Dr. Taussig's article in JAMA appeared on June 30, 1962, 7 months after the drug was removed from the market in West Germany.

*   *   *

In an effort to expedite the new drug application through FDA, the company had contacted the medical reviewer, Dr. Kelsey, in over 50 phone calls, visits, and letter requests.

The application had been submitted on September 12, 1960. In the weeks and months which followed, company representatives repeatedly remonstrated with Dr. Kelsey. They pointed to the fact that the drug had been in wide use in West Germany since 1957 and was well regarded there as a safe, useful medication.

*   *   *

The initial clue which aroused Dr. Kelsey's suspicion as to possible hazard from the pending drug came to her attention not through an organized information service, but through sheer happenstance. While looking for something else, she chanced on a letter to the editor in the *British Medical Journal.* The letter mentioned the possibility that thalidomide might be responsible for certain neurological symptoms in the feet and hands.

The *British Medical Journal* is, it may be noted, but 1 of over 5,000 medical serials in the world. Chance finding of an article in even the most prominent publications of the world's literature is like a lucky finding of the proverbial "needle in a haystack."

The chronology of events, as reconstructed by the subcommittee, shows that the original letter to the editor on peripheral neuritis appeared on December 31, 1960; a reply by the British company appeared on January 14, 1961. The first notation of the British discussion appeared in FDA's summary chronology as of a date a month later—February 23, 1961. At that time Dr. Kelsey requested additional information from the company.

In her request of February 23, 1961, Dr. Kelsey asked for "a *complete* list of investigators to whom the drug had been furnished," so as to check up on possible neurological effects. The company did not initially comply with FDA's request. It sent a list of only 56 investigators who had used the drug for a period of 4 months or longer.

*   *   *

On November 28, the West German Ministry of Health issued what Dr. Taussig characterized as "a firm but cautious statement that Contergan, the trade name for thalidomide, was suspected to be a major factor in the production of phocomelia. Women were warned not to take the drug. The announcement was carried on the front page of every newspaper, on the radio, and on television."

A week later, on December 5, 1961, the American company sent out a letter with only this modest warning:

DEAR DOCTOR: We have received information from abroad on the occurrence of congenital malformations in the offspring of a *few* mothers who had taken thalidomide (marketed in Canada as Kevadon) early in their pregnancies. It is impossible at this time to determine whether, in fact, there is any causal relationship.

However, until definitive information is available to us, as a precaution we are adding the following contraindication to the use of Kevadon:

Kevadon should not be administered to pregnant women nor to premenopausal women who may become pregnant.

We are actively following this matter and you will be advised when it is finally determined whether or not this precautionary step was necessary.

*   *   *

Although the drug never emerged out of investigational status in the United States, the company distributed such vast supplies as to raise serious doubt as to whether the company was "testing" or promoting the drug. The company sent 2½ million tablets to 1,267 investigators. This supply was so vast as to be capable of causing incalculable harm if the "investigational" drug turned out to be hazardous.

*   *   *

[T]he American company gave additional indications it was not too interested in "investigational" reports. A manual which it issued to its detail men who were to distribute the drug for "investigation" stated:

. . . the main purpose is to establish local studies whose *results will be spread among hospital staff members.* You can assure your doctors that *they need not report results if they don't want to,* but that we, naturally, would like to know of their results. Be sure to tell them that we may send them report forms or reminder letters *but these are strictly reminders and they need not reply.*

*   *   *

Hundreds of "investigators" failed, contrary to the traditions of science, to keep adequate records. They did not know which patient they had given the drug to, at what dosage or when.

One result was that later on, when the hazards became known, the investigators were unable to contact the patients.

Many doctors, however, did not contact the patients even though they did keep the patients' name and address. An FDA survey concluded that 259 of 1,258 M.D.'s interviewed took *inadequate* steps to contact patients who had been given the drug. Many of the 259 physicians felt that such action was unnecessary because of the length of time that had passed since the patient was given the drug; others had no records indicating which of their patients had received the drug.

The same FDA survey revealed that more than half of the physicians interviewed had *no record* of the quantities of the drug *returned* or *destroyed,* pursuant to the manufacturer's instructions.

*   *   *

[ii]
University of Miami
Procedure for Review of Research Projects
Involving Human Beings (1966) *

*   *   *

(9) After a committee has been assigned a project it will continue to maintain surveillance over it and to provide advice for the investigator in order to safeguard the rights and welfare of human subjects until the project is complete, discontinued, or assigned by the Executive Committee to a different committee either on its own motion or at the request of the committee which has been responsible. The extent and nature of the surveillance shall be determined by the committee upon the basis of giving primary attention to projects involving special risks or unusual conditions and shall be reflected in the minutes of the meeting at which the project is approved. In any event, there is to be a periodic review, which it is contemplated will be on a quarterly basis, of a sample of projects selected by the Executive Committee for review of procedures and conformity with policy. The progress of such review and surveillance shall be re-

---

* Reprinted by permission.

flected in minutes of the committee from time to time as action is taken.

(10) Each investigator is obligated to report to the committee which approved his project any unexpected developments so that they may be evaluated and the project reviewed by the committee.

(11) Each committee is expected to furnish to the investigator of any project assigned to the committee advice and consultation initially and from time to time during a project when appropriate to safeguard the rights and welfare of the individual.

(12) The Office of Assistant Dean for Research, School of Medicine shall maintain all files on projects and maintain a set of minutes of all committees, including the Executive Committee. Those files will be available for inspection and study by the panel and others having good reason to examine them.

*   *   *

NOTES

NOTE 1.

YALE REPORTS
ETHICS AND MEDICINE—CONTROL OF
HUMAN EXPERIMENTATION*

*   *   *

MR. CALABRESI: [D]oes the committee just review the project at the beginning, or do they keep an eye on it as it goes along and suggest times when the experiment ought to be terminated? Because it seems to me that that is as important a question, as data come in, especially in these complicated blind or double-blind experiments, to know at what point the same considerations which would make an experiment improper make it improper for an experiment to continue. Or for that matter to end an experiment too soon.

DR. KATZ: We have talked about it [but] we haven't done anything about this [problem]. It raises even more complicated issues because if you begin to supervise ongoing experiments and how they are being conducted—for example,

---

* A weekly broadcast review presented by Yale University and *WTIC*, March 3, 1968. Participating were Guido Calabresi, Professor of Law; Morton Kligerman, Chairman, Department of Radiology, (Yale Medical School); and Jay Katz, Professor (Adjunct) of Law and Psychiatry. Reprinted by permission.

whether what the experimenter tells us he will communicate to the patient, he actually does communicate—then one will have to institutionalize an extensive watchdog structure. . . .

MR. CALABRESI: But that's a rather different thing. . . . It is one thing to see whether the experimenter is telling you the truth, in terms of what he has communicated to the patient, and that may be hard and an unpleasant thing to police. The other thing is to say that either at given time intervals a report on the project is given to the committee or, if certain events occur, like serious harm to a certain number of patients involved in the experiment, that any of these things automatically should trigger a review of the experiment by people who are not involved in it and so who do not necessarily break the code or break the experiment by doing this.

DR. KLIGERMAN: I agree. Not only do I feel that there should be some lay persons aboard, but that the investigator should at some regular time, even once a year, send the results, a progress report, one page is all it takes, to the committee. I think that this would at least make him stop and think about what has happened. It would make him assess what he has done, and perhaps at an earlier time than he would have, had he not had to prepare such a report to the committee for review.

DR. KATZ: [S]ince I have been on the committee, I have not seen such progress reports. At least what we could do is to ask the experimenter that if anything happens which was not anticipated by the protocol, he should bring this to our attention immediately. . . . We could learn a great deal from such a procedure which would also aid us in reviewing future studies.

*   *   *

NOTE 2.

BERNARD BARBER, JOHN LALLY,
JULIA MAKARUSHKA, AND DANIEL SULLIVAN
THE STRUCTURE AND PROCESSES OF PEER
GROUP REVIEW*

*   *   *

The Public Health Service Regulation, "Protection of the Individual as a Research Sub-

---

* A preliminary version (1970) of *Experimenting with Humans: Problems and Processes of Social Control in the Bio-Medical Research Community.* New York; Russell Sage Foundation (forthcoming). Printed by permission of the authors who retain all rights.

ject," requires not only an initial review of all research protocols but continuing review. The regulation states that "the committee shall carry out interim review of all research in such a manner and at appropriate intervals in the light of apparent risks, existing administrative and supervisory organization, and other factors as to assure itself that its advice is being followed." . . . 24 per cent of the responding institutions report no continuing review at all. 36 per cent claim continuing formal review. 33 per cent report wholly or partly informal review. 6 per cent report that continuing review is given not by the peer review committee but by some institutional officials, such as department heads. The lack of wholly satisfactory continuing review is further evident in the fact that some of the institutions claiming continuing review, formal or informal, indicated in their responses to our question to be specific about what this continuing review consisted in that it was fairly perfunctory or operated only in some cases, not all. For example, a few respondents indicated that continuing review consisted in "informal discussion at lunch," or "through personal contact with researchers," or "as concern arises on the part of investigator, administrator, or senior faculty member." It is evident that procedures and practices for continuing review will have to be strengthened in many bio-medical research institutions using human subjects.

*   *   *

NOTE 3.

Liz Roman Gallese
Medical–Ethics Panels Are Set up to Resolve Dilemmas on Research*

*   *   *

In rare cases an ethics committee may have a physician-advocate peering over a researcher's shoulder to make sure all is well. In one big hospital, for example, a brain surgeon is seeking to use electrodes to stimulate the brains of patients undergoing surgery for various reasons.

The surgeon's project is based on discoveries that short bursts of electricity into certain parts of the brain can cause persons to "see" things, raising hopes that an artificial seeing device might someday be devised for the blind. As preliminary research, the surgeon intends to ask the patients, under local anesthesia, what they "see" as he stimulates their brains.

The hospital's ethics committee recently approved the project when the researcher clarified his intention that the electrodes be placed only on the surface of the brain. But the committee was deeply worried lest an electrode be pushed into the brain itself, a move that might cause permanent brain damage.

The project is approved, the committee stated, only so long as the physician-advocate in the case is present in the operating room to make sure an electrode doesn't penetrate into the patient's brain.

f.

Should Harm Be Assessed?

[i]
Wolf Wolfensberger
Ethical Issues in Research with Human Subjects*

*   *   *

Since the very question of experimental risk . . . appears so apt to arouse emotions that can becloud reason, conceptualization of the relation between certain types of research and experimental risks may be helpful. I propose that there are roughly three levels of research, and even though there is an underlying continuum most experiments with human subjects can probably be assigned to one of these levels.

In level-1 research, experimental activities and procedures are employed but are not consciously recognized or formally labeled as research. A considerable amount of the clinical management of human beings falls into this category. Many techniques of diagnosis and treatment, widely practiced in medicine, psychiatry, clinical psychology, social work, education, rehabilitation, and other human-management professions, lack adequate empirical validation and must be considered tentative and experimental. . . .

There appear to be three reasons why such activities are not recognized or labeled as research: (*i*) a certain hyperclinical type of practitioner finds it difficult to think of himself as being a researcher, and may even attach negative values to research activities; (*ii*) some experimentation loses its research identification be-

---

* *The Wall Street Journal* 1, col. 6, 17, col. 4 (April 14, 1971).

* 155 *Science* 47, 49–50 (1967). Copyright 1967 by the American Association for the Advancement of Science. Reprinted by permission.

cause of its sloppiness; and (*iii*) some experimental and ultimately nonvalidated procedures have been adopted so universally that they have lost their research identification.

There is no doubt that level-1 research can be risky to the subject. An invalidated medical treatment, like bloodletting as practiced in the 18th century, can be worse than no treatment at all. Is it really so inconceivable that some widely current but insufficiently validated human-management practices (psychotherapy, for example) may constitute the bloodletting of the 20th century?

Research at level 1 may also consist of the utilization of impersonal and grouped data collected in the course of routine and accepted operations of agencies. Thus school-enrollment, traffic-accident, and armed forces selection and rejection studies use information pertaining to individuals, group such information, and make it the substance of research. Such data are often collected without the knowledge or consent of the subjects and may or may not affect them.

Research at level 2 is clearly identified and conceptualized as research. Usually, but not necessarily, a distinct manipulation of subjects, individually or in groups, is entailed; at times it may be identified as research more by its "unnaturalness" than by anything else. A situation in which for several hours a subject has to push a button whenever a light appears on a screen (in a vigilance experiment, for instance is perceived quite differently from assignment to a dishwashing task as perhaps in a study of vocational-training practices. Regardless of the oddity of the task, a crucial characteristic of level-2 research is that it stays close to the mainstream of knowledge; the procedures employed are well tried, tend to be familiar at least to specialists, and are known to be harmless; the new knowledge sought is usually modest; and possible outcomes of the research can be fairly well described in advance. Most importantly, risk to the subject is very small, perhaps even smaller than in the often poorly conceptualized and planned and chaotically conducted level-1 research.

It is research at level 3 that tends to give rise to most of the ethical concern. Level-3 research is risky to the subject; either previous work has shown it to be risky or the procedures are novel and untried, and outcomes are less predictable. The fact that this kind of research may occasionally promise more substantial increments in knowledge is likely to lead to dilemmas.

Risk to the subject may exist at any level of research, but there is a very useful distinction between risk that is *intrinsic* to the experimental task and risk *extrinsic* to it. Intrinsic risk arises from the very nature of the task. For instance, a drug may trigger convulsions or allergic reactions; a spinal tap carries a low but definite risk of damage to the central nervous system; and sensory deprivation can result in disturbed behavior.

Extrinsic risk might be viewed as being little or not at all under the control of the experimenter, and not being ordinarily foreseeable; it might be subdivided into types *a* and *b*. Thus type-*a* extrinsic risk may refer to consequences for which the experimenter or his agency is legally liable, even though they comply most meticulously with ethical demands. For example, a subject may slip on the waxed floor of the experimental room, break his leg, and sue for compensation. Type-*b* extrinsic risk may refer to consequences for which the experimenter or his agency is not legally liable: a subject may be struck by a car as he leaves home on his way to the experiment.

Some extrinsic risks are difficult to classify, especially those arising from psychic processes within the subject, of which the experimenter has little or no knowledge. For instance, even the most innocuous research task may seem threatening to some subject; such a perceived threat can cause psychological stress, which in turn can result in physical harm. It is unlikely but conceivable that the mere request to serve as a subject in an "experiment" might lead to heart failure. I have in fact witnessed a breakdown in functioning in a mildly retarded teenager who was asked to leave class and spend a few minutes on an undemanding, simple, and utterly harmless task; it appeared that a "friend" had told him something to the effect that the psychologist was going to cut his head open.

Except in instances in which research involves only record data, the researcher can never state with certainty that a subject will not experience some kind of trauma. At best, he can estimate the level of probability of trauma if intrinsic research risks exist, or state that, if trauma occurs, it will occur because of the extrinsic risks.

*   *   *

[ii]
Robert J. Bazell
Food and Drug Administration—
*Is Protecting Lives the Priority?**

In January officials of the Food and Drug Administration (FDA) knew that the use of bottled intravenous feeding solutions manufactured by Abbott Laboratories had somehow led to an outbreak of blood poisoning and several deaths. Yet they took no action. In early March, the FDA found out that a large percentage of the Abbott solutions were contaminated with the infectious bacteria responsible for the blood poisoning. Yet they did not ban the products. They only recommended that certain precautions be taken when the solutions were given to patients. Not until 22 March did FDA recommend that hospitals stop using the Abbott products and then only after consumer-advocate Ralph Nader appeared on national television denouncing the agency for its failure to act.

The intravenous (I.V.) solutions (mostly combinations of dextrose and salts in water) are used in virtually every hospital to feed nutrients to critically ill patients. Until the ban Abbott Laboratories supplied 45 percent of the 250,000 bottles of I.V. solutions administered daily to patients in the United States.

*   *   *

A decision by FDA officials to ban any product involves complex consideration, many of them subjective. And from the vantage point of hindsight, the FDA can make an easy target for critics. Nevertheless, the case of Abbott's I.V. solutions involved enough irregularities and a sufficient number of deaths to warrant close scrutiny. . . .

*   *   *

The decision to remove a product from use rests . . . with the FDA. All through the investigation, George Blatt of FDA's Office of Compliance kept tabs on the CDC [Center for Disease Control] findings. Blatt does not believe that the relation discovered in January between the disease and the Abbott products warranted any action by the FDA and, indeed, FDA did nothing at the time.

"You don't take legal action against a

* 172 *Science* 41–43 (1971). Copyright 1971 by the American Association for the Advancement of Science. Reprinted by permission.

firm," Blatt told *Science*, "until you have evidence that can stand up in court. You have to define where the problem is. And all you had at the time was an association of the disease with the product." He emphasized, however, that the decisions regarding action against Abbott were made not by him, but by the Commissioner of Food and Drugs, Charles E. Edwards.

But, in spite of the illnesses and deaths resulting from the products, Edwards says he knew nothing of the problem. In an interview with *Science*, both Edwards and his associate commissioner for compliance, Sam Fine, insisted that the first they heard of the difficulties, other than what had been published in the *New England Journal of Medicine*, was 11 March. That was after the discovery of the contaminated bottle caps.

*   *   *

On 11 March representatives of Abbott, FDA, and CDC met in Atlanta. The next morning David Sensor, the director of CDC, Edward J. Ledder, the president of Abbott Laboratories, Surgeon General Jesse Steinfeld, and Commissioner Edwards met in Washington to discuss the problem. That afternoon Edwards and Sensor announced at a press conference that a ban was not feasible and that "special precautions must be taken . . . to reduce the risk of septicemia from the use of Abbott Laboratories' intravenous infusion products." The precautions included gentle removal of the bottle caps, changing of the I.V. apparatus every 24 hours, and watching for the first signs of blood poisoning.

*   *   *

In explaining his decision on 13 March not to ban the use of the contaminated solutions, Edwards told *Science*, "You've got to understand that all we had at that time was very preliminary data. We believed that the precautions could allow the solutions to be used safely." Edwards also emphasized that FDA didn't have accurate information about the availability of replacement products from Abbott's competitors. And since Abbott was supplying 45 percent of the critical solutions, he could not simply order hospitals to stop using the Abbott products. "We might have killed more people by banning the Abbott solutions than by allowing their use," added Fine.

Yet FDA officials acknowledge that they did not even check on the availability of solutions from other manufacturers until after the 13 March announcement. Thus while FDA met with Abbott on 12 and 13 March, Abbott's three competitors, Baxter Laboratories, Cutter Laboratories, and American Hospital Supply, heard from FDA a few days later. When on 19 March government specialists did complete a survey of the competitors, they concluded that, for the most part, hospitals' stocks of Abbott solutions could be replaced. "The reason for the delay," said Edwards, "was that we didn't know of the problem until 11 March. After that we acted as fast as possible."

Although the FDA had declared that the Abbott solutions could be used safely, the Army disagreed. On 15 March, the Army Surgeon General issued a worldwide notice ordering all Army medical facilities "to suspend from immediate use and issue all Abbott intravenous solutions." The Army and the FDA differed in their actions, according to one medical officer, because the Army wasn't depending solely on Abbott products. And "because in the military services we never take a chance with a product that might be faulty."

*   *   *

NOTE

M. B. VISSCHER
PUBLIC STAKE IN THE WISE CONTROL OF
CLINICAL INVESTIGATION*

*   *   *

. . . A drug which had been used in another country on some 300,000 human subjects for management of hypertension was found to have impressive anti-fibrillatory effects on the dog heart. The investigator carried out extensive toxicity studies in dogs at the dose levels required for the anti-fibrillatory effect and found no observable adverse effects. Lethal doses were many times the proposed therapeutic dosages. Application for permission to begin clinical studies was made, but numerous requirements for additional studies were laid down, including such stipulations as that possible local tissue injury at the site of intramuscular injection be fully investigated. Since the drug was intended to be used only in life-threatening situations, and

since the dogs employed in general toxicity studies had had intramuscular injections without gross evidence of local tissue damage, it seemed absurd to make these further studies as a prerequisite to clinical trial. If the drug were to be found to be clinically useful, it would actually be employed even if there were some damage to muscle at the site of injection because no satisfactory anti-fibrillatory drug is available today. After six months of delay, the Food and Drug Administration did grant permission to test the drug on humans, but months of time were lost, and the possible life-saving virtues of a drug which markedly raises the threshhold for ventricular fibrillation have been denied to the whole human race for those six months. A considerable amount of humans do die every day because of uncontrollable ventricular arrhythmias. Excessive caution has probably cost the lives of thousands of persons, simply by postponing the time at which a drug may become generally available.

*   *   *

g.
Should Societal Interests Be Considered?

[i]
Walsh McDermott
Comment on "Law as a System of Control"*

*   *   *

. . . While the public seems quite willing to accept that there are times in human experimentation when the interest of the individual cannot be paramount, it would probably not support the actual codification of that principle in either an administrative regulation or a statute. And these are the two forms of the law that have emerged to the forefront in this field of human experimentation. Attempts to create extralegal devices such as local committee review are likewise unsatisfactory. My objection to the committees is not that they perform no useful services, because they do provide such services of a limited sort; specifically, they serve to air the issue. But, as they are in effect self-appointed, they lack the authority to represent the interests of either the individual or society when these interests are in conflict in a particular case. For this reason they cannot be regarded as a

* V. Fattorusso, ed.: *Biomedical Science and the Dilemma of Human Experimentation.* Paris: Council for International Organizations of Medical Sciences 46, 49 (1968). Reprinted by permission.

* Paul A. Freund, ed.: *Experimentation with Human Subjects.* New York: George Braziller 218, 219–220 (1970). Reprinted by permission of the American Academy of Arts and Sciences.

major institutional form that meets the need; yet, they represent just about the only formal extra-legal structure that exists.

*   *   *

. . . I came to the conclusion that in medical research the problem of attempting to institutionalize the making of a judgment between the individual and society was basically unsolvable. Perhaps some day there might come to be a reasonably widespread, publicly voiced attitude on the individual vs. society issue that would permit appropriately flexible laws or administrative regulations. But until that presumably far-off day, as I saw it, we would simply have to live with the problem and handle it as best we could, by what must ultimately be arbitrary decisions. To ensure that these arbitrary decisions not be capricious, I could suggest only that we rely on the cultivated conscience of the experimenter, continuously reinforced by an organized effort to increase the local visibility surrounding each decision. Indeed, this seemed to me to be the chief role served by the local committees.

*   *   *

[ii]
Guido Calabresi
Reflections on Medical Experimentation
in Humans*

*   *   *

[P]erhaps the best general system of control would be the oft-suggested establishment of groups (hospital committees, say) that are sufficiently broadly based so that their judgment can reflect society's unspoken choice between present and future risks, and yet unofficial enough so that they do not seem to represent the government choosing to sacrifice the individual for the good of the collective. Society, in the form of the government, could retain its position as the protector of individual lives and step in mainly to establish stricter rules in areas where the unofficial groups had erred and allowed lives to be taken too blatantly or in a way that undermined our commitment to human dignity.

If hospital committees are to bear the main burden of overseeing experiments and experi-

* 98 *Daedalus* 387, 399–400 (1969). Reprinted by permission of Daedalus, Journal of the American Academy of Arts and Sciences, Boston, Massachusetts.

mental plans, if they are to be the principal instruments for balancing risks to present lives against future benefits, ways must be found of increasing the information that is available to these committees. It is not enough that they be made up of people of good will; their members must also be people who have available to them some sense of the balance that society desires between present and future lives. The difficulty here, of course, is that this sense cannot be given by government decrees, since that would involve society too clearly in the process of choosing against individuals. The sense of society's wishes must, instead, be brought to the committees through as many varied inputs as possible. In effect, the more the inputs of information and value judgments to the committees are broadened, the more the committees will seem to be doing no more than ratifying broad judgments inherent in the social system. In this way, the directness—the playing God by any single group—is reduced. This would be especially true if, in addition to the committees, there was not only some kind of market test (of the type I described) to be met, but also government intervention from time to time to protect individual lives by requiring more care than either the market or the committees deemed necessary.

The most obvious—but probably least important—method of broadening the input to the committees is by broadening the committees themselves. Many of these are now made up primarily of scientists from the very medical center where the research to be approved is to take place. The presence of scientists from other research centers and the presence of non-scientific members would certainly give the committees a greater sense of where the crucial balance is to be struck. My own guess is that while scientists from other medical centers would on occasion be stricter than local scientists in approving particular experiments, non-scientists on the committees would tend, on the whole, to approve some experiments that would not now be passed. This is especially true where the potential gains from an experiment are great, but the risks involved are also great. In such areas, I suggest, doctors are perhaps unduly hampered by fear of lawsuits (incidentally, the reduction of fear of such suits might be a side benefit of the kind of market compensation system I have described) and by the worthy tradition that, after all, the individual patient is in their care. Laymen, I believe, are less likely to be so emotionally concerned with either of these two factors and, hence, are more likely to give greater weight to society's long-run interest.

* * *

3.

In Reviewing Decisions and Consequences

a.

Through Public Scrutiny?

[i]
Guido Calabresi
Reflections on Medical Experimentation
in Humans*

* * *

. . . The best way of testing lay reaction to particular experiments—indeed, the best way of broadening the inputs to the committees—lies in . . . publication of the cases decided by the committees. Such cases could well be anonymous (at least at first). They could be collected and published in much the same way that decisions of courts are collected. The reports on any case could include, first, a factual part describing, among other things, the experience of the experimenter, the antecedent tests in non-human subjects, the major risks perceived, the scientific gains perceived possible, the availability of subsequent controls to limit the risks, the origin and life expectancy of the subjects, and the nature of the consent and the manner in which it was obtained; and, second, a jurisprudential section containing the decision of the committee (whether favorable or unfavorable), together with the principal arguments made for and against the decision reached.

Such published cases would soon become the subject of intense study both inside and outside the medical profession. Analyses in learned journals by lawyers, doctors, and historians of science would inevitably follow. These would undoubtedly re-argue the more important or path-breaking cases. If law cases are any guide, the analyses would sometimes conclude that the cases were wrongly decided, but frequently that they were rightly decided, and per-

---

* 98 *Daedalus* 387, 400–403 (1969). Reprinted by permission of Daedalus, Journal of the American Academy of Arts and Sciences, Boston, Massachusetts.

haps more frequently that they were rightly decided but for the wrong reasons. To the extent that Law Reviews consider themselves courts of last appeal beyond the highest courts in the land, so would the learned journals in which this *giurisprudenza* would be dissected. From all this, a sense of what society at large deems proper in medical experiments might well arise. This sense would, in turn, guide the committees and make their decisions more sophisticated. The result would not only be better thought out decisions, but also a more complex system of controls, which, in effect, took into account much broader sources of information as to societal values. In addition, the very existence of open criticism through published cases would reduce the finality of the judgment of any given committee. They might decide one case improperly, but the community would have the feeling that over time its judgments as to the proper balance of present risks against future gains would make itself felt. Moreover, this method of introducing community views would, at least in part, avoid the dangers of governmental rule-making, for at no given time would the community as such seem to be choosing to take an individual life for the general good. (Of course, the presence of published cases—even if anonymous—might make information available that could lead to lawsuits; one advantage of the compensation fund described earlier is that, since compensation would already be given to the injured subject, no lawsuits and hence no attribution of fault would occur.)

Three practical objections can be made to the publication of hospital committee decisions. The first is that such publication would destroy the confidentiality of research and might result in the pirating of good ideas. The second is that hospital committees do not now ask for any very definite indication of the possible scientific benefits perceived in an experiment, but concentrate only on the risks to the subjects and the experience and reputation of the experimenter. As a result, it is argued, publication would be of little use in establishing the balance between risks and benefits that the public at large desires. The third objection is that published hospital committee decisions would not reflect the actual facts before the committee. Committees, to protect themselves, would so emphasize those facts that favored their decision that the results reached would seem to be obvious in every case.

The first objection, if valid, can easily be met by providing for delay in publication until after the experiment itself is completed and published. Since the aim of publication is not to pass judgment on the particular experiment, but to encourage debate (for the guidance of future committees) on which experiments are desirable and which are not, delay in publication causes no particular problems. The important point is that real cases be examined; whether the examination takes place immediately or two years after an experiment is approved or forbidden matters relatively little.

The second objection is, I believe, misplaced. It may well be that most experiments involve sufficiently small risks so that, given the reputation of the experimenter and the type of consent obtained, no specific indication of benefits foreseen is needed to justify approving the experiment. In every case where this was so, the published opinion of the committee should indicate that. And I would expect that such judgments based on low risk and high reputation would find support among most commentators. If, however, a very high-risk experiment were either approved or turned down without an attempt to learn why the experiment seemed to the investigator to be worth doing, I would expect that there would be substantial criticism. Such criticism might well bring about a change in current practice and enable some experiments that would now be turned down, absent consideration of the possible benefits of the experiment, to take place. Conversely, other experiments that involved substantial risks might not be deemed worthwhile given their small possible benefits. Either response to societal desires made known through publication and criticism would be more desirable than blind approval or rejection of a dangerous experiment.

The final objection—that written committee decisions would not represent the true facts on which the decisions were based—would seem more damaging if a similar criticism could not be made of many court decisions; yet the usefulness of publishing legal opinions remains enormous. Commentators would soon become as adept at divining the issues involved in a hospital committee decision as are legal commentators at analyzing a judicial opinion. The informed criticism of both negative and positive decisions that would follow would, I venture to predict, lose no more from the fact that the opinions would, to some extent, be artificial and stylized than does the analogous legal criticism lose from the same defect in court opinions. Thus, publication, even if the opinions were to

some extent artificial, would remain a highly significant device for broadening hospital committee deliberations and thereby increasing and diversifying societal control of medical experiments.

* * *

[ii]
Louis L. Jaffe
Law as a System of Control*

* * *

How should the institutions of the law figure in furthering and protecting the interests implicated in human experimentation? The law as we know it is a system of decisional organs and their formal and informal products: the legislature (statutes), the executive-administrative (regulations and adjudication), and the courts (adjudication). Any of these in varying combinations can make law governing the conduct of the experimenter and the rights of the subject. There is not as yet much law explicitly dealing with human experimentation but the common law (by which we mean the law devised and administered by the courts) has developed and continues to develop doctrines that are applicable. . . .

The advantage of common law judicial control is its flexibility—a characteristic consonant with the presently fluid condition of ethical attitudes toward experimentation. *Ad hoc* judicial decisions, it is true, may mean a stiff judgment for damages against an individual who learns only after the event the precise application of the rules governing his conduct. . . .

* * *

The committee system is today part of a system of self-regulation, but it could and probably should become part of the legal system of control either generally or on a selective basis. This change could come about by statute, by administrative fiat, or by judicial decision. It would be going too far to require that there be a committee procedure in every experiment. Every medical intervention is to some degree experimental, and the physician in his practice is constantly faced with the challenge to use new drugs or new procedures. If he is a specialist, his interest in these will not be limited to their effect

---
* 98 *Daedalus* 406, 407–408, 412–416 (1969). Reprinted by permission of Daedalus, Journal of the American Academy of Arts and Sciences, Boston, Massachusetts.

in the particular case: He will be looking for guidance in the future. A general statutory requirement requiring institutional committees in any "experiment" would raise monstrous problems of interpretation, would unduly complicate medical practice, and would add unnecessary steps to experiments where the risks to the subject or patient are trivial. But as has been the practice with grants from the NIH, a governmental authority or a foundation might in specified instances require committee procedure for experiments funded by the grant.

Finally, a court exercising its common-law jurisdiction in a suit for damages could condemn experiments of high risk if there had been no committee approval of the protocol. To reach this result, the most likely recourse would be to the concept of negligence, which subjects the injury-producing action of an individual or corporate body to the test of "due care." It is particularly relevant that "due care" is a continually evolving concept. What was "due care" yesterday may not suffice today. In the famous case of the *T. J. Hooper*, 60 F.2d 737 (1932), Judge Learned Hand held that a vessel had violated the standard of due care because it was not equipped with a radio that would have given warning of approaching storms. It was no answer, said the judge, that radios had not been generally adopted. "Courts must in the end say what is required; there are precautions so imperative that even their universal disregard will not excuse their omission." Absorbed into the law in this way the committees and the procedures that they develop become a functioning part of the legal system of control.

*   *   *

Upon what principles will the experimenter govern his conscience, the committees exercise their sanctioning function, the administrative authorities establish the conditions of experimentation, and finally the courts test the validity of experimental intervention? We need not assume that the principles will be the same at all four levels, though they will rest on a common base. In fashioning the common law, the judges will ordinarily allow a considerable latitude for the exercise of conscience and skill. A committee may demand safeguards that the law does not require. It may, for example, require experiments to be performed by a group or demand that the therapeutic and experimental functions be kept separate and be performed by different

personnel. A court, on the other hand, would probably not impose such conditions even though it believed them to be wise. A committee might veto a project on the ground that it did not hold sufficient promise of fruitful results. It is unlikely that a court would feel qualified to make such a judgment, and, if the experimental subject had been fairly treated, it would not condemn the experiment. Thus, there is a significant area of discretion within which conscience and technical judgment are to be exercised.

Though there is almost no judge-made law dealing specifically with experimentation in the modern sense, it is nevertheless justifiable, indeed necessary, to extrapolate a common law based on the application of relevant legal concepts. There have been few lawsuits directly raising questions of the legality of experimentation and even now, with the vast amount of experimentation, resort to the courts is spasmodic. Thus, we cannot look to the common law judges for detailed prescriptions and proscriptions. Nevertheless, we must posit a common law as the ultimate legal guardian of the interests involved in experimentation. Where there is serious debate concerning the propriety or the necessity of certain procedures, where there is a real conflict of interests, an appeal to putatively relevant concepts of the common law provides authoritative standards for judgment.

*   *   *

Judges are sensitive to the ethos of the times. Our society places a high premium on scientific experimentation and the pursuit of knowledge. To a greater extent than was formerly true, judges will be conscious of the conflict of interests and will seek to give due weight to each of them in any case involving experimentation carried on pursuant to current standards of propriety. The courts, for example, have been willing to take account of the conditions of modern surgery in permitting a further operation without consent where unexpected and serious pathology turns up in the course of an operation performed under anesthesia. We should proceed on the hypothesis, therefore, that in framing our ethical principles the common law will be hospitable to procedures that recognize the social value of human experimentation without sacrificing the interests of patients and subjects.

*   *   *

NOTES

NOTE 1.

WALSH MCDERMOTT
COMMENT ON "LAW AS A SYSTEM OF CONTROL"*

*   *   *

What are the weaknesses of this approach of looking to the common law as our instrument for decision? Or, to put it differently, assuming the common law, fortified through extrapolation, is functioning with full effectiveness, how much of the problem remains unsolved? Several points have already been mentioned: human error or malperformance; no prospective decision in a particular case; and failure to remove the ultimate ethical responsibility from the investigator. As the last-named could not be accomplished by any institution presently conceivable, and as it by no means necessarily represents a desirable goal, its absence here is hardly an institutional failure.

One area in which the common-law approach might have a weakness as our sought-for institution would be that its advocacy of the interests of society in a particular experiment might not be specific, that is, framed in terms of that experiment, but would tend to be quite general.

For example, to what extent could the common law serve as a vigorous advocate of the best interests of society in a situation in which a powerful case for the social interest exists, yet to meet it demands the placing of an individual at an appreciable risk? One might argue that the common-law mechanism would perforce be doing this in every case, and in one sense this would be true. But in the personalized form of a lawsuit, the interest of society in the experiment itself is handled indirectly and might tend to become a side issue. By this I mean that a favorable decision based on "due care" might be very crudely paraphrased, "the physician meant well, he intended no injury, and he took due care to attempt to ensure that no injury occurred." This is clearly not quite the same as saying: "It was clearly in the best interests of society that this particular experiment be done because . . . this individual, through the hand of fate, was one of the few who would serve as a satisfactory subject; he gave his informed consent; and due care was taken to minimize the possibility of his suffering harm." I suppose that such an all-embracing decision is neither to be expected nor desired, because it would tend to get the judge into technical areas beyond his competence. Yet, its absence does mean that the common-law approach will not meet the whole need.

Another possible weakness is that extreme interpretations of due care itself could lead us into the same built-in contradictions that· are present, say, in the Helsinki Declaration. . . . [W]hile the physician *is* trained to weigh the probabilities of danger from off-setting risks, he is also trained to refuse to place his patient at *any* known risk *no matter how small the probability of danger* in the absence of a positive reason for doing so. Expressed differently, the fact that the probability of the occurrence of a known danger is extremely low is not in itself an ethical justification for placing the patient at risk. In an adversary proceeding involving the concept of due care, this "any known risk" principle might be invoked to establish a failure of due care.

The extent to which either of these two possible weaknesses will constitute problems cannot really be foreseen, because this approach through the common law has such a considerable degree of flexibility.

*   *   *

NOTE 2.

ALEXANDER M. BICKEL
COMMENT*

*   *   *

Because we know a little bit about medical experimentation at this time, I must raise a caution about collecting cases. The common law and other processes of adjudication out of which modes of behavior grow involve the resolution of manifest clashing interests. If we gathered information on how researchers have been behaving, we would be subject to the dangers of drawing from a process of adjudication in which we are self-interested. After all, committees passing on the research proposals are interested in furthering research. Mr. Jaffe says that

* Paul A. Freund, ed.: *Experimentation with Human Subjects.* New York: George Braziller 218, 222–223 (1970). Reprinted by permission of the American Academy of Arts and Sciences.

* *Proceedings of the Daedalus-NIH Conference on the Ethical Aspects of Experimentation on Human Subjects.* Boston: American Academy of Arts and Sciences 22 (1967). Reprinted by permission of the American Academy of Arts and Sciences.

the dynamic in favor of research is terrific. At no point in the process of quasi-adjudication is the interest of the individual, the subject, represented. Consequently, we might be misled and put that other interest aside. If we then attempted to look at the practice and perhaps formalize it, we would have minimized, if not excluded, the interest which we are here to analyze and assert.

*   *   *

[iii]
James Turner
The Chemical Feast*

The 1969 Ralph Nader Summer Study of the Food and Drug Administration's food protection activities was based on the conclusions of a preliminary report prepared during the summer and fall of 1968. . . . Based on interviews with present and former agency personnel, the preliminary report highlighted major problem areas in the FDA structure, including the control of cyclamates and other food additives, the failure of decision-makers to use scientific information effectively, and the misuse of food standards. In 1969 sixteen students or recent graduates (some of the 110 students who worked on the Nader Summer Studies that year) were divided into teams of two and assigned to research in depth each of ten identified problem areas, with two groups researching two related areas. . . .

The procedure of the Nader Summer Study Project was unique for a research effort. While the students spent many hours in the traditional library search for academic explanations of the problems they had discovered, the real heart of the project was the interviews with responsible agency officials and the collecting of official documents from them. In their four months of activity the sixteen members of the Nader team conducted over five hundred separate interviews, collected over ten thousand documents, and became regular fixtures in FDA libraries, reading rooms, and offices. Because of their daily presence at the agency, the students had an almost immediate impact upon FDA activities. The agency itself was eager to help. Commissioner Herbert L. Ley, Jr., and C. C. Johnson, his immediate superior in the Department of Health, Education, and Welfare, directed all employees to aid the investigation, and the Commissioner

and his staff made themselves available whenever possible to discuss information as it became available. They were glad to co-operate for their own reasons as well as simply to be helpful. In June, 1968, Theodore Cron, then Assistant FDA Commissioner for Information and Education and key adviser to Commissioner James Goddard, said in an interview that he welcomed the Nader investigation because he felt that several divisions of the agency were functioning badly and either intentionally or out of incompetence were providing the agency leadership with inaccurate or incomplete information. Many officials of the FDA who served under Dr. Ley seemed to share this view. The facts uncovered by the students supported it as well.

For the most part, the students who worked on the FDA investigation, both in 1968 and in 1969, began with faith in the quality of the American food supply but also with some skepticism, inspired primarily by (1) Ralph Nader's revelations in 1967 and 1968 that meat and poultry quality was not as high as had been widely assumed and (2) the realization that the FDA was a regulatory agency and therefore probably afflicted with the same bureaucratic density, inefficiency, and self-justification uncovered in other regulatory agencies brought under close scrutiny. It is fair to say that none of the students expected to find in the FDA the shocking disarray and appalling failure of responsibility that their investigations revealed almost daily. As the number of altered documents, misrepresented facts, and suppressed studies began to mount, the students' initial skepticism changed to a deep doubt about all the agency's activities and finally ended in the conviction that most agency efforts were a failure. The fact that most of the distortion and failure related directly to the safety or quality of food served to heighten their concern.

The first specific study the group completed concerned the Coca-Cola—Dr. Pepper fight to obtain a regulation that allowed the addition of caffeine to cola drinks and the Dr. Pepper drink without announcing the addition on the label. Agency documents showed that the overwhelming sentiment of the FDA officials involved in the decision was to require labeling. The record also showed strong reasons for following such a policy. But the first act of Commissioner James Goddard, taken four days after assuming office, was to sign a regulation that allowed the addition of caffeine without requiring that it be listed on the label. After spending ten days going over all the agency documents concerned with the decision, the student investigator involved spent the next days conducting interviews with all the responsible individuals, after which he said, "I will never be able to trust another government official again. Every one of these men lied about their involvement in the decision to one degree or another. If I hadn't had the records, I would have never known there had been any disagreement with the final regulation." The experience of many other students was similar if less dramatic.

Two students discovered that in a January, 1969 memo from Dr. Marvin Legator to Commissioner Ley a recommendation that the marketing of cyclamates be stopped had been deleted from the original memorandum by an intermediary without informing either the sender or the receiver of the memorandum. This discovery was immediately communicated to all parties concerned and was largely responsible for Dr. Ley's acknowledgment on October 18, 1969, that he had a communication problem in his Bureau of Science. Similarly, after Dr. Ley testified to a Congressional committee that his agency had conducted a number of studies, all of which showed that MSG was safe, a student contacted the FDA researchers mentioned and found that two of the four studies cited had not been undertaken and that two others had not been completed. These discoveries were then relayed orally to the individuals responsible. Six weeks later, after no effort had been made by the FDA to correct the erroneous testimony, a report of the incident was prepared for Ralph Nader to send to the Congressional committee involved, calling attention to the errors.

In December, 1968, the preliminary investigators discovered that FDA studies showed that a very high proportion of deformed chicken embryos came from eggs injected with cyclamates and cyclohexylamine, tending to confirm dangers suggested by studies showing genetic deformities in rats injected with cyclamates. For the next nine months scientists both inside and outside the FDA as well as the study team members tried to get the FDA to conduct some kind of official evaluation of these studies. At the end of September, 1969, Paul Friedman, an NBC news reporter from Washington, specifically asked a member of the study team about the state of cyclamate research at FDA and was informed of the chick embryo study along with other studies. He then arranged to interview the FDA personnel responsible for the studies and broadcast the results on the local Washington news and the Huntley-Brinkley network report. The result was nation-wide concern, which eventually led to the banning of cyclamates.

In various ways the results of the Nader group study were constantly communicated to the responsible officials within HEW. The purpose of the study was and is to contribute the effort of a group of concerned individuals to the solution of a major American problem—how to provide the highest quality, safest food at the most reasonable price to the American people. For this reason the students attempted at every opportunity to point out problems in need of attention and work toward solutions with agency personnel. In the course of this effort they discovered a kind of defeatist attitude which permeates every level of the FDA bureaucracy. There is little belief among the agency personnel that the FDA can really make any difference. Comments of various people associated with the FDA during the past ten years suggest how much frustration and despair grip the agency. . . .

*   *   *

Once the FDA's regulatory failures are seen as part of a general failure of protection for the public, reform of the FDA becomes only part of a more general problem. The public-interest activities of professionals supported by the activities of large groups of people are examples of actions to be taken as part of an overall campaign designed to make government more responsive to the real needs of the public. Legislative and regulatory actions will have to be undertaken in conjunction with the private activities of concerned citizens. One of the major failures of previous reforms was the belief that passing laws solved problems: this is rarely the case. However, it is often necessary to pass new laws as part of a more general attempt to solve a given problem. The same is true of the reorganization of all regulatory agencies. There will have to be new legislation passed to define more accurately the role to be played by the government in the food regulations area. The FDA will have to be reorganized so that it represents the public interest. The most important lesson learned during the Nader Summer Study of the FDA was the futility of trying to treat the FDA as an isolated organization. . . .

A spirit of concern about the future of America lives among a large segment of American youth. Many are trying in numerous and diverse ways to harness this spirit to the practical tools of change so that life for all Americans can be better. They have great hope, great energy, and with support from others a good chance of success.

*   *   *

However, none of it will succeed without the support and participation of the consuming public. Each individual consumer and every organization of consumers must make their dissatisfaction known from the local shop level to the national level of corporate managers and government officials. So little is now known about the particular abuses to which American people are subjected daily that it is often impossible to take corrective action. The Consumer Federation of America is organizing consumer chapters for the express purpose of finding abuses and planning action to correct them. Any group of local citizens, effectively organized, can provide a great deal of defense for themselves against the abuses of corporate insensitivity. Cities across the country are beginning to establish consumer-protection agencies which can be a focal point of effort on behalf of the public. Public action must be the primary part of the campaign to restore concern for the public interest in major American power centers, or the campaign will fail.

NOTE

CHRISTOPHER LYDON
NADER AND F.C.C. MEMBER CRITICIZE
KENNEDY CONSUMER AID PLAN*

Senator Edward M. Kennedy wants Congress to charter a new Public Counsel Corporation to represent the peoples' interest before Federal agencies.

But Ralph Nader, the consumer advocate, and Nicholas Johnson, a Federal communications commissioner, told the Senator today that a new organization might only compound the frustration of consumers.

All three men agreed this morning that the public commissions that were designed to represent the public interest had become some of the biggest obstacles to effective citizen participation in Government.

*   *   *

The Public Counsel Corporation Senator Kennedy has proposed would have a bipartisan board of 15 men and women, appointed by the

_____
* *The New York Times* 24, col. 1 (July 22, 1970). © 1970 by The New York Times Company. Reprinted by permission.

President and funded by Congress. It would have authority to intervene in specific cases or to propose fundamental reforms.

"Given the corporate domination of our national politics and government," Mr. Johnson commented on the Kennedy bill, "the question is whether any political appointee to an agency funded by the Government can do anything effective on behalf of people who are oppressed and manipulated by the large corporations. I think what you've done here is about as well as Government can do, but I don't know if it's good enough."

Mr. Nader, who has supervised a number of critical studies of the regulatory process and enlisted a corps of young "public interest" lawyers to challenge it, said it was important to get public funding for such efforts but that a new public counsel's office would be at best a beginning.

Mr. Nader said that the Nixon Administration's record in the consumer field was "woefully inadequate" and that it would be important to keep any new Public Counsel Corporation free of the Justice Department, which, he said, has become "anticonsumer" under Attorney General John N. Mitchell.

"The strongest case can be made," Mr. Nader proposed, "for actually requiring that the 300 top lawyers in Washington—already rich beyond the dreams of avarice—spend all their time representing the public interest. This is on the same level as telling people to stop what they are doing and put out fires, or stop what they are doing and fight an epidemic, or stop what they are doing and save the country."

b.

Through Professional Evaluation?

*CIOMS Roundtable Discussion
Comments on Editorial Censorship**

*   *   *

SIR JOHN ECCLES: In the problem of how you can educate or inform the whole of the medical community and other investigating human beings on these problems of ethics, there is another side to it that occurs to me, illustrated by certain journals now with regard to animal ex-

_____
* V. Fattorusso, ed.: *Biomedical Science and the Dilemma of Human Experimentation.* Paris: Council for International Organizations of Medical Sciences 94–95 (1968). Reprinted by permission.

perimentation. For example, *The Journal of Physiology* has certain strict regulations to the effect that experiments not conforming to certain standards governing the treatment of animals— avoiding unnecessary pain, for example—will not be published. This is true of experimental brain research also. I wonder whether a recommendation should not be made that scientific and medical journals should take action to prevent the publication of experimental investigations on human subjects which transgress the ethical principles that have been developed to safeguard the subject as a person. Such principles could be broadly interpreted, but at least they would alert the whole of the scientific medical community to the reality of the problem.

* * *

PROFESSOR FLORKIN: It means that research workers would not carry out a physiological experiment on animals when they could not publish the results, for the knowledge they gain thereby would be private to them and they want to make it available to the scientific public. In the present state of affairs, it is obviously impossible to find out whether people carry out experiments not conforming to ethical standards, but certainly it would be useful to recommend that research work should not be published when it offends against generally accepted rules. What is proposed is an initial cleaning-up operation.

PROFESSOR HALPERN: Since we are making publication dependent on something that seems to be a rule—the ethical rule—can we, as far as experiments on man are concerned, define such a rule in a way that will enable the editorial board to accept or reject the manuscript? The fact that we have no criteria would place an arbitrary weapon in the hands of the editorial board; would it not say that such and such work is ethically all right, such and such work not? How would you defend yourself if you submit a paper and it is refused? I state this problem, which Sir John Eccles will perhaps be able to elaborate on and give assurances about.

SIR JOHN ECCLES: It is quite clear from the discussion of today that no one can define the situation sharply. We have to go through a process of progressive education and we have to be alerted to the problem. The editorial boards of different journals will handle it in different ways, but this is all right too. Let them handle it. We want to alert them to the problem and gradually, I think, a degree of what might be called moral obloquy may descend upon the people who are doing unethical experiments. You cannot prevent these experiments being done, but gradually you can develop a conscience in investigators and in editorial boards, and this is at least one way to approach the problem. It is a process of what I should call "moral education."

* * *

MR. SABA: Since, as Professor Halpern has stressed, no ethical rules have been established, a prohibition of an absolute kind might have the effect of preventing knowledge from being spread. I wonder to what extent we should not differentiate between scientific information, which is an essential means of progress, and a recommendation. We should not recommend that experiments should be carried out in violation of professional ethical standards or what are generally considered as commonly accepted moral standards. But if scientific information has been obtained by an experiment carried out inadvisedly, would you prevent it from being disseminated?

* * *

NOTES

NOTE 1.

THE MASSACHUSETTS GENERAL HOSPITAL HUMAN STUDIES—GUIDING PRINCIPLES AND PROCEDURES*

Ordinarily data which have been unethically obtained will not be published. While the specific loss to medicine might be great, it is never as great in any reasonably conceivable circumstances as the moral loss sustained by medicine when unethically obtained data are published. Suppression of unethically obtained data will do much to curb the enthusiasm of the careless or the occasional unscrupulous investigator to carry on unacceptable practices. A parallel case can be seen in the Mapp decision of the United States Supreme Court, where it was recently ruled that evidence unconstitutionally obtained is never admissible in a court, however valuable the data might be in the pursuit of justice.

In the publication of experimental results it must be made unmistakably clear that the proprieties have been observed in the study. One of these proprieties is adequate disguise of the identity of the subject.

---

* Boston: The Massachusetts General Hospital 10 (2d ed., 1970). Reprinted by permission.

NOTE 2.

BRITISH MEDICAL RESEARCH COUNCIL MEMORANDUM ON CLINICAL INVESTIGATION*

* * *

A further matter to which the Council would draw attention is that of propriety in publication. It cannot be assumed that it will be evident to every reader that the investigations being described were unobjectionable. Unless such is made unmistakably clear misconceptions can arise. In this connection a special responsibility devolves upon the editors, and editorial boards, of scientific journals. In the Council's opinion, it is desirable that editors and editorial boards, before accepting any communication, should not only satisfy themselves that the appropriate requirements have been fulfilled, but may properly insist that the reader is left in no doubt that such indeed is the case.

* * *

NOTE 3.

T. F. FOX THE ETHICS OF CLINICAL TRIALS†

* * *

Speaking for one journal [*The Lancet*], I can say that, though we may not seem to be directly concerned in research, we too have our point of view. We do not *want* to publish information which, according to professional ethics, has been wrongly obtained; in fact we go so far as to believe that no use should ever be made of such information. To protect ourselves from publishing something we do not want to publish, we feel entitled to ask questions which must sometimes be more than a little irritating. Moreover, in line with the Medical Research Council, we think it advisable that, where criticism may arise, an author should avert it by explaining in his paper that the people on whom he experimented were true volunteers, or that valid consent was given on their behalf; and we reserve the right to refuse a paper unless such assurance is given. Finally, if we publish the paper, and one of our readers regards the assurance as inadequate, we will usually print his protest; for we think it professionally healthy that investigators should have to meet occasionally the public chal-

lenges of those who are troubled by their accounts of what they are doing.

* * *

NOTE 4.

JAY KATZ HUMAN EXPERIMENTATION*

[I]t would be unfortunate if data "improperly obtained" were not published. Such an editorial policy would maintain the low visibility of "unethical experimentation" and preclude not only review but also careful and constant appraisal of the conflicting values inherent in experimentation. Indeed, to make these problems even more visible and subject to our collective scrutiny, all clinical research papers submitted for publication should include in the section on *methods* a clear statement of how consent was obtained. . . .

c.

Through Governmental Action?

[i]

Statement of Edwin I. Goldenthal—
Acting Deputy Director, Office of New Drugs,
Bureau of Medicine,
Food and Drug Administration†

* * *

The New Drug Application for MER/29 was submitted by the William S. Merrell Company on July 21, 1959. I did not make the initial review of the application but was involved, in a supervisory capacity, with pharmacological application reviews of all New Drug Applications. Based on the pharmacology review of the application, FDA notified the drug's sponsor, in a letter dated September 14, 1959, that the application was incomplete because of a questionable margin of safety. We suggested a one-year oral study in rats and a three-month oral study in dogs, with one dosage level in each of these experiments selected with production of specific evidence of toxicity as a goal. Dr. F. Joseph Murray, Executive Assistant to the Director of Re-

---

* Memorandum MRC 53/649 (October 16, 1953). Reprinted by permission. *See* p. 847 *supra.*

† 28 *Medico-Legal Journal* 132, 139 (1960). Reprinted by permission.

---

* 275 *New England Journal of Medicine* 790 (1966). Reprinted by permission.

† Materials in this section are reprinted from *Competitive Problems in the Drug Industry—Hearings on the Present Status of Competition in the Pharmaceutical Industry before the Subcommittee on Monopoly of the Senate Select Committee on Small Business,* Part 10, Appendix V, 91st Congress, 1st Session (1969).

search of the William S. Merrell Company, by letter of September 24, 1959, to Dr. Jerome Epstein, the medical officer assigned this application, indicated his firm's disagreement with our conclusions. Dr. Murray maintained that the submitted animal data, particularly the results of the monkey study, showed MER/29 to have an "exceptionally good" margin of safety.

On October 6, 1959, Dr. Murray and another Merrell representative, Dr. William King, met with several members of the Division of Pharmacology to discuss the New Drug Application. I was present at that meeting. They advised us that they had some additional animal studies underway; specifically, a six-month dog study and a six-month rat study. They indicated that these tests were not mentioned in the initial NDA submission because no results had been obtained. We recommended that they administer the drug to one group of dogs for a minimum of three months, at the highest dose the dogs could tolerate, in an attempt to produce some evidence of toxicity.

We also recommended that they start an additional two groups of rats at dosage levels higher than those used in previous studies, and that treatment be continued for a period of one year.

In a letter to Dr. Epstein of October 13, 1959, Dr. Murray again asserted that the animal studies had demonstrated safety of MER/29, and stated: "We feel that the significance of the studies carried out in monkeys has been entirely overlooked."

On October 16, 1959, representatives of the William S. Merrell Company met with members of the Administration to discuss further the toxicological studies which we felt were necessary to support the safety of MER/29. They indicated they were planning to initiate a six-month dog study at dosage levels expected to produce toxicity and a rat study of twelve months' duration. In a letter dated November 6, 1959, the Administration acknowledged the firm's correspondence of September 24 and October 13, and said the results of the additional toxicity studies agreed upon would be reviewed when submitted.

On February 12, 1960, the firm submitted additional toxicity data on MER/29 consisting of results of three-month and nine-month studies in rats and a three- to six-month study in dogs. . . . I was concerned about the inherent toxic potential of the drug and the possible long term effects of elevated blood desmosterol. MER/29 was believed to reduce cholesterol levels by block-

ing the metabolic conversion of desmosterol to cholesterol. My recommendation was that the application should not be approved in the absence of satisfactory results from extensive, well-controlled clinical studies in which individuals received the drug for a period of several years. This was based on the high potential toxicity of the drug shown in the animal studies. By letter of February 29, 1960, Dr. Murray referred me to our telephone conversation in which adverse effects of MER/29 on the eyes of rats were discussed. He alleged that "the corneal changes have now been found in the control animals" and stated that the firm's consulting pathologist "feels that the changes are inflammatory," and not caused by the drug.

*   *   *

On March 31, 1960, FDA received personally from Dr. Murray, a tabulation of liver function tests. The firm continued to emphasize that an earlier toxicity study in monkeys, had likewise shown a total absence of toxicity from MER/29, and that monkeys being primates, were phylogenetically closer to man than either rats or dogs. Thus, he argued, the drug was safe under the conditions of use set forth in the New Drug Application. On April 19, 1960, FDA notified the William S. Merrell Company that the application was made conditionally effective and that the action allowing the application to become effective was based solely on the evidence of the safety of the drug. On May 12, 1960, FDA acknowledged receipt of the final printed labels and labeling and made NDA 12-066 fully effective, subject only to the terms set forth in the FDA letter of April 19, 1960.

My next involvement with this application was on November 7, 1961. I sent a memorandum to Dr. John Nestor, the medical officer then handling the application, in which additional data were reviewed. In light of reports of adverse reactions in humans, particularly the eye changes, the question had been raised as to whether or not the application should be suspended. While I agreed that the application should be suspended, I was not convinced that the new data submitted by the firm would be sufficient to support a revocation of the application. On November 13, 1961, various personnel within the Administration met to evaluate the situation and to decide on a course of action. The decision reached was that the drug should be removed from the market and the application suspended. In the absence of new clinical evidence that the drug was unsafe, however, this could not be done under the provisions of the Federal Food, Drug, and Cosmetic Act at that time. This question was reviewed with FDA scientists and the conclusion was reached that the available evidence would not support suspension action. On November 27, 1961, a drug warning letter was agreed upon by the William S. Merrell Company and FDA. This letter informed physicians of the incidence of cataracts and the necessity of early detection by slit lamp examination. It also advised that they be on the look out for hair changes, ichthyosis and other skin changes, depression of adrenocortical function, and other side effects associated with MER/29 therapy.

In March 1962, FDA was informed by a former employee of the firm that some parts of the chronic monkey data on MER/29 submitted to the Food and Drug Administration had been falsified. We were advised that one of the drug-treated monkeys had become ill and lost considerable weight during the latter part of the study and that a normal, untreated, healthy animal had been substituted. She stated that the report submitted to the FDA by the William S. Merrell Company, as part of the New Drug Application, had been modified to include data on this untreated monkey instead of the monkey receiving MER/29. There was also some question as to whether or not this sick monkey had been subject to autopsy.

It was decided that members of the Administration should visit the William S. Merrell Company to investigate this alleged falsification. On April 9, 1962, Dr. John Nestor of the Bureau of Medicine, Supervisory Inspector Thomas M. Rice, and I visited the firm's Cincinnati facilities and met with representatives of the firm. During the morning, a discussion was held regarding clinical experience with MER/29, particularly reports of the adverse effects. In the course of our discussion, we asked to see the raw data from the monkey studies. Pertinent laboratory records were made available to us. Our search for specific data was difficult because of the confusing manner in which these records had been kept. Upon reviewing some of their laboratory notebooks and weight charts, however, it became evident that the data were somewhat different from those submitted in the New Drug Application.

Discrepancies such as the following were uncovered: Notebooks and weight charts indicated that a marked loss of weight occurred in one monkey during the last five weeks of the reported study; the data submitted in the New Drug Application indicated that there was a weight increase of this monkey during that period. We could not find the record of autopsy for another monkey in this study. According to the NDA, a third monkey had received MER/29 for 16 months, whereas the firm's notebook and charts indicated that this monkey had received MER/29 for only 8 months. The laboratory records on three of the monkeys showed three different dates for the autopsy of these animals. Moreover, the autopsy dates given in the New Drug Application did not correspond to those found on the charts and notebooks. Delving further into the records, I discovered reports on another monkey which had been treated with MER/29, apparently as part of a second toxicity study in this species. Only one monkey study had been mentioned in the New Drug Application. The officials of the firm responsible for these studies were asked if they could explain the discrepancies. They had no immediate explanation.

Before leaving the firm that day, we were asked if we were satisfied with the results of our visit. We replied that while we had received the utmost cooperation, we had discovered some discrepancies in the monkey studies which had not been explained to our satisfaction. The senior officials of the firm indicated that they would discuss our findings with their personnel in an attempt to clarify the matter. We indicated that we would return on the following day.

On the morning of April 10, 1962, we again visited the firm. A conference was held with company representatives. An official told us that, although they had worked late into the evening, they were still unable to find any explanation for the discrepancies which we had noticed on the previous day. We met further with the officials of the firm who were directly involved with these studies and they, too, indicated they had been unable to explain the discrepancies.

On April 11, 1962, a memorandum summarizing our findings was sent to our Division of Regulatory Management. I indicated that we had found certain discrepancies between the chronic monkey studies submitted in Merrell's New Drug Application and those found in their laboratory records. We felt that these discrepancies did not represent an oversight on the part of the William S. Merrell Company, but constituted evidence of the submission of fraudulent and misleading data to the FDA. I indicated that the net effect of these misleading data was to make the drug appear less toxic to monkeys than was actually the case. These data were of particular significance at the time of our consideration of the NDA, when representatives of the William S. Merrell Company had vigorously maintained that evidence of safety obtained in these monkey studies outweighed any questionable findings in lower species, i.e., rats and dogs. It was apparent that the discrepancies uncovered in our visit supported the allegation by the former Merrell employee that fradulent monkey data had been submitted to the Food and Drug Administration.

On the basis of these findings, I recommended that the NDA be suspended. Moreover, I felt that sufficient evidence had been obtained to support prosecution of the William S. Merrell Company and the individuals involved and recommended such action.

On April 12, 1962, representatives of the firm met with FDA and advised us that they were immediately withdrawing MER/29 from the market. They requested that we suspend the New Drug Application. On May 22, 1962, a formal order suspending the New Drug Application for MER/29 was signed by the Commissioner of Food and Drugs.

Subsequently, as our investigation continued, we found that two of the reports of rat toxicity studies submitted in the New Drug Application contained falsified data. Regarding a six-week, two-dosage level study, the William S. Merrell Company reported in the NDA that four of the eight females at the high dosage (75 mg/kg) had died during the course of the experiment. Examination of Merrell's notebooks revealed that *no* females at that dosage level were alive at the end of six weeks. Seven of the female rats had died, and the eighth had been sacrificed. The firm's failure to report truthfully the results of this experiment resulted in further complications. Final organ weights and hematological values were reported in the NDA for these animals at the six-week period. In checking the firm's laboratory records, no organ weights or hematological values were found for these animals. This is not surprising since the animals did not survive for these determinations. The values which were reported were identical to those reported for rats in another study on MER/29— at a different dosage level and for a different duration.

In a second rat study, according to the New Drug Application, 20 rats per dosage group received MER/29 for three months. The NDA states that "In the rats receiving 40/mg/kg/day of MER/29, 8 out of 20 had grossly visible

opacity of the cornea. [T]here was also an associated conjunctivitis." The firm held that this was not a drug-induced phenomenon since it was also observed in control rats. When we checked their laboratory records, however, we found that actually 60 rats per dosage level had been administered MER/29. At the time of our review of the New Drug Application, we had no knowledge of these further studies.

These additional data, which were withheld by the William S. Merrell Company, established conclusively that MER/29 was capable of inducing cataract formation. After the three-month sacrifice, there were approximately 40 rats per dosage level still receiving MER/29. On March 28, 1960, approximately four months after the start of the experiment, and *before the New Drug Application was approved,* the eyes of the remaining rats were examined. The firm's notebooks state that the eyes of many of the rats receiving MER/29 "did not react to light or motion, therefore giving the appearance of being blind." At the highest dose level, 25 out of the 36 rats showed this blinding effect. Only 1 of the 38 control rats showed this effect. None of these data were submitted for inclusion in the New Drug Application. This omission is extremely serious since knowledge that MER/29 was causing cataracts in rats certainly would have caused the FDA to delay, and probably to withhold, permission to market the drug. As it developed, cataracts were one of the most disturbing features of toxicity which occurred in patients after the drug was released.

As early as November 1960, the William S. Merrell Company had been notified by another pharmaceutical firm, Merck, Sharp and Dohme, that MER/29 had shown extremely serious adverse effects in their experiments with rats and dogs; the drug had produced cataracts and other eye changes. Moreover, Merrell representatives had actually visited merck, Sharp and Dohme during January 1961, to examine the affected animals. No mention of these findings to the Food and Drug Administration was made by the William S. Merrell Company until January 2, 1962, when FDA and the William S. Merrell Company had received reports that this drug caused cataracts in human beings.

* * *

In this statement I have described my part in the MER/29 investigation and outlined the major aspects of those investigations insofar as my involvement was concerned. I feel that it can be concluded, from the evidence available, that the William S. Merrell Company withheld some important information and misrepresented other important information with the result that an unsafe drug was allowed to go on the market.

*   *   *

NOTES

NOTE 1.

E. F. van Maanen
The William S. Merrell Co.
Inter-Department Memo—May 5, 1959

*   *   *

I would like to request the respective Department Heads to go over their sections in the MER/29 brochure and to weed out extraneous material, such as windy descriptions of methods and results which were negative and are not contributing anything to clinical investigators. At the same time, add new material, particularly those experiments which indicate the safety of the compound as well as its mechanism of action.

In the toxicity section, I would like to request Dr. King to delete all material on the funny lymphocytes. I wonder also whether the reticulocyte change in the rat experiment needs the emphasis it has. Naturally, we should include our new chronic toxicity studies in monkeys.

*   *   *

NOTE 2.

The William S. Merrell Co.
Campaign Strategy—January 9–
February 17, 1961

*   *   *

Objective: To persuade "wait and see" G.P.'s and internists to prescribe MER/29 now for at least three patients.

Materials: MER/29 patient trial kit (10 per man); new case history brochure (150 per man); supplementary materials: *Archives of Internal Medicine* journal (Ruskin paper); direct mail and journal ad tear sheets.

It is no longer possible for you to "wait out" undecided doctors. The time for very definite forceful action is now. Such action is far and away your major responsibility this campaign.

By now you can identify the doctors not using MER/29. Yet, you know they should be. Very often, you know most of their reasons for not using it—cholesterol may not be atherogenic; desmosterol is a question mark; possible liver

toxicity; doesn't work; doesn't do anything fast enough; costs too much. Doctor "X" hasn't started using it yet. Are any of these legitimate? No! From our viewpoint: we know they aren't true, we know what MER/29 can do for a person who needs it, and we know they have not stopped top MER/29 salesmen. There is no point in trying to overcome each of these objections. That's the long way around.

The quick way to get the non-prescriber using MER/29 is to use every resource you have at your command to show him that he will be benefiting himself and his sick patients in a giant way just as soon as he uses MER/29. That's any doctor's hot button . . . and you must come down on it harder than ever before.

Yes, MER/29 works by lowering cholestorol—doctors know this. Now, show them what they don't understand well enough yet—just how much MER/29 can benefit their patients!

And, you can show any given doctor five benefits of MER/29 therapy in 5 minutes.

Here are two powerful tools placed at your disposal for this important job:

1. A field-tested structured presentation (with new selling aid).

2. The MER/29 patient trial program.

MER/29 Structured Detail

Doctor, when you are considering a course of therapy for a patient you must have good reasons for your selection. This is true in the case of MER/29. Knowing this and guessing that you have yet to decide in favor of MER/29, I would like to summarize today the important reasons why MER/29 should be a routine part of your treatment for patients with any manifestation of hypercholesterolemia.

First, MER/29 is a proven drug. It has been administered under controlled conditions to more than 2000 patients for periods up to three years. There is no longer any valid question as to its safety or lack of significant side effects. There is no longer any doubt about its ability to lower significantly the total sterol content of the human body.

But, here is what is most important. Here is the fact that recommends MER/29 for your routine use. You want to help sick people feel better while they are getting better—that is what is important to you. Mounting evidence makes it increasingly clear that MER/29, in some but certainly not all cases, affects for the better such manifestations of hypercholesterolemia as intermittent claudication, angina pectoris, myocardial infarction or ischemic ECG patterns.

As evidence of concurrent benefits obtained by lowering cholesterol in some patients, let me illustrate what I mean with some case histories which might parallel cases you see in your practice. . . .

(Insert at least two case histories—local if you can and as many as you can—until he gets restless in his chair!!!)

These results are occurring not because of some temporary change, but, as the Wilkins' group at Massachusetts Memorial Hospitals and others have pointed out, because MER/29 by lowering cholesterol may actually improve the adequacy of circulation.

*   *   *

Here's one that seems like a red hot idea for MER/29—if it's your style. It's from Tim Bowen, Charlotte, N.C. Aimed particularly at the "wait and see" physician, Tim's close goes something like this (we got it third hand):

Doctor, I can appreciate and admire your caution about any new drug, but MER/29 has been on the market almost a year now and was studied in thousands of patients for years before that. Its rate of use indicates that acceptance is broadening rapidly. Perhaps these words of Alexander Pope have some bearing to your consideration of MER/29: "Be not the first by whom the new are tried, nor yet the last to lay the old aside."

Lots of power there—can your style be bent just a bit to fit?

*   *   *

NOTE 3.

R. H. McMaster
The William S. Merrell Co.
Inter-Department Memo—April 19, 1960

Dr. Engelberg has made a verbal request for $500.00 to support his continued study of the effects of MER/29 on the lipoprotein fractions as assayed by the Codman technique using the ultracentrifuge. The results with the first two or three patients in whom this technique has been tried have been rather equivocal if not completely negative. Dr. Engelberg, however, is of the opinion that before any conclusions can be drawn, the experiment should be extended to include a larger group. He does not wish to subject these private patients to the expense of having these rather elaborate laboratory studies done and feels that The Wm. S. Merrell Company

should foot at least a part of the bill. He believes that $500.00 will cover the costs for cholesterol determinations and the separation of the high and low density lipoprotein fractions by ultracentrifuge in another ten to twelve patients.

Although it begins to appear that any report from this study may be a negative one, we may find that we are money ahead to keep Dr. Engelberg busy at it for a while longer rather than to take a chance on his reporting negatively on so few patients. As you are aware, the Codman technique is in some disfavor and certainly has never been generally accepted as providing for a true "atherogenic index" as claimed.

My personal recommendation is that the grant-in-aid be approved only to keep Dr. Engelberg occupied for a while longer.

NOTE 4.

Frank N. Getman
The William S. Merrell Co.
Inter-Department Memo—
October 24, 1961

*   *   *

Sherry Silliman and Fred Lamb have both advised me that a New Drug Application may not be suspended or revoked without a hearing —such hearings are not public. Apparently, however, the fact that a hearing is being called does become publicized.

. . . Silliman, of Norwich, said that the notice of hearing came after failure to reach agreement following a number of discussions with the FDA. According to him, news of the hearing was first published in Werble's "Pink Sheet," and he says Werble appears to have a good "pipeline" into the FDA. He added that the FDA does publish notices of hearings to be held. . . .

Going on with the Norwich case, the hearing technically is still in progress. All testimony on both sides was completed before the Examiner months ago. Briefs were filed in April, with no decision yet. Anticipating an adverse decision, Norwich plans an appeal to the courts. The product is still on the market and available to the physician. It has not been promoted in any way since the notice of hearing, and this was an agreement which Norwich made with the FDA. Naturally, sales have dropped drastically, but the product is still being prescribed by those physicians who have found it a very valuable drug. Norwich made its own publicity release to the public and to the stockholders after the notice of hearing had been received.

In the McNeil case, I know nothing more than what I have read in the "Pink Sheet," which stated McNeil sent out letters to MD's and drug wholesalers, setting in motion a "voluntary" recall program because of jaundice, hepatitis, and liver damage reports. As far as we can tell, McNeil, after conferences with Food and Drug in which a hearing was probably threatened, took this action rather than go through a hearing.

In the White Laboratories' Entecqual case, the Government seized the drug on the basis that representations in promotional material for MD's differed materially from the labeling claims permitted by the effective New Drug Application— in other words, false and misleading labeling. Apparently this followed a failure to agree with the FDA on appropriate disclosure of side effects and also an appropriate dosage exclusion limitation for children—these negotiations going on while the NDA was in effect. Other actions such as multiple seizures or a suspension of the NDA were being considered by the FDA before White withdrew the drug from the market.

This background is furnished in view of the request that I provide, in advance, a company statement in the event of government action. I told Art Boschen this morning that in view of our lawyers' advice on advance release it didn't seem necessary, but after tying the above factors together I am making the following suggestions:

In the event of rumor that the FDA is about to suspend the NDA:

"We have not received notice of any such hearing, as provided in the law. We are not in a position to comment until we do—if we do."

In the event of receipt of notice of hearing:

"The Wm. S. Merrell Company, Division of Richardson-Merrell Inc., has today received a notice of a hearing from the Federal Food and Drug Administration to determine whether its effective New Drug Application on MER/29 should be suspended. In our opinion such suspension would be unwarranted and unnecessary, and we believe that evidence presented at the hearing will sustain this position," stated H. R. Marschalk, president of Richardson-Merrell (or Frank Getman, president of The Wm. S. Merrell Company Division).

Let me know your final preference on who makes the announcement.

Admittedly, the letter announcement is extremely brief, but I am proposing it in this form for two reasons—the first is that the less said, the better, as long as it adequately covers our position—and secondly, it is hard to give added reasons until we get the notice of hearing, which is similar to a complaint and outlines the reasons why the NDA should be suspended. If it should be a claim we withheld evidence, that would call for one type of statement, whereas if it were based on certain kinds of toxicity, it would call for another.

*   *   *

NOTE 5.

FOOD AND DRUG ADMINISTRATION SUSPENSION ORDER—MAY 22, 1962

Wm. S. Merrell Company, Cincinnati, Ohio, the applicant for and the holder of effective New Drug Application No. 12-066 applying to MER/29 (triparanol) capsules, having requested the suspension of the effectiveness of said application, on the ground that clinical experience shows the drug is unsafe for use under the conditions of use upon the basis of which the application became effective, and thereby having waived Notice of Hearing as provided by Section 505(e) of the Federal Food, Drug, and Cosmetic Act, prior to such suspension;

The Commissioner of Food and Drugs, by virtue of the authority vested in the Secretary by the provisions of the Federal Food, Drug, and Cosmetic Act [Section 505(e); 52 Stat. 1052; 21 U.S.C. 355(e)] and delegated to the Commissioner by the Secretary (20 FR 1996) finds that clinical experience shows that MER/29 (triparanol) capsules are unsafe for use under the conditions of use upon the basis of which the application became effective;

Wherefore, on the foregoing finding of fact and the request of the applicant, the effectiveness of New Drug Application No. 12-066 applying to MER/29 (triparanol) capsules is suspended, effective May 22nd, 1962.

[ii]
Morton Mintz
*The Therapeutic Nightmare**

*   *   *

In March 1964, no-contest pleas were entered by the William S. Merrell firm to six of the nine counts in which it was named. Richardson-Merrell, named in the three remaining counts of the twelve-count indictment, pleaded nolo con-

---

* Boston: Houghton Mifflin Company 243–247 (1965). Copyright © 1965 by Morton Mintz. Reprinted by permission.

tendere to two. The same plea was entered by each of the scientists. Van Maanen had been named in nine counts, King in seven, and Werner in five. The pleas were consented to by the Department of Justice.

The count that Werner and Van Maanen did not contest, the fourth, was also one of the six to which the William Merrell firm pleaded no contest. . . .

Count two in the indictment was not contested by the third scientist, King, nor, again, by the William S. Merrell Company. The charges here were that the defendants "knowingly and willfully concealed and covered up, and caused to be concealed and covered up, by trick and scheme, material facts" in what purported to be "full reports of all investigations which were made by The William S. Merrell Company to show whether" MER/29 was safe. The true bill went on to specify that between mid-February and the end of March 1960 Werner and the Merrell firm withheld from FDA reports that certain investigations had been made, reports of results in some cases, and reports of adverse effects. Six investigations were described. In the first, all three of the female monkeys receiving daily 10 milligrams per kilogram of body weight (10 mg/kg) developed blood disorders, and one experienced ovarian changes. In the second, no evidence of recent ovulation was found in four female monkeys on 5 mg/kg per day. In the third, eight out of ten rats were dead seventeen days after being put on a dosage of 50 mg/kg per day, and the remaining two, whose dosage was cut in half, were dead a week later. In the fourth, female rats developed blood disorders. In the fifth, male and female rats that received 15 mg/kg of triparanol before and during cohabitation over a four-month period produced fewer offspring. In the sixth, pregnant rats dosed with 25 mg/kg per day had smaller litters; and among the newborn there was an increase in the death rate in the first twenty-four hours after birth.

Three months later, on June 4, the defendants appeared in United States District Court in Washington for sentencing. In behalf of Richardson-Merrell, Lawrence E. Walsh told the court:

All I can say is there certainly was no intention by this company or any of its employees to put on the market a dangerous drug. Whatever errors of judgment there were, this was not the intent.
I would say one further thing: That whatever these individuals did, they did what they thought they were doing on behalf of the company and, if there

must be punishment, we ask that it fall on the company and not on them.

Chief Judge Matthew F. McGuire agreed with Walsh, who is, incidentally, himself a former federal judge and deputy attorney general from 1957 to 1960. "That is the view I have taken," McGuire said. Speaking only of failure to comply with the law's requirements for full reporting on drug testing, he imposed the maximum fines allowed on the corporate defendants —$60,000 on William Merrell, and $20,000 on Richardson-Merrell, which in the fiscal year that ended a few weeks later had a consolidated net income of $17,790,000 on sales of $180 million, compared to $17,514,000 on sales of $170 million in the year ended June 30, 1963.

"I have taken the view," Judge McGuire said from the bench, "that responsibility in the background of this case is a failure, for want of a better term, of proper executive, managerial and supervisional control and that the responsibility of what happened falls on the company and its executive management. . . ." As vice president for research, Werner was presumably part of management. The Judge said, however, "I do not think, in this particular defendant's case, there was any willful violation of the statute." He placed Werner and his colleagues King and Van Maanen on probation for six months. Each had faced a maximum sentence of $10,000 and five years in prison.

Judge McGuire did not characterize the acts of withholding and falsifying data about a drug that was prescribed for hundreds of thousands of persons. Those who had expected him to express a sense of shock were disappointed. The sentences imposed on the scientists were unquestionably compassionate. What deterrent and educational impact they may have on others remains to be seen.

The pleas of nolo contendere, which the judge said were "tantamount to a plea of guilty," not only averted the publicity that would have accompanied a trial, but also precluded use of a trial record to civil litigants, who generally could not use the indictment or the pleas as evidence.

MER/29 was prescribed to an estimated 418,000 persons. According to Richardson-Merrell, "substantially less than 1 percent"—fewer than 4180, that is—were injured. The "classical triad" of injuries was usually operable cataracts in both eyes, loss or thinning of hair, and severe skin reactions. Among those who have claimed these and other injuries were between 400 and 500 persons whose approximately 175 lawyers pooled their resources, in a "MER/29 Group," to an extent believed without precedent in a product-liability case. The "Group," whose trustee is Paul D. Rheingold of New York, one of the lawyers who took Mrs. Jordan's deposition, has filed damage suits in 36 states and the District of Columbia.[6]

In the address made by Dr. Walter Modell in 1962 at the convention of the American Association for the Advancement of Science, he described "the pattern for disaster with new drugs: a short-sighted view of all effects; faulty experiments; premature publication; too-vigorous promotion; exaggerated claims; and careless use— in brief, a break in the scientific approach somewhere along the line." Perhaps this pattern was not cut to fit the MER/29 case precisely, but it comes close enough for a drug that physicians, in polls reported by the *Medical Research Digest,* had rated the most significant medical advance in medical therapy of 1960 and 1961.

d.

By Action of Subject?

[i]

Roginsky v. Richardson-Merrell, Inc.
378 F.2d 832 (2d Cir. 1967)

FRIENDLY, CIRCUIT JUDGE:

In this diversity action Sidney Roginsky sought to recover compensatory and punitive damages for personal injuries, primarily cataracts, from taking at his home in Pennsylvania a drug,

---

[6] In a letter to Senator Humphrey, Rheingold said that in addition to the "classical triad" of injuries there has been "a large number" of other reactions attributed to MER/29, even if less often involved. "These include," he wrote, "liver damage, spleen damage, personality change, diminished libido, impotence, damage to fingernails, sweat glands affected, vomiting and nausea, kidney damage, headaches, loss of normal circulation, pains in various parts of the body, anemia, gastrointestinal upset, ulcerative colitis, diminished adrenocortical function, and fatigue. Some of these, of course, may have only coincidentally occurred with the true reactions to MER/29."

Through April 1965 the outcome of civil damage suits brought by persons claiming to have been injured by MER/29 has varied. Some have been won, some lost, and some settled. On April 27 in San Francisco, a man who had suffered cataracts was awarded, after a seven-week jury trial, $175,000 in actual and $500,000 in punitive damages. The judgment, which was expected to be appealed, was reportedly the largest in a product-liability case in California history.

MER/29, developed by Richardson-Merrell Company for lowering blood cholesterol levels. Roginsky's was the first to be tried of some 75 similar cases now pending in the District Court for the Southern District of New York. Several hundred actions have been filed elsewhere, see Rheingold, "Products Liability—The Ethical Drug Manufacturer's Liability," 18 *Rutgers L. Rev.* 947—48 n. 4 (1964), in at least three of which trial courts have rendered large judgments for the plaintiffs.[3]

Although other theories of liability for compensatory damages had been advanced in the complaint, plaintiff withdrew all except negligence and fraud upon the Food and Drug Administration (FDA). Defendant moved for a directed verdict on all claims for injury by cataract as unsupported by sufficient proof of causation and on the fraud and punitive damage claims as unsupported by the evidence; the motions were denied. The judge instructed the jury it must first determine the issue of causation; if it found for the plaintiff on that, it should then pass upon the other issues, which he explained in a charge to which defendant took no exception. He helpfully submitted six separate questions: (1) causation, (2) negligence, (3) fraud upon the FDA, (4) amount of compensatory damages, (5) liability for exemplary damages, and (6) the amount thereof. The jury gave

---

[3] In *Toole* v. *Richardson-Merrell, Inc.* No. 524722, Superior Court, San Francisco County, Calif., the jury awarded $175,000 in compensatory and $500,000 in punitive damages, the latter of which the trial court reduced to $250,000 in the light of the other pending cases and the California rule requiring a reasonable relationship between compensatory and punitive damages. In *Ostopowitz* v. *Wm. S. Merrell Co.,* Supreme Court, Westchester County, N.Y., Jan. 4, 1967, the jury awarded $350,000 in compensatory and $850,000 in punitive damages to the injured party, and $5,000 to her husband for loss of services. The trial judge sustained the award of compensatory damages although plaintiff's cataracts had been successfully removed, but ordered a new trial unless she consented to a reduction of punitive damages to $100,000, the figure previously awarded in this case. See N.Y.L.J., Jan. 11, 1967, p. 21. In *Golden* v. *Richardson-Merrell, Inc.,* Civ. No. 5992, W.D.Wash., Apr., 7, 1966, appeal dismissed on stipulation of counsel, judgment on a verdict of $150,000 was rendered for a plaintiff who claimed the same injuries from taking MER/29 as does Roginsky. In two cases juries have returned verdicts for the defendant. See *Cudmore* v. *Richardson-Merrell, Inc.,* 398 S.W.2d 640 (Tex. Civ. App. 1965); *Lewis* v. *Baker,* 413 P.2d 400 (Or. 1966).

affirmative answers to all the questions relating to liability and fixed compensatory damages at $17,500 and punitive damages at $100,000, which the judge later declined to eliminate or reduce, 254 F.Supp. 430 (1966). . . . We affirm the award of compensatory damages but find that the evidence was not sufficient to warrant submission of the punitive damage issue to the jury.

*   *   *

We thus come to the issue of punitive damages, an issue of extreme significance not only in monetary terms to this defendant in view of the hundreds of pending MER/29 actions and to the plaintiff as well, but, from a longer range, to the entire pharmaceutical industry and to all present and potential users of drugs. Plaintiff, of course, does not claim that defendant intended to harm him; his contention is that defendant's negligence rose to such a level of irresponsibility or worse as to invite this extraordinary sanction.

*   *   *

The legal difficulties engendered by claims for punitive damages on the part of hundreds of plaintiffs are staggering. If all recovered punitive damages in the amount here awarded these would run into tens of millions, as contrasted with the maximum criminal penalty of "imprisonment for not more than three years, or a fine of not more than $10,000, or both such imprisonment and fine", 21 U.S.C. § 333 (b), for each violation of the Food, Drug, and Cosmetic Act with intent to defraud or mislead. We have the gravest difficulty in perceiving how claims for punitive damages in such a multiplicity of actions throughout the nation can be so administered as to avoid overkill. Judge Croake did all that he could here, instructing the jury that it "may consider the potentially wide effect of the actions of the corporation and, on the other hand. . . . the potential number of actions similar to this one to which that wide effect may render the defendant subject." Yet it is hard to see what even the most intelligent jury would do with this, being inherently unable to know what punitive damages, if any, other juries in other states may award other plaintiffs in actions yet untried. We know of no principle whereby the first punitive award exhausts all claims for punitive damages and would thus preclude future judgments; if there is, Toole's judgment in California, which plaintiff's brief tells us came earlier, would bar Roginsky's. Neither does it seem either fair or

practicable to limit punitive recoveries to an indeterminate number of first-comers, leaving it to some unascertained court to cry, "Hold, enough," in the hope that others would follow. While jurisprudes might comprehend why Toole in California should walk off with $250,000 more than a compensatory recovery and Roginsky in the Southern District of New York and Mrs. Ostopowitz in Westchester County with $100,000, most laymen and some judges would have some difficulty in understanding why presumably equally worthy plaintiffs in the other 75 cases before Judge Croake or elsewhere in the country should get less or none. And, whatever the right result may be in strict theory, we think it somewhat unrealistic to expect a judge, say in New Mexico, to tell a jury that their fellow townsman should get very little by way of punitive damages because Toole in California and Roginsky and Mrs. Ostopowitz in New York had stripped that cupboard bare, even assuming the defendant would want such a charge, and still more unrealistic to expect that the jury would follow such an instruction or that, if they didn't, the judge would reduce the award below what had become the going rate. There is more to be said for drastic judicial control of the amount of punitive awards so as to keep the prospective total within some manageable bounds. This would require, for example, a reduction of the instant $100,000 award to something in the $5000 $10,000 range, still leaving defendant exposed to several million dollars of exemplary damages. We perceive nothing in the New York decisions that would prevent our reducing a punitive damage award because of the large number of suits arising out of the same conduct by the defendant. But there is equally nothing to indicate that New York would follow such a course, and a state otherwise willing to impose such self-denying limits might be disinclined to do so until assured that others would follow suit.

Although multiple punitive awards running into the hundreds may not add up to a denial of due process, nevertheless if we were sitting as the highest court of New York we would wish to consider very seriously whether awarding punitive damages with respect to the negligent—even highly negligent—manufacture and sale of a drug governed by federal food and drug requirements, especially in the light of the strengthening of these by the 1962 amendments, 76 Stat. 780 (1962), and the present vigorous attitude toward enforcement, would not do more harm than good. A manufacturer distributing a drug to many thousands of users under government regulation scarcely requires this additional measure for manifesting social disapproval and assuring deterrence. Criminal penalties and heavy compensatory damages, recoverable under some circumstances even without proof of negligence, should sufficiently meet these objectives, see Note, supra note 6, 41 N.Y.U.L. Rev. at 1171, and the other factors cited as justifying punitive awards are lacking. Many awards of compensatory damages doubtless contain something of a punitive element, and more would do so if a separate award for exemplary damages were eliminated. Even though products liability insurance blunts the deterrent effect of compensatory awards to a considerable extent, the total coverage under such policies is often limited, bad experience is usually reflected in future rates, and insurance affords no protection to the damage to reputation among physicians and pharmacists which an instance like the present must inevitably produce. On the other hand, the apparent impracticability of imposing an effective ceiling on punitive awards in hundreds of suits in different courts may result in an aggregate which, when piled on large compensatory damages, could reach catastrophic amounts. If liability policies can protect against this risk as several courts have held, the cost of providing this probably needless deterrence, not only to the few manufacturers from whom punitive damages for highly negligent conduct are sought but to the thousands from whom it never will be, is passed on to the consuming public; if they cannot, as is held by other courts and recommended by nost commentators, a sufficiently egregious error as to one product can end the business life of a concern that has wrought much good in the past and might otherwise have continued to do so in the future, with many innocent stockholders suffering extinction of their investments for a single management sin.

However, the New York cases afford no basis for our predicting that the Court of Appeals would adopt a rule disallowing punitive damages in a case such as this, and the *Erie* doctrine wisely prevents our engaging in such extensive law-making on local tort liability, a subject which the people of New York have entrusted to their legislature and, within appropriate limits, to their own courts, not to us. Our task is the more modest one of assessing the sufficiency of the evidence within the framework of New York decisions on the award of punitive damages for recklessness. As to this, we are convinced that the consequences of imposing punitive damages in a case like the present are so serious that the New York Court of Appeals would subject the proof to particularly careful scrutiny.

* * *

. . . New York demands, as it might have to before punishing a defendant with fines similar to those imposed on a criminal charge, that the quality of conduct necessary to justify punitive damages must be "clearly established." *Cleghorn* v. *New York Cent. & H.R.R.R.*, 56 N.Y. 44, 48 (1874). Cf. *Hedrick* v. *Jebiley*, 198 N.Y.S. 2d 346 (N.Y. City 1960). As the Supreme Court has recently reminded us, the standard of proof "by clear, unequivocal and convincing evidence . . . is no stranger to the civil law." *Woodby* v. *I.N.S.*, 385 U.S. 276, 285, 87 S.Ct. 483, 17 L.Ed.2d 362 (1966), citing 9 *Wigmore*, Evidence § 2498 (3d ed. 1940). It would be hard to think of a situation more appropriate for invoking that standard than where the manufacturer of a new drug honestly believed to assist in prolonging human life is faced with claims for penalties by hundreds of plaintiffs running into millions of dollars, in addition to many millions more for damages sustained. We have little doubt that in such a case the New York Court of Appeals would require a judge to scrutinize the evidence in far closer detail before submitting punitive damages to a jury than it would on an issue of compensatory damages for negligence or breach of contract. If that prophecy should prove to be wrong, we would then be obliged to decide in future cases whether we nevertheless have power to impose a higher standard of proof for the award of punitive damages in a federal trial, cf. *San Antonio* v. *Timko*, 368 F.2d 983, 985 & n. 1 (2 Cir. 1966), as we surely would if we do.

The judgment as to compensatory damages is affirmed; the judgment as to punitive damages is reversed. No costs.

NOTES

NOTE 1.
TOOLE V. RICHARDSON-MERRELL, INC.
251 CAL. APP. 2D 689, 702–704,
60 CAL. RPTR. 398, 408–409 (1967)

SALSMAN, ASSOCIATE JUSTICE:

* * *

Section 355(b) of the Federal Food, Drug, and Cosmetic Act requires an applicant to submit ". . . full reports of investigations which have been made to show whether or not such drug is safe for use. . . ." As we have related in the statement of facts, reports submitted to the FDA by appellant in support of its application were in some respects false, and in other respects entirely failed to reveal the cataractogenic character of its drug as shown by its effect on rats and dogs. The trial court instructed the jury that if a party to this action violated section 355(b) ". . . a presumption arises that he was negligent," and at the same time called the jury's attention to the fact that the presumption, if found applicable, was not conclusive but could be overcome by a showing that, under all the circumstances, the violation was excusable or justifiable. (See *Alarid* v. *Vanier,* 50 Cal. 2d 617, 621, 327 P. 2d 897, and cases cited.)

Appellant contends the court's instruction was error in that no private cause of action arises because of a violation of section 355(b). (See *United States* v. *Gilliland,* 312 U.S. 86, 93, 61 S.Ct. 518, 85 1.Ed 598). In support of this contention appellant cites a 1933 proposal to include in the Federal Food, Drug, and Cosmetic Act a provision for a private right of action for damages for injury or death caused by violation of the act, and notes that this proposal was never adopted by the Congress. Appellant views this as a demonstration of congressional intent that no such private right of action exists. Respondent, however, did not attempt to state a cause of action for damages for breach of the federal statute. He stated a cause of action based upon alleged negligent conduct on the part of appellant which negligent conduct he asserted was the proximate cause of his injuries. In support of this cause of action, as well as others stated, he introduced a great deal of evidence by which he hoped to convince the jury that appellant had falsely stated the results of its tests of MER/29 on rats and dogs and hence had violated section 355(b). This was done, not to support a cause of action based upon the statute, but for the purpose of showing that appellant had violated statutory standards, thus raising a presumption of negligence on its part because of such conduct. This was entirely proper.

* * *

Appellant concedes that violation of the *labeling and marketing* provisions of the act may be shown to establish negligence, but argues there is a difference between violation of the labelling and marketing provisions and violation of the *reporting provisions,* because the labeling provisions of the statute are designed to protect the public, whereas the reporting provisions are concerned merely with raw data comprehensible only to scientists in the FDA. We find this argument unconvincing. The act is designed to protect the public as a whole and to keep dangerous and deleterious products from reaching the uninformed consumer. We see no logical distinction between the labelling provisions of the act on the one hand and the reporting provisions on the other, with respect to the class of persons to be protected or the harm to be prevented. Permission to market a drug depends in part at least upon an evaluation of test data submitted by an applicant. The submission of false and misleading reports of tests can only subvert the administrative decision, defeat the purposes of the act, and make the legend on the label a useless guide so far as protection of the public is concerned.

* * *

NOTE 2.
GOTTSDANKER v. CUTTER LABORATORIES
182 CAL. APP. 2D 602, 611–612,
6 CAL. RPTR. 320, 326 (1960)

DRAPER, J.:

* * *

Defendant strongly argues that public policy will best be served by denying recovery in warranty for "new" drugs. The argument is that development of medicines will be retarded if manufacturers are held to strict liability for their defects. While this argument might have merit if the warranty involved had to do with the mere failure of a medicine to cure or of a vaccine to prevent, it seems to be of but little weight where, as here, the warranty is limited to an assurance that the product will not actively cause the very disease it was designed to prevent. In any case, defendant's own argument is that the Legislature has indicated a full awareness of the problem by the statute (Health & Saf. Code, § 1623) providing that the distribution of blood and blood plasma is not a sale. If a sound public policy requires extension of this exception to biologics generally, or to polio vaccine specifically, the argument properly is one for the Legislature. For the courts to extend the legislative exemption would, in view of the statutory recognition of the problem, amount to judicial legislation.

* * *

[ii]
Irving Ladimer
Clinical Research Insurance*

*   *   *

Accepting the concept of participation in obligation in return for benefit deriving from bio-medical research, i.e. social responsibility, argues for accepting a *modus operandi* for removing the adversary attitude and proceeding whenever actual or potential injury develops. The magnitude and importance of the issues gravely affect the public interest. Scientific evaluation requires, at the clinical stage, the deliberate exposure of human beings, selected and available as test subjects. Although it is universally agreed that human volunteers—volunteers who have expressly or by implication consented to take part —may not be used unless every reasonable means has been taken to assure their safety, there is always the possibility of an untoward occurrence.

Assurance techniques for handling injury should be comprehensive, covering all aspects of participation for the patient or subject. They should also relieve the investigator of personal and economic jeopardy. Otherwise, there can be no proper expectation that volunteers or investigators will take part in such projects. This is not a vague threat or theoretical view.

In California, a fully equipped exposure chamber, specialized instrumentation and a team of investigators remained idle for years (1959–61) because the State found no legal basis for indemnifying or insuring the research hazards in a project requiring exposure to known air pollutants, thus placing liability on the investigator, and relegating the volunteers to legal action to recover. There was, moreover, no assurance that the investigator's personal malpractice policy would apply since such research did not clearly come within regular or standard medical practice. Even though the public authorities recognized the necessity for such research, there was no legislation or case law which, with certainty, provided direct protection to the volunteers or, in turn, supported the investigator or the public hospital if they chose to bear that responsibility. Thus, an injured volunteer would have no recourse but to sue for damages. Depending on the relationships, he might proceed against the

investigator and his staff; the hospital, agency or laboratory conducting the studies; the governmental department and perhaps the grantor or sponsor supplying the funds or approving the plan. The suit, following general practice and principle, would be based on demonstration of negligence or some other defect on the part of the investigator or sponsor. If the plaintiff won, payment might be due from any or all of the defendants.

It is submitted that this posture is both insufficient and unsuited to the nature and character of research. Studies on human beings, because they involve some intervention, exposure, manipulation or deprivation, are not intentional assaults and batteries which, in other contexts, properly call for recompense to account for the tort. It is equally inappropriate that a volunteer should have to face this prospect to be "made whole" to the extent that money and perhaps medical care can provide. Public interest programs, whether large or small, and human progress through medical science deserve comparable progressive methods to meet social responsibilities.

It is noteworthy that, within recent years, Federal agencies have, in appropriate cases, included funds as part of the research grant to defray liability costs. These are generally used to pay for liability insurance premiums. The National Institutes of Health has made such allowance. Under the 1957 Price-Anderson amendments to the Atomic Energy Act, the Commission may provide such insurance within its licensed or contract activities to cover catastrophic accidents, but Congress has made no similar provision for other hazardous programs. . . .

. . . The customary approach, however, has been to assume that some liability or malpractice policy is the answer. But, . . . the pay-off generally depends on proof of fault, whereas the likelihood of harm comes not so much from negligence of commission or omission but from the inherent nature of research. Chance factors, unknown elements, unanticipated actions and reactions and idiosyncratic responses are all too familiar gremlins that penetrate the fabric of the most closely knit research designs in clinical research. . . .

*   *   *

. . . It may be some time before the National Institutes of Health, to which this issue has been informally referred, will develop an answer.

---

* 16 *Journal of Chronic Diseases* 1229, 1230–1234 (1963). Reprinted by permission of Pergamon Press. Copyright 1963.

When it does, that answer may understandably be limited to the specific type of Federal sponsorship it offers. The problem, however, is not essentially different for the non-Federal institution or research hospital, the foundation, the voluntary health association and, of course, for the private pharmaceutical firms which support much of the drug testing. For them, particularly, in the aftermath of thalidomide and under the Drug Amendments of 1962 which require disclosure and patient consent in investigational drug trials, the necessity of sensible, fair and understandable protection is painfully obvious and menacingly present. The traditional umbrella-type of liability insurance, even if multiplied, does not meet the need.

Social cost. [S]ince the benefits of research redound to society, society should accept the responsibility for assuring that the investigator who proceeds with care and caution should not be inhibited in his research because of any inherent hazard. Likewise, the partner-subject—"clinical material" for the investigator—should not be placed at disadvantage, if injury should result directly from his participation. The cost of protection should therefore be considered a proper charge to the business of doing research, to be assumed by the sponsor, in much the same way as other administrative costs are borne by government or industry in production and service operations.

Entitlement based on relationship. Entitlement to recompense by the injured person should reasonably depend, in view of the current American research system and its implications, on the relationship of the parties and on the relationship or causal connection of the harm or loss to the clinical study. Simply put, an application of the workmen's compensation concept, rather than employer liability or malpractice, would seem feasible. Under this approach, the patient-subject, solely by being a recognized participant, would be eligible. Compensation would accrue upon establishing a cause-effect relationship between the clinical activity and the injury, harm or disability.

It would not be necessary to show fault, negligence or lack of caution, that is, to establish specific culpability. Several casualty insurance companies have recommended that claims for auto accidents, now so frequent and so difficult to attribute to one of the parties, be settled without attempting to judge fault.

Another solution, also avoiding the determination of culpability, is that of limited health and accident insurance written on each patient-volunteer. The occurrences of an accident or disability would then automatically invoke the stipulated benefits. The workmen's compensation form, however, is to be preferred since a sponsor or "employer" could carry such coverage for the entire research enterprise, effectively insuring all projects and participants with minimum administration.

Risks and contingencies. Assuming the conduct of studies under competent guidance and by qualified staff in approved research units (criteria could be established in cooperation with insurance carriers; this step could lead to an immeasurably useful secondary advantage in raising standards to achieve insurability) the contingencies could arise from (1) inherent risk or hazard of substances or procedures employed; (2) incidental or accidental events associated with, but not directly related to, the studies; and (3) peculiarities of the participants. It is essential, however, to cover all of these types, so as to avoid the need for distinguishing among them to establish maximum good faith and broad responsibility for any proximate occurrence. There is no great likelihood of self-inflicted injury or contributory negligence such as might rule out a plaintiff suing under a liability policy.

Consequences. The related consequences of an untoward event might include all or any of the following:

1. Illness or disability: direct or immediate; chronic; subsequent—physical, mental or social.
2. Death: immediate or subsequent.
3. Income loss: immediate or subsequent or potential.

These contingencies may arise at, during or following a study. Accordingly, the compensation, including medical service in broad aspect and cash payment, may be due at once or later and to the individual or dependent. An appropriate plan would therefore have to recognize that termination of a project or study would not necessarily terminate the need for protection. This consideration argues for use of some insurance system based on payment of premiums rather than on self-insurance, although the latter may well be feasible for a large, permanent research institution.

Service benefit. On the principle that the protection be commensurate with the need and character of such endeavor, appropriate insurance would seem to require *first,* immediate and sustained high quality medical care (physician's services, medication, hospitalization, after-care, if required, and rehabilitation when suitable) and *second*, cash compensation. Under this philosophy, there can be no "damages" of a windfall or exemplary nature or questionable payments for speculative costs and losses. The program should be such as fairly to encourage patient cooperation and volunteering by healthy subjects, for example, and not serve to demean medical research or to promise exorbitant returns.

In essence, protection as here considered is indeed the protection required—care and costs —not the gamble of win-or-lose all, which rarely gives the victim what he necessarily requires, even if he "wins," and certainly not if he loses.

Experience. There is no known actuarial experience which would indicate the costs of such a program. It can be reasoned, however, that absolutely and proportionately (that is, relative to the total cost of a clinical program) the cost will be small, not great.

First, there are actually very few compensable occurrences within the sphere of responsible research. Second, the sponsor's assumption of medical care to meet primary needs, often at the research premises, will tend to lessen out-of-pocket costs. Researchers will, in practice, want to follow such cases as part of their studies. Third, the adoption of such programs will tend to improve controls and designs. Fourth, and finally, the spirit and philosophy of such protection, which should be fully explained in advance as part of the consensual relationship, should serve to diminish rather than induce any questionable claims.

*   *   *

[*iii*]
Guido Calabresi
Reflections on Medical
Experimentation in Humans*

*   *   *

The basic [market device to supplement other systems of controlling experimentation] would be a compensation fund for subjects injured in unsuccessful experiments. A separate fund would exist at each medical center where experiments on humans were being undertaken. Moneys for the fund could come from two sources—income from successful results of pre-

* 98 Daedalus 387, 395–398 (1969). Reprinted by permission of Daedalus, Journal of the American Academy of Arts and Sciences, Boston, Massachusetts.

vious experiments, such as new marketable drugs, and grants from government or foundations based on the expectation that the researches undertaken would be more than worth the moneys used to compensate those subjects who were injured. The effect of such a fund— apart from compensating the victims, which may be desirable in itself—would be to stimulate greater analysis within each medical center of the possible benefits and risks a given experiment entails.

There are five principal difficulties with using such a fund in helping to control medical experiments. First, any compensation system is bound to be unacceptable if it directly or indirectly suggests that a doctor is at "fault" when a properly structured experiment fails. Second, often experiments may in a sense be successful, and yet the subject will nonetheless die or fail to recover completely. (He may have lived longer or as long as he would have had he been in the control group, and yet it may be difficult to show that his death was not due to the experiment.) Third, it may be hard to distinguish a subject in a medical experiment from the ordinary patient who, presumably, would not be compensated simply because the treatment chosen for him failed. Fourth, the institutions in which medical experiments are undertaken are typically charitable and, hence, not subject to market pressures in the usual sense. Fifth, the system may unduly hamper research in new or small medical centers. All of these difficulties are serious, but none is insurmountable.

The first three are best treated together since they all pertain to the fact-finding and administration needed to award compensation. A judicial system for deciding the issues seems totally inappropriate. It smacks too much of finding mistakes or wrongdoing and, as such, would be unacceptable. Accordingly, the best way of handling the issues would be for medical centers to institute such funds voluntarily and establish administrative boards to resolve questions of fact arising under the fund. It is to be hoped that the boards would be regional (so that no center could chisel on its own unlucky experiments) and staffed primarily by scientists. Since payments would, at least initially, be a matter of practice rather than contract, the findings of such panels would come to be regarded as final. (Ultimately, this practice would be likely to change as subjects came to expect payment, but by then the tradition and function of the panels would have been established and judicial review would probably not be harmful.) The boards would determine, first, whether the injured party was, in fact, a subject in an experiment or a member of a control group for such an experiment; and, second, whether he had suffered damage as a result of being a subject; and, finally, what the appropriate compensation would be under established schedules of damages.

Determination of whether the injured party was a "subject" could be made on the basis of something like the following criterion: Would the "subject's" own personal physician (responsible only for his patient's welfare and not for the advancement of knowledge) have recommended such a course of treatment—not only at the start, but throughout the course of the "experiment"—if he had available to him the information that the experimenters had (or would have had but for use of a double-blind experimental format)? It may be readily seen that this criterion may provide compensation for members of control groups as well as actual subjects. It also considers that a person may become a "subject"—that is, be treated in a fashion based on society's best interest rather than his own—not just at the beginning of an experiment, but anywhere along its course. For this reason, and to protect the possibility of double-blind experiments, the criterion deems relevant any knowledge that the experimenters would have had, but for the experimental format chosen.

Determination of damages would be difficult for the boards. But the issues are, in fact, no harder than those faced in establishing damages before non-expert groups, as is done throughout accident law. As such, there is no reason to discuss them here.

The problem of avoiding the stigma of fault or wrongdoing also does not come up in the hypothetical system described. I do not suggest that such funds be used in place of other controls over medical experiments on humans, but only as additional controls. It follows that all the experiments I am considering will have successfully gone through whatever procedures are established for examining and approving, in plan and design, any experiment involving human beings. Failure to carry out the experiment in accordance with the approved plan and negligence in carrying out the plan would not be issues to be decided by the panels set up to administer the compensation fund. The first would be subject to whatever sanctions were made part of the pre-experiment approval procedures. The second would remain, as it is now, a part of the law of malpractice. In neither case would such determinations be needed or even useful in deciding the issue of compensation from the fund.

The fourth difficulty in using a compensation fund as an added control on medical experiments in humans arises because such experiments are usually carried out in charitable institutions. Accordingly, it may be questioned whether financial pressures have the same effect on such institutions as they are said to have in competitive industries. Would the need to pay compensation for experiments that fail cause greater care within each institution in selecting experiments and experimenters, or would it simply put pressure on the institution to try only those experiments that have the greatest potential market payoff, regardless of the scientific importance of the results? There is no doubt that some pressure for marketable results would come from such a system. But the market is not the primary or even the secondary source of funds for such institutions. These sources are the government and charitable contributions, which would continue to give according to their judgment of the reputation of the institution and researcher involved. And reputations are based largely on past successful researches—quite apart from whether the past research got financial recognition in the market or only acclaim in the scientific community. It seems unlikely, therefore, that basic research of real promise would suffer from the existence of a compensation fund.

In fact, if one views research institutions as industries that have two possible markets for their products (one the industrial market, the other the scientific community), both of which reward successes handsomely in straight financial terms, the analogy to normal market control situations becomes quite striking. In each case, the payoff for success is notable, and the point of market control is to bring the real costs involved in trying something new to the attention of those who will decide whether the attempt is worth the risks.

The fifth problem with employing a compensation fund is the danger that research in new or small medical centers will be hampered. There is no doubt that it will. A new or small medical center must find an angel. It must convince someone that what it proposes to try is important enough to justify the potential compensation-liability as well as the cost of doing the experiment itself. But, I would suggest, this is precisely the point of the market control system. Not all medical research that involves risks to humans can be justified. One way of determining if it is justified is by seeing whether there is enough confidence in the proposed experiment or in the research center where the experiment would be carried out to fund payment not only for the test tubes and animals used, but also for the human beings who may suffer injury in the experiment. If there is not, it is a fair sign that the particular experiment is too risky (in relation to its possible beneficial results) to be tried by the particular research team or center. Professor Everett Mendelsohn of Harvard has suggested on various occasions that most significant pioneering research is, in fact, carried out by a very few people in a very few places. If this is so, requiring research centers to meet the full cost of experiments (including the cost of injuries to subjects) may be one of the least invidious ways of concentrating risky research among those who can do it best.

One may summarize the use of a compensation fund in the following way. Requiring compensation of injured subjects causes the full cost of research in humans to be placed on the research center. Accordingly, approval by the center of a particular experiment will require conscious consideration not only of the possible payoff (either in market or scientific terms), but also of the risks, converted to money, that the project entails. This may not deter many experiments, but it may cause those involved in the most risky or least useful ones to consider carefully whether the experiment is worth it, whether it is best done by those who propose to do it, and whether there is an alternative, and safer, way of obtaining approximately the same results. It may well be that all these considerations are already firmly in the minds of the experimenters. If so, nothing is changed by requiring compensation. But if researchers—like auto makers, coal-mine owners, and the rest of mankind—tend to consider costs and benefits a bit more carefully when money is involved, a useful added control device will have been imposed.

*   *   *

e.

By Action of Investigator?

The King v. Bourne
[1939] 1 K.B. 687

*   *   *

MacNaughten, J., in summing up the case to the jury, said: Members of the jury, now that you have heard all the evidence and the speeches of counsel, it becomes my duty to sum up the case to you and to give you the necessary directions in law, and then it will be for you to consider the facts in relation to the law as laid down by me, and, after consideration, to deliver your verdict. In a trial by jury it is for the judge to give directions to the jury upon matters of law, and it is for the jury to determine the facts; the jury, and the jury alone, are the judges of the facts in the case.

The charge against Mr. Bourne is made under § 58 of the Offenses Against the Person Act, 1861, that he unlawfully procured the miscarriage of the girl who was the first witness in the case. It is a very grave crime, and judging by the cases that come before the Court it is a crime by no means uncommon. This is the second case at the present session of this Court where a charge has been preferred of an offense against this section, and I only mention the other case to show you how different the case now before you is from the type of case which usually comes before a criminal court. In that other case a woman without any medical skill or medical qualifications did what is alleged against Mr. Bourne here; she unlawfully used an instrument for the purpose of procuring the miscarriage of a pregnant girl; she did it for money; 2£5s. was her fee; a pound was paid on making the appointment, and she came from a distance to a place in London to perform the operation. She used her instrument, and, within an interval of time measured not by minutes but by seconds, the victim of her malpractice was dead on the floor. That is the class of case which usually comes before the Court.

The case here is very different. A man of the highest skill, openly, in one of our great hospitals, performs the operation. Whether it was legal or illegal you will have to determine, but he performs the operation as an act of charity, without fee or reward, and unquestionably believing that he was doing the right thing, and that he ought, in the performance of his duty as a member of a profession devoted to the alleviation of human suffering, to do it. That is the case you have to try today.

It is, I think, a case, of first instance, first impression. The matter has never, so far as I know, arisen before a jury to determine in circumstances such as these, and there was, even amongst learned counsel, some doubt as to the proper direction to the jury in such a case as this.

The defendant is charged with an offense against § 58 of the Offenses Against the Person Act, 1861. That section is a re-enactment of earlier statutes, the first of which was passed at the beginning of the last century in the reign of George III. (43 Geo. 3, c. 58, s. 1.) But long before then, before even Parliament came into existence, the killing of an unborn child was by the common law of England a grave crime: see Bracton, Book III. (*DeCorona*), fol. 121. The protection which the common law afforded to human life extended to the unborn child in the womb of its mother. But, as in the case of homicide, so also in the case where an unborn child is killed, there may be justification for the act.

Nine years ago Parliament passed an Act called the Infant Life (Preservation) Act, 1929 (19 and 20 Geo. 5, c. 34). Sect. I, sub-s. I, of that Act provides that "any person who, with intent to destroy the life of a child capable of being born alive, by any wilful act causes a child to die before it has an existence independent of its mother, shall be guilty of felony, to wit, of child destruction, and shall be liable on conviction thereof on indictment to penal servitude for life: Provided that no person shall be found guilty of an offense under this section unless it is proved that the act which caused the death of the child was not done in good faith for the purpose only of preserving the life of the mother." It is true, as Mr. Oliver has said, that this enactment provides for the case where a child is killed by a wilful act at the time when it is being delivered in the ordinary course of nature; but in my view the proviso that it is necessary for the Crown to prove that the act was not done in good faith for the purpose only of preserving the life of the mother is in accordance with what has always been the common law of England with regard to the killing of an unborn child. No such proviso is in fact set out in § 58 of the Offenses Against the Person Act, 1861; but the words of that section are that any person who "unlawfully" uses an instrument with intent to procure miscarriage shall be guilty of felony. In my opinion the word "unlawfully" is not, in that section, a meaningless word. I think it imports the meaning expressed by the proviso in § I, sub-s. I, of the Infant Life (Preservation) Act, 1929, and that § 58 of the Offenses Against the Person Act, 1861, must be read as if the words making it an offense to use an instrument with intent to procure a miscarriage were qualified by a similar proviso.

In this case, therefore, my direction to you in law is this—that the burden rest on the Crown to satisfy you beyond reasonable doubt that the defendant did not procure the miscarriage of the girl in good faith for the purpose only of preserving her life. If the Crown fails to satisfy you of that, the defendant is entitled by the law of this land to a verdict of acquittal. If, on the other hand, you are satisfied that what the defendant did was not done by him in good faith for the purpose only of preserving the life of the girl, it is your duty to find him guilty. It is said, and I think said rightly, that this is a case of great importance to the public and, more especially, to the medical profession; but you will observe that it has nothing to do with the ordinary case of procuring abortion to which I have already referred. In those cases the operation is performed by a person of no skill, with no medical qualifications, and there is no pretense that it is done for the preservation of the mother's life. Cases of that sort are in no way affected by the consideration of the question which is put before you today.

*　　*　　*

I do not think it is necessary for me to recapitulate the evidence that has been given before you as to the reasons why Mr. Bourne in this case thought it right to perform the operation. You remember his evidence. The learned Attorney-General accepts his evidence as a frank statement of what actually passed through his mind. In view of the age and character of the girl and the fact that she had been raped with great violence, he thought that the operation ought to be performed. As I told you yesterday, and I tell you today, the question that you have got to determine is not are you satisfied that he performed the operation in good faith for the purpose of preserving the life of the girl. The question is, has the Crown proved the negative of that? If the Crown has satisfied you beyond reasonable doubt —if there is a doubt, by our law the accused person is always entitled to be acquitted—if the Crown has satisfied you beyond reasonable doubt that he did not do this act in good faith for the purpose of preserving the life of the girl, then he is guilty of the offence with which he is charged. If the Crown has failed to satisfy you of that, then by the law of England he is entitled to a verdict of acquittal. The case is a grave case, and no doubt raises matters of grave concern both to the medical profession and to the public. As I said at the beginning of my summing-up, it does not touch the case of the professional abortionist. As far as the members of the medical profession themselves are concerned—and they alone could properly perform such an operation —we may hope and expect that none of them would ever lend themselves to the malpractices of professional abortionists, and in cases of this sort, as Mr. Bourne said, no doctor would venture to operate except after consulting some other member of the profession of high standing.

You will give the matter your careful consideration, and if you come to the conclusion that the Crown has discharged the burden that rests upon it, your verdict should be guilty. If you are not satisfied of that, then your verdict should be not guilty.

*   *   *

Verdict Not Guilty.

CHAPTER TWELVE

Experimentation with Uncomprehending Subjects

The incapacity of uncomprehending subjects to participate in research decisions highlights two fundamental questions: When, if ever, should subjects be used for research without their own consent? What persons or institutions should be authorized to formulate, administer, and review rules about the participation of non-consenting subjects?

Investigators have strongly advocated the use of uncomprehending subjects, such as children, for some experiments in order to advance knowledge about the beginnings of life in general or childhood diseases in particular. Yet they have neither sought nor been given sufficient guidance on the permissible limits of such research.

The question of "permissible" experimentation emerges in this context for a number of reasons. First, unlike research with competent subjects in which the decision to conduct experiments has at least until recently rested with the investigator alone, the use of uncomprehending subjects requires the legal permission of the state which has assumed, though often failed to exercise, the role of *parens patriae* for the incompetent in society. However, the circumstances under which the state's permission must be obtained has never been well defined. This ambiguity has obscured the fact that the decision to experiment with uncomprehending subjects raises questions of public policy as well as scientific merit. Second, the dependent position of uncomprehending subjects has burdened the conscience of many investigators and led them to question the extent to which they should engage in such research. Since this topic is freighted with great anxiety, it is understandable that the participants have been unwilling or unable to consider carefully who should accept responsibility for the decision to experiment with uncomprehending subjects.

Although the cases presented in this chapter focus on children, the problems raised extend also to adults deemed intellectually or psychologically incapable of making understanding decisions about their own welfare. In studying these materials consider the following questions:

1.   What characteristics define the group (or groups) of uncomprehending patient-subjects?

2.   Should the use of uncomprehending patient-subjects, if permitted at all, be restricted to research which aims to cure their disease, seeks to aid in diagnosing their condition, or attempts to learn more about the disease from which they are suffering?

3.   Must these prospective benefits be intended for the individual subject or can they accrue to the group of which he is a part? If so, how and by whom should the group be defined?

4.   Should research be conducted with healthy uncomprehending subjects to supply more information about the "norms" for this group or to provide "controls" for an experiment?

5.   Who should be authorized to give permission for research on uncomprehending "volunteers" and patient-subjects? What general principles should guide such delegation of authority?

6.   Should "incompetent" patient-subjects who are institutionalized be included in, or be the primary source for, experiments?

a.   Does consent by relatives, the superintendent of the institution, or court-appointed guardians make a difference?

b.   Does participation by such subjects depend on whether non-institutionalized patient-subjects are available as an alternative?

7.   Under what circumstances should research not be permitted even with the consent of relatives or others acting on behalf of non-consenting patient-subjects?

8.   In the case of children, at what age or by what other criteria should they be considered "comprehending" patient-subjects?

9.   Should distinctions be made between research with subjects who do not consent and those who cannot consent?

A.

Case Studies of Children as Patient-Subjects

1.

Arthur J. Moss, Edward R. Duffie, Jr., and George Emmanouilides
Blood Pressure and Vasomotor Reflexes in the Newborn Infant*

The present investigation was undertaken to determine the intra-arterial pressure in normal full-term and premature infants during the early days of life. The effects of crying, of exposure to cold, and of postural tilting also were studied in order to appraise vasomotor reactivity.

*   *   *

Catheterization of the umbilical arteries was attempted in 113 normal newborn infants and was successfully accomplished in 100. In each case the procedure was discussed in detail with one or both parents followed by a written consent. Of the infants studied, 74 were full-term and 26 were prematurely born. The age at the time of study ranged from 1 to 77 hours. . . .

One of the umbilical arteries was isolated and a No. 5F nasogastric feeding tube was inserted and advanced into the aorta. This caused little discomfort and, with few exceptions, the infants appeared to be completely content. . . .

*   *   *

Cold pressor tests were made in 46 infants (29 full-term and 17 premature). This procedure was conducted as follows: 1 foot was immersed to the ankle in ice water at 4°C to 5°C for a period of 1 minute. The aortic pressure was recorded continuously during the immersion and at 30-second intervals thereafter for 2 to 5 minutes. Since the infant invariably cried when exposed to cold, 1 to 3 pretest immersions at 1-minute intervals were made until all signs of discomfort disappeared. This eliminated the complicating effects of crying and straining. . . .

The effect of posture (70° head-up tilt) on the arterial pressure was studied in 50 infants (27 full-term and 23 premature). The subjects were secured to a circumcision board with the upper extremities restrained in flexion and the lower extremities in extension. The board was tilted over the edge of the table with the catheter tip at the estimated level of the right atrium. Great care was taken to fix the fulcrum at this level. Tilting was accomplished within a second and usually did not cause any signs of discomfort. When it did, the test was repeated until a satisfactory pressure recording was obtained.

*   *   *

The results of this study indicate that newborn infants, whether premature or full-term, react to postural tilting in the same manner as do adults. This is submitted as further evidence that the vasomotor regulatory mechanisms are present and functional at birth and are independent of maturity.

*   *   *

NOTES

NOTE 1.

CLAUDE J. MIGEON, JEAN BERTRAND, AND PATRICIA E. WALL
PHYSIOLOGICAL DISPOSITION OF
4-C[14]-CORTISOL DURING LATE PREGNANCY*

*   *   *

The present work is an attempt to elucidate further the metabolism of corticosteroids during pregnancy. It was thought that radioactive cortisol might be useful since it would permit a dynamic study without interfering with the endogenous production of steroid.

If, following the injection of radioactive material to a mother, a large part of the dose were to cross the placenta, we had to be assured that the newborn would dispose of the compound as rapidly as do normal adults. Therefore, in a first step of the present study, we measured the urinary excretion of radioactivity during the 48-hour period following the administration of a minimal dose of 4-C[14]-cortisol (1.5×10^2 microcurie) to two newborns, 15 and 20 hours of age. Since . . . the 48-hour excretion of radioactivity was within normal limits, it was considered safe to proceed with the injection of mothers shortly before delivery.

The other subjects of the study were nine pregnant females, 20 to 38 years of age. An

---

* 32 *Pediatrics* 175–178 (1963). Reprinted by permission.

* 36 *Journal of Clinical Investigation* 1350 (1967). Reprinted by permission.

"elective, repeat caesarean section" was performed approximately at term and before onset of labor in all cases. . . .

* * *

NOTE 2.
A. M. RUDOLPH, J. E. DRORBAUGH,
P.A.M. AULD, A. J. RUDOLPH, A. S. NADAS,
C. A. SMITH, AND J. P. HUBBELL
STUDIES ON THE CIRCULATION IN THE
NEONATAL PERIOD—THE CIRCULATION IN THE
RESPIRATORY DISTRESS SYNDROME*

* * *

The purpose of the present study is to further delineate the changes in the circulation of infants with normal cardiovascular and pulmonary function and to determine whether a circulatory disturbance may be responsible for production of the syndrome of respiratory distress in certain newborn infants.

Studies of the circulation were conducted by means of cardiac catheterization in 28 newborn infants. These infants were carefully observed for evidence of respiratory distress, and were separated into three groups on the basis of the severity and duration of respiratory signs. Group I comprised 19 infants either with no signs of respiratory distress or with mild evanescent symptoms. Four of these babies showed unquestionable evidence of mongolism, and one was microcephalic. Eight of the 19 were infants of diabetic mothers. Their ages at the time of cardiac catheterization ranged from 2 to 34 hours. . . .

* * *

Group II consisted of nine infants with mild respiratory distress. All these were infants of diabetic mothers. Four infants were males and five, females. The ages at time of study varied from 2 to 11 hours. . . . Group III included 10 infants with severe respiratory distress. Seven of these infants were males and three, females. Five of this group were infants of diabetic mothers. Their ages at the time of catheterization were 3 to 21 hours. . . .

The decisions to perform studies on the infants were made only after careful clinical observation. Radiologic and electrocardiographic studies were carried out for all the infants with respiratory symptoms and for the majority of those with no respiratory distress. The procedure was performed after full discussion with and consent of at least one of the parents. . . .

In 15 newborn infants cardiac catheterization was attempted by inserting the catheter into the umbilical vein, with the aim of manipulating it through the ductus venosus into the inferior vena cava and then into the heart. In view of the tendency for the catheter to enter portal veins, with difficulty in maneuvering beyond the ductus venosus, the attempt was abandoned in five instances. In 10 infants, included in this report, the catheter could be manipulated into the heart, but in only 2 of these was it possible to pass the catheter into the pulmonary artery. In the remaining 28 infants, the catheter was inserted through the right saphenous vein in the groin. Under local procaine anesthesia, a small incision was made just below the groin and the saphenous vein was readily isolated. . . .

After the catheter was passed into the right atrium from the inferior vena cava, an immediate attempt was made to enter the superior vena cava. The catheter was then again withdrawn and manipulated into the right ventricle. A very careful continuous monitoring of the electrocardiogram was then conducted with the aid of an oscilloscope, and attempts were made to pass the catheter into the pulmonary artery. The catheter was rapidly withdrawn if ventricular ectopic beats were induced; consequently in only 22 instances was the pulmonary artery catheterized. In the other 16 instances the attempts to enter the pulmonary artery were abandoned in view of the induction of numerous ectopic beats during these manipulations.

* * *

2.

**Horst Bickel, John Gerrard, and
Evelyn M. Hickmans
Influence of Phenylalanine Intake
on Phenylketonuria***

In phenylketonuria phenylalanine accumulates in the blood and cerebrospinal fluid, probably because phenylalanine is not converted to a normal extent into tyrosine. On the assumption that this excessive concentration of phenyla-

* 27 *Pediatrics* 551–552 (1961). Reprinted by permission.

* 2 *The Lancet* 812–813 (1953). Reprinted by permission.

lanine (or perhaps of some breakdown product) is responsible for the mental retardation found in this condition we decided to keep a girl, aged 2 years, with phenylketonuria on a diet low in phenylalanine. She was an idiot and unable to stand, walk, or talk; she showed no interest in her food or surroundings, and spent her time groaning, crying, and banging her head. . . .

*   *   *

[A] gradual improvement in the child's mental state took place within the next few months: she learnt to crawl, to stand, and to climb on chairs; her eyes became brighter; her hair grew darker; and she no longer banged her head or cried continuously.

*   *   *

In view of the importance of establishing whether the clinical improvement noted (which depended at first largely on the observation of the mother) was real and due to the diet rather than to natural development, we decided to add L-phenylalanine 5 g. daily to the diet. This was added to the hydrolysate without the mother's knowledge, so that any change should be noted without bias.

A definite deterioration in the child's condition ensued, the mother reporting with distress that her daughter had lost in a few days all the ground gained in the previous ten months; that within six hours of starting the fresh supply of "food" the child had begun to cry and to bang her head as in the past, and within twenty-four hours could no longer stand and could scarcely crawl.

In view of the importance of obtaining adequate proof of the value of the special diet, at present very expensive, the mother agreed to a further similar trial in hospital, which permitted close correlation of clinical and biochemical findings and cinematographic records. After a period of observation on a low-phenylalanine diet, L-phenylalanine 4 g. daily was again added to the diet. Within twenty-four hours the patient became irritable and drowsy, lost interest in her food and surroundings, developed facial eczema, and salivated profusely. She also became ataxic and vomited repeatedly. By the sixth day she could no longer stand or crawl. The additional phenylalanine was then discontinued, and within three weeks she had almost completely recovered.

*   *   *

3.

**Robert M. Zollinger, Jr.,
Martin C. Lindem, Jr., Robert M. Filler,
Joseph M. Corson, and Richard E. Wilson
Effect of Thymectomy on
Skin-Homograft Survival in Children***

Recent investigations have indicated that the thymus gland has an important role in the initiation of immune potential in animals. Specifically, thymectomy in the neonatal period and thymectomy combined with total-body irradiation in adult animals have permitted prolonged survival of skin homografts. The latter principle has been utilized in an effort to prolong survival of human adult renal autografts. . . . There is no information available regarding neonatal thymectomy in man, but a study of the effect of thymectomy on skin homografts in immunologically competent children appeared practical from the point of view of clinical transplantation.

This is a report of data obtained from children, beyond the neonatal stage, undergoing major corrective heart surgery, in which the thymus is frequently dissected and partially removed for aortic-arch exposure. When desired, a complete thymectomy could be accomplished without increasing the hazards of surgery. Thus, an opportunity for the study of skin-homograft survival in patients having a carefully performed thymectomy was available for the first time.

Eighteen children of both sexes from three and a half months to eighteen years of age were chosen from among those operated upon at the Children's Hospital Medical Center for congenital heart disease. Eleven of these patients were randomly selected to have a total thymectomy whereas the remaining 7 had only a biopsy of the thymus and served as controls. At the conclusion of each heart operation a full-thickness skin homograft, approximately 1 cm. in diameter and obtained from an unrelated adult donor, was sutured in place on the chest wall.

The grafts were biopsied when initial gross evidence of rejection, such as edema, loss of pink color or failure to blanch with pressure, was apparent. When indicated serial biopsies were taken. . . .

. . . The mean rejection time of skin homografts in the totally thymectomized children was

---

* 270 *New England Journal of Medicine* 707–709 (1964). Reprinted by permission.

nine and four-tenths days, with a range of eight to thirteen days. The mean rejection time in the control group was ten and nine-tenths days, with a similar range. All rejections were fairly prompt, and the microscopical findings confirmed and closely correlated with the clinical observations. . . . No major complications occurred in the recovery periods. There was no gross infection delay in healing or prolongation of hospital stay in these patients.

*   *   *

In the neonatal animal the thymus has been linked to the production of small lymphocytes and to the development of lymphatic tissue. . . . Metcalf demonstrated a humoral "lymphocytosis stimulating factor" that originates in the thymus but has its effect on the cells in the peripheral lymphatic tissues. . . . Other investigators, however, believe that immunologically competent cells or their progenitors may originate in the thymus and migrate to the peripheral sites.

Thymectomy in laboratory animals, both neonates and adults, has resulted in lymphopenia, with a decreased number of small lymphocytes. In the adult the lymphopenia develops slowly over several months. In this study the total white-cell counts, the differentials and the total lymphocyte counts showed no consistent alteration. The period of elapsed time, however, was only ten to fourteen days.

*   *   *

Of interest has been the finding of cachexia in small animals thymectomized in the perinatal period. Many young children have undergone this procedure in the past during intrathoracic surgery, and no reports of a similar postoperative syndrome have appeared to date. It is true that some residual thymus has often been left behind, and the exact documentation of the amount of thymus removed is not available. This study was undertaken, therefore, with some historical reassurance as well as the plan to observe closely the growth and development of these children over the years. Since many young patients will continue to have at least partial thymectomy for vascular rings, tracheal compression and open-heart exposure it is doubly important that a known group of completely thymectomized persons be analyzed carefully. It is our specific plan to repeat the elements of this study after an interval of six to twelve months.

. . . No apparent difference in skin-homograft survival was noted between the two groups.

*   *   *

NOTES

NOTE 1.

BYRON H. WAKSMAN
THYMUS EXPERIMENTATION*

. . . A series of papers over the last two years has shown that the thymus has a key role in the development and maintenance of several types of immune function. . . . The clear-cut possibility that thymectomy, perhaps in combination with irradiation or "immunosuppressive" medication, can be used to prevent the rejection of homografts or the manifestations of diseases having an immunologic basis has created an atmosphere of optimism regarding the treatment of many surgical or medical conditions previously regarded as hopeless.

The proposal to use thymectomy as a therapeutic tool, however, must be tempered by the consideration that suppression of immune mechanisms, sufficient, for example, to prevent homograft rejection, must at the same time remove important defenses against infection. The unhappy consequences of immunologic deficiency have been vividly illustrated by many recent papers. It would hardly be appropriate to produce in the patient a condition analogous to agammaglobulinemia or perhaps to agammaglobulinemia with alymphocytosis to achieve a prophylactic or therapeutic result at any level less than lifesaving. It remains to be demonstrated whether it is possible to achieve a controlled intermediate degree of immunologic deficiency, sufficient to permit homograft survival but insufficient to lead to recurrent infection. Indeed, this question has not yet been satisfactorily answered at the level of experimentation in the laboratory animal.

One may properly question the philosophy underlying the use of agents or technics that affect immune responses in general to reduce the response to a specific antigen. Recent studies on specific acquired tolerance hold out the hope that it may soon be possible, by suitable treatment of adult subjects, to suppress permanently immunologic reactivity to specific antigens while immunologic responsiveness to unrelated anti-

---

* 270 *New England Journal of Medicine* 1018–1019 (1964). Reprinted by permission.

gens remains unimpaired. There is also a clear-cut possibility that, by manipulation of the thymus itself, it will be possible to achieve specific tolerance. This approach seems, on many grounds, preferable to what one may designate as the "nonspecific" approach.

With these facts in mind, one may well question the value and propriety of studies like that by Zollinger and his associates . . . in which total thymectomy was carried out as a purely experimental measure in subjects not having a disease to which this procedure is relevant. One may criticize the publication of data obtained at a time (immediately after thymectomy) when no positive finding could be anticipated, as noted in the authors' own discussion. One wonders whether the usual hazards, notably the possible transmission of serum hepatitis from graft donors and the unnecessary immunization against isoantigens, were sufficiently offset by the usefulness of the data obtained to be worth risking in these subjects. One may also ask if the long-term hazards, unknown at present, were duly noted and called to the subjects' attention. It seems pertinent to raise these questions at a time when the literature, especially in the field of transplantation, is being flooded with reports of human experimentation based in many cases on inadequate laboratory data and with insufficient attention to the long-term hazards.

NOTE 2.
R. M. ZOLLINGER, JR., M. C. LINDEM, JR.,
R. M. FILLER, J. M. CORSON, AND R. E. WILSON
ETHICS OF THYMUS EXPERIMENTATION*

The questions raised by Dr. Waksman . . . were considered by us and by our advisers. If one can set aside the scientific or moral rationalizations for performing thymectomies in human beings at the present state of knowledge the fact remains that thymectomies were and are being performed during various thoracic procedures. It was from this group that the patients of the study were chosen. The article unfortunately implied the creation of thymectomized patients whereas the patients were merely chosen from among the many who have total thymectomy as a necessary part of aortic exposure during cardiac surgery.

The skin-homograft donors were chosen carefully, and to date no case of hepatitis has

appeared in similar studies by several local investigators. In addition we believe the homografts introduced few new isoantigens beyond those received in the multiple transfusions required in open-heart surgery. In this setting the added hazards in this investigation were believed to be reasonable—not only because of the application of this study to transplantation but also because of its need in all cardiac and thoracic patients in whom thymectomy has been or may yet be done.

NOTE 3.
MELVIN LEWIS, AUDREY T. McCOLLUM,
A. HERBERT SCHWARTZ, AND JEROME A. GRUNT
INFORMED CONSENT IN PEDIATRIC RESEARCH*

*   *   *

Charles, a blind 7-year-old boy, was expected to die within the year from an inoperable brain tumor. Charles' mother gave consent for the boy to be hospitalized and subjected to endocrine studies that could not benefit him in any way. The justification for the studies was the possibility of their leading to earlier identification of brain tumors in other children.

The mother's motives in giving her consent for the studies were complex. She told the staff that she felt Charles' life would have been worthwhile if, through the studies, it led to knowledge that would benefit other children. This statement implied that her consent was partly a way of dealing with Charles' impending death (although Charles would die, the knowledge gained through him would live on) and partly a way of compensating for his loss (Charles would die so that other children might live). However, the statement also implied the existence of unconscious anger toward Charles, since it disregarded the severe stress to which the child would be subjected.

The psychological stress proved to be particularly severe since the medical procedure heightened the fears commonly experienced by a child at Charles' developmental stage—concern about body intactness and manipulation. Frequent venipunctures, necessary for the research, led to acute panic states in the child. Moreover, the usual means of dealing with such stress through play, visual, auditory and tactile experiences, and motor activity were denied to

---

* 270 *New England Journal of Medicine* 1314 (1964). Reprinted by permission.

* 16 *Children* 143, 147–148 (1969). Reprinted by permission.

Charles by his blindness and the imposed restraint necessary to the procedures.

When Charles was threatened with further restraint because reaching his difficult veins satisfactorily would require cutting through his skin, the investigator terminated the research.

*　　*　　*

4.

Howard E. Ticktin and Hyman J. Zimmerman Hepatic Dysfunction and Jaundice in Patients Receiving Triacetyloleandomycin*

Triacetyloleandomycin (TriA), a drug that has been introduced for the treatment of infection caused by staphylococcic and other gram-positive organisms, has been widely used, minimal toxicity being reported. Several isolated cases of jaundice in children receiving the drug have been observed. Robinson, however, has recently reported that in 5 of 48 patients who received TriA for fourteen days or longer elevated serum glutamic pyruvic transaminase values developed. These observations seem at variance with the previous reports of lack of side effects in patients receiving the drug for periods of sixty days or more.

The present study was undertaken in the attempt to determine the incidence and type of hepatic dysfunction relatable to the administration of TriA. This study demonstrates impaired hepatic function in over half and jaundice in 4 per cent of a group of patients receiving the drug for two weeks or longer.

The 50 patients studied included mental defectives or juvenile delinquents who had been inmates of Laurel Children's Center for two months or longer. There was no recognizable organic disease other than the mildly to moderately severe acne for which the drug was given. In none were there any systemic evidences of pyoderma. There were 38 males and 12 females, with ages ranging from thirteen to thirty-nine years. . . .

*　　*　　*

Eight patients, who had marked hepatic dysfunction, were transferred to the hospital for more intensive study. These included 6 in whom symptoms also developed. Two of the 6 patients

with symptoms (abdominal aching and anorexia) became jaundiced.

Liver biopsy was performed at the height of the dysfunction or jaundice, or both, in these 8 patients by the intercostal route with the use of the Menghini needle. In 4 of these patients it was repeated later.

A "challenge" dose of 1 gm., as four divided doses, was given on one day to 4 of the hospitalized patients, after their liver-function tests had returned to normal limits. . . .

. . . In all but 8 patients the tests of liver function yielded normal results at the beginning of the study. In 6 of these patients slightly abnormal bromsulfalein excretion was observed. . . .

Tests performed two weeks after the beginning of TriA administration revealed that in 54 per cent of the patients abnormal bromsulfalein excretion developed. . . .

In all these patients the abnormality was present, and in most cases greater, on retesting at three or four weeks after the beginning of therapy. Sixty-one per cent had abnormal bromsulfalein excretion. . . .

*　　*　　*

In 44 of the 50 patients there were no clinical evidences of reaction to the drug. Symptoms developed in only 6 patients, consisting of anorexia and mild aching in the epigastrium or right upper quadrant. In the 2 patients with overt jaundice dark urine and light stools were noted.

*　　*　　*

In the 4 patients in whom liver biopsies were obtained twice, the second specimens showed distinctly less abnormality than the first. In 2 the biopsy appeared almost normal. In the other 2 there was still distinct evidence of hepatocellular abnormality although cholestasis had disappeared.

Four patients were challenged with a 1 gm. dose of the drug after liver function had returned to normal. Within one or two days, hepatic dysfunction again developed in 3 of the 4. . . . Hepatic function returned to normal in all 3 patients within seven days after the challenging dose. . . .

The development of hepatic dysfunction in more than half the patients who received TriA for a period of two or more weeks seems reasonably ascribable to the administration of the drug. The sequence of normal hepatic function before administration of TriA, development of progressively worsening dysfunction as the drug was

---

* 267 *New England Journal of Medicine* 964–968 (1962). Reprinted by permission.

administered and the return to normal after its withdrawal strongly suggests that its administration was responsible for the development of the hepatic abnormality. This impression seems confirmed by the effect of a "challenge" dose, which, in 3 of 4 patients tested, again led to the development of abnormal hepatic function.

*   *   *

NOTES

NOTE 1.

MORE HUMAN GUINEA-PIGS*

Triacetyloleandomycin (TriA) is a derivative of the antibiotic oleandomycin and has a similar spectrum of action against staphylococci and other Gram-positive organisms. It has not been marketed in the United Kingdom as yet, but has been widely used in the U.S.A. as an alternative to penicillin or erythromycin. Until recently it was said to have few side-effects.

However, several isolated cases of jaundice have now been reported, and two enterprising physicians (H. E. Ticktin and H. J. Zimmerman) have published a study of 50 patients in whom the effects of this drug on the liver have been intensively examined. The patients concerned included "mental defectives or juvenile delinquents who had been inmates of Laurel Children's Center for two months or longer. . . ."

Ages of the patients ranged from 13 to 39 years and it is not stated to what extent they volunteered for the experiment or, in the case of the mental defectives, understood its purpose. There seems to be one or two lessons to be learnt from this study. The first is that liver toxicity from drugs may be like the iceberg, in which seven-eighths of the danger lies below the surface. The occasional case of jaundice may in fact indicate that large numbers of patients are suffering liver dysfunction which is only demonstrable by laboratory tests. The second is that it seems very questionable what value TriA has which would justify its use in view of this present information and the alternatives available. The third is that juvenile delinquency in the United States obviously carries hazards which many of us had not previously suspected. The pimpled gangster of today may find himself the bilious guinea-pig of tomorrow. It seems a little hard, perhaps, for a boy who has spent his formative years learning how to dodge flick-knives to

fall victim to intercostal perforation by the Menghini needle.

*   *   *

NOTE 2.

ROSS G. MITCHELL
THE CHILD AND EXPERIMENTAL MEDICINE*

*   *   *

[Throughout the nineteenth century very] few articles refer to parental permission for . . . studies, and there is seldom any expression of doubt about the morality of the work. Children from orphanages and "foundlings" were commonly used as subjects for these investigations. It is perhaps not surprising that this type of research was accepted unquestioningly, for infant and child mortality was still very high and methods of therapy were often drastic. Moreover, medicine had but recently emerged from an era in which children were little regarded, a world where foundlings were bought and sold and child labor was the rule. It is salutary to recall that a hundred years ago the American Society for Prevention of Cruelty to Animals was empowered by the courts to act in a case of cruelty to a child on the grounds that a child is an animal. A society for the prevention of cruelty to children was not founded until 1875—nearly ten years later. Against such a background, the use of orphans and foundlings for experiments would hardly have seemed to require permission or indeed justification.

With the advance of technology, research methods began to be more sophisticated. Techniques advanced from the mere withdrawal of blood to the injection of substances for experimental purposes. The first documented instance of this is probably the experiment by Oliver, who in 1894 injected crude extract of endocrine glands into his own son. After 1900, studies on the newborn infant began to increase, and these often involved the injection of chemicals such as fluorescein or experimental nutrients such as fat infusions. Fortunately at the same time there appears to have been some quickening of medical conscience, and the references to orphans and foundlings gradually diminished. Despite this, reports seldom referred to the obtaining of permission except curiously enough, from medical staff. Thus there were frequent acknowledgments in the early paediatric journals of the kindness

---

* 2 *British Medical Journal* 1536–1537 (1962). Reprinted by permission.

* 1 *British Medical Journal* 722, 725–726 (1964). Reprinted by permission.

of obstetric staffs in giving permission for experiments "on their cases"—a possessiveness which still exists to some extent to-day among doctors, as though the undertaking of medical care somehow conferred ownership of the patient on the physician.

* * *

5.

Office of Science and Technology Privacy and Behavioral Research*

Our society places a high value on the rights of the individual, among them the right to privacy. When the techniques and research methods of the behavioral scientist impinge on these rights, they pose a crucial question for the scientist and for society.

* * *

Some examples of research procedures that may harm the participant through a violation of his rights . . . may help to define the area of our concern:

1. In a study designed to discover the causes of personality qualities in children it was necessary to secure measures of the children's personalities. One device that has been widely used is the so-called sociometric measure which assesses certain personality characteristics of a child on the basis of judgments about him by his classmates. A set of statements about the child's behavior was prepared. Examples are: "He usually suggests a good idea for a new game." "He always gets mad when we don't do what he wants." "He can read better than anyone else in the class." The children were instructed to fill in the name of the child best described by each of these statements. By tabulating the answers given by all children in a class, it was possible to find out the peer judgment about various qualities of personality.

The problem of confidentiality did not enter this situation because the results were never seen by the children, their parents, or the teacher. However, the "sociometric method" invades privacy in the sense that it forces children to think about certain qualities of behavior shown by one another and to reach firm conclusions about what is "best" or "worst." The normal processes by which reputation develops were replaced by an artificial intervention:

2. In a series of experiments designed to discover the effects of a student's feelings of success or of failure at a particular task, the experimenter artificially induced feelings of success and failure in different groups of subjects. In the failure experiment, a subject was asked to learn a rather complex motor task and the experimenter expressed surprise at how slowly the subject learned, compared his performance unfavorably with that of other students, and expressed sympathy with him for his clumsiness. The net result was to induce in the subject a feeling of inferiority and of self-derogation. By the end of the experimental session, some subjects were depressed, brooding, and angry, and had lost a measure of self-esteem.

It is routine for an experimenter to explain the state of affairs following such an experiment. The subject can normally recover his usual level of self-esteem, but it is the responsibility of the experimenter to make sure that this recovery occurs. It should be added that the body of research of which this example is a part has led to a substantial modification of educational policy in America. The research showed clearly that the lowering of self-esteem and failure reduce learning ability. Educationally, the principle has been applied to modify teachers' schoolroom behavior in such a way that unsatisfactory performance can be challenged by means that avoid injuring the student's self-esteem.

* * *

6.

Kidney Transplantation in Identical Twins*

a.

Letter to Charles B. Barnes, Jr., President, Peter Bent Brigham Hospital from the Hospital's Attorneys

You have asked us on behalf of the Peter Bent Brigham Hospital [P.B.B.H.] for our opinion as to the civil and criminal liability of the hospital and its trustees, officers and employees upon the following assumed facts.

The parents of fourteen-year-old twins, one of whom has two diseased kidneys, enter into an agreement with a surgeon to perform a kidney transplant operation at the hospital. The operation contemplates the following acts: one surgeon

---

* Washington, D.C.: U.S. Government Printing Office 10–12 (1967).

* This study combines documents related to two kidney transplants performed in 1957; the names of the patients and their families have been changed.

removes one of the diseased kidneys from the ill twin while another surgeon removes a healthy kidney from the well twin. One of the surgeons then sews the healthy kidney into the ill twin. After a period of time, if all goes well with the ill twin, a second operation is performed to remove the second diseased kidney.

We understand that the twins must be identical and that the operation has, based on experience, a fair chance of preserving the life of the ill twin, whose disease would otherwise be fatal. It is also assumed that there is a danger that either or both of the twins may die on the operating table. The degree of danger can vary substantially. Moreover, removal of a healthy kidney from the well twin materially decreases his capacity to survive physical injury or disease involving the kidneys, since he no longer has a spare kidney upon which to rely if one should become injured or diseased.

We also assume that because of their age the twins do not understand the nature or consequences of the surgical procedure although a normal adult might be expected to do so. Further, we assume that it is difficult to explain the surgical procedures and that explanations may have the tendency to cause emotional strains which might prejudice the chances of a successful transplantation. Finally, we assume that there is no negligence on the part of anyone connected with the operations.

It is our opinion that upon these facts:

1. As a charitable corporation, the Peter Bent Brigham Hospital is immune from liability in this as in other situations involving possible torts.

2. With respect to the liability of any trustees, officers or agents of the hospital who participate in authorizing the procedure:

(a) The parents may give effective consent to the operation on the ill twin, i.e., a consent which is binding upon them and the ill twin.

(b) The parents have no power to give effective consent to the operation on the well twin, except insofar as the rights of the parents are concerned.

(c) The operation on the well twin may well be prohibited by the terms, if not the spirit, of the criminal statutes of this Commonwealth.

The Corporation's Freedom from Liability

Although there is no decision of the Massachusetts Supreme Judicial Court which deals squarely with the question whether a charitable corporation's immunity from tort liability extends to injuries resulting from intentional acts, the Court has never made any distinction in its opinions between such injuries and those resulting from negligence. Moreover, the various theories upon which the immunity rests are equally applicable to intentional and to negligent acts, and courts in other jurisdictions which still maintain the immunity have rejected any distinction based upon the character of the allegedly tortious act. See Annotation, 25 A.L.R. 2d 29, 52. Accordingly, there is no reason to believe that the Peter Bent Brigham Hospital would itself be held liable for the performance of a kidney transplantation at the hospital even if one assumes that under some circumstances the operation may be improper. Furthermore, since it is a corporation, the hospital cannot be guilty of crimes against the person. See *Commonwealth v. Proprietors of New Bedford Bridge,* 2 Gray 339, 345.

The immunity of the corporation from liability does not, of course, extend to the individuals who, either as trustees, officers or agents of the hospital, authorize or participate in the surgical procedure. The remainder of this opinion deals with the nature and extent of their liability.

The Civil Liability of Trustees, Officers and Agents

The legal problems in the kidney transplantation procedure are hardly less novel than its medical aspects. Needless to say, therefore, there are no authorities, judicial or otherwise, which are squarely in point. However, there are certain principles which have been established in more or less analogous situations which are helpful, if not definitive.

An attempt to state the basic rule governing this and other situations involving acts affecting the person of a minor is set forth in Section 59 of the American Law Institute's *Restatement of the Law of Torts.* While this statement has never been cited by the Massachusetts Supreme Judicial Court, neither has it been rejected. Furthermore, there is nothing in the decisions or opinions of the Court which is inconsistent with the rule as expounded by the Institute.

Section 59 states that:

(1) If a person whose interest is invaded is at the time by reason of his youth or defective mental condition, whether permanent or temporary, incapable of understanding or appreciating the consequences

of the invasion, the assent of such a person to the invasion is not effective as a consent thereto.

(2) The assent of a parent, guardian or other person standing in like relation to one described in Subsection (1) has the same effect as though given by the person whose interest is invaded, if such parent, guardian or other person has the power to consent to the invasion.

It was long ago established that a surgical operation for the benefit of a child constitutes an invasion of his person to which his parent does have the power to consent. Accordingly, assuming that both the ill twin and his parents assent to the operation by which diseased kidneys are removed and replaced by a healthy one, no liability will result from its performance.

The kidney transplantation presents a different question as far as the well twin is concerned. The operation which involves the removal of one of his kidneys, leaving him less capable of withstanding disease or injury, is clearly not an operation for his benefit. Whether such an operation constitutes an invasion of his person to which his parent has the power to consent is a question which neither the American Law Institute nor the decisions of the courts have answered. The best that can be found in the way of authority are statements which have appeared by way of dicta in court opinions. Unfortunately, even these provide no clear answer.

In *Bonner* v. *Moran*, 126 F. 2d 121 (D.C. Cir. 1941), the Court was called upon to decide whether a surgeon was liable to a minor for performing an operation which involved removing skin from his body and grafting it on the body of another patient. The youth had consented to the operation but no consent of either parent had been obtained. The Court held that the surgeon was liable to the minor for performing the operation. In its opinion, the Court said that the rule that a parent's consent is not necessary in an emergency, or where the minor is close to majority rests upon an assumption that the operation is for the minor's benefit. The Court went on to say that if the parent's consent had been obtained in the case before it, the action by the minor for assault and battery could not have been maintained.

There is no reason to believe that the Massachusetts Supreme Judicial Court would not have held, as the Court of Appeals for the District of Columbia did, that a surgical operation upon a minor which is not for his benefit and as to the nature and consequences which he has no clear understanding renders the persons performing it civilly liable in the absence of the consent of the parent. However, the question remains: Is the parent's consent sufficient if the minor, whether or not he expressed his assent, was incapable of understanding or appreciating the consequences of the operation? The dictum in the *Bonner* case would seem to indicate that the answer is "yes." However, that answer seems plainly inconsistent with statements of the Massachusetts Supreme Judicial Court. The cases in which the statements were made (*Banks* v. *Conant,* 14 Allan 497 and *Taylor* v. *Mechanics' Savings Bank,* 97 Mass. 345) were less closely analogous to the present situation on their facts. However they probably represent more reliable indicia of the attitude which our Court would take toward the problem presented than does the dictum in the *Bonner* case.

In each of the Massachusetts cases it was held that a parent could not recover money paid to an infant upon his voluntary enlistment in the Armed Forces. The court said by way of dictum in each instance that the parent could not require his son to enlist against the minor's wishes and that the money was paid to the son as an inducement "to undertake a service of an arduous and hazardous nature." In the American Law Institute's terms, the enlistment was an invasion of the minor's interest to which the parent had no power to consent.

If a parent has no power to make an effective decision regarding his child's enlistment because of the hazardous nature of the service, the conclusion seems inescapable that the parent likewise has no power to give effective consent to an operation which is both hazardous and personally detrimental to the child.

Criminal Liability of Trustees, Officers and Agents

The absence of effective consent is no less a matter of concern in attempting to weigh the possibility of criminal liability in connection with a kidney transplantation involving minor twins. Again, the problem is a novel one. Obviously, the minds of those concerned with the procedure would be free of the evil intention or moral turpitude usually associated with those acts which are defined and prohibited as crimes. In fact, the dominant motive for the procedure as a whole undoubtedly would be preservation of the life of the ill twin. Nevertheless, that purpose would be accomplished by inflicting upon the well twin a serious and permanent physical injury without benefit to himself and without his intelligent consent. Accordingly, there is serious danger that the procedure would involve criminal liability.

In summary, it is our opinion that any trustees, officers, or agents of Peter Bent Brigham Hospital who authorize or participate in kidney transplantations involving minor twins will become civilly liable to the well twin and subject to the possibility of criminal prosecution.

b.

Petition to Supreme Judicial Court of the Commonwealth of Massachusetts, Suffolk County

RESPECTFULLY represents your Petitioners:

1. That the Petitioners and Respondents are all the parties having or claiming any interest which might be affected by any declaration of the Court under these proceedings.

2. That the Petitioner, Gail Williams, is a resident of Sioux City, Iowa, and brings this Petition as mother and guardian of her minor children, Charles Williams, and John Williams. hereinafter mentioned in the Petition; and in behalf of said minor children as their next friend.

3. That the Respondents, namely, J. Hartwell Harrison, M.D., Joseph E. Murray, M.D., John P. Merrill, M.D., and Warren R. Guild, M.D., are practicing physicians in the Commonwealth of Massachusetts attached to the staff of the Peter Bent Brigham Hospital.

4. That the Respondent, Peter Bent Brigham Hospital, is a Massachusetts charitable corporation located in Boston in the County of Suffolk.

5. That the Respondent, Victoria M. Cass, is a physician and acting director of the respondent hospital and as such is charged with responsibility for the direction of the operation of the charitable functions of said hospital and has authority to determine whether or not the facilities of said hospital may be utilized by the physicians and surgeons attached to its staff for the performance of any operation which they desire to do in the course of their practice of medicine and surgery carried on by them for care and cure of their several patients.

6. That your Petitioner, Gail Williams, is the mother of Charles Williams and John Williams, two minor children born on November 28, 1943; that said minors are identical twins, one of whom has two diseased kidneys, the other of whom has two healthy kidneys.

7. That both said children are patients in respondent hospital in Boston, County of Suffolk, Commonwealth of Massachusetts, to undergo kidney transplantation operations to save the life of the sick twin, Charles Williams, who allegedly will die in the event that these operations are not performed.

8. That the said respondent physicians have successfully performed kidney transplantation operations on a number of identical twins, and are of the opinion that successful transplantation operations can be performed on Charles Williams and John Williams.

9. That your Petitioners, Gail Williams, Charles Williams and John Williams, have requested and urged the respondent physicians to perform said operations, which said Respondents agreed to perform on the conditions set forth in Paragraph 16, but now refuse to perform said operations because they have been advised by competent legal counsel that, as John Williams is a minor, he cannot consent to an invasion of his person which will deprive him of a well kidney, and that your Petitioner, Gail Williams, cannot legally consent to said operation because it is an invasion of the person of said John Williams which allegedly is not for his benefit.

10. That respondent physicians desire to utilize the facilities of respondent hospital to perform the kidney transplant operations described in Paragraph 7 and the Respondents, Victoria M. Cass and the Peter Bent Brigham Hospital, desire to permit said physicians to use said facilities and to allow them to have the assistance of nurses and others employed by said hospital for purposes of said kidney transplantation operations in the event that this Honorable Court shall determine that the Petitioner, Gail Williams, or a guardian of John Williams appointed by a Court with jurisdiction therefor, has the authority and power to grant formal consent which shall be binding upon the Petitioner, John Williams, and all persons claiming by, through, or under him and having any title whatsoever to claim damages for any loss or injury which they or said Petitioner, John Williams, may incur or suffer by reason of anything which may happen to the Petitioner, John Williams, in the course of said kidney transplantation operations and which consent shall absolve said Victoria M. Cass and said hospital and each of them, their agents, employees and servants and Respondents from any and all liability to them or to the Commonwealth or any public authority, whether by reason of common law or any statute of the Commonwealth.

11. That Respondents, Victoria M. Cass and the Peter Bent Brigham Hospital, therefore allege that all Petitioners are severally ready to grant consent as aforesaid, but unless and until this Honorable Court shall declare that consent may be legally given as aforesaid, said Respondents have been advised that they cannot conformably to law permit said operations to be performed on the premises of and with the use of the facilities of said hospital, all of which are subject to the direction of the Respondent, Victoria M. Cass. If this Honorable Court shall so declare, said Respondents will make such premises and facilities and employees whose assistance the respondent physicians desire available to them for purposes of said kidney transplantation operations upon the Petitioners, Charles Williams and John Williams.

12. That your Petitioners, Gail Williams, Charles Williams and John Williams, are capable of understanding and appreciating the consequences of these surgical operations.

13. That your Petitioner, John Williams, has been fully informed, and understands the nature of the operations and its possible consequences.

14. That there is risk of grave emotional impact upon your Petitioner, John Williams, if this operation is not performed and your Petitioner, Charles Williams, dies.

15. That the operation is necessary for the future well-being of your Petitioner, John Williams, and that in this respect performance of the operation will confer a benefit upon your Petitioner, John Williams, as well as your Petitioner, Charles Williams.

16. That the respondent physicians agreed with the Petitioner, Gail Williams, acting on behalf of her minor children, Charles Williams and John Williams, to perform said operations to save the life of said Charles Williams, but only in the event that consent to said operations could be given which would be legally binding upon said children.

17. That an actual controversy has arisen between the parties as to whether consent to said operations can be given by the Petitioner, Gail Williams, or by anyone else to said operations, which would be legally binding on said children.

WHEREFORE your Petitioners pray:

1. That the Court determine whether or not the Petitioner, Gail Williams, or anybody else can give consent to the operations mentioned in Paragraph 8, which will be legally binding on said Charles Williams and John Williams.

2. That the Court determine that your Petitioner, Gail Williams, have the right and authority to consent legally to said operations, or in the alternative, to authorize the Petitioner, Gail Williams, to consent to said operations or to appoint a guardian ad litem for said minor children to consent to said operations.

3. That this Honorable Court enter a binding declaration stating whether or not a document signed and sealed by John Williams, or by Gail Williams, or by any legally appointed guardian of John Williams, or by any other identified person wherein it shall be provided that by reason of the performance by the respondent physician or any of them or by any other practicing physician or surgeon attached to the staff of the Peter Bent Brigham Hospital of kidney transplant operations upon Charles Williams and John Williams upon the premises of the Peter Bent Brigham Hospital with the use of its facilities and with the assistance of its employees neither the Peter Bent Brigham Hospital nor its acting director, Victoria M. Cass, nor any agent, officer, employee or servant of either, shall be or become under any liability whatsoever by reason of any provision of the law of Massachusetts, whether common law or by statute, to the Commonwealth, to John Williams, or to any other person whomsoever will be effective to accomplish the said purpose.

4. For such other and further relief as to this Honorable Court may seem meet and proper.

c.

Psychological Report on John Williams

Patient was very cooperative and highly motivated to do well. His attitudes were excellent so that we can accept the results as representative of his personal functioning. He gives a history of eighth grade education, which he would have completed this year, were it not for his having to leave school to come to this hospital. He reports that his grades were "all right" and that he was not flunking any courses. Following graduation he has plans to take up carpentry. He works in his spare time at various jobs, which include baby sitting and waiting on tables.

In terms of his intelligence, he shows adequate functioning. His I.Q. is in the dull normal range; that is, 83, which in terms of competence places him within the perfectly acceptable range of understanding and judgment. If he were not competent to make decisions, 25 per cent of the general population would also be incompetent. This level of 83 is probably representative of his capacity, even though his education has undoubtedly been very poor. He shows great gaps in knowledge, for example, which are consistent with a poor educational background. In some mental functions he shows average ability, which suggests that he perhaps could have attained a higher score under an optimal educational setting.

I would say, therefore, that in terms of comprehension, judgment and intelligence, he is perfectly capable of making decisions. He has the capacity to grasp concepts consistent with his intelligence and should be treated as a competent, self-sufficient individual.

d.

Notes of Petitioners' Attorney on Court Hearing

John Williams took the stand and testified in substance that he is 14 years old. He knows that his brother Charles is ill with a kidney ailment. John stated he was willing to submit to the operation for the removal of a kidney from himself to be implanted in Charles.

Cross-examination was waived on behalf of the doctors but the attorney on behalf of P.B.B.H. asked John whether the doctors had said to him that they would take out one of his kidneys and put it into Charles, to which John said yes. The attorney asked John whether he knew the dangers. John said yes. He said he was willing to consent to the operation.

Dr. Warren Guild of Lexington, Massachusetts, was the next witness. . . . He is acting director of the Kidney Laboratory of P.B.B.H.

Dr. Guild has run tests on Charles and the well twin to determine the nature of the kidney problem, the heart condition and contents of blood vessels and the overall physical condition. He found that Charles' kidneys are two percent effective. As a result the heart action is not good. He also found that Charles is very anemic. In Dr. Guild's judgment Charles will die within a matter of weeks.

Dr. John Hartwell Harrison of Brookline took the stand. . . . He obtained his surgical training at P.B.B.H. and has been on the staff there and on the Harvard Medical School faculty for 21 years.

Dr. Harrison then testified as to the procedures that would be followed in the operations. At the time of the operation the well twin is in one operating room and the sick twin is in a contiguous operating room, with access between the rooms. The operations are done simultaneously and on a very rigid time control. Dr. Harrison takes out the kidney from the donor twin at the moment when Dr. Joseph Murray has prepared the blood vessels in the sick twin so that a grafting may be done. When the kidney is removed from the well twin, it is placed in a sterile basin and grafted as rapidly as possible so that the kidney may be without oxygen for as short a time as possible. Dr. Murray attaches the blood vessels to the kidney. Thereafter Dr. Harrison attaches the kidney to the urinary tract.

Removal of the sick kidneys from the ill twin depends upon the ill twin's condition. The doctors try to remove the kidneys as soon as possible but it all depends upon the ill twin's response and condition.

Dr. Harrison further stated that this operation has been done in three cases on adults. In no case so far has there been any problem experienced with the donor of the kidney. In the case of the donees two had no trouble, one had some troubles, but all are now well.

As to the seriousness of the operation, Dr. Harrison said it is a major operation and all major operations are serious. As a result, the donor would be going through a major operation.

On cross-examination Mr. Lyman [the attorney for Mrs. Williams] asked whether the operation is successful only on identical twins. Dr. Harrison stated that that was true. Mr. Lyman asked whether the subject matter of the operation had been explained to John, and Dr. Harrison said yes.

Mr. Wait [the attorney for the hospital] asked on cross-examination what John had been told. Dr. Harrison stated that John had been told that the kidney would be taken out and put into Charles. He was further asked what John's circumstances would be after the removal of the kidney. Dr. Harrison said that John's condition would be satisfactory but he would have only one kidney. He would have to be careful in the case of infection or traumatic troubles. In other words, if the kidney became infected or hurt as a result of an accident the consequences would be very serious. Mr. Wait summarized the testimony as: "It is like a car with one tire, without a spare." Mr. Wait then asked Dr. Harrison whether the explanation to John had been spelled out in words of one syllable. Dr. Harrison answered that the situation had not gotten to that point but would be before the operation was done. Mr. Wait asked whether technicians and nurses in the employ of the hospital would have to assist at the operation and whether the operation would take place at P.B.B.H., and Dr. Harrison said yes to both portions of the question.

Dr. Joseph Murray of Wellesley took the stand. He stated that he is a surgeon . . . and had been on the staff of P.B.B.H. and is on the teaching staff of Harvard Medical School faculty. His specialty is plastic surgery. He said he had heard Dr. Harrison testify and agrees completely with his statement as to procedure. Dr. Murray was asked whether he had explained to John about the taking out of a kidney and putting it into Charles. Dr. Murray said he had explained the situation and had done so prior to the time of making the experimental skin graft. The skin graft has already been done. Cross-examination was waived on behalf of the doctors and P.B.B.H.

Dr. Christopher Standish, a psychiatrist, testified. . . . He is an assistant professor of psychiatry at the Harvard Medical School and formerly was in a teaching position at Boston University Medical School and on the staff at Massachusetts Memorial Hospital.

He examined John and tried in the beginning to get to know John, to understand his level of intelligence and John's understanding of what was said to him. He also examined John's processes of thought to see whether he understood about the risks of the operation, what he thought about leaving school to come to P.B.B.H., what his thoughts are as to his brother's illness. Dr. Standish testified that he is of the opinion that John appreciates the situation with respect to Charles and what can be done by a transplant operation. Dr. Standish has tried to estimate what John's feelings are in the sense of whether there was indecision as to the choice of permitting taking of a kidney or not or whether John looked upon it as a sort of childish game. Dr. Standish has concluded that John has a firm conviction that he should permit the kidney to be taken. This conviction does not arise with the intent to please either himself (John) or his mother or anyone else. Apparently John found no need to justify the decision. John said in effect: Charles is my twin and if Charles dies it will be very

rough. Dr. Standish said that at that point in the conversation John had begun to weep.

Dr. Standish said that he had ascertained from John that in March he (John) was first told of the possibility that Charles might be saved by John's giving a kidney. John gathered that his mother and the doctor had been discussing the subject. Dr. Standish said that John said that his mother had told him (John) that the choice lay with John. John's first reaction was: Why give Charles a kidney when Charles has a good one? (It was apparently explained to John that the second kidney would become ill also, but Dr. Standish did not so testify.)

Dr. Standish said he tried to ascertain what pressures there might be on John in connection with the making of the decision. John had told him that the only pressures had been against his giving a kidney. His mother had told him (John) that people said that John would have to be away from school and in the hospital for some time and that he might be ill. Others had said that the doctors were experimenting. John apparently gave Dr. Standish the understanding that none of these remarks had made any impression upon him (John).

Dr. Standish examined how John had made up his mind. It appeared that John visited Charles with his mother. Thereafter the doctor (in Iowa apparently) explained the function of the kidney and that the kidney was getting worse. It was at this time that John decided to give a kidney to his brother Charles. There apparently was no conflict in John's mind and the decision apparently came naturally. John's present state of mind is that he must give the kidney. His state of mind is calm on the subject of the giving of the kidney. John's only question is apparently why the court is worried and wishes that the decision would be made quickly. He cannot understand why it is any of the court's business and wants to get the operation over with so that he can go back to school and his girl friend.

Dr. Standish said that he examined the relationship between John and Charles and gave two illustrations of how they conducted themselves together in the course of everyday life. From time to time Charles would take a girl to the movies. John would go to the same movie show alone. Part way through the performance Charles would excuse himself and would say to the girl that when he came back he would give a password so that she would know it was Charles (presumably because the movie theater was dark). Charles would then go out and would meet John. He would tell John the password. John would go back and give the password to the girl and spend the rest of the evening with the girl without her knowing that there had been a substitution. Another illustration: John would make a bet with some other boy. If John won the bet Charles would go and collect the bet and then John would turn up and say he had not been paid. A third illustration occurred in school. Charles and John sat side by side. At times Charles would be prepared in his lessons and John would not. On one occasion there was a poetry assignment. Charles had recited. Just before John was going to be called upon John asked permission to be excused from the room. While John was out of the room Charles would move into John's place. Then John would come back into the room and sit in Charles' place. The teacher would then call on Charles thinking that John was being called upon to recite. Charles being prepared, would recite on behalf of John and the teacher would be none the wiser.

In the light of the foregoing, Dr. Standish was asked what he thought the emotional effect would be on John if the operation could not be performed. Dr. Standish said he was of the opinion that John felt that the identity of the two twins had been destroyed because one had healthy kidneys and the other ill kidneys. Hence if John could give a healthy kidney to Charles, then each would have a healthy kidney. In other words, Dr. Standish felt that there would be a beneficial emotional result to John if he (John) was permitted to give the kidney to his brother.

I telephoned Dr. Harrison. He had not heard what the decree may contain. I told him what the Judge had indicated but that we could not count on it until the decree had been signed and the Judge had made his findings of fact. I further emphasized to Dr. Harrison that if the Judge did enter a decree permitting the operation, this decree would be in no way binding in any other case in which twins were involved and that we would have to go through precisely the same procedure.

e.

Findings, Rulings, and Order of the Supreme Judicial Court

This is a petition for a declaratory decree brought under G.L. (Ter. Ed.) c. 231A, inserted by St. 1945, c. 582, § 1 heard by me upon a statement of agreed facts and oral testimony.

Mrs. Gail Williams, and her husband Frank Williams, are the parents of Charles Williams and John Williams, born November 28, 1943. They have their domicile in Sioux City, Iowa. Mrs. Williams is guardian or temporary guardian of her minor children appointed by Probate Court within this Commonwealth. She brings this petition as mother, guardian, and next friend. She is the only parent of the children who is in Massachusetts and presently available here to consent to the operation as parent. Her husband has appeared in the proceedings and adopted the allegations and prayers of the petition.

The defendant physicians are highly skilled physicians and surgeons on the staff of the defendant Peter Bent Brigham Hospital and have performed several successful kidney transplant operations. The petitioners have requested that the defendant physicians perform a transplant operation transferring a healthy kidney from John Williams, who has two healthy kidneys, to his brother Charles whose two kidneys are diseased. John appears to be in good health, and medical opinion is that no unusual risks are involved to John beyond the inevitable risk of a major surgical operation and the hazards incident to having only one kidney in the event of later injury to that one kidney.

For a period of several months, it has been apparent that Charles' kidneys were in a seriously deteriorating condition and the possibility of a transplant operation has been under medical consideration. John has been giving thought to his action in the matter during this period. Charles is now suffering from an advanced kidney ailment which will result in his death in a relatively short period unless a kidney from his identical twin brother is transplanted in him successfully. Such an operation is the only hope of saving Charles' life. Although the operation could be postponed for a time, it has greater chance of success in saving Charles if performed before Charles' condition reaches an emergency state. This type of operation has been successful in the experience of the defendant physicians, when performed on identical twins. Preliminary tests indicate that John and Charles are identical twins.

John testified before me. He is a boy of fourteen with good understanding and intelligence. He has been fully informed of and understands the nature of the operation and its possible risks and consequences. He has talked with a donor of a kidney in a similar operation. The mother of the boys has also been informed of the possible consequences and understands them. She consents to the operation. John and his mother desire that the operation take place and John's consent to it is the result of his own decision, free from pressure or coercion, made with admirable courage, generosity, and appreciation of the factors involved.

I find the facts stated above. I also find upon the testimony of John and of a qualified psychiatrist, who has examined John at length, (1) that if this operation is not performed and Charles dies, there is danger of serious emotional impact upon John, (*Brown* v. *Board of Education,* 347 U.S. 483, 493–494), and (2) that, because the risk of emotional disturbance will be reduced and because of the probability that John will be enabled by the operation to have the continued companionship of his twin brother, John will receive a benefit from the operation, and (3) that the operation, if the doctors decide to perform it, is necessary to John's future welfare and happiness.

This petition presents a proper case for a declaratory decree. Section 9 of c. 231A provides that such a petition as this lies "to remove, and

to afford relief from, uncertainty and insecurity with respect to rights, duties, status and other legal relations. . . ." It further provides that c. 231A should be liberally construed. Because of the fact that the defendants have been advised that they may become liable to the well twin in tort or suffer criminal prosecution if they operate or be liable in contract if they fail to operate, they are unwilling to undertake it. I am of opinion that an actual controversy has arisen so that a justiciable question is presented.

. . . I rule, as a matter of law, that it is proper for the defendant surgeons with the assistance of the defendant, the Peter Bent Brigham Hospital, its agents, and servants, to perform the operation described in the petition and the agreed statement of facts with the consent of the petitioner, Gail Williams, and her husband Frank Williams, and of John, and of Charles, if he is able to give it, without incurring any civil liability to John or to Charles or any criminal prosecutions.

*   *   *

B.
Appraising the Role of the Participants*

1.

In Formulating Policy

a.

Deciding about Choice of Subjects?

[i]
Bonner v. Moran
126 F.2d 121 (D.C. Cir. 1941)

GRONER, C. J.: This is an action for damages for assault and battery. There was a verdict and judgment for the defendant (appellee). The facts are these: Appellant, a colored boy residing in Washington city, was at the time of the events about to be stated 15 years of age. His cousin, Clara Howard, who lived in North Carolina, had been so severely burned that she had become a hopeless cripple. She was brought to Washington by her aunt, who was also the aunt of appellant, and taken to the charity clinic in the Episcopal Hospital, where she was seen by appellee, a

_____
* This appraisal section focuses on uncomprehending subjects. For a fuller exposition of the factors requiring appraisal, consult section D of Chapter Eleven, beginning at p. 818 *supra*.

physician specializing in plastic surgery. Appellee advised that a skin graft would help her, provided the blood of the donor matched. After a number of unsuccessful efforts to match her blood, the aunt persuaded appellant, then a student in junior high school, to go with her to the hospital for the purpose of having a blood test. His blood matched, and the aunt telephoned appellee, who came to the hospital and performed the first operation on appellant's side. His mother, with whom he lived, was ill at the time and knew nothing about the arrangement. After the operation, appellant returned home and while there advised his mother that he was going back to the hospital to have his side "fixed up." Instead, he remained and in the subsequent operations a tube of flesh was cut and formed from his arm pit to his waist line, and at the proper time one end of the tube was attached to his cousin in the effort to accomplish her relief. The result was unsatisfactory, because of improper circulation of the blood through the tube. Accordingly, the tube was severed, after appellant had lost a considerable amount of blood and himself required transfusions. The tube of flesh was later removed and appellant was released from the hospital. From beginning to end, he was there nearly two months.

There was the usual amount of contradictory evidence as to what occurred prior to the first operation and during the period when appellant was in the hospital. We notice this only for the purpose of saying that there was sufficient evidence, if believed by the jury, to show that appellant's mother never knew the nature of the operations or consented to them. At the close of all the evidence, appellant's counsel asked the court to instruct the jury that, before appellee could have the right to perform the operation, he must first have obtained the consent of appellant and of appellant's parents. The court declined so to instruct, but on the contrary told the jury that if they believed that appellant himself was capable of appreciating and did appreciate the nature and consequences of the operation and actually consented, or by his conduct impliedly consented, their verdict must be for the defendant. The decisive question on the appeal is the correctness of this charge to the jury.

*   *   *

. . . Here, as we have already seen, the question is whether the consent of a boy 15 years of age dispenses with the necessity of consent by his parents. The trial court decided that it did. In this the court followed Section 59 of the Law Institute *Restatement of the Law of Torts.* There it is stated that, if the child is capable of appreciating the nature, extent, and consequences of the invasion, his assent prevents the invasion from creating liability, even though the assent of the parent is expressly refused. The institute rule is bottomed on the principle that the very nature of rights of personality is freedom to dispose of one's own person as one pleases. But even if this conclusion be granted, it overlooks the infancy exception to such a rule. In deference to common experience, there is general recognition of the fact that many persons by reason of their youth are incapable of intelligent decision, as the result of which public policy demands legal protection of their personal as well as their property rights. The universal law, therefore, is that a minor cannot be held liable on his personal contracts or contracts for the disposition of his property. . . . Hence it is not at all surprising that, generally speaking, the rule has been considered to be that a surgeon has no legal right to operate upon a child without the consent of his parents or guardian.

There are, of course, exceptions to the rule.

One of them is in cases of emergency, when obviously an operation is necessary; others perhaps in cases in which the child has been emancipated, or where the parents are so remote as to make impracticable the obtaining of their consent in time to accomplish proper results. And where the child is close to maturity, it has been held that the surgeon may be justified in accepting his consent. But in all such cases the basic consideration is whether the proposed operation is for the benefit of the child and is done with a purpose of saving his life or limb. The circumstances in the instant case are wholly without the compass of any of these exceptions. Here the operation was entirely for the benefit of another and involved sacrifice on the part of the infant of fully two months of schooling, in addition to serious physical pain and possible results affecting his future life. This immature colored boy was subjected several times to treatment involving anesthesia, blood letting, and the removal of skin from his body, with at least some permanent marks of disfigurement.

*   *   *

As we have already indicated, the question here is different from that in any of the cases to which our attention has been drawn, for here we have a case of a surgical operation not for the benefit of the person operated on but for another, and also so involved in its technique as to require a mature mind to understand precisely what the donor was offering to give. We are constrained, therefore, to feel that the court below should, in the circumstances we have outlined, have instructed that the consent of the parent was necessary. Undoubtedly, the case from the doctor's standpoint is a hard one. At all times he was rendering, without compensation, his skill and professional services to alleviate pain and suffering. Doubtless this fact weighed with the jury, who regarded his activities in the matter as impelled wholly by humane and charitable motives. But by his own testimony it clearly appears that he failed to explain, even to the infant, the nature or extent of the proposed first operation. As to those which followed, he claims, and we assume correctly, that the matter was fully explained. And there is evidence that during the ensuing progress of the experiment the mother, too, was apprised of her son's heroism and gloried in the newspaper notoriety which followed, and which, as nearly as we can gather, resulted in public contributions of money for the boy's future education. Whether this attitude of the mother was a sufficient ratification, we have no need to decide, since that question is not now in the case. However, if on a new trial the evidence in this respect is substantially the same, the question whether there was consent by ratification should be submitted to the jury under appropriate instructions. And if, after the mother learned of the preliminary operation, she made no objection thereto but publicly expressed her pride in her son's courage and without remonstrance allowed him to return for the completion of the experiment, such action on her part would be tantamount to consent by implication; and that, in the circumstances, would be sufficient.

On the whole case, we are of opinion that there was error in giving the instruction objected to, and in refusing to instruct that the consent of the parent was necessary.

Reversed and remanded for a new trial.

NOTES

NOTE 1.

British Medical Research Council Responsibility in Investigations on Human Subjects*

*   *   *

The situation in respect to minors and mentally subnormal or mentally disordered persons is of particular difficulty. In the strict view of the [English] law parents and guardians of minors cannot give consent on their behalf to any procedures which are of no particular benefit to them and which may carry some risk of harm. Whilst English law does not fix any arbitrary age in this context, it may safely be assumed that the Courts will not regard a child of 12 years or under (or 14 years or under for boys in Scotland) as having the capacity to consent to any procedure which may involve him in an injury. Above this age the reality of any purported consent which may have been obtained is a question of fact and as with an adult the evidence would, if necessary, have to show that irrespective of age the person concerned fully understood the implications to himself of the procedures to which he was consenting.

In the case of those who are mentally subnormal or mentally disordered the reality of the consent given will fall to be judged by similar criteria to those which apply to the making of a will, contracting a marriage or otherwise taking decisions which have legal force as well as moral and social implications. When true consent in this sense cannot be obtained, procedures which are of no direct benefit and which might carry risk of harm to the subject should not be undertaken.

Even when true consent has been given by a minor or a mentally subnormal or mentally disordered person, considerations of ethics and prudence still require that, if possible, the assent of parents or guardians or relatives, as the case may be, should be obtained.

Investigations that are of no direct benefit to the individual require, therefore, that his true consent to them shall be explicitly obtained. After adequate explanation, the consent of an adult of sound mind and understanding can be relied upon to be true consent. In the case of children and young persons the question whether purported consent was true consent would in each case depend upon facts such as the age, intelligence, situation and character of the subject and the nature of the investigation. When the subject is below the age of 12 years, information requiring the performance of any procedure involving his body would need to be obtained incidentally to and without altering the nature of a procedure intended for his individual benefit.

*   *   *

NOTE 2.

William J. Curran and Henry K. Beecher Experimentation in Children*

*   *   *

One of the authors (H.K.B.) has been in correspondence with the British Medical Research Council concerning this statement. He asked for further information regarding the legal precedent or authority upon which the "strict view" of English law was based, since no legal citations had been provided in the original statement. The inquiry was referred to Sir Harvey Druitt, KCB, who answered by letter dated Dec. 16, 1968. Sir Harvey has allowed us to refer to and to quote from his letter. First, he writes that the legal position taken in the statement of the Research Council was based upon his advice. He then continues, "I am confident about

* Report of the Medical Research Council for 1962–63 (Cmnd. 2382) 23–24 (1963). Reprinted by permission.

* 210 *Journal of the American Medical Association* 77, 81 (1969). Reprinted by permission.

the correctness of that statement, but I cannot cite any statute or decided case which is exactly in point." The letter concludes with the following summary paragraph:

It follows from the foregoing that a parent's right to assault his child is in law strictly limited. No doubt the parent has the right to consent to a doctor carrying out upon his child medical procedures which are thought to be for the child's benefit. But I am confident that the parent has no legal authority to consent to medical procedures being carried out on his child for the advancement of scientific knowledge or for the benefit of humanity, if those procedures "are of no particular benefit to" the child and "may carry some risk of harm."

* * *

NOTE 3.

R. E. W. FISHER
CONTROLS*

It is a matter for regret that the use of normal children (or children suffering from some irrelevant disease) as controls in clinical research appears to be increasing.

No medical procedure involving the slightest risk or accompanied by the slightest physical or mental pain may be inflicted on a child for experimental purposes unless there is a reasonable chance, or at least a hope, that the child may benefit thereby.

If this is true—and I hope that there are few doctors in this country who would disagree—then it must surely be difficult to justify the use of two hydrocephalic infants reported in the paper by Dr. Doxiadis and his colleagues, and the use of a normal control by Dr. Bickel and his colleagues. Both papers appeared in your issue of October 17.

It may be, of course, that there were some good reasons for the use of these children which have not been made clear. If so, the authors owe it to themselves to explain.

NOTE 4.

K. S. HOLT
CONTROLS†

It is quite reasonable that Dr. Fisher should raise the question of the use of normal children or children suffering from some irrelevant dis-

ease as controls in clinical research. There are extreme opinions on both sides, but I feel most of us adopt a policy between the two—somewhere in the grey between the rather theoretical white and black. My own working policy, which differs slightly from that expounded by Dr. Fisher in the second paragraph of his letter, is that no procedure should be carried out involving risk or discomfort without a reasonable chance of benefit to that child *or other children;* and this principle was followed throughout our work. The crux of the matter is contained in the last sentence of Dr. Fisher's letter—we owe it to ourselves to explain our actions. Surely we all weigh these matters most carefully in our own consciences.

NOTE 5.

AMERICAN MEDICAL ASSOCIATION
ETHICAL GUIDELINES FOR CLINICAL
INVESTIGATION*

* * *

Minors or mentally incompetent persons may be used as subjects [in nontherapeutic situations primarily for the accumulation of scientific knowledge] only if:
i. The nature of the investigation is such that mentally competent adults would not be suitable subjects.
ii. Consent, in writing, is given by a legally authorized representative of the subject under circumstances in which an informed and prudent adult would reasonably be expected to volunteer himself or his child as a subject.

* * *

NOTE 6.

PRINCE v. MASSACHUSETTS
321 U.S. 158, 170 (1944)

MR. JUSTICE RUTLEDGE delivered the opinion of the Court:
[Appellant and her nine year-old niece, of whom she was custodian, were devout Jehovah's Witnesses. For allowing her niece to sell the sect's literature publicly, appellant was convicted under state statutes which prohibited "boys under twelve and girls under eighteen" from selling newspapers and magazines "in any street or public place" and also prohibited others from per-

---

* 2 *The Lancet* 993 (1953). Reprinted by permission.
† 2 *The Lancet* 993 (1953). Reprinted by permission.

* *Opinions and Reports of the Judicial Council.* Chicago: American Medical Association. 9–11 (1969). Reprinted by permission. *See* pp. 845–846 *supra.*

mitting such children to engage in these activities. She attacked the statutes' validity on equal protection and freedom of religion grounds.]

* * *

. . . Parents may be free to become martyrs themselves. But it does not follow they are free, in identical circumstances, to make martyrs of their children before they have reached the age of full and legal discretion when they can make that choice for themselves. . . .

* * *

NOTE 7.

DAVID DAUBE
TRANSPLANTATION—ACCEPTABILITY OF
PROCEDURES AND THE REQUIRED LEGAL
SANCTIONS*

* * *

Children should on no account be donors, and there should be no cheating by maintaining, for example, that the child would suffer a trauma if he were not allowed to give his twin a kidney or whatever it might be. The psychologist who alleged this danger is presumably identical with the one whose little daughter did not eat. He asked her what she wanted and she said "Daddy, I want a worm;" so he went into the garden and got a worm. She said "No, it must be a hairy one;" so he went again and got a hairy one. She then said "It must be cooked," so he cooked it. She said "Daddy, you must eat half it it;" he overcame his nausea and ate half of it. Then she burst into tears and said "That was the half I wanted!" The likelihood of a trauma, incidentally, will be greatly lessened if the law leaves not the shadow of a doubt that a transplantation is here out of the question: the case will then be no different from where a twin dies from pneumonia—bad enough, but with no scope for offer of a sacrifice, disappointment, self-torture.

I would, however, advocate extending the age of consent of donors downwards to roughly the age of conscription; that is why I referred to children in this context instead of to minors. I believe I owe this idea to Professor Woodruff with whom I discussed the subject a few years

_____
* G. E. W. Wolstenholme and Maeve O'Connor, eds.: *Ethics in Medical Progress—With Special Reference to Transplantation.* Boston: Little, Brown and Co. 198–199 (1966). Reprinted by permission of J. & A. Churchill, London.

ago. From an age when we encourage or even compel a person to lay down his life for his country, he should also be allowed to make a potential sacrifice for a near relation. This would mostly be seventeen or eighteen years. Of course, conscription does not exist everywhere: there are countries which do not contemplate war. I suppose marriage might count as an equivalent, which would give us about the same age. A friend observed to me that refusal to allow children to give organs will hamper medical progress. If this is so, it is regrettable, but medical progress must then be hampered; it might be impeded more seriously if the prohibition were not enforced and if, after some mishap, there were an indiscriminate public reaction. Anyway I do not believe anyone has the right to dispose of an organ from the body of a living child simply because this is a child.

* * *

[ii]
*The Editors of the British Medical Journal
Experiments on the Fetus**

The statement by Mr. Norman St. John-Stevas that "aborted live fetuses have been sold for medical experiments" has understandably caused some consternation. In a few words it raises at least three issues of great concern to the medical profession. These are, firstly, the use of living human organisms, not merely their tissues, for experiments; secondly, the sale of them; and, thirdly, the medical context. . . .

. . . That to save a mother's life or preserve her health one "human life" in that sense must on occasions be sacrificed is the justification for terminating pregnancy or even (though very rarely nowadays) destruction of the baby during parturition. But a clear implication of this ethical precept is that a distinction must be drawn between fetal tissues and the fetus as a living organism: the doctor's ethical obligations are different in the two circumstances. The use of tissues would not seem to raise any special problems, and the question of consent by the mother hardly arises if cells from disorganized fetal tissues that would otherwise be incinerated are used for experimental purposes. But what of a living fetus, removed by hysterotomy after perhaps several months' development?

_____
* 1 *British Medical Journal* 433–434 (1970). Reprinted by permission.

The question when human life begins is if anything more difficult than the much-discussed problem of when it ends. Yet the time may now have come when it must be seriously considered in relation to experiments in fetal physiology. . . .

A legally recognized human life is protected by the law of murder. That law protects only human beings who have been born alive—that is (in England), totally extruded from the body of the mother and having a circulation independent of the mother. Legal authorities give little assistance when considering the degree to which the criminal courts might interfere in the conduct of experiments on a fetus. Nor does the Infant Life (Preservation) Act of 1929 provide a definite answer. That Act created the offence of child destruction committed by anyone who wilfully causes a child to die "before it has an existence independent of its mother," and so it would probably not apply to a fetus killed after a short existence linked to a machine. But in any event the offence is committed only if the child was "capable of being born alive." While the Act provides that evidence of 28 weeks of gestation or more shall be prima facie proof that the child was capable of being born alive, it does not provide that this is the only possible evidence of that fact. Consequently, until science has advanced so far that it can be proved that a particular fetus was capable of being reared by machine to a fully independent life, the criminal law seems unlikely to intervene to protect its life provided it was lawfully detached from the mother.

* * *

The rearing of fetuses from a previable state to one of independent life is no longer a remote possibility, while the experimental work that must precede it has been carried out for some time on animals. Though the sale of fetuses, if it has ever been conducted, must surely be summarily condemned, thorough discussion of the ethical and legal aspects of the work itself is greatly needed and should be initiated soon, perhaps jointly by the B.M.A. and the Royal College of Obstetricians and Gynaecologists. The government is to set up an advisory group "to consider the ethical, medical, social, and legal implications of using fetuses or fetal material in research," and meanwhile the Department of Health has informed approved abortion clinics that they must not supply fetuses for research purposes. The general public must be heard on these debatable issues, and the medical profession has an obligation to assist lay people to understand the medical implications as well as to formulate its own collective thoughts. . . .

b.

Deciding about the Ambit of Experimentation?

Leon R. Kass
Freedom, Coercion, and Asexual Reproduction*

* * *

Our first experience with nuclear transplantation in human beings will almost certainly come on a small scale. The first attempt to clone a man will be an entirely voluntary undertaking on the part of a few people. No social coercion will be required; on the contrary, government and law need contribute only silent acquiescence.

Consider a likely first case. A husband and wife, each a carrier of a debilitating recessive genetic disease wish to have a child. They are unwilling to run the risk of having a child with the disease, a risk facing them in normal procreation. The husband is opposed to adoption; the wife very much wants to bear her own child. Knowledgeable about asexual reproduction by means of nuclear transplantation, they ask the experimental geneticist and his obstetrical colleagues to provide them with a child by cloning either husband or wife. The geneticist sees a natural marriage between his scientific interest in the outcome of the transplantation and his desire to help the couple have a healthy child. Confident as a result of much success in cloning chimpanzees, and encouraged by his opportunity to do good, he decides to risk the first human experiment.

What issues of freedom and coercion are raised by such a case? The existence of the technique of nuclear transplantation permits the couple to have a child without fear that it will acquire the disease for which they are both carriers. The right to procreate is for this couple a right they are not fully free to exercise: they are inhibited by a proper anxiety. Nuclear transplantation offers a new opportunity, and thus enhances their freedom. In the absence of societal and legal prohibitions, they will be free to use their new freedom. Should the law remain silent? It can be

* Unpublished manuscript 9–16, 21–24 (1970). Printed by permission of the author, who retains all rights.

argued that the use of nuclear transplantation in this instance, or in any other instance, should be prohibited, not because of any evil present in this case but because of evils likely to result from the widespread practice of cloning. In other words, the first case can be considered objectionable not in itself but for what it might lead to. Yet one can argue, on the other hand, that the possibility or even likelihood of future abuses of a technological development does not justify preventing the use of a technique on a proper scale, for proper ends, by appropriate men. . . . In considering these arguments we may agree that the likely social and moral costs of future widespread use and abuse need to be weighed in deciding about the first case. We might even insist that methods for controlling future use be developed before we permit first use. Nevertheless, an appropriate verdict would seem to require an evaluation of the merits of the specific case itself, setting to one side its importance as a precedent.

In my view, this hypothetical first attempt to clone a man—or any other proposed first case—can be criticized on ethical grounds even when it is considered singly and apart from its importance as a first case. Any moral assessment of this procedure, no less than of any other procedure, must consider the person on whom it is performed, in this case, the unborn child-to-be that develops from the egg with transplanted nucleus. In other words, the attempt to clone a man is an experiment on a human subject, albeit a potential one, and as such, should conform to our standards of ethical experimentation, standards which at minimum require the free consent of the human subject. My previous statement that "the first attempt to clone a man will be an entirely voluntary undertaking" was misleading. It can never be entirely voluntary; the will of one of the participants, a participant of at least equal rank despite his merely potential existence, can never be consulted. That the asexually reproduced individual might give consent in retrospect—or at least would not protest his origin—would be insufficient to establish the morality of performing the transplantation in the first place.

On first glance, it might seem that the argument just presented calls into question the morality of normal procreation. However, without minimizing the responsibility of parents for bringing a child into the world, we can recognize that normal procreation is never an experiment performed to produce *that particular* child. (Prop-

erly understood, procreation is not an experiment at all, despite its uncertain outcome; the distinction is between generating and making, between nature and art). In the language of genetics, all parents are responsible for the decision to generate a new genotype, but not for the particular genotype generated. Any child born naturally can perhaps legitimately complain about his having been generated without his consent, but he cannot hold his parents responsible for his particular genotype. Such a claim might justly be made by a person with genetic disease whose parents had foreknowledge that exercise of their right to procreate would result in a diseased child. If we acknowledge the justness of this claim where chance has played a large role and where probably only a single gene is involved, how much more just the claim against complete determination of genotype without consent?

The arguments made here do not speak to and hence do not weigh against interventions *in utero*, even genetic engineering *in utero*, where such interventions are for the purpose of correcting specific diseases or defects found to be present in the fetus. These interventions would be forms of therapy, and as such would be subject to the ordinary ethical standards of medical practice in children and in others incapable of giving their own consent. . . .

*   *   *

What are the reasons for asserting that the consent of the clonant cannot be assumed, for the above first case or for any other first case? What are the likely and legitimate grounds of his possible retrospective objection? In short, what's wrong with cloning? One issue is that of identity and individuality. The problem can be illustrated by exploiting the ambiguity of the word "identity": the clonant may experience serious concerns about his identity (distinctiveness) because his genotype, and hence appearance, stands in a relationship of identity (sameness) to another human being.

The natural occurrence of identical twins does not weaken an attack on the artificial production of identical humans; there are many things which occur by accident that ought not to be done by design (Who would justify the deliberate creation of an earthquake or the deliberate production of birth defects?) In fact, the problem of identity faced by identical twins should instruct us and enable us to recognize how much greater the problem might be for someone who was the "child" (or "father") of his twin. I cannot improve upon Paul Ramsey's reflections on this subject:

Growing up as a twin is difficult enough anyway; one's struggle for selfhood and identity must be against the very human being for whom no doubt there is also the greatest sympathy. Who then would want to be the son or daughter of his twin? To mix the parental and the twin relation might well be psychologically disastrous for the young. Or to look at it from the point of view of parents, it is an awful enough responsibility to be the parent of a son or daughter as things now are. Our children begin with a unique genetic independence of us, analogous to the personal independence that sooner or later will have to be granted them or wrested from us. For us to choose to replicate ourselves in them, to make ourselves the foreknowers and creators of every one of their genetic predispositions, might well prove to be a psychological and personally unendurable undertaking. For an elder to teach his "infant copy" is a repellent idea not because of the strangeness of it, but because we are althogether too familiar with the problems this would exponentially make more difficult.*

* * *

Fabrication is a second major issue. Is it not reasonable to suppose that the first clonant might resent the trademark "Made by the Departments of Genetics and Obstetrics, Brave New University School of Medicine"? Can we assert the natural right of an individual not to be manufactured? Again, we face a strange question, one which could not have been imagined in earlier discussions of natural rights.

This question needs to be clarified by emphasizing that the issue of fabrication goes far beyond any similar issue attending artificial insemination or even "test-tube fertilization." Both of these techniques are sexual, even if only in the genetic sense. The particular genotype which results is the product of chance, even if both egg and sperm are taken from selected donors. Cloning is manipulation with a vengeance; it means the virtual elimination of chance. . . .

* * *

To return to our cloned individual. To claim for him or for us the right to an indeterminate origin is not merely a sentimental preference for "the natural" or "the accidental." On the contrary, it reflects a prudent judgment about alternative unpredictable masters. The right not to be

manufactured protects the individual against the far greater capriciousness of the human artificer.

* * *

c.

Deciding about Harm?

Susan W. Gray
Ethical Issues in Research
in Early Childhood Intervention*

In a sense this paper . . . examine[s] the ethical issues involved in research on the effects of planned intervention early in a child's life. In another sense, however, I am presenting here a somewhat personal account of over a decade of involvement in intervention research with young children from low-income families. . . .

* * *

Intervention research . . . imposes some special characteristics of its own. It is necessarily longitudinal—that is, it takes place over a considerable period of time. Typically many changes, some intentional and others not, are introduced into the system—the child and his world. The objectives are apt to relate to motivational characteristics and also to various facets of intellectual competence. Thus, the program may touch not only the persons who are its specific targets but also those with whom they live and associate. The effects are intended to be lasting and substantial. . . .

A decade ago developmental "interveners" were seldom questioned about their motives and general intentions. It was usually taken for granted that a program that had clear implications for human welfare originated from positive motives. Today questions arise, particularly from members of minority groups, concerning such motivation. The majority of these questions have little to do with methods of research, but rather with intervention as such, whether in a service or a research program. . . .

Some objections center on the rights of parents. There is certainly no question from the legal standpoint that the parent is completely responsible for the child and has a full right to grant *or* withhold consent for the preschool child's participation in any program—up to a point. . . . The more difficult question perhaps is whether the parents' rights extend to decision-making with respect to the intervention program itself and in-

---

* Paul Ramsey, *Fabricated Man.* New Haven: Yale University Press 71–72 (1970).

---

* 18 *Children* 83–89 (1971). Reprinted by permission.

clude the right to dictate the program's methods and goals. This is not an easy issue to resolve. . . .

Other questions go beyond the parents' rights. One criticism leveled at developmental interveners these days is often put this way: How do you dare to work simply with young children when the basic problem is the entire social system?

This question, of course, implies a certain lack of distinction between a child development worker's professional role and his civic role. Asking a developmental intervener to work to change the whole social system is about as inappropriate as asking a thoracic surgeon why he does not give up the practice of lung surgery and instead work on outlawing cigarettes and certain pollutants in the atmosphere. The answer must be that it is highly appropriate for the professional person to engage in social action in his role as a citizen, but to expect him to devote his entire time to such efforts ignores the ethical imperative for using most productively his particular competence in promoting human welfare.

*   *   *

In his civic role the citizen-scientist can appropriately work to change the social system or environment that has created some of the problems to which his research addresses itself. In his scientific role, his first concern ethically should be to carry on his research to the best of his ability.

Another broad issue that comes under the general questioning by the public today has to do with the goals and values of the intervener. The issue typically is brought up by members of minority groups or persons who see themselves as spokesmen for minority groups. Many of their questions are highly relevant. The usual accusation is that interveners are promoting a white middle-class model of what is appropriate behavior when dealing with other ethnic groups. Obviously, intervention programs can confound, or can be perceived as confounding, elements of social class and race, for the representation of minority groups—especially the black, the Spanish-speaking, and the American Indian—in the low-income segment of the population is disproportionately high.

Developmental interveners are often accused of working with a theoretical model based on an assumption of deficiency in the subject. In theory we all speak about cultural differences; in practice many of us are concerned with cultural deficiencies. Today these terms are laden with emotion and provoke bitter criticism. In a sense the accusation is just.

There are two ways, however, to look at cultural deficiencies. One is to take the view that a given culture simply tends to be deficient; some cultures are better—presumably in God's eyes —than others. Few social or behavioral scientists would defend such a stand. The other view, a broader one, emphasizes cultural differences among segments of our society but looks at and attempts to remedy the "deficiencies" of a given subculture in relation to a specific societal demand. If we accept the point of view that the technological civilization of the 1970's rewards the person who can read more than the person who cannot read, then we have a case for intervening to correct a specific deficiency—if a person wishes to take advantage of these rewards. Some subcultures have child-rearing practices that make learning to read more of a problem for their children than it is for children generally. . . .

The issue of cultural differences versus cultural deficiencies is, of course, confounded with the failure to distinguish the differences in social class. A few years ago a great deal of professional attention was being directed towards the concept of a "culture of poverty." Those who espouse this concept believe that patterns of coping develop in extreme poverty and that certain of these patterns are institutionalized—that is, they are adaptive to living in poverty but may be maladaptive to moving out of poverty. . . .

*   *   *

The confounding of social class differences with true cultural differences has led to problems in planning intervention programs and in observers' interpretations of these programs. How we resolve these problems is probably going to depend in part upon our view of how we should deal with cultural differences.

We could follow the old American philosophy of a melting-pot society. Today, however, many minority groups are becoming less and less willing to be melted down. We could ignore cultural differences—a rather unsatisfactory approach since it does not work. We could use cultural differences to build a bridge for meeting the demands of the larger society.

This last approach is the one used by many of the more carefully planned intervention programs. The child is taken "where he is." His first reading materials, for example, are based upon experiences that are familiar to him. So far so good; most interveners would "buy" this in relation to certain skills and areas of understanding that are regarded as necessary for a person to have in our ever-contracting globe. The problem is how far interveners should go in this direction.

The more thoughtful intervention programs today, as well as the general trends in our society, seem to reflect a move toward a degree of "cultural pluralism." Ideally, under cultural pluralism many different groups live in the same society with mutual respect, and mobility from group to group is possible not only over an extended period of time but also immediately.

*　　*　　*

My suggestion for resolving these issues is certainly not unique, but it is one with which I can live. It is that an appropriate goal in intervention programs is to make possible more options for the individual in his childhood and in adulthood.

One of the most characteristic aspects of poverty is that the poor have no options. The extremely poor must live hand to month, day by day, because they are at the mercy of external circumstances; they cannot take advantage of opportunities nor can they plan ahead. In a very different way, certain cultures tend to restrict individual experiences regardless of socio-economic class. Take, for example, the Amish. In the view of the "old order" Amish, education should be simply teaching the child to read well enough to read the Bible and to cipher well enough to figure simple quantities on the farm. There is some evidence that the Amish children experience adjustment problems in school because of the discrepancies between the school's and their families' values. The way of life of the old order Amish has much to recommend it, but many people would question a view of education that systematically limits the options for the coming generation.

A society that maximizes options may be one having a degree of cultural pluralism but enough commonality in the education of the young to make a range of choices available to all. This approach should not be regarded as based on a belief that the schools and society are always right or that early childhood intervention alone can resolve their problems. Clearly, throughout society, including the schools, many changes are needed to widen the options for young people. The research intervener, however, may appropriately make his scientific contribution by developing knowledge that can be used to improve the ability of young children and their parents to take advantage of these options as they become available or to open up more options themselves.

*　　*　　*

Let us look now at some specific ethical principles. Paramount among these is the importance of remembering that in intervention research *you can't do just one thing.* In attempting to make relatively large and enduring changes in a child and his world, we generally take as the point of entry the child himself, although we may take the mother and child together. However, no matter what the point of entry, when one is trying to make profound changes in a system, one must work with due regard to all the aspects of that system, including the relationships involved. Furthermore, one cannot ethically terminate an intervention program without making whatever provision possible for some type of continuation or sustaining treatment. Herein lies the reason for the increasing emphasis in intervention programs on work with parents and for the establishment of Follow Through programs to pick up in the first grade where Head Start leaves off.

Another principle is the avoidance of the invasion of privacy. . . . What one family regards as intrusion may be interpreted simply as friendly interest by another family. A person can easily learn not to pry; it is not so easy to identify the line between intrusion and an appropriate interest in the concerns of the person with whom one is working.

Another problem associated with the invasion of privacy is that work with young children and parents from poverty-stricken homes is good newspaper copy. [I]t is difficult to provide public recognition of the needs of the poor without some invasion of privacy, particularly by local news sources. Our solution, not always successful, has been to avoid all publicity until a study has been completed. We have, however, felt an obligation to communicate findings that might be helpful to others, always avoiding the release of any identifying data. It is not always possible, however, to avoid premature publicity. The only solution we have found is to work with reporters of local newspapers and TV stations to try to help them understand why it is important to withhold publicity at a particular time.

Another important ethical principle—one not always honored—is to show respect for the dignity of the individual, whether a little child or an adult. This seems obvious. But persons with a strong middle-class bias are not always able to respect persons whose ways are different from their own. It is not always easy for an inexperienced, middle-class worker to hide an aversion to clutter or to conceal annoyance over complete apathy in the face of a solvable problem. Consequently, a research director must exercise extreme caution in selecting staff members, to be sure that they can show true respect.

*　　*　　*

A well-known ethical principle requires that "informed consent" be obtained from the child's parents and from the child himself if old enough to understand. . . .

Much of our research is carried on with children who are far too young to understand. The answer, we say, is to inform and get counsel from the parent, by which we usually mean the mother. Well and good, but how can one really inform the parent if the parent has very limited understanding of the principles of child development? Still, one must try to give the parent as great an understanding of the goals and methods of the program as possible. If the principle of informed consent were applied literally, however, most intervention research would have to cease.

My own answer to the dilemma of informed consent is this: intervention researchers should inform the mother as best they can and then should work with her over a period of time to make more options available to her in her interactions with her child. Of greatest importance, perhaps, are efforts to help the mother increase her understanding of and competence in carrying out the acts that will　be instrumental in achieving her own goals for the child.

Thus, informed consent in intervention research involves a collaborative approach. It also involves another principle: one must be very careful not to raise false hopes. The best guide is complete honesty with the parent.

Another ethical dilemma facing the developmental intervener derives from the discrepancies in the values between generations. We know next to nothing of the future of the infants with whom we work. . . . Since the future is largely unknown, the major emphasis of an educational program for any human being might well be placed on the development of the qualities and characteristics that make learning possible. Perhaps the only thing we know about life 20 years from now is that the competencies required of people will be different from those required today.

*　　*　　*

d.

Deciding about Interests of Science and Society?

[i]

The Editors of the New England Journal of Medicine
"Judgment Difficult"*

*　　*　　*

Since infants and young children cannot be expected to comprehend the procedures to which they may be subjected, parental permission has been accepted as a substitute for that of the subject, and the World Medical Association's Draft Code of Ethics on Human Experimentation . . . provides that parents should have complete freedom to make decisions on behalf of children. One may even question the moral legitimacy of such freedom and, in the light of present knowledge of the way in which parental responsibility is sometimes discharged, this could sometimes be of little value in protecting the human rights of the individual. Children in institutions and not under the care of relatives, according to the Code, should not be the subject of human experiment. Certainly a procedure must be really innocuous in most cases and relatively so in the remainder, and the expected reward in terms of potential benefit to the individual and all mankind must be the greater, the greater the risk; the desired end should always be of sufficient value to justify the means. . . .

[ii]

Ross G. Mitchell
The Child and Experimental Medicine†

*　　*　　*

The former practice of subjecting "charity children," orphans, or mentally defective children to procedures which would be considered undesirable for more fortunately placed children is wholly objectionable and morally indefensible. By the same token, however, there is no fundamental reason why children in hospital should be considered ineligible, since no unethical experiment should be contemplated in any case. There are certain disadvantages in this practice, however, apart from the obvious scientific one that children in hospital are seldom "healthy." The

---

* 269 *New England Journal of Medicine* 479 (1962). Reprinted by permission.

† 1 *British Medical Journal* 722, 725–726 (1964). Reprinted by permission.

hospital is a friendly and homely place to the paediatrician and others who spend their lives in it, but it may be terrifying to some young children, who appear docile and cooperative but are really fearful and resentful. Unnecessary investigation must be kept to a minimum in such children, so that they are generally unsuitable for experimental investigation unless this is essential for their recovery. On the other hand, many older children really enjoy life in hospital and are pleased to be the center of attraction in the ward. After years of working in children's wards, one learns to recognize the different reactions of children and the meaning of different sorts of behavior—this is one further attribute of the paediatrician as investigator, that he knows which patients are emotionally suited to participation in experimental research. Special care must be taken, of course, that children in hospital are not used in preference to other more suitable children simply because they are accessible, and the difficulties inherent in obtaining observations on healthy control subjects must be faced squarely, even at the cost of greatly increased effort and expense.

. . . Sometimes it is suggested that experiments of doubtful propriety are permissible on babies with severe malformations. To me, this is an affront to the whole concept of the individual as a person, and I do not believe that any experiment should be carried out on a malformed child which would place the malformed child in a separate category, thus creating two types of human being and paving the way for Hitlerian ideas of inferior beings.

*   *   *

2.
In Administering Research

a.

Who Should Participate, within What Structure, in State Regulation?

[i]
Strunk v. Strunk
445 S.W. 2d 145 (Ky. 1969)

OSBORNE, JUDGE.

The specific question involved upon this appeal is: Does a court of equity have the power to permit a kidney to be removed from an incompetent ward of the state upon petition of his committee, who is also his mother, for the purpose of being transplanted into the body of his brother, who is dying of a fatal kidney disease? We are of the opinion it does.

The facts of the case are as follows: Arthur L. Strunk, 54 years of age, and Ava Strunk, 52 years of age, of Williamstown, Kentucky, are the parents of two sons. Tommy Strunk is 28 years of age, married, an employee of the Penn State Railroad and a part-time student at the University of Cincinnati. Tommy is now suffering from chronic glomerulus nephritis, a fatal kidney disease. He is now being kept alive by frequent treatment on an artificial kidney, a procedure which cannot be continued much longer.

Jerry Strunk is 27 years of age, incompetent and through proper legal proceedings has been committed to the Frankfort State Hospital and School, which is a state institution maintained for the feeble-minded. He has an I.Q. of approximately 35, which corresponds with the mental age of approximately 6 years. He is further handicapped by a speech defect, which makes it difficult for him to communicate with persons who are not well acquainted with him. When it was determined that Tommy, in order to survive, would have to have a kidney the doctors considered the possibility of using a kidney from a cadaver if and when one became available or one from a live donor if this could be made available. The entire family, his mother, father and a number of collateral relatives were tested. Because of incompatibility of blood type or tissue none were medically acceptable as live donors. As a last resort, Jerry was tested and found to be highly acceptable. This immediately presented the legal problem as to what, if anything, could be done by the family, especially the mother and the father, to procure a transplant from Jerry to Tommy. The mother as a committee petitioned the county court for authority to proceed with the operation. The court found that the operation was necessary, that under the peculiar circumstances of this case it would not only be beneficial to Tommy but also beneficial to Jerry because Jerry was greatly dependent upon Tommy, emotionally and psychologically, and that his well-being would be jeopardized more severely by the loss of his brother than by the removal of a kidney.

Appeal was taken to the Franklin Circuit Court where the chancellor reviewed the record, examined the testimony of the witnesses and adopted the findings of the county court.

A psychiatrist, in attendance to Jerry, who

testified in the case, stated in his opinion the death of Tommy under these circumstances would have "an extremely traumatic effect upon him" (Jerry).

The Department of Mental Health of this Commonwealth has entered the case as amicus curiae and, on the basis of its evaluation of the seriousness of the operation as opposed to the traumatic effect upon Jerry as a result of the loss of Tommy, recommended to the court that Jerry be permitted to undergo the surgery. Its recommendations are as follows:

It is difficult for the mental defective to establish a firm sense of identity with another person and the acquisition of this necessary identity is dependent upon a person whom one can conveniently accept as a model and who at the same time is sufficiently flexible to allow the defective to detach himself with reassurances of continuity. His need to be social is not so much the necessity of a formal and mechanical contact with other human beings as it is the necessity of a close intimacy with other men, the desirability of a real community of feeling, an urgent need for a unity of understanding. Purely mechanical and formal contact with other men does not offer any treatment for the behavior of a mental defective; only those who are able to communicate intimately are of value to hospital treatment in these cases. And this generally is a member of the family.

In view of this knowledge, we now have particular interest in this case. Jerry Strunk, a mental defective, has emotions and reactions on a scale comparable to that of normal persons. He identifies with his brother Tom; Tom is his model, his tie with his family. Tom's life is vital to the continuity of Jerry's improvement at Frankfort State Hospital and School. The testimony of the hospital representative reflected the importance to Jerry of his visits with his family and the constant inquiries Jerry made about Tom's coming to see him. Jerry is aware he plays a role in the relief of this tension. We, the Department of Mental Health, must take all possible steps to prevent the occurrence of any guilt feelings Jerry would have if Tom were to die.

The necessity of Tom's life to Jerry's treatment and eventual rehabilitation is clearer in view of the fact that Tom is his only living sibling and at the death of their parents, now in their fifties, Jerry will have no concerned, intimate communication so necessary to his stability and optimal functioning.

The evidence shows that at the present level of medical knowledge, it is quite remote that Tom would be able to survive several cadaver transplants. Tom has a much better chance of survival if the kidney transplant from Jerry takes place.

Upon this appeal we are faced with the fact that all members of the immediate family have recommended the transplant. The Department of Mental Health has likewise made its recommendation. The county court has given its approval. The circuit court has found that it would be to the best interest of the ward of the state that the procedure be carried out. Throughout the legal proceedings, Jerry has been represented by a guardian ad litem, who has continually questioned the power of the state to authorize the removal of an organ from the body of an incompetent who is a ward of the state. We are fully cognizant of the fact that the question before us is unique. Insofar as we have been able to learn, no similar set of facts has come before the highest court of any of the states of this nation or the federal courts. The English courts have apparently taken a broad view of the inherent power of the equity courts with regard to incompetents. Ex parte *Whitebread* (1816), 2 Mer. 99; 35 E.R. 878, L.C. holds that courts of equity have the inherent power to make provisions for a needy brother out of the estate of an incompetent. This was first followed in this country in New York, *In the Matter of Willoughby,* a Lunatic, 11 Paige 257 (NY 1844). The inherent rule in these cases is that the chancellor has the power to deal with the estate of the incompetent in the same manner as the incompetent would if he had his faculties. This rule has been extended to cover not only matters of property but also to cover the personal affairs of the incompetent. . . .

*   *   *

. . . Testimony in this record shows that there have been over 2500 kidney transplants performed in the United States up to this date. The process can be effected under present techniques with minimal danger to both the donor and the donee. Doctors Hamburger and Crosneir describe the risk to the donor as follows:

This discussion is limited to renal transplantation, since it is inconceivable that any vital organ other than the kidney might ever be removed from a healthy living donor for transplantation purposes. The immediate operative risk of unilateral nephrectomy in a healthy subject has been calculated as approximately 0.05 per cent. The long-term risk is more difficult to estimate, since the various types of renal disease do not appear to be more frequent or more severe in individuals with solitary kidneys than in normal subjects. On the other hand, the development of surgical problems, trauma or neoplasms, with the possible necessity of nephrectomy, do increase the long-term risks in living donors; the long-term risk, on this basis, has been estimated at 0.07 per cent. These data must, however, be considered in the light of statistical life expectancy which, in a healthy 35-year-old adult, goes from 99.3 per cent to 99.1 per cent during the next five succeeding years; this is an increase in risk equal to that incurred by driving a car for 16 miles every working day (Merrill, 1964). The risks incurred by the donor are therefore very limited, but they are a reality, even if, until now, there have been no reports of complications endangering the life of a donor anywhere in the world. Unfortunately, there is no doubt that, as the number of renal transplants increases, such an incident will inevitably be recorded.*

* * *

We are of the opinion that a chancery court does have sufficient inherent power to authorize the operation. The circuit court having found that the operative procedures in this instance are to the best interest of Jerry Strunk and this finding having been based upon substantial evidence, we are of the opinion the judgment should be affirmed. . . .

STEINFELD, JUDGE (dissenting):

Apparently because of my indelible recollection of a government which, to the everlasting shame of its citizens, embarked on a program of genocide and experimentation with human bodies I have been more troubled in reaching a decision in this case than in any other. My sympathies and emotions are torn between a compassion to aid an ailing young man and a duty to fully protect unfortunate members of society.

The opinion of the majority is predicated upon the authority of an equity court to speak for one who cannot speak for himself. However, it is my opinion that in considering such a right in this instance we must first look to the power and authority vested in the committee, the appellee herein. KRS 387.060 and KRS 387.230 do nothing more than give the committee the power to take custody of the incompetent and the possession, care and management of his property. Courts have restricted the activities of the committee to that which is for the best interest of the incompetent. . . . The authority and duty have been to protect and maintain the ward, to secure that to which he is entitled and preserve that which he has. . . .

* * *

The majority opinion is predicated upon the finding of the circuit court that there will be psychological benefits to the ward but points out that the incompetent has the mentality of a 6-year-old child. It is common knowledge beyond dispute that the loss of a close relative or a friend to a 6-year-old child is not of major impact. Opinions concerning psychological trauma are at best most nebulous. Furthermore, there are no guarantees that the transplant will become a surgical success, it being well known that body rejection of transplanted organs is frequent. The life of the incompetent is not in danger, but the surgical procedure advocated creates some peril.

* * *

Unquestionably the attitudes and attempts of the committee and members of the family of the two young men whose critical problems now confront us are commendable, natural and beyond reproach. However, they refer us to nothing indicating that they are privileged to authorize the removal of one of the kidneys of the incompetent for the purpose of donation, and they cite no statutory or other authority vesting such right in the courts. The proof shows that less compatible donors are available and that the kidney of a cadaver could be used, although the odds of operational success are not as great in such a case as they would be with the fully compatible donor brother.

I am unwilling to hold that the gates should be open to permit the removal of an organ from an incompetent for transplant, at least until such time as it is conclusively demonstrated that it will be of significant benefit to the incompetent. The evidence here does not rise to that pinnacle. To hold that committees, guardians or courts have such awesome power even in the persuasive case before us, could establish legal precedent, the dire result of which we cannot fathom. Regretfully I must say no.

NOTE

WILLIAM J. CURRAN
A PROBLEM OF CONSENT—KIDNEY
TRANSPLANTATION IN MINORS*

During 1957 the Supreme Judicial Court of Massachusetts issued three highly significant opinions in declaratory judgment proceedings in a developing area of medical science: the homo-transplantation of functioning tissue. . . .

* * *

---

* Hamburger and Crosneir, "Moral and Ethical Problems in Transplantation," in *Human Transplantation* 37 (Rapaport and Dausset ed. 1968).

---

* 34 *New York University Law Review* 891, 893–898 (1959). Reprinted by permission.

In each of the three cases, the court relied on the testimony of a psychiatrist. . . . The use of psychiatric evidence in support of a finding such as this is similar to the method used in the famous school segregation case, *Brown* v. *Board of Education,* where the Supreme Court was strongly impressed with the evidence of the bad psychological and cultural effect of "separate but equal" school facilities on Negroes in the South. The use of this technique in *Brown* has received generally praiseworthy comment, but the writer cannot help but recall the masterly critique of this portion of the segregation decision by Edmond Cahn. Professor Cahn questioned the value of much of the "scientific proof" produced by the social scientists in their famous special brief in that case. . . . Many years before, [Charles C.] Moore issued similar complaints about the "new science" of psychology and what he felt to be its much too ambitious claims to usefulness in the courts. Basically, he said the psychologists were merely offering common sense in technical jargon, a common sense which had been used in the courts for years. One can see the same objections being made to the psychiatric opinions in the kidney transplant cases. It hardly seems that psychiatric evidence is necessary to convince anyone that a healthy identical twin would suffer a grave emotional impact on the death of his twin brother. This statement does, of course, rest on an important assumption on which psychiatric opinion may be valuable. It assumes that the donor twin is within normal intelligence levels and experiences normal emotional responses. And yet, every lawyer knows that courts make their own judgments on issues of this type every day without expert testimony. In the kidney transplant cases, for example, the justice presiding at each hearing determined for himself by questioning of the donor twin whether or not the twin was intelligent enough to understand the nature and consequences of the operation and fully and freely consented to it. This determination was equally as difficult and as technical as the question of sustaining a "grave emotional loss" on the death of the sick twin.

*   *   *

In the instant case, we see a rather unique involvement of community and professional judgments in a narrow issue, *i.e.,* whether a minor should be allowed to donate a kidney to a twin sibling under very serious circumstances. The family and both twins are involved and must understand and consent. The hospital and the surgeons are vitally concerned. The court steps in as a "community" representative, more or less, and it relies on another professional judgment, that of a psychiatrist, in reaching its conclusion. The ubiquitous declaratory judgment procedure is used to accomplish this result, and with, as is becoming more and more usual in these proceedings, no real controversy or likelihood of litigation between the parties.

*   *   *

. . . What would the situation be if the twins were willing to go through with the operation, but the parents refused? . . . In the ordinary case of parental refusal to allow medical procedures on their children, many states have legislation allowing a state agency, usually a Child Welfare Department, to take temporary custody of the child as a "neglected child" for a period sufficient to obtain the needed treatment. These statutes are limited to cases of very serious emergency treatment, however. It is doubtful that they would cover taking custody of the healthy twin unless some theory of benefit such as that suggested in these opinions prevailed.

[W]e keep coming back to the issue of a lack of direct therapeutic benefit to the healthy twin. We might have been more satisfied had the court met it more directly. Actually the benefit found by the court with the aid of the psychiatric evidence is more the prevention of possible detriment than it is the conferring of a positive gain. As life will have it, this is brought to mind most strongly today by the fact that of the transplants attempted in these cases only one has survived to this date. The younger children who received the kidneys . . . died some months after the operations.

*   *   *

[ii]
Joseph D. Cooper
*Creative Pluralism—Medical Ombudsman**

The clamor for practical application of discoveries of biomedical knowledge grows louder. Medical researchers are being told they must release the secrets of their laboratories to physi-

---

* *Research in the Service of Man—Hearings on Biomedical Development, Evaluation of Existing Federal Institutions before the Subcommittee on Government Research of the Senate Committee on Government Operations,* 90th Congress, 1st Session 46–61 (1967).

cians for the public benefit. This poses quite a problem for the research community which must ask itself: What are we holding back?

The situation is not an unexpected one. Sooner or later, an impatient public was bound to ask for delivery on promises made recurringly that the conquest of innumerable diseases would be achieved quickly if only enough were spent in a hurry.

*   *   *

. . . In our haste to win the medical wars—society's haste—and to enjoy promised fruits of conquest, we are adventuring beyond prudent limits of risk. The hope becomes the theory which leads to selective discovery of evidence to support the wish, while contrary evidence which might slow the pace is ignored or rationalized away. This naturally stems from single-minded advocacy which sometimes has led to great gains, but more often has blocked or retarded action along other avenues of progress.

What is wrong is the absence of mechanisms for obliging proponents of action to offer evidence, in reasonable depth, to independent judges who do not have causes to espouse. Consequently, it has been too easy for bold new programs in the medical sector to come into being without scientific bases for promises or hope that benefits could or would materialize. Once activated these new programs become irreversibly committed because of public promises, dependence of program personnel on continuity of support, and force of legislation.

As an example of prematurity and the lack of constructive challenge which once was more dominant in scientific discourse, I will discuss the national program to prevent a rare disease called phenylketonuria, a disease which often results in mental retardation.

*   *   *

Phenylketonuria, more commonly called PKU, is a genetically acquired disease commonly associated with mental retardation, although some phenylketonuric babies grow up to be normal or bright without treatment. Apart from, or in addition to, retardation, the child may have postural peculiarities, convulsive or jerking movements, and a characteristic musty body odor, among other symptoms. PKU belongs to a disease category called "inborn errors of metabolism". . . .

For the symptomatic child and its parents, PKU is a calamity. For society generally, PKU

is a rare disease. The incidence of the disease is estimated, on the high side, about 1 out of every 10,000 births. On the low side, the incidence has been estimated at 1 in 25,000 or lower. A true figure cannot really be given due to errors of diagnosis which may yield either false positives or false negatives and to difficulties of projecting statistically from small samples. . . .

The institutional population of phenylketonurics is also relatively rare, having been estimated at considerably less than 1 percent (0.793 percent). . . .

Why, one may ask, is this disease so much in the public view, despite its relative rarity? The reasons mainly are these:

1. Universally, mothers are fearful of having a child with a birth defect. . . .

2. Close to 6 million Americans are mentally retarded in varying degree. Mental retardation is the single largest category of childhood disease. . . . A broad base of missionary interest is to be found, therefore, among parents and lay voluntary groups.

3. A medical breakthrough in PKU and other metabolic disorders associated with retardation was hailed both symbolically and practically as an opening wedge—as a gain which would be followed by other breakthroughs which eventually would reduce the incidence of mental retardation. A national PKU crusade was therefore organized by voluntary health agencies, working through government agencies and state legislatures, partly to control this disease and partly to bolster the spirits of those who seek anxiously for additional gains.

4. There existed a small but active group of physicians and medical researchers who had begun to build investigational interests and careers around the phenomena of the "inborn errors of metabolism." Some—not all—of the more actively disposed of these medical personalities involved themselves in the promotion of the PKU program. They became the advisers to legislators, government administrators, and voluntary health organizations. Out of the fusion of their own professional convictions and career interests emerged a professional evangelism.

5. The public was eager for delivery of new medical breakthroughs which it had been promised and for which it had been primed through the successive miracles of the sulfonamides, antibiotics, and poliomyelitis vaccines. . . .

I shall review now some of the things known about PKU. Phenylketonuria is a metabolic defect transmitted genetically as a Mendelian recessive factor. This disease was first recognized and described in 1934. Detection at birth was difficult because the development of the child with phenylketonuric symptoms progresses quite normally during the first few months of life. Thereafter, intellectual growth is retarded. This is believed to be caused by the failure of a liver enzyme to metabolize the amino acid phenylalanine whose excessiveness in the bloodstream causes brain damage.

For some years after this disease had been defined and was made recognizable, medical science could offer little more than identification and explanation. A major advance which permitted widespread screening economically was the development of a simple urine test. This test was not wholly satisfactory because the presence of phenylpyruvic acid, a spillage byproduct of the excessive phenylalanine, was not readily detectable until the baby reached 6 to 8 weeks of age. At that time it was no longer under hospital control and less amenable to screening and the commencement of dietary control. Prompt therapeutic management during the first weeks of life is believed by many to be essential to prevent development of a brain lesion, the cause of retardation. Robert Guthrie, of Children's Hospital, Buffalo, developed a blood test which utilized only a few drops of blood taken by simple puncture from the baby's heel when it is only 4 or 5 days old. This afforded hospital control of the procedure. It is at the heart of today's mass screening programs which have been instituted in many states.

The development which really fired the imagination, which offered the hope of cure not only for PKU retardees but for other victims of inborn errors of metabolism, was the reported impression that a special diet, low in phenylalanine, apparently prevented or limited the retardation of intellectual growth and other phenylketonuric symptoms. From a public health standpoint, therefore, the formula for action seemed clearcut: put every newborn child through a PKU screening test and then take all who are found to be PKU positive and put them on the special diet. This is the simplistic model now widely adopted for the detection and treatment of PKU. It is the model which it is hoped will be useful in the treatment of many other metabolic disorders.

The belief that effective control of a genetic disorder—of PKU—has been achieved was electrifying. The bandwagon quickly took on a heavy load—several voluntary health agencies, several

federal agencies, and medical researchers, among others. "PKU" became a household word. Interest in screening for other metabolic diseases was heightened. . . .

People soon began discussing a new problem: What would happen when salvaged PKU patients grew up and procreated? Would they then add to the pool of defective genes in the total population? This, however, was a deferrable problem to be faced later. Meanwhile, in relatively short order, 37 states, as of November 1966, passed PKU screening laws. The American Medical Association also endorsed screening programs, as had other groups, but it did not favor legislative requirements for them.

Thus, the consensus was that an excellent medical model was available for the management of PKU and that screening and treatment should proceed accordingly. Only here and there were voices raised in protest against the legislative approach. Even fewer scientific challenges were expressed as to the validity of the medical model. I use the word "expressed" deliberately, because as I explored the PKU program I was to learn that many who had doubts had not expressed them. I also learned that the source of consensus was traceable to a rather small group of people who were in substantial agreement among themselves. The same people appeared time after time on professional programs throughout the country. They reinforced each other in their convictions, sincerely and earnestly held.

* * *

The evidence of a faulty medical model I will now present covers diagnostic validity and reliability, control and effects of treatment, and readiness of the PKU program to be put into a service status for the public.

The diagnostic finding of a high phenylalanine content in the blood does not in itself establish the infant as phenylketonuric. Neither does the finding of a low serum phenylalanine level necessarily predict the absence of PKU. Guthrie and associates reported that about 85 percent or more of presumed positives turned out to be false positives. Presumably, the false positives are eliminated through use of confirmatory tests, but the literature offers no assurance that existing tests, used generally, will exclude all false positives. . . .

The blood phenylalanine test is given in the hospital before discharge of the newborn; usually when 4 days old. The recommended procedure is that all infants be tested again at age 4 weeks, so that false positives and false negatives might then be rechecked. What happens to those babies who were put on low phenylalanine diets very early? How does a later test reveal them to be false positives or false negatives if already on diet? What happens to non-PKU children falsely diagnosed so to be? It has been suggested that when put on low phenylalanine diets, their own body proteins break down through catabolic action to release blood phenylalanine intake whereas more would actually be needed.

While Dr. Guthrie has reported, on the one hand, that 85 percent of his initial positive screenings are false upon recheck, other investigators have . . . claimed that the Guthrie test has a potential of 53 percent false negatives. So, on the one hand the test pulls in too many babies, and, on the other, it is claimed to bypass too many.

One of the problems with which we are here confronted is that the most meager data have been used in projecting the incidence of disease, the validity and reliability of diagnostic screens and the clinical value of the dietary treatment. The efficacy of the dietary substance used to feed PKU babies, Lofenalac, was originally demonstrated through experience with only six cases as a basis for obtaining FDA approval in 1958.

The trouble is in the difficulty of collecting enough new cases in any one clinical center to provide an adequate statistical base for study. Thus, the last time I checked on experiences in the District of Columbia, which has a screening program, only one confirmed case had been found in 2 years.

* * *

Consider the reactions of the parents who are told that their children are or might be retarded and will require additional tests over a period of time which will narrow the field down to only a fraction of those screened out. How does the imparting of this information change their lives? What traumata are thereby induced and at what cost? Even as to children who are eventually adjudged to be PKU-negative, are the lingering doubts in parents' minds ever dispelled?

* * *

One of the more recent uncertainties is whether "Phenylketonuria" is a single disease or a spectrum or collection of many different diseases each of which would require its variant of treatment. This is a matter for more profound conjecture than it has been given, particularly in view of our tendency to identify diseases and their cures through rather simplistic models.

Consequently, children who test out to be phenylketonuric, in terms of blood chemistry, may grow up to be normal in all respects. Under present screening and treatment procedures, they would be put on a diet which might very well do them harm. On the other hand, some children who develop normally on a PKU diet might have developed even more normally without the diet.

A factor which impairs the ability of scientists to conduct research, even to know whether or not the low phenylalanine diet is beneficial, is that when an entire universe—all babies who show up as PKU positives—is put on the diet, no control groups are left for comparison. We do not know whether any children under dietary management who do not become retarded would have remained normal under ordinary diets. Untreated children with high phenylalanine levels have been found with intelligence in the normal and high normal range.

* * *

Earlier, I mentioned the widely held belief that diagnosis and treatment within the first weeks of life are important in order to prevent brain damage. Some recent work by Fuller, a psychologist of New York, suggests otherwise. She found that, taking all phenylketonurics (within her study) as a group, the earlier they were placed on the low phenylalanine diet, the less impaired they were. This would possibly support the views on early diagnosis and treatment, but let us face that one further after looking at some more of Fuller's findings.

Some PKU babies started on early control showed marked retardation. On the other hand, some children started on the diet after 3 years of age—long after brain damage should have occurred—showed great improvement to the point of little or no retardation. Furthermore, in a study of siblings on PKU diets, a significant proportion started at a later age showed better improvement than their sisters or brothers who were started at younger ages.

The implications are profound. It is not improbable that measured improvement is in part, at least, the result of an intervention factor —the giving of individual attention to children who previously had been abandoned by society —rather than to biochemical effects of withholding an amino acid from the diet. The intervention factor, which may in this case be response to attention and training, is known among psychologists as the "Hawthorn effect."

* * *

. . . Now I will take up problems of treatment, especially as related to child safety. Very little attention has been given to deleterious effects of treatment, including the incidence of death attributable to induced dietary insufficiency. Other side effects and complications of the PKU diet, which consists solely of an unpalatable preparation from which phenylalanine has been removed include skin lesions, refractory anemia, bone changes, vomiting, lethargy, appetite failure, poor weight gain, retarded growth, and miscellaneous symptoms of malnutrition.

Recently, investigators found that the immune responses of PKU children to certain infectious diseases were lowered by dietary treatment. Wooley has argued that PKU patients saved from idiocy might become schizophrenic when taken off their diets later in life. The Food and Drug Administration informed me it had no knowledge of deaths. The Children's Bureau informed me it had no evidence of fatalities occurring as a result of treatment. Yet references to treatment-induced death are indeed to be found in the medical literature.

* * *

A reported case of death, as an example, was attributed to megaloblastic anemia of nutritional origin. A phenylketonuric infant was started on a low-phenylalanine diet at age 2 weeks, suffered serious setbacks resulting in three hospital readmissions, and died at age 7 months. The reference to this death was published in a bibliography of the Children's Bureau.

As a commentary on public attitudes, one must observe that if any drug company were actively promoting the PKU program, which is not the case, it would be hoisted on the nearest lamppost if deaths were involved.

One of the problems in treatment, related to adverse reactions, is the need for exquisite balancing of nutrient intake to metabolic changes in the growing infant and child. Phenylalanine is an essential amino acid. It is necessary for growth, repair of tissues, and physical survival. The blood content or serum phenylalanine levels must be checked regularly to guide dietary management.

* * *

From all experience—even poor experience—lessons ought to be taken. One big lesson from the PKU situation is that one should not commit any major endeavor on a broad scale without first having undergone pilot testing. Inevitably, such testing leads to correction of assumptions and procedural techniques. We did not have this in the PKU program. Rather, the cry went out that society owed it to every child to have a PKU test at birth and that it would be unethical to deprive any child of the dietary treatment once he had been diagnosed as phenylketonuric.

Just how the PKU program was determined to be service-ready ought to be examined, in order to learn more lessons therefrom. Mandatory PKU screening first became law in Massachusetts. As near as I can determine, universal screening was originally introduced in order to find cases for research programs, although I am sure the researchers must have felt this would also lead to public benefit.

At no point, however, has the public ever been told that the PKU program is still mainly investigational and that almost the entire population of newborn infants has been converted into a national laboratory of clinical research with attendant risks. Few physicians and hardly any parents have been made aware of these risks and of all the reasons for screening.

The claim has been made that the physician is still free to decide the course of treatment for the patient, the infant. Theoretically this may be so, but the specter of the malpractice suit must exert a powerful stimulus to prescribe in accordance with the cultural mores for these are what influence the court. Already, there have been two malpractice suits in which physicians have been charged with failure to treat.

The inauguration of screening programs was well along when the Committee on Fetus and Newborn of the American Academy of Pediatrics published the following criteria for screening of newborn infants for metabolic disease:

1. Does the seriousness of the disorder justify screening?
2. Is therapy for the disease in question available?
3. Is there a clearly identifiable segment of the population with an increased incidence of this disease?
4. Is it possible to perform reliable screening during the first few days of life?
5. Can the screening test be performed in a routine service laboratory?

6. Is the test acceptable to the physician and to a majority of parents?

7. Is the cost of the test acceptable?

8. Are there acceptable medical facilties prepared to confirm diagnosis and consult about the institution of therapy?

*   *   *

To underscore the state of confusion as regards PKU and to show how sharply opinions are divided even with the American Academy of Pediatrics, the following is quoted from a heretofore unpublished report of its Committee on Nutrition to the Children's Bureau, dated July 30, 1965:

1. The objectives and ways and means for implementing such wide-scale screening programs remain to be evaluated as do the methods for following through of patients with heritable metabolic diseases detected by such programs.

2. The beneficial effects of good dietary management of any of the heritable metabolic diseases, detected in these programs or elsewhere, have yet to be proven unequivocally. Under the circumstances, the committee felt that caution was indicated in launching widespread screening programs until practical therapeutic programs, the effects of which are predictable in the majority of children participating, have been designed.

3. It must be demonstrated with certainty that any normal children who receive these restrictive diets through inadvertence or because of misdiagnosis will not suffer irreparable neurological or physical damage.

*   *   *

[A]lthough most of this discussion has pertained to PKU, I am less interested in that rare phenomenon than in how decisions are made affecting public health and welfare. The PKU affair happens to be a well-contained example of how not to proceed. It also enables us to derive lessons from establishment workings, for there happens to be a PKU establishment.

*   *   *

The PKU establishment embraces lay and professional personalities in academic institutions, hospitals, public health departments, the federal government, and voluntary health agencies. It has erred, I believe, in not submitting itself to the discipline of independent critique—in not opening the channels of doubt and criticism. The principal federal agency involved is the Children's Bureau. Of course, it has been involved in PKU establishment affairs and has, I believe, committed errors of its own, but to be

critical of it on that score would be unfair. The Children's Bureau has done a tremendous job in developing clinical programs and aids in the area of mental retardation, overshadowing the PKU activity in importance.

The Children's Bureau is to be commended, in fact, for its efforts to promote constructive dialog through numerous symposia in which divergent points of view have often been expressed. Nevertheless, the Children's Bureau has been dominated as to PKU by a small group of outside program proponents who have also been the source of guidance of federal and state legislators, who have dominated the professional literature, who have advised lay voluntary groups, and who have been the main recipients of federal grants for PKU activity. I criticize none of the members of this establishment individually, but collectively there seems to be a fair case for saying that their mutual enthusiasm has led them to block outside challenges to unbridled program execution beyond the state of knowledge.

*   *   *

Reversal is hard to achieve in the government, because it implies lack of good judgment. This is unfortunate. As we move more deeply into the inner fastnesses of medical science, we had better be prepared to reverse gears without implications of dishonor.

*   *   *

What do I propose?

1. *As to mechanisms of advice:*

Any one solution, such as some independent ombudsman or office of review in the executive or legislative branches, would be insufficient. Rather, we need a return to old-fashioned scientific pluralism. We need open, constructive conflict of ideas from which truth may emerge. We should not discourage advocacy, dissidence, and special pleading. One approach is to dilute the concentration of advisory sources. The same people or program sources should not at once guide legislative and executive branches, from within and without, while also dominating voluntary and professional society channels. Let us round out our pluralisms and at least occasionally have some spirited debates over both ends and means, right out in the open.

2. *As to program choice and priorities:*

The making of choice becomes more difficult as more is learned about situations and problems. On the whole, reliance must be placed on the professional judgments of the experts and the administrators. Legislators must also play a part in choice, for they thereby bring in the popular view—provided it is really that—as opposed to the dominance of professionalism. Yet choice must be subject to criteria-based review, taking into account total needs and total resources. Thus, if PKU programs are still investigational, should we not limit their scope while resources are deployed to improvements in more prevalent areas of mental retardation?

3. *As to application of knowledge:*

Before particular disease targets are selected for widespread preventive or therapeutic application, there must first be a base of adequate knowledge derived through fundamental and controlled clinical research. Consistent with advances in clinical experience protracted pilot tests should be conducted in one or more states under controlled, scientifically modeled conditions, in order to derive adequate experience. Progressively, as wider field trials are conducted under varying conditions, independent medical judges without personal cause should evaluate progress. Then, assuming that the program demonstrates its worthiness, it should be expanded at a rate consistent with the development of adequate clinical and laboratory facilities and professional manpower.

The public should be fully informed as to whether a program is investigational or service-ready. Evaluations against criteria of benefit should be continuous.

The need for developing informational bases as prerequisites for action is just as important in all other areas of public medicine, whether in the regulation of drugs or in the extension of medical services to the public.

4. *As to legislative prescription of medical practice:*

Legislative enactments of medical practice should be limited to assuring good practice, to protecting the public against hidden or unseen external hazards, and to protecting the rights of patients, especially the incompetent. Laws cannot specify action, when individuals are biochemically and biosocially unique and when the knowledge of medicine undergoes constant change. Laws cannot substitute for the professional judgments of physicians.

*   *   *

NOTE

STANDARD DIET FOR PKU MAY IMPAIR INTELLIGENCE*

By producing profound malnutrition, treatment of phenylketonuria in early life with the standard low-phenylalanine diet may cause, rather than prevent, permanent intellectual impairment, a Canadian investigator reported . . . to the Society for Pediatric Research.

A more liberal allowance of phenylalanine and protein to insure satisfactory growth and development appears to result in improved functioning, said Dr. William B. Hanley, of the University of Toronto.

*   *   *

Dr. Hanley and co-workers in Toronto became "dissatisfied" with the results of low-phenylalanine diet therapy about two and a half years ago when they observed that nearly all phenylketonurics started on the diet in the first few months of life had poor weight gain and linear growth and some showed evidence of serious malnutrition. Moreover, ultimate I.Q.'s were not as high as had been anticipated despite early diagnosis and seemingly adequate treatment.

"Studies of children in underdeveloped countries had revealed that protein malnutrition in early infancy may produce intellectual impairment," Dr. Hanley said. "We wondered whether our treatment was producing mental retardation by too vigorous restriction of phenylalanine and protein."

When dietary therapy of PKU was introduced a decade ago the aim was to maintain fasting serum phenylalanine within a normal range of 1 to 3 mg. per 100 ml., he recalled. Subsequently values of up to 6 mg. per 100 ml. were allowed since it was felt the original limitation might be too strict.

But Dr. Hanley and associates found that 3 of 19 children put on either regimen within the first six months of life had required hospitalization for severe illness between four and nine months, showing classic signs of malnutrition, deficient growth, hypoproteinemia, and anemia. The other 16 showed less severe "but definite and prolonged evidence of malnutrition."

*   *   *

* *Hospital Tribune* 1, 18 (June 3, 1968). Reprinted by courtesy of *Hospital Tribune*.

[E]ffects of early malnutrition on mental development were . . . longer-lasting, Dr. Hanley said. Four are definitely retarded, eight are rated "dull normal" and two are of "borderline" intelligence. Only five are mentally normal.

* * *

b.

Who Should Participate, within What Structure, in Professional Regulation?

[i]

Protocol for Clinical Studies to Be Approved by the Yale Medical School Clinical Investigation Committee (1969) *

Title of project	Evaluation of Drug Therapy in Hyperkinetic Behavior
Chief Investigator	Daniel S. Rowe, M.D.
Other Investigators	Frederic P. Anderson, M.D., Ethelyn H. Klatskin, PH.D., John V. Federico, M.D., Gary R. Wanerka, M.D.
Description of Study	1) *General goals and pertinence*
	2) *Procedures*
	3) *Possible hazards to the subjects*

Children with hyperkinetic behavioral disturbances have long represented a problem of management to the physician faced with their care. Previously employed pharmacological, environmental, and therapeutic approaches have not been wholly successful in management of this entity. The pharmacological approach, however, offers the best opportunity of achieving a positive impact in this area.

The goal of this study is to evaluate the effectiveness of two different drug regimens and counseling as opposed to counseling and placebo medication. The effect will be measured by the evaluation of hyperactivity, attention span, behavior, and aggressiveness before and during the course of the study.

Sixty patients between 7 and 10 years of age will be selected from the out-patient pediatric services of the Yale-New Haven Medical Center and from the educable, retarded children in classes of local school systems. The prospective patients, all of whom will be in the I.Q. range 60–80, will be evaluated by a clinic pediatrician and psychologist to adjudge whether each prospective patient fulfills the criteria for the hyperactive behavior syndrome. Patients with sei-

_____
* Reprinted by permission of the investigator who retains all rights.

zure disorders, chronic renal or hepatic disease, history of allergy, or sensitivity to the benzodiazepines or amphetamines will be excluded.

The sixty patients selected for the study will be divided into three treatment groups. The groups will receive *d*-amphetamine and placebo, *d*-amphetamine and diazepam, and placebo, respectively. The study will be double blind. Patients will be seen semimonthly and evaluated for the effects of the medication. For this purpose, report forms for the physicians, parent, and teacher will be utilized. At the completion of the study period data will be statistically reviewed.

Side effects which may be anticipated with diazepam include drowsiness, ataxia, and dizziness; with *d*-amphetamine include appetite loss, irritability, increased hyperactivity, epigastric distress, and wakefulness. These will be recorded. In most instances these are dose related and may be avoided by dosage adjustment.

Why must this study be done in humans?
To assess the effect in the group most in need. Non-human subjects are not applicable to this study.

Subjects for the Study
(*Approximate number, type of subject, how consent is to be gained, medical supervision*). *Subjects under age 21 must have parental consent.*

Sixty patients, selected from the out-patient pediatric service at the Yale-New Haven Medical Center and educable, retarded children in classes of local school systems. Consent will be gained through direct contact with the parent and explanation of the study and goals. All patients will be under the medical supervision of the pediatricians involved in the study.

* * *

PATIENT CONSENT FORM FOR PARTICIPATION IN A CLINICAL INVESTIGATION PROJECT

YALE UNIVERSITY SCHOOL OF MEDICINE
YALE-NEW HAVEN HOSPITAL

Description of Project: The project being undertaken, and the one for which your child is a prospective participant, is to evaluate the use of specific drugs in the management of hyperkinetic behavior. Children with this type of behavior characteristically are those who are overactive, difficult to manage, tend to be disruptive in the school classroom, and have short attention spans.

Children with this pattern of activity have long represented a most difficult management problem for the physician faced with their care. Previous programs of drugs, counseling, and psychiatric management have not proved to be completely successful. At this time, we are planning to study the effects of several newer drugs employed in this area of concern.

Of course, in any study employing and evaluating medications, not all patients will be receiving the drug. In order to have a means of comparison, some patients will be receiving a placebo, or "sugar pill," which would resemble the real medication. Eventually, however, all children would benefit from any positive results which might emerge from the study. If we are able to prove that there is a benefit from the use of these medications, then, of course, all participants would be able to use the drug. During the course of the study even the physicians involved will not know which patients are actually receiving the drugs; thus there will be no bias in the interpretation of the results.

The drugs being used are both available commercially and no longer in the "experimental" stage of testing. Of course, as with any medication, there can be undesirable side effects. One of the drugs in diazepam (Valium), which on occasion can cause drowsiness, dizziness, and instability of gait; the other drug is *d*-amphetamine (Dexedrine), which on occasion can cause appetite loss, increase in overactivity, irritability, and wakefulness. In the case of both drugs, such side effects can easily be controlled simply by reducing the dosage. We will be making a careful effort to prevent any side effects from occurring.

Authorization: I have read the above and agree to the participation of _____

_____

_____ (name or names and how related) _____
in the project described above. Its general purposes, potential benefits, and possible hazards and inconveniences have been explained to my satisfaction.

_____
Signature

_____
Date

_____
(Physician)

[*ii*]
Melvin Lewis, Audrey T. McCollum,
A. Herbert Schwartz, and Jerome A. Grunt
*Informed Consent in Pediatric Research**

*   *   *

In view of the difficulties involved in determining the meaning of informed consent, we suggest the following safeguards for children being considered for participation in medical research:

1. The nature of the research design and all risks to the child should be assessed by a review committee that includes pediatric investigators who are not involved in the research as well as the pediatric investigator who is to conduct the study. This will provide safeguards against the investigator's inevitable bias and gaps in knowledge.

2. The review committee should include a professional person especially equipped to assess the psychological risks to the child. This person would have to be aware of those areas of development especially vulnerable to impairment at the child's developmental stage, have the interviewing skill required for assessing the child's degree of vulnerability, and understand the kinds of stress likely to be provoked by the research procedures.

3. The investigator should have a series of personal interviews with the parents and at times with the child to build a relationship of trust, and establish an understanding of the research goals and methods and of the risks involved.

4. When the investigator lacks the skill or experience necessary for preparing the parents and the child for the research, correcting their misconceptions about it, and dealing with the child's reactions as the admission date approaches, a social worker and a psychiatrist may be called upon to help fulfill these functions, in supplementary preadmission interviews.

5. The investigator, research director, nurse, social worker, and psychiatrist should plan in advance for the child's care in the hospital since special arrangements may be required to prevent impaired development.

6. The research team should include a pediatrician, nurse, child psychiatrist, child psychologist, or social worker to provide a continuing evaluation of the psychological reactions of

_____
* 16 *Children* 143, 148 (1969). Reprinted by permission.

the child and his parents to the research procedures and to train research personnel in the early recognition of emotional stress and ways of dealing with it.

7. The activities of all the staff members on the research team should be coordinated in regularly held interdisciplinary conferences.

8. Follow-up care should be provided to deal with whatever reactions to the research procedures may occur after the child's discharge from the hospital.

9. Parents and staff members should have an understanding of what parts of the psychological information revealed during the research are to be shared with other members of the staff and what parts will remain in confidence; and all staff members should understand the need for discretion in divulging such information.

c.

Should Research Design and Scientific Merits Be Evaluated?

Nancy Bayley
Implicit and Explicit Values in Science as
Related to Human Growth and Development*

*   *   *

. . . Leon Yarrow is now [studying] the effects on the infant of separation from the mother. A number of psychologists and psychiatrists hold that such separation is likely to have devastating effects on the infant's development. There are others who question the great importance to the infant of the changes in mother-figures. When there is the possibility of damage to the child as would be the case if the first-named group of theorists is correct, we do not just set up an experiment in which, say, we induce a group of mothers to exchange babies. We can, however, test the hypothesis without making such a drastic experiment. We can find conditions in which the child, by force of circumstances, is separated from his mother. What Yarrow has done is to seek out such cases and to study them by observation in their homes. Through the cooperation of adoption agencies, he is able to observe infants who live in foster care homes with the foster mother before the change to an adoptive home, and then to observe them with the adoptive mother afterward. The effect

of the child's age on the nature of his adjustment to change is studied by comparing those who were placed at different ages during the first year: before 3 months, 3 to 6, 6 to 9, and 9 to 12 months of age. The babies can also be compared according to the kinds of mother-child relations that are established, and according to their emotional adjustment in the two or three years subsequent to adoption. Another group of babies placed directly in adoptive homes, from the hospital, is being studied, as adoptive controls.

*   *   *

d.

Should Consent Be Supervised?

[*i*]
William McD. Hammon, Lewis L. Coriell,
and Joseph Stokes, Jr.
Evaluation of Red Cross Gamma Globulin
as a Prophylactic Agent for Poliomyelitis*

The principal purpose of the experiment . . . was to determine whether gamma globulin, as prepared for and furnished by the American National Red Cross for measles prophylaxis, would protect against the paralytic manifestations of poliomyelitis when administered in reasonable dosage before the onset of illness. A secondary purpose was to determine, if protection were afforded, the duration of protection in the dosage selected for the experiment. . . .

*   *   *

This study appeared to have considerable, immediate importance, since epidemiological studies had led to no hope of control in the near future by breaking the infection chain. Furthermore, no active immunizing agent was available, and no specific therapeutic drug or antibiotic was known, while the incidence of paralytic poliomyelitis appeared to be increasing. Information obtained from animal experiments suggested strongly that human gamma globulin might give temporary protection. It was available in limited quantities and could be produced in much larger amounts. Since the effectiveness of gamma globulin in man could be determined only through actual administration to human beings and since its safety had been previously determined through use in well over one million cases of measles and hepatitis, a

---

* *Merrill-Palmer Quarterly* 121–126 (Spring 1956). Reprinted by permission.

* 150 *Journal of the American Medical Association* 739–747 (1952). Reprinted by permission.

human field test under suitably controlled conditions was believed to be indicated.

* * *

For reliable evaluation of results, essentially alternate controls to receive an inert, safe material resembling gamma globulin would be necessary. Only this type of test would withstand critical scientific scrutiny and be accepted universally as a final evaluation. If all volunteers were inoculated with gamma globulin, the uninoculated group could not serve as comparative controls for many reasons. Fear, motivating volunteering, would bring a higher proportion of children from areas or groups known to be most heavily exposed. Economic, social, and racial differences might readily influence response to public clinics. These and other factors would render the two groups dissimilar. Better cooperation in reporting suspected cases would probably occur among the inoculated than the uninoculated, and our own clinicians as well as physicians of the community could not entirely avoid being influenced in making a diagnosis in questionable cases if they knew that the patient had received an injection of gamma globulin. Thus, bias could not be avoided. Furthermore, among those not receiving injections at the clinics, an unknown number might receive injections of gamma globulin from others, so the control group would not be entirely uninoculated, as planned.

Almost every conceivable variation to avoid "control" inoculations was suggested and carefully considered, but had to be ruled out as endangering the success of the test. This was the most debated problem in planning, because it introduced a novel approach in evaluating immunization in man. It was readily recalled that, had typhoid and rabies vaccines been originally tested in this manner, years of uncertainty might have been saved and we might not be in our present, unenviable quandary regarding the efficacy of these immunizing procedures after a great many years of routine application. . . .

In order that no member of the team could be biased by a knowledge of what was injected and that no favoritism or yielding to pressures to obtain the active material for selected children could occur, it was decided to arrange a random distribution of all the vials when they were packed and to give each child the first unit of inoculum presenting in the box in order of serial number and packaging. All units would look alike, and the serial number of the lable

would be the only means of identification. Fifty units of the same size would be packed in a box, 25 of gamma globulin and 25 of control inoculum, all numbered serially as a single series. . . . In this way gamma globulin and control groups should be comparable, and no knowledge of the type of agent used could influence the mother, physician, or consultant in reporting, hospitalizing, or making a final diagnosis, or the physical therapist in grading the degree of muscle involvement.

* * *

The consent form to be signed by the parent would be carefully worded with legal assistance. It should explain accurately the purpose and procedure of the study. It would be printed in the newspapers and read over the radio so that all parents could be fully informed and understand what they would sign before coming to the clinic. We were anxious that everyone would understand that half the children would receive control material. The text of the consent form was as follows:

FORM OF CONSENT

I have been informed that Dr. William McD. Hammon, Professor of Epidemiology of the Graduate School of Public Health of the University of Pittsburgh, with the financial support of the National Foundation for Infantile Paralysis, Inc., and with the cooperation of the _____ County, and _____ State Health Departments, has inaugurated in _____ County, _____ a project which aims at the injection of a large number of children for test purposes in connection with the study of Infantile Paralysis and its causes and remedies. For the purpose of that test, it is proposed that a solution of gamma globulin or a solution of specially prepared gelatin be injected into a buttock of each of the children. The method of identifying the substance injected into each child is such that the person administering the injection does not know which one is being used at the time. To assist this project, I hereby consent that either one of the preparations above mentioned may be injected into the buttock of my child

_____
(Name of Child)
Signed: _____
(Father or Mother)

_____
(Relationship to Child)

_____
(City or Town)

Witness: _____
Date: _____

* * *

THE ROLE OF THE PARTICIPANTS IN ADMINISTRATION 997

Following selection of a city for a field trial and after obtaining the support of all official agencies and medical groups, a public announcement of the decision would be made. The widest possible local publicity would be desirable at this time. Press and radio releases would be prepared in advance to insure that full and factual information be available. At a special conference of reporters, editors, radio, and television program directors from this city and any nearby larger city with significant local coverage, this material would be released and fully discussed. The date of opening the clinics, their locations, hours of operation, the age group of children to be included, and the estimated closing day of clinics would be announced. So that the scientific aspects and background of the study would be appreciated by the press, radio, and others, we would try to anticipate and answer through previously prepared and mimeographed releases all questions that might arise.

It was believed that since parents were being asked to bring their children for an unusual type of test, every attempt should be made to explain completely all scientific details of the project and to withhold nothing. National publicity would be avoided whenever possible, since it could not contribute to the success of the local study and might hinder subsequent studies in other areas. However, it was realized that wire services would pick up the story, and national publicity could not be avoided. Local leaders of the women's organizations of the community would be approached to recruit a large group of women volunteers to assist in the clinics.

* * *

The public attendance at the clinics was so much greater than expected that several changes had to be made at the end of the first day. The house-to-house canvass was called off, since it was obviously unnecessary. Since almost every syringe and needle was used on the first day, instead of half as planned, provisions had to be made to wash, repack, and autoclave all 1,800 every night. The nearest autoclaves of adequate size were in Salt Lake City, nearly 50 miles away.

Instead of running for five or six days as planned, all clinics were closed in three and one-half days, because the supply of biologicals was exhausted. . . . Hundreds of people were turned away when the clinics were closed on the fourth day. There were indications that 75 to 90 percent of the population had planned to partici-

pate and would have done so had supplies been adequate. . . .

* * *

[ii]
Liz Roman Gallese
Medical–Ethics Panels Are Set Up to Resolve
Dilemmas on Research*

* * *

In cases involving young children, especially those who are mentally retarded and unable to understand a research project, obtaining patient consent is all but impossible. . . . The consent of both young patients and their parents is often required. Yet research with such children is practically the only way to obtain certain scientific information.

The ethics committee at [the] Massachusetts General [Hospital] recently wrestled with this dilemma. Scientists know that certain types of cancer trigger a high level of calcium in the blood that can kill the patient far faster than the cancer itself. They also suspect that the amount of calcium in a person's blood may be at least partly regulated by calcitonin, a recently discovered hormone produced by the thyroid gland. This opens the possibility of using calcitonin to control calcium levels and thus greatly prolong the patient's life. Scientists also suspect that calcitonin may have other and as yet undefined therapeutic values.

But first scientists are trying to nail down the fact that calcitonin does indeed control calcium and how it does so. To prove this, the scientists need a group of normal children whose thyroids produce calcitonin and a group of children without thyroids producing this hormone so that the two groups can be compared.

Dr. Alberto Hayek, a Harvard University researcher who is working on the calcitonin study, proposed using mentally retarded children in an institution affiliated with Massachusetts General for the group without thyroids. This upset the ethics committee. During a committee meeting to consider Dr. Hayek's written proposal, members posed question after question.

"Why does he wish to use mentally retarded children?" one ethics committee member asked.

"Why use institutionalized children, who

* *The Wall Street Journal* 1, col. 6; 17, col. 3 (April 14, 1971). Reprinted by permission of *The Wall Street Journal*.

constitute a captive group?" another member asked.

"Can't other subjects be found who are intelligent enough to give consent to the study?" a third member asked.

The committee framed its questions in a letter.

In a written reply to the committee and in a later interview, Dr. Hayek said other subjects aren't suitable.

"Only one in every 30,000 babies is born without a thyroid gland and more than half of these have an IQ far less than 90. The result is that many of the members of this very tiny group are in institutions for the mentally retarded. There is virtually no place else to find them."

Dr. Hayek also emphasized that the study, while tedious, would pose very little risk to the children. The project involves three-hour calcium infusions into the bloodstream and blood samples taken every half hour to check calcitonin levels so doctors can assess the relationships between the two chemicals.

The ethics committee finally agreed to approve the project but only after appointing a physician-advocate—a move that is increasingly being used at research hospitals.

The physician-advocate, who is not one of the researchers, is named to represent the children's interests. His duty is to make sure that full information is given to parents when their consent is asked, that undue risks are avoided and that every safety precaution available is taken. He can withdraw the patients he represents from a research project if he thinks they are taking too great a risk.

* * *

NOTE

THE MASSACHUSETTS GENERAL HOSPITAL HUMAN STUDIES—GUIDING PRINCIPLES AND PROCEDURES*

During the course of the first years that this small guide was put to use, it became apparent that the problem of protecting the rights and welfare of children and other incompetent individuals had not been given sufficient attention. . . . As a result and in line with the intent of the Trustees' Advisory Committee on Research and the Individual . . . the guidelines have been re-

---

* Boston: The Massachusetts General Hospital 6, 8–9, 11–12 (2d ed., 1970). Reprinted by permission.

vised by the Committee in agreement with suggestions by the Committee on Research and its Subcommittee on Human Studies.

* * *

A. *Studies for the benefit of others, with no direct benefit for the subject involved*

* * *

3. When a procedure is not for the diagnosis or treatment of his own condition, this must be made clear to the patient. When the subject of the study is a child or an incompetent individual, informed consent must be obtained from parents or legal guardian. If the subject has reached an age of understanding, every effort must be made to obtain his consent as well. In this context a subject under sixteen years of age will be considered a child.

* * *

6. A safeguard is to be found in the practice of having at least two professionally qualified persons involved in experimental situations: First there is the physician or other person concerned with the care of the subject; his primary interest is the subject's welfare. It is of utmost importance in experimental situations involving children or incompetent individuals that this person serve as the subjects' advocate. Second there is the investigator whose interest is the sound conduct of the investigation. Perhaps too often a single individual attempts to encompass both roles.

* * *

B. *Experimental diagnosis or therapy for the direct benefit of the patient whether or not there is benefit for others*

* * *

5. It is recognized that certain forms of psychological testing of achievement may involve subjects who are children and that in such testing, informed consent may unduly bias the result. Since these tests as a rule are for the benefit of the subject, strict adherence to the requirement for informed consent may not be justified. In times of uncertainty, review by the investigator's peers would be in order.

C. *Volunteers, normal and patient*

* * *

3. An individual cannot soundly volunteer for an experiment unless he first understands

what he is volunteering for, as well as the degree of inconvenience and risk involved. Here again the problems raised by studies of normal children must be considered with special care. Informed consent of parents or guardian and, if feasible, of subjects must be obtained. If such would unduly bias the study or if other uncertainties exist, review by the investigator's peers would be in order.

e.

Should Harm Be Assessed?

[i]
Ross G. Mitchell
The Child and Experimental Medicine*

* * *

. . . When deciding whether an experiment is justifiable, the old question: "Would you subject your own child to this?" is still a good yardstick for most moderately minded people. It should be remembered, however, that some zealots may be prepared to submit their own families to indignities which the average man would consider excessive. The experiment referred to above, in which Oliver injected his own son with a crude extract of endocrine glands, is a well-known example.

* * *

[ii]
C. Henry Kempe
The Battered Child and the Hospital†

* * *

At least 700 children are killed every year in this country by their parents or parent surrogates. Thousands more are permanently injured, physically or mentally. In the week before this article was prepared, nine young victims of serious abuse were seen here at Colorado General Hospital, and it is a rare week indeed in which four or five new cases do not come to our attention. From some of our early work on case-finding, it is our impression that at least 15 percent of all children under age five who come into the emergency room fall into the battered category. Data such as these suggest that the problem of the abused child and the

* 1 *British Medical Journal* 722, 725–726 (1964). Reprinted by permission.
† *Hospital Practice* 44 (October 1969). Reprinted by permission.

abusing parent is one of the most important "epidemic" diseases in the U.S.

* * *

3.
In Reviewing Decisions and Consequences

a.

Through Public Scrutiny?

Statement of Representative
Cornelius E. Gallagher—
September 29, 1970*

* * *

I want to welcome you here today to our hearing into Federal responsibility in promoting the use of amphetamines to modify the behavior of grammar school children. The indications are that these drugs are now being widely employed to ameliorate the effects of what is called minimal brain dysfunction (MBD) in children. One of our witnesses today has been quoted as saying that the use of this type of therapy will "zoom" from its current usage in approximately 200,000 to 300,000 American children today.

These amphetamines, such as Dexedrine and Ritalin, apparently do not act the same in children as they do in young adults, according to some authorities. Instead of being "speed" and accelerating the individual's activity pattern, proponents of the program claim that amphetamines slow down the child and make him controllable both in the classroom and at home. This use of stumulants to calm children termed hyperactive is called the "paradoxical effect" and it is but one of the many paradoxes which this hearing is designed to explore. Let me list a few contradictory implications.

First, and a distressingly obvious paradox, is the effect of accelerating this use of amphetamines on our extensive national campaign against drug abuse. From the time of puberty onward, each and every child is told that "speed kills" and that amphetamines are to be avoided. Yet, this same child has learned that Ritalin, for example, is the only thing which

* Materials in this section are reprinted from *Hearings on Federal Involvement in the Use of Behavior Modification Drugs on Grammar School Children before a Subcommittee (The Right to Privacy Inquiry) of the House Committee on Government Operations*, 91st Congress, 2d Session 1–74 (1970).

makes him a functioning member of the school environment and both his family and his doctor have urged the pills on him.

*   *   *

Second, I am very concerned [that] the fact that the child . . . has been undergoing drug therapy becomes a permanent part of the child's school record, to be recalled and available to anyone who wishes to see it. We may well break the child's MBD-induced hyperactive behavior pattern, but by freezing on the record the fact that it took drugs to do it, we cast a cloud of suspicion over the child's future. . . .

A third paradoxical effect is directly related to the jurisdiction of this subcommittee of the Committee on Government Operations. We are charged with the responsibility of determining whether Federal funds are spent in an economical manner and whether the operations of Federal agencies are conducted efficiently. We have learned that Federal funds have been used to support various experimental programs and studies concerning the use of drugs to treat learning disabilities in children. Assisted by this infusion of tax dollars, it has become apparent that biochemical medication and an alteration of the learning environment is considered as part of a "new wave" approach to public education in the United States by many persons both in and out of the Government.

Not only has this issue never been subjected to full public discussion and understanding, but I am deeply concerned about the possibility that an overreliance on drug therapy could spread far beyond its apparently valid applications and thus denigrate the novel learning methods which have also been explored by the use of Federal funds. In so many areas which the Privacy Subcommittee has explored, we have seen a dependence on quick and inexpensive solutions offered by the new technology without adequate attention being paid to the slower and perhaps more costly methods which would preserve the sanctity of human values and the precious resources of the human spirit.

This point is made well in a telegram I received recently from a parent who lists 10 drugs given his child in one year. He says, "Testing proved child creatively gifted, no classroom available. My state has hundreds of gifted and creative children on prescribed drugs as result of refusal to provide proper education facilities."

And here we come to what is perhaps the greatest paradox in this entire program and why I am convinced that public discussion must take place before the use of behavior modification drugs "zooms." As the father of four, I am well aware of the occasional frustrations which come from the fact that children do not simply sit quietly and perform assigned tasks. Based on my personal experience, I believe that children learn with all their senses, not just with their eyes and ears. For childhood is an exploratory time and the great energy of children propels them into situations which may look frivolous or counterproductive to more restrained adults, but which are the sum and substance of the child's learning experience. I do not think I am overstating the case when I say that the learning environment for the young child is the total environment and every experience is a learning experience.

Obviously, this unstructured passion for all the events in a child's world is regarded as unruly and disruptive, particularly in overcrowded classrooms. I fear that there is a very great temptation to diagnose the bored but bright child as hyperactive, prescribe drugs, and thus deny him full learning during his most creative years.

While we intend to hear from the Food and Drug Administration about the legal guidelines for the use of such drugs in children and the warnings they require to be printed on the packages, I am deeply concerned about the mislabeling of the child and packaging an ill-conceived program as an answer to our ills in the education of our children.

In addition, are there reliable medical guidelines which can be universally and absolutely applied to separate the normally active child from a clinically diagnosed hyperactive child?

*   *   *

Public men must investigate the uses of science and research and decisions must not be made solely on the expertise of those connected with a new technology. In the past we have tried to excise the potentially toxic elements from the beneficial tonic of technology; that is the purpose of this hearing today.

Before calling our first witness, I want to place in the hearing a portion of the preliminary report I received last Friday, September 25, from the General Accounting Office. This shows almost $3 million in Federal funds have been expended solely by the National Institute of

Mental Health in grants in the conduct of research of learning disabilities and, as part of each study, behavior modification through the use of drugs.

This document, focusing only on grant awards by the NIMH of the Department of HEW shows nine grants totaling nearly $3 million. Of that figure, the General Accounting Office reports $965,000 has been granted since the beginning of 1970.

*   *   *

NOTES

NOTE 1.

TESTIMONY OF DR. THOMAS C. POINTS,
DEPUTY ASSISTANT SECRETARY FOR HEALTH
AND SCIENTIFIC AFFAIRS, HEW, AND
DR. RONALD LIPMAN, CHIEF, CLINICAL
STUDIES SECTION, FDA—SEPT. 29, 1970

*   *   *

DR. POINTS: Hyperkinesis is recognized by the medical community as one of the more common behavior disorders of childhood which, when diagnosed by a competent physician or medical team, lends itself to safe and effective drug treatment, given, of course, adequate medical supervision. While this treatment should not be "forced" upon the parent, neither should it be denied to those children whose parents willingly give permission for such treatment. In most cases, proper drug treatment will provide symptomatic relief and will reduce the personal unhappiness of the child while enabling him to profit from the educational experience and from other forms of therapy such as psychotherapy, family counseling, and remedial reading.

While it seems clear that there is some diagnostic heterogeneity in children labeled as hyperkinetic, this syndrome, in addition to the key symptom of overactivity, usually includes many of the following symptoms: short attention span, low frustration tolerance, aggressive-hostile behavior, and hyperexcitability. The syndrome is frequently accompanied by impairment in perception, conceptualization, language, and memory. A neurological examination typically reveals minimal signs of neurological impairment.

Most clinicians feel that the hyperactivity per se is outgrown by adolescence. However, the few follow-up studies that have been reported suggest that hyperkinetic children who have not received treatment and/or whose treatment

has been limited to either individual or group psychotherapy show as adults, a disproportionately high incidence of diagnosed psychoses and sociopathic personality. Conversely the percentage of hyperkinetic children whose adjustment was characterized as evidencing "no psychiatric disease" (21 percent) was quite low relative to a matched control group (60 percent). It should be noted that the hyperkinetic children comprising this sample of roughly 250 children were not mentally retarded, nor were they psychotic at the time of the original diagnosis.

*   *   *

The present consensus of expert opinion regarding the treatment of hyperkinetic children is that Ritalin (methylphenidate) and Dexedrine (dextroamphetamine) are the drugs of choice. Although Ritalin and Dexedrine are considered stimulants, they have a calming and quieting effect in hyperkinetic children in striking contrast to their exciting, stimulating effect in adults. Given under competent medical supervision, these drugs are regarded as safe and clinically effective in a very high percentage of hyperkinetic children. While children report that they feel better when receiving these drugs, we are aware of no evidence to suggest any feeling of euphoria and no evidence to suggest that these drugs are addicting in children.

The therapeutic efficacy of the stimulant drugs is evidenced both behaviorally (there is reduced overactivity, impulsiveness, temper outbursts, aggressiveness) and on such cognitive tasks as arithmetic, spelling, paired-associate learning, recognition, maze learning, etc. This improvement is obvious to the physician, parents, teachers, peers, and to the child himself. Moreover, there is evidence to suggest that the stimulant drugs do not "dull" the child or decrease his activity level in appropriate situations such as free play; rather these drugs enable the child to sit still and attend in those situations, such as in the classroom, where this behavior is both appropriate and, indeed, necessary if the child is to profit from the education experience and not become a school dropout.

*   *   *

MR. GALLAGHER: How do you select the children?

DR. LIPMAN: Children are typically referred either from the report of the parent seeking help for the child, from the child's physician or pediatrician, or on the recommendation of a teacher and then the child may go through the route of seeing the school psychologist and then being referred on.

None of these studies are done directly in the school system.

MR. GALLAGHER: What qualifications would a teacher have to make this kind of diagnosis to nominate a child for this kind of study?

DR. LIPMAN: I think typically what may happen is the teacher will see that the child is extremely inattentive in class, extremely restless. The child is not performing up to the level of intellectual ability that the child has.

The child seems personally unhappy, unable to get along with his or her peers. The child is continually in motion, continually getting into things, and in general their academic performance does not come up to what their intellectual abilities would suggest it should.

MR. GALLAGHER: Couldn't it also be similarly a result of a poor teacher or a bright child who is beyond the point of concentration because the class is dull?

DR. LIPMAN: I would say that the role of the teacher is not to diagnose the medical syndrome.

MR. GALLAGHER: But that is where the child begins the treatment, diagnosed by some teacher, isn't that a fact? It comes from the public school system, as opposed to a parent who may take a child to a doctor?

DR. LIPMAN: I think the role of the teacher is really a referral function. That the diagnosis should be properly made by a skilled medical person or a medical team.

*   *   *

MR. GALLAGHER: . . . The thing in these programs that troubles me is the number of children involved. How many children would you say today are being treated—we have seen quoted a figure of some 200,000 to 300,000 children. Would that be correct? More? Less?

DR. LIPMAN: Well, if you restrict it to amphetamine and to Ritalin, I would say that figure is probably high. It would probably be closer to about 150,000 to 200,000. That is just a rough estimate. . . .

*   *   *

MR. GALLAGHER: Then further you state, "I think the results of the last few years of research will soon reach the nation's doctors. The pediatricians will begin using them." In effect,

what will happen is it will zoom as word of its success spreads throughout the nation's medical community.

Where do you think it will zoom to 5 years from now?

DR. LIPMAN: I didn't use the term "zoom." I said it would probably increase.

MR. GALLAGHER: I think your enthusiasm led to the word "zoom."

DR. LIPMAN: I guess really some evidence that we have indicates that child psychiatrists tend to be using more of the stimulant drugs than pediatricians. I think the more recent studies that are well controlled and meet scientific standards have strengthened the earlier clinical reports and I think as the scientific validity of the treatment of children with hyperkinesis with the stimulant drugs as part of their total treatment program becomes better known and better accepted by the medical community, that there probably will be some increase. Now, where it will go, I don't know.

MR. GALLAGHER: Do you think that it should be allowed to increase or zoom or whatever word we want to use, on the basis of the follow-up studies which involve, as I recall, some 250 children out of 200,000 or 150,000 or 300,000, whatever is the correct figure? Are we justified at this point in further funding the use of amphetamines for children?

DR. LIPMAN: . . . I think we need more knowledge in these areas and I think the studies that we are currently supporting are directed to developing that knowledge.

*   *   *

MR. GALLAGHER: If we don't have it, then should the program be allowed to grow? This is one of the points of our inquiry. If there is not this amount of scientific dedication around at this time, why are we allowing this to grow in the proportion that it appears—to use your own words here, whatever they indicate—if we don't have any real follow-up studies in light of all of the evidence that we do have of the effect of the drug culture on American children today?

DR. LIPMAN: Well, the follow-up study by Conners which is the only one I can really talk to with any—

MR. GALLAGHER: Yes, but Dr. Conners has been involved in this for some time. He is obviously a dedicated scientist to this thing. Where do we have some other dedicated scientist who may question this? This is the point. An adversary development may well produce a more valid opinion, no matter how dedicated the people may be. Are we doing any of that before we begin to zoom?

*   *   *

MR. GALLAGHER: In these studies that you have concluded and Dr. Conners' study, what is the addiction percentage of children in these programs, or the dependency percentage? Say out of 150,000 children?

DR. LIPMAN: As I mentioned, Mr. Gallagher, the results of Dr. Conners' study are still preliminary, in the first 67 cases he examined, there have been no instances of diagnosed alcoholism or drug addiction.

MR. GALLAGHER: Sixty-seven out of 150,000. That is all we have looked at? That is not a real basis to give additional millions of dollars to these programs, if all we know is 67, and when the whole bulk of the medical industry is trying to tell us, and all parents are trying to say, that amphetamines are so widely used they become the basis of addiction.

*   *   *

MR. WYDLER: I want to go back to something more fundamental here so I can get a point clear in my mind.

We are giving some school children these drugs. What is the purpose of it?

Is it to make that child learn better or more?

Is it to make it easier for his classmates to learn more because he becomes more amenable to the learning process and less disruptive, or is it to help the teacher possibly control the class?

For what purpose are we giving these drugs to children in school? ...

DR. POINTS: ... It is mainly to improve their learning.

*   *   *

MR. WYDLER: What evidence do we have that that has worked?

DR. POINTS: There are several reports over the years that in these true hyperkinetic children, their arithmetic improves, and so forth.

These true hyperkinetic diagnosed children, treated with these drugs, have increased their learning capacities and improved their social adjustment.

*   *   *

MR. ROSENTHAL: ... What percentage of our children suffer from MBD?

DR. LIPMAN: The estimates we have are from 3 to 10 percent of those up to 12 years of age.

*   *   *

NOTE 2.

STATEMENT OF JOHN HOLT,
EDUCATIONAL CONSULTANT AND
LECTURER AT HARVARD UNIVERSITY—
SEPTEMBER 29, 1970

One of my concerns has been the lack of real knowledge as to the nature and effects of the use of these drugs. What actually happens when a child is given these drugs? A mother brings a child to a doctor and says, "Doctor, my child is doing this or that, he won't sit still at meals, he fights with other children, he doesn't pay attention to me when I talk, et cetera, et cetera." Does the doctor himself observe any of this behavior? He does not. Does he have any way of knowing the history of the child and the mother, whether there is anything in her way of dealing with the child that might cause the child's behavior? He does not.

Does he fulfill his minimum responsibility as a physician by giving the child a thorough enough physical examination to be reasonably sure that there is not some other somatic cause for the child's behavior—bad hearing or sight, other body malfunctions, muscular or nervous injury, tension, pain, hypoglycemia, protein or vitamin deficiency, allergies, glandular disturbances? In the cases I have heard of, he does not. Does he test in any way the hypothesis that it might be something other than brain damage in the child that is causing the mother to describe him as she does? For the most part, he does not.

Might not one of the causes be the fact that we take lively, curious, energetic children, eager to make contact with the world and to learn about it, stick them in barren classrooms with teachers who on the whole neither like nor respect nor understand nor trust them, restrict their freedom of speech and movement to a degree that would be judged excessive and inhuman even in a maximum security prison and that their teachers themselves could not and would not tolerate? Then, when the children resist this brutalizing and stupefying treatment and retreat from it in anger, bewilderment, and terror, we say that they are sick with "complex and little-understood" disorders, and proceed to dose them with powerful drugs that are indeed complex and of whose long-run effects we know little or nothing, so that they may be more ready to do the asinine things the schools ask them to do.

*   *   *

Given the fact that some children are more energetic and active than others, might it not be easier, more healthy, and more humane to deal with this fact by giving them more time and scope to make use of and work off their energy?

In addition to the educational questions, there are two other areas that we must consider. First, the social response of the child, and second, the kinds of pressure that the parents are subjected to.

In the first instance, what I think we can say, and with great certainty, is that if we think a child is strange, treat him as if he were strange, and tell him he is strange, he will begin to think of himself as strange and will act more and more strangely. I have known some such children myself. They often talked and acted as if they had a license to act crazy, to do what other children were embarrassed or ashamed or forbidden to do. This, in turn, added to their reputation of strangeness, and so around in a vicious circle.

Further, in a community where parents are under enormous pressure to have their children look well and do well, in school and everywhere else, where people justify their lives through their children's accomplishments, the parents of these children are out of the rat race, off the hook. Other people might have to agonize—"What have I done? What must I do?"—when their son or daughter has failed in school, misbehaved, and broken windows. But not these other parents, for they have the perfect answer—their child has a medical label, so it is not their fault, there is nothing for them to do about it, and how lucky it is that there are these experts here to look after their poor darlings. Everyone is taken care of, except, of course, the child himself, who wears a label which to him reads clearly enough "freak," and who is denied from those closest to him, however much sympathy he may get, what he and all children most need—respect, faith, hope, and trust.

* * *

NOTE 3.
TESTIMONY OF DR. JOHN E. PETERS, CHILD STUDY CENTER, UNIVERSITY OF ARKANSAS MEDICAL CENTER— SEPTEMBER 29, 1970

* * *

MR. GALLAGHER: . . . What we are really doing is looking at the total effect on our children.

DR. PETERS: My concern is not the general-

ity of our children but these particular children that these parents bring to me. This is my concern.

MR. GALLAGHER: We have a broader responsibility to the children of our country. What a doctor recommends is the doctor's business, but not when our government is sponsoring it.

* * *

MR. GALLAGHER: Do you feel the diagnostic procedure used today is sufficient and adequate?

DR. PETERS: I think it is clear to us, particularly in, say, the middle-class home where the nutrition and the psychological environs have been what we might call healthy. I think it sometimes is not clear in the culturally deprived. We do not know which it is.

MR. GALLAGHER: But you feel that you can at least detect it and properly diagnose it as this, as MBD. Can a country doctor do this?

DR. PETERS: If I had the chance to teach him, yes.

* * *

MR. GALLAGHER: In your judgment then, is more research required in this area or do you feel we have adequate knowledge now to properly train and carry out the treatment?

DR. PETERS: Well, I think we have adequate knowledge to treat as we are now, but I think we need much more research because we need to know much more about what is going on in the brain, what is happening in these children, what is different about them, how the medication is affecting them, and more than anything we need other educational approaches as ways of handling them too.

* * *

b.

Through Professional Evaluation?

[i]
Report of the Conference on the Use of Stimulant Drugs in the Treatment of Behaviorally Disturbed Young School Children*

On January 11–12, 1971, the Office of Child Development and the Office of the Assistant Secretary for Health and Scientific Affairs, Department of Health, Education, and Welfare, called a conference to discuss the use of stim-

---

* Daniel X. Freedman, M.D., Chairman. Washington, D.C.: Department of Health, Education, and Welfare (1971).

ulant medications in the treatment of elementary school-age children with certain behavioral disturbances. In convening the conference, the Office of Child Development was aware of public concern about the increasing use of stimulant medications (such as dextroamphetamine and methylphenidate) in treating so-called hyperkinetic behavior disorders. Were these drugs— so widely misused or abused by adolescents and adults—truly safe for children? Were they properly prescribed or were they used for youngsters who, in fact, need other types of treatment? Is emphasis on medications for behavior disorders misleading? Might this approach tempt many to oversimplify a complex problem, leading to neglect of remedial social, educational or psychological efforts on the part of professionals, parents, schools and public agencies?

In order to clarify the conditions in which these medications are beneficial or harmful to children, to assess the status of current knowledge, and to determine the best auspices for administering these drugs to children, a panel of fifteen specialists was invited to meet in Washington. The panelists were from the fields of education, psychology, special education, pediatrics, adult and child psychiatry, psychoanalysis, basic and clinical pharmacology, internal medicine, drug abuse and social work. The panel's task was to review the evidence of research and experience and to prepare an advisory report for professionals and the public.

*   *   *

We know little about definitive causes. The disorder has been ascribed to biological, psychological, social or environmental factors, or a combination of these. There is speculation that the core set of symptoms—those affecting control of attention and motor activity—may have their origin in events taking place before the child is born, or during the birth process, or they may be related to some infection or injury in early life. The neurological and psychological control of attention is an important but incompletely researched topic, as are the nutritional, perinatal and developmental factors. Thus, in many instances, it is not yet possible even to speculate as to original causes.

Usually, the excessive activity and attentional disturbances are less apparent after puberty. Specialists citing experience and some fragmentary research data believe that treatment enables many to lead productive lives as adults, while severely afflicted children who remain untreated may be significantly at risk for adult disorders. Extensive research is still required on these points. Because the ages of 5 to 12 are crucial to the child's development and self-image, treatments which permit the child to be more accessible to environmental resources are warranted and useful.

In diagnosing hyperkinetic behavioral disturbance, it is important to note that similar behavioral symptoms may be due to other illnesses or to relatively simple causes. Essentially healthy children may have difficulty maintaining attention and motor control because of a period of stress in school or at home. It is important to recognize the child whose inattention and restlessness may be caused by hunger, poor teaching, overcrowded classrooms, or lack of understanding by teachers or parents. Frustrated adults reacting to a child who does not meet their standards can exaggerate the significance of occasional inattention or restlessness. Above all, the normal ebullience of childhood should not be confused with the very special problems of the child with hyperkinetic behavioral disorders.

The diagnosis is clearly best made by a skilled observer. There unfortunately is no single diagnostic test. Accordingly, the specialist must comprehensively evaluate the child and assess the significance of a variety of symptoms. He considers causal and contributory factors—both permanent and temporary—such as environmental stress. He distinguishes special dysfunctions such as certain epilepsies, schizophrenia, depression or anxiety, mental retardation or perceptual deficiencies. The less severe and dramatic forms of hyperkinetic disorders also require careful evaluation. Adequate diagnosis may require the use not only of medical, but of special psychological, educational and social resources.

*   *   *

We will now turn to various concerns about hazards and abuses when stimulant medications are used for children. For example, concern has been expressed that the medical use of stimulants could create drug dependence in later years or induce toxicity. This subject touches on the rights of the child to needed treatment, as well as risks to both the child and the public, and requires continued intensive scrutiny.

One should not confuse the effects of intravenous stimulants and the high dosages used by drug abusers with the effects or the risks of the low dosages used in medical therapy. In the dosage used for children, the questions of acute or chronic toxicity noted in the stimulant abuser are simply not a critical issue. Unwanted mental or physical effects do rarely appear in children; cessation of therapy or adjustment of dosage quite readily solves the problem.

Thirty years of clinical experience and several scientific studies have failed to reveal an association between the medical use of stimulants in the pre-adolescent child and later drug abuse. Physicians who care for children treated with stimulants have noted that the children do not experience the pleasurable, subjective effects that would encourage misuse. They observe that most often the child is willing to stop the therapy, which he views as "medicine." Thus, the young child's experience of drug effects under medical management does not seem to induce misuse. The medical supervision may "train" him in the appropriate use of medicines. . . .

* * *

It is sometimes suggested that treated children may not be able to learn normal responses and master adjustments to the stresses of everyday life. These fears are understandable but are not confirmed by specialists who have experience with the conditions and the situations in which medications are properly used. For the correctly diagnosed child, these medications—if they work at all—facilitate the development of the ability to focus attention and to make judgments in directing behavior. Such children can acquire the capacity to tolerate and master stress. The medications, in these circumstances, help "set the stage" for satisfactory psychological development.

The hyperkinetic behavioral disturbance is a form of disorganization that creates great stress in the afflicted child. The use of therapeutic stimulants for this disturbance should not be equated with the misuse of medication aimed at allowing a normal child or adult to avoid or escape the ordinary stresses of life.

Under no circumstances should any attempt be made to coerce parents to accept any particular treatment. As with any illness, the child's confidence must be respected. The consent of the patient and his parents or guardian must be obtained for treatment. It is proper for school personnel to inform parents of a child's behavior problems, but members of the school staff should not directly diagnose the hyperkinetic disturbance or prescribe treatment. The school should initiate contact with a physician only with the parents' consent. When the parents do give their approval, cooperation by teach-

ers, social workers, special education and medical personnel can provide valuable help in treating the child's problem.

* * *

Pharmaceutical companies producing stimulants or new medications which may become useful for hyperkinetic disorders have a serious obligation to the public. These medicines should be promoted ethically and *only* through medical channels. Manufacturers should not seek endorsement of their products by school personnel. In the current climate, society can best be served if industry refrains from any implicit urging that nonspecialists deal with disorders and medications with which they are unfamiliar. Professionals and the news media can play useful roles by not pressing for treatments in advance of their practical availability.

Our society has not as yet found complete solutions to the problem of the delivery of special health care. When available treatments cannot be confidently and appropriately delivered by physicians, they are perhaps best withheld until such treatments can be provided—especially with milder dysfunctions. This is not to say that severely afflicted hyperkinetic children should not or cannot receive available medical treatment. But until systems of continuing professional education and ready access to consultants are financed and perfected, some judgment about the pace at which unfamiliar treatments can be widely fostered is required. Finally, we must recognize that it is not only the scarcity of trained personnel, but factors such as poverty and inadequate educational facilities which prevent accessibility to individualized treatment.

In preparing this report, the committee was repeatedly struck by our lack of information in many crucial areas. The facts are that children constitute well over half our population, but receive a disproportionately low share of skilled research attention. We have noted the difficulties in arriving at accurate methods of diagnosis and the importance of launching careful longitudinal and follow-up studies. The investigation of causal factors lags. Such factors as perinatal injury, environmental stress or the development of the neurological and psychological controls of attention require study. Variations in different socioeconomic and ethnic groups must be considered in order to arrive at better definitions of behavior properly regarded as pathological. All such research efforts would have aided us in assessing the numbers of affected children and in recommending designs for more effective treatment programs.

Clinical pharmacologists have repeatedly found that drugs may act differently in children than in adults. To use medicines of all kinds effectively in children, more specialists must be trained in drug investigation—pharmacologists who can develop basic knowledge about the action of drugs in the developing organism. There is the obvious need for better and more precisely targeted drugs for the whole range of severe childhood behavior disorders. This requires intense research and training efforts. Such efforts provide the means for developing, testing and delivering better treatment programs. There is a similar need for research in the techniques of special education and also a need to make these techniques available to children who can benefit. It would appear to be a sound federal investment to conduct such research and training.

In summary, there is a place for stimulant medications in the treatment of the hyperkinetic behavioral disturbance, but these medications are not the only form of effective treatment. We recommend a code of ethical practices in the promotion of medicines and candor, meticulous care and restraint on the part of the media, professionals and the public. Expanded programs of continuing education for those concerned with the health care of the young, and also sustained research into their problems are urgently needed.

* * *

[ii]
Stephen Goldby
Experiments at the Willowbrook State School*

You have referred to the work of Krugman and his colleagues at the Willowbrook State School in three editorials. In the first article the work was cited as a notable study of hepatitis and a model for this type of investigation. No comment was made on the rightness of attempting to infect mentally retarded children with hepatitis for experimental purposes, in an institution where the disease was already endemic.

The second editorial again did not remark on the ethics of the study, but the third sounded a note of doubt as to the justification for extending these experiments. The reason given was that some children might have been made more susceptible to serious hepatitis as the result of the

administration of previously heated icterogenic material.

I believe that not only this last experiment, but the whole of Krugman's study, is quite unjustifiable, whatever the aims, and however academically or therapeutically important are the results. I am amazed that the work was published and that it has been actively supported editorially by the *Journal of the American Medical Association.* . . .

* * *

. . . Is it right to perform an experiment on a normal or mentally retarded child when no benefit can result to that individual? I think that the answer is no, and that the question of parental consent is irrelevant. In my view the studies of Krugman serve only to show that there is a serious loophole in the Draft Code [of the World Medical Association], which under General Principles and Definitions puts the onus of consent for experimentation on children on the parent or guardian. It is this section that is quoted by Krugman. I would class his work as "experiments conducted solely for the acquisition of knowledge," under which heading the code states that "Persons retained in mental hospitals or hospitals for mental defectives should not be used for human experiment." Krugman may believe that his experiments were for the benefit of his patients, meaning the individual patients used in the study. If this is his belief he has a difficult case to defend. The duty of a pediatrician in a situation such as exists at Willowbrook State School is to attempt to improve that situation, not to turn it to his advantage for experimental purposes, however lofty the aims.

* * *

If Krugman and Giles are keen to continue their experiments I suggest that they invite the parents of the children involved to participate. I wonder what the response would be.

NOTES

NOTE 1.

THE EDITORS OF THE LANCET
REPLY TO GOLDBY*

Dr. Goldby asks *The Lancet* a question it ought to have faced long ago. The journal's eagerness to discuss all the events in the elucida-

---

* 1 *The Lancet* 749 (1971). Reprinted by permission.

* 1 *The Lancet* 749 (1971). Reprinted by permission.

tion of the spread of hepatitis left it exposed to these criticisms, which we accept. The Willowbrook experiments have always carried a hope that hepatitis might one day be prevented there and in other situations where infection seems almost inevitable; but that could not justify the giving of infected material to children who would not directly benefit. Dr. Krugman and Dr. Giles argue that "the artificial induction of hepatitis implies a 'therapeutic' effect because of the immunity which is conferred." It is hard to accept that view, even when applied to a school where a very high proportion of children will, in existing conditions, be infected anyway.

NOTE 2.

SAUL KRUGMAN
EXPERIMENTS AT THE
WILLOWBROOK STATE SCHOOL*

Dr. Stephen Goldby's critical comments about our Willowbrook studies and our motives for conducting them were published without extending us the courtesy of replying in the same issue of *The Lancet.* Your acceptance of his criticisms without benefit of our response implies a blackout of all comment related to our studies. This decision is unfortunate because our recent studies on active and passive immunization for the prevention of viral hepatitis, type B have clearly demonstrated a "therapeutic effect" for the children involved. These studies have provided us with the first indication and hope that it may be possible to control hepatitis in the institution. If this aim can be achieved, it will benefit not only the children, but also their families and the employees who care for them in the school. It is unnecessary to point out the additional benefit to the world-wide populations which have been plagued by an insoluble hepatitis problem for many generations.

* * *

. . . Viral hepatitis [at Willowbrook] is so prevalent that newly admitted susceptible children become infected within 6 to 12 months after entry in the institution. These children are a source of infection for the personnel who care for them and for their families if they visit with them. We were convinced that the solution of the hepatitis problem in this institution was dependent on the acquisition of new knowledge leading to the development of an effective immunizing

agent. The achievements with smallpox, diphtheria, poliomyelitis and more recently measles represent dramatic illustrations of this approach.

It is well known that viral hepatitis in children is milder and more benign than the same disease in adults. Experience has revealed that hepatitis in institutionalized, mentally retarded children is also mild, in contrast with measles which is a more severe disease when it occurs in institutional epidemics involving the mentally retarded. Our proposal to expose a small number of newly admitted children to the Willowbrook strains of hepatitis virus was justified in our opinion for the following reasons: 1) they were bound to be exposed to the same strains under the natural conditions existing in the institution, 2) they would be admitted to a special, well-equipped and well-staffed unit where they would be isolated from exposure to other infectious diseases which were prevalent in the institution; namely, shigellosis, parasitic infections and respiratory infections. Thus, their exposure in the hepatitis unit would be associated with less risk than the type of institutional exposure where multiple infections could occur; 3) they were likely to have a subclinical infection followed by immunity to the particular hepatitis virus; and 4) only children with parents who gave informed consent would be included.

The statement by Dr. Goldby accusing us of conducting experiments exclusively for the acquisition of knowledge with no benefit for the children cannot be supported by the true facts.

NOTE 3.

JOAN P. GILES
HEPATITIS RESEARCH AMONG
RETARDED CHILDREN*

No man has yet known absolute right or absolute wrong. We are grateful to those who would have us review, to examine our ethics. Let us go back.

The institutional problem does not begin with endemicity and its morbid toll. It begins with heredity, pre- and postnatal infection, pre- and postnatal trauma. So do its ethics. The compounding of moral decisions that precede institutionalization gives us pause. The geneticist, weighing adverse chance with fact and figures, advises that a handicapped child should not be conceived; the parents, informed, accept or re-

---

* 1 *The Lancet* 966–967 (1971). Reprinted by permission.

* 1 *The Lancet* 1126 (1971). Reprinted by permission.

ject such advice. The therapeutic abortionist, equally fundamental, equally weighing adverse chance with fact and figures, advises that a handicapped fetus should not be born; the parents, informed, accept or reject such advice. The obstetrician, knowledgeable though fallible, makes decisions according to his best judgment; the parents, informed, accept or defer to his decisions. The pediatric surgeon must do the same, weighing knowledge and success against adverse chance; the parents, informed, accept or reject his advice. The physician, religious leader or social worker who advises removal of the retarded child from the home his presence disrupts must weigh the repercussions of moral responsibility. The parents who accept this advice must answer to their conscience. In each case the skilled, the knowledgeable physician, informs, advises; in each case, from before conception to day of admission to an institution, it is the parents who ultimately decide: an awesome precedent. The physician does not make the moral judgment. He stands by, ultimately human, to accept or reject parental decision. If he cannot accept, he refers. If he accepts, he acts.

*   *   *

We too are dealing with facts, with adverse chance, with, to be specific, our problem: endemicity of hepatitis. We too must await the ultimate parental decision: controlled or uncontrolled exposure, immunity safely by design through minimal disease, or by natural endemic exposure, ill-timed perhaps, with the adverse chance of complicating with respiratory disease, shigellosis, Coxsackie or Echo viruses—the compounded infections which threaten survival. We are physicians, dedicated to life, to support, to teach, to grow with our knowledge, to offer more because of this knowledge; and because of overwhelming circumstances we knew that action was warranted. We too believe that it is the duty of the pediatrician to attempt to improve the situation. Put back the knowledge gained and we must deal, in conscience, with ignorance. This too begets reaction. We could have stepped over disease and been blamed for not caring. As a matter of record instead we have slowly and carefully advanced. The population has been among the earliest to have been vaccinated against measles and rubella, and soon shigellosis. Now the encouragement of promise against serum hepatitis.

Yet are we faced with the conflict to truths. The ethical relativism, honest and honorable

within the environment we are dedicated to serve, is questioned. The truth is that our conscience does not inhabit a germ-free area and the children were sick upon it. Our actions are dissected by words and the result is fatuous.

A farmer may pull up corn seedlings to destroy them, or he may pull them up to set them in hills for better growing. How then does one judge the deed without the motive?

We are advised to improve the situation; of what is the situation but a child (and retarded at that), and a virus (whose only constancy is its love-affair with the human host), and society (who puts them together and departs)? In our honesty we cannot separate the child from the situation of which he is an integral part: both cause and effect. To do so is a trick of words.

And what of knowledge? A physician brings to the care of a patient all the knowledge of which he is possessed (much of it born of controversy now forgotten), and learns from each patient to whom he ministers. In our honesty, we have learned. We cannot separate knowledge from the child, no more than deed from motive, or child from situation.

*   *   *

Now examine the accusation that "infected material" is injected into children, and let us discuss knowledge, and *degree* of infectivity, and resultant gain. Yes gain, and to the child. For the half-truth of the accusation is that we proceed blind and wanton for our own unspeakable advantage. The thought shames us for here is proof that you have never known us, that you have not come the three thousand miles to know what you condemn, nor walked with us even the first mile. For here is truth: you cannot clinically tell the newly admitted child from the child injected, at the height of response, from the child whose response is over, except for the fact that those who have been with us longer, by virtue of our care, are better adjusted, better nourished, and more scheduled within their capabilities. And immune, and this is a measurable fact. Your assumption is of illness. We have seen more reaction to countless vaccines than to the procedure we have so carefully controlled.

Truth is many things: the truth of parents, realistic after trial; the truth of critics, idealistic and apprehensive of what they have not seen and do not know; there is the truth of those whose judgment has led to action, and the truth, acknowledged, that there are no absolutes. There is the final truth that above all else man must help man, and the knowledge that each may approach by a different path, in conscience.

NOTE 4.

THE EDITORS OF THE JOURNAL OF THE AMERICAN MEDICAL ASSOCIATION PREVENTION OF VIRAL HEPATITIS— MISSION IMPOSSIBLE?*

Letters to the editor of *Lancet* harshly criticized Krugman and his colleagues for their studies. . . . One writer (Goldby) was "amazed that the work was published and that it has been actively supported editorially by the *Journal of the American Medical Association*. . . ." In pious tone, *Lancet's* editor supported Goldby's view. . . .

*   *   *

This issue of *The Journal* carries the most recent report from Krugman's group and, as it turns out, *Lancet's* editor would have been well advised to keep his pen away from paper. The evidence is now in; viral hepatitis, type B (MS-2) can be prevented by active immunization induced by inoculation of an inactivated preparation of MS-2 serum.

Mission accomplished!

c.

Through Governmental Action?

*Medical Notes in Parliament
Ethics of Clinical Investigation*†

The conduct of clinical trials in hospitals and the right of the patient to be informed and to give or withhold his consent were discussed in the House of Commons on February 16. It was raised by MR. STEPHEN SWINGLER (Newcastle-under-Lyme, Lab.). . . . He put forward two principles: medical experiments on patients should not be conducted unless there was a chance of patients benefiting; and clinical experiments in hospitals should not be conducted unless the consent of the patients had been freely given. . . .

In the Bristol case, he said, penicillin was administered to newly born babies for the purely scientific purpose of observing their reaction to penicillin and to establish the properties of the preparations. The penicillin was not required by

---

* 217 *Journal of the American Medical Association* 70–71 (1971). Reprinted by permission.

† 1 *British Medical Journal* 546–547 (1955). Reprinted by permission of the editor.

the babies, and there was no question of its having any beneficial effect on the babies. It had been established by the Minister of Health on inquiry that the consent of the parents was not sought. In his opinion, even if consent had been given, the experiment was ethically dubious. [I]n the same issue of the *Journal* in which the experiment was reported there was a report of a speech by a distinguished doctor to a meeting of the Royal Society of Medicine about the uses and abuses of antibiotics, in which he was reported to have said that a doctor should think twice before prescribing the first-ever dose of penicillin to any patient.

*   *   *

MAJOR W. J. ANSTRUTHER-GRAY (Berwick and East Lothian, Con.) was concerned that all consideration of the parents appeared to have been overlooked. He quoted extracts from the *Journal* report, and said that he had no doubt the experiment was quite harmless. There was a note at the foot of the article in which a lot of people were thanked. But the parents were not only not thanked, they were not even consulted.

MR. IAN MACLEOD, Minister of Health, said it was admitted that the consent of the parents should have been asked for. The people responsible, who were of the greatest authority and competence, regretted very much—as he did—that that was not done. What the House was discussing was whether such experiments were proper, and whether any action should be taken by the Minister in these matters. He disagreed with Mr. Swingler's proposition that it would be wrong and unethical for any clinical investigation to be carried out which would not immediately benefit the person concerned. If it was to add to future knowledge he did not see how that could be so. The reward to those who tried to catch the common cold at the Salisbury research unit was not that they would derive direct benefit themselves, but that the general pool of knowledge might be increased and others helped in the future. The answer to Mr. Swingler, therefore, was that babies yet unborn might benefit from this continued thrusting forward to new frontiers.

There were two propositions with which he thought most of the House would agree. First, there was bound to be clinical investigation and experiment. If that were not so, knowledge of surgery and medicine would not have changed over the centuries. Second, only the clinician in charge could say what was right and proper and what safeguards were needed in the action he took. Mr. Swingler had asked, in questions on February 14, that before further clinical experiments on children were undertaken the nature of such experiments should be reported to the Ministry of Health so that the medical staff of the Ministry could ensure that there were adequate safeguards against harmful effects; and also that the Minister should issue a directive to hospital management committees on the ethical principles involved. That was in his (Mr. Macleod's) view a wrong conception of the duty of the Minister of Health. He thought it would be wholly improper for him to try to lay down what ethical and medical principles should govern the conduct of professional men in the work they undertook at hospitals.

In this instance there was undertaken an experiment which all those concerned, who were of the highest capability, were quite certain was completely harmless. If a small child of his, or a child of any age, was in hospital, and he was told by people of the standing, for example, of professor of medicine and child health at the university concerned, "We are interested to know the effects of a perfectly safe clinical investigation; it may very well be that we can learn from what is done, and as a result can drive still lower the infant mortality rate," he would be more than ready to give his consent.

The common sense of the matter was that where a clinician intended to undertake an investigation which was so novel as to amount to an experiment he would be wise to seek consent from the patient or parent for what was proposed. But he was absolutely convinced that it would be quite wrong for a Minister of Health to issue directives on a matter that was essentially one of medical ethics to those concerned. He was sure it was best to leave the matter to the profession, and not to have a lay Minister interfering in a matter that was very precious to those professionally concerned.

MR. SWINGLER said he appreciated why the Minister should resist the idea that he should himself go into this matter and issue a directive. But in view of the complexity of the situation, did he not think it was the duty and responsibility of the heads of the medical profession to give some ethical guidance? As it had been brought to his attention that there were cases where, for example, consent had not been obtained, and where experiments were being conducted which had nothing to do with actual treatment, would he not use his good offices to ask the heads of the medical profession to give some guidance on that?

MR. MACLEOD said that was a very different matter and one with which he was in some sympathy. If he had the slightest reason to believe that the position was not fully understood, then he would informally—and it could only be informally in a matter like this—draw the attention of those responsible to what had been said. The Medical Research Council sent out a confidential memorandum rather on those lines. If he had any reason to believe that the position was not completely clear, and that it was desirable for these things to be drawn to the attention of those responsible, then of course he would not object at all to what he might call an informal notification from himself. Of one thing he was clear: no directive must come from the Ministry of Health on a matter of this delicacy.

*   *   *

CHAPTER THIRTEEN

Experimentation with Captive Subjects

The prosecutors at Nuremberg maintained that the use of political and military prisoners for experimental purposes constituted a "crime against humanity." The defense tried to meet this argument by presenting evidence, especially from American sources, of the longstanding practice of enlisting prisoners in research projects. Heated exchanges ensued about the capacity of any captive person to participate in research on a truly voluntary basis.

From these debates emerges a broader and more basic question for the entire human experimentation process: What persons or institutions should be authorized to formulate, administer, and review decisions to allow investigators to recruit subjects who are vulnerable to external pressures? Since these subjects are usually the "captives" of state institutions, the decision to experiment with them, as with uncomprehending subjects, must be grounded in public policy and cannot be left solely to the discretion of investigators. Although the case materials in this chapter focus primarily on prisoners, the issues they raise apply in varying degrees to other captive groups, *e.g.* soldiers, the economically disadvantaged, and persons in hospitals and other non-penal institutions.

In studying these materials, consider the following questions:

1. What groups should be defined as "captive" for research purposes? Is vulnerability to "external pressures" the most important cause for concern?

2. Should external pressures be taken as a characteristic common to all human activity and thus deemed of no special significance to decisions in human experimentation?

3. To what extent are external pressures strengthened or weakened by making rewards for participation in an experiment explicit or leaving them implicit?

4. If permitted, should the use of captive patient-subjects be restricted to research which aims to benefit them or attempts to learn more about the conditions which made them members of the captive group?

5. Should captive subjects be permitted to participate in research if non-captive subjects could be selected instead?

6. If research is permitted on captive groups generally, should any sub-group be specifically excluded from participation in research?

7. What impact might the widespread use of prisoners for research have on the administration of justice?

A.
Case Studies of Prisoners and Soldiers as Patient-Subjects

1.

Richard P. Strong
Vaccination against Plague*

Although the question of protective inoculation against plague has received considerable attention during the past few years and prophylactics for the disease have been recommended . . . apparently no successful experiments have been made on human *vaccination* against the malady—i.e., protective inoculation in which the living attenuated pest bacillus has been employed. . . . In 1781, Samoilowitz, a Russian physician, inoculated himself with plague pus, suffered a mild attack of the disease, and so became immune. Therefore, he recommended that a lint compress previously saturated with the pus from a plague bubo be bound upon the arm of the person to be immunized. The skin of the individual was not to be abraded. Other observers attempted similar experiments; but many of these resulted disastrously; thus, Cerutti performed such inoculations on six persons, five of whom died of plague. Because of these results this method of immunization obviously was soon abandoned and has not since been employed. . . .

* * *

In 1902 and 1903 Kolle and Otto inoculated eighteen guinea pigs subcutaneously with an attenuated culture of the pest bacillus. The organism was an old laboratory culture in which the

* 1 *Phillipine Journal of Science* 181, 184–187 (1906). Reprinted by permission.

reduction of the virulence had, in some unknown manner, taken place during its growth on artificial media. Buboes, which later discharged and healed and in the pus from which a few bacilli were present, developed in the animals, but they showed no other evidence of sickness and subsequently entirely recovered. The animals were reinoculated two, three, and eight months later with one-twentieth to one-fiftieth dose of a pest culture (of which one one-hundredth dose represented the fatal dose for a normal guinea pig). Seven of the animals remained alive.

* * *

In December of the past year (1904) Kolle and Otto in further detail reported upon the immunization of guinea pigs with the attenuated pest bacillus. Among thirty-four of these animals immunized with such a culture, of which none died during the process of immunization, twenty-one were reinoculated with a virulent organism one to four months after their vaccination, and of this number sixteen (76 per cent) remained alive, and five died. Nine other guinea pigs were inoculated with the avirulent culture, and at the same time with plague immune serum; all proved to be immune upon reinoculation with the virulent pest bacillus. The organism with which these vaccination experiments were performed possessed so little virulence that from two to three living, agar slant cultures, when injected into a guinea pig of 250 grams' weight, did not cause the death of the animal. . . .

* * *

In the present paper it is merely my desire to call attention to the fact that vaccination in man can with safety be performed with attenuated cultures of the living plague organism, and therefore only the human inoculations undertaken with one strain of this bacillus will be referred to. The organism in question possesses so little virulence that in a series of twelve guinea pigs and thirty monkeys inoculated with from one to two entire agar slant cultures, not one succumbed from the effects of the inoculation. It was with this culture that the first experiments were performed in human beings. Since I believe that the guinea pig is an equally if not even a more susceptible organism than man to the pathogenic action of the plague bacillus, it was presumed that, if this animal could invariably withstand the action of such large amounts as two whole agar slant cultures of the organism, much smaller quantities could be inoculated into human beings with safety, and, indeed, before performing the experiments on man, I felt thoroughly convinced of this fact; nevertheless, the human inoculations were performed as carefully and with as much deliberation as possible.

*　　*　　*

The first injections were carried on upon prisoners under sentence of death; in the first case one-hundredth dose of the attenuated culture was inoculated subcutaneously without any noticeable effect. After ten days, ten other individuals were innoculated with the same dose, in order to demonstrate that no special natural immunity against the plague organism had been existent in the first instance. In this manner the amount of living organisms given was gradually increased, a single person being first inoculated with the larger dose and then, after it had been observed that no unfavorable effects occurred, from five to ten other persons were also treated with the same amount of the vaccine. This method of procedure was adopted in order to minimize the danger of inoculating a very susceptible individual with a dose which might prove disastrous. It was argued that if ten persons selected at random withstood the inoculation of a certain amount of the organism without developing unfavorable symptoms, a single individual, also selected at random, could probably receive a slightly larger dose without great danger. In this manner as mentioned the dose was gradually increased until one whole agar slant was inoculated. No attempt has been made to inject a larger amount of the organism, since

from experiments performed on animals it has been concluded that a sufficient immunity in man will probably result from an inoculation of this quantity. Up to the present time forty-two persons have been injected with this large dose (one twenty-four hour agar slant culture) of the living bacillus, and, although the inoculations which I include in this report were all performed more than two months ago and the individuals treated have been under constant surveillance, I have no accident to report.

Surprising as it may seem, the injection of these large amounts of the living plague organism have not given rise to any very severe reactions. . . .

*　　*　　*

NOTE

RESEARCH ON THE KINETICS OF THE GERMINAL EPITHELIUM IN MAN

In an article published in 1964,* Heller and Clermont reported their investigation of "the dynamic processes taking place in the seminiferous epithelium of man." The study was conducted with eight previously vasectomized "inmate volunteers" at the Oregon State Penitentiary who ranged in age from 20 to 42 years. When Dr. Heller analyzed his subject population, he found that

they were a rather uniformly mixed group of northern Europeans. They were Irish, Scots, English, and French mixed (and one French Canadian). We are now looking for other volunteers from other racial groups. I found a splendid full-blooded American Indian volunteer, and the preliminary studies suggest that at 16 days and at 31 days he falls right where he should be. I have a negro volunteer at present. Other ethnic groups are absent from the Oregon State Penitentiary; I cannot find anybody with a full-blooded semitic background. There are no Japanese, there are no Chinese, but there are many of Filipino origin and we are searching for such a volunteer.

Bilateral testicular biopsies were performed by first administering local novocaine anesthesia (the testes remaining uninjected). After the scrotal skin had been incised, a 0.5–1.0 cm cut was made in the tunica "and the testicular tissue was separated from the tunica by lateral undercuts. External pressure on the testis was avoided.

---

* Carl G. Heller and Yves Clermont: "Kinetics of the Germinal Epithelium in Man." G. Pincus, ed.: 20 *Recent Progress in Hormone Research.* New York: Academic Press 545 (1964).

Due to internal pressure, the underlying seminiferous tubules protruded above the tunica and were severed by a stroke of a razor blade parallel to the surface of the testis."

To determine the duration of the spermatogenic process, radioactive thymidine (thymidine-H³) was introduced directly into the testicular matrix. This procedure was first tested in rats before being applied to men. The injection sites were marked by a black silk suture to facilitate their identification for subsequent repeated biopsies.

In another experiment, a normal healthy subject was injected intramuscularly with 4000 I.U. of chorionic gonadotropin every second day for thirty-five days. Subsequently 10 mc. of thymidine-H³ was injected intratesticularly and some time later a biopsy was obtained.

The authors concluded "that neither a steroidal hormone nor chorionic gonadotropin has affected the rate of development of the germ cells; the rate of spermatogenesis in man therefore appears to be a biological constant in confirmation of Ortavant's conclusion derived from . . . studies on the ram."

2.

**Arthur L. Mattocks and Charles C. Jew
Assessment of an Aversive "Contract"
Program with Extreme Acting-Out
Criminal Offenders***

*   *   *

The drug succinylcholine (Anectine) has been widely used during recent years by medical practitioners as a muscle relaxant in proper dosages. Succinylcholine, when injected intravenously, results in a brief muscle paralysis and respiratory arrest. Administered in sufficient dosage, the patient goes through a sensation of suffocation similar to drowning although he remains fully conscious of the experience (temporary paralysis and apnea). This experience, to some, can be a highly frightening experience which psychologists would term "aversive."

*   *   *

Concerned with the inability to prevent self-destructive and/or assaultive behavior among extreme acting-out patients despite psychotherapy, phenothiozine tranquilizers, anti-depressant

_____
* Unpublished manuscript (1971). Printed by permission of the authors who retain all rights.

drugs, therapeutic milieu, electro-shock therapy and other resources, a program of Anectine treatment as a last resort was initiated at the California Medical Facility [CMF] in January, 1967. The first case was a patient who had continued inexorably to mutilate himself and imperil his life by swallowing six- to nine-inch sharpened metal wires which required multiple laparotomies. He then persistently reopened his laparotomy wounds and shoved pieces of wood and metal under his skin. The use of Anectine treatment prevented the patient from harming himself for many weeks which led to the continuation of the program to handle similar patients who posed a constant serious threat to themselves (self-mutilation, suicidal attempts) or to others (assaults on other inmates or staff) for whom all available treatments within the institution have been exhausted and failed to alter their behavior. The conceptual scheme was to develop a strong association between any violent or dangerous acting-out behavior and the drug Anectine (and its frightful consequences) such that it would be an effective suppressant to further contemplation or commission of these acts.

The Anectine program was begun in January, 1967 and continued until April, 1968. During that time, sixty-four inmates participated by signing a treatment contract with the institution's Special Treatment Board.[†] The aversive cues

_____
[†] . . . On five patients, consent was not received from the patient himself, but was granted by the institution's Special Treatment Board. Thus, these five patients were included in the treatment program against their will.

*   *   *

It is interesting to note that although only five of those interviewed in the present study were signed up involuntarily for the aversive treatment program, eighteen indicated they involuntarily signed the treatment contract indicating that they felt some implied pressure to do so in the doctor's request. Related to this is the fact that a sizable number of the patients perceived the motive of the doctor as one of punishing them even though the medical staff exerted efforts to assure the patients that this was not to punish but to help the patient control his own behavior. While the staff was successful in convincing a majority of the subjects interviewed of their helpful intentions, it is clear that in the environmental context, and with the experiential background of the subjects in the type of population used in this study, such efforts are not apt to meet with total success.

*   *   *

of the drug were described by the medical staff as each individual become involved in the program. The contract emphasized that he would receive an Anectine injection *if, and only if,* he indulged in behavioral acts such as (1) violently attacking others, (2) serious self-mutilation, or (3) suicidal attempts, but he would receive no injection if he did not commit such acts. It was therefore up to him whether he ultimately would receive an injection since this was determined by his own behavior.

As it will be seen later in the study, only a small portion of the patients involved in the program actually had violated their contracts and received Anectine injections. The actual administration followed closely the patients' acting-out behavior. Because the administering procedure is also a crucial part of the aversive program, it is outlined here as it was described by one of the medical staff administering the program:

Our technique is simply to administer 20 to 40 mg. of succinylcholine intravenously with oxygen and an airway available, and to counsel the patient while he is under the influence of the drug that his behavior is dangerous to others or to himself, that it is desirable that he stop the behavior in question, and that subsequent behavior of a nature which may be dangerous to others or to himself will be treated with similar aversive treatments. During the entire time, oxygen is administered so that there is no danger of anoxia and . . . there is no pain accompanying the procedure, only cessation of respiration for a period of approximately two minutes duration. We have been very careful to explain to all individuals involved that they will suffer no permanent ill effects, that the treatment is safe as long as it is given by competent medical personnel, that it will not cause pain, and that at all times they will be supervised closely so that they need not worry about ill effects of the treatment.

How severe is the Anectine experience from the point of view of the patient? Sixteen likened the experience to dying. Three of these compared it to actual experiences in the past in which they had almost drowned. The majority described it as a terrible, scary, experience. Nearly all of these subjects based their descriptions not only upon what the doctor had told them, but either on personal experience or the first-hand description from patients who had had an Anectine injection. Again, two patients denied the experience bothered them at all, and two were noncommittal. It would seem therefore that the perception of the aversive consequence by the patients was of sufficient severity to warrant consideration of this factor as a possible explanation for the inhibition of aggressive behavior. [From an earlier draft of the same paper.]

Most of the sixty-four patients in the program were housed in the acute treatment area due to their recurring pattern of extreme and potentially dangerous behavior both to themselves and others. Nearly all could be characterized as angry young men who directed their anger impulsively outwards in attacks on others, or inwardly towards themselves, or exhibited both types of behaviors at various times. The average age of the subjects was twenty-five years and the mean time at the institution was fifteen months. The frequency and repetition with which they engaged in these dangerous behaviors cannot be overstated. Examples of violent behavior of two of the patients read as follows:

He was a twenty-four-year-old committed to prison for murder 2nd originally, who, while he was in the county jail, hanged his cell partner. On being sent to the California Department of Corrections he was placed in an adjustment center where he engaged in self-mutilative efforts which gained him admission to the institution hospital. While there he murdered another time (a defenseless psychotic prisoner) and was sent forthwith to us for psychiatric observation while he was waiting to stand trial. His stay at our institution was without self-mutilation or assault under the promise of Anectine treatment and he received no treatments.

Another patient under the treatment program was considered by institution officials as very dangerous. He had killed one man and assaulted another with a bayonet (commitment offense). During his stay in the institution he accumulated twenty-three violations of rules necessitating thirteen placements in administrative segregation and/or isolation. He had threatened officers and recently "stabbed" another inmate a few days ago.

Three months prior to the termination of the program, an evaluation strategy was developed by the CMF Research Unit to assess the impact of the Anectine program. The evaluation goals were to determine: (1) whether Anectine had an impact in inhibiting the continued repetition of suicidal, homicidal, and self-mutilative behavior(s), (2) whether a generalization effect will occur leading to the overall reduction of undesirable behavior, including those not specified within the treatment contract, and (3) whether the response to Anectine differs according to the type of commitment offense of the patient.

At the time of the data collection most of the patients had been under the Anectine "contract" for at least three months. Considering the frequent repetition of aggressive behavior among this population, the results shown tend to suggest Anectine is highly effective in inhibiting the commission of "contract" behavior in that only twenty-eight percent (18) of the population had received one or more injection of Anectine. Seventy-two percent (46) had not committed any of the specified acts and did not receive an injection of Anectine. This constitutes an improvement in that they fulfilled the treatment contract. While there is no way in which one can accurately estimate the number of assaults, stabbings, self-mutilations, and suicidal attempts inhibited through the use of the Anectine program, a fact not to be ignored is that fifty-seven percent of the patients were able to be assigned later to a psychiatric program or sufficiently stabilized for transfer to other prisons for programming.

Indeed, at the time of the evaluation, sixteen of the participants had been transferred to other penal institutions for programming. The remaining thirty-five were interviewed and their disciplinary records reviewed. . . .

*   *   *

A most unexpected result from the Anectine program data is the differential effect it has upon different types of criminal offenders, which came to light through comparing increases and decreases in disciplinary infractions among offense types. Patients who committed "crimes against persons" (i.e., robberies, homicides, assault, sex, rapes) responded entirely differently to the Anectine program than patients who committed crimes against property (fraud, theft, tax evasion, etc.) The former offense types tended to decrease while the latter tended to increase the overall number of disciplinary infractions as a result of the Anectine "contract."

*   *   *

This type of program seems to be particularly useful in institutions where the concern is to inhibit highly dangerous behavior through the temporary application of an aversive stimulus in which more effective alternatives are not to be found. However, extreme caution needs to be exercised in the use of Anectine because more knowledge is certainly needed to understand the subsequent anxiety and the side effects derived from its usage, especially the "paradoxical" effects of punishment in which the use of aversive stimuli may increase the rate of the punished behavior when the aversive stimulus is removed. In addition, not everyone in the program had considered the Anectine program "aversive." In subsequent interviews with some of the patients

who received Anectine injections, several indicated that they enjoyed undergoing the Anectine experience. In a similar vein, nine persons not only did not decrease but had actually exhibited an increase in their overall number of disciplinary infractions. Thus, careful selection as to who may be included in programs of this nature seems mandatory because the application of aversive stimuli to inhibit one or a series of behaviors may be highly effective to some patients, ineffective for some, and for still others may stimulate an increase in behaviors which the aversive stimuli were intended to inhibit.

3.

William R. Brink, C. H. Rammelkamp, Jr., Floyd W. Denny, and Lewis W. Wannamaker
Effect of Penicillin and Aureomycin on the Natural Course of Streptococcal Tonsillitis and Pharyngitis*

The problem of determining the efficacy of therapy of acute streptococcal infections of the upper respiratory tract is difficult, for these infections are of short duration and are usually not severe. Only by controlled studies in which an attempt is made to quantitate the occurrence of symptoms, physical signs and fever is it possible to conclude that this disease has been affected favorably. The present study was undertaken to determine the relative efficacy of penicillin and aureomycin in the treatment of group A hemolytic streptococcal respiratory infections. For this purpose 475 patients with exudative tonsillitis or pharyngitis were studied by clinical, bacteriologic and serologic methods.

The investigation was conducted in Francis E. Warren Air Force Base, Wyoming, between March 8 and April 30, 1949. During the period of study streptococcal respiratory infections were epidemic with rates of ten to thirteen hospitalized cases per 1,000 men per week.

All patients admitted to the base hospital with respiratory symptoms or fever were examined within a few hours by a physician from the Streptococcal Disease Laboratory. If exudate of any degree was observed on the tonsils or pharyngeal mucosa, the patient was admitted to the study ward. Selection for the treated and control groups was determined by the air force serial number. While penicillin was being eval-

* 10 *American Journal of Medicine* 300–308 (1951). Reprinted by permission.

uated, patients whose serial numbers ended in an even digit received intramuscular injections of procaine penicillin. . . . Patients whose serial number ended in an odd digit served as controls and received no treatment.

One week after concluding the study of penicillin, aureomycin therapy was employed. Patients with serial numbers ending in the digits one and three were given no specific treatment. All other patients with exudative tonsillitis and pharyngitis received one gram of aureomycin. . . .

While in the hospital the patients received no antipyretics but were given small doses of codeine for severe headache.

*   *   *

There was a total of 198 patients who received no treatment; 197 received penicillin and 80 were treated with aureomycin.

*   *   *

The relative frequency of feverishness, headache and loss of appetite was similar in the three groups; sore throat, however, occurred somewhat less frequently in those who received penicillin than in the other two groups. This was also associated with a decreased incidence of tenderness of the cervical lymph nodes in the patients who later received penicillin. There was a distinct difference in the incidence of edema of the soft palate, the control group exhibiting less swelling of the palate and uvula than the group receiving aureomycin or penicillin.

*   *   *

. . . Penicillin or aureomycin treatment resulted in a more rapid disappearance of symptoms than occurred in the control group of patients. Aureomycin was more effective than penicillin although the differences were not marked. The prevalence of anorexia was about equal in the three groups throughout the period of observation. Nausea and vomiting were especially prevalent among those patients receiving aureomycin, 51 per cent having these complaints. In the untreated group 35 per cent complained of nausea or vomiting during the course of the illness. Loose stools occurred in 45 percent of the patients receiving aureomycin whereas only 15 per cent of the control group exhibited this symptom.

Treatment instituted early in the course of illness resulted in a more rapid recovery than when therapy was delayed. . . . Patients treated

with aureomycin within the first twenty-four hours of onset of illness no longer complained of sore throat after the fourth day whereas on the sixth day 8 per cent of the control group still had this symptom. Penicillin therapy instituted after the first twenty-four hours of illness resulted in only a slightly more rapid disappearance of sore throat than occurred in those who received no treatment.

. . . Following treatment with either aureomycin or penicillin there was no marked improvement in the physical signs. However, in almost every instance individuals receiving treatment improved somewhat more rapidly than those serving as controls. Aureomycin appeared more effective than penicillin in this regard, but the differences cannot be considered significant.

*   *   *

Suppurative complications were unusual. There were ten (5 per cent) patients with peritonsillar cellulitis in the control group, thirteen (6.5 per cent) in the group receiving penicillin and four (5 per cent) in the group treated with aureomycin. In two of the patients being treated with penicillin peritonsillar cellulitis developed after therapy was instituted.

The number of patients in whom signs of otitis media developed is not known but 6.5 per cent of the control group complained of an earache beginning twenty-four hours or more after hospitalization. This is in contrast to 2 per cent of the patients treated with penicillin and 1 per cent of the aureomycin-treated group in whom earache developed after the institution of treatment.

There were seven instances of definite acute rheumatic fever developing within ten to thirty-five days following the acute streptococcal illness. Five of these patients were in the control group which received no treatment and two developed in patients treated with penicillin. No rheumatic fever occurred in those patients treated with aureomycin. No instance of acute nephritis was observed.

*   *   *

The fact that acute rheumatic fever developed in only two patients receiving penicillin and five patients of the control group suggests that penicillin may prevent rheumatic fever. The two cases occurring following penicillin were the only instances observed in a much larger study of 698 patients treated with this drug and is in contrast to seventeen instances of the disease among 702 controls who received no specific therapy. This study established that penicillin is an effective agent in the prevention of rheumatic fever when administered during the preceding acute streptococcal infection. The fact that no case of rheumatic fever followed the acute infections treated with aureomycin suggests this drug may also prevent the subsequent development of acute rheumatic fever.

*   *   *

B.
Appraising the Role of the Participants*

1.

In Formulating Policy

a.

Deciding about Choice of Subjects?

[i]

*John D. Arnold, Daniel C. Martin,
and Sarah E. Boyer
A Study of One Prison Population
and Its Response to Medical Research†*

*   *   *

It will be our goal to discuss the act of volunteering for medical research and its relationship to the social structure of the prison system. From previous studies, it was noted that communication between potential volunteers in prison and the experimenters, who belong to free society, was an obvious problem. In general, members of prison groups have a low verbal ability. The type of language of the prison inmates is very often specialized. Along with the technical difficulties overlying the use of language, the usual difficulties with informed consent are accentuated in the prison setting. Additionally, information originating in free society is often considered suspect by the prison population. A great many explanations can be called on to account for this, but for our purpose, it is important simply to recognize that a credibility gap does exist.

In a recent study of a prison population, we found two major factors contributing to the availability of a subject: the type of prison and the value scale of the prisoner. It is difficult for members of the free-living society to visualize the condition of most penal institutions. [I]t is necessary to understand the general condition of prisons in order to examine more closely the volunteer and the volunteering process. The second portion of our study concerns itself with the value scale by which prisoners judge risk, reward and social merit.

We have analyzed the inmate's views of the prison system in this study (county jail), as well as his view of other prison systems (federal and state penitentiaries) in which he has also resided.

The federal prisons, according to our inmates, are the best run institutions. Prison discipline is usually good, and the aberrant behavior of prisoners seen in other prisons is less common. Inmates also indicate that federal prisons offer more opportunities for employment during incarceration and that many federal institutions have active and intensive rehabilitation programs.

The prisons in the state systems vary widely. Some are considered to be well run, while others are described as chaotic and dangerous. The long-term character of imprisonment in the state system leads to the development of certain social phenomena. In the state prisons there is a tendency toward the formation of powerful social cliques. Admission to these influential social groups depends almost entirely upon individual behavior. Street relationships have little or no influence on a prisoner's membership in an organized social clique. Preservation of street relationships within the state penitentiary system is often difficult. Prisoners rank state institutions as good when they offer job opportunities and when the prison supervision is effective. Prisons considered chaotic and dangerous are those where supervision is lax or indifferent.

The county and city jail systems have a character quite different from that of either the state or federal prisons. In county and city prisons, street associations are often a binding

---

* This appraisal section focuses on captive subjects. For a fuller exposition of the factors requiring appraisal, consult section D of Chapter Eleven, beginning at p. 818 *supra*.

† 169 *Annals of the New York Academy of Sciences* 463–469 (1970). © The New York Academy of Sciences, 1970. Reprinted by permission.

social force. In county jails, street relationships are sometimes transferred intact from the street to a given area of the jail. Depending upon the orientation and size of the jail, these street relationships can become powerful forces operating within the institution. Membership in these cliques, unlike the cliques in state prisons, is dependent entirely upon whom the prisoner knew while he was on the streets. If a prisoner in a county jail has no friends from the street serving time with him, he more than likely will find himself considered an outcast by the organized groups. Such outsiders are subject to the whims and sometimes the abuse of the clique.

Supervision in county jails often is less effective than it is in the other groups of prisons. Because of inadequate supervision, the powerful cliques are difficult to control. Effective supervision is further hampered by the poor physical facilities typical of many of our county jails. Perhaps of greatest importance is the fact that very little constructive activity is normally provided in county jails. As a result of so much inactivity, there is less competition for the time and interest of the prisoners. Therefore, medical research in these institutions is given a competitive advantage.

The medical research conducted in the county jail of this study falls into two general categories. The first includes all of those studies concerned with the treatment of malaria, and it is referred to by staff and prisoners alike as the "malaria project." The second category is concerned with a variety of drugs and their effect on certain body functions. This group, taken collectively, is always called "the drug studies." Prisoners who volunteer for either type of research must meet certain criteria before they can be accepted for any of the studies.

Eligibility requirements were set up by the project director and the jail warden. These considerations include the kind of crime committed, the type of previous convictions, and the time remaining on the prisoner's sentence. Prisoners who volunteer for either type of research must have received their sentences and have at least six months of jail time remaining. Volunteers are individually screened by the project director to see if they meet all the physical requirements of the project.

A prisoner who volunteers and is accepted for the research project moves into the special project area. This area differs from the other parts of the jail because the volunteers are treated more like members of a free society. Clean linens are provided, beds instead of bunks are installed, the quality of the food is better, and food is available to the volunteers 24 hours a day.

During the past five years several studies of our prison population have been conducted. Our most recent study was developed in three phases designed to examine the attitudes and motivation of prisoners toward volunteering. Phase I includes open-ended in-depth interviews of a group of 14 volunteers. From these data a semistructure interview schedule was developed. During Phase II, this interview was administered to all of our volunteers ($N=13$) on all of the research projects during the first week of April, 1969. Phase III consisted of interviews conducted with 15 prisoners from all areas of the jail who had no present or previous affiliations with any of the research studies. The data for this paper are drawn primarily from our most recent study. However, we have used supporting information taken from previous clinical research conducted during the past 12 years of work, including six years in a state prison and six years in a county jail.

We had assumed that living conditions in the other areas of the jail would influence a prisoner's decision to volunteer. During the open-ended interview conducted in the beginning of this study, the volunteers were asked to describe the living conditions in the jail. Their remarks, taken collectively, described the jail living conditions as "impossible situations." When asked if this influenced their decision to volunteer for medical research, more than 50 percent indicated that their decision to volunteer was based in part on their desire for better living conditions.

It was an assumption of our present study that street relationships would be an influential factor in the volunteering process. In an attempt to establish a correlation between street relationships and volunteering, the volunteer subjects were asked how many inmates they then knew were people they had formerly known in the streets. Only three prisoners in our sample had known any of the other prisoners from the street. These three respondents did not consider this relationship a strong one. Further questioning of our volunteer subjects indicated that the majority of them considered themselves "loners."

The loner, by definition, had not belonged

to any organized group. According to our study, the outcasts from the street cliques often sought membership in the only group that would take them—the research project. In effect, the medical research project provided a new environment.

There is another force operating within the prison system that influences medical research. This additional force is far less acceptable than inadequate supervision, constructive use of time, living conditions, or street associations. This less acceptable force is the general level of fear that exists in many city and county and state prisons. One of the more graphic descriptions of this was given by Davis, who studied sexual assaults in a county jail. This prison also had a medical research project that provided a haven from fear, as well as offering financial and other rewards.

* * *

Our volunteers stated that it was safer in the research project than it was elsewhere in the jail. In the volunteers' words, "You could trust people on the project," and, "There was less tension among the volunteers than among the other prisoners." The volunteers felt they could go to sleep in the research project without being afraid someone would "bust you in the head" or "set fire" to their bunks while they slept. All of the prisoners who did not volunteer, but who knew about the research project, agreed that there was probably less tension on the project than there was in their tanks. When asked why they believed this to be true, volunteers and nonvolunteers agreed that it was because the prisoners on medical research had something constructive to do with their time. As one volunteer said, "We are too busy to get into trouble." Seventy-five percent of the volunteers said that being on the project had helped keep them out of trouble while they were in jail.

Value Scales

One of our special interests has revolved around the problems of the value scale by which prisoners judge risk, reward, and social merit. To some degree, prisoners have their own value scale for the things that compete for their time. This is so because they have relatively few competing proposals. In their arid existence, some activities that are of little interest to free-living individuals are highly regarded by prison inmates. This fact alone gives every time-use proposal that is offered to their group a stronger

appeal than it might have among free-living groups.

There is an element in their way of life that we have also considered. That element is risk taking. This consideration is not unusual, for many of these men are dedicated professional criminals. Their professional lives are often devoted to activities that expose them to personal risk. The form and amount of risk taken by them is rarely seen among free-living people. To the degree that volunteering requires risk taking, certain inmate groups may endow this activity with status. This may be especially true if there is actual physical danger in the activity.

The prison inmate has two standards of risk. One applies to the period of incarceration (short-term risk) and the other applies to the time he is free-living (long-term risk). There is something about the state of imprisonment or the environment of a prison that alters a subject's view of risk. For instance, 12 of a group of 13 volunteers indicated that the apparent risk of adverse physical effects had little negative influence on their decisions to volunteer as long as they were in jail. In some instances, it constituted an attraction for volunteering. On the other hand, when confronted with a hypothetical experiment with the same risk considerations as that of the malaria project, of these same volunteers, only eight indicated that they would not be willing to face these same risks when free-living. Most of the free-living people whom we have interviewed would also not accept risks of this magnitude.

There is a small proportion of our volunteers that has included the element of risk in their life styles. From another group of 14 volunteers, three inmates expressed *no* concern about long-term risks, because they rarely planned ahead for anything. As an example, one prison volunteer indicated he would volunteer for anything, regardless of the risk. As a professional thief, he regarded life as just one long chance. Because of this attitude, he viewed his long-range survival with much doubt.

This last group of prisoners is the exception, rather than the rule. However, both of our volunteer groups demonstrated rather curious behavior with regard to family consultation concerning their volunteerism. If they informed their family, they always minimized the risk. They did this even though they themselves had a high estimate of adverse physical effects. When questioned about this discrepancy, they usually ndicated that it was immaterial whether or not here would be a recurrence of their malaria as long as they were under the protection of the program. This introduced another factor that plays a major role in volunteerism. This is the factor of a substitute parent.

One of the most striking factors influencing concern about risk was the protection provided by the research team. There develops by the volunteer an almost parental view of the research physician. In part, the research team has replaced the real family. Many prisoners would say, "I would do anything the doctor tells me to." Not only does this relationship remain strong in prison, but it tends to carry over after discharge. Some discharged prisoners attempt to use members of the research team for moral and medical support after leaving prison.

Money is as important in most jails as it is outside them. However, the value scale is different because money is much more difficult to obtain. In some jails money is contraband, but it undoubtedly circulates in all penal systems. Having money during one's incarceration enables one to buy certain privileges that are otherwise unavailable. But the need for money is most acute at the time a prisoner is to be released. The adjustment to a free-living society is made with greater ease when the returning prisoner has some financial independence. With rare exceptions, no provision has been made for the prisoner in terms of financial support. His first problem is to make a score soon after discharge. It is a fairly common consensus inside the prison that a return to crime, at least briefly, is the only way to manage during the early discharge period.

At present, one alternative to scoring is to be a prison volunteer. This provides the individual with a chance to gain financial independence for the critical period immediately following his release. Even with these opportunities, money earned by the volunteer is often spent while the inmate is in jail, and the inmate still leaves jail penniless. To whatever degree money may diminish the pressures on a newly discharged inmate to commit a crime, the payment for participation in medical research should be considered as a possible help in crime prevention.

Another prison force leading to participation in medical research is, surprisingly enough, the desire to do something worth while. It takes very little search of the *curriculum vitae* of these men to realize how little they have done for fam-

ily, friends, and society. A large proportion of those interviewed expressed a desire to make a positive contribution to society. The opportunities to satisfy this wish are often limited by the prisoner's dearth of skill.

In one part of this study volunteers were asked to respond to a set of statements by indicating those phrases that most clearly described their own feelings about volunteering. This group indicated that their participation in the malaria project would be a direct help to the servicemen in Vietnam. Several of the volunteers had been in military service or had relatives in it, and they felt they were making a positive effort toward eventual control of malaria. Others on the project stated that since they had experienced malaria, they would be able to help members of their family or friends if there would ever to be an "outbreak of malaria" in the United States. It mattered little to them that there is no real likelihood of this happening. All of the volunteers interviewed, with the exception of three, felt that by volunteering they were doing something worth while. Volunteerism, therefore, offers them a sense of satisfaction, and this feeling is frequently expressed by the volunteers both before and after an experiment.

One other aspect of the study concerned the fringe benefits of volunteering. The volunteers were divided in their opinions regarding this issue. Half of our prisoners believed that by volunteering for medical research, they had improved their chances for obtaining a job once they were released from prison. Only a very few of this group felt that volunteering had increased their opportunity for early paroles. Examination of nonvolunteers indicated that they held the same views concerning the fringe benefits of volunteering. Ninety-two percent of the group indicated that the experience as human subjects would have no bearing on their life styles once they were again members of the free society.

In this study we made no attempt to chart the steps in the decision-making process. We asked our volunteer subjects how they had first learned about the research project. Most of them had heard about the project either from other inmates or from the nurses who went around and asked for volunteers. The volunteers were asked to try to remember what the other inmates had told them about the project. Remarks from the other inmates regarding the project could be placed on a continuum ranging all the way from "they kill people down on malaria" to "medical research is the best way to do your jail time." The volunteers were asked what effect these remarks had on their decisions to volunteer. All of the volunteers, with one exception, indicated that the remarks of the other prisoners had no influence on their decisions to volunteer. Again, this is probably because this particular sample was made up of loners.

Although at various times we have had volunteers only from the "loners," this is not invariably so. At other times the jail cliques have strongly supported the program. At these times we can almost always identify the role of a single enthusiast who has great personal influence over a group of inmates. As we have indicated earlier, these groups are usually built around the street relationships.

If strong figures can turn on the flow of volunteers, they can also turn it off, except for those men whom we have called "loners."

We are also interested in knowing if the decisions to volunteer were made quickly, or if the prisoners thought for a long time before deciding.

About half of our group made up their minds to volunteer for medical research the same day they heard about the project. When asked if this decision had been an impulsive one, most of the volunteers responded that it had been made on impulse. Those volunteers who took a month or longer to make up their minds did not consider their decisions impulsive, but, on careful analysis, the long delays were often due to the fact that the prisoners were waiting for their jail time. We could conclude that decisions were very rapidly arrived at for most volunteers.

*   *   *

[ii]
Daniel C. Martin, John D. Arnold,
T. F. Zimmerman, and Robert H. Richart
Human Subjects in Clinical Research*

*   *   *

[This] study attempted to determine why prisoners did or did not volunteer as subjects in a search for new antimalarial drugs and the extent to which they understood the element of

_____
    * 279 *New England Journal of Medicine* 1426, 1427–1428 (1968). Reprinted by permission.

risk involved. Subjects of the motivation study were selected from inmates who had previously been asked to volunteer for the Malaria Project at the Jackson County Jail, Kansas City, Missouri.

The procedure originally used to enlist volunteers for the Malaria Project had been consistent with each prisoner. Inmates with sentences of one year or less were approached by a physician—one of the authors. He carefully explained the Malaria Project, the need for human subjects and the probable risks involved for the subjects. Each inmate was told that he would be paid for his participation but that he could expect no reduction of his sentence.

After the project had been explained in detail, inmates wishing to volunteer were examined to ascertain whether their current state of health permitted participation. Those determined to be in reasonably good physical and emotional health were given an "informed-consent" form to read. If they agreed to the conditions set forth in that document, they signed the consent form. To this point, all inmates who were approached had received the same initial explanation. However, those who volunteered continued to receive detailed information regarding the project, whereas nonvolunteers did not. During their extensive contact with the volunteers in the course of the project, the physicians continued to explain the element of objective risk (which was minimal). The process of the disease itself was explained in simple terms, and the discomfort that the volunteers would experience during the illness was carefully detailed.

In the present motivation study, two groups of inmates were interviewed. The inmates who served as volunteers in the Malaria Project (36 in number) comprised the first group. All had been ill with malaria and had been treated successfully. Inmates who could have volunteered for the project but did not (24 in number) made up the second group. The interviews and evaluations of the sample were carried out by behavioral scientists who were not involved in the clinical investigations of drugs and malaria.

The responses of these two groups (total of 60) were compared regarding their comprehension of the Malaria Project (that is, of the risks involved and the chances of being cured) and their reasons for volunteering or refusing.

The results of this pilot investigation pose more questions than they resolve. Inmates who had participated in the Malaria Project understood the nature of the disease and its probable threat to human life no better and no worse than those who had not volunteered. This occurred in spite of the fact that the volunteers had signed the "informed-consent" document and had continued to receive detailed information throughout the program. Although the physicians had repeatedly explained what the objective risks would be (and they were minimal), more than 60 per cent of the volunteers continued to describe the project in terms of "high risk."

The informed-consent procedure assumes that in reaching their decision, volunteers attempt to understand the information provided, consider the alternatives that have been explained and only then give free assent. The results of this short study indicate that the act of volunteering does not necessarily result from so logical a process. The volunteers' comprehension of the risks is little different from that of nonvolunteers, and, where it does vary, it is certainly not more accurate. Furthermore, very few in either group cited risk as a consideration in their decision. It becomes apparent that there are other issues involved in the decision to volunteer.

Both groups uniformly expressed belief in the importance of clinical research designed to discover new and better "cures" for disease. About half the participants gave "altruism," and the other half money, as the major reason for volunteering. One quarter of those who mentioned money gave "altruism" as a second reason. Nearly all the nonvolunteers believed that volunteering for such an enterprise was an "act of courage." Although nonparticipants gave a wide variety of personal reasons for not volunteering, they stated or implied respect for those who did volunteer.

The almost universal respect among nonvolunteers for those who did volunteer may offer some clue to the other group's reasons for volunteering. Although society at large regards prison life as having low status and few privileges, a system of privileges and status does operate within the prison itself. In a county jail, however, the opportunities to assert one's superiority are few, and those that do exist are open to a limited number of inmates. Projects like the malaria experiment provide many with a real chance to demonstrate their importance, not only to other inmates but to the "square Johns," and it is possible that this consideration takes precedence

over the weighing of risk and benefit implied by the informed-consent procedure.

* * *

NOTES

NOTE 1.
HOUSE OF DELEGATES OF THE AMERICAN MEDICAL ASSOCIATION RESOLUTION ON DISAPPROVAL OF PARTICIPATION IN SCIENTIFIC EXPERIMENTS BY INMATES OF PENAL INSTITUTIONS (1952) *

WHEREAS, During recent years, numerous medical and scientific experiments and research projects have been conducted partly or wholly in federal and state penal institutions; and

WHEREAS, Volunteers among the inmates of such institutions have been permitted to participate in scientific experimental work and to submit to the administration of untested and potentially dangerous drugs; and

WHEREAS, Some of the inmates who have so participated have not only received citations, but have in some instances been granted parole much sooner than would otherwise have occurred, including several individuals convicted of murder and sentenced to life imprisonment; and

WHEREAS, The Illinois State Medical Society's delegation to the American Medical Association's clinical session whole-heartedly supports research and progress in the fight against disease but does believe that persons convicted of vicious crimes should not qualify for pardon or early parole in this manner; now therefore be it

RESOLVED, That the House of Delegates of the American Medical Association express its disapproval of the participation in scientific experiments of persons convicted of murder, rape, arson, kidnapping, treason, or other heinous crimes, and also urges that individuals who have lost their citizenship by due process of law be considered ineligible for meritorious or commendatory citation; and be it further

RESOLVED, That copies of this resolution be transmitted to the Surgeons General of all federal services, the governors of all states, all officials of state and federal penal institutions and parole boards.

* *Digest of Official Actions.* Chicago: American Medical Association 617–618 (1959). Reprinted by permission.

NOTE 2.

ETHICAL COMMITTEE OF THE WORLD
MEDICAL ASSOCIATION
DRAFT CODE OF ETHICS ON
HUMAN EXPERIMENTATION (1961) *

* * *

Experiments not done for the benefit of the subject (whether healthy or ill) of the experiment, but solely for acquiring knowledge, should be conducted under the most stringent safeguards, as follows:

(a) The subject of the experiment should be in such a mental, physical, and legal state as to be able to exercise fully his power of choice.

(b) No doctor should lightly experiment on a human being when the subject of the experiment is in a dependent relationship to the investigator, such as a medical student to his teacher, a patient to his doctor, a technician in a laboratory to the head of his department.

(c) Prisoners of war, military or civilian, should never be used as subjects of experiment.

(d) Civilians detained in any place as a result of military invasion or occupation, or for administrative or political reasons, should never be used for human experiment.

(e) Persons retained in prisons, penitentiaries, or reformatories—being "captive groups"—should not be used as subjects of experiment; nor persons incapable of giving consent because of age, mental incapacity, or of being in a position in which they are incapable of exercising the power of free choice.

(f) Persons retained in mental hospitals or hospitals for mental defectives should not be used for human experiment.

[iii]
Charles Black, Jr.
Constitutional Problems in Compulsory
"National Service"†

. . . Proposals for compulsory non-military service by young people show a considerable variety among themselves, and this variety gives to any constitutional discussion a tentative and very general character. But those proposals which I have seen would in some way require that those

_____
* 2 *British Medical Journal* 1119 (1962). Reprinted by permission.
† *Yale Law Report* 19–21 (Summer 1967). Reprinted by permission.

young men, or perhaps even those young people, who are not selected for military service, enter, for a period of two or three years, some other kind of national, state or community training or service.

It may be needless to say that only the *compulsory* feature of these proposals raises serious constitutional issues. I cannot think that our Constitution inhibits us from tendering opportunities to our young people; the constitutional problems—and the very serious problems of policy—arise when we consider saying to these young people that they must accept one of the tendered opportunities or go to jail.

There is the Thirteenth Amendment. It seems, at first reading, that a distinction between "involuntary service," which is certainly the thing proposed, and "involuntary servitude," which the Thirteenth Amendment forbids, is too delicate to live in a constitutional atmosphere. . . .

To this principle there have been admitted, necessarily, exceptions based on history. The clearest and most important of these is the military draft. At this point I would suggest to you that the root-idea to which we ought to recur, in dealing with any suggested analogy from the draft, is that, in our public policy and in our constitutionalism, military service is and ought to be a striking, even a startling, exception, and not a thing which can readily be used for founding arguments by analogy. If one uses the military draft as an analogical basis for other invasions of personal freedom, then it seems evident that almost anything can be justified. Time forces me to make this point assertively, without briefing it, but I nevertheless emphasize it and commend it to your consideration. Either military service is an exception, a clearly delimited exception, from which analogical and *a fortiori* arguments may not be made, or there are few if any practical constitutional restraints in the government's dealing with our persons, whether we are 18, 8 or 80.

* * *

. . . In some manner or another, the military draft itself might be used to coerce, indirectly but effectively, participation in the National Service program. You can imagine the different ways in which this might be done—by holding up the military draft as a threatened alternative to entry, by drafting all who ceased to cooperate after they had entered, and so on. It might even be suggested, though I hope it will not be, that Congress could provide for a universal draft, and then in effect parole those not needed in or really eligible for military service into civilian work groups.

Even this might not work. If the subterfuge were palpable enough (and anything so large-scale would be hard to conceal) the courts might not swallow it. But it is true that the Supreme Court ought to and traditionally does defer to Congress on the nature and size of the military establishment, and some use of the military draft to coerce non-military service might be devised, so sophisticated as to force the Court to go along with it.

I suggest to you that such a development would be most unfortunate. The use of mere fictions for supporting a course of action which very probably would violate the Thirteenth Amendment is a thing which it seems we ought to reject simply on hearing the issue stated. Or, at another and more realistic level, if it can reasonably be thought that this "National Service," standing in the open, would violate the Thirteenth Amendment, then the least Congress ought to do is to put it in the open, without protecting fictions, so that the processes of law may determine on the merits, unembarrassed by presumptions suitable only to real military determinations, whether the claim of unconstitutionality has substance.

*   *   *

b.

Deciding about Societal Interests and Priorities?

Jack Kevorkian
Capital Punishment or Capital Gain*

Experimentation on human beings has, of necessity, been limited to volunteers during normal times whether it involves prisoners or others. However there is always a limit in such cases which curtails the means to any medical end, which detracts from the total of knowledge which might be obtained from the undertaking.

———
* 50 *Journal of Criminal Law, Criminology and Police Science* 50–51 (1959). Reprinted by special permission of the Journal of Criminal Law, Criminology and Police Science (Northwestern University School of Law). Copyright © 1959.

Capital punishment as it exists today offers a golden opportunity to break those limits by introducing into the situation an involuntary factor without destroying the necessary safeguard of consent. I propose that a prisoner condemned to death by due process of law be allowed to submit, by his own free choice, to medical experimentation under complete anesthesia (at the time appointed for administering the penalty) as a form of execution in lieu of conventional methods prescribed by law. After his choice has been made, let the condemned deliberate at his leisure, and have professional consultation at his request, and even let him reverse his decision within the week before the date set for execution.

The experiments should be very seriously outlined and should deal with questions that can be investigated under usual clinical circumstances on laboratory animals. They should be submitted from research scientists of many nations to an agency of the United States composed of reputable researchers who would select those deemed exceptionally promising. The same agency would then arrange for the research team to travel to the nation in which a prisoner has chosen to die under anesthesia. Thus the medical genius of all civilized nations can participate in a program of benefit to us all.

The medical, legal, and moral principles involved can best be discussed by considering the advantages and disadvantages to the parties concerned.

The disadvantages:

(1) For the condemned there is none. The choice is entirely his.

(2) For medicine, too, there is none. Physicians could not be executioners because their aim is not to kill but to learn. Ultimate death could be induced by an overdose of anesthetic given by a layman.

(3) For law one might say that the plan ostensibly tampers with the formality of law which stipulates executions in a prescribed manner. However, the plan simply offers a new form of execution which promises much more than the bleak aim of ending a criminal's life.

(4) For society it would mean tax dollars to run the agencies. But these costs need not be great, and a few human experiments would make allocations of funds for much animal work now in progress a complete waste of time and money.

The advantages:

(1) To the condemned it allows the dignity inherent in being permitted to decide how he

is to die. The only immediate rewards he can expect are the feeling of utility through death and the avoidance of a potentially harsh death (in contrast to non-condemned volunteers who usually anticipate special consideration at parole hearings). Furthermore, it would actually lengthen the condemned's life and create hitherto unthinkable "thirteenth" and even "fourteenth" hour chances of commutation.

(2) For medicine it would mean rapid progress in those fields where animal work cannot help (for one example, anatomy of the human brain). It also would make available a final and indispensable means of screening every new drug, device, or procedure before ultimate trial on sick patients.

(3) Law would acquire another beneficent aspect of enormous potential good to humanity. The plan would detract somewhat from the purely negative nature of capital punishment per se engendered by law.

(4) For society this proposed "judicial euthanasia" for the first time introduces the concept of recompensing into a matter now of pure vengeance. It offers a means of restoring some honor to the family of the condemned and of imparting positive significance to the death of his victim if he be a murderer. And it offers the ultimate means of assuring all of us and our descendants of improving health and lengthening life.

The plan differs markedly from the Nazi crimes of World War II which, in themselves, were wartime atrocities under the auspices of a demented government. The victims were unjustifiably condemned under makeshift "laws" on racial or political grounds; they were not asked for consent and were not anesthetized. The medical objectives were frivolous—the scientists sadistic.

The pros and cons of capital punishment are not at all involved in my proposal. My only contention is that so long as it is practiced, and wherever it is practiced, there is a far more humane, sensible, and profitable way to administer it. I have substantiated this through interviews with two men now facing electrocution, one of whom eloquently confirmed it in writing. Whether or not the plan is practicable on a worldwide basis remains to be seen. But it is feasible, and I hope that one of the states of our country which endorses capital punishment will legally allow a condemned man the *choice* and thereby set an example for the world to follow.

c.

Deciding about Harm?

Daniel C. Martin, John D. Arnold,
T. F. Zimmerman, and Robert H. Richart
Human Subjects in Clinical Research*

*   *   *

The first phase of the study dealt with personal willingness to volunteer. Persons interviewed were arbitrarily drawn from fairly well defined groups that had been identified in terms of general socio-economic criteria. The subjects interviewed were clients of the Helping Hand (a Nazarene Mission) and other welfare recipients, maids and janitors, skilled maintenance men, policemen and firemen and professionals—that is, scientists, lawyers and educators. A sixth group, prisoners from the Kansas City Municipal Farm, was also included in the study. All subjects were interviewed privately and assured that their comments would be kept in confidence.

The study took the form of a simulated enlistment of volunteers for medical research. The subjects were aware that the experiments proposed were hypothetical. Each respondent was asked to volunteer for participation in each of four "experiments" investigating malaria, new-drug toxicity, the common cold and air pollution (poisons). In this last hypothetical procedure, the volunteer would exhale air into a machine that measured "enzyme efficiency."

These four "experiments" were selected because they presented the subject with different degrees of personal risk, different time demands, varying requirements for interrupting family or employment obligations and different degrees of social importance. It was expected that these differences would be apparent to the subjects.

The subjects were first asked to volunteer for participation in each of the four experiments in the sequence listed above. Little or no explanation was offered, but all questions were answered. After he had volunteered or refused to volunteer for each of the four, the subject was interviewed further. Regarding each experiment separately, the respondent was first asked what he knew about the disease. Those who had refused were also asked whether they would volunteer after receiving more detailed information, what they thought of those who were willing to volunteer and what inducements it would take to get

* 279 *New England Journal of Medicine* 1426, 1428–1429 (1968). Reprinted by permission.

TABLE 1
Willingness of Several Social Groups to Volunteer

Volunteer Group	Malaria		Drugs		Cold		Air pollution		Group Totals
	yes	no	yes	no	yes	no	yes	no	
Prisoners	40	20	44	16	49	11	50	10	60
Low income*	7	19	9	17	10	16	17	9	26
Fire & police	3	37	5	35	11	29	28	12	40
Professionals	0	28	1	27	2	26	26	2	28

* Welfare recipients & maintenance personnel.

them to volunteer. All respondents were then asked whether medical experimentation using human subjects was worthwile, and where subjects should come from. . . .

Table 1 shows the frequency of volunteering for the various groups. Several groups have been merged because they gave similar reasons for volunteering or refusing to volunteer.

Table 1 clearly indicates that the hypothetical conditions elicit similar responses from all groups, in that each group shows least willingness to volunteer for the malaria experiment and a willingness that increases proceeding to "drugs" to "cold" and to "air pollution." It is inferred that the respondents perceive the four experiments in terms of differing degrees of risk or inconvenience or both. Even the prisoner group, generally inclined to volunteer for "everything," is least likely to volunteer for malaria and most likely to volunteer for the "air-pollution test," with gradations between. The evidence indicates that the four hypothetical experiments presented in the interview are responded to in low-to-high scalar fashion from malaria to air-pollution test.

Whereas all respondents are least likely to volunteer for malaria and most likely to volunteer for air-polution tests, social groups having different socioeconomic characteristics are not equally willing to volunteer. It can be inferred from these data that people of lower socioeconomic circumstances show the greatest willingness to participate as subjects in clinical studies. In proceeding up the socioeconomic scale, willingness to participate greatly diminishes, except for the task (poison test) perceived as involving least risk or inconvenience.

The data were also organized along dimensions of age, sex, living conditions (with whom

do they live) and race. Examination of data by age and race shows no difference in any regard. When the prisoner group is extracted from the total, it appears that the sex of the respondent and the living arrangements do determine his willingness to volunteer.

*   *   *

In the tests that were perceived as having higher risk or discomfort, *women* demonstrate a significantly higher willingness to volunteer as human subjects. Both men and women perceive the requirements of the four tasks in scalar fashion. Experiments involving malaria are least likely, and air-pollution test most likely, to acquire volunteers, with gradations between.

*   *   *

In all experimental groups there is a significantly greater willingness to volunteer when the potential volunteer is not obligated to others. The closeness of that obligation seems to make a difference in willingness to volunteer. When subjects have only themselves to be concerned about, volunteering is relatively frequent. When they have obligations to others who are not "immediate" family, they demonstrate a lesser willingness. Willingness is lowest when the potential volunteer is responsible for spouse and children.

It should be noted at this point that all six groups uniformly agreed on the importance of human participation in medical research. For the most part, all groups indicated an understanding of the difficulties encountered in attempts to discover better ways to treat disease. They also spoke sensibly about the risks human subjects take in participating in such efforts. With the exception of the professional group, those interviewed tended to emphasize what might be called the theme of "human responsibility."

*   *   *

2.

In Administering Research

a.

Who Should Participate, within What Structure, in State Regulation?

[i]
Committee Appointed by Governor
Dwight H. Green of Illinois
Ethics Governing the Service of Prisoners
*as Subjects in Medical Experiments**

During the war the Governor of the state of Illinois and the Department of Public Safety permitted prisoners in one of the state penitentiaries in Illinois to serve voluntarily and without any prior promise of a pardon or a reduction of sentence in prison as subjects in medical experiments. These experiments were designed to find a better preventive and curative treatment of malaria. The question has arisen of giving a reduction of sentence in prison as a reward for such service in addition to that ordinarily allowed because of good conduct.

The expression "reduction of sentence in prison" is used to indicate that under the parole system the total sentence is not reduced since the prisoner is subject to the regulations of the Parole Board after parole, his activities are supervised and the board may return him to prison. A prisoner is not subject to parole or a reduction of sentence in prison until the minimum duration fixed by court has been served in the case of sentences for an indeterminate period (e.g., ten to twenty years) when the maximum is less than life and in the case of sentences for a definite term of years but not including life.

The committee was appointed by the Governor to advise the Department of Public Safety relative to the ethical principles governing the conditions under which prisoners may be (a) permitted to serve as subjects for medical experiments and (b) granted a reduction of sentence in prison as a reward for such service.

*   *   *

---

* A. C. Ivy, M.D., Chairman. 136 *Journal of the American Medical Association* 447–458, 461–465 (1948). Reprinted by permission.

It would appear likely that a reduction of sentence in prison as a recognition for service in a medical experiment is consonant with the statutory "good time," "merit time" and "industrial credits" provisions of the parole system.

Prisoners render meritorious services in prison, such as working in a barber shop, the kitchen, the shoe shop or furniture shop, and this service is rewarded. The rendering of such service is encouraged by the warden and his administrators, and service as a subject in a medical experiment may be similarly encouraged and rewarded.

Since one of the purposes of the parole system is reformative, the reformative value of serving as a subject in a medical experiment should be considered. Serving as a subject in a medical experiment is obviously an act of good conduct, is frequently unpleasant and occasionally hazardous and demonstrates a type of social consciousness of high order when performed primarily as a service to society. The extent to which the service of a prisoner in an experiment is motivated by good social consciousness on the one hand and by the desire for a reduction of sentence in prison on the other is a matter for consideration in the case of each prisoner.

Regardless of a prisoner's motives for volunteering for an experiment, a habitual criminal or a prisoner who has committed a notorious or heinous crime should not be considered an acceptable volunteer for a medical experiment.

The most important requirement for the ethical use of human beings as subjects in medical experiments is that they be volunteers. Volunteering exists when a person is able to say "yes" or "no" without fear of being punished or of being deprived of privileges due him in the ordinary course of events.

A reduction of sentence in prison, if excessive or drastic, can amount to undue influence. If the sole motive of the prisoner is to contribute to human welfare, any reduction in sentence would be a reward. If the sole motive of the prisoner is to obtain a reduction in sentence, an excessive reduction of sentence which would exercise undue influence in obtaining the consent of prisoners to serve as subjects would be inconsistent with the principle of voluntary participation.

It is not considered a function of this committee to determine where the reward becomes excessive. This is a matter to be considered in relation to each prisoner and the nature of the experiment.

Obviously no one may make representations to a prisoner concerning the extent and types of reward which may accrue as a result of his service as a subject in a medical experiment.

NOTE

RICHARD R. WILLEY
EXPERIENCE IN DESIGN, CONDUCT, AND
EVALUATION OF RESEARCH*

*   *   *

The motivation for prisoners' volunteering as subjects for research is also complex. I have heard Dr. Reuben Gustavson recount the days of the antimalarial testing at Joliet State Prison, in Illinois, about the time of World War II. He described the preparations that were made for the use of prisoners: the possible outcomes of the research were explained to them, the risks were explained, the possibility of sickness or death was explained. When the call went out for volunteers, a reasonable number responded. The research went along well until one prisoner died, obviously from the effects of the experimentation. The experimenters, at this point, expected the worst, anticipating that the volunteers would disappear. Much to their surprise, the number of volunteers increased markedly! It is rather interesting to reflect on why this might have occurred, what it was that was really motivating these men.

*   *   *

[ii]
Department of the Army
Use of Volunteers as Subjects of Research†

1. *Purpose.* These regulations prescribe policies and procedures governing the use of volunteers as subjects in Department of the Army research, including research in nuclear, biological, and chemical warfare, wherein human beings are deliberately exposed to unusual or potentially hazardous conditions. These regulations are applicable world-wide, wherever volunteers are used as subjects in Department of the Army research.

2. *Definition.* For the purpose of these regulations, unusual and potentially hazardous conditions are those which may be reasonably expected to involve the risk, beyond the normal

call of duty, of privation, discomfort, distress, pain, damage to health, bodily harm, physical injury, or death.

3. *Exemptions.* The following categories of activities and investigative programs are exempt from the provisions of these regulations:

   a. Research and nonresearch programs, tasks, and tests which may involve inherent occupational hazards to health or exposure of personnel to potentially hazardous situations encountered as part of training or other normal duties, e.g., flight training, jump training, fire drills, gas drills, and handling of explosives.

   b. That portion of human factors research which involves normal training or other military duties as part of an experiment, wherein disclosure of experimental conditions to participating personnel would reveal the artificial nature of such conditions and defeat the purpose of the investigation.

   c. Ethical medical and clinical investigations involving the basic disease process or new treatment procedures conducted by the Army Medical Service for the benefit of patients.

4. *Basic Principles.* Certain basic principles must be observed to satisfy moral, ethical, and legal concepts. These are—

   a. Voluntary consent is absolutely essential.

*   *   *

   b. The number of volunteers used will be kept at a minimum. . .

   c. The experiment must be such as to contribute significantly to approved research and have reasonable prospects of yielding militarily important results essential to an Army research program which are not obtainable by other methods or means of study.

   d. The experiment will be conducted so as to avoid all unnecessary physical and mental suffering and injury.

   e. No experiment will be conducted if there is any reason inherent to the nature of the experiment to believe that death or disabling injury will occur.

   f. The degree of risk to be taken will never exceed that determined to be required by the urgency or importance of the Army program for which the experiment is necessary.

---

* 169 *Annals of the New York Academy of Sciences* 509 (1970). © The New York Academy of Sciences, 1970. Reprinted by permission.
† Army Regulation No. 70–25 (1962).

g. Proper preparations will be made and adequate facilities provided to protect the volunteer against all foreseeable possibilities of injury, disability, or death.

h. The experiment will be conducted only by scientifically qualified persons. . . .

i. The volunteer will be informed that at any time during the course of the experiment he will have the right to revoke his consent and withdraw from the experiment, without prejudice to himself.

j. Volunteers will have no physical or mental diseases which will make the proposed experiment more hazardous for them than for normal healthy persons. This determination will be made by the project leader with, if necessary, competent medical advice.

k. The scientist in charge will be prepared to terminate the experiment at any stage if he has probable cause to believe, in the exercise of good faith, superior skill, and careful judgment required of him, that continuation is likely to result in injury, disability, or death to the volunteer.

l. Prisoners of war will not be used under any circumstances.

5. *Additional safeguards.* As added protection for volunteers, the following safeguards will be provided:

a. A physician approved by the Surgeon General will be responsible for the medical care of volunteers. The physician may or may not be the project leader but will have authority to terminate the experiment at any time that he believes death, injury, or bodily harm is likely to result.

b. All apparatus and instruments necessary to deal with likely emergency situations will be available.

c. Required medical treatment and hospitalization will be provided for all casualties.

d. The physician in charge will have consultants available to him on short notice throughout the experiment who are competent to advise or assist with complications which can be anticipated.

6. *Approval to conduct experiment.* It is the responsibility of the head of each major command and other agency to submit to the Surgeon General a written proposal for studies which come within the purview of this directive. The proposal will include for each study the name of the person to be in charge, name of the proposed attending physician, and the detailed plan of the experiment. The Surgeon General will review the proposal and forward it with his comments and recommendations on medical aspects to the Chief of Research and Development for approval. When a proposal pertains to research with nuclear, biological, or chemical agents, the Chief of Research and Development will submit the proposal, together with the Surgeon General's review, to the Secretary of the Army for approval. No research with nuclear, biological, or chemical agents using volunteers will be undertaken without the consent of the Secretary of the Army.

7. *Civilian employees.* When civilian employees of the Department of the Army volunteer under this program, the following instructions will be observed:

a. Any duty as a volunteer performed during the employee's regularly scheduled tour of duty will be considered as constructive duty for which straight time rates are payable. Time spent in connection with an experiment outside the employee's regularly scheduled tour will be considered as voluntary overtime for which no payment may be made nor compensatory time granted. The employee will be so informed before acceptance of his volunteer services.

b. Claims [are authorized to be] submitted to the Bureau of Employees' Compensation, U.S. Department of Labor, because of disability or death resulting from an employee's voluntary participation in experiments. . . .

*   *   *

b.

Who Should Participate, within What Structure, in Professional Regulation?

[i]
Robert E. Hodges and William B. Bean
The Use of Prisoners for Medical Research*

*   *   *

. . . Because we needed [volunteers] urgently, we held a conference with officials of both pris-

* 202 *Journal of the American Medical Association* 513, 514–515 (1967). Copyright 1967 by the American Medical Association. Reprinted by permission.

ons, members of the Board of Control which governs these institutions, and physicians from several departments of the College of Medicine and the university hospitals. As a result of this conference, a working arrangement was agreed upon verbally. The physician who wished to send volunteers was to send a written request to the warden who would then ask for those inmates who wished to participate in a particular project. We knew that this procedure was not specifically permitted by law but neither was it specifically prohibited. But the law did permit the hospitalization of prisoners at the university hospitals for treatment of medical illness.

For a time things went well. As a result of this arrangement, we were able to conduct and complete many useful investigations. As time went by, new state officials were puzzled about this arrangement. On one occasion, the state attorney general was asked to rule upon the legality of our operation. In his judgment, it was not legal for us to accept prison volunteers for medical research. Accordingly, we discontinued use of prisoners for research purposes for two years. During this time, we sought and obtained enactment of a specific law permitting the use of prisoners for medical research at the university hospitals. This law states:

The Board of Control may send to the hospital of the medical college of the state university inmates of the Iowa state penitentiary and the men's reformatory for medical research at the hospital. Before any inmate is sent to the medical college, he must volunteer his services in writing. An inmate may withdraw his consent at any time.

Since enactment of this law, we have availed ourselves of this valuable opportunity to conduct clinical investigation in healthy volunteers under ideal investigative conditions.

One of the chief advantages of this arrangement is that it permits selection of men of any given age, height, and weight. By screening, the investigator can select persons who have a specific disorder, such as diabetes mellitus or hypertension. He can select subjects with any characteristic that might commonly be found within a prison population. These subjects can then be hospitalized in the metabolic ward under combined prison and research discipline or in the clinical research center under similar supervision for the time necessary to complete an experiment.

*   *   *

Once a faculty member has decided upon a

project, he presents his proposal to a research committee of the College of Medicine. Following the committee's evaluation and approval, the dean sends a note of approval to the investigator who establishes liaison with the prison authorities by calling or writing the director of penal institutions in the Board of Control and sends a copy of the message to the warden of the prison. . . . After the proposal has been approved by the Board of Control, the warden is authorized to present to the men a simple explanation of the type of study to be conducted and to provide an opportunity for volunteers to make themselves known. From these volunteers, the prison authorities select a suitable group of men who are not emotionally ill, nor habitually unreliable, nor otherwise unsuited for the project. Usually the authorities provide a select group of volunteers which is about double the number requested by the investigator. The investigators, along with the head nurse of the metabolic ward and other authorized personnel, then visit the prison for the purpose of explaining in detailed yet simple language the nature of the investigation, the risks involved, and the manner in which the study will be conducted. The volunteers are then given an opportunity to withdraw or to ask additional questions before accepting. After the final selection is made, the men are transported by prison authorities to the university hospitals where they are hospitalized either on the metabolic ward or on the clinical research ward. In no instance are prison research subjects housed on the open wards. After they arrive at the hospital, they are given an additional detailed briefing and an opportunity to ask additional questions. Then they sign a consent form and undergo the customary detailed history and physical examination followed by appropriate laboratory tests.

. . . For their participation in research activities, they receive no reduction of their sentences nor any favoritism regarding paroles. We do, however, send a letter to the warden at the termination of each experiment expressing our appreciation for the inmate's participation in the study. It is possible that this letter in the prisoners file may favorably influence the parole board.

Since our first patient, who was an unofficial volunteer, we have accepted a total of 224 prisoners for medical research at university hospitals. Only a few of these represent "repeaters" since we try to avoid selecting a man more than once. . . . Of the total, ten have escaped. Most of the escapees were subjects for the medical experiment who had been selected rather hastily at the insistence of an investigator; hence prison officials had not been given ample opportunity to make their usual careful selection.

The level of compliance by prisoners with research rules and regulations has been surprisingly high. They have eaten strange diets, swallowed tubes, submitted to repeated venipunctures, and participated in a wide variety of physiological tests with a commendable degree of good humor and cheerfulness. Although any man may leave the study to return to the prison if he so desires, this has happened in very few instances. . . . We feel that the use of prison volunteers for medical research is justified and highly desirable for the investigator, for the subjects, and for society. It not only permits the conduct of human investigation under ideal circumstances, but it enables the participants to feel that they are serving a useful function as indeed they are.

*   *   *

NOTE

Thomas E. Starzl
Ethical Problems in Organ Transplantation—A Clinician's Point of View*

*   *   *

[P]enal volunteers [for organ donation] had been accepted in our Colorado hospitals under conditions that it was thought would fully insure the protection of their individual rights and permit their complete freedom of choice, objectives that in principle may have been less realistic than with the identical twin minors. In any event, there is every reason to believe that this practice, however equitably handled in a local situation, would inevitably lead to abuse if accepted as a reasonable precedent and applied broadly. For these reasons, and because the donor motivation that characterizes proper intrafamilial transplantation could not be said to exist except in the most idealized and universal sense, the acceptance of criminal volunteers was permanently discontinued at the University of Colorado 1½ years ago.

*   *   *

Community Research Review Committee Requirements for Research Involving the Black Community*

Preamble

In a time when the research findings of social and biological scientists are being used increasingly to justify political and legal decision-making, it is imperative that all parties responsible for research projects that may involve such extra-theoretical and -methodological uses pay careful attention to these issues in the planning, conduct and reporting of their research.

Since the major consequences of political and legal decisions of a social nature descend upon members of this country's black communities, the need for vigilance in the conduct of research in black communities is most acute.

Members of the black community do not believe that a large majority of social science investigators who conduct research projects in black communities are sensitive to the many extra-theoretical or -methodological issues that their research necessarily entails. More than that, members of the black community do not believe that most of these investigators are sensitive to cultural nuance which is a necessary input to any well-conceived and conducted research in the black community.

If an investigator obtains results that for one reason or another are inaccurate, or if the results of his investigations are used by people in powerful positions to effect abhorrent policies, the investigator may find his professional reputation tarnished, but the people who are recipients of the false conclusions or abhorrent policies may find their lives, psychologically and physically, in extreme danger.

"Academic freedom," "scientific objectivity" are ivory tower terms that are applicable to ivory tower activities. But, when these ivory tower practitioners step out into the world of people and begin to deal with human lives, they must accept a *pronounced* shift in the balance sheet of "Rights and Responsibilities"—away from the former and toward the latter.

When investigators use human beings in their research, they are *required* to provide assurances of ethical and moral treatment for these subjects. Furthermore, these investigators are re-

---

quired to abide by all Civil Rights statutes as they may apply in the conduct of their research. Members of the black community feel we need such assurances also. We further feel that we need to have a working, first hand relationship with all research conducted in our community to insure the faithful, steadfast adherence to our interest in self-preservation.

However, all research conducted in the black community is not academic. A vast amount of money directly from political sources is spent on projects and programs in the black community. These programs themselves are often not research in the sense of data gathering and analysis. However, funding sources like to know how well or productive their grant or program dollars are spent. Evaluation is the inevitable consequence.

The black community can no longer allow foreign parties uncontrolled access rights. Every viable institution or entity in this country maintains the right of ultimate control. We of the black community feel that such control is critical to our collective survival, and further, to our ability to formulate the concepts and experiences which will move us toward a collectively liberated future.

Pursuant to the issues raised above, we have organized and adopted the following set of principles as guidelines for the conduct of all research in the black communities of the greater Boston areas.

Guidelines

1. A Committee composed of Black agencies, organizations, professional groups, and individuals from the Black Community, representing 25,000 Black people, was established by the Boston Black United Front as the Community Research Review Committee (CRRC). The CRRC's function is to review research being conducted or proposed in the Black Community, and to determine whether, in its judgment, such research and/or its implications will be in the best interests of the Black Community.

2. All research grant proposals that intend to use Black subjects and/or facilities in the Black Community are subject to review and approval by the CRRC *before* any such research may begin, and are subject to continuing approval by this Committee.

3. All research conducted in the Black Community must involve Black personnel at significant positions of authority. The role of such Black staff would, of course, vary with different kinds of projects and investigations, but must include significant involvement in the *design and development* of the study. Generally, the primary role would be to protect the interests of the Black Community.

*   *   *

5. Those research projects approved for operation in the Black Community will necessitate monitoring of all project activities for their duration.

    a. Approved Black staff, as well as consultants, must be involved in all aspects of the study including:

        (1) design and development of the study

        (2) implementation of the study

        (3) monitoring of the study

        (4) analysis and interpretation of the results

        (5) preparation and publication of reports, papers, talks, etc., based on the research data.

    b. Copies of all data, subsequent analyses, and relevant materials must be available for deposit with the CRRC as these become available. The confidentiality of such materials will be maintained by the CRRC.

*   *   *

    d. After analyzing the data, summarizing the results, and preparing a preliminary final report, but *before* disseminating any such information to the funding source, or to the professional or lay public, the principal investigator must:

        (1) circulate a copy of the proposed report to the CRRC for review and comment, criticism, and, if necessary, rebuttal. If the principal investigator has the report independently reviewed of his own initiative, such reviews must be included with the report when it is sent to the CRRC.

        (2) agree to include (under separate authorship) *as part of the final report and as part of any subsequent publication of the findings,* a critical presentation of any alternative interpretations of major findings which cannot be reconciled with the principal investigator's main finding.

6. The monitoring activities imposed on the CRRC by the operation of a project in the Black Community are substantial. Therefore, the expenses of the monitoring are to be borne by each project in question. These expenses, not to

exceed ten percent (10%) of the total project funds, are calculated on a project by project basis.

*   *   *

[iii]
Harvard Medical School
Rules Governing the Participation of
Medical Students as Experimental Subjects*

The participation of medical students as experimental subjects in research studies has raised practical and philosophical problems difficult to resolve. Misunderstandings have arisen, owing in part to inadequate communication and in part to the complex nature of the issues involved.

In discussing this situation, the principles that should govern the employment of human beings as research subjects, the motivations of medical students in volunteering, the educational implications, the matter of financial remuneration, the protection of health, the conflict with scheduled studies, the moral and legal responsibilities of the investigator and of the Medical School, and the advisability of the centralization of all pertinent records, have all been considered by the Administrative Board and the Faculty of Medicine.

After extensive study of these points, the University Health Services and the Dean's Office formulated the following policies and procedures, which have been unanimously approved by the Administrative Board and supported by the Faculty of Medicine.

Statement of Policy
1. The guiding principle in considering the participation of medical students as subjects in experiments is the belief that no student should be exposed to risk as far as his health and well-being are concerned.
2. A student's time should not be invaded to the extent of creating conflicts with his scheduled work.
3. Inasmuch as motivation should stem from an opportunity to learn and to contribute, rather than from a financial inducement *per se*, payment should not ordinarily be made to the student for participating as a subject in an experiment. This does not preclude remuneration for collaborating in a research project nor for participation in programs in which a student may be employed during vacation

periods, or under special circumstances at other times during the academic year, or as a Student Research Fellow.
4. The contact between investigator and student is recognized as an excellent opportunity for the investigator to demonstrate to the student both his personal responsibility for the student's health and safety and an active interest in furthering the student's education.

Procedure
In order to simplify and to standardize the participation of medical students as experimental subjects, the following administrative procedure has been established for the mutual benefit of the student, the investigator, and the Medical School.
1. Each project must be approved by the head of the department, of which the investigator is a member. This provision specifically shall include approval of the desirability of the proposed study, the details of the experimental protocol, and the use of medical students as subjects. It shall imply, in addition, the assumption of responsibility for any medical expenses that the student may incur as a consequence of participation.
2. Subsequent to such approval, a detailed protocol must be submitted to the Director of the Medical Area Health Service and to the Dean's Office. In experiments involving the use of radioactive materials, a copy of the protocol shall be submitted also to the Secretary of the Committee on Medical Research in Biophysics.
3. Following review and commentary by these parties, the protocol must be presented to the Administrative Board for discussion and for approval or disapproval of student participation.
4. If approved, the investigator must explain the details of the project to the medical student in advance, and must refer him to the Health Service for medical clearance before beginning the experiment. The result of the Health Service's examination shall be sent in writing to the investigator.
5. The Health Service must maintain records of the research projects in which medical students participate. These records shall include dosages of drugs or radioisotopes used on each individual and the total body irradiation received. In addition, the investigator must report to the Health Service concerning any significant medical observations that are made during the course of a given experiment.

---

* Memorandum from George Packer Berry, M.D., Dean (1968). Reprinted by permission.

c.

Should Research Design and Scientific Merits Be Evaluated?

Norval Morris
Impediments to Penal Reform*

*   *   *

It has recently become fashionable to stress our lack of knowledge of the relative efficacy of our various treatment methods and I do not wish on this occasion to retrace that melancholy story. The central question eludes us: which treatment methods are effective for which types of offenders and for how long should they be applied for optimum effect? . . . At last, however, there is widespread verbal agreement (if not action) that we must critically test our developing armamentarium of prevention and treatment methods, and that to do so requires testing by means of controlled clinical trials. Follow-up studies, association analysis, predictive attributes analysis— no matter how sophisticated other research techniques we apply, we cannot escape the need for direct evaluative research by means of clinical trials. And this leads me to the next impediment to penal reform—clinical trials themselves raise important ethical issues that demand consideration.

*   *   *

There is . . . a respectable and reasonable ethical argument against clinical trials of correctional treatment methods which must not be burked in our enthusiasm for the acquisition of knowledge. It runs like this: Terrestrially speaking man is an end in himself; he must never be sacrificed to some self-appointed superman's belief that knowledge about man's behavior is of greater value than respect for his human rights. This is particularly true if the sacrifice is made without his uncoerced and fully informed choice. The explorer may, choosing thus freely, risk his life in the pursuit of knowledge. The citizen may, under certain controlled conditions, risk his life and physical well-being in furtherance of medical experiments. But when hint of coercion, or restraining or unduly influencing pressures appear, it is (choose your epithet) sinful, unethical, socially unwise, to permit such sacrifice of the individual to the supposed collective good. The argument shifts, of course, in wartime; but then

---

* 33 *University of Chicago Law Review* 627, 646–653 (1969). Reprinted by permission.

the threat to the collectivity is seen as the overwhelming value.

Put in less pretentious terms, the proposition is: given that our knowledge is exiguous, nevertheless, we must at all times act in the way that within that knowledge is thought best for the individual we are treating. When the problem of his treatment raises (as it does generally in relation to criminal sanctions) the issue of the proper balance between the community's need for protection from him and people like him, and his treatment needs if he is to be reestablished as a member of society, conforming sufficiently to avoid criminal conduct, the same principle holds true; we are never justified in applying other than our best judgment concerning that balance for the sake of experimentation aimed at expediting the acquisition of knowledge of how to handle like cases in the future.

It is my view that the ethical argument against clinical trials is not convincing and that, given certain safeguards, it is entirely appropriate, indeed essential, for evaluative research projects of this type to be built into all new correctional developments. The two safeguards that I have in mind may not in perpetuity solve the problem, but they do at least provide sufficient protection of human rights for many decades of correctional research.

First, we do not have to apply such research techniques at the stage of judicial sentencing; they can well operate within the sentence that the judge has determined to be the just and appropriate sentence. Secondly, by applying a principle which might be called the principle of "less severity," abuse of human rights can be minimized.

Experiment at the judicial stage is not necessary since correctional sanctions already include wide diversities of treatment within the judicially imposed sentence. A defined term of imprisonment may in any one state involve a commitment to possibly extremely different types of institutions having substantially different reformative processes and with appreciably different degrees of social isolation. And given the operation of discretionary release procedures, including parole, most prison sentences permit widely differing periods of incarceration. Likewise, a sentence of probation can lead to a close personal supervision or to the most perfunctory experience of occasional reporting. The range of subtreatments within each correctional treatment is thus very wide; so wide that ample room for evaluative clinical research into these subtreatments exists without interference with judicial processes. Of course, as information relevant to sentencing emerges from such administratively created clinical trials, it will be fed back into the judicial process and will then create new opportunities for further evaluative research. And knowledge will grow without experimentation at the judicial level.

"Less severity" is the other safeguard. By this I mean that the new treatment being studied should not be one that is regarded in the mind of the criminal subjected to it, or of the people imposing the new punishment, or of the community at large, as more severe than the traditional treatment against which it is being compared. To take a group of criminals who otherwise would be put on probation and to select some at random for institutional treatment would be unjust; conversely, to select at random a group who would otherwise be incarcerated and to treat them on probation or in a probation hostel would seem to be no abuse of human rights. Applying this principle it is possible to pursue many decades of valuable evaluative research.

There are many methodological problems in evaluative research. I do not wish to deal with them now, but rather to continue to focus on these ethical issues. Have these two principles of administrative rather than judicial experimentation and "less severity" sufficiently disposed of the ethical problems? Let us probe this question by the classroom method of a hypothetical case. Last night this problem was on my mind when I went to sleep and I had a dream which still troubles me. I dreamt that I observed and heard a conversation between a furious burglar sitting in his cell and a garrulous social scientist. Physically, each was a Lombrosian stereotype, and their speech too was a caricature of what one would expect from their widely different backgrounds and experiences. I cannot precisely recall their words, and perhaps it is a mercy that neither the sociologese nor the scatological blasphemy have remained in my mind. I can, however, describe the situation in which they found themselves and, later, in less colorful terms than theirs, tell you the substance of their conversation.

In my dream I saw the furious burglar sitting in his cell. He was part of our control group. The experiment had been impeccably and carefully designed. We desired to test the wisdom of releasing a defined group of offenders some three months earlier than they would otherwise be released by sending them to a recently established halfway house where daily they would go out to work and where their evenings and leisure time would be devoted to guided group interaction, using the most modern techniques, and to other processes designed for their easier and more effective resettlement into the community. This relatively new type of facility had been legislatively and administratively established as an "experiment" which, as you know, is the name of all new penal developments. This experiment differed from the usual experiment in that the social scientists were allowed to make it an experiment.

The group of offenders thought suitable for this new type of treatment had been carefully delineated in terms of their personalities and background. Since the halfway house could accommodate only twenty people it became necessary to discover how many such offenders would be found in the prison system. A careful assessment of the prison population and cautious predictions of its likely future shape led to the view that there were at any one time forty prisoners precisely matching the criteria for selection for this new treatment facility. It was therefore decided that the diagnostic center would be responsible for the selection of the prisoners who fell and might fall within this category; that they would be given a code number; and that chance would be allowed to condition whether a man fell within the T group, and would go to the new halfway house, or the C group, and would be treated just as he would have been had the facility not been built. It was, of course, early and necessarily decided that the C group must never know this had happened and that the T group must never know that they were part of a controlled experiment—though, of course, it would be clear to them that new opportunities were being given to them. They must believe that they were given these opportunities because the staff of the diagnostic center had convinced the parole board of their peculiar suitability for the halfway house. They might prefer to believe that they had conned the diagnostic center and the parole board, this being an even better belief, experimentally speaking. My furious burglar fell within the C group. My social scientist had been garrulous indeed, and a series of indiscretions had led to his revealing this fact to the burglar. That is why the burglar was furious.

FB (Furious Burglar): You mean you're holding me here because of some . . . experiment!

GSS (Garrulous Social Scientist): Yes.

FB: Why didn't you tell me?

GSS: It would spoil the experiment . . . the Hawthorne effect, you know.

FB: Habeas corpus? What chance?

GSS: That is a somewhat difficult question. I am told that it has some constitutional aspects to it. To my knowledge the matter had never been tested. You should ask our Legal Aid Division.

FB: Wasn't it tested in the Nuremburg Trial?

GSS: Everyone knows that was different.

FB: How different?

GSS: Well, you see, the Nazi experimentation met our criterion that the decision must be administrative and not judicial but it did not meet the important and to my mind determinative criterion; that is, the new treatment we are testing must be, in our eyes, and in your eyes, and in the eyes of all right-minded members of the community, a lesser infringement on freedom, a lesser suffering, than the traditional punishment against which it is being tested and which would otherwise be applied to everyone. You have not lost anything; twenty people just like you have gained, but you have not lost. And think what good you do for others. We will learn how to develop better release procedures; earlier release for some is a likely result; crime will be diminished. You should be thanking me, not complaining.

FB: I'm complaining. Obfuscate it as you will, because of your . . . experiment, I'm here. Have I an action in false imprisonment against you, or the warden, or the governor?

GSS: That too is a matter for our Legal Aid Division but I don't think you do. We have not increased the maximum of your legally prescribed punishment in any way. Why are you complaining? You had a fifty per cent chance of getting out three months ago; we were quite fair; without us you would have had no chance.

FB: You lie. The halfway house would have been set up whether you had anything to do with it or not. The prison administrators are not conned by you social scientists; that's just the way they get federal subsidies. I know and you know that I am peculiarly suited to release to a halfway house and that I can talk well to the parole board and that if you had kept your white coat out of it I would have had at least an eighty per cent chance of being sent to that halfway house. By grouping me with those other thirty-nine and tossing coins, you reduced my chances to fifty per cent. Surely it must be clear to you that it is

thirty per cent likely that I am here because of your . . . experiment.

GSS: All of us must suffer in the cause of science, you know. Your error lies in failing to appreciate that men must fall into categories for purposes of social research, they cannot be seen entirely as individuals, and we treated you fairly as part of your appropriate category.

And then the garrulous social scientist stalked out of the cell mumbling, "How else will we ever learn?" and slammed the cell door shut behind him, which awakened me. The dream continues to trouble me. I think there were one or two more things that the garrulous social scientist should have said in his own defense, but I am not sure that they are finally convincing. He should have pointed out the randomness of the whole edifice of correctional sanctions. He might well have stressed that repeated studies over the past forty years have beyond a doubt established the gross irrational variations in sentencing practice, even within the same courthouse, and should have tried to persuade the burglar that this type of experimentation was one effective way of acquiring knowledge relevant to the elimination of such unjust disparities. He might have more strenuously argued that the need to devise treatments suitable to categories of individuals sometimes of necessity involves an insufficiently fine balancing of differences between them, and that the burglar's differences from the other thirty-nine in the punishment control group were so slight as to be immeasurable in the macrocosm of the sentencing and punishing jungle. I think he should have tried more diligently to persuade the burglar of the need for such groupings of individuals, if knowledge of rational treatment methods is ever to be acquired. I doubt that he would have succeeded, and I am convinced that it is unwise to employ a garrulous social scientist.

Some have suggested that one way of avoiding this dilemma is, in an experiment of this type, to have arranged that both the treatment and the control groups obtained an advantage over the traditional punishment. That is, that in the previously considered experiment, twenty should be sent to the halfway house three months before their otherwise planned release and twenty should be completely released at the earlier time. Though this minimizes the ethical problem, it does not eliminate it. Now the furious burglar who is complaining is to be found in the halfway house bewailing the fact that he is under the degree of control that he is there. And also, it becomes a different experiment, and it will be necessary if effective knowledge is to be gained from the experiment to compare both our freely released group and our halfway house group with some control group still in the institution if the maximum knowledge is to be gained from the experiment—and they have cause for complaint.

*   *   *

In conclusion, let me say that it is my position that the ethical difficulties in empirical evaluation research are so slight as not to constitute a serious impediment to it. I confess that I feel happier when such projects test differences of practice within existing treatments, so that no burglar will bother to be furious, but I know that is no answer. My final reason for not being persuaded by the furious burglar, even in his precise situation, is this: the whole system of sanctions, from suspicion to arrest to trial to sentence, punishment, and release is now so full of irrational and unfair disparities that marginal arguments of the type the furious burglar produces are to me lost in the sea of injustice from which in the long run we can only be saved by these means. Yet I remain on his side to the extent that I abhor experimental design which is not anxiously perceptive of these ethical problems and does not do its utmost to minimize them.

*   *   *

d.

Should Consent Be Supervised?

[i]
Louis Jaffe
*Law as a System of Control**

*   *   *

There appears to have crept into the thinking of some people the notion that the motivation of a consenting subject should be disinterested, that he should be acting for the benefit of mankind. There is a disposition, for example, to scrutinize closely the motivation of prisoners and to exclude their use because their presumptive motive is self-interest. This line of thinking seems to me to reflect an excessive ethical fastidiousness. (It may also possibly proceed from a subcon-

scious impulse to glorify the enterprise—which, it is thought, might be sullied by the participation of unworthy persons.) But assuming that the experiment otherwise satisfies professional standards, the only requirement, in my opinion, is that no "undue" advantage be taken of the subject. A prisoner, even a patient, may be under pressures to consent not present in the situation of a citizen at large or a stranger. But those pressures should not be accounted an undue advantage. A prisoner, for example, may consent in order to give meaning to his life or because he hopes (though no promise has been given) to receive favorable treatment. A stranger may consent because he is paid, because he seeks excitement, or because he has a problem. Indeed, the motivation of consent is so complex, so various, and so obscure that it defies determination.

From the point of view of the experiment, the motivation of the subject is irrelevant unless his psychology is a factor in the experiment. From the subject's point of view, there is no lack of respect in allowing him to decide to participate for what seem to him to be sufficient reasons. He must be treated fairly, and the touchstone of fairness is, for the most part, what in retrospect will seem fair to him. Indeed fairness is at the heart of the whole consent problem, at least from the point of view of the subject or the patient.

. . . Assuming that the subject has the requisite minimum of intelligence, presumptively what he thinks is fair suffices to justify the experimental action. Both law and morals disapprove of the use of certain tactics in securing consent—such as falsification, failure to state crucial facts, and undue pressure. What is "undue" is a function of the situation. We can decide (as, for the most part, we have) that to seek the consent of a prisoner is not undue despite the presence of pressures absent in the case of the citizen at large. He must not, however, be threatened with adverse consequences if he refuses, and for this reason his refusal should not be of record. Let us admit that problems arise in part because there are disturbing contradictions in the prison situation itself. But that statement characterizes almost any life situation, and for that reason it may be the path of wisdom to focus on the simplicities. Experimentation on prisoners offers advantages to the experimenter, to the prisoner, and to the public. It offends, I believe, only a very few persons. . . .

*   *   *

* 98 *Daedalus* 406, 423–425 (1969). Reprinted by permission of Daedalus, Journal of the American Academy of Arts and Sciences, Boston, Massachusetts.

[ii]
Edmond Cahn
*Drug Experiments and the Public Conscience**

* * *

Reasonable compensations for serving as subjects are entirely warranted provided they do not operate to purchase or coerce an unwilling consent, particularly from those who are poor or in hospital wards or derelict. It is clearly wrong to purchase the consents of prisoners by offering them a release or parole or any equivalent inducement that exercises a coercive effect. There is not much to say for a society that sends a burglar to prison for ten years and gives him to understand that he can be free in five if he subjects himself to medical experiments.

* * *

3.

In Reviewing Decisions and Consequences

a.

Through Public and Professional Scrutiny?

[i]
*Drug Investigation Committee of the
Medical Association of the State of Alabama
The Use of Prisoners for Drug
Trials in Alabama†*

* * *

It appears that the Southern Food and Drug Research, Inc. has been operating a research program in the Alabama Prison System since 1962 with the approval of Commissioner Frank Lee and the Alabama Board of Corrections. The president of Southern Food and Drug Research . . . is Dr. Austin R. Stough who is a graduate of the University of Oklahoma and of the Medical College of the University of Tennessee. He conducted research programs in the Oklahoma prison system before coming to Alabama. Dr. Irl Long who was previously in general practice in Montgomery and who is still prison physician for Kilby Prison is associated with Dr. Stough

in providing medical direction for Southern Food and Drug Research.

The original emphasis for Southern Food and Drug Research was on a plasmapheresis program but this was discontinued in 1964 following an outbreak of hepatitis which involved 376 prisoner participants with three deaths. (A Public Health Service investigation showed that the outbreak was definitely linked with the plasmapheresis program and a significant break in aseptic technique was found which accounted for this.) In 1963, however, the Food and Drug Administration set for the various drug houses much stricter standards for drug testing and these included a greatly increased demand for Phase I testing (Phase I testing is that done on healthy humans after completion of the animal experimental work). As a result, proficient investigators with adequate facilities were in considerable demand and Southern Food and Drug Research then concentrated its attention in this area.

Over the years since then, the drug houses seem to have been generally satisfied with what was done in Alabama and the Food and Drug Administration has had no specific complaints although they queried the number of investigations being done at any one time as being perhaps too many for adequate medical supervision by the limited medical staff of Southern Food and Drug Research. Internal control over the program by the Board of Corrections and its officers appears to have been limited in amount with the medical member of the board (Dr. McLaughlin) briefly reviewing the protocols for each new drug trial and occasionally mentioning them to members of the Board.

Membership on the Board of Corrections is not a full-time position. With their primary interest to attend to, it could not be expected that members of this board be completely and constantly aware of every transaction affecting the prison system at a given time. A busy physician could not devote the time required to properly evaluate the protocols without neglecting his private patients.

The Commissioner and his wardens apparently gave Dr. Stough and his group ready cooperation with very few questions being openly asked. The prison physicians for the other two prisons involved in the drug testing program (Dr. Edwards at Tutwiler and Dr. Mracek at Draper) generally required that they be kept advised of new drug-testing programs in their own prisons when they were initiated.

* * *

* Paul Talalay, ed.: *Drugs in Our Society.* Baltimore: The Johns Hopkins Press 225, 263 (1964). Reprinted by permission.
† Tinsley R. Harrison, M.D., Chairman (1969). Reprinted by permission.

In January, 1969, the *Montgomery Adver-tiser-Journal,* over the byline of Mr. Harold E. Martin (Editor and Publisher), launched a series of attacks at the drug-testing program being conducted in Alabama prisons. In addition to hinting at excessive profits being made at the expense of the health of the prisoners by Southern Food and Drug Research, certain additional medically oriented accusations were made:

1. Although the inmates signed a waiver they were not told of the possible effects of tests while the prisoners' strong need for extra money largely invalidated the requirement of informed consent.
2. Physical examinations were not being performed before each program as required in some protocols.
3. A doctor was not present during many of the potentially critical periods of reaction.
4. Some of the experiments left the men too sick to perform their regular duties.
5. Prison inmates drew blood and performed other technical procedures.
6. The contrast between the facilities for the private concern's testing program and the extremely inadequate facilities available for treating sick prisoners was shocking.
7. A number of quite serious reactions had occurred among prisoners but these had received little attention.
8. The administration of the program, with prisoners sometimes giving false histories and not taking the medicine provided for them, made the results of the testing program somewhat unreliable.

The newspaper articles were not entirely negative and they did point out that needed research was carried out, inmates did receive money to buy cigarettes and other needs, and the Prison Welfare Fund received some monies which could be used for programs that the state did not provide. (At Kilby and Draper twenty percent of the money paid to the prisoners went to the Prison Welfare Fund.) The newspaper suggested that the entire program be placed under the authority and supervision of the University of Alabama Medical School, that the participants be properly remunerated, that profits from the program should go for improvements in the prison system, that the testing program be so scheduled as not to interfere with the work or training at the prison, that the participants be clearly informed of possible dangers involved in the program, that the controls over the program provide for good scientific evaluation and that

good medical supervision be exercised at all times.

Following this adverse publicity which carried distinct connotations of laxity on the part of the Board of Corrections and possible dishonesty on the part of certain of their senior employees, the Board of Corrections adopted the following resolution:

That the Chairman be authorized to appoint a committee of two or more persons qualified to determine from a medical standpoint, and not connected with the Board of Corrections, to investigate any drug-testing programs conducted in the state prisons, to determine whether the programs are properly supervised to protect the health of the participants, both in testing and in the event of any aftereffects of the testing, to determine whether any prisoners are being abused in any way, and to report to the board their findings.

Upon receipt of this request, this committee was appointed by the governing body of the medical association. This report constitutes our findings.

* * *

1. Prison Testing Facilities

* * *

At Kilby Prison a list was seen of prisoners who had been selected by Southern Food and Drug Research from their records as being suitable subjects for a new test which was being started that morning. No person in the prison system had any hand in selecting this initial list. From about 60 names which had been submitted, the warden had deleted about ten because, so he advised us, these persons could not be spared by their division heads from their official prison occupation. Most of the remaining 50 prisoners had been called into the testing room in the prison that morning in groups of about six persons. While blood was being taken from them (apparently for laboratory testing) they had received a rapid explanation of the purpose of the test (there was considerable variation in the understanding of what had been said), with the statement that the drug being tested was safe and, should the laboratory tests be satisfactory, they would be asked to sign a waiver-consent form. All this had seemingly been done by technicians with no physician being present as far as could be determined. Two of the four prisoners who were interviewed indicated that they had never been examined by a physician while they were in the prison although they had been on several drug trials. One of these prisoners told of tests with an anti-hypertensive drug which had had to be discontinued after three weeks (the trial was supposed to run for four weeks) because of severe reactions among those taking the pills. He himself had hung on to the end although he had been feeling very ill and had not complained of this illness, because it would have meant his losing the pay which he was hoping to receive for his participation. The majority of the prisoners interviewed indicated that the only reason they participated in the drug trials was because of the money which they were paid.

*   *   *

Conditions in the so-called hospital at Kilby were appallingly bad and would not have been acceptable fifty years ago, let alone today. One felt that a little extra effort and a little additional money would have made a tremendous difference if only the drive had been there. The importance of this hospital at Kilby is that it turned out later that persons having severe reactions to any of the drug trials in any of the prisons were transferred to this hospital for more intensive care.

*   *   *

The situation in Draper was similar to that which had been found at Kilby, though not as bad. The difference was probably related to the dedication of the prison physician and to the strong sense of responsibility of the warden. There was no question here but that inmates had been used as technicians until very recently, while severe drug reactions were not being given the attention (medical or experimental) which their condition deserved. Supervision for patients who had been "stopped up" in the special room constructed by Southern Food and Drug Research appeared to be almost entirely non-medical in nature and no really adequate provision had been made for any serious, unexpected, severe reaction. Once again, it appeared that most of the prisoners were volunteering purely for monetary reasons and were staying on the tests even after disturbing reactions had occurred simply to be paid more....

Your committee believes that, by and large, the research studies completed and published in highly respected journals by staff members of Southern Food and Drug Corporation represent creditable, useful, and practical contributions to medical science. However, this good should not be permitted to hide the manifest defects in the present system.

The Board of Corrections with its physician member has naturally assumed that any doctor conducting experimental studies on human subjects would take the utmost precautions to safeguard the health of such subjects. Their confidence has been gravely abused.

*   *   *

This committee was confronted with a seeming conflict of interest when it viewed the dual role of Dr. Irl Long serving as both senior prison physician and as an officer of Southern Food and Drug Research. Even Dr. Long readily acknowledged that a potential conflict of interest could exist. This unconscionable situation, regardless of reason, should never have been permitted to come into existence. This situation places all persons concerned in an untenable position exemplified by the necessity for the investigation.

*   *   *

3. Drug-House Relationships

Reputable drug firms are concerned with developing and producing effective, safe medications. Their record in carrying out this function is unassailable. In their search for new therapeutic agents they maintain an impressive laboratory operation with a competent, highly trained research staff....

*   *   *

In the present instance there is no reason to believe that the pharmaceutical firms failed to act in good faith or failed to discharge their responsibility to the general public to develop safe effective therapeutic agents. They contracted with approved clinical investigators to carry out approved research projects. However, there are some points for possible criticism: (1) There may have been a too superficial monitoring of the clinical work which they support. (2) They demonstrated some lack of discretion in selection of their Phase I investigator. Thus, there was a need to consider the number of projects to which the prospective investigator was already committed. (3) Their initial conference sessions may not have provided for adequate grounding of the investigator in all the significant basic properties of the test material, a particularly important point when the limited training in basic pharmacology of both clinical investigators (Drs. Stough and Long) is considered.

That the drug manufacturers are interested in conducting and supporting research programs of quality is confirmed by a consideration of two clinical programs established and operated by two of the major firms, the Upjohn Company and Parke-Davis at the Southern Michigan State Prison. These programs involved an initial expenditure of perhaps one half million dollars for facilities and are generally believed to be first class, both in providing for optimum safety and welfare of the human subjects and in providing dependable clinical data.

There is no reason to doubt that excellent programs are desired by the drug manufacturers or that they would support such programs. Despite this, both the drug firms and FDA have given tacit approval to the research in Alabama prisons, and approval based on their confidence in the reliability of data so obtained. It should be noted, however, that neither is primarily concerned with the rights and welfare of the institutionalized research subject. There is within the body of the law some provision for protecting the welfare and rights of prisoners used as research subjects, but in the absence of sufficient funds and some watchdog mechanism, these rights may be abused. There is the justifiable view that the drug manufacturer is not abandoning any moral or ethical responsibility in assuming that the welfare of institutionalized human subjects used in testing its products will be adequately underwritten by the administrators of the institutions or by other state agencies, boards, or commissions charged with that responsibility. . . .

*   *   *

Implications

Our investigations have shown substantial defects in the drug-testing program as administered at present in Alabama prisons. This does not, however, change our opinion that drug trials using prisoners can and do serve an essential purpose. They benefit the nation and provide the prisoner with an opportunity to contribute something back to society, to earn some extra needed money and to improve living conditions in the prisons through a well-developed welfare fund. In addition, a well-conducted drug-testing program would provide extra medical coverage for prisoners with the possibility of the early diagnosis and treatment of disease and better diagnostic facilities than might otherwise be available. Actually this has frequently happened in Alabama.

Considering the present situation we regard it as being distinctly unsatisfactory. The pris-

oners' welfare is not being adequately safeguarded and the validity of the drug trials themselves must occasionally be seriously in doubt. The chief deficiencies are undoubtedly the lack of an adequately trained staff, the lack of sufficient interest in the prisoner as a patient, the lack of medical supervision, the unique pressure toward signing a "consent form" because of the need for money, unsatisfactory conditions for the treatment of those prisoners who do fall ill and the lack of any adequate peer review of protocols which are submitted. For the staff and facilities which are available, there is no question but that far too many trials are being conducted at the same time. Thus, at the time of our visit it appeared that no fewer than seven separate trials were being conducted in the three prisons we visited.

. . . The work of Dr. Stough and, to some extent, Dr. Long, is bluntly unacceptable. Others seem to have been involved more through innocent acceptance than through anything else. In retrospect it is easy to see that a request to the State Health Officer for an adequate control inspection might have saved a lot of grief, but this overlooks reality.

It is only right that prisoners, as wards of the state, should *in the absence of a drug-testing program,* receive medical care of the same general quality as that received by the average citizen of the state.

We believe that with very little help from the state, a sincere attempt has been made at Atmore prison to give this level of medical care. The dedicated physician providing this care has paid not only with time and at the probable price of his own health but, in part, out of his own pocket. It is totally wrong that a physician should, because of his dedication be forced to meet an obligation that should rest firmly on the shoulders of the tax payers of Alabama.

Where *there is a drug-testing program* the obligation is different. Here the responsibility is to provide the quality of care that a volunteer ordinarily receives at a first-class research institution. The fact that the volunteer is a prisoner does not alter this. . . .

*   *   *

Alternatives

[W]e are faced with the dilemma of "right" versus "right." It is certainly "right" that new drugs should be evaluated before release to the general public; it is "right" that this evaluation should be meaningful—that is, it should be done in a thorough, scientific manner by competent individuals. It is "right" that the individual who is to participate in the trial (whether he is a prisoner or not) should do it purely on voluntary basis with full knowledge of the hazards involved.

In this area we are to be guided by the principles outlined in the Nuremberg Code, the Declaration of Helsinki, and the American Medical Association's Ethical Guidelines for Clinical Investigation. . . . It is "right" that the prisoner with few rights of any kind should receive at least the average medical care available to free citizens, and be protected from those who might abuse his position and sometimes his ignorance to the detriment of his health for experimental purposes. It is certainly good if not right that prisoners be given a chance to earn some money (especially considering the pittance they receive otherwise in the Alabama Prison System). It is also good that prisoners so motivated may enhance their self-esteem by making a positive contribution to the general public welfare by participating in a medical research program. . . .

If there is so much right and good about the program, it is also right that [it] should be regulated and be well run by reputable free enterprise (such as ethical drug firms presumably do in Michigan) or by nonprofit research organizations as long as the research is monitored adequately by the officially designated commission or regulatory board. . . .

A foundation established by a state institution such as a major university could serve as a functional unit with laboratories and other necessary fixed facilities and with clerical and administrative staff directed by a clinical pharmacologist qualified to conduct human drug research. This foundation would be under control of a board of appointees qualified in medico-legal aspects of human experimentation, with the foundation director serving as permanent chairman. The controlling board would be charged with the responsibility of reviewing all protocols from pharmaceutical firms, or others submitting clinical research projects, assessing hazards inherent in the projects and critically evaluating the safeguards to be provided. The controlling board would also be responsible for seeing that all research subjects were aware of hazards and entered the programs voluntarily.

To protect themselves from any possible imputation of a "conflict of interest," the controlling board of the responsible foundation might advantageously appoint a Prison Experimental Review Committee to advise them on any potential risk to the health of the prisoners. The members of this committee should not be related to the research foundation and might include a competent practicing physician appointed by the Board of Censors, a lawyer nominated by the Attorney General, and a designee of the State Health Officer. Since our suggestion does not envisage a monopoly for the responsible foundation (though the bulk of research investigations would be channeled through them) the proposed committee could also advise with regard to other groups which wish to conduct their own research in the Alabama prison system.

* * *

Summary

It is the unanimous opinion of this committee that the drug-testing program is almost essential and should be continued for the benefit of the prisoners and society in general. However, as presently conducted the program does not provide adequate safeguards for the health of the prisoners and leaves something to be desired in quality of results obtained. . . .

Early in our report, we likened our task to that of observing and commenting upon a "play" in a theater. Perhaps it is not inappropriate to pursue that analogy.

It has been our privilege to sit on the front row. We have observed a drama that has displayed certain minor aspects of comedy and many features of melodrama. But the major impact has been that of tragedy. There has appeared, over and over again, conflict between right and right.

From our posts of vantage we have watched the entrances and the exits of the characters and the unfolding of the plot of this drama, we have constantly asked ourselves one question: "Who if anyone, is the villain in the play?"

From time to time we have made tentative judgments as indicated earlier in this report, but our final judgment indicates that our search has been successful and that the greatest villain has been identified. At times, he brazenly occupied the spotlight; at others he has been seen flitting in the shadows. More often his presence has been felt even while he remained hidden in the wings. That villain is human nature. The same character is also the knight in shining armour, the hero of the play.

[ii]
Walter Rugaber
Prison Drug and Plasma Projects
*Leave Fatal Trail**

The Federal Government has watched without interference while many people sickened and some died in an extended series of drug tests and blood plasma projects.

The profits generated by these activities have gone to an enterprising contractor for the nation's biggest pharmaceutical manufacturers.

The immediate damage has been done in the penitentiary systems of three states. Hundreds of inmates in voluntary programs have been stricken with illness and serious disease. An undetermined number of the victims have died.

In a broader sense, countless millions of American consumers have been involved.

Potentially fatal new compounds have been tested on prisoners with little or no direct medical observation of the results.

Prisoners failed to swallow pills, failed to report serious reactions to those they did swallow, and failed to receive careful laboratory tests.

These studies have generated data that have in turn been used to justify the sale of drugs at prescription counters across the country.

This forbidding trail has been marked out by an Oklahoma-born physician named Austin R. Stough and corporations in which he owns a substantial interest. Despite his importance in two vital fields, he is practically unregulated in either.

As a general practitioner who reports no formal training or education in pharmacology, he is said to have conducted between 25 per cent and 50 per cent of the initial drug tests in the United States.

The 59-year-old doctor, whose companies have been blamed for the repeated use of dangerous methods and inadequate equipment, is estimated to have produced the plasma for about a fourth of an important byproduct that is widely used to protect people exposed to infectious diseases.

These prison-based enterprises have regularly incurred local disfavor. Dr. Stough was evicted from one prison by the Oklahoma authorities in 1964. He was forced out of an Arkansas prison by officials there in 1967. One of

---

* *The New York Times* 1, col. 5; 20, col. 1 (July 29, 1969). © 1969 by The New York Times Company. Reprinted by permission.

his corporations is now under orders to close down prison operations in Alabama.

But Dr. Stough (rhymes with HOW) is said to retain financial interests in some private blood banks in Birmingham and Dallas, and he is known to be seeking connections with prison systems in new areas.

He can do so freely. He has incurred no penalties, and dissatisfaction with his performance in one state has not prevented a repetition of it in another.

The Federal Government and the pharmaceutical industry—the two forces with enough broad power to compel safe practices from state to state—have maintained a general indifference at every turn.

Several agencies within the Department of Health, Education, and Welfare have known the details of Dr. Stough's plasma collections and drug tests for years. They have not curtailed them.

*   *   *

The Division of Biologics Standards, a unit of the National Institutes of Health that is responsible for the regulation of blood products, recently asserted that the safety of plasma donors was not its concern.

Several major pharmaceutical manufacturers have recognized that some of the methods employed by Dr. Stough were extremely dangerous. They continued to support him with large sums of money.

An executive of Cutter Laboratories once acknowledged, for instance, that gross contamination was apparent in the areas where the largest blood plasma operations were conducted. The rooms were "sloppy," he observed.

When a Government doctor asked why Cutter continued to reward such an enterprise with hundreds of thousands of dollars' worth of business, the executive explained that the Stough group enjoyed crucial "contacts" with well-placed officials.

These contacts involved, among other things, the payment of sizable retainers to influential lawyer-legislators and the establishment of "partnerships" for a number of prison physicians who remained on the public payrolls.

*   *   *

On March 25, 1962, the inmates at McAlester began lining up to participate in a medical procedure called plasmapheresis. Under it, a unit of whole blood is drawn and the plasma, a fluid that makes up about 55 per cent of the blood, is taken out.

The remaining cells are reinjected. That was the critical step on Sept. 19, 1962, when one of Dr. Stough's technicians processed an inmate named Tommy Lee Knott, 47, an illiterate prisoner with a long criminal record.

Knott's blood type was O-positive, but he subsequently charged in a lawsuit that after the plasma had been drawn off, the technician pumped another man's cells, which happened to be A-negative, back into his veins.

Unfortunately for Knott, his liver, lungs, brain, kidneys and other organs were injured, his nervous system underwent shock, and his weight dropped 58 pounds in 17 days.

In suing Dr. Stough and two associates for $270,000 in damages, Knott also reported that the incompatible blood had caused a double hernia, permanent secondary anemia and a 10 per cent reduction in life expectancy.

The defendants managed to settle out of court for $2,000 after Knott, who had been removed from the penitentiary for treatment, went off on a crime spree that landed him in a small-town jail.

Only three months after this inauspicious episode, Dr. Stough embarked on an ambitious expansion effort. The financial rewards inherent in his initial plasmapheresis program would now be greatly multiplied.

He brought his plasma operation to Kilby Prison, a drab institution near Montgomery, Ala., in December, 1962, and in the following year he began drawing blood in two more of the state's prisons, Draper and Atmore.

*   *   *

As a measure of his grip on the market at about this time, a Government source calculated that Dr. Stough's plasma would produce 193,970 cubic centimeters of hyperimmune gamma globulin solution monthly.

Since only about 800,000 cubic centimeters of this type of plasma product were distributed each month throughout the United States, Dr. Stough's output was the source of practically a fourth of the entire national supply.

"With demand exceeding supply," a Government doctor wrote of the boom, "inquiries were made in other states concerning the possibility of opening plasmapheresis centers in other . . . prisons."

A certain style had developed. In Oklahoma, Dr. Stough himself was the prison physi-

cian. The salary of $13,200 a year was inconsequential by his standards, but the standing it gave him within the prison was invaluable.

So, in Alabama, he awarded Dr. Irl R. Long, the senior prison physician, a financial interest in the program. Until a few weeks ago, Dr. Long simultaneously received a salary of $942 a month from the state.

A committee of the Alabama Medical Association remarked in a report issued earlier this year that "this unconscionable situation, regardless of reason, should never have been permitted to come into existence."

The prison physician in Arkansas, Dr. Gwyn Atnip, was paid $20,000 a year for his work in the plasma program there. As a desperately needed doctor among the inmates, he received $8,000 annually from the state.

Dr. Stough also lined up political support outside the prisons, a tactic that demonstrated its importance when members of the Oklahoma Legislature began to ask whether his penitentiary operations were sanctioned by law.

One of Dr. Stough's most vehement opponents was Gene Stipe, then a State Senator. But early in 1963 Senator Stipe changed sides and successfully pushed a bill that firmly established the physician's standing in the prison.

Later it was discovered that at about the time this change of direction occurred and the saving law was enacted, Mr. Stipe, a lawyer, began to receive a $1,000-a-month retainer from the concern headed by Dr. Stough.

A spokesman for the organization asserted that the money was for legal services only. Mr. Stipe agreed. Henry Bellmon, then Governor, expressed displeasure but noted that the state had no applicable conflict-of-interest law.

*   *   *

The factors pertinent to Dr. Stough's activities included a lack of medical attention (it bordered on the nonexistent in Arkansas), an absence of records, and an atmosphere of isolation and secrecy.

Still, Dr. Stough's trail remains vivid at each significant turn, and its progress behind the high walls of Kilby Prison serves to illustrate the type of infection that was spread through four other institutions.

By April, 1963, five months after Dr. Stough had opened his plasmapheresis center at Kilby, the incidence of viral hepatitis, an often fatal disease of the liver, was climbing sharply.

From none or one or two cases a month,

the disease now rose to more than 20 in a single period. Moreover, the outbreaks held generally firm between 10 and 15 a month through the following November.

The rates then soared again. There were 29 cases in December, 22 in January, 1964, 23 in February, 27 in March, and 27 in April. A tenth of the prison population had been admitted to the Kilby hospital.

Joe Willie Tifton, 46, died on March 18. Emzie B. Hasty, 42, died on April 14. Charlie C. Chandler Jr., 31, died on April 16. David Mc-Cloud, 27, died on May 22. Each death was attributed to infectious hepatitis.

Little bits and pieces then began to leak to the outside world. A penciled note from one inmate said, "They're dropping like flies out here."

But a prison spokesman said:

"The doctors are quite confident that there is no connection between the plasma program and the cause of hepatitis and jaundice."

*   *   *

The exact number of hepatitis cases in the five prisons was never established and is never likely to be. Too many medical histories vanished, too many were never completed, and too many were improperly kept by "inmate doctors."

Some 544 cases were firmly established, and that conservative figure is the one most often used. But the communicable disease center records also contain estimates of more than 800 and evidence that the figure could run to more than 1,000.

The number of deaths is similarly undetermined. In addition to at least the four in Alabama, there were reports of at least one in Arkansas and at least one in Oklahoma.

The dimensions of the disease were more clearly and precisely stated in sets of percentages, or "attack rates," that measured the incidence of hepatitis among those who gave plasma and those who did not.

At Kilby, for example, 28 per cent of the men who participated in Dr. Stough's program came down with the disease. For those who did not take part, the rate was only 1 per cent.

The rate for participants in one of the barracks at Kilby was 39.1 per cent. At the four other centers, the illness struck between 20 per cent and 26 per cent of the donors and from 0.9 per cent to 1.8 per cent of the nondonors.

The Federal investigators, reflecting scientific caution, initially referred to the prison cases as "illnesses associated with jaundice". . . .

*   *   *

The single physician employed by the Food and Drug Administration to investigate drug tests throughout the United States has visited Dr. Stough's operations twice, an agency spokesman said.

Some citizens tend to think of the agency as an eternally vigilant organization, and in his dealings with local officials and newspapermen Dr. Stough has turned this misapprehension to advantage.

"They [F.D.A. officials] love to close people down," he said in the brief telephone conversation in which he refused to grant an interview. "So if I was off-color, they'd be on me like a hawk."

"That's one of the reasons the [Alabama Corrections] Board wasn't concerned," explained Frank Lee, the state's commissioner. "We knew they [F.D.A. officials] came in here and looked into the operation."

Dr. Herbert L. Ley, Jr., the F.D.A. Commissioner, branded Dr. Stough's assertion "a non sequitur."

The Food and Drug Administration's lone medical inspector is alert to "flagrant" dishonesty, and there have been men who tested drugs on nonexistent people and who produced imaginary results.

But an inspection is limited mostly to checking data that have been submitted to the sponsoring drug company to insure that it agrees with data sent to the agency. There is little or no effort to look behind the figures.

"Our responsibility is not the direct supervision of the [drug] investigators," Dr. Ley said in an interview. "Our responsibility is to evaluate the data that come in to us. We can't be omnipotent or omniscient."

While the agency has never found occasion to reprimand Dr. Stough, its inspector, Dr. Alan B. Lisook, did make some "suggestions" earlier this year about "the lack of medical supervision of patients."

"We told him we thought there should be more supervision," Dr. Lisook said, "and he admitted there was not as much as he would like because of the volume of drugs being tested."

This was virutally an acknowledgement by Dr. Stough that more tests had been undertaken than could be adequately overseen, but the F.D.A. did not require change.

The agency "frowns" on insufficient supervision, Dr. Ley said, but under present policies there are no specific minimum standards. In the gray area that results, frowning is about the limit.

Since between 25 per cent and 50 per cent

of the phase one studies have been concentrated in Dr. Stough's hands, Dr. Ley was asked whether volume alone—quality aside—concerned his agency.

"It's a red flag; there's no question about that," he replied. But the commissioner explained that neither law nor regulation permitted the agency to force a cutback in the number of studies assigned to a single man.

There is no step short of outright disqualification for obvious misconduct, Dr. Ley said. That is an action the F.D.A. has taken no more than a dozen times in its history.

The drug companies contend there is a shortage of investigators, and Dr. Ley said that while he believed there were enough to study the "really new drugs," he wanted to avoid charges that the agency blocked progress.

"It's harder to get a driver's license in the United States than it is to get fatal drugs," complained Dr. William M. O'Brien, an associate professor of preventive and internal medicine at the University of Virginia. He added:

"To get a driver's license you have to take tests, show you know how to drive, and so on. For drugs, you just walk in the door and say, 'I'm an M.D. I want to test drugs.' It's fantastic. It's unbelievable."

It is difficult to measure the precise sums of money that the pharmaceutical industry has poured into Dr. Stough's operations, but a number of reliable clues are available.

Operating within at least nine separate corporations, the major one of which is Southern Food and Drug Research, Inc., Dr. Stough has a gross income in a good year probably approaching $1-million.

He has not carried a high overhead. His net income in Alabama in 1967 was nearly $300,000 (on a $500,000 gross), and his profit before taxes in Arkansas in 1966 was about $150,000.

* * *

NOTE

WALTER RUGABER
F.D.A. WILL REQUIRE DRUG TEST REVIEW*

. . . A Federal agency said today that it would move to halt abuses in tests of new drugs. It announced that it would impose requirements for the direct review of studies within prisons and other institutions.

Dr. Herbert L. Ley, Jr., Commissioner of the Food and Drug Administration, disclosed the plans for stricter controls and other enforcement measures during testimony before a Senate monopoly subcommittee.

He said the agency would soon publish formal proposals to establish committees that would examine preliminary plans for drug tests and monitor the evaluation work itself.

These groups will be made up of physicians, lawyers, clergymen and other professionals, Dr. Ley said, and will be appointed by institutions where much of the initial testing is carried out.

The committee will be expected to have no connection with the pharmaceutical manufacturer seeking to have the drug approved for sale and no connection with the evaluator paid to conduct the tests, he said.

* * *

The local review committees that Dr. Ley suggested would fit somewhere between the present system and a more extensive reform advocated by Senator Gaylord Nelson, the subcommittee chairman. Senator Nelson, a Wisconsin Democrat, recently introduced legislation to take the management of drug testings away from the manufacturers and give it to the Federal Government.

Senator Nelson asked, as an example, how the "peer group" provision could have prevented a case of gross fraud reported by Dr. Ley today. An unidentified doctor in upstate New York falsified data in drug tests.

The Commissioner conceded that the proposed arrangement would not cover individuals operating on their own and that this represented a "remaining loophole." The review committees would not be "a sole cure," he said.

He also acknowledged under questioning that it was "unusual" for 14 pharmaceutical concerns to have sought out "a general practitioner in a small New York State community" to conduct tests on 45 drugs.

[iii]
*The Editors of the New England Journal
of Medicine
Typhoid in Volunteers**

* * *

Reported in this issue are the values of amino acids in the serums of patients in whom

* *The New York Times* 1, col. 2; 32, col. 3 (August 13, 1969). © 1969 by The New York Times Company. Reprinted by permission.

* 278 *New England Journal of Medicine* 332–333 (1968). Reprinted by permission.

typhoid fever was induced. [The subjects were seventeen healthy inmates of the Maryland House of Corrections.] . . . The primary overall aim of the studies was to appraise the efficacy of typhoid vaccine for use in our military personnel. . . .

* * *

In 1948 field trials, involving volunteers who exposed themselves in endemic areas, demonstrated that antibiotics would prevent scrub typhus fever. Basic immunologic principles were firmly established. . . .

Carefully designed studies conducted during the past 10 years have defined the human dose of *Salmonella typhosa* needed to produce disease and have shown that typhoid vaccines are of low protective value. The cooperation of more than 400 healthy volunteers has provided the data regarding typhoid vaccine; the infected men recovered promptly, and there have been no important complications or sequelae, nor has the carrier state developed. Volunteers have been infected only when testing of animals, including primates, failed to yield meaningful data.

Field trials can yield interpretable results if properly conducted. They place heavy demands, however, on resources and health manpower. Limitations also include lack of information about the size of the infecting dose, its relation to host resistance and natural variations in virulence. Volunteer trials with induction of typhoid fever have permitted the following goals over and above those attainable by field trials: measurement of duration of vaccine protection; evaluation of immunity in nonendemic areas; appraisal of effect of various antigenic fractions in small numbers of vaccines; measurement of the effect of combinations of vaccines and of booster doses; evaluation of the protection against varying doses of the infecting bacilli; simultaneous appraisal of the physiologic and biochemical abnormalities of the blood and intestinal tract that help to clarify pathogenesis; analysis of the immune response and its influence on the presence of typhoid bacilli in the feces and blood; information on the nature of the protective antibodies; and reduction in the time and costs of vaccine evaluation. In addition to these considerable benefits, experience derived from volunteer studies provides invaluable guidance for better planning of field trials and interpretation of the results.

NOTE

Lawrence A. Kohn
Experimental Typhoid in Man*

The apologetic editorial in the February 8 issue fails to relieve the *Journal* of the onus of having published the article on "Whole-Blood Amino Acids in Experimentally Induced Typhoid Fever in Man." It is unfortunate that this type of study is conducted, but even more so that the *Journal* should announce the results, which incidentally are of limited value since the food intake of the subjects was not apparently standardized. Even with available drug treatment, typhoid fever is not free of immediate or delayed risks. The paper in itself gives no assurance that there were no ill effects; the editorial comment must have been based on generalizations or on data not presented.

Other responses to infection might be studied experimentally in man: the dyspnea of lobar pneumonia, the chemical changes in the spinal fluid in meningitis; and the nature of the natural defenses against poliomyelitis and how to modify them. These analogies are farfetched, but the principles outlined in the editorial do not convince one that this study was either more justified or more necessary. The *Journal* could well have refused it space.

b.

By Action of Subject?

The People ex. rel. *Blunt v. Narcotic Addiction Control Commission*
58 Misc. 2d 57, 295 N.Y.S. 2d 276, aff'd.,
251 App. Div. 456, 296 N.Y.S. 2d 533 (1968).

Hyman Korn, J.: The relator Rudolph Blunt, by way of a writ of habeas corpus, seeks his release from Rikers Island on the grounds that the New York State Narcotic Addiction Control Commission, hereinafter referred to as NACC, has failed to provide rehabilitative treatment for his drug addiction.

A hearing was held pursuant to a direction of this Court and extensive testimony was adduced with respect to the issue raised by the relator.

Relator was convicted of a misdemeanor on October 17, 1967. Though such violation would ordinarily have subjected him to punishment for no more than one year at the penitentiary, as a

_____
* 278 *New England Journal of Medicine* 739 (1968). Reprinted by permission.

convicted addict, he was committed to the custody of the NACC for an indefinite period not to exceed 36 months (Mental Hygiene Law, §208). He is presently at Rikers Island in the custody of the Addiction Service Agency, hereinafter referred to as ASA. This agency administers the narcotics program in the City of New York for criminal addicts under a contract entered into between the State of New York and City of New York.

Specifically it is relator's contention that he is being treated in no different manner than the other nonaddict inmates at the prison. Testimony offered by the relator was to the effect that he and the other committed criminal addicts live and work with nonaddict prisoners and are subject to the same prison routine and regulations as their nonaddict cellmates. However, where the nonaddict cellmates are released within one year, relator and other criminal addicts may be held for a period of 36 months.

*   *   *

The respondent seriously contests relator's claim and asserts that there is presently on Rikers Island a bona fide and meaningful program under which effective rehabilitative treatment is afforded to the committed criminal addict.

*   *   *

There is no question that confinement of relator for a period in excess of that provided for in the Penal Law could not be based purely on his status as an addict. Justification for holding him in custody for a maximum period of three years may be predicated solely on the basis that such additional term is required to effect treatment for his addiction. Absent such rehabilitative treatment, his continued confinement became purely custodial and is legally untenable.

At the outset, it should be noted that it is not for this court to determine the nature of the treatment to be given nor the facilities to be furnished. The commission, with its expertise in the field, ought to be left to determine the method of care and treatment best suited for achieving its established purpose. It is only where the court finds that the treatment offered is so meaningless, that as a matter of law it is really no treatment or where the claim of treatment is a mere pretext to keep an addict in custody, that the court is under a duty to intercede on the addict's behalf. . . .

Upon a review of the facts in this case, the court is not prepared to find that the narcotic program presently offered by the ASA is totally without merit. However, the evidence adduced does show serious flaws in the present approach to the problem. Though millions have been spent in setting up this program, the results have not been too encouraging. To date, only 20 to 25 criminal addicts have been provisionally designated as rehabilitated. A critical problem which seriously threatens the program's success is the refusal by the committed addicts to participate. [O]ver 50 per cent of the addicts presently in custody by their own choice do not take part in its rehabilitative plan and receive no other treatment or therapy. [T]here is little, if any, professional attention given during the initial motivational phase of the agency's program. Major responsibility for making the very vital first phase work is placed upon addict-group leaders who themselves are in the same program. They in turn are supervised by a director and assistant director who are former addicts. Well-meaning as they may be, these persons have little, if any, formal education. Except for some scientific jargon they may have gleaned during their own treatment, they seem to operate to a large extent on their own intuition. . . .

*   *   *

[W]hatever its present shortcomings, New York State's new and revolutionary approach to drug addiction and crime should be given every chance to succeed. Some addicts are participating in the city program and some progress has been shown. The experimental nature of this program is obvious, and trial and error must be permitted if an effective and efficient program is to be evolved. The courts should not thwart the legislative purpose in enacting article 9 of the Mental Hygiene Law by prematurely interfering in its mechanics. For the reasons stated, relator's writ is dismissed.

NOTE

SKINNER V. OKLAHOMA
316 U.S. 535 (1942)

MR. JUSTICE DOUGLAS delivered the opinion of the Court:

*   *   *

The statute involved is Oklahoma's Habitual Criminal Sterilization Act. That Act defines an "habitual criminal" as a person who, having been convicted two or more times for crimes "amounting to felonies involving moral turpitude" either in an Oklahoma court or in a court of any other state, is thereafter convicted of such a felony in Oklahoma and is sentenced to a term of imprisonment in an Oklahoma penal institution. Machinery is provided for the institution by the Attorney General of a proceeding against such a person in the Oklahoma courts for a judgment that such person shall be rendered sexually sterile. . . .

*   *   *

[T]he instant legislation runs afoul of the equal protection clause, though we give Oklahoma . . . large deference. . . . We are dealing here with legislation which involves one of the basic civil rights of man. Marriage and procreation are fundamental to the very existence and survival of the race. The power to sterilize, if exercised, may have subtle, far-reaching and devastating effects. In evil or reckless hands it can cause races or types which are inimical to the dominant group to wither and disappear. There is no redemption for the individual whom the law touches. Any experiment which the state conducts is to his irreparable injury. He is forever deprived of a basic liberty. . . . When the law lays an unequal hand on those who have committed intrinsically the same quality of offense and sterilizes one and not the other, it has made as invidious a discrimination as if it had selected a particular race or nationality for oppressive treatment. . . . Sterilization of those who have thrice committed grand larceny, with immunity for those who are embezzlers, is a clear, pointed, unmistakable discrimination. Oklahoma makes no attempt to say that he who commits larceny by trespass or trick or fraud has biologically inheritable traits which he who commits embezzlement lacks. . . . In terms of fines and imprisonment, the crimes of larceny and embezzlement rate the same under the Oklahoma code. Only when it comes to sterilization are the pains and penalties of the law different. The equal protection clause would indeed be a formula of empty words if such conspicuously artificial lines could be drawn. . . .

*   *   *

Reversed.

MR. CHIEF JUSTICE STONE, concurring:

*   *   *

Science has found and the law has recognized that there are certain types of mental deficiency associated with delinquency which are inheritable. But the state does not contend—nor can there be any pretense—that either common knowledge or experience, or scientific investigation, has given assurance that the criminal tendencies of any class of habitual offenders are universally or even generally inheritable. In such circumstances, inquiry whether such is the fact in the case of any particular individual cannot rightly be dispensed with. Whether the procedure by which a statute carries its mandate into execution satisfies due process is a matter of judicial cognizance. A law which condemns, without hearing, all the individuals of a class to so harsh a measure as the present because some or even many merit condemnation is lacking in the first principles of due process. . . .

MR. JUSTICE JACKSON, concurring:

*   *   *

I . . . think the present plan to sterilize the individual in pursuit of a eugenic plan to eliminate from the race characteristics that are only vaguely identified and which in our present state of knowledge are uncertain as to transmissibility presents other constitutional questions of gravity. This Court has sustained such an experiment with respect to an imbecile, a person with definite and observable characteristics, where the condition had persisted through three generations and afforded grounds for the belief that it was transmissible and would continue to manifest itself in generations to come. *Buck v. Bell,* 274 U.S. 200.

There are limits to the extent to which a legislatively represented majority may conduct biological experiments at the expense of the dignity and personality and natural powers of a minority—even those who have been guilty of what the majority define as crimes. But this Act falls down before reaching this problem, which I mention only to avoid the implication that such a question may not exist because not discussed. On it I would also reserve judgment.

CHAPTER FOURTEEN

Experimentation with Dying Subjects

The decision to use dying patients as research subjects is one of the most controversial an investigator can make. Persons suffering from terminal illness present many of the same problems as those encountered in the previous two chapters—like children, their ability to make informed decisions is often either impaired or disregarded, and, like soldiers and prisoners, they are not really free but are the "captives" of their disease, their physicians and hospital, and their enforced isolation. It is therefore not surprising that some commentators flatly oppose the use of the dying as subjects. On the other hand, investigators argue that meaningful research on some fatal diseases can be conducted only on those suffering from these diseases, that terminally ill patients are often eager to receive innovative treatment, and that participation in research may make their final period of life worthwhile.

The issues raised in this chapter have of late taken on added significance because organ transplantation usually involves dying patients, both as recipients and as donors. Moreover, experimental organ surgery has raised a host of troublesome new questions revolving around the criteria and procedures for determining death as well as for choosing potential recipients and donors.

In studying these materials, consider the following questions:

1. Should research on dying persons be permitted?
2. If research is permitted, who ought to set its limits and balance the risks against the potential benefits to the patient and to society?
3. Since the prolongation or termination of life has social, legal, moral, psychological,

and religious ramifications, what considerations enter into the choice of adopting firm standards or of allowing decisions to be made on a case-by-case basis?

4. Since the length of life can increasingly be extended by a variety of experimental means, how, to what extent, and to whom should opportunities be provided to terminate such experiments?

A.
Case Studies of the Dying as Research Subjects and Organ Donors

1.

James A. Helmsworth, Johnson McGuire, and Benjamin Felson
Arteriography of the Aorta and Its Branches by Means of the Polyethylene Catheter*

As the scope of vascular and thoracic surgery is extended, detailed information concerning abnormal morphology of the major vessels is of more than academic interest. For example, knowledge of the length of the constricted segment in aortic coarctation and of the exact relations of the vessels in arteriovenous aneurysm in the neck enables the surgeon to plan accurately an effective operative procedure. Similarly, the differentiation between a mediastinal tumor and an aneurysm may be the determining factor for exploration of the chest.

* * *

The catheter was the most important item of equipment used in this method. A standard woven ureteral catheter was used in several of the early cases but the advantage of its radiopacity was outweighed by the disadvantage of the thickness of its wall. Catheters made of polyethylene tubing were employed because of the experience of others and proved more satisfactory. Lengths of from 50 to 75 cm. were prepared. . . .

* * *

The arteries selected for this study were the brachial and the ulnar collateral at the level of the transverse crease of the elbow, and the femoral in the middle third of the thigh below the origin of the profunda.

After preparation of the skin, anesthesia was produced by local infiltration. The artery

* 64 *American Journal of Roentgenology* 196–200, 210–212 (1950). Reprinted by permission.

was exposed through a small incision and a 2 cm. segment mobilized by ligation and division of the fine branches. It was essential that the field be entirely free of ooze and that the vessel segment be without hematoma in the adventitia. After a looped sling of ligature silk had been placed about the proximal and distal extremities of the segment, the artery was opened by a transverse incision estimated to be slightly longer than the diameter of the catheter to be inserted. The catheter, filled with heparinsaline solution (70 mg. of heparin to 1 liter of physiological saline) and free of bubbles, was then inserted and advanced toward the heart as tension on the proximal looped sling was relaxed. To prevent the formation of a thrombus within the catheter or about its tip, it was necessary to keep a stream of heparin solution flowing slowly through the catheter. The catheter was advanced until its tip was estimated to be near the desired site of injection. Under roentgenoscopic control the opaque medium, diodrast or neo-iopax, was injected slowly into the catheter until it opacified the tip. The catheter was then advanced or withdrawn to the site of injection. The patient was placed in the position best suited for roentgenographic demonstration of the artery. A fraction of a cubic centimeter of the contrast substance was then injected as a test for sensitivity.

The injection of the contrast medium was made as rapidly as possible with the 50 cc. syringe. This step was carefully timed and usually required from 0.7 to 1.8 seconds. The volume injected varied from 8 to 30 cc. and the Potter-Bucky roentgenogram was usually made as the last cubic centimeter was ejected from the syringe. . . .

During withdrawal of the catheter the artery was irrigated with a liberal quantity of heparin solution. When it had been determined that no thrombus was present proximal or distal to the incised segment the artery was repaired. . . . In several instances repair of the brachial artery was impossible, and ligation and division of this artery was carried out. A simple approximation of the skin margins completed closure of the wound. Anticoagulant was administered only during the examination, as described above. With this method visualization of the aorta and its major branches was undertaken.

* * *

In the present attempt at coronary arteriography preliminary experiments were carried out on 5 unselected mongrel dogs. . . .

Attempts at coronary arteriography were then made on 6 patients. In 4, no filling was obtained. Visualization of some of the circulation was obtained in the other 2 cases, which follow.

CASE I. B. K., a white female, aged eighty-eight, was admitted on February 23, 1949, in coma following a cerebral accident. A history of coronary occlusion one year earlier was obtained from the family. The patient remained deeply comatose throughout her stay in the hospital. On March 10, under local anesthesia, catheter No. 2 was inserted through the left brachial artery into the proximal portion of the ascending aorta. With the patient in the left posterior oblique position 12 cc. of 70 per cent diodrast was injected in 0.5 second. A Potter-Bucky film was obtained at the end of the injection. The procedure was repeated five times. Immediately following the last injection the patient suddenly developed an arrhythmia and, despite emergency treatment, died. Autopsy showed marked cerebral softening, marked arteriosclerosis of the coronary arteries, and an old thrombosis of an anterior coronary branch near the cardiac apex. The coronaries were otherwise patient. There was no evidence that the catheter had traumatized the ascending aorta and no anatomic cause of the sudden death was apparent.

Review of the roentgenograms . . . showed the tip of the catheter in the ascending aorta at the level of the aortic valve. Two of the five films revealed filling of the right coronary artery and its branches, but no filling of the left.

CASE II. L. Z., a white male, aged seventy-four, was admitted on February 19, 1949, in a stuporous condition. A diagnosis of multiple myeloma was established. On March 3, with the patient obviously moribund and deeply comatose, catheter No. 2 was inserted through the right brachial artery into the proximal ascending aorta. Ten cubic centimeters of 75 per cent neo-iopax was injected in about 0.7 second with the patient in the left posterior oblique position. The roentgen exposure was made as the injection was completed. The procedure was repeated six times using between 5 and 10 cc. of the contrast substance with each injection. The catheter was re-

moved and the artery repaired. The patient's condition did not appear to change immediately following the procedure but he died six hours later. Autopsy revealed multiple myeloma and lobular pneumonia. The coronary vessels and aorta showed arteriosclerosis of a moderate degree. The coronary ostia were not narrowed. Again, evidence of trauma to the aorta was lacking.

* * *

Although Cases I and II died following the procedure, it should be noted that in both instances the patients were already moribund, and that multiple injections of contrast agent were administered. In Case I the death must be attributed to the arteriography, but in Case II the procedure was probably not at fault. Failure to visualize the coronaries occurred in a number of the attempts in these 2 patients. It is possible that the failures were due to the relatively small quantity of the agent used. Further studies of this problem are being made.

* * *

The most important consideration in a procedure of this type is its effect upon the patient. One death, in a woman aged eighty-eight who was already moribund, was directly attributable to the procedure. Another patient developed convulsions immediately after the injection of contrast medium, but recovered. A third patient, who was semicomatose at the time of the procedure, became excited for a brief period following the injection.

Experience with this method has yielded certain information concerning these reactions. In the first place, there have been no serious symptoms attributable to the procedure of catheterization itself. In some of the earlier attempts vasospasm, unaccompanied by pain, occurred in the extremity and continued up to thirty-six hours. In every instance this followed the use of a catheter which was too large. In later studies, in which smaller catheters were used, this complication was not encountered, even though repeating the injections sometimes meant that the catheter remained in the artery from thirty to ninety minutes. Thrombosis of the incised artery did not occur when the artery was sutured and even when ligation of the brachial [artery] was performed no sequelae developed. In one patient the right brachial artery was catheterized on two occasions six days apart, using the same incision. The radial pulse remained normal after both procedures and no complications arose. Bleeding was never a problem since the contraction of the artery sealed the opening of the vessel around the catheter.

*   *   *

The one fatality occurred after the injection of 70 per cent diodrast while the other 2 cases developed symptoms following the use of 75 per cent neo-iopax. In all 3 instances concentrated medium might have entered the cerebral circulation and, as noted by Broman and Olson, cerebral damage might well have been responsible for the reactions. . . .

It is imperative to weigh the dangers of the procedure against the value of the information obtained. Although the present study was basically experimental, the resulting information was often important in the management of the patient and could not have been obtained by completely safe conventional methods. If its dangers can be reduced or eliminated, as by improving the contrast medium, arteriography may prove of value in the elucidation of diseases of the aorta and its major branches.

*   *   *

2.

Howard R. Bierman, Earl R. Miller, Ralph L. Byron, Jr., Kenneth S. Dod, Keith H. Kelly, and Daniel H. Black Intra-Arterial Catheterization of Viscera in Man*

The afferent artery from which a neoplasm obtains its blood supply represents a route of attack on such growth, with diagnostic and possibly therapeutic implications. . . .

*   *   *

If the major artery leading to a specific organ could be isolated to the exclusion of other viscera, not only could that specific organ be visualized roentgenographically, but also various chemotherapeutic agents could be administered in high concentration directly to neoplastic lesions involving this organ. Furthermore, such an isolation of the arterial supply of such an organ in vivo would enable the employment of this method for many pharmacological and

---

* 66 *American Journal of Roentgenology* 555–567 (1951). Reprinted by permission.

physiological studies. In the search for clinical methods by means of which the afferent artery to deep-seated neoplasms could be reached, the feasibility of intra-arterial catheterization of viscera was explored. This communication reports the development of the method.

Materials and Methods

The investigations were carried out by a team of a surgeon, radiologist, internist and anesthetist. Radiopaque, intracardiac catheters, 100 to 150 cm. long, No. 6 to No. 9F with a fixed curve at the tip, were used.

The technique was first tried on cadavers. . . .

Twenty-eight arterial catheterizations were then performed on 24 patients with metastases from various neoplastic diseases. The procedure in its entirety, including the hazards, risk and experimental nature, was explained fully to each patient and an unqualified agreement was obtained in all cases.

Catheterization technique. The procedure in adults is carried out under routine preoperative medication and local procaine anesthesia. The 3 children in this series had a general anesthetic; the 2 eldest had nitrous oxide and the fourteen-month-old received ether. The artery is exposed in the supraclavicular area and loops of *thin*, flexible rubber tubing or rubber bands are placed around the vessel above and below the site for the opening of the artery. . . . A 2 mm. longitudinal incision is made through the wall of the artery with a small scalpel and the tip of the catheter is inserted. . . . The catheter is filled with saline containing 2 mg. per 100 cc. of heparin before insertion, and this solution is kept running slowly through the catheter during the procedure. . . .

After insertion into the artery, the catheter is guided by roentgenoscopy. . . . The catheter is advanced into the aortic arch via the innominate artery . . . and into the descending aorta. . . .

To enter the celiac artery, the tip of the catheter is pointed anteriorly as it descends to the aortic hiatus at the level of the diaphragm. . . . The injection of 5 cc. of 70 per cent . . . diodrast visualizes the vascular pattern of the hepatic, left gastric, and splenic arteries and their branches. . . .

The superior mesenteric, inferior mesenteric, renal . . . middle sacral, iliac, hypogastric, and gluteal vessels . . . have been similarly catheterized. . . .

Tumor masses in the neck may prevent satisfactory exposure of the carotid arteries. To reach the carotids, subclavians, and their branches under these circumstances, the brachial, ulnar, and femoral arteries have been employed. . . .

After completion of the procedures with the catheter in place, the catheter is withdrawn under roentgenoscopic control and the arterial incision is closed with arterial silk suture after milking the artery from both ends to remove any thrombi that may be present. The wound is closed in routine fashion.

*   *   *

Complications

Four complications have been encountered. There was a wound infection in one case . . . with subsequent hemorrhage three weeks after catheterization. In this case the exposure of the carotid artery had to be performed through a large lesion of mycosis fungoides which, despite rigorous cleansing, probably was not completely sterile. The erosion in the artery was sutured, but was followed within thirty-six hours by a left hemiplegia, with later recovery of motion in the face and lower extremity. Approximately eight weeks later hemorrhage again ensued and the carotid was ligated without significant change in the patient.

The second complication during the procedure occurred in a male, aged sixty-five with carcinoma of the larynx, metastatic to the neck with a hypertension of 170/110, arteriosclerotic heart disease, and chronic nephritis (non-protein nitrogen 59 mg. per cent). The patient developed a left hemiplegia five minutes after the procedure started and after the injection of only 11 cc. of 35 per cent diodrast. He died four days later. The right cerebral hemisphere was found to be infarcted, probably due to the marked arteriosclerosis of the right carotid artery together with compression of the artery by the tumor mass, as the head was moved to the left during the procedure, and perhaps aided by arterial spasm from the diodrast.

In a third case . . . the physician holding the rubber bands about the artery became confused in the dark of the roentgenoscopic room and somehow switched the clamps so that tension was exerted downward on the upper tubing and upward on the lower tubing, resulting in twisting the artery into a knot and completely shutting off the blood flow through the right common carotid. Complete left hemiplegia appeared twelve hours later.

The fourth complication occurred in a moribund male, aged fifty-six, with marked arteriosclerosis, syphilitic aortitis, aortic insufficiency and widespread metastatic adenocarcinoma. The blood pressure in the right arm was 90/0 and 160/70 in the left. The catheter was inserted into the left brachial artery at the mid-humeral level. Twelve hours later the forearm and hand were cyanotic, cold and cadaveric. The patient continued to fail progressively and died forty-eight hours after nitrogen mustard was administered into the aortic arch and a thrombus was found just above the cut-down site.

*   *   *

Discussion

The technique of intra-arterial catheterization has proved to be a feasible procedure. However, it must be undertaken with a calculated risk. . . .

The injection of a 70 per cent diodrast solution usually, but not always, causes the patients to complain of a burning sensation along the course of the vessels with somatic reference. The position of the catheter may often be confirmed in this manner.

While four serious complications in a group of 24 patients would appear to give a high incidence, it is not prohibitively high considering the initial effort in this direction, mostly on critically ill patients with far advanced neoplastic illnesses. The complications of wound infection (Case I) and surgical error (Case III) are avoidable and have been corrected. From our further experience it is now almost certain that the complication in Case II was in all likelihood due to a diodrast reaction which together with the marked arteriosclerosis and large metastatic tumor was sufficient to cause cerebral anoxia. The fourth complication occurred before we instituted the milking of the artery from both ends to remove any thrombi that may have occurred during the procedure. Since that time no further complications of this sort have been noted.

New techniques encounter difficulties until they are perfected. Since the complications noted were all amenable to improvement, as has been shown in the later catheterizations, it would appear that this procedure has some value for the purpose stated.

*   *   *

3.

R. H. Johnson, A. C. Smith, and J. M. K. Spalding
Oxygen Consumption of Paralysed Men Exposed to Cold*

When a mammal is exposed to a cold environment its metabolism increases and there may be a progressive increase in activity of skeletal muscle . . . leading eventually to shivering. In small mammals metabolism also increases in tissues other than skeletal muscles . . . but it is uncertain whether this is so in larger mammals including man. . . . The oxygen consumption of five subjects whose skin was cooled for 80–210 min was measured. Two subjects were healthy men, one had almost complete paralysis of skeletal muscle due to poliomyelitis and two were unconscious and were studied before and after receiving a muscle relaxant.

Subjects. Subjects R. H. J. (28 years; 69 kg; 175 cm) and A. C. S. (45 years; 64 kg; 163 cm) were healthy men. Subject G. W., male, 34 years, had had poliomyelitis 2½ years before and was completely paralysed below the neck except that he was capable of slight movement of the right toes. He was entirely dependent upon intermittent positive pressure respiration (IPPR) which he received from a Radcliffe Respiration Pump . . . through a cuffed tracheostomy tube . . . which provided an air-tight seal in the trachea. His autonomic nervous system was intact as judged clinically and by the response of the arterial blood pressure to Valsalva's manoeuvre and by observations on central venous pressure and venous distensibility. He received no drugs.

Subject E. H., male 68 years, had been unconscious for 3 months after hypotension and anoxia associated with an abdominal operation elsewhere. He had been emphysematous for several years and after the operation could not breathe adequately. He received artificial respiration in the same way as subject G. W. His autonomic nervous system was imperfect, for the response of the aterial blood pressure to Valsalva's manoeuvre showed little evidence of reflex vasoconstriction. The following autonomic responses, however, were normal: he did not have postural hypotension; on cooling one arm there was vasoconstriction in the opposite hand, as indicated by a reduction in heat flow from the pulp of the finger, measured with heat-flow

* 169 *Journal of Physiology* 584–587, 590 (1963). Reprinted by permission.

disks; when his trunk was heated with a radiant-heat cradle there was normal vasodilatation in his hands measured in the same way, and sweating tested with Quinizarin was normal. His metabolic rate was first examined without his having received any drugs, and then whilst receiving paralysing doses of D-tubocurarine. (Heights and weights are not available for the patients receiving IPPR.)

Subject M. M., male (17 years; 54 kg; 170 cm) had been unconscious for 12 months after a severe closed head injury. He normally breathed spontaneously. The same tests of the autonomic nervous system were performed as in subject E. H. Sweating was slightly greater on the right than the left side of the body, but other tests gave normal results. In particular the response of the arterial blood pressure to Valsalva's manoeuvre, to changes of posture and to noise were normal.

*   *   *

Skin temperature was measured at one point on the abdomen with a thermocouple. Body temperature was measured in subject R. H. J. with a mercury thermometer in the mouth, in A. C. S. with a thermocouple in the rectum, and in G. W., E. H., and M. M. with a thermocouple in the oesophagus. Oesophageal temperature reflects changes in arterial blood temperature. Temperatures of room air and of the gas in the Benedict Roth spirometer were measured with mercury thermometers.

Procedure. Observations were made over a 10-min cycle which was repeated continuously throughout the experiment. Minute 1 (approximately); the subject breathed oxygen through the closed circuit. Minutes 2 and 3; he breathed the oxygen-air mixture through the open circuit. . . .

Minutes 4–6; the subject's oxygen consumption was measured with the closed circuit. . . . Minutes 7–10; the subject breathed the oxygen-air mixture. The skin, body and room temperatures were measured.

In each subject this cycle of observations was continued for 40–80 min while the subject was recumbent and covered with blankets. The blankets were then removed and fans played cool air on the subject for 80–210 min and the observations were continued. The subject was then covered with blankets or warmed with a heat cradle and further observations were made during the recovery period.

When the normal subjects R. H. J. and

A. C. S. were cooled there was pilo-erection and sporadic shivering. "Skin" temperature fell to 24–26° C, deep temperature rose slightly and O_2 consumption and CO_2 output increased. When the subjects were warmed these changes were reversed. When subject G. W. (who had had poliomyelitis) was cooled, there was pilo-erection and his teeth chattered. "Skin" temperature fell to a minimum of 17.6° C. Oesophageal temperature fell by 1.5—1.8° C and O_2 consumption and CO_2 output did not rise and may have fallen. . . . When subjects E. H. and M. M. (who were unconscious) were cooled without receiving any drugs there were pilo-erection and sporadic shivering, and O_2 uptake and CO_2 output increased. When they received paralysing doses of muscle relaxants (D-tubocurarine, E. H.; gallamine, M. M.) there was no shivering and no rise in O_2 consumption or CO_2 output.

These findings indicate that, under the conditions of our observations, an increase in O_2 uptake and CO^2 output occurred when men with active skeletal muscles were cooled. It did not, however, occur in men whose skeletal muscles were paralysed. This was true whether the paralysis was due to poliomyelitis or muscle relaxants (D-tubocurarine or gallamine).

* * *

. . . Our results are consistent with the view that in man the increase in metabolism on cooling for periods up to 3½ hr occurs solely in skeletal muscles.

4.

Renato Cavaliere, Enrico C. Ciocatto, Beppino C. Giovanella, Charles Heidelberger, Robert O. Johnson, Mario Margottini, Bruno Mondovi, Guido Moricca, and Alessandro Rossi-Fanelli
Selective Heat Sensitivity of Cancer Cells*

Numerous laboratory and clinical reports scattered throughout the literature strongly suggest a remarkably selective destructive effect of heat against cancer cells that could be systematically exploited for therapeutic purposes.

* * *

Patients with large, recurrent or single meta-

* 20 *Cancer* 1351, 1360–1361, 1364–1369, 1373 (1967). Reprinted by permission of the American Cancer Society.

static cancers localized in an extremity offer an excellent opportunity to study the effect of localized high temperature treatment because of the availability of amputation as an alternative form of therapy if the disease were not well controlled or the limb irreparably damaged. Isolation perfusion with extracorporeal circulation for localized high-dose chemotherapy of tumors of the extremities has become an established technique, which has been adopted for the present study; however, in this case no drugs were perfused and the perfusate fluid was heated. Studies on the isolated dog hind limb have indicated that a temperature of 42 to 44° C (107 to 111° F) for two hours can be tolerated without major damage.

* * *

We are reporting on the first 25 high-temperature perfusions that were performed in 22 patients at the Regina Elena Institute, of which 18 were done via the iliac, six via the axillary and one via the brachial vessels. . . . The total perfusion times ranged between 2 hours, 7 min to 8 hours, 5 min, with the duration of adequate temperatures (above 40° C) in the tumor from 50 minutes to 6 hours, 50 min.

The tumors in this series included 12 sarcomas, seven melanomas, two squamous cell carcinomas of the skin and one metastatic leiomyosarcoma from the uterus. . . .

* * *

Intensive postoperative care was required, especially during the first 5 days. The patients required multiple transfusions of whole blood, plasma, fluids, electrolytes, hydrocortisone, mannitol, cardiac supportive therapy, antibiotics, multiple vitamins and physiotherapy. Operative interventions were required in a few patients. These procedures included tracheotomy, amputation, vascular repair, incision and drainage, debridement, skin grafting and embolectomy.

Complications: Eight of the 25 perfusions were accomplished without complications, which were often multiple. Second degree burns occurred in six patients, one of which was serious. Death occurred in six patients within 15 days postoperatively: One died of a myocardial infarction at 12 hours; one patient died of shock one day after perfusion at a tumor temperature of 49° C due to a thermometer failure (subsequently, two independent thermometer systems were always used); one died at 3 days from a transfusion reaction; another at three days from septicemia; one at 5 days from a "crushed limb syndrome" from kidney failure probably caused by the total regression of a massive tumor; and one from an embolus on the fifteenth day. . . .

Response: . . . A complete gross disappearance of the tumor was obtained in 10 of the 22 patients; a 20 to 80 per cent decrease in tumor volume was observed in five patients (good response), no response was seen in three patients (of which two received inadequate temperatures) and in four cases the response could not be evaluated for various reasons. Microscopically, a total necrosis of the tumor with no viable cells visible in any of the sections examined was obtained in eight patients; seven of these patients are alive and free of disease at the present time and one died of the "crushed limb syndrome."

Histologically an excellent response as indicated by a very massive necrosis, but no visible nests of viable tumor cells, was observed in eight patients; all of these had recurrences of their tumors. Microscopically no response was observed in three patients and the response could not be evaluated in three. In the present series malignant melanomas appear to be the most responsive to high temperature perfusion.

Most of these patients had a poor prognosis since 14 of 22 had recurrent disease prior to high-temperature perfusion. At present, 12 of the 22 patients are alive and free of the disease over intervals ranging from 3 to 28 months after perfusion; however, in this group eight had other forms of therapy subsequent to the perfusion, including two amputations that were required by the loss of a functional limb due to total destruction of bone and total regression of the osteogenic sarcoma; four amputations due to tumor recurrence; one recurrence that was amputated and followed by x-ray therapy and one recurrence that was treated with x-ray therapy. One patient is currently alive with disease and two have been lost to follow-up. In spite of the advanced status of their diseases, only one of the patients that responded to the perfusion has died of metastatic disease.

* * *

The method of high-temperature perfusion of advanced cancers of the extremities has demonstrated the clinical feasibility of heat treatment. Nevertheless, the procedure is far from ideal. It is hazardous and there were numerous complications which have declined with experience. . . .

The incidence of therapeutic effects of high-temperature perfusion and degree of response to it was considerably greater than those produced by the conventional regional perfusions with short-acting chemotherapeutic agents; however, in many cases it was necessary to amputate the limb after treatment (only in case 1 as a complication of the perfusion) because of the destruction of the tumor and consequent loss of a functional limb or because of recurrences when a second high-temperature perfusion was impractical or refused. In the three patients that received a second perfusion one tumor disappeared totally and has not recurred 17 months after the second perfusion and two patients had recurrences 2 months after the second treatment.

Of the 25 high-temperature perfusions in 22 patients there were 10 total gross disappearances of tumor and eight microscopic total necroses. It seems rather unlikely that the mechanical act of perfusion or the supportive therapy, i.e., cortisone and transfusions, contributed appreciably to the therapeutic results but these possibilities cannot be ignored.

Deaths from complications occurred rather early in the series but with experience and more aggressive post-perfusion supportive therapy the mortality was diminished. Local complications were also diminished by the early abandonment of tourniquets and infrared heating. The death of patient 8 from a "crushed limb syndrome" following total regression of a massive tumor suggests that large tumors should be reduced surgically before high-temperature perfusion is carried out. The possibility of combining high-temperature perfusion with chemotherapy obviously deserves exploration. The present study and its current extension to additional cases will serve as a baseline for the evaluation of such combined treatments.

* * *

This method of high-temperature treatment obviously has limitations and at present is indicated in patients with primary or recurrent malignant tumors of the limbs for whom the only alternative therapy would be amputation, which often does not prevent metastases. The fatal risks and complications encountered in the earlier cases have been gradually overcome but this method should be attempted only by highly qualified and experienced clinicians. The selective destructive effect of high temperature on neoplastic cells suggests the possibility of combining this treatment with a local excision of the tumor when this is feasible. It is evident that future progress in this field will come from total-body high-temperature treatment. We are now in the process of developing techniques towards this end. . . .

5.

Eric Kast
LSD and the Dying Patient*

*   *   *

While observing patients during the final months of life, one can see certain defense mechanisms developing in an attempt either to structure death and subsequent "existence" or to deny all possibility of death and assume an eerie positivism which seems surrealistic in character. The usual approach to death is by a combination of both, and it seems to take an extraordinary toll in a person's ability to relate to his environment and communicate with his family. He becomes isolated and is deprived, to a large extent, of his ability to realistically and deeply experience these last months or weeks of greatest importance in his life. Therefore, interference seems justified if it enables the patient to see and feel with greater intensity. Of course, such medicinal interference must not tamper with the patient's religious ideas and must have the latitude to permit any philosophic interpretation. This study attempts to explore LSD as a means of increasing the perceptive powers of the dying patient. Lysergic acid diethylamide (LSD) has been reported to enhance the depth of feeling without structuring the individual's interpretation of these increased feelings. Increased communication lessens suffering and isolation and there is always the possibility that increased perception may enable the patient to penetrate, to some extent, the mysteries of cessation of existence.

To explore the means of making the last months of a patient less distressful is the second purpose of this study. . . .

*   *   *

Eighty patients suffering from terminal malignant disease with an estimate life expectancy of weeks or months were selected. Only patients who had been informed of their diagnosis were included. An interview was conducted in

which the patient's condition and prognosis were discussed, and he was invited to participate in this investigation. It was emphasized that there was no curative value in LSD.

*   *   *

No placebo control was used because of the obvious and immediate differentiation of LSD from placebo by the patient as well as the observer. After the interview we gave 100 meg of LSD hypodermically to insure uniformity of absorption. A trained observer was at the patient's bedside until the termination of the experiment. Upon the appearance of fear, panic, or the desire to rest, the patient was given 100 mg. of chlorpromazine intramuscularly which induced sleep within 30 minutes. The patients were interviewed daily for the subsequent three weeks. . . .

As expected, the overall improvement rate of gravely ill patients after 100 meg of LSD administration was considerable during the first eight or ten hours. About half of the patients became upset around six hours after administration, and the experience was terminated with chlorpromazine at that time. Only ten patients were able to tolerate the experience for more than ten hours without having some frightening image that necessitated termination. However, contrary to our previous experience only 10 per cent or eight patients did not wish to repeat the administration, compared to 33 per cent in our previous study in which the experience was not terminated and the patients were permitted to experience the whole gamut of feelings, even when the frightening images made their appearance. The relatively high percentage of patients whose experience was terminated can be accounted for by the fact that these were debilitated patients who tired easily.

Thus it seems that an avoidance of the tiring and, at times, the frightening images can add to the patient's willingness to repeat the experience.

Seventy-two patients gained a special type of insight 'from this experience: This "insight" was a greater lucidity and tridimensionality with which they viewed events in and around themselves. Through this insight, communication was greatly facilitated, both between observer and patient and among the patients themselves. It also created a sense of cohesion and community among patients, excluding those who did not "know" the experience. This greatly enhanced the morale and self-respect of the patients involved.

---

* 26 *Chicago Medical School Quarterly* 80–82, 86 (Summer 1966). Reprinted by permission.

Only seven patients felt that the experience in some way interfered with the privacy of their religious and philosophical ideas. These were the patients who experienced strong hallucinatory or frightening images, and whose experience had to be terminated early. It is interesting to note that the unstructured question, "did it go too far?" was universally understood. The 12 patients responding positively were among those with frightening images whose experience had to be terminated early.

While the depression returned to a certain extent, a definite lifting of the mood was noted for approximately two weeks. . . .

* * *

During and after LSD administration, acceptance and surrender to the inevitable loss of control were noted; and this control is anxiously maintained and fought for in non-drugged patients. LSD administration apparently eases the blow which impending death deals to the fantasy of infant omnipotence, not necessarily by augmenting the infantile process, but by relieving the mental apparatus of the compelling need to maintain the infantile fantasy. Parallel to the general improvement in the patient's feelings, mood and conflict situation, sleep patterns improved for approximately 12–14 days.

The results of this study seem to indicate that LSD is capable not only of improving the lot of pre-terminal patients by making them more responsive to their environment and family, but it also enhances their ability to appreciate the subtle and aesthetic nuances of experience. . . .

* * *

6.

**James D. Hardy, Carlos M. Chavez,
Fred D. Kurrus, William A. Neely,
Sadan Eraslan, M. Don Turner,
Leonard W. Fabian, and Thaddeus D. Labecki
Heart Transplantation in Man***

Heart transplanation has interested many investigators. [I]n the spring of 1963, Webb and the senior author considered that the laboratory and clinical heart work justified a planned ap-

---

* 188 *Journal of the American Medical Association* 1132–1139 (1964). Reprinted by permission.

proach directed toward eventual heart transplantation in man. This objective, a natural outgrowth of transplantation research, was cleared with the administrative officials of the University Medical Center.

* * *

As the laboratory work continued and animal heart transplants came to exceed 200 in number, considerable reflection was devoted to a definition of the clinical circumstances under which heart transplantation might be ethically carried out. . . .

* * *

During the last weeks of December, 1963, a number of patients considered by their physicians to be in absolutely terminal heart failure were admitted and served to sharpen the orientation of the surgical group. . . .

. . . One patient was admitted to the emergency room "moribund" from acute myocardial infarction, but he recovered. Another patient admitted in deep shock from myocardial infarction improved considerably, only to die abruptly. No time would have been afforded in which to make the most meager preparations for cardiopulmonary bypass using a disposable bag oxygenator, even had a suitable donor been available. Still other similar instances made it clear that the recipient must be dying of long-standing heart disease, in which the downward course had been progressive and inexorable to a clearly discernible terminal collapse. In such a situation, the transplant would offer some possibility of life prolongation, as opposed to certain death otherwise.

As with clinical lung transplantation previously performed, specific written protocols had been drawn up for the donor team and for the recipient team, and these had been distributed as confidential information to all personnel who might be immediately involved in a transplant.

* * *

By this stage of the program it had become abundantly clear that unless one were willing to halt mechanical support of respiration in a potential donor, it would be exceedingly unlikely that a potential recipient would die during the time a patient dying of myocardial insufficiency and shock could be kept on the pump oxygenator. Since we were not willing to stop the ventilator, we had concluded that a situation might arise in which the only heart available for transplantation would be that of a lower primate. Following a visit to New Orleans to examine at first hand the surprising but remarkable results achieved in maintaining survival of functioning primate heterotransplants using immunosuppressive drugs, we had purchased two large chimpanzees for possible use as kidney donors when no human donor kidney was available. Routine studies of these animals performed using anesthesia had included chest x-ray, ECG, blood grouping and chemistries, blood volume, and cardiac output. . . .

* * *

On Jan. 21, 1964, a 68-year-old white man was referred to the surgical service with gangrene of the lower portion of the left leg. He had had hypertensive cardiovascular disease for many years for which he had been taking digitalis and diuretics. Two nights earlier he had been admitted to his community hospital in a comatose state and with no detectable blood pressure. At that time rapid atrial fibrillation had been recorded, and vasopressor drugs in high dosage had been required to elevate the blood pressure to a systolic level of 100 mm Hg. By the following morning, however, it was possible to maintain his blood pressure level with minimal vasopressor drug therapy. The sensorium had cleared slightly, but it was not determined whether his impaired mental state was secondary to previous shock with hypoxia imposed upon an already atherosclerotic cerebral vascular bed, or to an intracranial vascular accident, or to the fact that the blood pressure level remained abnormally low for this previously hypertensive patient. He was able to move all four extremities, but such motion was limited. The bifurcation of the left common femoral artery had been explored while using local anesthesia in an attempt to restore blood flow in the left lower leg and a clot suggestive of an embolus had been removed, but without improvement in blood flow.

When his condition had stabilized, he was referred to the University Hospital for amputation of the gangrenous left lower leg and further management.

Examination revealed a large man of approximately the stated age of 68 years who was in a stuporous or semicomatose condition and who responded only to painful stimuli. The grossly irregular cardiac rhythm was again identified by an ECG as atrial fibrillation and the blood pressure in this previously hypertensive individual fluctuated at a systolic level of be-

tween 90 and 110 mm Hg. It was uncertain how much digitalis he had received, but the medical consultant now initiated all the usual measures available for support of the heart, whose failing capacity was reflected in the marked arrhythmia, cardiomegaly, relative hypotension, and dependent edema. Since the respiratory effort was inadequate in depth and irregular, a tracheostomy was performed and mechanical ventilatory assistance was initiated. This reduced the degree of cyanosis and appeared to somewhat improve his general condition.

The following day his total clinical condition was essentially unchanged, although the rate of urine secretion had increased. Use of vasopressor drugs had been required intermittently to support the blood pressure at a systolic level of 100 mm Hg. Meanwhile, the condition of the gangrenous portion of the left lower leg had further deteriorated, and it was decided to perform brisk amputation of this portion of the extremity under analgesia achieved through minimal anesthesia administered through the tracheostomy tube. This amputation was quickly completed without detectable effect on the patient's general condition.

Cardiac Evaluation.—By noon of Jan. 23 the formal report of the cardiologist was available. . . .

The conclusions of the cardiologist were as follows: "From the cardiovascular standpoint, the situation is unequivocally critical due to myocardial failure and apparent multiple emboli arising from the left atrium or ventricle. By all rules, life expectancy can be measured in the case in hours only."

In view of this opinion, which was concurred in by members of the transplant team, the possibility of heart transplantation was raised. There was in the recovery ward a young man near death from irreversible brain damage who might serve as a suitable donor, and the responsible relatives of the heart patient were apprised of the situation. They were well aware that death was imminent and were willing to have heart transplantation performed in the event of a terminal collapse. The written permission stated that the undersigned understood that, although many hearts had been transplanted in animals in our laboratory and elsewhere, no heart had ever been transplanted in man. The factors weighing against long-term success of the transplant were acknowledged. Furthermore, at this point the possibility of using a lower primate heart, raised at the time of the operation on the previous patient one week earlier, was made a part of the permission that was to be signed. It was not expected that this need come to pass, but experience with the previous case had underscored the fact that, for a homotransplant to succeed, the donor and the recipient must "die" at almost the same time; although this might occur, the chances that both prospective donor and prospective recipient would enter fatal collapse simultaneously were very slim. The properly signed permission was witnessed by three persons who were not members of the transplant team.

*   *   *

At approximately 6 PM the prospective recipient went into terminal shock, with a systolic blood pressure of 70 mm Hg and virtual apnea without the continued use of mechanical ventilation through the cuffed tracheostomy tube. Death was clearly imminent, and it was obvious that if heart transplantation were to be performed it must be done at once. Meanwhile, the condition of the prospective donor was not such that death appeared to be immediately imminent. At this time a tranquilizing drug was given to the larger of the two chimpanzees. This animal weighed 96 lb., considerably less than the heart patient, but his cardiac output had been measured at 4.25 liters per minute. . . . The cardiac output of the prospective recipient had been measured at 3.6 liters per minute prior to the terminal collapse; this output was certainly not at a normal level for a man of his size, but it had been sufficient to sustain a systolic blood pressure level of from 90 to 110 mm Hg. Should the primate heart be used, the artificial ventricular pacemaker could be employed to produce a relatively rapid rate in order to increase the minute output of the large venous return.

The patient was moved to the operating room while being maintained on ventilation by the anesthesiologist. . . . He was quickly prepared and draped, and at approximately 7:30 PM the heart was exposed through the usual median sternotomy incision; a femoral artery was simultaneously exposed to receive the arterial return catheter. . . . By this time, approximately 20 minutes of operating time had elapsed, and the blood pressure afforded by the extremely rapid and irregular heart beat was intermittently obtainable at only 40 mm Hg systolic despite all supportive measures employed by the anesthesiologist. The caval catheters were inserted through purse-string sutures in the lateral wall of the right atrium. Effective heart action ceased at about this time, not to be resumed even as the blood pressure was raised to a level of 100/60 mm Hg by the extracorporeal circuit. . . .

The Decision.—The decision that the work in animals should lead eventually to clinical exploration had been made almost a year before and this posed no problem, although the clinical occasion had developed sooner than had been anticipated. But now a second, and in many ways a far more difficult, decision of critical importance had to be faced. The patient was on cardiopulmonary bypass and the prospective human donor lingered on in the recovery ward. The larger chimpanzee had already been anesthetized in an adjacent operating room. The decision had to be made either to discontinue cardiopulmonary bypass and allow the patient to die, or to transplant the primate heart. At this point both teams were assembled in the main operating room to consider the matter. The major factors weighed in the decision were essentially three: (1) The senior author had been impressed at first hand by the surprising degree of at least early clinical success that had been achieved with chimpanzee kidney transplants, and certainly a vigorous organ for transplantation would be available if the chimpanzee heart were used. In contrast, failure of a cadaver heart to beat following transplantation might be due to antemortem changes, a failure which could not be properly assessed. (2) Clinical transplantation of another nonpaired organ, the liver, under otherwise hopeless conditions, had been accepted as justifiable by us and apparently by many other physicians. (3) An extracorporeal apparatus for extended cardiac support had justifiably been used in a heart patient in a terminal condition. The fact that total success could hardly have been expected with this less than final model of such equipment was no reason that such a beginning should not have been made under the circumstances.

Nevertheless, regardless of the positive factors in favor of proceeding with the heterotransplant, it was appreciated that psychological problems were involved. The clinical transplantation of a human heart might prompt controversy, and the clinical transplantation of the primate heart was even more likely to arouse controversy. Even so, it was felt that to perform this transplant, under the specific set of circumstances which existed at that instant, was well within ethical and moral boundaries. Thus, the five primary team members were individually polled and their votes made a matter of record. Four voted to proceed and the fifth abstained. The first author believed that the circumstances justified the heterotransplant, and from this point on the transplantation proceeded smoothly.

Donor Preparation.—Thoracotomy was quickly performed under sterile conditions and the heart of the primate was exposed. His body temperature had drifted downward to 32 C (89.6 F) and he was now heparinized. . . . The heart was briefly perfused with a cold, heparinized Ringer's lactate solution through which oxygen had been bubbled to increase the pO_2. After the primate blood had been removed, the perfusion fluid was changed to cold oxygenated blood, administered by gravity flow, with the heart remaining submerged in cold Ringer's lactate solution. A slow and satisfactory ventricular fibrillation developed.

The Recipient.—Meanwhile, the still heart of the recipient was excised. . . . The total body perfusion was proceeding smoothly, the blood pressure was satisfactory, and the patient's pupils were not unduly dilated, indicating that irreversible brain damage did not necessarily exist.

The continuously perfused donor heart was sutured in place. . . .

The coronary sinus perfusion catheter was removed and the aorta was unclamped approximately 45 minutes from the beginning of the actual insertion of the donor organ. The time was now 9 PM, and the patient had been on total bypass for slightly more than one hour. The blood from the pump oxygenator quickly rewarmed the transplanted heart, and a strong ventricular fibrillation was developed and recorded by camera. A single shock with the pulse defibrillator produced complete cardiac arrest, which was followed by a regular and forceful beat at a rate of approximately 80 per minute. This was a most gratifying development, since it had been agreed that this must represent the minimal acceptable degree of success.

*   *   *

It was soon apparent that the smaller heart would not be able to handle the large venous return, unless its rate was increased. For this reason, and to prevent problems referable to heart block postoperatively, the electrodes of a ventricular pacemaker were sutured to the left ventricle. Just at this stage, 0.5 mg of digoxin (Lanoxin) was given intravenously, producing a pulsus bigeminus which was broken by turning up the amplitude of the pacemaker which had

been set at a rate of 100 beats per minute. Meanwhile, the left ventricular vent had been removed and the bypass support greatly reduced. At 9:45 PM all perfusion catheters were removed. . . .

The primate heart paced at a rate of 100 beats per minute was able to maintain a blood pressure ranging from 60 to 90 mm Hg. Unfortunately, as time passed, the heart became increasingly unable to handle the large venous return. By 11 PM, approximately one hour after the removal of the bypass catheters, the heart was judged incapable of accepting the large venous return without intermittent decompression by manual cardiac massage. Further support was abandoned, even though a weak and regular beat continued. The azathioprine that was to be injected intravenously at the close of the operation to suppress the immune response had not been given.

What Was Accomplished.—First, it was found that the heart could be effectively preserved for one hour while being transplanted into man. . . . Second, the suture techniques widely employed for heart transplantation in experimental laboratories were adequate and otherwise acceptable. Third, a regular and forceful beat was promptly restored following defibrillation with a single weak shock of the pulse defibrillator. . . . Fourth, the transplanted heart reacted immediately to intravenously administered digoxin, as reflected in relative heart block with pulsus bigeminus. The cardiac pacemaker readily broke through this arrhythmia when the current was increased.

It was also apparent that the heart of the lower primate, at least at the chimpanzee level, is not quite large enough to support the circulatory load of the adult human being.

*   *   *

Public Announcement.—[B]y the time the operation was over, almost 25 persons, many of them physicians, had gained entrance to the operating suite on one pretext or another, despite the fact that a doorkeeper had been placed at the only unlocked entrance. Clearly, the news would shortly be disseminated and, to announce the bare facts accurately, the director of public information decided to release a short statement. In accord with usual Medical Center policy, no member of the transplant team was to grant any interview, release any illustrative material, or be photographed, except under the formal auspices of national medical meetings. This was strictly adhered to.

Unfortunately, the first release resulted inadvertently in the need to permit another. The initial announcement did not specify that a chimpanzee heart had been used; this was to be divulged at the Sixth International Transplantation Conference a few days later. However, when it was announced in a distant city that the donor heart had been taken from a living human being, the situation had to be clarified. At this point, the university officials decided to halt piecemeal news leaks by one final announcement which included the membership of the transplant team.

* * *

The general discussion which the heart transplant stimulated has had, with other factors, a penetrating influence on and within the transplantation movement. Many are reassessing their positions, reappraising their guidelines. We ourselves underestimated the extent and the vigor of the debate which was to center around the use of clinical transplants—especially the use of lower primate organs. We believed then and we believe at this writing that the insertion of the chimpanzee heart, under the conditions which existed at that moment, was well within the bounds of medical ethics and morality. While the transplant did not function for as long a period as we had hoped, a great deal was learned, and this will render continuing laboratory studies more meaningful.

NOTES

NOTE 1.

OPERATIVE PERMIT*

I hereby give full permission for left leg amputation and heart surgery on Boyd Rush. I understand that any clots present will be removed from the heart to stop them from going to still more arteries of his body. I further understand that his heart is in extremely poor condition. If for any unanticipated reason the heart should fail completely during either operation and it should be impossible to start it, I agree to the insertion of a suitable heart transplant if such should be available at that time.[†] I further understand that

hundreds of heart transplants have been performed in laboratories throughout the world but that any heart transplant would represent the initial transplant in man.

Signed (for family) *Mrs. J. H. Thompson*
(sister)

* * *

NOTE 2.
SURGEONS CHEER RISING TRANSPLANT SCORE*

At the second International Congress of the Transplantation Society, the atmosphere was pervaded by the sweet smell of success. . . . The big news of the conference, said Nobelist Peter B. Medawar, was that kidney transplants are no longer news. He predicted that heart grafts would reach the same point before the next transplant congress two years from now.

The bulk of the program dealt with experimental work and basic research, but the tenor of the meeting reflected what Dr. Medawar called "the year of the surgeon." For many, the high point of the conference came when Dr. Denton Cooley presented his patient Louis John Fierro, who four months before had been near death with repeated bouts of congestive heart failure. With a teen-age heart beating in his 54-year-old chest, the chunky used-car salesman strode up the four steps to the stage, shook his surgeon's hand, and gave a triumphant wave in response to the congress audience's applause.

Exactly a week later, Dr. Cooley would perform his 11th human heart transplant—an operation that has catapulted transplant surgery into the era of multiple organ preparation grafts. He and his colleagues at St. Luke's Hospital in Houston transplanted a heart-lung preparation, including both whole lungs, from a dead anencephalic child into a two-month-old recipient, a girl, who had a persistent A-V shunt and defective mitral and aortic valves. She was near to death's door with congestive heart failure and severe pulmonary vascular disease.

Because of this combination of defects, a hospital spokesman said, Dr. Cooley decided that "a heart transplant alone would not suffice. So the heart and attached lung were transplanted."

Breathing with the aid of a respirator, the child regained consciousness following the operation, then quickly lapsed into coma. She died of cardiac arrest 14 hours after surgery.

---

* James D. Hardy and Carlos M. Chavez: "The First Heart Transplant in Man—Historical Reexamination of the 1964 Case in the Light of Current Clinical Experience," 1 *Transplantation Proceedings* 717, 721 (1969). Reprinted by permission.

[†] "The possibility of using a lower primate heart was acknowledged in discussion with the recipient's relatives, should the anticipated death of the patient with massive brain injury not occur." *Ibid.*

* *Medical World News* 26–27 (September 27, 1968). Copyright 1968, McGraw-Hill, Inc. Reprinted by permission.

Another participant was Dr. James Hardy of the University of Mississippi, who suffered severe censure when he transplanted a chimpanzee heart into a man in 1964.

Dr. Hardy reclaimed his place as the world's first cardiac transplanter by showing his heretofore self-suppressed filmed record of that historic occasion. But in the light of acute failure in that case and two subsequent ones elsewhere, Dr. Hardy and the other panelists agreed that, at least for the time being, heart xenografts are unworkable.

*   *   *

Several of the surgeons expressed the fear that delayed rejection would place the now surviving heart patients in jeopardy in the not too distant future. This dismal outlook is based in part on experience with kidney transplants. According to the tissue-typing pioneer Paul Terasaki of UCLA, who did all the histocompatibility studies for the Houston heart transplants, recipients of mismatched kidney grafts do well for a year or so but tend to die off two or three years later at a more rapid rate than those who are well matched. All but one of the Texas heart recipients turned out to have been poorly matched. Oddly enough, rejection occurred in the well-matched exception and killed the patient.

In bridging the antigen gap, antilymphocyte globulin (ALG) has established itself—at least for the next few years—as an important part of the immunosuppressive armamentarium. By a show of hands, the heart transplant panelists indicated that they all use it. But Dr. Thomas Starzl, who has achieved excellent results in kidney and liver transplants at the University of Colorado, reported that a trial with refined ALG on 13 kidney patients had resulted in three deaths and five rejections. Like Dr. Michael DeBakey, he is now attempting a "blitzkrieg approach" of giving larger doses of ALG at the outset, with the hope of avoiding long-term use of the agent.

*   *   *

NOTE 3.

BLAIBERG—VICTORY OR DEFEAT?*

The death of Dr. Philip Blaiberg on August 17 in Cape Town, South Africa, fixes the longest survival of a heart-transplant recipient at 593 days—19½ months. The 60-year-old retired dentist had been kept alive by the heart of a 24-year-

* *Medical World News* 14–15 (September 5, 1969). Copyright 1969, McGraw-Hill, Inc. Reprinted by permission.

old factory worker since Jan. 2, 1968, when Dr. Christiaan Barnard performed the transplant, his second and history's third.

*   *   *

"The autopsy report isn't complete yet," [Dr. Christiaan Barnard] told MWN, "but I think that the cause of death is quite clear. It's extensive myocardial damage due to acute and chronic rejection."

*   *   *

[H]is condition had come full cycle. By the time of his final admission to the hospital, he was carrying a heart more than two thirds destroyed by the relentless rejection process. "He was back to the point where he was before we did the transplant," Dr. Barnard said. "I think that in Dr. Blaiberg we were unfortunate to have two acute rejection episodes. When this happens, even if you reverse the episode, there's a certain amount of permanent damage."

During the more severe bout with rejection in July 1968, a second transplant was considered and Dr. Blaiberg consented to having it done if necessary. But with the final illness, Dr. Barnard felt the opportunity no longer existed. "By the time he really needed it, his renal function had deteriorated and he had very bad arteriosclerosis, marked weakness in the legs, and muscle wasting. The autopsy showed that one renal artery and both femoral arteries were occluded. He also had a patch of pneumonia in his right lung."

*   *   *

Dr. Barnard is completely satisfied with the original operation and subsequent course taken. "We are sad that it is all over now, but we did far better than we expected."

Other heart surgeons and immunologists are not so certain. The frequency of heart transplants has dropped off sharply from a peak of 26 last November; since April, no more than four have been done in any month. The total number of heart transplants recorded by the American College of Surgeons is 143 in 141 recipients, of whom 29 are living, 21 of them surviving more than six months. Of the total, U.S. surgeons have performed 84 in 82 recipients, of whom 19 survive, 13 for more than six months.

A number of surgeons have said that with the death of the longest-surviving patient and with a continuing decline in the percentage of survivors, it is time for a reappraisal of heart transplantation. The Montreal Institute of Cardiology team headed by Dr. Pierre Grondin, which has done nine of the 15 Canadian heart transplants, suspended its work early this year to study such factors as the importance of tissue matching and immunosuppressive regimens and has not yet resumed transplant operations. Of the 56 teams that have done heart transplants, no more than ten are still active.

Dr. Barnard strongly disagrees about the need for reassessment now. "I can't understand why Dr. Blaiberg's death should make any difference," he says. "Dr. Blaiberg did much better than we anticipated, or than anybody anticipated. People were predicting that he wouldn't last 14 days, 17 days, two months, three months, a year."

Far more significant, he feels, is that the total survival time of his five transplant patients, of whom two are still alive, is 1,101 days. "That means that the average survival time of these patients is 220 days. Now Dr. Norman Shumway has figured that the average life expectancy of patients at the same stage of illness who don't get transplants is 30 days, so there's more than a 700 per cent improvement already."

* * *

Dr. [C. Walton] Lillehei adds: "Though I'm more encouraged than ever, I'm sure potential recipients have become discouraged. The problem now is not so much a lack of donors but recipients. We've been turned down about six to eight times in the past three months."

Dr. Lillehei also blames the transplant slowdown in part on "some surgeons who jumped on the bandwagon without the background or psychological make-up to do developmental work in this area. Those who get discouraged easily have dropped out, though."

Dr. Adrian Kantrowitz of Maimonides Medical Center in Brooklyn concurs. "Those who've viewed heart transplants as experimental all along and have anticipated the problems are going on with it," he says. He and his team expect to perform more transplants, but their tissue-matching standards will be more stringent. "We'll want at least a B-minus match," he declares.

NOTE 4.
TESTIMONY OF DR. CHRISTIAAN BARNARD—
MARCH 8, 1968*

SENATOR CURTIS: [T]he young lady whose heart was transplanted into Mr. Washkansky's body received artificial respiration.

DR. BARNARD: Yes, sir.

* * *

SENATOR CURTIS: Who made the decision to discontinue the use of the machine?

DR. BARNARD: The neurosurgeons and neurologist. Those are a group of four doctors—

SENATOR CURTIS: Now, that coincided with the time you were ready to begin the surgery?

DR. BARNARD: Yes, sir; that is correct.

SENATOR CURTIS: It did not necessarily coincide with the time they made the decision that she was going to die?

DR. BARNARD: This was a few hours later.

SENATOR CURTIS: So the machine was continued and stopped, not in relation to the time that the knowledge was available that she would not live, but it was continued to a time and stopped at a time to fit in with the schedule of the heart transplant to another person?

DR. BARNARD: That is correct.

SENATOR CURTIS: And her surgeons made that decision?

DR. BARNARD: The doctors who were caring for her, as she was a patient who had severe brain damage, and therefore was cared for by the neurologist and the neurosurgeons.

SENATOR CURTIS: Did they represent the recipient of the heart?

DR. BARNARD: No; they were only representing the donor. Their names are not on this team that you see published as the transplant team.

* * *

_____

* National Commission on Health Science and Society—Hearings on S.J. Res. 145 before the Subcommittee on Government Research of the Senate Committee on Government Operations, 90th Congress, 2d Session 74–75 (1968).

B.

Appraising the Role of the Participants*

1.

In Formulating Policy

a.

Deciding about Societal Interests and Priorties?

What Price Transplanted Organs?†

The last desperate 16 days of heart transplant recipient Mike Kasperak's life at the Palo Alto-Stanford Hospital cost $28,845.83. Care for Everett C. Thomas, one of the six patients to survive more than four weeks among the world's first 21 heart recipients, is expected to cost $25,000 by the time he is discharged from St. Luke's Hospital in Houston.

Cardiovascular surgeons tend to agree, says Dr. Theodore Cooper, director of the National Heart Institute, "that it costs $20,000 for the care of cardiac transplant patients in the immediate intraoperative period until the cardiovascular status is stabilized. Thereafter, it takes another several hundred dollars a day to manage the patient and deal with the immune phenomenon."

Such sums are astronomic to the average American. Multiplied by the estimated 5,000 potential transplant recipients a year, the total bill for new hearts would come to a staggering $100 million annually. . . .

*　　*　　*

Where does the money for transplants come from in the U.S., where the government does not generally pay a citizen's medical bills? In the initial stages of a new procedure, funds stem mostly from grants made by the National Institutes of Health or private foundations.

Over the past five years, for example, the NIH has contributed about $2 million for the cardiac assist and transplant research carried out by Dr. Adrian Kantrowitz at Brooklyn's Maimonides Medical Center. And since 1959, the American Heart Association has given

$437,960 to Dr. Norman E. Shumway and his research team at Stanford University.

*　　*　　*

Some of the same factors—enormous amounts of lab work, heavy drug costs, and intensive care—go into the high costs of transplanting other organs. At the University of California Medical Center in San Francisco, the average kidney transplant costs $11,753, plus another $2,000 to $3,000 for the hospital care of live donors. And in Denver, at the University of Colorado Medical Center, the prices of five recent kidney transplants ranged from $3,057 to $31,663, with an average of $12,070.

*　　*　　*

None of the figures from university medical centers includes professional fees. Like Colorado's Dr. Thomas E. Starzl, most surgeons transplanting kidneys in a university setting are full-time, salaried faculty members. And even though they may charge fees for other types of surgery—such money usually goes into a fund for educational and other uses—the university men generally have waived professional charges in kidney operations up to now.

"Kidney transplantation is a research procedure," says Dr. Samuel L. Kountz, associate professor of surgery and chief of transplant surgery at the University of California's San Francisco medical center. If the men who do the transplants were to be compensated on a fee-for-service basis, he estimates, "it would probably add $2,000 or $3,000 to the cost—if you could find doctors willing to work that hard."

*　　*　　*

A bill now in Congress would provide up to $30 million a year in federal aid for the establishment and operation of new, badly needed kidney centers. Although it is part of a $1-billion program proposed last year by a White House-appointed committee, the bill lacks Administration support. PHS Surgeon General William H. Stewart told a Senate subcommittee in March that such a program would require "drastic curtailment or abandonment of many other health programs."

A massive kidney care campaign would have to compete for dollars with the federal program

---

* This appraisal section focuses on dying subjects. For a fuller exposition of the factors requiring appraisal, consult section D of Chapter Eleven, beginning at p. 818 *supra*.

† *Medical World News* 28–29 (June 28, 1968). Copyright 1968, McGraw-Hill, Inc. Reprinted by permission.

for artificial heart research and development. About $8 million in National Heart Institute money was spent on this project in fiscal 1967. But Dr. Frank W. Hastings, chief of the artificial heart program, estimates that a fully implantable artificial heart is at least five years away from clinical trials. Meanwhile, Congress is threatening to wield an ax on federal research funds in general.

[A]nother problem confronting the prospective kidney program is the controversy over medical priorities. Is it more important to improve the quality of specialized care for the few or to deliver more general care to the many? Sen. Walter F. Mondale (D-Minn.), who is proposing a national commission to study the issues involved in transplants, puts it this way: "A public commitment of $1 billion could buy enough kidney dialysis centers to serve 25,000 persons in the next decade—or it could provide ambulatory care of a general nature for 1.2 million poor people."

NOTES

NOTE 1.

Henry K. Beecher
Ethical Problems Created by the
Hopelessly Unconscious Patient*

. . . Inevitably, with more and more bold and venturesome and commendable attempts to rescue the dying, more and more patients will accumulate in the hospitals of the land —patients who can be kept "alive" only by extraordinary means, in whom there is no hope of recovery of consciousness, let alone recovery to a functioning, pleasurable existence, and all this at a cost of $25,000 to $30,000 per patient per year. Burdensome as this cost is, it is the lesser of two. Another cost: if the average hospital stay is two weeks, the irretrievably unconscious patient then occupies space that could have been used by 26 others in a year's time. There are today great delays in hospital admissions owing to bed shortages, even of patients with cancer. A life could be lost owing to delay in getting definitive hospital care—lost because a bed was occupied by a hopeless patient.

It seems clear that the time has come to reexamine this situation. Money *is* human life; so

---

* 278 *New England Journal of Medicine* 1425, 1429 (1968). Reprinted by permission.

are available hospital beds. The money spent to maintain unconscious and hopelessly damaged persons could be used to restore those who are salvageable. What are our privileges and responsibilities in this confusing situation? What decisions must we make about this "striving officiously to keep alive"? It must be borne in mind that "hopeless" when established by a killing disease is often not the same thing as "hopeless" resulting from a recent accident. Astonishing recoveries have occurred in the latter case. A five-year-old boy, for example, was submerged for 22 minutes in a Norwegian river at a temperature of −10° C and still recovered.

It must be remembered that such advances as were employed in this case are sometimes the result of intensive, even desperate efforts to alleviate the condition of the hopelessly ill. There *is* profit for mankind sometimes in the prolongation of dying, justified as it can be by concern for the specific sick man. The rights of the individual and the rights of society are interrelated.

NOTE 2.

Leon R. Kass
Caveat on Transplants*

*   *   *

The development of borrowed and artificial vital organs presents a new instance of an old problem: how to distribute scarce resources justly. Medical care is a scarce resource; quality care, especially so. Is large-scale transplantation the best use of these limited resources?

Is it just that 30 doctors perform a heart transplant while the ordinary medical problems of the indigent go untended because of a shortage of physicians? The treatment of a child's streptococcal sore throat is less spectacular than the replacement of the heart, but the former can prevent the development of rheumatic heart disease and thereby obviate the possible need for a future transplant.

I am not suggesting that Drs. Barnard, Kantrowitz and their colleagues give up their surgical virtuosity for a career in pediatrics or public health. But I am arguing that the public planning and expenditures for medical development be guided by a concern for the health of the entire community. Decent health for the majority of

---

* *The Washington Post* B-1, col. 5 (January 14, 1968). © 1968, *The Washington Post*. Reprinted by permission.

our people should not be sacrificed to our infatuation with technological progress.

*   *   *

b.

Deciding about the Ambit of Experimentation?

Hans Jonas
Philosophical Reflections on
Experimenting with Human Subjects*

*   *   *

[P]atients should be experimented upon, if at all, *only* with reference to *their* disease. Never should there be added to the gratuitousness of the experiment as such the gratuitousness of service to an unrelated cause. This follows simply from what we have found to be the *only* excuse for infracting the special exemption of the sick at all—namely, that the scientific war on disease cannot accomplish its goal without drawing the sufferers from disease into the investigative process. If under this excuse they become subjects of experiment, they do so *because,* and only because, of *their* disease.

Experiment as part of therapy—that is, directed toward helping the subject himself—is a different matter altogether and raises its own problems, but hardly philosophical ones. As long as a doctor can say, even if only in his own thought: "There is no known cure for your condition (or: You have responded to none); but there is promise in a new treatment still under investigation, not quite tested yet as to effectiveness and safety; you will be taking a chance, but, all things considered, I judge it in your best interest to let me try it on you"—as long as he can speak thus, he speaks as the patient's physician and may err, but does not transform the patient into a subject of experimentation. Introduction of an untried therapy into the treatment where the tried ones have failed is not "experimentation on the patient."

Generally, there is something "experimental" (because tentative) about every individual treatment, beginning with the diagnosis itself; and he would be a poor doctor who would not learn from every case for the benefit of future cases, and a poor member of the profession who

* 98 *Daedalus* 219, 241–243 (1969). Reprinted by permission of Daedalus, Journal of the American Academy of Arts and Sciences, Boston, Massachusetts.

would not make any new insights gained from his treatments available to the profession at large. Thus, knowledge may be advanced in the treatment of any patient, and the interest of the medical art and all sufferers from the same affliction as well as the patient may be served if something happens to be learned from his case. But this gain to knowledge and future therapy is incidental to the bona fide service to the present patient. He has the right to expect that the doctor does nothing to him just in order to learn.

In that case, the doctor's imaginary speech would run, for instance, like this: "There is nothing more I can do for you. But you can do something for me. Speaking no longer as your physician but on behalf of medical science, we could learn a great deal about future cases of this kind if you would permit me to perform certain experiments on you. It is understood that you yourself would not benefit from any knowledge we might gain; but future patients would." This statement would express the purely experimental situation, assumedly here with the subject's concurrence and with all cards on the table. In Alexander Bickel's words: "It is a different situation when the doctor is no longer trying to make [the patient] well, but is trying to find out how to make others well in the future."

But even in the second case of the nontherapeutic experiment where the patient does not benefit, the patient's own disease is enlisted in the cause of fighting that disease, even if only in others. It is yet another thing to say or think: "Since you are here—in the hospital with its facilities—under our care and observation, away from your job (or, perhaps, doomed), we wish to profit from your being available for some other research of great interest we are presently engaged in." From the standpoint of merely medical ethics, which has only to consider risk, consent, and the worth of the objective, there may be no cardinal difference between this case and the last one. I hope that my medical audience will not think I am making too fine a point when I say that from the standpoint of the subject and his dignity there is a cardinal difference that crosses the line between the permissible and the impermissible, [under the] principle of "identification". . . . Whatever the rights and wrongs of any experimentation on any patient—in the one case, at least that residue of identification is left him that it is his own affliction by which he can contribute to the conquest of that affliction, his own kind of suffering which he helps to alleviate in others; and so in a sense it is his own cause. It is totally indefensible to rob the unfortunate of this intimacy with the purpose and make his misfortune a convenience for the furtherance of alien concerns. The observance of this rule is essential, I think, to attenuate at least the wrong that nontherapeutic experimenting on patients commits in any case.

NOTE

HENRY K. BEECHER
RESEARCH AND THE INDIVIDUAL—
HUMAN STUDIES*

* * *

The remarkably increased average length of life indicates that the time of dying has been greatly postponed. Even the characteristics of dying often differ from those of earlier years. The changes have been brought about by a variety of factors: antibiotics, potent drugs, intravenous fluids, transfusions, pain suppression, and artificial and transplanted organs. Sometimes the ancient prerogatives of the patient—his right to be let alone and to die in comfort and dignity—seem to be overlooked. Individuals who may die suddenly or who seem to be in imminent danger of death should not, under ordinary circumstances, be chosen as subjects for experimentation, however harmless the planned procedure may be. Obviously, if death occurs during such an experiment, it could cast a shadow over a potentially valuable agent or useful technique, not to mention placing the investigator in an unhappy predicament where, although innocent, he may have the appearance of guilt.

* * *

[T]hose who are in imminent danger of death should not ordinarily be subjected to experimentation, except as part of a therapeutic effort to save their lives. An exception to this can be found in the irreversibly comatose individual who may be used as an organ donor under certain rigid circumstances. Occasionally one encounters reports wherein the term *hopelessly incurable* seems to be used to justify dangerous experimentation. It is not the physician's prerogative to make or to profit from such dubious judgments. . . .

* * *

---

* Boston: Little, Brown and Co. 44, 85 (1970). Reprinted by permission.

c.

Deciding about Choice of Subjects?

[i]
Henry K. Beecher
Ethical Problems Created by the Hopelessly
Unconscious Patient*

* * *

Starzl has spoken of "the declining curve of life," implying that as the end approaches there is less and less life in the individual, and that a quantitative factor is present—a sort of death by inches. To a certain point this is supportable in that all organ and nerve centers do not become irreversibly damaged simultaneously: consciousness as a brain function is often irretrievably destroyed months before the respiratory and vasomotor centers fail. At the same time one can share Schreiner's discontent and insist that "a coordinating vital principle exists which is either there or not there." The moment of death can only be approximated.

From ancient times down to the recent past it was perfectly clear when the respiration and heart stopped that the brain would die in a few minutes, so that the obvious criterion of a heart in standstill as synonymous with death was accurate enough. This is no longer the case when modern resuscitative and supportive measures are involved. These improved activities can now restore "life" as judged by the ancient standards of persistent respiration and continuing heartbeat, even when there is not the remotest possibility that consciousness will be recovered after massive brain damage. In other situations "life" can be maintained only by means of artificial respiration and electrical stimulation of he heartbeat, in temporary bypass of the heart or, in conjunction with these things, reducing with cold the body's oxygen requirement.

* * *

. . . When is death, what is death, what is life? It is self-evident that there is no simple answer to what life is. One can submit that life is the ability to communicate with others. If this ability is lost in permanent unconsciousness, the future will surely confirm that that man is dead. One can make a considerable case that if a physician judges his patient's ability to communicate as lost beyond retrieval through permanent un-

---

* 278 *New England Journal of Medicine* 1425–1427 (1968). Reprinted by permission.

consciousness, he not only may, but *must,* declare the man dead.

When is death? The traditional compulsive urge to know and record the exact moment of death is not useful, except sometimes for legal purposes. What usually matters is not the time of death, but the time when a physician undertook to declare the patient dead.

So much for general comments; now we come to specifics in an attempt to decide how death is exhibited. As mentioned, there is the incontrovertible fact that when the circulation ceases the brain dies within five minutes under ordinary circumstances. Various workers have striven to go beyond this basic situation. For example, according to Schreiner, "Some biologists (unrealistically) accept one minute of E.E.G. silence as incontrovertible proof of death. Others accept three minutes or five minutes." Alexandre states that a flat electroencephalogram alone is not an adequate criterion of death, and he does "[not] think five minutes would be enough anyway." Hamburger reports that "at least two cases in Paris were observed to have a flat E.E.G. for several hours, followed by complete recovery; in both cases the coma was due to severe barbiturate poisoning." Alexandre states that air embolism during heart surgery can lead to a flat encephalogram with recovery. Murray asks if a flat electroencephalogram for four to six hours along with the other conditions set down by Alexandre (enumerated below) would be enough to indicate incontrovertible evidence of death. Alexandre objects that one cannot wait six hours if the object is kidney transplantation, for falling blood pressure would have led to conventional death and an unsatisfactory kidney for transplantation. Starzl doubts if any member of his transplantation team would accept a person as dead as long as there was a heartbeat. If there was a mistake in evaluating the "living cadaver," he continues, removal of a kidney should not necessarily lead to death. The taking of single organs such as the liver is a different matter. He asks if any physician would be willing to remove an unimpaired organ before the circulation had stopped. In transplantation of a kidney one's reliance would depend on a kind of "statistical morality": the severity of the operation itself in such desperately injured persons would doubtless have an appreciable death rate—if the subjects were alive. Alexandre, in Belgium, has in nine cases used unconscious patients with head injuries, whose hearts had not stopped, as kidney donors

for transplantation. "Five conditions were always met in these nine cases: (1) complete bilateral mydriasis; (2) complete absence of reflexes, both natural and in response to profound pain; (3) complete absence of spontaneous respiration, five minutes after mechanical respiration had been stopped; (4) falling blood pressure, necessitating increasing amount of vasopressive drugs; (5) a flat E.E.G." Some have spoken of taking organs from a dying person. "I would like to make it clear [says Alexandre] that, in my opinion, there has never been and never will be any question of taking organs from a dying person who has "no reasonable chance of getting better or resuming consciousness." The question is of taking organs from a dead person, and the point is that I do not accept the cessation of heart beats as the indication of death"....

Revillard looks for Alexandre's five signs and adds two others: interruption of blood flow in the brain as judged by angiography (he assumes that this is a better sign of death than a flat electroencephalogram); and ("of less value") the absence of reaction to atropine. He does not agree with Alexandre that the blood pressure inevitably falls at once. He finds that it sometimes stabilizes at a satisfactory level for transplantation for several hours.

Calne states bluntly that Alexandre was "in fact removing kidneys from live donors." He believes that "Any modification of the means of diagnosing death to facilitate transplantation will cause the whole procedure to fall in disrepute with the entire profession."

Alexandre and Calne agree that two separate teams should be involved in deciding these matters, one concerned with resuscitating the patient and the other with an interest in donor possibilities. Schreiner differs; he does "[not] believe that mechanical separation of two teams and the problems of the surgeon's disrepute are really germane to the philosophical problem.... The moral problem can't be settled on the basis of what might happen to a reputation.... This question of deciding death transcends the problems of transplantation." Schreiner concedes that, if cadaver transplants become available by "updating" death and do as well or nearly as well as organs from live donors, the morality of continuing to use transplants from live, unrelated donors is open to question.

These matters have been presented in some detail to show the differences of opinion and uncertainty among experts who have given much thought to the as yet unresolved question of what is truly death.

* * *

[ii]
Ad Hoc Committee of the
Harvard Medical School
A Definition of Irreversible Coma*

Our primary purpose is to define irreversible coma as a new criterion for death. There are two reasons why there is need for a definition: (1) Improvements in resuscitative and supportive measures have led to increased efforts to save those who are desperately injured. Sometimes these efforts have only partial success so that the result is an individual whose heart continues to beat but whose brain is irreversibly damaged. The burden is great on patients who suffer permanent loss of intellect, on their families, on the hospitals, and on those in need of hospital beds already occupied by these comatose patients. (2) Obsolete criteria for the definition of death can lead to controversy in obtaining organs for transplantation.

Irreversible coma has many causes, but *we are concerned here only with those comatose individuals who have no discernible central nervous system activity.* If the characteristics can be defined in satisfactory terms, translatable into action—and we believe this is possible— then several problems will either disappear or will become more readily soluble.

More than medical problems are present. There are moral, ethical, religious, and legal issues. Adequate definition here will prepare the way for better insight into all of these matters as well as for better law than is currently applicable.

An organ, brain or other, that no longer functions and has no possibility of functioning again is for all practical purposes dead. Our first problem is to determine the characteristics of a *permanently* nonfunctioning brain.

A patient in this state appears to be in deep coma. The condition can be satisfactorily diagnosed by points 1, 2, and 3 to follow. The electroencephalogram (point 4) provides confirmatory data, and when available it should be utilized. In situations where for one reason or another electroencephalographic monitoring is not available, the absence of cerebral function has to be determined by purely clinical signs, to be described, or by absence of circulation as judged by standstill of blood in the retinal vessels, or by absence of cardiac activity.

1. *Unreceptivity and unresponsivity.*— There is a total unawareness to externally applied stimuli and inner need and complete unresponsiveness—our definition of irreversible coma. Even the most intensely painful stimuli evoke no vocal or other response, not even a groan, withdrawal of a limb, or quickening of respiration.

2. *No Movements or Breathing.*—Observations covering a period of at least one hour by physicians are adequate to satisfy the criteria of no spontaneous muscular movements or spontaneous respiration or response to stimuli such as pain, touch, sound, or light. After the patient is on a mechanical respirator, the total absence of spontaneous breathing may be established by turning off the respirator for three minutes and observing whether there is any effort on the part of the subject to breathe spontaneously. (The respirator may be turned off for this time provided that at the start of the trial period the patient's carbon dioxide tension is within the normal range, and provided also that the patient had been breathing room air for at least 10 minutes prior to the trial.)

3. *No reflexes.*—Irreversible coma with abolition of central nervous system activity is evidenced in part by the absence of elicitable reflexes. The pupil will be fixed and dilated and will not respond to a direct source of bright light. Since the establishment of a fixed, dilated pupil is clear-cut in clinical practice, there should be no uncertainty as to its presence. Ocular movement (to head turning and to irrigation of the ears with ice water) and blinking are absent. There is no evidence of postural activity (decerebrate or other). Swallowing, yawning, vocalization are in abeyance. Corneal and pharyngeal reflexes are absent.

As a rule the stretch of tendon reflexes cannot be elicited; i.e., tapping the tendons of the biceps, triceps, and pronator muscles, quadriceps and gastrocnemius muscles with the reflex hammer elicits no contraction of the respective muscles. Plantar or noxious stimulation gives no response.

4. *Flat Electroencephalogram.*—Of great confirmatory value is the flat or isoelectric EEG.

---

* Henry K. Beecher, M.D., Chairman. 205 *Journal of the American Medical Association* 337– 339 (1968). Reprinted by permission. [The committee, all members of the faculty of Harvard University, included ten physicians, one theologian, one historian, and one lawyer.]

We must assume that the electrodes have been properly applied, that the apparatus is functioning normally, and that the personnel in charge is competent. We consider it prudent to have one channel of the apparatus used for an electrocardiogram. This channel will monitor the ECG so that, if it appears in the electroencephalographic leads because of high resistance, it can be readily identified. It also establishes the presence of the active heart in the absence of the EEG. We recommend that another channel be used for a noncephalic lead. This will pick up space-borne or vibration-borne artifacts and identify them. The simplest form of such a monitoring noncephalic electrode has two leads over the dorsum of the hand, preferably the right hand, so the ECG will be minimal or absent. Since one of the requirements of this state is that there be no muscle activity, these two dorsal hand electrodes will not be bothered by muscle artifact. The apparatus should be run at standard gains $10\mu v/mm$, $50\mu v/5mm$. Also it should be isoelectric at double this standard gain which is $5\mu v/mm$ or $25\mu v/5mm$. At least ten full minutes of recording are desirable, but twice that would be better.

It is also suggested that the gains at some point be opened to their full amplitude for a brief period (5 to 100 seconds) to see what is going on. Usually in an intensive care unit artifacts will dominate the picture, but these are readily identifiable. There shall be no electroencephalographic response to noise or to pitch.

All of the above tests shall be repeated at least 24 hous later with no change.

The validity of such data as indications of irreversible cerebral damage depends on the exclusion of two conditions: hypothermia (temperature below 90 F [32.2 C]) or central nervous system depressants, such as barbiturates.

The patient's condition can be determined only by a physician. When the patient is hopelessly damaged as defined above, the family and all colleagues who have participated in major decisions concerning the patient, and all nurses involved, should be so informed. Death is to be declared and *then* the respirator turned off. The decision to do this and the responsibility for it are to be taken by the physician-in-charge, in consultation with one or more physicians who have been directly involved in the case. It is unsound and undesirable to force the family to make the decision.

*　　*　　*

It is recommended as a part of these procedures that judgment of the existence of these criteria is solely a medical issue. It is suggested that the physician in charge of the patient consult with one or more other physicians directly involved in the case before the patient is declared dead on the basis of these criteria. In this way, the responsibility is shared over a wider range of medical opinion, thus providing an important degree of protection against later questions which might be raised about the particular case. It is further suggested that the decision to declare the person dead, and then to turn off the respirator, be made by physicians not involved in any later effort to transplant organs or tissues from the deceased individual. This is advisable in order to avoid any appearance of self-interest by the physicians involved.

It should be emphasized that we recommend the patient be declared dead before any effort is made to take him off a respirator, if he is then on a respirator. This declaration should not be delayed until he has been taken off the respirator and all artificially stimulated signs have ceased. The reason for this recommendation is that in our judgment it will provide a greater degree of legal protection to those involved. Otherwise, the physicians would be turning off the respirator on a person who is, under the present strict, technical application of law, still alive.

*　　*　　*

NOTES

NOTE 1.

GEORGE P. FLETCHER
LEGAL ASPECTS OF THE DECISION
NOT TO PROLONG LIFE*

*　　*　　*

If one were to have a legal standard endorsing the physician's decision not to prolong life, should the standard be limited to the case of a doomed comatose patient with a flat EEG reading? Consider how this case blends so gradually into many related cases. First, there is the case of the doomed comatose patient who still shows some signs of brain activity. Does this patient *deserve* prolongation of life? Neither he nor his brother with a flat EEG reading can enjoy the beauties of life on earth. Why should we keep them alive? Secondly, compare the case of the doomed but conscious patient who can perceive

---

* 203 *Journal of the American Medical Association* 65, 68 (1968). Reprinted by permission.

the world about him but who suffers from excruciating pain. Is the fact of consciousness and the fact of an EEG reading sufficient to say that this man must be kept alive? In analyzing the physician's legal obligation to prolong a patient's life, we should keep in mind the infinitely graduated spectrum from the clear cases to the cases that are far from clear. . . .

*   *   *

It will not do for the medical profession to demand that we lawyers devise a legal definition of death. There might be many uses of a legal definition of death; one might wish to know the time of death to apply rules on the disposition of the decedent's estate. But this is not what medical practitioners have in mind. It seems that they should like to have a clear standard for deciding when and when not to render aid to their dying patients. Sweden's Dr. Crafoord has proposed that a patient be declared legally dead when his EEG reading is flat. The standard is clear and easy to apply, but it is morally insensitive. Should one totally disregard all the other factors: the likelihood of recovery, the family's financial position, the patient's expressed wishes, other demands on hospital facilities and the attending physician's time? Even if we could formulate a just resolution of these conflicting factors today, would it be a resolution that would remain fair in the face of medical innovation? It surely would not. What one regards as excessive and extraordinary today might well become commonplace in a few years. A legal standard of death, which would define the limits of the doctor's duty to his patient, would be an overly rigid solution to a problem that changes dimensions with each medical innovation.

NOTE 2.
CARL E. WASMUTH AND BRUCE H. STEWART
MEDICAL AND LEGAL ASPECTS OF HUMAN
ORGAN TRANSPLANTATION*

*   *   *

Recently, physicians from the Karolinska Institute received international attention when they removed a kidney from a 40-year-old dying woman and transplanted it into the recipient. The donor had suffered a cerebral hemorrhage and was brought into the neurosurgical clinic in

a comatose condition. Her condition had been pronounced hopeless. While she could not, herself, be asked to consent to the removal of the kidney, the operation was performed with her husband's approval. She died in a respirator two days after operation. Professor Crafoord defended the action and the principle. He said that he and his staff had previously agreed that in cases in which irreparable damage to the central nervous system had occurred, and in which the prognosis with 100 per cent certainty be deemed hopeless, the possibility could be considered of removing a kidney for transplantation before what is currently interpreted as "death" had occurred. It was his opinion that if the physician were to wait until death, in the conventional sense, the possibility of a successful transplantation would have decreased tremendously. The position taken by the Swedish physicians is based upon a liberal interpretation of the definition of death. In their particular case, neither respiration nor circulation had ceased and the patient was not, according to the information at hand, dependent upon either of these mechanical means for support. The brain may have been irreversibly damaged, although neither respiration nor circulation had failed.

*   *   *

NOTE 3.
J. B. BRIERLEY, J. H. ADAMS, D. I. GRAHAM,
AND J. A. SIMPSON
NEOCORTICAL DEATH AFTER CARDIAC ARREST—
A CLINICAL, NEUROPHYSIOLOGICAL, AND
NEUROPATHOLOGICAL REPORT OF TWO CASES*

*   *   *

It is now generally accepted that a patient who has suffered severe brain damage—e.g., as a result of head injury, cerebrovascular accident, or cardiac arrest—whose electroencephalogram (E.E.G.) is isoelectric (strictly defined), who is totally areflexic and whose respiratory and therefore cardiac function depends upon mechanical ventilation is already dead. It is less well appreciated that, in the specific situation of cardiac arrest, spontaneous respiration, coordinated movements, and also reflex activities at brainstem and spinal-cord levels may return in occasional cases despite the persistence of an isoelectric E.E.G. In this situation the critical clinical ques-

---

* 14 *Cleveland-Marshall Law Review* 442, 467 (1965). Reprinted by permission.

* 2 *The Lancet* 560, 564–65 (1971). Reprinted by permission.

tion is whether consciousness and intellectual activity will or will not be restored.

Patients with cardiac arrest and irreversible brain damage rarely survive for more than a few days, but in the two cases reported here unconsciousness with an isoelectric E.E.G. persisted for five months after cardiac arrest [at which time the patients died following pulmonary complications]. In case 1, eye-opening, yawning with associated movements, spontaneous respiration, and certain reflex activities at brainstem and spinal-cord levels were present; while in case 2 the resumed central nervous activity was restricted to spontaneous respiration and certain brainstem and spinal-cord reflexes. In both cases, neurophysiological investigations led to the conclusion that the neocortex was dead while certain brainstem and spinal centres remained intact. Subsequent detailed neuropathological analysis confirmed this prediction in each case.

*   *   *

These two cases permit, probably for the first time, a precise definition of "cortex death" as a sequel of cardiac arrest. "Cortex death," or preferably "neocortical death," implies a persistently isoelectric E.E.G. and the absence of sensory evoked responses in the neocortex, together with the resumption of spontaneous respiration and of certain brainstem reflexes.

In contrast, "brain death" or "total brain death" implies a persistently isoelectric E.E.G. and the absence of any reflex activity and of spontaneous respiration, so that cardiac function depends upon the continuation of mechanical ventilation. . . .

*   *   *

In case 2 spontaneous respiration and brainstem reflex activity were resumed a few minutes after the cardiac arrest. In case 1, brainstem and spinal reflex activity were demonstrable on the 2nd day, although mechanical ventilation had to be maintained for 17 days. Thereafter the clinical state of the two patients was identical. On the 6th day, neurophysiological investigations in case 1 established death of the neocortex and the preservation of certain reflex activities up to the level of the geniculate bodies. It cannot be overemphasised that the subsequent neuropathological examination in case 1 confirmed in detail the predictions based upon the neurophysiological assessment "in vivo."

In the specific context of cardiac arrest, we consider that the existence of irreversible neocortical destruction can be established within a few days of the arrest provided that drugs with a central depressive effect are not being given. If any element of doubt should then remain, neocortical death could be confirmed by the appropriate neuropathological examination of a biopsy specimen (a 1–1:5 cm. cube) taken from the posterior half of a cerebral hemisphere.

Once neocortical death has been unequivocally established and the possibility of any recovery of consciousness and intellectual activity thereby excluded, the question must be asked, although this patient breathes spontaneously, is he or she alive? The decision whether or not to continue intensive care in the present era of organ transplantation is contingent upon the answer to this question. However, where a definition of death is concerned "This is a general problem, prima facie not at all particularly associated with transplantation." Perhaps the most important consideration is the suffering imposed upon the relatives by a person with whom they can no longer communicate but who breathes without the aid of a machine.

According to the Ad Hoc Committee of the Harvard Medical School, a person who resumes spontaneous respiration after cardiac arrest, yet exhibits an isoelectric E.E.G., is to be regarded as "alive," while another surviving the same accident, also with an isoelectric E.E.G. but whose cardiac function depends upon mechanical ventilation, may be regarded as "dead." Clearly this distinction between "alive" and "dead" attaches cardinal importance to the function of respiration and none to those higher functions of the nervous system that demarcate man from the lower primates and all other vertebrates and invertebrates.

Thus, according to the [Harvard Medical School] both the present patients would be regarded as "alive," although the neurophysiological assessment, made during life, that the neocortex was dead in each, was confirmed by the neuropathological examinations.

These two cases, together with the two of Lewis which survived for 22 days and 2¼ years, may be regarded as products of the present era of intensive care and they may not long remain unique. Their documentation in clinical and neuropathological terms represents a challenge to any definition of life that is unconcerned with the functional and structural integrity of the neocortex.

[iii]

Cape Town Symposium
Experience with Human Heart Transplantation*

* * *

PROFESSOR BARNARD: . . . I think many a man in the terminal stages of heart failure (and you have often had patients with severe pain and they have said, "please let me die") who is really sick and has a poor blood supply to the brain from poor cardiac output, would say: "Oh please leave me alone, I want to die." But I don't think that the patient can decide whether he wants to die or not. I think that as doctors our duty is to give the patient all the therapy and all the treatment that is available to us. To say that the patient must have a will to live—I don't quite understand that. I think that he is very severely ill, that he just does not have the will to live.

DR. GRONDIN: Dr. Barnard, I think we could correct this. You are right, the patient may not at this terminal stage have the will to live; but I think if we replace this statement by that of a stable personality, it is a broader term and it eliminates some of the hysterical individuals we sometimes meet.

PROFESSOR BARNARD: Well, that is, of course, not the patient being examined at that stage by a psychiatrist, to decide whether he now has a stable personality; you must go into his background and find out from that whether he has a stable personality. But I would ask you, Dr. Grondin, would you turn down a patient and say: "No, you must die, because you don't have a stable personality"?

DR. GRONDIN: I think one should elaborate further, Dr. Barnard. There are some patients who, because of their psychiatric status, are not worth saving and we have all had this experience in cardiac surgery. Sometimes we ask ourselves the question: "Was it worth all that effort?" and even though it is a very difficult. . . .

PROFESSOR BARNARD: I would hate to make that decision myself.

DR. GRONDIN: Between who is fit and who is unfit, yes, but as a general statement, there are really some individuals who will never be able to take the post-operative care and the post-operative seclusion that a heart transplant involves.

DR. KANTROWITZ: I am not sure, Dr. Grondin, that I would agree. I don't take the attitude that

I make decisions about whether a patient can receive the best treatment available on the basis of his emotional stability or whether he hated his mother. I don't think that has anything to do with the fact that this patient is suffering from an organic lesion that is correctible, and that I can do something about it. I think that making decisions about treatment on the basis of the patient's emotional stability is very dangerous and I don't think doctors should become involved in it.

PROFESSOR BARNARD: I want to ask the psychiatrists: when they have a patient who is mentally deteriorated to the stage where he defaecates in bed and eats his faeces and is certainly not a worthwhile citizen, if that man develops pneumonia, will they stop treating that man and allow him to die?

DR. GRONDIN: Are you asking a psychiatrist or are you asking me?

DR. CACHERA: In Paris now, for renal transplants patients who are selected for a graft are examined before operation by a psychiatrist. The conclusion of the psychiatrist plays a role in the final selection of the potential recipient.

PROFESSOR BARNARD: Well, do you think that's correct?

DR. GRONDIN: I do think that it is correct, Dr. Barnard. Let me give you an example that you certainly will agree with. In the heart valve surgery cases there are a lot of patients that you know will never be able to follow an anticoagulant regime adequately, and this has become a problem with heart valve replacements. I know of several patients who, because of their inability to follow such simple rules as taking pills every day, and watching their prothrombin levels, have died of embolism; and there is certainly a lower limit of intelligence and co-operation on the part of the patient that you must require, if you are going to embark upon such an operation.

PROFESSOR BARNARD: But I know of patients who have had infections due to their inability to take antibiotics, who have died—so do you stop their treatment?

DR. GRONDIN: No, but I think you must admit that between giving antibiotics, and undergoing a heart transplant, there is a big difference.

PROFESSOR BARNARD: So, actually you are just making things easier for yourself.

DR. GRONDIN: No, I think we are thinking of the patient—the patient who will have a heart transplant will need a close follow-up and needs to be intelligent enough to understand his situation and how to cope with it. Doctors who treat diabetic

———
* H. A. Shapiro, ed. New York: Appleton-Century-Crofts 266–273 (1968). © 1969, Butterworth & Co. (South Africa) Ltd. Reprinted by permission.

patients require from them a minimum of intelligence and understanding. I am not talking about emotionally disturbed patients. I am talking about the mentally deteriorated patient.

DR. KANTROWITZ: I think we are on very dangerous ground. We all, I am sure, make these decisions about whether one should operate on a patient—for replacement of a mitral valve or for incision of a carbuncle—on the basis of examining and assessing the total patient—this is called being a doctor, and we do the best that we can. I don't believe that the psychiatrists, for whom I have great respect, are in the best position to assess the total problem, particularly when it is organic—when the major problem, the condition that is bringing about the patient's death, is an organic problem which is amenable to the surgical approach. I think the surgeons should make the decision whether or not to operate.

DR. GRONDIN: But we are not talking about who makes the decision, we are talking about a minimum requirement in the selection of a recipient. It was mentioned earlier when we discussed this topic that we would like a patient with a reasonably stable personality; not only that, but also with an understanding of what is going on, and it has been rewarding for survivors of heart transplants to see how well they behave, in spite of the somewhat miserable social and emotional conditions which they endure in the recovery period.

DR. ROSS: Mr. Chairman, I think Dr. Schrire has something to say, and I think we would like to hear some audience participation.

PROFESSOR SCHRIRE: This discussion has clarified very clearly the difference between surgeons and physicians. You have a whole group of surgeons who have been talking about the patient's selection and so on. The surgeon sees the patient, by and large, when he is presented as a problem as to whether he should operate or not. He doesn't look at the patient over a period of years and years during which the average doctor or cardiologist gets to know this patient. By the time a heart transplant patient is transferred for surgery, generally the physicians or cardiologists have seen him over a period of many, many years, usually 10–15 years. No surgeon has lived with his patient before the operation. Although Professor Barnard has certainly said many times he wouldn't turn down patients—it is very obvious why. We turn down patients every day of the week, but he would be horrified. I agree absolutely with Dr. Grondin. We turn down patients all the time who cannot take anticoagulants. We

never present them to our surgeons. Many of our problem cases never come to the surgeons. The physician lives with his patients for years and years, before and after the operation, and that's why I was very concerned initially.

I don't agree with Dr. Kantrowitz. I think that I would not refer patients for a major procedure, such as a heart transplant, which is completely unknown territory, if the patient is, for example, a depressive who hasn't the least bit of interest in life, whom you can only keep alive by giving him drugs; and you only know these patients if you live with them for a long time. I don't think it is fair for the surgeon to make the decision, without the advice of physicians (it need not be cardiologists) who know their patients.

DR. PIERCE: One of the most gratifying experiences in the renal transplant patients, is to see the transformation in the personalities and the outlook of patients, once their organic problem has been corrected. Many of these patients have had many years of decreasing capacity. If one would look at them and say what their potential might be, it would be easy to grossly underestimate their possibilities. I remember very clearly a man who was withdrawn, who could barely get out of bed, whose limbs were so thin that, if you can imagine it, some of the other patients who were in not too different a situation, poked fun at him. Well, after this man's transplant, he became an outgoing individual, he regained his interest in reading, in studying and in doing things, and you wouldn't recognize him as the same person.

It is true that there are patients with difficult personalities and low intelligence levels which can greatly magnify the problems of management, but I would like to submit that, in the present state of knowledge, it is very difficult to predict in which patients this will prove to be an insurmountable obstacle.

PROFESSOR BARNARD: I think that is very important, because even when Professor Schrire sees his patient for the first time, the man already suffers from heart disease and his personality and outlook on life must be changed as a result of that.

Jim, let me ask you a question. You have been working with the psychiatry department to select patients for many, many years now—how many have you turned down because their brains are not suitable?

DR. PIERCE: Well, some of our best results in terms of rehabilitation have been in patients whose intelligence levels were not too high. I should point out that, in children and patients who do not have normal intelligence, one has to take a special precaution to ensure that they take their immunosuppressive drugs every day. This means that another individual who is responsible has to give them the medicine and see that they take it.

PROFESSOR BARNARD: But that also applies to the treatment of diabetes with insulin.

DR. PIERCE: That's correct. It is a point in management and not to say that we can't operate on children because they are not responsible in taking their medicines—the mother just has to give it to them, that's all.

PROFESSOR BARNARD: Yes, but Professor Schrire says that the patient can't take his anticoagulants, so you must turn him down for surgery. He would also say, then, I won't give insulin to a man who has got diabetes because I am not sure he will take his insulin.

PROFESSOR SCHRIRE: I didn't say so. I must impress upon Professor Barnard, and others here, that conditions that occur in the United States of America do not necessarily apply to every other country in the world. There is just not the available help for them and one has to take this into account.

*   *   *

DR. KANTROWITZ: . . . I am not sure that Professor Schrire is right. Professor Schrire has taken a point of view which is not unusual. Many internists who deal frequently with their patients over prolonged periods of time, make decisions affecting their patients' welfare, their living or dying. Now Dr. Barnard has pointed out that if a cardiac patient is referred to his room the decision is made unemotionally; after all, if you don't see the patient every week, you are not so likely to be emotionally involved with him. You may not want to take the chance of exposing this patient to an operation which admittedly carries a risk. I maintain, as Dr. Barnard does, that such decisions are much better made by a group of doctors who have had a great deal of experience in making them, and are not emotionally involved with the patient.

I believe, sir, that you do your patients a disservice by not sending your patients to a group of men who will make an unemotional decision.

DR. ZERBINI: I believe that the selection of the patient must be done by a team, a large team of cardiologists, surgeons, psychiatrists and so on.

DR. KANTROWITZ: Yes, but no psychiatrist. No rabbi, no priest and no psychiatrist.

DR. ZERBINI: We have one, but the decision for the indication of surgery must be done at a meeting of all these people together, not only the surgeon and not only the cardiologist, but the group.

DR. GRONDIN: Dr. Zerbini, I think you have touched the right point. The decision to operate on such a patient does not only belong to the surgeon, nor does it only belong to the cardiologist. I think it has to be a decision taken by a team of doctors.

DR. KANTROWITZ: And I don't think it belongs to a man who is emotionally involved and is not qualified. The decision whether this patient will benefit by a heart operation should be made by people who are qualified in heart surgery.

DR. GRONDIN: Oh, no question about that.

DR. MOWBRAY: I just wanted to say, if Dr. Kantrowitz is talking about an unemotional group of people selecting patients and he considers that, at the moment, he is one of an unemotional group of cardiac surgeons, I cannot agree.

PROFESSOR BARNARD: We have Dr. van der Spuy, who is the head of the Cardio-Thoracic Unit at one of our universities in Pretoria, who would like to say something.

DR. GRONDIN: Dr. van der Spuy, I think I would like you to conclude this discussion.

DR. VAN DER SPUY: I sincerely hope that I will, if you all agree with me.

The thing that has been occupying my mind here is the selection of the recipient—the whole problem in this congress actually turned to rejection. We have been talking about the psychiatric aspect as far as the recipient is concerned, except that we haven't been talking about rejection. Now the thing that I want to know is this, and this concerns the recipient vitally, should we tell the recipient that this is a palliative operation? We have been hearing about so many patients waiting and so many patients that we are going to operate on, as if we are going to cure them. We are only going to prolong their lives, in a small percentage (as the position stands now) for a few weeks or a few months. What about informing the patient? If we are absolutely honest with the patient, then all my objections fall flat; but, as far as I am concerned, the essence of the whole thing is this, that we must take the patient and his relatives into our trust and say, this is the problem—now do you agree to have an operation?

PROFESSOR BARNARD: I think you must treat the patient the same way in which you would treat a patient who has a carcinoma of the lung—which is also really a palliative operation in most cases.

DR. VAN DER SPUY: I think, reading from press reports and patients approaching one, that patients think this operation is curative. They ask me: "Is this chap going to live; is he going to reach the age of 80 years?" We know beforehand that this patient is doomed, according to our present knowledge. I believe that we are misinforming our future patients. We are not gaining the confidence of our future patients, because we are probably, for our own benefit, for the personal benefit, for the egoist each one of us is, we are withholding the essence of the whole matter—this patient will probably be dead in a few months' time. Thank you.

DR. GRONDIN: There is no doubt in the patients' minds, because they read the newspapers and they know that the longest survival so far is 6 months. When we propose a heart transplant to an intelligent patient, he knows very well that there have not been any long-term survivals but, even though we look upon a heart transplant at this moment as a palliative procedure, it might prove to be curative and provide a long-term cure.

When one talks about rejection, one might say that one is implanting a foreign heart, and the body has to accept it. I think, from the psychiatric point of view also, that there should not be any rejection to the operation. . . .

*   *   *

NOTE

PIETRO CASTELNUOVO-TEDESCO
CARDIAC SURGEONS LOOK AT TRANSPLANTATION
—INTERVIEWS WITH DRS. CLEVELAND, COOLEY,
DEBAKEY, HALLMAN AND ROCHELLE*

*   *   *

There are also problems of conscience in relation to the donor, however much an attempt may be made to rationalize them. Dr. Cooley recalls, "Well, I was worried because I was taking the heart out of the donor while it was still beating and putting it over here, and that meant the cadaver over there was completely wiped out. No question of life or death! I satisfied myself completely that death was in the process at the time we removed the heart and I didn't worry

about those things. I didn't worry whether the donor was dead or alive. . . . My concern was primarily with the recipient and everyone. . . .— the public, most physicians—were more concerned with protecting the rights of the donor. Well, to me the donor was dead. He didn't have any real rights . . . [except those] exercised by his relatives and next of kin, but the one who really had some rights was the recipient. Therefore, we wanted to see that he got the best chance to live and there are ways one could jeopardize his chances by, say, . . . trying to satisfy everyone that this donor was completely wiped out and waiting until the heart was almost at the point of cessation entirely. Then you say, okay, now we'll take it out and put it over here. So you are giving the recipient a badly abused organ, which is not fair to that recipient." Dr. Hallman described similar feelings even more starkly, ". . . it gives you the impression that you have . . . influence over life and death . . . When . . . [we] take the heart out of a donor, we've gone through the medico-legal procedures that . . . [say that] the patient is legally dead when the brain is dead but yet you are the one who makes the final blow and takes out the heart and this is a peculiar feeling the first time you do it . . . I guess just like an executioner who has to pull the switch on the electric chair because it's his job. It bothers him the first time, but the more times he does it, the less it bothers him. . . . This was upsetting to me personally the first time I did it, but the more I did it the easier it became . . . But the first time you do it you have the feeling as if you are killing the patient. The only justification that one can have for doing [it] is that the patient is for all practical purposes . . . dead and that everybody has agreed to this. . . ."

*   *   *

[iv]
Paul H. Blachly
*Can Organ Transplantation Provide an
Altruistic–Expiatory Alternative to Suicide?**

*   *   *

When President Eisenhower was sustaining repeated heart attacks, at least 20 persons offered their own hearts for transplant. At other transplant centers this same sort of offer has been made for persons unknown to the donor. Public solicitations for kidney donors have been successful in San Francisco. Dr. Harrison Sadler at

* Pietro Castelnuovo-Tedesco, ed.: *Psychiatric Aspects of Organ Transplantation. 3 Seminars in Psychiatry* 5, 13 (1971). Reprinted by permission of Grune & Stratton, Inc.

* 1 *Life-Threatening Behavior* 6, 8–9 (1971). Reprinted by permission.

the Langley Porter Institute has been impressed by the salutary effect of such organ donation on the life pattern of unrelated donors. He describes a woman leading a meaningless anhedonic existence who after organ donation experienced a satisfying sense of well-being and ability to feel satisfaction in interpersonal relationships. There are other reports that kidney donors generally experienced a sustained feeling of satisfaction and of being "noble."

Could it be that sacrifice has a psychotherapeutic potential that we have overlooked? Sacrifice seems quite uncommon in our culture, unless one wishes to consider our periodic wars. We know that some suicidal persons view their actions as sacrifice.

* * *

Suicide seems to diminish during periods when major sacrifices are demanded, as in times of war. It is in such circumstances that the intensity of egoism and anomie is diminished as the individual participates in a common social goal.

Now we can come back to our unreachable egoistic-anomic suicidal person. Is it possible, then, that such highly individualistic suicidal persons could follow the route that sacrifice has followed in history and could be induced to give a partial sacrifice for a total human sacrifice? If such a partial sacrifice could satisfy an altruistic purpose, then not only would benefit accrue to the suicidal person but also to the physically ill person who would be restored to health through such sacrifice. What psychotherapist has ever suggested to a depressed person that he donate a pint of blood?

It is often said that we can not give love until we have received it. I suspect there is another population, one which rarely seeks psychotherapy, which can not accept love until it has given. I suspect that Dr. Sadler's patient who could not deal with persons in a satisfying way until she had given one of her lifesaving kidneys found that she could think of herself as a lovable person only after she had given part of herself.

It would seem to make sense, then, for a suicide prevention service to use as one resource a mobile organ bank. A mobile organ bank might be a group of persons who are willing to donate various organs so that others might live. Those who might want to donate their heart (suicide) could likely be encouraged in most cases to give a partial sacrifice such as a kidney

or regular blood donation. The time required for the thorough immunological studies the surgeons need could be used for thorough psychiatric evaluation and treatment. At the University of California San Francisco Medical Center a waiting period of two to three months is imposed between the time of offering donation and actual surgery, which permits time for careful assessment of motivation.

It is, of course, true that certain donors seek to donate because of the dramatic attention-seeking rewards; but how do these people differ from those who commit suicide for the same reason? Does it not reflect an emotional need that might be best resolved through the psychiatric attention possible in an organ bank?

Dr. Sadler feels that the act of giving in itself is not sufficient for permanent improvement if the donor has insufficient "ego strength" or cannot make a transference to the institution or transplant team. History reveals that sacrifice is a periodically repeated behavior; except for blood donation this is impossible with organ donation. Apparently the process of organizing groups of persons who have donated organs is already underway, which may provide the kind of postdonation support that is sometimes necessary. The organ bank conducted on a group basis should provide benefits superior to those of the isolated donor giving to an isolated recipient in that it reinforces the group solidarity, decreasing the egoism and anomie.

It may turn out that efforts to prevent suicide may best be achieved through means that do not emphasize the word "suicide." Opportunities to save the lives of others through sacrifice of part of oneself offered to a population of potentially altruistic but anomic, egoistic persons might prove more successful than offers of psychological "help" or "therapy." Unlike help or therapy such a sacrifice could enhance the person's sense of dignity and self-determination, while permitting him to rejoin the human race on his own terms.

It is hard to deal with the inevitable case who, despite all therapeutic effort, would continue to insist upon suicide. Until our mores change to permit such a person to end his own life in a dignified way that would permit utilization of his organs, we will continue to insist that he not do it, thus permitting continuation of the present wasteful idiosyncratic methods. One would think that the stigma that the friends and relatives attach to a suicide would be much lessened if they knew several persons would live as a result. Perhaps it is premature to ask whether it is immoral for a person not to give an organ if another person can thereby live.

* * *

NOTE

BELDING H. SCRIBNER
ETHICAL PROBLEMS OF USING ARTIFICIAL
ORGANS TO SUSTAIN HUMAN LIFE*

* * *

[I]f I knew that I had a fatal disease I would seriously consider volunteering to donate one of my kidneys while I was still well. As far as death is concerned, I would like to be able to put into my will a paragraph urging that when my physician felt that the end was near, I be put to sleep and any useful organs taken prior to death. . . . I think the ethical and legal guidelines should be devised to permit me and others to volunteer in these ways.

* * *

d.
Deciding about the Delegation of Authority to Control, Review, and Reformulate the Process?

[i]
*National Conference of Commissioners on
Uniform State Laws
Uniform Anatomical Gift Act†*

An act authorizing the gift of all or part of a human body after death for specified purposes.

SECTION 1. (*Definitions*)
(a) "Bank or storage facility" means a facility licensed, accredited or approved under the laws of any state for storage of human bodies or parts thereof.

---

* 10 *Transactions of American Society for Artificial Internal Organs* 209, 211 (1964). Reprinted by permission.
† Final Draft as approved on July 30, 1968. The National Conference of Commissioners on Uniform State Laws is composed of law professors, lawyers, and judges, representing every state, whose function is to help make state laws more uniform and up-to-date. This Act was the product of three years of intensive study by a special committee of the conference. Earlier drafts of the Act were reviewed by medical and scientific groups, including the Committee on Tissue Transplantation of the Division of Medical Sciences of the National Research Council.

(b) "Decedent" means a deceased individual and includes a stillborn infant or fetus.
(c) "Donor" means an individual who makes a gift of all or part of his body.
(d) "Hospital" means a hospital licensed, accredited or approved under the laws of any state and includes a hospital operated by the United States government, a state or a subdivision thereof, although not required to be licensed under state laws.
(e) "Part" includes organs, tissues, eyes, bones, arteries, blood, other fluids and other portions of a human body, and "part" includes "parts."
(f) "Person" means an individual, corporation, government or governmental subdivision or agency, business trust, estate, trust, partnership or association or any other legal entity.
(g) "Physician" or "surgeon" means a physician or surgeon licensed or authorized to practice under the laws of any state.
(h) "State" includes any state, district, commonwealth, territory, insular possession, and any other area subject to the legislative authority of the United States of America.

SECTION 2. (*Persons Who May Execute an Anatomical Gift*)
(a) Any individual of sound mind and 18 years of age or more may give all or any part of his body for any purposes specified in section 3, the gift to take effect upon death.
(b) Any of the following persons, in order of priority stated, when persons in prior classes are not available at the time of death, and in the absence of actual notice of contrary indications by the decedent, or actual notice of opposition by a member of the same or a prior class, may give all or any part of the decedent's body for any purposes specified in section 3.
(1) the spouse,
(2) an adult son or daughter,
(3) either parent,
(4) an adult brother or sister,
(5) a guardian of the person of the decedent at the time of his death,
(6) any other person authorized or under obligation to dispose of the body.
(c) If the donee has actual notice of contrary indications by the decedent, or that a gift by a member of a class is opposed by a member of the same or a prior class, the donee shall not accept the gift. The persons authorized by subsection (b) may make the gift after death or immediately before death.

(d) A gift of all or part of a body authorizes any examination necessary to assure medical acceptability of the gift for the purposes intended.

(e) The rights of the donee created by the gift are paramount to the rights of others except as provided by section 7(d).

SECTION 3. (*Persons Who May Become Donees, and Purposes for Which Anatomical Gifts May Be Made*)

The following persons may become donees of gifts of bodies or parts thereof for the purposes stated:

(1) any hospital, surgeon, or physician, for medical or dental education, research, advancement of medical or dental science, therapy or transplantation; or

(2) any accredited medical or dental school, college or university for education, research, advancement of medical or dental science or therapy; or

(3) any bank or storage facility for medical or dental education, research, advancement of medical or dental science, therapy or transplantation; or

(4) any specified individual for therapy or transplantation needed by him.

SECTION 4. (*Manner of Executing Anatomical Gifts*)

(a) A gift of all or part of the body under section 2(a) may be made by will. The gift becomes effective upon the death of the testator without waiting for probate. If the will is not probated, or if it is declared invalid for testamentary purposes, the gift, to the extent that it has been acted upon in good faith, is nevertheless valid and effective.

(b) A gift of all or part of the body under section 2(a) may also be made by document other than a will. The gift becomes effective upon the death of the donor. The document, which may be a card designed to be carried on the person, must be signed by the donor, in the presence of 2 witnesses who must sign the document in his presence. If the donor cannot sign, the document may be signed for him at his direction and in his presence, and in the presence of 2 witnesses who must sign the document in his presence. Delivery of the document of gift during the donor's lifetime is not necessary to make the gift valid.

(c) The gift may be made to a specified donee or without specifying a donee. If the lat-ter, the gift may be accepted by the attending physician as donee upon or following death. If the gift is made to a specified donee who is not available at the time and place of death, the attending physician upon or following death, in the absence of any expressed indication that the donor desired otherwise, may accept the gift as donee. The physician who becomes a donee under this subsection shall not participate in the procedures for removing or transplanting a part.

(d) Notwithstanding section 7(b), the donor may designate in his will, card or other document of gift the surgeon or physician to carry out the appropriate procedures. In the absence of a designation, or if the designee is not available, the donee or other person authorized to accept the gift may employ or authorize any surgeon or physician for the purpose.

(e) Any gift by a person designated in section 2(b) shall be made by a document signed by him, or made by his telegraphic, recorded telephonic or other recorded message.

SECTION 5. (*Delivery of Document of Gift*)

If the gift is made by the donor to a specified donee, the will, card, or other document, or an executed copy thereof, may be delivered to the donee to expedite the appropriate procedures immediately after death, but delivery is not necessary to the validity of the gift. The will, card or other document, or an executed copy thereof, may be deposited in any hospital, bank or storage facility or registry office that accepts them for safekeeping or for facilitation of procedures after death. On request of any interested party upon or after the donor's death, the person in possession shall produce the document for examination.

SECTION 6. (*Amendment or Revocation of the Gift*)

(a) If the will, card or other document or executed copy thereof has been delivered to a specified donee, the donor may amend or revoke the gift by:

(1) the execution and delivery to the donee of a signed statement, or

(2) an oral statement made in the presence of 2 persons and communicated to the donee, or

(3) a statement during a terminal illness or injury addressed to an attending physician and communicated to the donee, or

(4) a signed card or document found on his person or in his effects.

(b) Any document of gift which has not been delivered to the donee may be revoked by the donor in the manner set out in subsection (a) or by destruction, cancellation, or mutilation of the document and all executed copies thereof.

(c) Any gift made by a will may also be amended or revoked in the manner provided for amendment or revocation of wills, or as provided in subsection (a).

SECTION 7. (*Rights and Duties at Death*)

(a) The donee may accept or reject the gift. If the donee accepts a gift of the entire body, he may, subject to the terms of the gift, authorize embalming and the use of the body in funeral services. If the gift is of a part of the body, the donee, upon the death of the donor and prior to embalming, shall cause the part to be removed without unnecessary mutilation. After removal of the part, custody of the remainder of the body vests in the surviving spouse, next of kin or other persons under obligation to dispose of the body.

(b) The time of death shall be determined by a physician who attends the donor at his death or, if none, the physician who certifies the death. This physician shall not participate in the procedures for removing or transplanting a part.

(c) A person who acts in good faith in accord with the terms of this Act, or under the anatomical gift laws of another state (or a foreign country) is not liable for damages in any civil action or subject to prosecution in any criminal proceeding for his act.

(d) The provisions of this Act are subject to the laws of this state prescribing powers and duties with respect to autopsies.

SECTION 8. (*Uniformity of Interpretation*)

This Act shall be so construed as to effectuate its general purpose to make uniform the law of those states which enact it.

*   *   *

[ii]
State of Kansas
*An Act Relating to and Defining Death**

*   *   *

A person will be considered medically and legally dead if, in the opinion of a physician, based on ordinary standards of medical practice, there is the absence of spontaneous respiratory

and cardiac function and, because of the disease or condition which caused, directly or indirectly, these functions to cease, or because of the passage of time since these functions ceased, attempts at resuscitation are considered hopeless; and, in this event, death will have occurred at the time these functions ceased; or

A person will be considered medically and legally dead if, in the opinion of a physician, based on ordinary standards of medical practice, there is the absence of spontaneous brain function; and if based on ordinary standards of medical practice, during reasonable attempts to either maintain or restore spontaneous circulatory or respiratory function in the absence of aforesaid brain function, it appears that further attempts at resuscitation or supportive maintenance will not succeed, death will have occurred at the time when these conditions first coincide. Death is to be pronounced before artificial means of supporting respiratory and circulatory function are terminated and before any vital organ is removed for purposes of transplantation.

These alternative definitions of death are to be utilized for all purposes in this state, including the trials of civil and criminal cases, any laws to the contrary notwithstanding.

*   *   *

NOTE

Ian McColl Kennedy
The Kansas Statute on Death— An Appraisal*

*   *   *

[T]he lip service paid by the courts to outdated concepts of death . . . can create havoc in the law, in the light of medical developments. But the changes that must come should be brought about through case law, through recognition by the courts, in cases before them, of the prevailing medical opinion as the law. Legislation may make for certainty, but at what cost to future flexibility? For, in an area as fast moving as this, the flexibility to respond to further medical developments must be the keystone of the law, and this is not an attribute usually associated with legislation. [W]hat reason can there be for legislating? The answer often put forward is that the doctor will never know where he stands in the absence of firm guidelines and will always

---

* House Bill No. 1961, approved March 17, 1970; Sessions Laws of Kansas, Ch. 378 (1970).

* 285 *New England Journal of Medicine* 946–947 (1971). Reprinted by permission.

be in fear of litigation arising from an act of his that, although medically entirely valid, by the existing standards is still of only doubtful legality. But, of course, this is no real answer. Let us have guidelines by all means. They are essential. But let them be set down by the medical profession, not by the legislature, so that the body best equipped to evaluate and examine them can always have them under review, rather than depend on the time-consuming and often whimsical processes of the legislature. Now, this recommendation presupposes the existence of a strong professional body able to control and sanction anyone who practices that profession. The British model of the British Medical Association comes to mind: a self-regulating body to which matters of practice can safely be left since it has wide powers of sanction and is not afraid to use them. The American medical profession is not at all as well regulated. My view is that it should remedy this lack with all speed. In the absence of responsible self-regulation and the setting and enforcing of proper standards, the task will be assumed by some other body, most probably the legislature. If one accepts, as I do, that the matters properly within the competence of a profession should be dealt with by that profession, whose views would then be accepted, if it could be shown that they were informed and objectively arrived at, the intervention of the legislature is regrettable.

. . . Furthermore, whatever changes may from time to time become necessary can be made by the simple act of the courts' giving recognition to the then prevailing views of the profession. When I speak of "consensus view" and "prevailing views of the profession," it may appear that to appeal to such a consensus ignores the fact that I stress throughout that this is a fast-changing scientific area. There is an answer to this doubt. At any given time a wide range of opinions may be held by doctors. Only some, however, will gain the approval of the vast majority of doctors, after being discussed and debated in the usual ways. These opinions, and there need not necessarily be only one view, would represent the consensus of informed opinion. As has been argued it may well be that the profession should look for ways of giving some kind of "official approval" to certain views, so that doctors who then continue to follow unacceptable ideas will be in breach of the required standards of conduct and thus liable to sanction.

*   *   *

2.

In Administering Research

a.

Who Should Participate, within What Structure, in State Regulation?

[i]
Advisory Group on Transplantation Problems Advice on the Question of Amending the Human Tissue Act 1961*

*   *   *

Kidney transplantation has reached the development stage and is an established therapeutic measure. Grafting of other organs is still in the research phase. It may well be that in the course of time surgeons will be able to use this technique on a wider scale as a means for saving life by grafting other organs, but the best working assumption seems to be that the rate of development will not be uniform.

*   *   *

[T]wo fundamental objectives are to be achieved. First, each individual's right to decide whether he would wish his organs to be used after death must be respected. Second, transplant teams should have a readier and greater supply of organs. The courses open fall into two categories: options of action, and options of reinforcement to follow through changes.

(a) OPTIONS OF ACTION

(*i*) *No change.* If the law can properly be interpreted in the interests of transplantation (that is, if the "person lawfully in possession" can be taken to mean the hospital or its officers for the critical time, if the "reasonable enquiry as may be practicable" can be held to be a flexible commonsense statement that doctors should try to obtain the consent of relatives but that practicability must pay regard to the extremely limited time available, and if "surviving relatives" can be taken to mean those in the immediate degrees of kinship), then it could be said to be tolerable from the point of view of surgeons

---

   * Sir Hector MacLennan, M.D., Chairman. National Health Service (Cmnd. 4106). London: Her Majesty's Stationery Office 3, 6–8 (1969). Reprinted by permission. [The advisory group, appointed by the Health Ministers, consisted of five physicians, a nurse, a theologian, a lawyer, a social scientist, a journalist, and a businessman.]

engaged in transplantation to leave the law as it is. The merit of taking no action would appear to be flexibility; its disadvantages, the lack of clarity in which the general public and the professions would continue to find themselves and the risk of legal action against doctors who had acted in good faith. . . .

(ii) *Limited amendment*. By this is meant removing the ambiguities in the Human Tissue Act. It would imply clarifying that the "person lawfully in possession" was the hospital authority during the time between death and the time when next of kin or executors claim the body; defining the persons with a right to be consulted who should be the next of kin; and defining the minimum procedure of enquiry.

(iii) *Double contract*. By this is meant a single public and central register for both consents and objections recorded during life. This would have the advantage, from the point of view of the public, of recording their wishes either way, and of indicating the movement of public opinion to the further end of enabling the authorities to judge when any further action might be acceptable. Its great disadvantage is the uncertain position of those who neither expressed an objection to their organs being used after death, nor indicated that they would be willing to donate parts of their body. It could, however, be associated with limited amendment ((ii) above).

(iv) *Contracting out*. Provided that an effective mechanism for recording objection exists, this means that surgeons should be able to remove organs unless there were definite indications that the deceased had objected. The Group is advised that this would require a change in the law, but understands that certain other countries (Denmark, Sweden, Israel, Italy and France) have legislation in this sense. Implementation would depend on public acceptance and on there being a register of information as in double contract to which transplant teams could have speedy access.

(b) REINFORCEMENT

(i) *Publicity*. The public needs information as to the procedures under existing law on the use of human tissue and on the certification of death. If it were decided that the basis of the law must remain as "contracting in" the progress of transplantation would depend upon enrolling donors. Government sponsorship would be needed, and also delicacy of touch. The form of presentation should lay emphasis on the fact that the donation of an organ can save life. How-

ever, while making it clear that this is a decision for the individual, the Health Ministers could properly make it clear that, in their view, this would be a laudable act.

(ii) *Identification of potential donors or objectors*. This would have to be durable, immediately recognisable, and unique. Ideally, the identification would be carried on the person at all times. In the longer run, the public may come to accept the desirability of carrying medical record cards with details of some other factors, *e.g.*, allergy, of importance in a medical emergency. The uses of such a card are being considered by the Standing Medical Advisory Committee. Voluntary addition of a record of willingness or unwillingness to use of organs after death would help to put this question in perspective. A decision depends on other factors and may not be favorable yet.

(iii) *Enrolment of cohorts*. The Group is advised that a person of years mature enough to form a proper judgment and of sound mind can give consent to the use of organs after death just as consent can be given to operations at age 16. This opens the way to approaches to groups of young people at school, college or university. If contracting in were to be the basis, this means might produce better results than unselective encouragement aimed at the general public.

(iv) *The right to object*. The individual or his parent or guardians should have a right to object which must be made effective. If a register of objections is kept, the public must be aware of it and have access to it. There would be a need for publicity and postage-paid cards readily available at public offices so that the individual might contract out by the stroke of a pen, upon giving his personal details. In addition, it would be necessary to provide for automatic exemption of persons who could not give a valid consent such as persons under 16 and mentally disordered.

* * *

NOTES

NOTE 1.

RENAL TRANSPLANTATION BILL*

* * *

2. It shall be lawful to remove from the body of a human person, duly certified as dead, any kidney or kidneys required for the direct

---

* See 762 *Parliamentary Debates, H.C.* (5th ser.) 810 (1968).

purpose of saving the life of another sick human being, unless there is reason to believe that the deceased during his lifetime had instructed otherwise.

3. Section 2 of this Act does not apply to any person who is:—

(a) mentally insane, or

(b) mentally handicapped, or

(c) below the age of 18, or

(d) 65 years old or more than that age, or

(e) deprived of his liberty by the conviction and judgment of a court, or

(f) a permanent resident of a hostel, home, or institution for the aged, the disabled, or the handicapped.

4. For the purposes of section 2 of this Act, a death certificate must be signed by not less than two medical practitioners, one of whom shall have been registered for at least five years, but neither of them shall be the surgeon conducting the renal transplantation.

5. For the purpose of section 2 of this Act, the qualified medical practitioner responsible for the welfare and safety of the donor or potential donor must be a person other than the qualified medical practitioner responsible for the welfare and safety of the recipient or potential recipient.

6. No person shall be under any duty, whether by contract or by any statutory or other legal requirement, to participate in any treatment authorised by this Act, to which that person has a conscientious objection.

7.—(1) The Minister of Health shall within three months of the passing of this Act establish a Central Renal Registry wherein any objector to the transplant of his kidney may duly register his objection in a form to be decided by the Minister.

(2) Information as to any objection duly registered in the Registry shall be available on demand to any hospital in the United Kingdom of Great Britain and Northern Ireland, and shall be treated as sufficient evidence of an instruction for the purposes of section 2 of this Act.

* * *

NOTE 2.

ALFRED M. SADLER, JR., BLAIR L. SADLER,
E. BLYTHE STASON, AND DELFORD L. STICKEL
TRANSPLANTATION—A CASE FOR CONSENT*

* * *

[T]he Uniform Anatomical Gift Act prepared by the Commissioners on Uniform State

---

* 280 *New England Journal of Medicine* 862, 866 (1969). Reprinted by permission.

Laws represents a responsible and realistic model for reform that not only is badly needed but will be widely accepted. We further believe that, *when obtaining organs or tissue for transplantation, the fundamental principle of informed consent should be maintained, and that, if the present consent framework is adequately streamlined and modernized (as is done in the Uniform Anatomical Gift Act), the principal legal constraints will be eliminated without compromising other important rights and sensitivities.*

* * *

. . . Dukeminier and Sanders . . . suggest that the principles of consent and voluntary donation should be discarded in favor of allowing tissue removal by a physician without his having to give notice to anyone. They propose that a surgeon should be allowed to remove cadaver organs "routinely . . . unless there were some objection entered before removal. The burden of action would be on the person who did not want the organs removed to enter his objection." Under this system, the donor could object during life to the taking of his organs after death. The next of kin could also object to the use of a deceased's organs before removal, provided that the deceased did not specifically authorize donation.

The question, as they see it, is where the burden of action should rest: with the surgeon to obtain consent, or with the next of kin to object. They believe that only by shifting the burden to the next of kin will an adequate quantity of organs be obtained.

This argument is dubious for several reasons. The first is that, in the system proposed, the burden actually remains with the responsible surgeon to assure himself that no objection has been raised either by the deceased himself before death or by the next of kin after death. To absolve himself of this burden adequately would require an inquiry tantamount to obtaining consent itself.

Moreover, it is certain that there are some people who would object to tissue use on religious grounds (as recognized by Dukeminier and Sanders) or because of other beliefs. Such people, if not immediately available at the time of death of a relative, might object strongly and vigorously after the fact. They could forcefully argue that, because they did not know of the demise of their next of kin, they could not exercise their authority to enter an objection to tissue removal. Any system based on this premise would need to include a method of registering objection in a manner to make this information readily available to the interested surgeon. Otherwise, grave constitutional questions, such as the abridgement of religious freedom or the denial of due process, could invalidate the system. . . .

Dukeminier and Sanders assert that the "bereaved survivors usually do not want to know what has happened to the body of the deceased in the hospital" and to ask a relative of someone who is about to die "for the kidneys may seem a ghoulish request." We submit that current medical practice strongly shows that this kind of request is usually not offensive when properly presented and the need sensitively raised. . . . Not to be told of such a removal or to be informed only after the fact would be "ghoulish" indeed.

As further support for their argument of telling nothing to the next of kin, they cite an example of a detailed description of autopsy procedures or embalming technics as being the usual practice in obtaining permission for autopsy. These authors confuse the obtaining of adequate "informed consent" for such procedures with a detailed technical explanation of them. One asks for an autopsy but does not describe the fine points of the procedure in intimate detail. Similarly, one asks for permission to remove an organ for transplantation without enumerating every nuance of surgical technic. Properly informed consent is admittedly difficult to define, but a discussion of it must be based on currently accepted medical practice.

*   *   *

[ii]
Compulsory Removal of Cadaver Organs*

The proliferation of heart transplants within the last eighteen months has raised the hopes of those suffering from organic diseases. At the same time, the publicity accompanying these operations has focused public attention on the need for a supply of healthy organs. . . . A possible solution may be a statute which authorizes the compulsory removal of cadaver organs. . . .

*   *   *

The fifth amendment to the United States Constitution and similar provisions in most state constitutions, require the payment of "just compensation" whenever the government takes property for a public use. The questions to be considered here are, first, whether the involuntary

removal of cadaver organs constitutes a taking of property for public use; and, second, what amount will satisfy the just compensation requirement.

One of the most vexing problems in eminent domain cases involves the concept of "taking." Whether a particular governmental act requires compensation will often turn on the label which the court will place on such an act. If the act constitutes a taking, compensation will have to be paid; if it amounts to a regulation, no compensation is required.

[A] physical invasion of private property has always constituted a taking. The entire interest affected by the condemnation need not be taken; even when the physical invasion is so minor as to be "practically trifling," a valid claim for compensation will be found. The involuntary removal by the state of cadaver organs, therefore, would appear to involve an exercise of the government's eminent domain powers rather than a regulatory measure. . . .

*   *   *

[C]onsidering the state's interest in preserving lives, it is difficult to conceive of a court invalidating an organ removal statute because no "public use" is present. The basic purpose of the public use requirement—to prevent governmental excesses by disallowing condemnation where the object is a purely private gain—would not be disserved by a statute under which all of society stands to gain. [A]lthough no more than one person could receive a particular organ, every member of the public would have a right to receive cadaver material if he were in need of it.

. . . The last, but perhaps the thorniest issue . . . concerns "just compensation." [T]he next of kin appears to have a compensable claim whenever the deceased's organ is removed; the question is, how is this claim to be assessed?

Traditionally, when the property taken has an ascertainable market value, this value has been employed to determine the amount of compensation. When no market value exists, the courts have allowed the "intrinsic" value of the property to be shown. This value may be determined by considering such criteria as age of property, condition, location, original cost and adaptability. A variation of this rule is the "value to the owner test," which takes into account the owner's personal use for the property.

Unfortunately the market, intrinsic, and personal value tests are all basically tests of economic value and are practically impossible to

* 69 *Columbia Law Review* 693, 695–696, 699–703, 705 (1969). Reprinted by permission.

apply to commodities such as cadaver organs which have never been bought and sold. . . .

*   *   *

. . . The involuntary removal of the organs, will, at least in the beginning, inflict a disproportionate burden on some individuals. Although the burden is in the form of an injury to the emotions of the next of kin, the law has traditionally carved out a special niche for this kind of emotional distress. Thus, although mental anguish is not an item of damages in most breach of contract actions, it has been compensable when the breach occurred in a contract for burial.

Similarly, the involuntary removal of a cadaver organ should entitle the next of kin to compensation. Since the exact amount would be difficult to ascertain, the statute itself should provide for it. It would be relatively simple, for example, to set a schedule of fees—perhaps varying in amount with the nearness of the relationship between the survivor and the deceased.

Freedom of Religion

The first amendment forbids the enactment of laws which "prohibit" the free exercise of religion. At least one article has suggested that a compulsory removal statute may pose "grave constitutional problems respecting freedom of religion." And it is likely that some religious sects will be able to show that their doctrines command them to bury the dead intact.

Statutes which run afoul of the free exercise clause may burden religious practices either directly or indirectly. . . . Direct infringement occurs when a law forbids the individual to engage in practices which are required by his religious beliefs. One of the best known cases involving such a statute was *Reynolds* v. *United States.* At issue was the conviction of a Mormon under a statute which prohibited polygamy in federal territories. Although Mormons were *required* at that time to practice polygamy under "penalty [of] damnation" the Court upheld the conviction. After consideration of the adverse social consequences of polygamy, the Court held that no exception need be made for those motivated by religious belief.

*   *   *

An indirect infringement on free exercise, on the other hand, occurs when a statute makes it more difficult or expensive to be faithful to a set of beliefs, although no religious practices are proscribed. The test which the Supreme Court applies when determining the validity of such a statute was set out in *Braunfeld* v. *Brown.* In *Braunfeld,* an Orthodox Jewish merchant contended that a Sunday closing law forced him to choose between forsaking his faith by keeping his business open on Saturday or going out of business. The Supreme Court found that a burden was clearly placed on free exercise, but it held, nevertheless, that the statute was constitutional. The Court established the following rule:

[I]f the State regulates conduct by enacting a general law within its power, the purpose and effect of which is to advance the State's secular goals, the statute is valid despite its indirect burden on religious observance unless the State may accomplish its purpose by means which do not impose such a burden.

*   *   *

Assuming that legitimate religious objections were raised to the application of a compulsory organ removal statute, it is clear that the kind of burden created by such a law would be a direct one. If an individual believed that his faith required that he be buried intact, the statute would not merely make it difficult or expensive to follow this religious command; it would make it impossible. In determining the statute's validity the courts would look to the state interest in bringing about the desired result of the statute. Presumably, this would involve a finding that a state could reasonably see a need for a large supply of organs and that procurement of cadaver material is a proper area of state concern. There can be no doubt that both findings could eventually be made. However, the problem with a statute of this type is that although it directly burdens religious practices, it does not reflect any state policy in favor of eliminating these practices. Therefore, exceptions need not thwart state policy. In this way the statute resembles those which indirectly burden free exercise and, perhaps, will be made subject to the same test of validity. If that is the case, the states adopting such a law would have to show that they could not obtain an adequate number of organs without treading on religious practices.

*   *   *

The ultimate resolution of this issue will not be easy; the competing interests are unusually strong and emotion-laden. A legislature should not, however, hide behind the Constitution and fail to face the essentially ethical question presented. Neither the first nor fifth amendment is a bar to the compulsory taking of organs. Whether enough public support could be mustered to pass such a law is an open question. . . . The burden rests on the medical profession to acquaint the public with the acuteness of the problem. The point must be made that a death resulting from the unavailability of an organ is neither inevitable nor must it be viewed simply as a statistical occurrence. It must be seen for what it is in fact: a senseless tragedy which could be avoided by overcoming needlessly restrictive taboos. . . .

NOTE

CODE OF VIRGINIA
AUTHORITY OF CHIEF MEDICAL EXAMINER
OR DEPUTIES TO PROVIDE ORGANS FOR
TRANSPLANT (1970)

§ 19.1–46.1 In any case where a patient is in immediate need for an internal organ as a transplant, the Chief Medical Examiner or his deputies where a decedent comes under their jurisdiction, who may provide a suitable organ for transplant and there is insufficient time to contact the next of kin of the decedent in order to maintain the viability of the organ to be transplanted, and no known objection by the next of kin is foreseen by the Chief Medical Examiner or his deputies . . . may in their discretion where providing the organ for transplant will not interfere with subsequent course of the investigation or autopsy provide such organ on the request of the transplanting surgeon.

b.

Who Should Participate, within What Structure, in Professional Regulation?

[i]
Liz Roman Gallese
Medical–Ethics Panels Are Set Up
to Resolve Dilemmas on Research*

*   *   *

In some cases . . . researchers trying to achieve medical breakthroughs are coming into sharp conflict with ethics committees worried about patients' welfare. After several years of conflict, Dr. Adrian Kantrowitz, a noted heart surgeon, left Maimonides Medical Center in Brooklyn late last year for Sinai Hospital in De-

---

* *The Wall Street Journal* 1, col. 6; 17, col. 3 (April 14, 1971). Reprinted by permission of *The Wall Street Journal.*

troit. With him went a group of 20 surgeons, nurses and researchers and $2,500,000 of federal funds for heart research.

"I was ready to perform a heart transplant a year or so before Dr. Christiaan Barnard (the South African physician)," Dr. Kantrowitz says. But the Maimonides ethics committee refused to grant approval because "it had never been done before," Dr. Kantrowitz contends. When the committee finally approved the proposal about a year later, he says, Dr. Barnard had already done the world's first heart transplant, on Dec. 3, 1967. Dr. Kantrowitz did his first heart transplant three days after Dr. Barnard's operation.

Dr. Jacques Sherman, acting director of Maimonides, denies Dr. Kantrowitz's description of events and says his transplant proposal was approved a year or so before he performed the operation.

Another and more recent clash at Maimonides involved Dr. Kantrowitz's attempts to use a mechanical pump to aid in bringing heart attack patients out of shock. The mechanical pump was to supplement the heart's own pumping action.

"There's usually a 95 per cent mortality rate for these patients, but I was able to bring 60 per cent of them out of shock," although not all of them survived, Dr. Kantrowitz says. After initial experiments, the Maimonides ethics committee rejected further work "because I couldn't save all my patients," Dr. Kantrowitz says.

Again Dr. Sherman of Maimonides differs. He says the ethics committee rejected the research only at first because the proposal failed to contain an adequate definition of heart patients in shock. He adds that once the proposal was rewritten, it was approved.

*   *   *

NOTES

NOTE 1.

LYMAN A. BREWER, III
CARDIAC TRANSPLANTATION—AN APPRAISAL*

*   *   *

The great difficulty in obtaining donors for cardiac transplantation makes the future of cardiac transplant appear to be very limited. When one considers the fact that about a million people die of heart disease each year in this country, the potential need for cardiac trans-

---

* 205 *Journal of the American Medical Association* 691–692 (1968). Reprinted by permission.

plants appears to be great. Yet many of them would not be suitable subjects for this surgery. And too, if cardiac transplantation develops beyond the present experimental stage and becomes one of proved worth, then enormous moral problems would arise: Who would get the seldom available transplant? This is a problem that should be solved by clinicians and not lay groups. In emergency and disaster situations, the doctors traditionally decide who should be operated on first, who should receive the blood transfusion, or special attention, and so forth. Thus, there has always been a reliance upon the basic wisdom and integrity of the physician. Lay boards, the clergy, government commissions, and hospital administrators will be less well qualified to make these awesome decisions.

*   *   *

In the last analysis, it is preferable that the medical profession control circumstances under which cardiac transplants are performed. Rigid laws passed by the legislature, rules laid down by legal and clerical boards or other lay groups, might becloud rather than clear the atmosphere. The medical profession should seek and be cognizant of the opinions of these other segments of society so that no phase of the problem will be overlooked. However, the sine qua non of the practice of medicine is integrity of the physician and the surgeon in treating the patient. Without it, the filling-in of forms and reports to comply with rigid rules and to justify the operative procedure is meaningless. . . .

*   *   *

NOTE 2.
FRED ANDERSON
WHO WILL DECIDE WHO IS TO LIVE?*

*   *   *

Physicians maintain that uniquely medical questions are involved here, that they should be answered by those whom training and professional insight have equipped to provide the correct answers. In the exercise of their duty they feel that they are hampered by the intrusions of lay people (chiefly journalists and lawyers) who misunderstand both the high standards of medical practice involved and the unique qualities of judgment that physicians possess. . . . But in

choosing between two housewives with defunct kidneys, who are in the same general state of health, is a physician more competent than a layman to select one for dialysis? Even the medical staff at one Seattle hospital does not think so; there, a lay panel decides.

As needless as the encroachment may seem, if we are to establish decision-making procedures that point to the best use of the advances of medical science, physicians must face more and more challenges to their absolute right to decide. What to physicians may appear to be the most specialized advances, thus definitely medical in nature, may present society with the broadest kind of fundamental problems. This is not to say that after policy decisions are argued out in committees, on public forums and if necessary before legislatures, that a committee should decide whether to turn off respirators. Nothing could be worse than to bureaucratize and diffuse decisions even more than they already are in this early team-age society. But there are ways to educate individual decision-makers, or to threaten them, or to encourage them to consult a variety of persons before shouldering individual responsibility.

The opinion of the Harvard committee on brain death is not clearly right or wrong; the question is still open, and before it can be answered adequately the best thoughts of many, including theologians, philosophers, economists and jurists, along with physicians, must be heard. . . .

*   *   *

NOTE 3.
DELFORD L. STICKEL
MEDICOLEGAL AND ETHICAL ASPECTS
OF ORGAN TRANSPLANTATION*

*   *   *

. . . The usual approach to . . . difficult decisions is that of consultation to obtain more than one medical opinion, and in some circumstances it is legally required that multiple concurring opinions be documented. Further medical and scientific advances conceivably will eventually reduce the determination of time of death to a simple set of criteria that will be applicable to all pronouncements of death. If such criteria are generally established and used in everyday medical practice as the standard basis for pronouncing

* The New Republic 9, 10 (April 19, 1969). Reprinted by permission of The New Republic. © 1969, Harrison-Blaine of New Jersey, Inc.

* 169 Annals of the New York Academy of Sciences 362, 365–366 (1970). © The New York Academy of Sciences, 1970. Reprinted by permission.

death and are widely accepted legally and by the general public, then the exercise of judgment will be less crucial than it presently is. Until such criteria are developed, however, there appears to be no alternative to securing and documenting multiple concurring medical opinions to support the judgment rendered in situations deemed at present to be too crucial to be left to one person. In practice, it is difficult to document multiple opinions in situations that arise on short notice, as is the case with many vital organ donations; but such difficulties probably are surmountable.

As a backup of consultation prior to the fact, review after the fact is common practice in hospitals. Examples, of course, are clinicopathological conferences, review of surgical cases by tissue committees, deaths and complications conferences, and case reviews in service or departmental conferences. Such retrospective case reviews undoubtedly exercise a favorable influence on the quality of medical judgment and patient care. It may be appropriate now to add a hospital committee for the review of the terminal care and the determination of time of death of patients who actually became or who were considered as possible vital organ donors. Ideally, such a committee should include representation of the transplant team, the physician who attended the donor as a patient, and physicians with responsibility for neither donor nor recipient.

*   *   *

NOTE 4.

LEO ALEXANDER
ETHICAL AND LEGAL BASE LINES FOR
PROFESSIONS AND COMMUNITY*

*   *   *

[T]he great safeguard in the thousands of years since Hippocrates has been the mutual approval and dependence of the physicians on the medical scientists. . . . Now, apparently, we have lost this safeguard.

At one time I thought it was due to the intervention of a third party—the state or organizations such as drug companies—and the intrusion of their interests. Are we now asking for other third-party intrusion? We evidently want to balance one third-party intrusion, the governmental and the commercial interest, with another

third-party intrusion, somebody who can look over our shoulders and give us their advice.

[T]he one person who I believe bears the ethical crux in this situation, and who should never be asked, is the patient's relative. Such a request would place an intolerable burden of guilt upon him. Dr. Visscher has pointed out very clearly the problem of relatives' urging the doctor to "pull the plug." I believe this is dangerous, and I would stand above that. I believe that such a decision must be made by the doctor, alone with his God and his conscience.

As a psychiatrist, I can say that if relatives ask him to pull the plug, he must never do it on that basis. That would place a burden of lifetime guilt upon them. No person will be able to bear that. The doctor must have the courage to bear that guilt if he ever chooses to do as suggested, in view of the tenets of our sacred profession.

At one time the doctor was supposed to have direct authority from the Lord, just like the priest, and, I think, very rightfully, because there are certain decisions a doctor must have the courage to make by himself.

In my own personal practice, I've taken care of many people. I never actually "pulled the plug;" it was never necessary, because death always comes soon enough. There are some impatient relatives, naturally, but I wouldn't play along with them at all. . . . But certainly the last person I would ever let make a decision is a relative; that would be dangerous.

In other words, if I were ever tempted to pull out the intravenous apparatus, it would be to save the patient's veins; I would never let the relatives believe otherwise; that would be a great mistake. . . .

NOTE 5.

FRANCIS D. MOORE
GIVE AND TAKE*

*   *   *

[T]here is always the ethical and humane problem involved in the exploration of any new field of medical or surgical treatment. Mortality has been very high in certain kinds of homotransplantations. It is not enough to tell the patient that "there is no other hope." If he is in full possession of his faculties, he should be given a clear picture of the hazards involved, and allowed to

* 169 *Annals of the New York Academy of Sciences* 334–335 (1970). © The New York Academy of Sciences, 1970. Reprinted by permission.

* Garden City, N.Y.: Doubleday and Co., Inc. 166 (1964). Reprinted by permission of W. B. Saunders Co.

join in the decision. Yet under no circumstances should the final decision be left in the hands of the patient; he has not the education, background, nor dispassionate view necessary to make a decision in his own best self-interest. The doctor must take the time and trouble to help educate the patient far enough along the road, so that when the patient joins in the decision, he does so with some idea of the alternatives. It is up to the doctor to advise, and to seek the patient's consent.

* * *

NOTE 6.

Leon R. Kass
A Caveat on Transplants*

* * *

Although there have always been deaths that occurred because the physician was occupied with another patient, the health of an individual has rarely depended necessarily on the demise of another. This has acutely troubled physicians involved in kidney transplants. One surgeon, whose work involves a search for potential donors of kidneys for his clients, said of himself: "I am the vulture hiding at the foot of the bed."

However, most doctors will more or less easily accommodate this tension. They are prepared by their familiarity with death, by their sound judgment about when dying is irreversible and by their clear sense of the value of transplantation.

The dying patient and his family have different problems. Is everything reasonable being done to save the patient, to return him to a more than vegetating condition? Confidence of the patient in his doctor and in his chances for recovery are important for the patient's will to recover and sometimes for the recovery itself. Even when —or perhaps especially when—recovery is impossible, it would be reprehensible to add to the pain and grief the suspicion that the dying patient was being sacrificed for his value as spare parts.

Joshua Lederberg has clearly stated the problem: "We must preserve the confidence of every patient that his physician's dedication to his welfare is uncontaminated by the patient's utility as a biological resource for some other, possibly worthier patient."

---

* *The Washington Post* B-1, cols. 2–3 (January 14, 1968). © 1968, *The Washington Post*. Reprinted by permission.

But we must go further than Lederberg. We must consider the consequences of transplantation of vital organs for society at large. Lederberg expresses a concern for the preservation of confidence; he is discussing the image of the doctor. I would add that we must insure that the confidence remains deserved, that we must also preserve the truthfulness of that image. We must see to it that no doctor indeed sacrifices his patient's welfare for the sake of his utility as a source of spare parts.

That such practices might be likely under tyrannical regimes is of course obvious, but our society is not immune. Consider the possibility that a high-ranking Government official suffers a massive heart attack and requires a new heart to survive. Might not even the best of physicians be tempted to ease up on the treatment of a critically ill patient deemed less worthy?

Is it too far-fetched to imagine that people might be asked to step forward and volunteer their organs under these circumstances? If no volunteers were available, would mercy-killing or murder be excusable in order to provide a new heart for the statesman? If we are willing to send men involuntarily to their death in battle for the welfare of their country, is it not conceivable that we may someday expand that notion of the general welfare to include the health of our leaders?

* * *

[ii]
Executive Committee of the International Society of Cardiology Statement on Announcement of Cardiovascular Experiments*

Since the time of Hippocrates, the medical profession has preserved the ethics governing the extent of the information conveyed to the public at large and the way in which it is conveyed. With the availability today of modern media for mass communication there is a greater need to ensure that such information is spread in a responsible manner.

We deplore the fact that in recent times medical and surgical experiments have become matters of public entertainment and even sensationalism. Such a trend can only bring discredit to the profession as a whole and indirectly misrepresent to the public, who are not in a position to judge the implication of such developments,

---

* *News from the International Society of Cardiology* 8–9 (July 1968). Reprinted by permission.

the dangers and limitations inseparable from such procedures in their initial phase.

While it is not possible to control the behaviour of those who seek instant publicity, the Council of the International Society of Cardiology feels that a lead must be given by responsible members of the profession. One method of ensuring more ethical behaviour and avoiding extremes of anxiety or misplaced hope is to suggest strongly that no new procedures, either medical or surgical, are released to the lay press before being published in the reputable medical journals after full scientific evaluation.

* * *

NOTE

RENÉE C. FOX
A SOCIOLOGICAL PERSPECTIVE ON ORGAN
TRANSPLANTATION AND HEMODIALYSIS*

* * *

The degree and kind of attention that the mass media have accorded to organ transplantation has served a number of functions. It has publicized the need for live and cadaver donors, introduced the lay public to the new conception of "brain death," and helped families and local communities to raise funds for prospective organ recipients. In the opinion of at least one investigator, by dramatizing unsolved medical problems, most notably rejection reactions and tissue typing, the press has helped to interest more researchers to work in these areas. However, the extensive, often theatrical coverage of transplantation has also created certain problems for the medical profession and for the recipients and donors involved. It has invaded the confidentiality and privacy to which the physician and patient, individually and collectively, are ethically entitled. It has encouraged physicians, or put them under pressure, to report their clinical trials to the lay public before submitting them to the trained judgment and criticism of colleagues through channels such as professional publications. In the eyes of some physicians, it has facilitated self-advertising, competition, and commercialized behavior on the part of certain members of the profession in ways that many feel violate the universalism, disinterestedness, and collectivity-orientation of the medical and scientific community. Furthermore, numerous

medical spokesmen have expressed the opinion that the publicity transplantations have received may have "misled" the general public in two key regards. On the one hand, it may have given them a "too optimistic" impression of the present state and promises of transplantation; on the other, by excessively emphasizing the role of the physician as a "taker of organs," it may have undermined public trust in his function of healer and guardian of life. ("Can anyone ever again be sure that physicians will do all that can be done to save him rather than regard him as a potential spare-parts supermarket?")

c.

Should Research Design and Scientific Merits Be Evaluated?

[i]
*Board on Medicine of the National Academy of Sciences
Statement on Cardiac Transplantation**

Progress in medicine depends largely on the cautious extension to man of a body of carefully integrated knowledge derived from programs of basic and developmental research in the laboratory. Extension to man is itself an investigative process that must meet the same meticulous scientific standards that obtain in the laboratory, and the extension can appropriately be started only when the total body of knowledge has reached a certain point. It is clear that this point has been reached in the case of cardiac transplantation.

* * *

[I]t is the considered view of the Board on Medicine of the National Academy of Sciences

* 169 *Annals of the New York Academy of Sciences* 406, 421–422 (1970). © The New York Academy of Sciences, 1970. Reprinted by permission.

* Walsh McDermott, M.D., Chairman. 18 *News Report of National Academy of Sciences* 1–3 (March 1968). Reprinted by permission. [The National Academy of Sciences is an organization of distinguished scientists and engineers devoted to the furtherance of science and its use for human welfare. Although it is not a government agency, it is called upon by its Congressional charter of 1863 to serve as an official adviser to the federal government in matters of science and technology. The Board on Medicine was formed by the Academy in November 1967 to study the social functions of medicine. It is composed of two biologists, a biophysicist, a psychologist, two economists, a lawyer, a nurse, and fourteen physicians, among them the president of the American Medical Association, the director of the National Institutes of Health, and a number of medical school deans.]

that, for the present, cardiac transplantation should only be carried out in those institutions in which all of the following criteria can be met:

1. The surgical team should have had extensive laboratory experience in cardiac transplantation, and should have demonstrated not only technical competence but a thorough understanding of the biological processes that threaten functional survival of the transplant, i.e., rejection and its control. Investigators skilled in immunology, including tissue typing and the management of immunosuppressive procedures, should be readily available as collaborators in the transplantation effort.

2. As in any other scientific investigation, the overall plan of study should be carefully recorded in advance and arrangements made to continue the systematic observations throughout the whole lifetime of the recipient. The conduct of such studies should be within an organized framework of information exchange and analyses. This would permit prompt access by other investigators to the full positive and negative results. Thus the continued care of each recipient would be assured the continuing benefit of the most up-to-date information. Such an organized communication network would also permit the findings to be integrated with the work of others and assist in the planning of further investigative efforts. In this way, it would be possible to ensure that progress will be deliberate and that the experience from each individual case will make its full contribution to the planning of the next.

3. As the procedure is a scientific investigation and not as yet an accepted form of therapy, the primary justification for this activity in respect to both the donor and recipient is that from the study will come new knowledge of benefit to others in our society. The ethical issues involved in the selection of donor and recipient are a part of the whole complex question of the ethics of human experimentation. This extremely sensitive and complicated subject is now under intensive study by a number of well-qualified groups in this country and abroad. Pending the further development of ethical guidelines, it behooves each institution in which a cardiac transplantation is to be conducted to assure itself that it has protected the interests of all parties involved to the fullest possible extent.

Rigid safeguards should be developed with respect to the selection of prospective donors and the selection of prospective recipients. An independent group of expert, mature physicians— none of whom is directly engaged in the transplantation effort—should examine the prospective donor. They should agree and record their unanimous opinion as to the donor's acceptability on the basis of the evidence of crucial and irreversible bodily damage and imminent death. Similarly the prospective recipient should be examined by an independent group of competent physicians and clinical scientists including a cardiologist and an expert in immunology. In this instance the consulting group should also record their opinion as to the acceptability of the recipient for transplantation on the basis of all the evidence including the presence of far advanced, irreversible cardiac damage and the likelihood of benefit from the procedure.

Enumeration of the above criteria is based on the conviction that in order to obtain the scientific information necessary for the next phase in this form of organ transplantation, only a relatively small number of careful investigations involving cardiac transplantation need be done at this time. Therefore, the Board strongly urges that institutions, even though well equipped from the standpoint of surgical expertise and facilities but without specific capabilities to conduct the whole range of scientific observations involved in the total study, resist the temptation to approve the performance of the surgical procedure until there has been an opportunity for the total situation to be clarified by intensive and closely integrated study.

NOTE

Lyman A. Brewer, III
Cardiac Transplantation—An Appraisal*

* * *

The scientific data accumulated concerning the cardiac transplant should be released first through regular medical channels, medical journals and meetings, and not handed out to the lay press for prior presentation.

Because cardiac transplantation is technically no more difficult than some current cardiac operations, many cardiac surgeons may be tempted to perform this procedure, since it is well within their technical grasp. This being true, it is hoped that the operation will never be performed as a status symbol to the surgical team or hospital embarking on this surgery. Nothing

---

* 205 *Journal of the American Medical Association* 691, 692 (1968). Reprinted by permission.

would cause more discredit to the procedure in particular and to surgery in general than the precipitous plunging of many surgical teams in the United States and throughout the world into this type of surgery with its high mortality and uncertain future. Certainly, however, at this stage of development of this operation, it is inadvisable to have a regulating board to determine the surgical and research capabilities of the surgical team and institution. Rather should the innate ethical and surgical good sense and temperate professional restraint in each cardiac group prevail.

* * *

[ii]
Allen S. Fox
Heart Transplants—Treatment or Experiment*

Time magazine [29 Dec.] quotes Christiaan Barnard, with regard to the Washkansky heart transplant, as follows: "I wouldn't like to call this operation an experiment—it was treatment of a sick patient. Although Washkansky died, I don't think we have any evidence that transplantation is not good treatment for certain heart diseases." There are serious reasons to question the validity of the first of these assertions; the second is not much more than a general expression of faith.

Two different kinds of problems must be solved before transplantation surgery may be regarded as treatment rather than experiment. The first is that of surgical technique. . . . Actual performance of the Washkansky operation was not needed to know that Barnard and his associates, or other similar groups, had reached the point in experience, skill, daring, and sophistication to carry it out with technical success.

The second problem, that of overcoming the genetic barrier to transplantation, is the more critical one. . . .

There are ways . . . of minimizing the histocompatibility barrier. Matching of red blood cell types is elementary. Matching with respect to transplantation antigens is more pertinent to this discussion. This is most conveniently accomplished by the detection of individual leukocyte antigens with suitable isoimmune antiserums (leukocyte typing) or by the use of matching tests such as mixed leukocyte cultures (MLC typing). The results of both of these kinds of

tests are at least partially predictive of transplantation success. . . .

Although a full scientific report of the Washkansky case is not yet available, sufficient information has been provided by the press to make an evaluation with respect to this second problem. The importance of the sex difference between donor and recipient cannot be evaluated. Apparently red blood cell typing was performed in advance of the operation. Apparently, also, limited leukocyte typing was performed, but not until after the operation had been initiated. One may infer from press reports that MLC or other matching tests were not performed. Obviously no prior attempt was made to match donor and recipient with respect to transplantation antigens. There is every indication from available information that they were actually incompatible, as most unrelated donor-recipient combinations would be if chosen at random.

Under these circumstances massive immunosuppression and radiation were judged to be required and were applied. It is not surprising, therefore, that the patient died of pneumonia. One must conclude that the histocompatibility problem was not dealt with in the Washkansky case, even within available limits. The operation should not be justified as treatment, and if it was an experiment it must be judged as premature and poorly designed. . . .

* * *

d.

Should Consent Be Supervised?

[i]
He Had a New Heart for a Week and Didn't Know It*

The 23-year-old, happy-go-lucky cowboy had journeyed hundreds of weary miles east from Brazil's harsh Mato Grosso plateau. Dressed in rags one morning last April, pain hammering at his heart, João Ferreira da Cunha joined hundreds of poor who arrive daily between 4 A.M. and 6 A.M. at São Paulo's Hospital das Clínicas for free treatment.

A highly qualified surgical team, including one doctor who had worked at Dr. Christiaan Barnard's side for a week in South Africa, picked the cowboy out of the throng for South America's first heart transplant, performed May 26th.

But, medical observers close to the scene now contend, the illiterate da Cunha agreed to the operation without beginning to comprehend its nature or seriousness. A week afterwards, sitting up in his bed and strumming his guitar, he heard a news broadcast detailing the recovery of a celebrity with his name. The young patient turned to his nurse and asked, "Who is the radio talking about?" The nurse replied, "Why, it is you!" Da Cunha was amazed.

*   *   *

Fully informed consent was impossible in da Cunha's case, say his doctors. Asked whether the team could give him a new heart, he said, "Yes, anything to stop the pain," apparently without understanding at all what the operation meant.

Afterwards, still unaware of his precarious condition, da Cunha joyously rose from his bed on June 17th and walked about his hospital room. His heart went into fibrillation almost immediately. After repeated crises, he died on June 22nd. Autopsy disclosed that his body had not rejected the heart. Rather, a clot had formed in an iliac vein, had been carried to the right ventricle, and lodged in the bifurcation of the pulmonary trunk, causing heart failure.

*   *   *

[T]he Brazilian surgeons point out at the same time that no ethical questions are raised by da Cunha's lack of informed consent. If a man is incapable of understanding an operation he vitally needs, they say, there is no choice but to proceed. And there has been no outcry in the Brazilian medical community. In an underdeveloped nation, illiteracy and ignorance are common. Besides, add the surgeons, da Cunha was psychologically better off not knowing and worrying about his risks.

*   *   *

[ii]
Barney G. Glaser and Anselm L. Strauss
Awareness of Dying*

*   *   *

Our conception . . . of a patient's response to direct disclosure is based largely on our inter-

---

* Chicago: Aldine Publishing Co. 122–123, 130–132, 185–193 (1965). Copyright © 1965 by Barney G. Glaser and Anselm L. Strauss. Reprinted by permission of Aldine · Atherton, Inc.

views with patients, doctors, and nurses in the cancer wards of a Veterans' Administration Hospital. In this hospital the normal procedure is to tell every patient the nature of his illness; as a result, many patients are told of a fatal illness.

By and large the patients in these wards are in their middle or late years, of lower-class status, and in destitute circumstances. Since their case is free, they are captive patients—they have little or no control over their treatment, and if they do not cooperate their care may be stopped. If a man goes "AWOL" the hospital is not obliged to readmit him, or if it does readmit him, it can punish him by denying privileges. Because the patients lack financial resources, they typically have no alternative to their current "free" care, and lower-class status accustoms them to accepting or to being intimidated into following orders from people of higher status. Since these captive lower-class patients cannot effectively threaten the hospital or the doctors, the rule at this hospital is to disclose terminality regardless of the patient's expected reaction. . . .

*   *   *

Disclosure of fatal illness to patients in this hospital has two major characteristics. First, the patient is told that he is certain to die, but not when he will die. . . .

Second, the doctors typically do not give details of the illness, and the type of patient under consideration usually does not ask for them. Primarily, this is a problem of communication: a doctor finds it hard to explain the illness to a working-class patient, while lack of familiarity with the technical terms, as well as a more general deference to the doctor, inhibits the patient's impulse to question him. In addition, not giving details is a tactic doctors use to avoid or cut down on talk with the patient and to leave him quickly. . . .

*   *   *

Some patients accept their fatal illness but decide to *fight* it. Unlike denial behavior, this fight indicates an initial acceptance of one's fate together with a positive desire to somehow change it. . . .

*   *   *

The search for a way to fight the fatal illness can . . . lead a patient into a clinical experiment. If he does not win his own battle, he at least may help future patients with theirs. The chance to contribute to medical science does not, however, sustain the motivation of *all* research patients. Some, realizing things are hopeless for themselves and finding the experimental regime too rigorous to bear, try to extricate themselves from the experiment. If the doctors decide to carry on anyway, these patients sometimes interfere with the experiment by pulling tubes out, by not taking medicine, or by taking an extra drink of water. Some attempt auto-euthanasia.

* * *

Although it contradicts the usual priorities in patient care, a patient dying in a medically "interesting" way, or suffering from an "interesting" condition, may receive special attention as an object of study and as a teaching "case." This increased attention does not necessarily make the unaware patient suspicious. He may feel that his chances of recovery are improved by the attention of so many doctors. The unaware family, too, may become very hopeful when they find numerous experts concerned with the patient's condition.

Hope for the patient wanes, however, and even turns to high suspicion if his case is so "interesting" that the doctors decide to keep him alive "for the rest of the semester" and start applying various kinds of equipment to prolong life. Medical equipment can be one of the surest indicators to patients and families that death is certain, but is being delayed. Once aware of dying, the patient may then have to ask for his own death, to put a stop to undue prolonging. A nurse told of a patient who was "kept alive for over three weeks on a pacemaker for teaching purposes." This was so hard on both the patient and her family that the patient, knowing she would die, told the doctor to stop the pacemaker. She was dead within thirty-six hours.

* * *

The goal of recovery, with its high priority for the doctor's attention, can be reinstated, at least provisionally, by enrolling the dying patient in a clinical research project. In general, the basic legitimate condition for this proposal is the doctor's absolute certainty that, given present knowledge, there is "nothing more to do" for the patient in any available hospital. (For patients with sufficient personal financial resources, "available" hospitals may include those in Brit-

ain, France, and Germany.) At this time, the family and patient must be presented with the facts of "nothing more to do," even if they were hitherto unaware. Then they are given the alternative: to risk the research with its promise of recovery, however slight. The negative side effects of the treatment or drug are not always presented. If the patient is adult and sentient, he must consent in writing; otherwise a family member must consent. Sometimes, however, "captive" patients are put on a study drug unawares. Parents who "donate" their child often do so without letting the child know that he is dying, so that the closed awareness context is maintained, at least in the beginning.

Recruitment into research is timed according to the current type of death expectation and the availability of a testable treatment. Among patients in the "nothing more to do" phase there are more potential research *cases* than research experiments. A cancer patient, for instance, certain to die, may have been lingering for months when a new chemical drug to be tested is sent from the National Institutes of Health to the hospital; the patient is then asked to be a research case, with, if necessary, an attendant change in his awareness. Unaware patients and families may be converted to awareness for naught, if they do not agree to the experiment. The longer a patient lives in the "nothing more to do" phase, the more likely it is that an effort to recruit him for research purposes will occur which may alter his own and his family's awareness.

On the other hand, sometimes an experiment requires waiting until a particular dying patient has reached the "nothing more to do" phase. Having watched the patient closely, until they are virtually certain of his impending death, doctors negotiate with patient or family immediately to try a new drug or a transplant, for example....

* * *

For patients who are *not* to be recruited for research, however, especially when experiments with a high probability of saving the patient are going on at the hospital, doctors have a stake in maintaining a closed awareness context for both patient and family. For, if the family became aware that the patient was certain to die, they might demand that the patient be given the experimental drug or that the new machine be tried. Since for most experiments, resources are limited, there are not enough chances to go around. This situation becomes even more difficult for the doctors when the news media make known that a new machine or drug with great promise is being tested. In a university medical center, of course, both the facilities for research and the pressure to give a patient a chance to participate are much greater than they are elsewhere.

A patient can also volunteer for basic rather than clinical research. In basic research the objective is to find possible cures, not to test potential ones, so there is no implicit change back to the goal of recovery. Yet for a lingering patient the hope is always present that "his" project will succeed in finding a cure, and he will be the first subject to recover. Thus, some people volunteer to continue their dying at the National Institutes of Health, for example, where basic research is done along with clinical research.

In clinical research, the chief drawback for all concerned is that it takes time, and this means that for some patients life will be unduly prolonged. Once committed to the research, the patient and his family are expected to see it through to the end. Certainly most research doctors are highly committed; generally, their attitude was, "If it is a study, we go all out." One doctor did say, "If a patient is in the study and *near death,* we provide ordinary treatment. Don't use extra measures just because they are in the study. If he is in agony, I wouldn't keep a man alive just because of a study."

Nurses, on the other hand, tend to go along with research in the beginning, but their collective mood in response to undue prolonging is "Why not let him die?" When the doctors continue to prolong the patient's life, the nurses often feel frustrated by their helplessness in being unable to let him die. Occasionally they refuse to acknowledge the legitimacy of the research effort—the well-being of future patients—suspecting that the research patient is really being exploited for personal career purposes, and making statements like: "They keep them alive until the research report is written." Yet, the nurses remain helpless since, as one put it, "Usually you hate to say anything like, 'Why not let him die?' "

Resolution of this problem of unduly extending research patients' lives often depends on the awareness context. If the patient is unaware, as in the case of a child committed by his parents, or a comatose adult, then family members must decide. This is not an easy decision to make, because often they can see the possible benefit to future patients and so feel morally obligated to

allow an indefinite prolonging. As one nurse said, "The mother felt obligated, if it teaches them something."

Aware patients react to prospective prolonging according to their death expectation—whether they think of themselves as lingering (time of death unknown) or believe that without excessive staff effort they would die quickly. A patient who thinks he will linger anyway may expect the research to make a possibly uncomfortable fate less so; hence he will probably stay with the study. But if he feels that the research is increasing his discomfort, he may ask to be released from it so that he can live out his last weeks in comfort. A patient, who is aware that without research medication or equipment he will die quickly, must weigh this against the pain of having his life prolonged, and decide accordingly. Again, this is a difficult decision to make, and a patient's intention to remain in the study is always subject to reversal.

Because the equipment necessary to prolong life may be so elaborate, many research patients readily become aware that death would come within a few hours or days if they were not in the project. Thus, when prolonging becomes very painful, the patient is apt to lose any moral commitment to the research he might have had, abandon any prospect of recovery, and want simply to be left alone to die. A basic principle in clinical research is that a subject should be allowed to withdraw when he feels that continuation is mentally and physically impossible. But this principle is most appropriately applied to clinical research patients who are either not certain to die, or who are expected to linger on fairly comfortably for weeks or months. They have a moral right to save themselves discomfort; imminent death is not the issue.

A patient expected to die quickly if released from the experiment, on the other hand, may find it difficult to get out of the research if he is not in undue pain. The doctors' point of view may be that his comfort, to be attained through his imminent death, is less important than the success of the experiment if it can be achieved in a few more days or a week. A patient in this situation can withdraw most easily by having his family request it, but family members are not always willing to do this. Much as they might like to help the patient, they may be influenced by the potential benefits to medicine in prolonging his life, or they may still harbor the hope that recovery is a real possibility. If the patient negotiates for dismissal, doctors, who tend to be highly committed to the research, usually try to persuade him to go on with the research, using the idea that it is better than immediate death.

A patient who succumbs to a doctor's argument, however, may have second thoughts after the doctor leaves and try to take measures into his own hands, in spite of his personal obligation to the doctor and the potential benefits to mankind. One research patient, having recovered from the side effects of chemotherapy, was sent back for more. He asked the nurse to remove his restraints, and she agreed, saying they would be ordered back on in the morning. The patient nodded that he understood. After the nurse left the room, he wrote on a slate that he didn't want to go back for more treatment and pulled his catheter out. When the nurse returned, she found him in a pool of blood. She did, however, keep him from killing himself.

Nurses who adhere to the "let him go" belief, based on the comfort goal, try to help the research patient. They may ask the doctor indirectly why he does not let the patient die, by asking why he is prescribing a treatment—for example, tracheotomy or more blood—that will prolong life. The doctor's reply is likely to be on the order of "because he needs it!" So the nurse either must ask directly, "Why not let him die?" or must carry out her tasks of helping to prolong the patient's life, with no satisfactory answer. Other nurses—only a few—simply walk out, indicating they will not give the treatment or prepare the patient. In reply one doctor said to a departing nurse: "I think we ought to give him the blood right now!" One nurse felt morally obligated to help a patient in his struggle if he said he wanted out. She said, "When he tells me that I want to die, it is at this point that I would go right up to the doctors and say, 'Let him die.' "

As we have noted, the research proposal itself may disclose to the patient that he will die, and the change of awareness sometimes induces depression. In part, however, the proposal reinstitutes the recovery goal, and this carries a "lift" for patients whose awareness has just been transformed, as well as for those who are already aware. Indeed, an apparent reprieve often does occur in the first days or weeks of the experiment: tumors go down, transplants work, the progress of the cancer is halted, and so on. But often the new treatment eventually fails, the patient's awareness is transformed back to the "nothing more to do" phase, and his depression is all the worse because he has lost a renewed hope. . . .

3.
In Reviewing Decisions and Consequences

a.

Through Governmental Action?

*Trial to Test MD's Role in Death of Heart Donor**

The physician's role in the death of a heart transplant donor is being challenged in a Milwaukee court.

Lloyd G. Johnson, 23, has been charged with manslaughter in the death of Robert E. Buelow, 30 . . . following a fight in which Buelow struck his head on the pavement, receiving severe brain damage. Buelow was kept alive by artificial means and later his heart was transplanted into the body of Mrs. Elizabeth Anick, 49 . . . by physicians at St. Luke's Hospital, Milwaukee.

*   *   *

Johnson's attorney indicated he would maintain Johnson struck Buelow in self-defense after Buelow swung at him.

The defense also is expected to raise the question of who is acutally to blame for the death of the mortally injured heart donor—the man who caused the initial injury or the physicians who removed his heart?

Thomas Dougherty in the district attorney's office commented that the case poses some complex medical and legal questions, but he stressed that the physicians performing the operations and the hospital definitely "are not on trial."

He explained Helen Young, MD, county medical examiner, was notified by the heart surgeons of the impending operation. Dr. Young was called in before the transplant was conducted, and she talked with District Attorney David Cannon, he said. Dr. Young also participated as an observer during the actual transplant surgery.

. . . Dougherty said the official finding was that Buelow died of severe skull fracture and cerebral hemorrhage. He said the prosecutor's office does not anticipate any finding in court that the cause of death was anything other than the trauma by the blow and fall of the victim to the ground.

If the cause of death cannot be tied to the trauma, Dougherty said, there is little doubt that there is adequate foundation for the state's

---

* *AMA News* 2 (November 11, 1968). Reprinted by permission.

charge of injury by conduct regardless of life, for which the penalties are the same as manslaughter.

*   *   *

NOTE

MAN KEPT ALIVE AS KIDNEY DONOR*

At an inquest here tonight on a man who received severe head injuries in a brawl last month, a jury was told that he was kept alive for 24 hours on a respiratory machine so that one of his kidneys could be taken for transplanting in another man who was dying from kidney trouble.

The jury decided that the removal of the man's kidney had nothing to do with his death, which they accepted had been caused by brain injuries, and returned a verdict of manslaughter against Henry Hall. [He] was committed to Durham Assizes by the Coroner . . . to answer a charge of causing the death of John David Potter . . . .

Hall . . . was alleged to have admitted in a statement that he had butted Potter twice in the face. Potter had fallen backwards on to his head.

Dr. R. H. Appleby, of Newcastle General Hospital, said that about 14 hours after admission Potter stopped breathing. He was put on the machine for 24 hours.

Dr. Appleby said in his opinion when Potter ceased breathing on June 16 he had virtually died, though from the legal point of view it would be correct to say he died when the heart ceased beating and the circulation ceased to flow on June 17.

Mr. John Swinney, consultant neurological surgeon at the hospital, said he was told that Potter was technically dead and sought permission from Mrs. Potter for consent for removal of the kidney for transplanting. This was given. The Coroner said that he was asked for consent which he gave, but he had supposed that the kidney would be taken after the man's death.

*   *   *

After the kidney had been removed, the respirator was turned off and there was no spontaneous breathing or circulation. Had there been no intention of taking the kidney there would have been no point in putting Potter on the machine.

*   *   *

---

* *The London Times* 9, col. 3 (July 26, 1963). Reprinted by permission.

After the inquest, Mr. Swinney said the kidney was given to a man aged 30, who died three weeks after the operation from cerebral haemmorhage. Mr. Swinney said he felt the case had advanced medical research and that the operation could be regarded as a success.

b.

Through Public Scrutiny?

[i]

*John D. Arnold, Thomas F. Zimmerman, and Daniel C. Martin
Public Attitudes and the Diagnosis of Death**

*   *   *

By and large, there was little public concern about the subtleties involved in the diagnosis of death until the cardiac transplant became a reality. During most of the 20th century, the public has shown a nearly complete acceptance of the prevailing professional practice in regard to the diagnosis of death. This has not always been the case. If one examines the literature of the 19th century, it becomes apparent that the *diagnosis* of death has concerned a fairly large number of writers. A prominent example of this is Poe's essay on premature burial. In addition, it is possible to cite several hundred pamphlets and tracts written between 1700 and 1900 on the fallibility of the diagnosis of death. These collectively provide testimony to the existence of a public apprehension about premature burial.

The reason for this concern had to do with specific cases which came to the attention of the public. . . . T. M. Montgomery reports on the moving of the Fort Randall Cemetery in 1896:

We found among these remains, two that bore every evidence of having been buried alive. The first case was that of a soldier that [*sic*] had been struck by lightning. Upon opening the lid of the coffin, we found that the legs and arms had been drawn up as far as the confines of the coffin would permit. The other was a case of death resulting from alcoholism. The body was slightly turned, the legs were drawn up a trifle and the hands were clutching the clothing. In the coffin was found a large whisky flask. Nearly 2 per cent of those exhumed here were no doubt victims of suspended animation.

Alexander Wilder, MD, in a pamphlet entitled "Burying Alive, a Frequent Peril," mentions several cases:

---

* 206 *Journal of the American Medical Association* 1949, 1950–1954 (1968). Reprinted by permission.

One, a six-year-old boy who was exhumed after 25 years and found to have the arms bent over the skull, one leg drawn up and the other bent over it. Another case is of a man, 35, who was buried 48 hours after the diagnosis of death from scarlet fever. He was exhumed two months later. The coffin was found to have the glass front shattered, the bottom kicked out and the sides sprung. The body lay face downwards, the arms were bent and in the clenched fists were handfuls of hair.

The following notes appear in an 1877 issue of the *British Medical Journal.*

A correspondent at Naples states that the Appeals Court has had before it a case not likely to inspire confidence in the minds who look forward with horror to the possibility of being buried alive. It appeared from the evidence that some time ago, a woman was interred with all the usual formalities, it being believed that she was dead, while she was only in a trance. Some days afterwards, when the grave in which she had been placed was opened for the reception of another body, it was found that the clothes which covered the unfortunate woman were torn to pieces, and that she had even broken her limbs in attempting to extricate herself from the living tomb. The Court, after hearing the case, sentenced the doctor who had signed the certificate of decease, and the major who had authorized the internment each to three month's imprisonment for involuntary manslaughter.

Actually very little is known of the accuracy of the several methods of diagnosing death either in the 19th century or the 20th century. Except for the electrocardiogram and the electroencephalogram, it appears that medicine has acquired no new tools for determining the functional state of organs critically important in the diagnosis of death. Although the EEG and the ECG are new and sophisticated supplements to the old techniques, they are not often used today in the diagnosis of death. Except in the very recent past, medical education has appeared to be relatively indifferent to this problem. . . .

*　　*　　*

[O]f a group of hospital interns and residents, who were graduates of approximately 15 medical schools, not one could remember having been instructed in medical school concerning the requirements for the diagnosis of death. One young intern on his first real test asked the nurse for instructions.

*　　*　　*

Unlike the situation in the 19th century, the 20th century practice of embalming all persons pronounced dead has served to remove any mistakes from public view. In the 19th century, it was the public view that aroused concern. In fact, this concern may have been one of the factors leading to the introduction of embalming. In America, embalming is almost universal, although not legally required. In Europe, embalming is not so widespread, but postmortem medical examinations are. . . .

*　　*　　*

It is believed useful to make systematic attempts to assess public concern and to involve the public in a dialogue about the vital issues raised by new concepts dealing with the diagnosis of death. To this end, two preliminary studies of public attitudes and perceptions were made to give perspective to historical data. . . .

*　　*　　*

1. The public is giving thought to the issues of how death is determined. In the samples of opinion surveyed, 69 per cent responded that they had thought frequently or occasionally about the topic prior to the time of interview. There is evidence the information emanating from the mass media regarding heart transplants had stimulated much of this thought.
2. The public thinks of death in terms of cessation of cardio-pulmonary functions. Two thirds of individuals surveyed thought that death occurred when the heart stopped or breathing has ceased or both. Only 9 per cent thought of death in terms of irreversible loss of cerebral function. . . .
3. The public has an inaccurate concept of the mechanics associated with diagnosing death. This inference is supported by two types of findings. First, there is some confusion about who is responsible for saying a person is dead. While all people that were involved in the assessment thought that physicians or the coroner or both were responsible, there was considerable variation. Some individuals felt that only the decision of one physician was required, others said two or more physicians must agree. Still others responded that both a physician and the coroner must make the determination. A few individuals indicated that the coroner alone is responsible. . . .

*　　*　　*

Except for the medical examiner system, the coroner need only be 21 years of age and an American citizen.

Ninety-two percent of people questioned thought that a death certificate is required for embalming. In actual practice . . . this is not the case. As new life-support techniques increase the need for precision in the pronouncement of death, the dissonance between practice and perception will become an increasingly important factor.

4. The public will desire consensus about the practices of death pronouncement. This is supported by historical evidence, as well as by the individuals surveyed. A subsample of people were given an explanation of the importance of changing the method of determining death in the specific case of the single-organ transplant. Potential margins of error and problems were discussed. That "the rules of the game be made very clear to everybody" sums up well the response. Furthermore, there was evidence that the diagnosis of death in light of new technology should be regarded as more than a medical problem. Because of the far-reaching social implications, the individuals surveyed see the issue in a social framework.

*   *   *

[ii]
Statement of Senator Walter F. Mondale,
Minnesota—March 7, 1968*

. . . I think these hearings will constitute a classic document of statements and of discussion in this field which will be unique in our nation's literature, and from which could flow not only the creation of this commission, but also advancement of medical science; an improvement of health care; and a far more responsible and rational handling of the moral and social dimensions which undoubtedly exist as a part of those developments.

*   *   *

[T]hese advances and others yet to come [raise] grave and fundamental ethical and legal questions for our society—who shall live and who shall die; how long shall life be preserved and how shall it be altered; who shall make decisions; how shall society be prepared.

*   *   *

---

* Materials in this section are reprinted from *National Committee on Health Science and Society— Hearings on S.J. Res. 145 before the Subcommittee on Government Research of the Senate Committee on Government Operations,* 90th Congress, 2d Session (1968).

[T]his society is in a constant race to keep up with advancing technologies, understand them, and see that they are put to constructive use. We have been too late, too secret, and too superficial in too many cases.

*   *   *

. . . I have seen first hand the techniques that are used to develop this new technology; the sorts of things that must be done; the indispensable freedom that the researcher and the health practitioner must have. But I do not see any conflict of interest between a rational study of this issue, the taking of important, rational steps, and the preservation of this fundamental function. Indeed, I see them as complementary. The notion that somehow ignorance of what medical technology is producing protects the scientist better than public understanding is one which I am unable to accept.

I think the medical professional has a right to ask us to give him the resources and the elbow room he needs to fulfill his function. But I think that same professional must understand that society has a stake in what he is doing, and that society must know not only what he is doing, but the implications of his efforts.

*   *   *

Shortly after I came to the Senate, a bill was introduced which, in my opinion, would have sharply restricted animal research. At the University of Minnesota I think it is fair to say that we have gone very far in this field, and there has been a remarkable dividend, to human health and to animal health, from the experimentation that has occurred there. That is one of the reasons for our advance in transplantation technology.

Doctors from the university came to me and said, "Senator, this is a very, very serious thing. The public does not understand this problem. They think it is a case of mutilating dogs. They do not understand it. And if we are not careful, we are going to destroy one of the basic sources of medical knowledge, and new medical knowledge."

I listened to them and I said, "You are right." And I introduced legislation to protect against the inhumane treatment of dogs, and to provide funds to assist in the proper care, treatment, and feeding of animals, including dogs, but at the same time to leave the medical profession free to do the experimentation that it needs— humane research.

But I think there is something instructive there. I think what it tells us is that those who really believe in advancing medical knowledge have far more to gain from public understanding than public ignorance. That was an emergency situation. We could have taken steps in this field. Fortunately, I think we came up with a measure that was workable.

But I would hope the medical profession would approach these hearings not as a risk or a danger, but as an opportunity to put their work in proper perspective; to promote public knowledge of what they are doing; and to foster what I am sure will be broadened and more sophisticated public support.

* * *

NOTES

NOTE 1.

TESTIMONY OF DR. ADRIAN KANTROWITZ, DIRECTOR OF SURGICAL SERVICES, MAIMONIDES MEDICAL CENTER, BROOKLYN, NEW YORK— MARCH 7, 1968

* * *

In recent months, the pioneering achievements of Dr. Christiaan Barnard and others in the field of human heart transplantation have attracted understandable—if sometimes lamentably confused—attention. Public interest in the phenomenon of transplantation of organs from one human being to another has tended to obscure the at least equally bright promise of what we call heart-assist devices. I think we should bear in mind that such devices are likely to be even more important than transplantation in the future treatment of human heart disease.

Be that as it may, both paths of experimentation have already led to substantial achievement. Both must be followed with maximum energy, creativity, and skill by persons now in the work and by others who, it is hoped, will be drawn to it.

* * *

[N]o constructive purpose is served by representing the first human heart transplantation procedures as a sudden breakthrough, as if the idea had sprung full-blown from someone's brain and was perhaps a product of ill consideration as well as inspiration. The operations were breakthroughs only if a clinical trial—a forward step —can be adorned with so grandiose a label.

* * *

This brings me to a second focus of confusion—the question of whether experimental heart surgery contains ethical, moral, social, legal, economic, and political problems of a quality or magnitude never before encountered. As you know, this question has been raised on innumerable occasions not only in the general press but in journals of science and medicine. I am grateful that the subcommittee has invited comments.

The ethics of heart transplantation or of the implantation of a heart-assisting device are, first of all, the ethics of medicine, the ethics of reverence for human life. Where implantation of a heart-assisting device is contemplated the ethical problem is summarized in a few words: can the patient survive by any other known means? If the answer is affirmative, the physician recognizes that the patient is not a candidate for experimental use of a heart-assisting device. But if the patient is beyond the help of established procedures, it is entirely ethical to try to save his life with an experimental heart-assisting device which has demonstrated its effectiveness in animals.

The same process of ethical thought determines a patient's candidacy for heart transplantation. The process is not different from that which takes place in the mind of the physician prior to deciding whether a patient is an appropriate candidate for some new drug. Will anything else probably help the patient? Will the new drug expose the patient to unnecessary risk? Obviously, no surgeon would consider removing a human being's heart and replacing it with another except as a last-ditch effort to save life, all other possibilities having been exhausted.

* * *

Clinical trials are a far cry from the final accomplishment of a fully tested and substantiated procedure. As trials they are undertaken in the knowledge that failure is inherent in risk—and risk is synonymous with trial. And trials need the most searching scrutiny and review by the medical investigator's peers. The tradition of conducting these trials in a careful, orderly fashion, and of awaiting scientific evaluation before proceeding further is of vital importance to the public, and is hardly served by premature, over-emphatic publicity.

On the other hand, the public has the right to information about projects for which it pays the bills. Furthermore, biomedical research could hardly have achieved the levels of governmental and private support to which it has become accustomed if the press had not been attentive to interesting developments in years gone by.

But does the public need to know at 2:45 A.M. what may have happened in a surgical amphitheater at 2:43? And need the scientific investigator pause at the most stressful point in his effort to save life, need he then become a television personality, a sage, an answerer of sensational questions? Does this serve the public well? I think not.

* * *

SENATOR HARRIS: You view the transplantation of the human heart as experimentation at this stage, or is it a therapeutic procedure, or does it depend upon the particular case?

DR. KANTROWITZ: I do not think there is any question, Senator, about this. Not only in my opinion, but in the opinion of all of us who have done this procedure in humans, this is a highly experimental procedure. It is far from worked out to the point where it should be offered to the public. . . . It should be done—no question about this—it must be done—this is no longer a choice —it will be done, whether it is going to be done here or in South Africa or in Paris or Moscow— it is going to be done. It is a procedure that is going to be explored, and quite properly should be explored.

* * *

We are stepping into areas in the development of medicine where a certain amount of courage and boldness is necessary for success. I do not think this is really different than in any other business. I am sure this is true in your own affairs, where courage and boldness are needed. I am not sure committees have established a reputation for courage and boldness. They apparently survive much better being careful, not taking any chances.

But this is not the way progress is made. At least in my estimation. Progress is made by people who have some understanding of the problem, and enough courage to have the willingness to fail, because failure is part of success; it is part of the scientific process. My main concern is that a committee should not set up guidelines without the help of that segment of the medical profession which has some experience in developing these kinds of things. . . .

* * *

NOTE 2.
TESTIMONY OF DR. CHRISTIAAN BARNARD,
DIRECTOR OF SURGICAL RESEARCH,
MEDICAL SCHOOL, UNIVERSITY OF CAPE TOWN,
CAPE TOWN, SOUTH AFRICA—MARCH 8, 1968

* * *

[I]f you mean by this commission that you should have a qualified group of doctors belonging to that institution where the transplant is being done, then I could say I have nothing further to say, because this is done all over the world where transplantations are done. They have a group of doctors qualified and understanding the problems of organ transplantation which decide whether a patient should be selected for a transplant of such an organ, and decide on the various legal and medical aspects of this operation—and moral.

* * *

But if you are trying to set up a commission which is different from the one that I have indicated, I must say that I think you are seeing ghosts where there are no ghosts. If I am in competition with my colleagues of this country, which I am not, and were I completely selfish, then I would welcome such a commission, because it would put the doctors who embark on this type of treatment so far behind me, and hamper the group of doctors so much that I will go so far ahead that they will never catch up with me.

* * *

SENATOR RIBICOFF: [T]his has become a public issue because the public is paying the cost —society as a whole is paying the general costs. . . .

Now, who makes the decision? Should one doctor or a team of doctors be the sole ones to make the decisions as to who lives or dies?

DR. BARNARD: [L]et me give you something to compare that with.

Who pays for the cost of war? The public. Who decides where the general should attack and how he should attack? . . .

* * *

. . . The general is qualified to make that decision. And, therefore, he is qualified to spend the public's money the best way he thinks it is fit to spend it.

You cannot have control over these things. You must leave it in the people's hands who are capable of doing it.

SENATOR RIBICOFF: So not only the operation, but the person who would be the donee, in your opinion, should be left entirely to the medical team?

DR. BARNARD: Yes, sir.

* * *

Senator, by wanting to set up a commission, you must have one of two reasons. Either you are seeing new problems, or you are not satisfied with the way the doctors have handled problems in the past. That is the only reason you can ask for a commission.

SENATOR MONDALE: Don't you think some of the questions that have been asked today could profit by a further exploration by a responsible commission?

DR. BARNARD: But have you in our report of our cases—have you found any questions that could be explored by a commission, and could be clarified by a commission?

SENATOR MONDALE: Well, we have gone into the question of, when can a heart be made available, what should be the rights of the donor to select the donee. If there are only a limited number of transplants possible and a much larger number of people who will live or die, who receives the benefit of having his life being saved, with surgery that costs, by your estimates $30,000 each, and maybe $45,000 in the United States? How are those economic problems solved? Is there enough money being poured into this research to accelerate it, so that we can save more lives? What about the degree to which we are making these skills available more widely? What about the necessary facilities and the rest? Don't you believe these problems are the appropriate issues for the public to be concerned about?

DR. BARNARD: Well, I think that you are now mentioning problems which I think a commission would handle very well, as deciding to give money for research, and problems like that. But I think we must distinguish between what this commission is going to do. Is this commission going to decide on medical problems, and how the various transplant teams should handle a medical problem? If you ask me whether I think a commission should be necessary for that, I would disagree. But if you think that one should have a commission to decide whether money

should be poured into research because we now have these new techniques, and this may need more money, and aspects like that, I would agree that there you need a commission; but not to help the doctor to make his decision.

* * *

. . . Commissions have been set up to decide on various medical advances in the past. These commissions . . . have hampered the progress of medicine in nearly every case where such commissions intervene; because they were not qualified to deal with the various aspects.

SENATOR MONDALE: I would like you to comment on one other issue—and once again, I mean it in the finest sense.

There is a quotation from one of the great clergy of our country that relates to the surgery that you performed in South Africa. I would like to quote from Rabbi Raskus who said this:

Is it all right to have the heart of a Negro inside you, beating for you, giving you life, but not all right to have him live next door? Is it perfectly permissible to use the kidneys of Negroes for one's welfare, but then to deny them the rights of employment and the opportunity to better their minds through education and protect their right to the pursuit of happiness?

* * *

DR. BARNARD: You see, sir, the statement that you have just read has been made by a man who does not understand medicine. And that is why he raises this issue. Because to a medical doctor, there are no boundaries, and we do not know any boundaries. And therefore we do not think along the lines that he has thought. For me to have taken out the heart of a colored man and put it into a European body was not an issue at all, because there was no difference for me between the two. And this is the danger you run into, when you have people making statements and deciding on things to be done they are not qualified to do.

* * *

NOTE 3.

TESTIMONY OF DR. OWEN H. WANGENSTEEN, PROFESSOR EMERITUS OF THE UNIVERSITY OF MINNESOTA MEDICAL SCHOOL, MINNEAPOLIS, MINNESOTA—MARCH 8, 1968

* * *

Senator, I was a little worried by your letter in which you indicated . . , you had written to

200 people interested in the field; that you were going to study the problem and to suggest to the President and to the Congress directives which would do something for the field.

Now, if you mean support of research, that is good. I share Dr. Barnard's concern and worry over getting people into this field on the fringes, who do not really know much about the heart of the problem—the conscionable, dedicated, experienced people who are working day by day with the problem—these are the people who can speak knowledgeably and who can and must be trusted.

* * *

. . . If you are thinking of theologians, lawyers, philosophers, and others to give some direction here for the ongoing and for the development in this field, I cannot see how they could help. I would leave these decisions to the responsible people doing the work.

* * *

I think it is about like peeling an apple. The fellow who holds the apple can peel it best. I cannot conceive of 20 people holding an apple, and a man trying to get in there to peel it.

SENATOR MONDALE: . . . I think there is also an assumption underlying some of the testimony that medicine has an option by which the public can be prevented from participating in these problems.

Is that in fact the case? Or is it to be assumed that the public will be involved, and rather an issue whether they will be involved in a sophisticated, responsible way, or whether we will be acting out of ignorance or prejudice, because of the absence of a responsible approach. . . .

* * *

NOTE 4.

TESTIMONY OF CHIEF JUDGE DAVID L. BAZELON, U.S. COURT OF APPEALS FOR THE DISTRICT OF COLUMBIA CIRCUIT, MARCH 28, 1968

* * *

[S]ome mechanism will be needed for recording all these decisions. The impulse for this idea came from a session I attended at a large university general hospital on a Monday morning at 9 o'clock, when . . . they were to decide which of seven patients who were in need of dialysis would get the three places. And the decision was made that morning to select them. I was allowed to sit in on this meeting. The heads of the staff of the hospital were there. After they had gotten through with their discussion, which took about an hour and a half, they turned to me and said "What values do you bring from your end of the society that you think would bear upon these questions?" I was a little shaken by what I had just been through. I said "I have no wisdom except . . . the decision you made today should not be made behind those closed doors. Those doors ought to be open."

They said you mean we should have people in here who are not doctors or professionals?

I said—"No, make the decision now, you have to make it now. But let everybody know about it, let everybody know what went into it. Was it because he could pay money, or was it because he was young, or was it because he had a family, or was it because he was going to make a contribution to society—whatever was involved in deriving the decision."

Over time the public is going to react to this —but they are not going to know with that door closed.

* * *

Table of Cases

Table of Authors

Table of Books, Articles and Other Sources

1127

Subject Index

Rates of, 741
Use of drugs during, 420–22, 756–57, 919–21, 957–58
see also Birth Control
Prenatal diagnosis, 492, 505
Primitive cultures
Studies of, 381–82, 417–18
Principle of less severity, 336
Prisoners
As donors, 1034, 1046–49
Compensation of
financial, 303, 1023, 1041
reduction of sentence, 303, 1030–31, 1033, 1041
Condemned prisoners as subjects, 1015, 1027–28, 1041
Consent by special treatment board, 1016
Consent by subjects, 303, 306, 1024–25, 1028–30, 1040
Drug trials with, 1041–49
Experimentation with, 34–36, 292–306, 335–36, 378, 450–51, 1014–18, 1020–34, 1038–52
Experimentation with correctional treatment methods, 378, 450–51, 1016–18, 1037–40
Living conditions of, 1020–21
Random assignment of, 335–36, 378
Review committees for research with, 904, 1049
Selection as subjects, 1025, 1026, 1032–33, 1034
Sterilization of, 1051–52
Values of, 1022–23
Privacy
And personality tests, 355–57, 591–94, 964; *see also* Psychological studies
Invasion of, 326, 328, 347–48, 384–87, 406–07, 409–11, 723–24, 964, 981
Marital, 468–70, 556
Of jurors, 72ff
Psychological aspects of, 627
Right to, 79–80, 326–30, 432–33, 555, 730, 964
exceptions to, 723–24
historical aspects of, 329–30, 381, 405
legal aspects of, 329–30, 409–11
pursuit of knowledge versus, 341–42, 351
see also Confidentiality
Professions
Compulsory membership in, 191
Control over experimentation, 1004–07, 1041–46; *see also* Review Committees
Editorial control of, 934–36, 1007, 1010
Ethics of, 191ff, 222, 225–28, 333–36, 384, 493; *see also* Ethics

Lay control over, 196–97, 225–29, 231–35
Nature of, 186–91, 203–207
Protection of, 191–96, 206–228
Relationship to society, 186ff, 210–11, 222–29
Role in delaying innovation, 913
Sharing power with laymen, 230–34
Training of, 186, 425
Trust in, 186–87
see also, Lawyers; Physicians
Progesterone
Studies with, 732
Progress
And interests of community, 728–32
As a value, 124–27, 128, 130, 134–35, 487–88, 511
Relative value of, 148
Science as tool for, 122–24
Social cost of, 148, 184
Prolonging life
Choice of patient, 551–52, 709, 711
Desire to cease, 709–11
Family's role in, 711
Legal responsibility, 710–14
Means of, 706
Mitigation of pain, 707
Obligation for, 706
Psychological aspect of, 708–09
see also Euthanasia
Prostitution, *see* Sexual relations
Psilocybin, *see* Hallucinogen studies
Psychological and psychiatric studies, 142–46, 336–38, 352–69, 389–404, 419–20, 423–24, 444–48, 493, 591–94, 632–33
Deception in, 357–58, 406, 423–24, 427–32
Psychological interactions
Of investigator and subject, 206, 216–17, 222–25, 229–30, 387
Psychologists
Ethical standards of, 314–15, 423–24, 592
Psychopathology
Among organ donors, 646–47
Among research volunteers, 622–24
Studies of, 336–38, 444–98
Psychotherapy
As behavior control, 444
Homosexuality in, 470–82
Models of interaction in, 230–31, 637
Sexual intercourse in, 466–68, 493
Publications concerning research
As obligation of scientist, 425–26
Censorship of, 413–14, 493–94, 934–36
Credit to subjects in, 629
Ethics in, 346–52, 381–82, 408–09, 411–14, 418–19, 935ff, 1096–97